Comprehensive Pharmacy Review for NAPLEX

Eighth Edition

Comprehensive Pharmacy Review for NAPLEX

Eighth Edition

EDITORS

Leon Shargel, PhD, RPh

Alan H. Mutnick, PharmD, FASHP, RPh

Paul F. Souney, MS, RPh

Larry N. Swanson, PharmD, FASHP, RPh

Wolters Kluwer | Lippincott Williams & Wilkins
Health

Philadelphia • Baltimore • New York • London
Buenos Aires • Hong Kong • Sydney • Tokyo

Acquisitions Editor: Sirkka Howes
Product Manager: Michael Marino
Marketing Manager: Joy Fisher-Williams
Design Coordinator: Teresa Mallon
Production Services: Absolute Service, Inc.

Eighth Edition

351 West Camden Street
Baltimore, MD 21201

Two Commerce Square
2001 Market Street
Philadelphia, PA 19103

Printed in China

9 8 7 6 5 4 3 2 1

Library of Congress Cataloging-in-Publication Data

Comprehensive pharmacy review for NAPLEX / editors, Leon Shargel ... [et al.]. — 8th ed.
p. ; cm.
Comprehensive pharmacy review for North American Pharmacist Licensure Examination
Includes index.
Rev. ed. of: Comprehensive pharmacy review / editors, Leon Shargel ... [et al.]. 7th ed. c2010.
ISBN 978-1-4511-1704-2 (pbk.)
I. Shargel, Leon, 1941- II. Comprehensive pharmacy review. III. Title: Comprehensive pharmacy review for North American Pharmacist Licensure Examination.
[DNLM: 1. Pharmacy—Examination Questions. QV 18.2]

615'.1076—dc23

2012020144

DISCLAIMER

Care has been taken to confirm the accuracy of the information present and to describe generally accepted practices. However, the authors, editors, and publisher are not responsible for errors or omissions or for any consequences from application of the information in this book and make no warranty, expressed or implied, with respect to the currency, completeness, or accuracy of the contents of the publication. Application of this information in a particular situation remains the professional responsibility of the practitioner; the clinical treatments described and recommended may not be considered absolute and universal recommendations.

The authors, editors, and publisher have exerted every effort to ensure that drug selection and dosage set forth in this text are in accordance with the current recommendations and practice at the time of publication. However, in view of ongoing research, changes in government regulations, and the constant flow of information relating to drug therapy and drug reactions, the reader is urged to check the package insert for each drug for any change in indications and dosage and for added warnings and precautions. This is particularly important when the recommended agent is a new or infrequently employed drug.

Some drugs and medical devices presented in this publication have Food and Drug Administration (FDA) clearance for limited use in restricted research settings. It is the responsibility of the health care provider to ascertain the FDA status of each drug or device planned for use in their clinical practice.

To purchase additional copies of this book, call our customer service department at **(800) 638-3030** or fax orders to **(301) 223-2320**. International customers should call **(301) 223-2300**.

Visit Lippincott Williams & Wilkins on the Internet: http://www.lww.com. Lippincott Williams & Wilkins customer service representatives are available from 8:30 a.m. to 6:00 p.m., EST.

CCS0812

Preface

This eighth edition of *Comprehensive Pharmacy Review* reflects the continuing evolution of pharmacy practice and educational requirements. The main objective of the book is to provide a comprehensive study guide for pharmacy students and other candidates who are preparing for the North American Pharmacist Licensure Examination (NAPLEX). This volume represents the contributions of more than 50 specialists who provide wide expertise in pharmaceutical science, pharmacy practice, and clinical pharmacy. Their contributions to *Comprehensive Pharmacy Review* assure that this review guide is accurate and current as well as written in a comprehensible manner for students, teachers, and practitioners alike. This review publication, along with the separate booklet of simulated NAPLEX exams (Comprehensive Pharmacy Review Practice Exams, 8th edition), provides both guidance and test practice for NAPLEX candidates.

The current pharmaceutical education provides greater career opportunities for pharmacists than ever before. Pharmaceutical education, including pharmaceutical science and practice, must prepare pharmacy practitioners for the future. Among the many career choices for pharmacists include work in academic pharmacy, community pharmacy, long-term care, and consulting pharmacy, including hospice and home care, pharmaceutical and health care distributors, pharmaceutical industry, professional trade organizations, uniformed (public health) services, federal and state governments, hospital and institutional practice settings, managed care pharmacy, and other settings. Moreover, pharmacists are actively involved in health care. Examples include counseling and medication therapy, disease state management, and screening programs such as diabetes, hypertension, and high cholesterol along with the more traditional role of dispensing medication and educating patients. Many students enroll in pharmaceutical education programs that are combined with a business (MBA), research (PhD), or law (JD) degree to provide opportunities in various pharmacy-related professions and other challenging fields.

Comprehensive Pharmacy Review is principally written for NAPLEX candidates. However, the book is also intended for a broader audience of pharmacy undergraduates and health professionals who seek detailed summaries of pharmacy subjects. A wide range of topics central to the study of pharmacy—chemistry, pharmaceutics, pharmacology, pharmacy practice, drug therapy—is organized to parallel the pharmacy curriculum and presented in outline form for easy use. The *Comprehensive Pharmacy Review* may be used as a quick review (or preview) of essential topics by a diverse group of readers, including

- **Matriculating pharmacy students.** The organization and topical coverage of *Comprehensive Pharmacy Review* are such that many pharmacy students will want to purchase it in their first professional year and use it throughout their pharmacy education to prepare for course examinations.
- **Instructors and preceptors.** *Comprehensive Pharmacy Review* also functions as an instructor's manual and a reference for teachers and tutors in pharmacy schools. Chapter outlines can be used to organize courses and to plan specific lectures.
- **Professional pharmacists.** *Comprehensive Pharmacy Review* offers practitioners a convenient handbook of pharmacy facts. It can be used as a course refresher and as a source of recent information on pharmacy practice. The appendices include prescription dispensing information, common prescription drugs, and general pharmacy references.
- **Foreign pharmacy graduates.** *Comprehensive Pharmacy Review* provides a source of current information on pharmaceutical science, pharmacy practice, and clinical pharmacy for foreign pharmacy graduates who may be candidates for the Foreign Pharmacy Graduate Equivalency Examination (FPGEE). The appendices include prescription dispensing information, common prescription drugs, and general pharmacy references.

WHAT'S NEW IN THIS EDITION

The continuing evolution of pharmacy practice is reflected by the licensure examinations developed by the National Association of Boards of Pharmacy (NABP) to assess the competence of pharmacy candidates. For this reason, we have requested and have been given permission by NABP to reproduce the competency statements for the NABP examination (NAPLEX) in the front matter of this edition of *Comprehensive Pharmacy Review*.

Because of the significant advances in drug therapy since the publication of the last edition, this edition has been revised to reflect the current educational and competency requirements for a successful career in pharmacy. Many of the chapters have been revised to represent the latest understanding of disease and therapeutic management. New chapters, such as Pain Management Including Migraines, Hepatic Disorders, Pediatrics, Geriatrics, Women's Health have been added to reflect the needs of special populations. The addition of the chapter, Biostatistics and Medical Literature Evaluation provides a basis for the evaluation of new therapeutic moieties that will be marketed in the future.

ORGANIZATIONAL PHILOSOPHY AND CHAPTER STRUCTURE

The organization of the eight edition reflects the current undergraduate pharmacy curriculum. Pharmaceutical Sciences (Chapters 1–18), contains subject matter pertaining to the basic science of pharmacy. Pharmacy Practice (Chapters 19–64), contains subject matter for the practice of pharmacy with emphasis on pharmaceutical care. Each chapter of the book contains topic outlines and practice questions according to the pharmacy school curriculum.

At the front matter of this book, you'll find guidelines for taking a test and an introduction to the NAPLEX exam, including the actual NAPLEX blueprint. The appendices of this book are compilations of handy reference tables.

Contributors

S. Thomas Abraham, PhD
Associate Professor of Pharmacology and Toxicology
Department of Pharmaceutical Sciences
Campbell University College of Pharmacy and Health Sciences
Buies Creek, North Carolina

Michael L. Adams, PharmD, PhD
Assistant Professor of Medicinal Chemistry
Department of Pharmaceutical Sciences
Campbell University College of Pharmacy and Health Sciences
Buies Creek, North Carolina

Loyd V. Allen Jr., PhD
Professor Emeritus
College of Pharmacy
University of Oklahoma
Oklahoma City, Oklahoma
Editor-In-Chief
International Journal of Pharmaceutical Compounding
Edmond, Oklahoma

Teresa M. Bailey, PharmD, BCPS, FCCP
Department of Pharmacy Practice
Ferris State University College of Pharmacy
ProMed Family Practice
Portage, Michigan

Connie Lee Barnes, PharmD
Professor
Director, Drug Information Center
Department of Pharmacy Practice
Campbell University College of Pharmacy and Health Sciences
Buies Creek, North Carolina

Caryn Domenici Belisle, RPh
Pharmacy Manager, Sterile Products and Robotics Service
Department of Pharmacy Services
Brigham and Women's Hospital
Boston, Massachusetts

Brooke Bernhardt, PharmD, BCOP
Clinical Pharmacy Specialist, Hematology/Oncology
Texas Children's Hospital
Houston, Texas

Lawrence H. Block, PhD, RPh
Professor of Pharmaceutics
Division of Pharmaceutical Sciences
Mylan School of Pharmacy
Duquesne University
Pittsburgh, Pennsylvania

James A. Boyd, PharmD, MBA
Associate Professor and Director
Joint PharmD/MBA Program
Campbell University College of Pharmacy and Health Sciences
Buies Creek, North Carolina

K. Paige D. Brown, PharmD
Assistant Director of Experiential Education
Assistant Professor of Pharmacy Practice
Campbell University College of Pharmacy and Health Sciences
Buies Creek, North Carolina

Todd A. Brown, MHP, RPh
Clinical Instructor and Vice Chair
Department of Pharmacy Practice
Bouve College of Health Sciences School of Pharmacy
Northeastern University
Boston, Massachusetts

Marcia L. Buck, PharmD, FCCP, FPPAG
Clinical Pharmacy Coordinator, Children's Hospital
Associate Professor, Pediatrics
School of Medicine
Clinical Associate Professor
School of Nursing
University of Virginia Health System, Department of Pharmacy Services
Charlottesville, Virginia

Robert Cisneros, PhD
Associate Professor
Department of Pharmacy Practice
Campbell University College of Pharmacy and Health Sciences
Buies Creek, North Carolina

Valerie B. Clinard, PharmD
Associate Director, Drug Information
Assistant Professor, Pharmacy Practice
Campbell University College of Pharmacy and Health Sciences
Buies Creek, North Carolina

Dean S. Collier, PharmD, BCPS
Assistant Professor
Department of Pharmacy Practice
University of Nebraska Medical Center
Clinical Pharmacist
Department of Pharmacy Practice
The Nebraska Medical Center
Omaha, Nebraska

Stephen C. Dragotakes, RPh, BCNP
PET Nuclear Pharmacy
PET Pharmaceutical Production Manager
Division of Nuclear Medicine and Molecular Imaging
Department of Radiology
Massachusetts General Hospital
Boston, Massachusetts

Elise Dunzo, PhD
Director, Clinical Pharmacology and Pharmacokinetics
Applied Biopharmaceutics, LLC
Raleigh, North Carolina

Alice C. Engelbrecht, PharmD
Clinical Coordinator for Pharmacy Clinical Services
Oklahoma University Medical Center
Oklahoma City, Oklahoma

John Fanikos, RPh, MBA
Director of Pharmacy Business
Department of Pharmacy Services
Brigham and Women's Hospital
Boston, Massachusetts

Robert B. Greenwood, RPh, PhD
Associate Dean of Academic Affairs
Professor of Pharmaceutical Sciences
Campbell University College of Pharmacy and Health Sciences
Buies Creek, North Carolina

James B. Groce III, PharmD, CACP
Professor, Department of Pharmacy Practice
Campbell University College of Pharmacy and Health Sciences
Clinical Assistant Professor of Medicine, Department of Medicine
University of North Carolina School of Medicine
Clinical Pharmacy Specialist—Anticoagulation
Department of Pharmacy
Cone Health
Greensboro, North Carolina

Rebekah R. Arthur Grube, PharmD, BCPS
Pharmacist Consultant
Charlotte, North Carolina

Terri S. Hamrick, PhD
Associate Professor
Department of Pharmaceutical Sciences
College of Pharmacy and Health Sciences
Campbell University
Buies Creek, North Carolina

Charles Herring, PharmD, BCPS, CPP
Associate Professor, Campbell University
College of Pharmacy and Health Sciences
Clinical Pharmacist, Adult Medicine Team
Downtown Health Plaza of Baptist Hospitals
Winston-Salem, North Carolina

Manish Issar, PhD
Assistant Professor of Pharmacology
College of Osteopathic Medicine
Western University of Health Sciences
Pomona, California

Alan F. Kaul, PharmD, MS, MBA, FCCP
President
Medical Outcomes Management, Inc.
Sharon, Massachusetts
Adjunct Professor of Pharmacy
Department of Pharmacy Practice
University of Rhode Island College of Pharmacy
Kingston, Rhode Island
Adjunct Professor of Pharmacy Practice
Department of Pharmacy Practice
School of Pharmacy
Massachusetts College of Pharmacy and Health Sciences
Boston, Massachusetts

Kevin P. Keating, MD
Director, Cardiothoracic Surgical ICU
Department of Surgery
Hartford Hospital
Hartford, Connecticut
Assistant Professor of Surgery
Department of Surgery
University of Connecticut School of Medicine
Farmington, Connecticut

Julie J. Kelsey, PharmD
Clinical Pharmacy Specialist
Women's Health and Family Medicine
Department of Pharmacy Services
University of Virginia Health System
Charlottesville, Virginia

D. Byron May, PharmD, BCPS
Professor
Department of Pharmacy Practice
Campbell University College of Pharmacy and Health Sciences
Buies Creek, North Carolina
Clinical Specialist in Adult Internal Medicine
Department of Pharmacy
Duke University Hospital
Durham, North Carolina

David I. Min, PharmD, MS, FCCP
Professor
Department of Pharmacy Practice and Administration
Western University of Health Sciences, College of Pharmacy
Pomona, California

Alan H. Mutnick, PharmD, FASHP, RPh
Corporate Director/Clinical Services
Catholic Health Partners
Cincinnati, Ohio

Andrew J. Muzyk, PharmD
Assistant Professor
Department of Pharmacy Practice
Campbell University College of Pharmacy and Health Sciences
Buies Creek, North Carolina
Clinical Pharmacy Specialist
Department of Pharmacy
Duke University Hospital
Durham, North Carolina

Eric C. Nemec, PharmD, BCPS
Clinical Assistant Professor
Department of Pharmacy Practice
Western New England University
Springfield, Massachusetts
Informatics Specialist
Department of Pharmacy
Holyoke Medical Center
Holyoke, Massachusetts

Jeffrey P. Norenberg, PharmD, BCNP, FASHP, FAPhA
Professor, Chair, Radiopharmaceutical Sciences Program
College of Pharmacy, University of New Mexico
Albuquerque, New Mexico

Roy A. Pleasants II, PharmD
Associate Professor
Department of Pharmacy Practice
Campbell University College of Pharmacy and Health Sciences
Buies Creek, North Carolina
Clinical Assistant Professor
Division of Pulmonary Medicine
Duke University School of Medicine
Durham, North Carolina

John J. Ponzillo, PharmD
Critical Care Pharmacist
St. John's Mercy Medical Center
Saint Louis, Missouri

Robert A. Quercia, MS, RPh
Editor and Co-Coordinator of Focus Column Formulary Journal
Medical Editor, University of Connecticut/Hartford Hospital
Evidenced-based Practice Center
Hartford, Connecticut
Adjunct Associate Clinical Professor
University of Connecticut School of Pharmacy
Storrs, Connecticut

Azita Razzaghi, RPh, PharmD
Associate Director
Pharmacovigilance
Genzyme Corporation
Cambridge, Massachusetts

Gurvinder Singh Rekhi, PhD
Director, Research and Development
Elan Drug Delivery, Inc.
Gainesville, Georgia

Gerald E. Schumacher, PharmD, MS, PhD
Professor of Pharmacy, Emeritus
Bouve College of Health Sciences School of Pharmacy
Northeastern University
Boston, Massachusetts

Leon Shargel, PhD, RPh
Manager
Applied Biopharmaceutics, LLC
Raleigh, North Carolina
Affiliate Associate Professor
Department of Pharmaceutics
School of Pharmacy
Virginia Commonwealth University
Richmond, Virginia
Adjunct Associate Professor
School of Pharmacy
University of Maryland
Baltimore, Maryland

Penny S. Shelton, PharmD, CGP, FASCP
Vice-Chair, Experiential and Continuing Education
Associate Professor, Department of Pharmacy Practice
Campbell University College of Pharmacy and Health Sciences
Buies Creek, North Carolina

Jennifer D. Smith, PharmD, CPP, BC-ADM, CDE, C-TTS
Associate Professor
Department of Pharmacy Practice
Campbell University College of Pharmacy and Health Sciences
Buies Creek, North Carolina
Clinical Pharmacist Practitioner
Wilson Community Health Center
Wilson, North Carolina

Paul F. Souney, MS, RPh
Vice President
Medical Affairs and Pharmacotherapy Management
Medical Outcomes Management, Inc.
Sharon, Massachusetts

Linda M. Spooner, PharmD, BCPS with Added Qualifications in Infectious Diseases
Associate Professor of Pharmacy Practice
Department of Pharmacy Practice
Massachusetts College of Pharmacy and Health Sciences
School of Pharmacy-Worcester/Manchester
Worcester, Massachusetts
Clinical Pharmacy Specialist in Infectious Diseases
Department of Pharmacy
Saint Vincent Hospital
Worcester, Massachusetts

Gilbert A. Steiner, PharmD
Associate Professor
Department of Pharmacy Practice
Campbell University College of Pharmacy and Health Sciences
Buies Creek, North Carolina

Larry N. Swanson, PharmD, FASHP, RPh
Professor and Chairman
Department of Pharmacy Practice
Campbell University College of Pharmacy and Health Sciences
Buies Creek, North Carolina

Ryan S. Swanson, PharmD, RPh
Clinical Pharmacist
Kerr Drug
Fuquay-Varina, North Carolina

Heather A. Sweeney, PharmD, RPh
Clinical Manager
Pharmaceutical Distribution
Cardinal Health
Cincinnati, Ohio

Barbara Szymusiak-Mutnick, BS Pharm, MHP, RPh
Home Infusion Pharmacist
Walgreen Home Infusion Pharmacy
Centerville, Ohio

Tina Harrison Thornhill, PharmD, FASCP, CGP
Associate Professor
Department of Pharmacy Practice
Campbell University College of Pharmacy and Health Sciences
Buies Creek, North Carolina
Clinical Specialist, Geriatrics and Acute Rehabilitation
Wake Forest Baptist Health
The Sticht Center on Aging and Rehabilitation
Winston-Salem, North Carolina

Jenny A. Van Amburgh, PharmD, FAPhA, BCACP, CDE
Associate Clinical Professor and Assistant Dean for Academic Affairs
Department of Pharmacy Practice
Bouve College of Health Sciences School of Pharmacy
Northeastern University
Boston, Massachusetts
Director of Clinical Pharmacy Services & Clinical Pharmacist
Clinical Pharmacy Services
Harbor Health Services, Inc.
Dorchester, Massachusetts

Christopher Vitale, PharmD
Clinical Pharmacist
Clinical Informatics Research and Development
Partners Healthcare System
Wellesley, Massachusetts

Susanna Wu-Pong, PhD
Associate Professor
Director, Pharmaceutical Sciences Graduate Program
Dean's Office
Virginia Commonwealth University
Richmond, Virginia

Anthony E. Zimmermann, BS, PharmD
Professor and Chair
Department of Pharmacy Practice
College of Pharmacy
Western New England University
Springfield, Massachusetts

Contents

Additional Chapters Published Online at thePoint.lww.com

Taking a Test

One of the least attractive aspects of pursuing an education is the necessity of being examined on the material that has been presented. Instructors do not like to prepare tests, and students do not like to take them.

However, students are required to take many examinations during their learning careers, and little, if any, time is spent acquainting them with the positive aspects of tests and with systematic and successful methods for approaching them. Students perceive tests as punitive and sometimes feel as if they were merely opportunities for the instructor to discover what the student has forgotten or has never learned. Students need to view tests as opportunities to display their knowledge and to use them as tools for developing prescriptions for further study and learning.

While preparing for any exam, class and board exams as well as practice exams, it is important that students learn as much as they can about the subject they will be tested and are prepared to discover just how much they may not know. Students should study to acquire knowledge, not just to prepare for tests. For the well-prepared student, the chances of passing far exceed the chances of failing.

MATERIALS NEEDED FOR TEST PREPARATION

In preparing for a test, most students collect far too much study material, only to find that they simply do not have time to go through all of it. They are defeated before they begin because either they cannot get through all the material, leaving areas unstudied, or they race through the material so quickly that they cannot benefit from the activity.

It is generally more efficient for the student to use materials already at hand—that is, class notes, one good outline to cover and strengthen all areas and to quickly review the whole topic, and one good text as a reference for complex material that requires further explanation.

Also, many students attempt to memorize far too much information, rather than learning and understanding less material and then relying on that learned information to determine the answers to questions at the time of the examination. Relying too heavily on memorized material causes anxiety, and the more anxious students become during a test, the less learned knowledge they are likely to use.

ATTITUDE AND APPROACH

A positive attitude and a realistic approach are essential to successful test taking. If the student concentrates on the negative aspects of tests or on the potential for failure, anxiety increases and performance decreases. A negative attitude generally develops if the student concentrates on "I must pass" rather than on "I can pass." "What if I fail?" becomes the major factor motivating the student to run from failure rather than toward success. This results from placing too much emphasis on scores. The score received is only one aspect of test performance. Test performance also indicates the student's ability to use differential reasoning.

In each question with five alternatives, of which one is correct, there are four alternatives that are incorrect. If deductive reasoning is used, the choices can be viewed as having possibilities of being correct. The elimination of wrong choices increases the odds that a student will be able to recognize the correct choice. Even if the correct choice does not become evident, the probability of guessing correctly increases. Eliminating incorrect choices on a test can result in choosing the correct answer.

Answering questions based on what is incorrect is difficult for many students because they have had nearly 20 years of experience taking tests with the implied assertion that knowledge can be displayed only by knowing what is correct. It must be remembered, however, that students can display knowledge by knowing something is wrong, just as they can display it by knowing something is right.

PREPARING FOR THE EXAMINATION

1. **Study for yourself.** Although some of the material may seem irrelevant, the more you learn now, the less you will have to learn later. Also, do not let the fear of the test rob you of an important part of your education. If you study to learn, the task is less distasteful than studying solely to pass a test.

2. **Review all areas.** You should not be selective by studying perceived weak areas and ignoring perceived strong areas. Cover all of the material, putting added emphasis on weak areas.
3. **Attempt to understand, not just to memorize, the material.** Ask yourself: To whom does the material apply? When does it apply? Where does it apply? How does it apply? Understanding the connections among these points allows for longer retention and aids in those situations when guessing strategies may be needed.
4. **Try to anticipate questions that might appear on the test.** Ask yourself how you might construct a question on a specific topic.
5. **Give yourself a couple days of rest before the test.** Studying up to the last moment will increase your anxiety and cause potential confusion.

TAKING THE EXAMINATION

1. Be sure to pace yourself to use the test time optimally. You should use all of your allotted time; if you finish too early, you probably did so by moving too quickly through the test.
2. Read each question and all the alternatives carefully before you begin to make decisions. Remember, the questions contain clues, as do the answer choices.
3. Read the directions for each question set carefully. You would be amazed at how many students make mistakes in tests simply because they have not paid close attention to the directions.
4. It is not advisable to leave blanks with the intention of coming back to answer questions later. If you feel that you must come back to a question, mark the best choice and place a note in the margin. Generally speaking, it is best not to change answers once you have made a decision. Your considered reaction and first response are correct more often than are changes made out of frustration or anxiety.
5. Do not let anxiety destroy your confidence. If you have prepared conscientiously, you know enough to pass. Use all that you have learned.
6. Do not try to determine how well you are doing as you proceed. You will not be able to make an objective assessment, and your anxiety will increase.
7. Do not become frustrated or angry about what appear to be bad or difficult questions. You simply do not know the answers; you cannot know everything.

SPECIFIC TEST-TAKING STRATEGIES

Read the entire question carefully, regardless of format. Test questions have multiple parts. Concentrate on picking out the pertinent key words that will help you problem-solve. Words such as *always*, *all*, *never*, *mostly*, *primarily*, and so forth play significant roles. In all types of questions, distractors with terms such as *always* or *never* most often are incorrect. Adjectives and adverbs can completely change the meaning of questions—pay close attention to them. The knowledge and application of grammar often are key to dissecting questions.

MULTIPLE CHOICE QUESTIONS

Read the question and the choices carefully to become familiar with the data provided. Remember in multiple choice questions, there is one correct answer and there are four distractors, or incorrect answers. (Distractors are plausible and possibly correct, otherwise they would not be called distractors.) They are generally correct for part of the question but not for the entire question. Dissecting the question into parts helps eliminate distractors.

Many students think that they must always start at option A and make a decision before they move to option B, thus forcing decisions they are not ready to make. Your first decisions should be made on those choices you feel the most confident about.

Compare the choices with each part of the question. To be wrong, a choice needs to be incorrect for only part of the question. To be correct, it must be totally correct. If you believe a choice is partially incorrect, tentatively eliminate that choice. Make notes next to the choices regarding tentative decisions. One method is to place a minus sign next to the choices you are certain are incorrect and a plus sign next to those that potentially are correct. Finally, place a zero next to any choice you do not understand or need to come back to for further inspection. Do not feel that you must make final decisions until you have examined all choices carefully.

When you have eliminated as many choices as you can, decide which of those that remain has the highest probability of being correct. Above all, be honest with yourself. If you do not know the answer, eliminate as many choices as possible and choose reasonably.

Multiple choice questions are not as difficult as some students make them. There are two general types of multiple choice questions, including (1) the more traditional single answer type question in which the candidate must decide one of five choices (a, b, c, d, or e) and (2) the combined response ("K" type) multiple choice question, which is shown next. In this case, these are the questions for which you must select from the following choices:

A if **only I** is correct
B if **only III** is correct
C if **I and II** are correct
D if **II and III** are correct
E if **I, II, and III** are correct

Remember that the name for this type of question is *multiple true–false* and then use this concept. Become familiar with each choice and make notes. Then concentrate on the one choice you feel is definitely incorrect. If you can find one incorrect alternative, you can eliminate three choices immediately and be down to a 50–50 probability of guessing the correct answer. If choice A is incorrect, so are choices C and E; if choice B is incorrect, so are choices D and E. Therefore, you are down to a 50–50 probability of guessing the correct answer.

After eliminating the choices you are sure are incorrect, concentrate on the choice that will make your final decision. For instance, if you discard choice I, you have eliminated alternatives A, C, and E. This leaves B (III) and D (II and III). Concentrate on choice II and decide if it is true or false. (Take the path of least resistance and concentrate on the smallest possible number of items while making a decision.) Obviously, if none of the choices is found to be incorrect, the answer is E (I, II, III).

GUESSING

Nothing takes the place of a firm knowledge base; but having little information to work with, you may find it necessary to guess at the correct answer. A few simple rules can help increase your guessing accuracy. Always guess consistently if you have no idea what is correct—that is, after eliminating all that you can, make the choice that agrees with your intuition or choose the option closest to the top of the list that has not been eliminated as a potential answer.

When guessing at questions that present with choices in numeric form, you will often find the choices listed in an ascending or descending order. It is generally not wise to guess the first or last alternative because these are usually extreme values and are most likely incorrect.

USING A PRACTICE EXAM TO LEARN

All too often, students do not take full advantage of practice exams. There is a tendency to complete the exam, score it, look up the correct answer to those questions missed, and then forget the entire thing.

In fact, great educational benefits could be derived if students would spend more time using practice tests as learning tools. As mentioned previously, incorrect choices in test questions are plausible and partially correct, otherwise they would not fulfill their purpose as distractors. This means that it is just as beneficial to look up the incorrect choices as the correct choices to discover specifically why they are incorrect. In this way, it is possible to learn better test-taking skills as the subtlety of question construction is uncovered.

In addition, it is advisable to go back and attempt to restructure each question to see if all the choices can be made correct by modifying the question. By doing this, you will learn four times as much. By all means, look up the right answer and explanation. Then, focus on each of the other choices, and ask yourself under what conditions, if any, they might be correct.

SUMMARY

Ideally, examinations are designed to determine how much material students have learned and how that material is used in the successful completion of the examination. Students will be successful if these suggestions are followed:

- Develop a positive attitude and maintain that attitude.
- Be realistic in determining the amount of material you attempt to master and in the score you hope to attain.
- Read the directions for each type of question and the questions themselves closely, and follow the directions carefully.
- Bring differential reasoning to each question in the examination.
- Guess intelligently and consistently when guessing strategies must be used.
- Use the test as an opportunity to display your knowledge and as a tool for developing prescriptions for further study and learning.

Board examinations are not easy. They may be almost impossible for those who have unrealistic expectations or for those who allow misinformation concerning the exams to produce anxiety out of proportion to the task at hand. Examinations are manageable if they are approached with a positive attitude and with consistent use of all of the information the student has learned.

Michael J. O'Donnell

Introduction to the NAPLEX

After graduation from an accredited pharmacy program, the prospective pharmacist must demonstrate the competency to practice pharmacy. The standards of competence for the practice of pharmacy are set by each state board of pharmacy. NAPLEX—The North American Pharmacist Licensure Examination—is the principal instrument used by the state board of pharmacy to assess the knowledge and proficiency necessary for a candidate to practice pharmacy. The National Association of Boards of Pharmacy (NABP) is an independent, international, and impartial association that assists member boards and jurisdictions in developing, implementing, and enforcing uniform standards for the purpose of protecting the public health. NABP develops examinations that enable boards of pharmacy to assess the competence of candidates seeking licensure to practice pharmacy. Each state board of pharmacy may impose additional examinations. The two major examinations developed by NABP are

- The North American Pharmacist Licensure Examination (NAPLEX)
- Multistate Pharmacy Jurisprudence Examination (MPJE)

Foreign pharmacy graduates must pass the Foreign Pharmacy Graduate Equivalency Examination (FPGEE) as part of the Foreign Pharmacy Graduate Equivalency Certification process. Foreign-educated pharmacists awarded FPGEC certification is considered to have partially fulfilled eligibility requirements for licensure in those states that accept the certification.

A description of these computerized examinations and registration information may be found on the NABP website online at http://www.nabp.net. Before submitting registration materials, the pharmacy candidate should contact the board of pharmacy for additional information regarding procedures, deadline dates, and required documentation.

The NAPLEX is a computer-adaptive test. These questions measure *the prospective pharmacist's ability to measure pharmacotherapy and therapeutic outcomes, prepare and dispense medications, and implement and evaluate information for optimal health care*. The computer adaptive exam tests a candidate's knowledge and ability by assessing the answers before presenting the next test question. If the answer is correct, the computer will select a more difficult question from the test item pool in an appropriate content area; if the answer is incorrect, an easier question will be selected by the computer. The NAPLEX score is based on the difficulty level of the questions answered correctly.

NAPLEX consists of 185 multiple choice test questions. In the past, 150 questions were used to calculate the test score. The remaining 35 items served as pretest questions and do not affect the NAPLEX score. Pretest questions are administered to evaluate the item's difficulty level for possible inclusion as a scored question in future exams. These pretest questions are dispersed throughout the exam and cannot be identified by the candidate.

A majority of the questions on the NAPLEX are asked in a scenario-based format (i.e., patient profiles with accompanying test questions). To properly analyze and answer the questions presented, the candidate must refer to the information provided in the patient profile. Some questions appear in a stand-alone format and should be answered solely from the information provided in the question.

NAPLEX Blueprint

THE NAPLEX COMPETENCY STATEMENTS

All NAPLEX questions are based on competency statements that are reviewed and revised periodically. The NAPLEX Competency Statements describe the knowledge, judgment, and skills that the candidate is expected to demonstrate as an entry-level pharmacist. A complete description of the NAPLEX Competency Statements is published on the NABP website and is reproduced, with permission of NABP. A strong understanding of the Competency Statements will aid in your preparation to take the examination.

Area 1 Assess Pharmacotherapy to Assure Safe and Effective Therapeutic Outcomes (Approximately 56% of Test)

- **1.1.0** Identify, interpret, and evaluate patient information to determine the presence of a disease or medical condition, assess the need for treatment and/or referral, and identify patient-specific factors that affect health, pharmacotherapy, and/or disease management.
- **1.1.1** Identify and assess patient information including medication, laboratory, and disease state histories.
- **1.1.2** Identify patient-specific assessment and diagnostic methods, instruments, and techniques and interpret their results.
- **1.1.3** Identify and define the etiology, terminology, signs, and symptoms associated with diseases and medical conditions and their causes and determine if medical referral is necessary.
- **1.1.4** Identify and evaluate patient genetic, biosocial factors, and concurrent drug therapy relevant to the maintenance of wellness and the prevention or treatment of a disease or medical condition.
- **1.2.0** Evaluate information about pharmacoeconomic factors, dosing regimen, dosage forms, delivery systems and routes of administration to identify and select optimal pharmacotherapeutic agents for patients.
- **1.2.1** Identify specific uses and indications for drug products and recommend drugs of choice for specific diseases or medical conditions.
- **1.2.2** Identify the chemical/pharmacologic classes of therapeutic agents and describe their known or postulated sites and mechanisms of action.
- **1.2.3** Evaluate drug therapy for the presence of pharmacotherapeutic duplications and interactions with other drugs, food, and diagnostic tests.
- **1.2.4** Identify and evaluate potential contraindications and provide information about warnings and precautions associated with a drug product's active and inactive ingredients.
- **1.2.5** Identify physicochemical properties of drug substances that affect their solubility, pharmacodynamic and pharmacokinetic properties, pharmacologic actions, and stability.
- **1.2.6** Evaluate and interpret pharmacodynamic and pharmacokinetic principles to calculate and determine appropriate drug dosing regimens.
- **1.2.7** Identify appropriate routes of administration, dosage forms, and pharmaceutical characteristics of drug dosage forms and delivery systems to assure bioavailability and enhance therapeutic efficacy.
- **1.3.0** Evaluate and manage drug regimens by monitoring and assessing the patient and/or patient information, collaborating with other health care professionals, and providing patient education to enhance safe, effective, and economic patient outcomes.
- **1.3.1** Identify pharmacotherapeutic outcomes and end points.
- **1.3.2** Evaluate patient signs and symptoms and the findings of monitoring tests and procedures to determine the safety and effectiveness of pharmacotherapy. Recommend needed follow-up evaluations or tests when appropriate.
- **1.3.3** Identify, describe, and provide information regarding the mechanism of adverse reactions, allergies, side effects, iatrogenic, and drug-induced illness, including their management and prevention.

(2) If a child's dose (5 mL) of a cough syrup contains 10 mg of dextromethorphan hydrobromide, what mass of drug is contained in 240 mL?

$$\frac{240\text{ mL}}{5\text{ mL}} = \frac{x\text{ mg}}{10\text{ mg}}$$

$$x = \frac{240 \times 10}{5} = 480\text{ mg}$$

(3) If the amount of dextromethorphan hydrobromide in 240 mL of cough syrup is 480 mg, what would be the volume required for a child's dose of 10 mg?

$$\frac{x\text{ mL}}{240\text{ mL}} = \frac{10\text{ mg}}{480\text{ mg}}$$

$$x = \frac{10 \times 240}{480} = 5\text{mL}$$

(4) How many milligrams of dextromethorphan base (molecular weight = 271.4) are equivalent to 10 mg of dextromethorphan hydrobromide (molecular weight = 352.3)?

$$\frac{x\text{ mg}}{10\text{ mg}} = \frac{271.4}{352.3}$$

$$x = 10 \times \frac{271.4}{352.3} = 7.7\text{ mg}$$

b. **Mixed ratios**. Some pharmacists use mixed ratios (in which dissimilar units are used in the numerator and denominator of each ratio) in their proportion calculations. Such computations generally give correct answers, providing the conditions in which mixed ratios cannot be used are known. A later example shows mixed ratios leading to failure in the case of dilution, when inverse proportions are required. For **inverse proportions**, similar units must be used in the numerator and denominator of each ratio. Following is an example of a mixed ratio calculation using the previous problem.

$$\frac{480\text{ mg}}{10\text{ mL}} = \frac{240\text{ mg}}{x\text{ mL}}$$

$$x = 240 \times \frac{10}{480} = 5\text{ mL}$$

The **same answer** is obtained in this example whether we use proper ratios, with similar units in numerator and denominator, or mixed ratios. This is not the case when dealing with inverse proportions.

3. **Inverse proportion**. The most common example of the need for inverse proportion for the pharmacist is the case of **dilution**. Whereas in the previous examples of proportion the relationships involved direct proportion, the case of dilution calls for an inverse proportion (i.e., as volume increases, concentration decreases). The necessity of using inverse proportions for dilution problems is shown in this example.

If 120 mL of a 10% stock solution is diluted to 240 mL, what is the final concentration? Using inverse proportion,

$$\frac{120\text{ mL}}{240\text{ mL}} = \frac{x\%}{10\%}$$

$$120 \times \frac{10}{240} = 5\%$$

As expected, the final concentration is one-half of the original concentration because the volume is doubled. However, if the pharmacist attempts to use direct proportion and neglects to estimate an appropriate answer, the resulting calculation would provide an answer of 20%, which is twice the actual concentration.

$$\frac{120\text{ mL}}{240\text{ mL}} = \frac{10\%}{x\%}$$

$$240 \times \frac{10}{120} = 20\%\text{ (incorrect answer)}$$

Likewise, the pharmacist using mixed ratios fails in this case

$$\frac{120 \text{ mL}}{10\%} = \frac{240 \text{ mL}}{x\%}$$

and

$$10 \times \frac{240}{120} = 20\% \text{ (again, incorrect answer)}$$

B. Aliquot. A pharmacist requires the aliquot method of measurement when the **sensitivity** (the smallest quantity that can be measured with the required accuracy and precision) of the measuring device is not great enough for the required measurement. Aliquot calculations can be used for measurement of solids or liquids, allowing the pharmacist to realize the required precision through a process of measuring a multiple of the desired amount, followed by dilution, and finally selection and measurement of an aliquot part that contains the desired amount of material. This example problem involves weighing by the aliquot method, using a prescription balance.

A prescription balance has a sensitivity requirement of 6 mg. How would you weigh 10 mg of drug with an accuracy of ± 5% using a suitable diluent?

1. First, calculate the least weighable quantity for the balance with a sensitivity requirement of 6 mg, assuming ± 5% accuracy is required.

$$\frac{6 \text{ mg}}{x \text{ mg}} = \frac{5\%}{100\%}; x = 120 \text{ mg (least weighable quantity for our balance)}$$

2. Now it is obvious that an aliquot calculation is required because 10 mg of drug is required, whereas the least weighable quantity is 120 mg to achieve the required percentage of error. Using the least weighable quantity method of aliquot measurement, use the smallest quantity weighable on the balance at each step to preserve materials.
   - **a.** Weigh 12 × 10 mg = 120 mg of drug.
   - **b.** Dilute the 120 mg of drug (from step **a**) with a suitable diluent by geometrical dilution to achieve a mixture that will provide 10 mg of drug in each 120-mg aliquot. The amount of diluent to be used can be determined through **proportion**.

$$\frac{120 \text{ mg drug}}{10 \text{ mg drug}} = \frac{x \text{ mg total mixture}}{120 \text{ mg aliquot mixture}}$$

$$x = 1440 \text{ mg total mixture}$$

$$1440 \text{ mg total} - 120 \text{ mg drug} = 1320 \text{ mg diluent}$$

   - **c.** Weigh 120 mg (1/12) of the total mixture of 1440 mg that will contain the required 10 mg of drug, which is 1/12 of the 120 mg.

II. SYSTEMS OF MEASURE.

The pharmacist must be familiar with **three systems** of measure: the **metric system** and two common systems of measure (the **avoirdupois** and **apothecaries'** systems). The primary system of measure in pharmacy and medicine is the metric system. Most students find it easiest to convert measurements in the common systems to metric units. A table of conversion equivalents is provided and should be memorized by the pharmacist (see Appendix B). The metric system, because of its universal acceptance and broad use, will not be reviewed here.

A. Apothecaries' system of fluid measure. The apothecaries' system of fluid measure is summarized in Appendix B.

B. Apothecaries' system for measuring weight. The apothecaries' system for measuring weight includes units of grains, scruples, drams, ounces, and pounds (see Appendix B).

C. Avoirdupois system of measuring weight. The avoirdupois (AV) system of measuring weight includes the grain, ounce, and pound. The grain is a unit common with the apothecaries' system and allows for easy conversion between the systems. The avoirdupois pound, however, is 16 AV ounces in contrast to the apothecaries' pound that is 12 apothecaries' ounces (see Appendix B).

D. Conversion equivalents. See Appendix B.

In answering this one question, the first two types of problems listed beforehand have been solved, while exhibiting two methods of solving percentage problems—namely, by **dimensional analysis** and **proportion**.

b. For an example of the **third type** of percentage w/v problem, determine what volume of syrup could be prepared if we had only 8 g of magnesium carbonate. Use proportion to find the total volume of syrup that can be made using only 8 g of magnesium carbonate. If we have 10 g of magnesium carbonate in 1000 mL of solution, then, according to the recipe, 800 mL of solution can be prepared using all 8 g of the drug.

$$\frac{10\text{ g}}{1000\text{ mL}} = \frac{8\text{ g}}{x\text{ mL}};\ x = 800\text{ mL}$$

B. Percentage volume in volume (v/v). Percentage v/v indicates the number of milliliters of a constituent in 100 mL of liquid formulation. The percentage strength of mixtures of liquids in liquids is indicated by percentage v/v, which indicates the parts by volume of a substance in 100 parts of the liquid preparation. The **three types** of problems that are encountered involve calculating **percentage strength**, calculating **volume of ingredient**, and calculating **volume of the liquid preparation**. Using the same tolu balsam syrup formula from earlier, we'll now work a percentage v/v problem.

What is the percentage strength v/v of the tolu balsam tincture in the syrup preparation? By proportion, we can solve the problem in one step.

$$\frac{50\text{ mL tolu balsam tincture}}{x\text{ mL tolu balsam tincture}} = \frac{1000\text{ mL syrup}}{100\text{ mL syrup}};\ x = 5\%$$

C. Percentage weight in weight (w/w). Percentage w/w indicates the number of grams of a constituent per 100 g of formulation (solid or liquid). Solution of problems involving percentage w/w is straightforward when the total mass of the mixture is available or when the total mass can be determined from the available data. In calculations similar to those for percentage w/v and v/v, the pharmacist might need to solve several types of problems, including determination of the weight of a constituent, the total weight of a mixture, or the percentage w/w.

1. **How many grams of drug substance should be used to prepare 240 g of a 5% w/w solution in water?**
   - **a.** The first step in any percentage w/w problem is to attempt identification of the total mass of the mixture. In this problem, the total mass is, obviously, provided (240 g).
   - **b.** The problem can be easily solved through **dimensional analysis**.

$$240\text{ g mixture} \times \frac{5.0\text{ g drug}}{100\text{ g drug}} = 12\text{ g}$$

2. When the total mass of the mixture is unavailable or cannot be determined, an **extra step** is required in the calculations. Because it is usually impossible to know how much volume is displaced by a solid material, the pharmacist is unable to prepare a specified volume of a solution given the percentage w/w.

   How much drug should be added to 30 mL of water to make a 10% w/w solution? The volume of water that is displaced by the drug is unknown, so the final volume is unknown. Likewise, even though the mass of solvent is known (30 mL × 1 g/mL = 30 g), it is not known how much drug is needed, so the total mass is unknown. The water represents 100% − 10% = 90% of the total mixture. Then, by proportion, the mass of drug to be used can be identified.

$$\frac{30\text{ g of mixture (water)}}{x\text{ g of mixture (drug)}} = \frac{90\%}{10\%};\ x = 3.33\text{ g of drug required to make a solution}$$

   The **common error** that many students make in solving problems of this type is to assume that 30 g is the total mass of the mixture. Solving the problem with that assumption gives the following incorrect answer.

$$\frac{x\text{ g drug}}{10\text{ g drug}} = \frac{30\text{ g mixture}}{100\text{ g mixture}};\ x = 3\text{ g of drug (incorrect answer)}$$

D. Ratio strength. Solid or liquid formulations that contain low concentrations of active ingredients will often have concentration expressed in **ratio strength**. Ratio strength, as the name implies, is the expression of concentration by means of a ratio. The numerator and denominator of the ratio indicate grams (g) or milliliters (mL) of a solid or liquid constituent in the total mass (g) or volume (mL) of a solid or liquid preparation. Because **percentage strength** is essentially a ratio of parts per hundred, conversion between ratio strength and percentage strength is easily accomplished by proportion.

1. **Express 0.1% w/v as a ratio strength.**
   a. Ratio strengths are by convention expressed in reduced form, so in setting up our proportion to solve for ratio strength, use the numeral 1 in the numerator of the right-hand ratio as shown:

$$\frac{0.1\text{ g}}{100\text{ mL}} = \frac{1\text{ part}}{x\text{ parts}}; = 1000\text{ parts, for ratio strength of 1:1000}$$

   b. Likewise, conversion from ratio strength to percentage strength by proportion is easy, as seen in the following example. Keep in mind the definition of percentage strength (parts per hundred) when setting up the proportion.
2. **Express 1:2500 as a percentage strength.**

$$\frac{1\text{ part}}{2500\text{ parts}} = \frac{x\text{ parts}}{100\text{ parts}}; x = 0.04\text{, indicating 0.04\%}$$

E. **Other concentration expressions**

1. **Molarity** (M) is the expression of the number of moles of solute dissolved per liter of solution. It is calculated by dividing the moles of solute by the volume of solution in liters.

$$M_A = \frac{n_A}{\text{solution (L)}}$$

2. **Normality.** A convenient way of dealing with acids, bases, and electrolytes involves the use of equivalents. One equivalent of an acid is the quantity of that acid that supplies or donates 1 mole of H^+ ions. One equivalent of a base is the quantity that furnishes 1 mole of OH^- ions. One equivalent of acid reacts with one equivalent of base. Equivalent weight can be calculated for atoms or molecules.

$$\text{Equivalent weight} = \frac{\text{atomic weight or molecular weight}}{\text{valence}}$$

The **normality** (N) of a solution is the number of gram-equivalent weights (equivalents) of solute per liter of solution. Normality is analogous to molarity; however, it is defined in terms of equivalents rather than moles.

$$\text{Normality} = \frac{\#\text{ equivalents of solute}}{\#\text{ liters of solution}}$$

3. **Molality** (m) is the moles of solute dissolved per kilogram of solvent. Molality is calculated by dividing the number of moles of solute by the number of kilograms of solvent. Molality offers an advantage over molarity because it is based on solvent weight and avoids problems associated with volume expansion or contraction owing to the addition of solutes or from a change in temperature.

$$m_A = \frac{n_A}{\text{mass}_{\text{ solvent (kg)}}}$$

4. **Mole fraction** (X) is the ratio of the number of moles of one component to the total moles of a mixture or solution.

$$X_A = \frac{n_A}{n_A, n_B, n_C \ldots}, \text{ where } X_A + X_B + X_C + \ldots = 1$$

VI. DILUTION AND CONCENTRATION.

If the amount of drug remains constant in a dilution or concentration, then any change in the mass or volume of a mixture is inversely proportional to the concentration.

A. **Dilution and concentration problems can be solved by the following:**

1. Inverse proportion (as mentioned earlier)
2. The equation $\text{quantity}_1 \times \text{concentration}_1 = \text{quantity}_2 \times \text{concentration}_2$

2. Calculate the equivalent weight (Eq wt) of KCl.

$$\text{Eq wt} = \frac{\text{mol wt}}{\text{valence}} = \frac{74.5}{1} = 74.5 \text{ g}$$

3. Determine the milliequivalent weight, which is 1/1000 of the equivalent weight.

$$\text{mEq wt} = 74.5 \text{ g}/1000 = 0.745 \text{ g or } 74.5 \text{ mg}$$

Now that we know the milliequivalent weight, we can calculate by dimensional analysis and proportion the concentration in percentage in a fourth step.

4. 0.0745 g/mEq × 2 mEq = 0.149 g of drug

$$\frac{0.149 \text{ g drug}}{1 \text{ mL}} = \frac{x \text{ g drug}}{100 \text{ mL}}; x = 14.9 \text{ g}/100 \text{ mL} = 14.9\%$$

How many milliequivalents of Na^+ would be contained in a 15-mL volume of the following buffer?

$Na_2HPO_4 \cdot 7H_2O$		180 g
$NaH_2PO_4 \cdot H_2O$		480 g
Purified water	a.d.	1000 mL

For each salt, the mass (and milliequivalents) must be found in a 15-mL dose.

$$\text{mol wt } Na_2HPO_4 \cdot 7H_2O \text{ (disodium hydrogen phosphate)} = 268 \text{ g}$$
$$\text{Eq wt} = 268/2 = 134 \text{ g}$$
$$1 \text{ mEq} = 0.134 \text{ g or } 134 \text{ mg}$$

$$\frac{180 \text{ g}}{x \text{ g}} = \frac{1000 \text{ mL}}{15 \text{ mL}}; x = 2.7 \text{ g of disodium hydrogen phosphate in each 15 mL}$$

$$2.7 \text{ g} \times \frac{1 \text{ mEq}}{0.134 \text{ g}} = 20.1 \text{ mEq of disodium hydrogen phosphate}$$

$$\text{mol wt } NaH_2PO_4 \cdot H_2O \text{ (sodium biphosphate)} = 138 \text{ g}$$
$$\text{Eq wt} = 138 \text{ g}$$
$$1 \text{ mEq} = 0.138 \text{ g}$$

$$\frac{480 \text{ g}}{x \text{ g}} = \frac{1000 \text{ mL}}{15 \text{ mL}}; x = 7.2 \text{ g of sodium biphosphate in each 15 mL}$$

$$7.2 \text{ g} \times \frac{1 \text{ mEq}}{0.138 \text{ g}} = 52.2 \text{ mEq of sodium biphosphate}$$

$$20.1 \text{ mEq} + 52.2 \text{ mEq} = 72.3 \text{ mEq of sodium in each 15 mL of solution}$$

B. **Milliosmoles (mOsmol).** Osmotic pressure is directly proportional to the total number of particles in solution. The milliosmole is the unit of measure for osmotic concentration. For nonelectrolytes, 1 millimole represents 1 mOsmol. However, for electrolytes, the total number of particles in a solution is determined by the number of particles produced in a solution and influenced by the degree of dissociation. Assuming complete dissociation, 1 millimole of KCl represents 2 mOsmol of total particles, 1 millimole of $CaCl_2$ represents 3 mOsmol of total particles, etc. The ideal osmolar concentration can be calculated with the following equation.

$$\text{mOsmol/L} = \frac{\text{wt of substance in g/L}}{\text{mol wt in g}} \times \text{number of species} \times 1000$$

The pharmacist should recognize the difference between **ideal** osmolar concentration and **actual** osmolarity. As the concentration of solute increases, interaction between dissolved particles increases, resulting in a reduction of the actual osmolar values.

C. **Isotonic solutions.** An **isotonic** solution is one that has the same osmotic pressure as body fluids. **Isosmotic** fluids are fluids with the same osmotic pressure. Solutions to be administered to patients should be isosmotic with body fluids. A **hypotonic** solution is one with a lower osmotic pressure than body fluids, whereas a **hypertonic** solution has an osmotic pressure that is greater than body fluids.

1. **Preparation of isotonic solutions.** Colligative properties, including freezing point depression, are representative of the number of particles in a solution and are considered in preparation of isotonic solutions.
   a. When 1 g mol wt of any nonelectrolyte is dissolved in 1000 g of water, the freezing point of the solution is depressed by 1.86°C. By proportion, the weight of any nonelectrolyte needed to make the solution isotonic with body fluid can be calculated.
   b. Boric acid (H_3BO_3) has a mol wt of 61.8 g. Thus, 61.8 g of H_3BO_3 in 1000 g of water should produce a freezing point of 1.86°C. Therefore, knowing that the freezing point depression of body fluids is −0.52°C,

$$\frac{-1.86°\text{C}}{-0.52°\text{C}} = \frac{61.8\ \text{g}}{x\ \text{g}};\ x = 17.3\ \text{g}$$

   and 17.3 g of H_3BO_3 in 1000 g of water provides a solution that is **isotonic**.
   c. The degree of dissociation of electrolytes must be taken into account in such calculations. For example, NaCl is approximately 80% dissociated in weak solutions, yielding 180 particles in a solution for each 100 molecules of NaCl. Therefore,

$$\frac{-1.86°\text{C} \times 1.8}{-0.52°\text{C}} = \frac{58\ \text{g}}{x\ \text{g}};\ x = 9.09\ \text{g}$$

   indicating that 9.09 g of NaCl in 1000 g of water (0.9% w/v) should make a solution isotonic. Lacking any information on the degree of dissociation of an electrolyte, the following **dissociation values** (i) may be used:
   (1) Substances that dissociate into two ions: 1.8
   (2) Substances that dissociate into three ions: 2.6
   (3) Substances that dissociate into four ions: 3.4
   (4) Substances that dissociate into five ions: 4.2
2. **Sodium chloride equivalents.** The pharmacist will often be required to prepare an isotonic solution by adding an appropriate amount of another substance (drug or inert electrolyte or nonelectrolyte). Considering that isotonic fluids contain the equivalent of 0.9% NaCl, the question arises, how much of the added ingredient is required to make the solution isotonic? A **common method** for computing the amount of added ingredient to use for reaching isotonicity involves the use of **sodium chloride equivalents.**
   a. **Definition.** The sodium chloride equivalent represents the amount of NaCl that is equivalent to the amount of particular drug in question. For every substance, there is one quantity that should have a constant tonic effect when dissolved in 1000 g of water. This is 1 g mol wt of the substance divided by its dissociation value (i).
   b. **Examples**
   (1) Considering H_3BO_3, from the last section, 17.3 g of H_3BO_3 is equivalent to 0.52 g of NaCl in tonicity. Therefore, the relative quantity of NaCl that is equivalent to H_3BO_3 in tonicity effects is determined as follows:

$$\frac{\text{mol wt of NaCl}/i\ \text{value}}{\text{mol wt of H}_3\text{BO}_3/i\ \text{value}} = \frac{58.5/1.8}{61.8/1.0}$$

   Applying this method to atropine sulfate, recall that the molecular weight of NaCl and the molecular weight of atropine sulfate are 58.5 and 695 g, respectively, and their i values are 1.8 and 2.6, respectively. Calculate the mass of NaCl represented by 1 g of atropine sulfate (*Table 1-2*).

$$\frac{695 \times 1.8}{58.5 \times 2.6} = \frac{1\ \text{g}}{x\ \text{g}};\ x = 0.12\ \text{g NaCl represented by 1 g of atropine sulfate}$$

Table 1-2 SODIUM CHLORIDE (NaCl) EQUIVALENTS

Substance	NaCl Equivalent
Atropine sulfate (H_2O)	0.12
Boric acid	0.52
Chlorobutanol	0.24
Dextrose (anhydrous)	0.18
Ephedrine hydrochloride	0.29
Phenacaine hydrochloride	0.20
Potassium chloride	0.78

(2) An example of the practical use of sodium chloride equivalents is seen in the following problem:

How many grams of boric acid should be used in compounding the following prescription?

Rx	phenacaine hydrochloride	1%
	chlorobutanol	0.5%
	boric acid	q.s.
	purified water, a.d.	60.0 mL
	make isotonic solution	

The prescription calls for 0.3 g of chlorobutanol and 0.6 g of phenacaine. How much boric acid is required to prepare this prescription? The question is best answered in four steps:

(a) Find the mass of sodium chloride represented by all ingredients.

$0.20 \times 0.6 = 0.120$ g of sodium choloride represented by phenacaine hydrochloride

$0.24 \times 0.3 = \underline{0.072}$ g of sodium chloride represented by chlorobutanol

0.192 g of sodium chloride represented by the two active ingredients

(b) Find the mass of sodium chloride required to prepare an equal volume of isotonic solution.

$$\frac{0.9 \text{ g NaCl}}{100 \text{ mL}} = \frac{x \text{ g NaCL}}{60 \text{ mL}}; x = 0.540 \text{ g of sodium chloride}$$

in 60 mL of an isotonic sodium chloride solution

(c) Calculate, by subtraction, the amount of NaCl required to make the solution isotonic.

0.540 g NaCl required for isotonicity
0.192 g NaCl represented by ingredients
0.348 g NaCl required to make isotonic solution

(d) Because the prescription calls for boric acid to be used, one last step is required

$$\frac{0.348 \text{ g}}{0.52} \text{ (sodium chloride equivalent for boric acid)} = 0.669 \text{ g of boric acid to be used}$$

Study Questions

Directions for questions 1–30: Each question, statement, or incomplete statement in this section can be correctly answered or completed by **one** of the suggested answers or phrases. Choose the **best** answer.

1. If a vitamin solution contains 0.5 mg of fluoride ion in each milliliter, then how many milligrams of fluoride ion would be provided by a dropper that delivers 0.6 mL?

(A) 0.30 mg
(B) 0.10 mg
(C) 1.00 mg
(D) 0.83 mg

2. How many chloramphenicol capsules, each containing 250 mg, are needed to provide 25 mg/kg/d for 7 days for a person weighing 200 lb?

(A) 90 capsules
(B) 64 capsules
(C) 13 capsules
(D) 25 capsules

3. If 3.17 kg of a drug is used to make 50000 tablets, how many milligrams will 30 tablets contain?

(A) 1.9 mg
(B) 1900 mg
(C) 0.0019 mg
(D) 3.2 mg

4. A capsule contains ⅛ gr of ephedrine sulfate, ¼ gr of theophylline, and $\frac{1}{16}$ gr of phenobarbital. What is the total mass of the active ingredients in milligrams?

(A) 20 mg
(B) 8 mg
(C) 28 mg
(D) 4 mg

5. If 1 fluid ounce of a cough syrup contains 10 gr of sodium citrate, how many milligrams are contained in 10 mL?

(A) 650 mg
(B) 65 mg
(C) 217 mg
(D) 20 mg

6. How many capsules, each containing ¼ gr of phenobarbital, can be manufactured if a bottle containing 2 avoirdupois ounces of phenobarbital is available?

(A) 771 capsules
(B) 350 capsules
(C) 3500 capsules
(D) 1250 capsules

7. Using the formula for calamine lotion, determine the amount of calamine (in grams) necessary to prepare 240 mL of lotion.

calamine	80 g
zinc oxide	80 g
glycerin	20 mL
bentonite magma	250 mL
calcium hydroxide topical solution	sufficient quantity to make 1000 mL

(A) 19.2 g
(B) 140.0 g
(C) 100.0 g
(D) 24.0 g

8. From the following formula, calculate the amount of white wax required to make 1 lb of cold cream. Determine the mass in grams.

cetyl esters wax	12.5 parts
white wax	12.0 parts
mineral oil	56.0 parts
sodium borate	0.5 parts
purified water	19.0 parts

(A) 56.75 g
(B) 254.24 g
(C) 54.48 g
(D) 86.26 g

9. How many grams of aspirin should be used to prepare 1.255 kg of the powder?

Aspirin	6 parts
phenacetin	3 parts
caffeine	1 part

(A) 125 g
(B) 750 g
(C) 175 g
(D) 360 g

10. A solution contains 1.25 mg of a drug per milliliter. At what rate should the solution be infused (drops per minute) if the drug is to be administered at a rate of 80 mg/hr? (1 mL = 30 drops)

(A) 64.00 drops/min
(B) 1.06 drops/min
(C) 32.00 drops/min
(D) 20.00 drops/min

11. The recommended maintenance dose of aminophylline for children is 1.0 mg/kg/hr by injection. If 10 mL of a 25-mg/mL solution of aminophylline is added to a 100-mL bottle of 5% dextrose, what should be the rate of delivery in mL/hr for a 40-lb child?

(A) 2.30 mL/hr
(B) 8.00 mL/hr
(C) 18.90 mL/hr
(D) 18.20 mL/hr

12. For children, streptomycin is to be administered at a dose of 30 mg/kg of body weight daily in divided doses every 6 to 12 hrs. The dry powder is dissolved by adding water for injection, in an amount to yield the desired concentration as indicated in the following table (for a 1-g vial).

Approximate Concentration (mg/mL)	Volume (mL)
200	4.2
250	3.2
400	1.8

Reconstituting at the lowest possible concentration, what volume (in mL) would be withdrawn to obtain a day's dose for a 50-lb child?

(A) 3.40 mL
(B) 22.73 mL
(C) 2.50 mL
(D) 2.27 mL

13. The atropine sulfate is available only in the form of 1/150 gr tablets. How many atropine sulfate tablets would you use to compound the following prescription?

atropine sulfate	1/200 gr
codeine phosphate	¼ gr
aspirin	5 gr
d.t.d.	#24 capsules
Sig:	1 capsule p.r.n.

(A) 3 tablets
(B) 6 tablets
(C) 12 tablets
(D) 18 tablets

14. In 25.0 mL of a solution for injection, there are 4.00 mg of the drug. If the dose to be administered to a patient is 200 μg, what quantity (in mL) of this solution should be used?

(A) 1.25 mL
(B) 125.00 mL
(C) 12.00 mL
(D) None of the above

15. How many milligrams of papaverine will the patient receive each day?

R_x	papaverine hcl	1.0 g
	aqua	30.0 mL
	syrup tolu, q.s. a.d.	90.0 mL
	Sig:	1 teaspoon t.i.d.

(A) 56.0 mg
(B) 5.6 mg
(C) 166.0 mg
(D) 2.5 mg

16. Considering the following formula, how many grams of sodium bromide should be used in filling this prescription?

R_x	sodium bromide	1.2 g
	syrup tolu	2.0 mL
	syrup wild cherry, q.s. a.d.	5.0 mL
	d.t.d.	#24

(A) 1.2 g
(B) 1200.0 g
(C) 28.8 g
(D) 220.0 g

17. How many milliliters of a 7.5% stock solution of $KMnO_4$ should be used to obtain the KMnO needed?

$KMnO_4$, q.s.
Distilled water, a.d. 1000 mL
Sig: 2 teaspoons diluted to 500 mL yield a 1:5000 solution

(A) 267.0 mL
(B) 133.0 mL
(C) 26.7 mL
(D) 13.3 mL

18. The formula for Ringer's solution follows. How much sodium chloride is needed to make 120 mL?

R_x	sodium chloride	8.60 g
	potassium chloride	0.30 g
	calcium chloride	0.33 g
	water for injection, q.s. a.d.	1000 mL

(A) 120.00 g
(B) 1.03 g
(C) 0.12 g
(D) 103.00 g

19. How many grams of talc should be added to 1 lb of a powder containing 20 g of zinc undecylenate per 100 g to reduce the concentration of zinc undecylenate to 3%?

(A) 3026.7 g
(B) 2572.7 g
(C) 17.0 g
(D) 257.0 g

20. How many milliliters of a 0.9% aqueous solution can be made from 20.0 g of sodium chloride?

(A) 2222 mL
(B) 100 mL
(C) 222 mL
(D) 122 mL

21. The blood of a reckless driver contains 0.1% alcohol. Express the concentration of alcohol in parts per million.

(A) 100 ppm
(B) 1000 ppm
(C) 1 ppm
(D) 250 ppm

22. Syrup is an 85% w/v solution of sucrose in water. It has a density of 1.313 g/mL. How many milliliters of water should be used to make 125 mL of syrup?

(A) 106.25 mL
(B) 164.10 mL
(C) 57.90 mL
(D) 25.00 mL

23. How many grams of benzethonium chloride should be used in preparing 5 gal of a 0.025% w/v solution?

(A) 189.25 g
(B) 18.90 g
(C) 4.73 g
(D) 35.00 g

24. How many grams of menthol should be used to prepare this prescription?

R_x	menthol	0.8%
	alcohol, q.s. a.d.	60.0 mL

(A) 0.48 g
(B) 0.80 g
(C) 4.80 g
(D) 1.48 g

25. How many milliliters of a 1:1500 solution can be made by dissolving 4.8 g of cetylpyridinium chloride in water?

(A) 7200.0 mL
(B) 7.2 mL
(C) 48.0 mL
(D) 4.8 mL

26. The manufacturer specifies that one Domeboro tablet dissolved in 1 pint of water makes a modified Burow's solution approximately equivalent to a 1:40 dilution. How many tablets should be used in preparing ½ gal of a 1:10 dilution?

(A) 16 tablets
(B) 189 tablets
(C) 12 tablets
(D) 45 tablets

27. How many milliosmoles of calcium chloride ($CaCl_2 \cdot 2H_2O$ – mol wt = 147) are represented in 147 mL of a 10% w/v calcium chloride solution?

(A) 100 mOsmol
(B) 200 mOsmol
(C) 300 mOsmol
(D) 3 mOsmol

28. How many grams of boric acid should be used in compounding the following prescription?

Phenacaine HCl 1.0% (NaCl eq = 0.17)
Chlorobutanol 0.5% (NaCl eq = 0.18)
Boric acid, q.s. (NaCl eq = 0.52)
Purified H_2O, a.d. 30 mL
Make isotonic solution
Sig: 1 drop in each eye

(A) 0.37 g
(B) 0.74 g
(C) 0.27 g
(D) 0.47 g

29. A pharmacist prepares 1 gal of KCl solution by mixing 565 g of KCl (valence = 1) in an appropriate vehicle. How many milliequivalents of K^+ are in 15 mL of this solution? (atomic weights: K = 39; Cl = 35.5)

(A) 7.5 mEq
(B) 10.0 mEq
(C) 20.0 mEq
(D) 30.0 mEq
(E) 40.0 mEq

30. A vancomycin solution containing 1000 mg of vancomycin hydrochloride diluted to 250 mL with D_5W is to be infused at a constant rate with an infusion pump in 2 hrs. What is the rate of drug administration?

(A) 2.08 mg/min
(B) 8.33 mg/min
(C) 4.17 mg/min
(D) 16.70 mg/min
(E) 5.21 mg/min

2

Pharmaceutical Principles and Drug Dosage Forms

LAWRENCE H. BLOCK

I. INTRODUCTION.

Pharmaceutical principles are the underlying physicochemical principles that allow a drug to be incorporated into a pharmaceutical **dosage form** (e.g., solution, capsule). These principles apply whether the drug is extemporaneously compounded by the pharmacist or manufactured for commercial distribution as a **drug product**.

A. The finished **dosage form** contains the active drug ingredient in association with nondrug (usually inert) ingredients (**excipients**) that make up the **vehicle**, or **formulation matrix**.

B. The **drug delivery system** concept, which has evolved since the 1960s, is a more holistic concept. It embraces not only the drug (or prodrug) and its formulation matrix, but also the dynamic interactions among the drug, its formulation matrix, its container, and the physiologic milieux of the patient. These dynamic interactions are the subject of **biopharmaceutics** (see Chapter 3).

II. INTERMOLECULAR FORCES OF ATTRACTION

A. **Introduction**. The application of pharmaceutical principles to drug dosage forms is illustrated when drug dosage forms are **categorized** according to their **physical state**, **degree of heterogeneity**, and **chemical composition**. The usual relevant states of matter are **gases**, **liquids**, and **solids**. Intermolecular forces of attraction are weakest in gases and strongest in solids. Conversions from one physical state to another can involve simply overcoming intermolecular forces of attraction by adding energy (heat). Chemical composition can have a dramatic effect on physicochemical properties and behavior. For this reason, it is necessary to distinguish between **polymers**, or **macromolecules**, and more conventional (i.e., smaller) molecules, or **micromolecules**.

B. **Intermolecular forces of attraction**. Because atoms vary in their electronegativity, electron sharing between different atoms is likely to be unequal. This asymmetric electron distribution causes a shift in the overall electron cloud in the molecule. As a result, the molecule tends to behave as a **dipole** (i.e., as if it had a positive and a negative pole). The dipole associated with each covalent bond has a corresponding **dipole moment** (μ) defined as the product of the distance of charge separation (d) and the charge (q):

$$\mu = q \times d$$

The molecular dipole moment may be viewed as the vector sum of the individual bond moments.

1. **Nonpolar** molecules that have **perfect symmetry** (e.g., carbon tetrachloride) have dipole moments of zero (*Figure 2-1*).

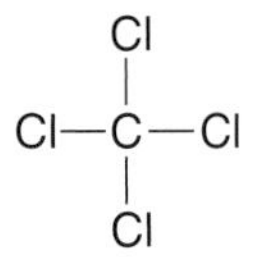

Figure 2-1. The carbon tetrachloride molecule.

2. **Polar** molecules are **asymmetric** and have nonzero dipole moments.
3. When **dipolar** molecules approach one another close enough—"positive to positive" or "negative to negative"—so that their electron clouds interpenetrate, **intermolecular repulsive forces** arise. When these dipolar molecules approach one another so that the positive pole of one is close to the negative pole of the other, molecular **attraction** occurs (**dipole–dipole interaction**). When the identically charged poles of the two molecules are closer, **repulsion** occurs.

C. **Types of intermolecular forces of attraction** include the following:
1. Nonpolar molecules do not have permanent dipoles. However, the instantaneous electron distribution in a molecule can be asymmetric. The resultant transient dipole moment can induce a dipole in an adjacent molecule. This **induced dipole-induced dipole interaction** (**London dispersion force**), with a force of 0.5 to 1 kcal/mol, is sufficient to facilitate order in a molecular array. These relatively weak electrostatic forces are responsible for the liquefaction of nonpolar gases.
2. The transient dipole induced by a permanent dipole, or **dipole-induced dipole interaction** (**Debye induction force**), is a stronger interaction, with a force of 1 to 3 kcal/mol.
3. **Permanent dipole interactions** (**Keesom orientation forces**), with a force of 1 to 7 kcal/mol, together with Debye and London forces, constitute **van der Waals forces**. Collectively, they are responsible for the more substantive structure and molecular ordering found in liquids.
4. **Hydrogen bonds**. Because they are small and have a large electrostatic field, hydrogen atoms can approach highly electronegative atoms (e.g., fluorine, oxygen, nitrogen, chlorine, sulfur) and interact electrostatically to form a hydrogen bond. Depending on the electronegativity of the second atom and the molecular environment in which hydrogen bonding occurs, hydrogen bond energy varies from approximately 1 to 8 kcal/mol.
5. **Ion–ion, ion–dipole, and ion-induced dipole forces**. **Positive–negative ion interactions** in the solid state involve forces of 100 to 200 kcal/mol. Ionic interactions are reduced considerably in liquid systems in the presence of other electrolytes. **Ion–dipole** interaction, or **dipole induction by an ion**, can also affect molecular aggregation, or ordering, in a system.

III. STATES OF MATTER

A. **Gases**. Molecules in the gaseous state can be pictured as moving along straight paths, in all directions and at high velocities (e.g., mean velocity for H_2O vapor: 587 m/sec; for O_2: 440 m/sec), until they collide with other molecules. As a result of these random collisions, molecular velocities and paths change, and the molecules continue to collide with other molecules and with the boundaries of the system (e.g., the walls of a container holding the gas). This process, repeated incessantly, is responsible for the **pressure** exhibited within the confines of the system.
1. The interrelation among **volume (V)**, **pressure (P)**, and the **absolute temperature (T)** is given by the **ideal gas law**, which is the equation of state for an ideal gas:

$$PV = nRT$$
$$PV = (g/M)RT$$

where n is the number of moles of gas—equivalent to the number of grams (g) of gas divided by the molecular weight of the gas (M)—and R is the **molar gas constant** (0.08205 L atm/mole deg).
2. Pharmaceutical gases include the **anesthetic gases** (e.g., nitrous oxide, halothane). **Compressed gases** include oxygen (for therapy), nitrogen, and carbon dioxide. **Liquefiable gases**, including certain **halohydrocarbons** and **hydrocarbons**, are used as propellants in **aerosol products** (**pressurized packaging**), as are compressed gases, such as nitrous oxide, nitrogen, and carbon dioxide. Ethylene oxide is a gas used to sterilize or disinfect heat-labile objects.
3. In general, as the temperature of a substance increases, its **heat content**, or **enthalpy**, increases as well.
   a. Substances can undergo a change of state, or phase change, from the solid to the liquid state (**melting**) or from the liquid to the gaseous state (**vaporization**).
   b. **Volatile liquids** (e.g., ether, halothane, methoxyflurane) are used as inhalation anesthetics. Amyl nitrite is a volatile liquid that is inhaled for its vasodilating effect in acute angina.
   c. **Sublimation** occurs when a solid is heated directly to the gaseous, or vapor, state without passing through the liquid state (e.g., camphor, iodine). Ice sublimes at pressures below 3 torr. The process of **freeze-drying**, or **lyophilization**, is a form of vacuum drying in which water is

removed by sublimation from the frozen product. It is an especially useful process for drying aqueous solutions or dispersions of heat- or oxygen-sensitive drugs and biologicals (e.g., proteins, peptides).

d. The reverse process (i.e., direct transition from the vapor state to the solid state) is also referred to as sublimation, but the preferred term is **deposition**. Some forms of sulfur and colloidal silicon dioxide are prepared in this way.

4. The intermolecular forces of attraction in gases are virtually nonexistent at room temperature. Gases display little or no ordering.

B. **Liquids**. The intermolecular forces of attraction in liquids (**van der Waals forces**) are sufficient to impose some ordering, or regular arrangement, among the molecules. **Hydrogen bonding** increases the likelihood of cohesion in liquids and further affects their physicochemical behavior. However, these forces are much weaker than **covalent** or **ionic** forces. Therefore, liquids tend to display short-range rather than long-range order. Hypothetically, although molecules of a liquid would tend to aggregate in localized clusters, no defined structuring would be evident.

1. **Surface and interfacial tension**

a. Molecules in the bulk phase of a liquid are surrounded by other molecules of the same kind (*Figure 2-2A*). Molecules at the surface of a liquid are not completely surrounded by like molecules (*Figure 2-2B*). As a result, molecules at or near the surface of a liquid experience a net inward pull from molecules in the interior of the liquid. Because of this net inward intermolecular attraction, the liquid surface tends to spontaneously contract. Thus, liquids tend to assume a spherical shape (i.e., a volume with the minimum surface area). This configuration has the least free energy.

b. Any expansion of the surface increases the free energy of the system. Thus, **surface free energy** can be defined by the work required to increase the surface area A of the liquid by 1 area unit. This value is expressed as the number of millinewtons (mN) needed to expand a 1-m^2 surface by 1 unit:

$$\text{work} = \gamma \times \Delta A$$

where ΔA is the increase in surface area and γ is the **surface tension**, or **surface free energy**, in mN m^{-1}—equivalent to centimeter-gram-second (CGS) units of dynes cm^{-1}. At 20°C, water has a surface tension of 72 mN m^{-1}, whereas *n*-octanol has a surface tension of 27 mN m^{-1}. Thus more work must be expended to expand the surface of water than to expand the surface of *n*-octanol (i.e., to proceed from a given volume of bulk liquid to the corresponding volume of small droplets).

c. At the **boundary**, or **interface**, between two immiscible liquids that are in contact with one another, the corresponding **interfacial tension** (i.e., free energy or work required to expand the interfacial area) reflects the extent of the intermolecular forces of attraction and repulsion at the interface. When the interface is between two liquids, substantial molecular interaction occurs across the interface between the two phases. This interaction reduces the imbalance in forces of attraction within each phase. The interfacial tension between *n*-octanol and water is reduced to 8.5 mN m^{-1} from 72 mN m^{-1} (γ air/water). This reduction indicates, in part, the interfacial interaction between *n*-octanol and water.

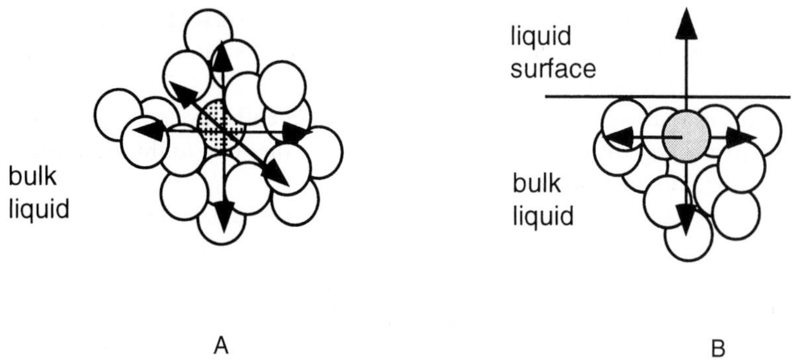

Figure 2-2. A. Molecules in the bulk phase. **B.** Molecules at the surface of a liquid.

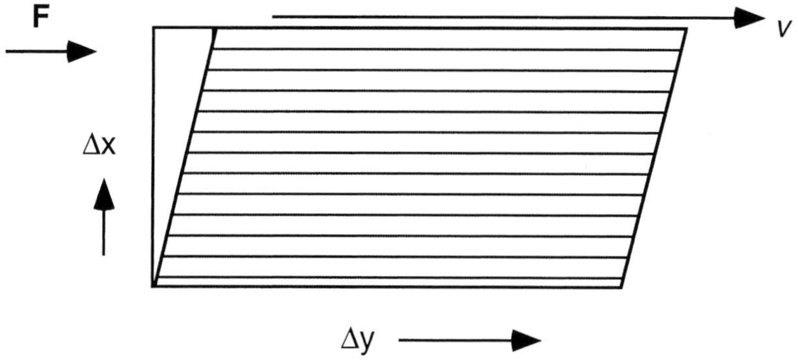

Figure 2-3. Liquid flow.

2. The flow of a liquid across a solid surface can be examined in terms of the **velocity**, or rate of movement, of the liquid relative to the surface across which it flows. More insight can be gained by visualizing the flow of liquid as involving the movement of numerous parallel layers of liquid between an upper, movable plate and a lower, fixed plate (*Figure 2-3*). The application of a constant force (F) to the upper plate causes both this plate and the uppermost layer of liquid in contact with it to move with a velocity $\Delta y/\Delta x$. The interaction between the fixed bottom plate and the liquid layer closest to it prevents the movement of the bottom layer of liquid. The **velocity** (v) of the remaining layers of liquid between the two plates is proportional to their distance from the immovable plate (i.e., $\Delta y/\Delta x$). The **velocity gradient** leads to deformation of the liquid with time. This deformation is the **rate of shear**, dv/dx, or D. **Newton** defined flow in terms of the ratio of the force F applied to a plate of area A—**shear stress** (τ)—divided by the velocity gradient (D) induced by τ:

$$\frac{F}{A} = \eta\frac{dv}{dx}$$

or

$$\frac{\tau}{D} = \eta$$

The proportionality constant η is the coefficient of **viscosity**. It indicates the resistance to flow of adjacent layers of fluid. The reciprocal of η is **fluidity**. Units of viscosity in the CGS system are dynes $cm^{-2}s^{-1}$, or poise. In the SI system, the units are Newtons $m^{-2}s^{-1}$, which corresponds to 10 poise. The viscosity of water at 20°C is approximately 0.01 poise, or 1 centipoise (cps), which corresponds to 1 mN $m^{-2}s^{-1}$ or 1 mPa • s (milliPascal second).

a. Substances that flow in accordance with the equation in III.B.2 (Newton's law) are known as **Newtonian substances**. Liquids that consist of simple molecules and dilute dispersions tend to be **Newtonian**. For a Newtonian fluid, a plot of shear stress as a function of shear rate (a **flow curve** or **rheogram**) yields a straight line with a slope of η (*Figure 2-4, Curve 1*).

b. **Non-Newtonian substances** do not obey Newton's equation of flow. These substances tend to exhibit **shear-dependent** or **time-dependent viscosity**. In either case, viscosity is more aptly termed **apparent viscosity** because Newton's law is not strictly obeyed. Heterogeneous liquids and solids are most likely non-Newtonian.

(1) **Shear-dependent viscosity** involves either an *increase* in apparent viscosity (i.e., **shear thickening** or **dilatancy**) (*Figure 2-4, Curve 3*) or a *decrease* in apparent viscosity (i.e., **shear thinning** or **pseudoplasticity**) (*Figure 2-4, Curve 2*) with an increase in the rate of shear. Shear thickening is displayed by suspensions that have a high solid content of small, deflocculated particles. Shear thinning is displayed by polymer or macromolecule solutions. **Plastic**, or **Bingham body**, behavior (*Figure 2-4, Curve 4*) is exemplified by flocculated particles in concentrated suspensions that show no apparent response to low-level stress. Flow begins only after a limiting yield stress (**yield value**) is exceeded.

(2) **Time-dependent viscosity**

(a) The yield value of **plastic** systems may be time dependent (i.e., may depend on the time scale involved in the application of force). **Thixotropic** systems display shear-thinning behavior but do not immediately recover their higher apparent viscosity

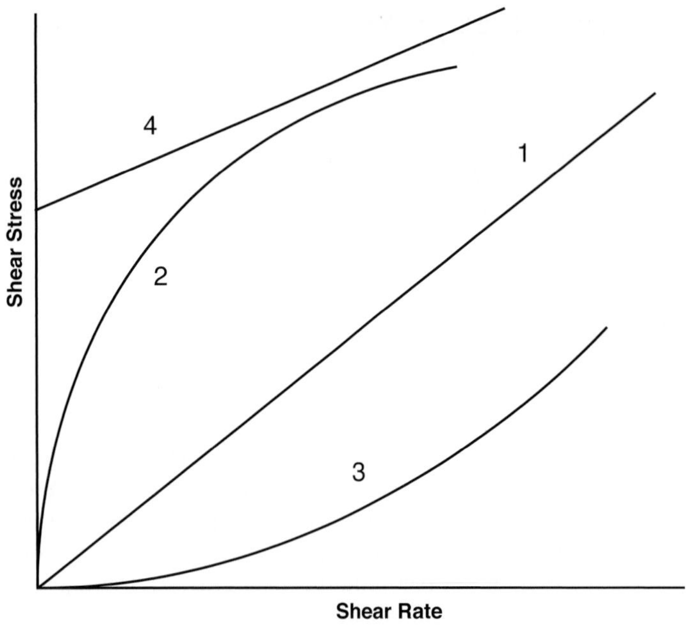

Figure 2-4. Non-Newtonian flow curves.

when the rate of shear is lowered. In a thixotropic system, structural recovery is relatively slow compared with structural breakdown.

(b) **Thixotropy** occurs with heterogeneous systems that involve a three-dimensional structure or network. When such a system is at rest, it appears to have a relatively rigid consistency. Under shear, the structure breaks down and fluidity increases (i.e., **gel–sol** transformation).

(c) **Rheopexy** (**negative thixotropy**, **or antithixotropy**) occurs when the apparent viscosity of the system continues to increase with continued application of shear up to some equilibrium value at a given shear rate. These systems display a **sol–gel** transformation. One explanation for antithixotropic behavior is that continued shear increases the frequency of particle or macromolecule interactions and leads to increased structure in the system.

C. Solids. Intermolecular forces of attraction are stronger in solids than in liquids or gases. Molecular arrangements in solids may be characterized as either crystalline or amorphous.

1. **Crystalline solids** have the following attributes:
   - **a.** Fixed **molecular order** (i.e., molecules occupy set positions in a specific array)
   - **b.** A distinct melting point
   - **c.** **Anisotropicity** (i.e., their properties are not the same in all directions), with the exception of cubic crystals
2. **Amorphous solids** have the following attributes:
   - **a.** Randomly arranged molecules with the short-range order typical of liquids
   - **b.** No melting points
   - **c.** **Isotropicity** (i.e., properties are the same in all directions)
   - **d.** Less thermodynamic stability than the corresponding crystalline solid and therefore more apt to exhibit chemical and physical instability, increased dissolution rate, etc.
3. **Polymorphism** is the condition wherein substances can exist in more than one crystalline form. These **polymorphs** have different molecular arrangements or crystal lattice structures. As a result, the different polymorphs of a drug solid can have different properties. For example, the melting point, solubility, dissolution rate, density, and stability can differ considerably among the polymorphic forms of a drug. Many drugs exhibit polymorphic behavior. Fatty (triglyceride) excipients (e.g., theobroma oil, cocoa butter) are recognized for their polymorphic behavior.
4. The incorporation of solvent molecules into the crystal lattice of a solid results in a molecular adduct known as a **solvate** or **hydrate** (the latter term is used when water is the solvent). In general, solvates or hydrates exhibit different solubilities and dissolution rates than their unsolvated/anhydrous counterparts.

5. **Melting point and heat of fusion**. The melting point of a solid is the temperature at which the solid is transformed to a liquid. When 1 g of a solid is heated and melts, the heat absorbed in the process is referred to as the **latent heat of fusion.**

D. **Phase diagrams and phase equilibria**. A **phase diagram** represents the states of matter (i.e., solid, liquid, and gas) that exist as temperature and pressure are varied (*Figure 2-5*). The data arrays separating the phases in *Figure 2-5* delineate the temperatures and pressures at which the phases can coexist. Thus, gas (or vapor) and liquid coexist along "curve" *BC*, solid and liquid coexist along "curve" *AB*, and solid and gas (or vapor) coexist along "curve" *DB*. Depending on the change in temperature and pressure, **evaporation** or **condensation** occur along curve *BC*, **fusion** or **melting** along curve *AB*, and **sublimation** or **deposition** along curve *DB*. The three "curves" intersect at point *B*. Only at this unique temperature and pressure, known as the **triple point**, do all three phases exist in equilibrium. (The triple point for water is 0.01°C and 6.04 $\times$ 10^{-3} atm) Continuing along curve *BC*, to higher temperatures and pressures, one ultimately reaches point *C*, known as the **critical point**, above which there is no distinction between the liquid and the gas phases. Substances that exist above this critical point are known as **supercritical fluids**. Supercritical fluids such as carbon dioxide (critical point, 30.98°C and 73.8 atm) often exhibit markedly altered physicochemical properties (e.g., density, diffusivity, or solubility characteristics) that render them useful as solvents and processing aids in the production of pharmaceuticals and drug delivery systems.

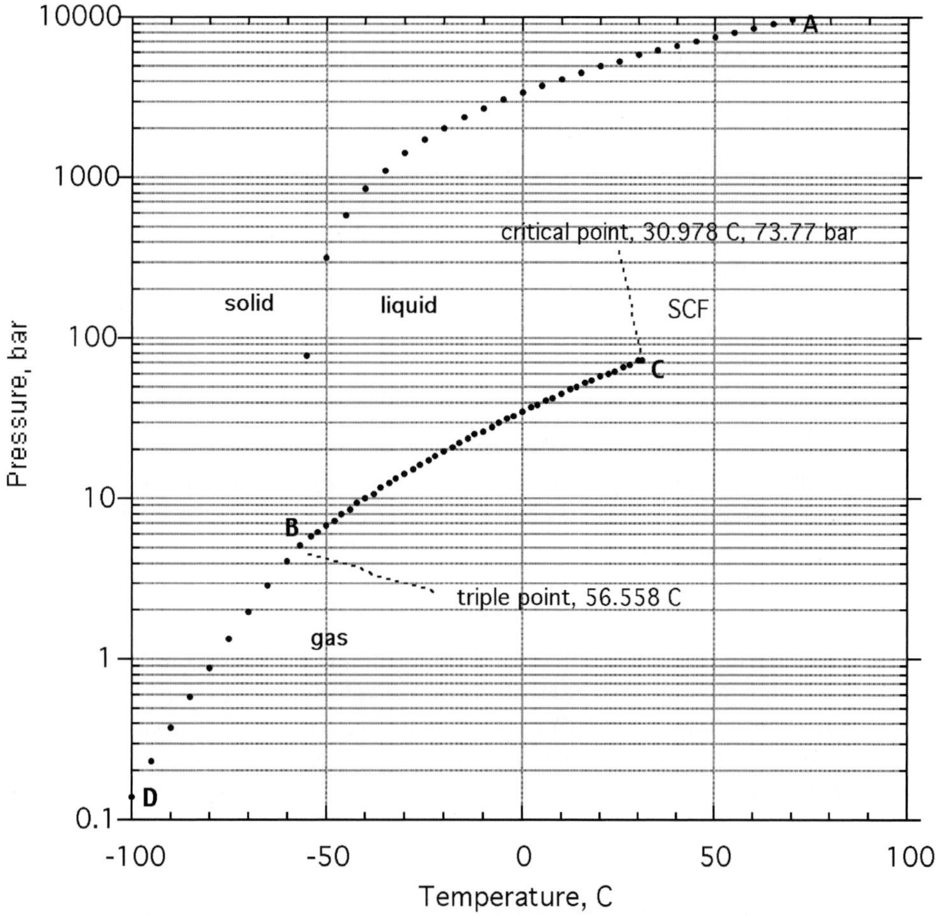

Figure 2-5. Phase diagram for CO_2 showing the variation of the state of matter as pressure and temperature are varied. The solid state exists in the region *ABD*; the liquid state, in the region *ABC*; and the gas state, in the region to the right of curve *CD*. *B* corresponds to the triple point, the pressure and temperature at which all three phases coexist. *C* corresponds to the critical point, the pressure and temperature above which the liquid and gas phases are indistinguishable.

IV. PHYSICOCHEMICAL BEHAVIOR

A. **Homogeneous systems**

1. A **solution** is a homogeneous system in which a **solute** is molecularly dispersed, or dissolved, in a **solvent**. The solvent is the predominant species. **Saturated solutions** are solutions that, at a given temperature and pressure, contain the maximum amount of solute that can be accommodated by the solvent. If the saturation, or solubility, limit is exceeded, a fraction of the solute can separate from the solution and exist in equilibrium with it.
   a. **Solutes** can be gases, liquids, or solids, and nonelectrolytes or electrolytes.
      (1) **Nonelectrolytes** are substances that **do not form ions** when dissolved in water. Examples are estradiol, glycerin, urea, and sucrose. Their aqueous solutions do not conduct electric current.
      (2) **Electrolytes** are substances that **do form ions** in solution. Examples are sodium chloride, hydrochloric acid, and atropine. As a result, their aqueous solutions conduct electric current. Electrolytes are characterized as **strong** or **weak**. Strong electrolytes (e.g., sodium chloride, hydrochloric acid) are **completely ionized** in water at all concentrations. Weak electrolytes (e.g., aspirin, atropine) are **partially ionized** in water.
   b. The **colligative properties of a solution** depend on the total **number of ionic and nonionic solute molecules in the solution**. These properties depend on ionization but are **independent of other chemical properties of the solute**.
2. **Colligative properties** include the following:
   a. **Lowering of vapor pressure**. The **partial vapor pressure** of each volatile component in a solution is equal to the product of the mole fraction of the component in the solution and the vapor pressure of the pure component. This is **Raoult's law**:

$$P_A = P_A^0 \times x_A$$

where P_A is the partial vapor pressure above a solution in which the mole fraction of the solute A is x_A and P_A^0 is the **vapor pressure** of the pure component A. The vapor pressure is the pressure at which equilibrium is established between the molecules of A in the liquid state and the molecules of A in the gaseous (vapor) state in a closed, evacuated container. The vapor pressure is temperature dependent, but independent of the amount of liquid and vapor. Raoult's law holds for ideal solutions of nonelectrolytes. For a **binary solution** (i.e., a solution of component B in component A)

$$\frac{P_A^0 - P_A}{P_A^0} = (1 - x_A) = x_B$$

The lowering of the vapor pressure of the solution relative to the vapor pressure of the pure solvent is proportional to the number of molecules of solute in the solution. The actual lowering of the vapor pressure by the solute, Δp_A, is given by

$$\Delta p_A = (P_A^0 - p_A) = x_B P_A^0$$

   b. **Elevation of the boiling point**. The **boiling point** is the temperature at which the vapor pressure of a liquid equals an external pressure of 760 mm Hg. A solution of a nonvolatile solute has a higher boiling point than a pure solvent because the solute lowers the vapor pressure of the solvent. The amount of elevation of the boiling point (ΔT_b) depends on the concentration of the solute:

$$\Delta T_b = \frac{RT_0^2 M_1 m}{1000 \times \Delta H_{vap}} = K_b m$$

where K_b is the molal boiling point elevation constant, R is the molar gas constant, T is absolute temperature (degrees K), M_1 is the molecular weight of the solute, m is the molality of the solution, and ΔH_{vap} is the molal enthalpy of vaporization of the solvent.

   c. **Depression of the freezing point**. The **freezing point**, or melting point, of a pure compound is the temperature at which the solid and the liquid phases are in equilibrium under a pressure of 1 atmosphere (atm). The freezing point of a solution is the temperature at which the solid phase of the pure solvent and the liquid phase of the solution are in equilibrium under a pressure of 1 atm. The amount of depression of the freezing point (ΔT_f) depends on the molality of the solution:

$$\Delta T_f = \frac{RT_0^2 M_1 m}{1000 \times \Delta H_{fusion}} = K_f m$$

where K_f is the molal freezing point constant and ΔH_{fusion} is the molal heat of fusion.

d. Osmotic pressure. Osmosis is the process by which solvent molecules pass through a semipermeable membrane (a barrier through which only solvent molecules may pass) from a region of dilute solution to one of more concentrated solution. Solvent molecules transfer because of the inequality in chemical potential on the two sides of the membrane. Solvent molecules in a concentrated solution have a lower chemical potential than solvent molecules in a more dilute solution.

(1) **Osmotic pressure** is the **pressure** that must be applied to the solution to prevent the flow of pure solvent into the concentrated solution.

(2) Solvent molecules move from a region where their **escaping tendency is high** to one where their **escaping tendency is low**. The presence of dissolved solute lowers the escaping tendency of the solvent in proportion to the solute concentration.

(3) The **van't Hoff equation** defines the osmotic pressure π as a function of the number of moles of solute n_2 in the solution of volume V:

$$\pi V = n_2 RT$$

3. Electrolyte solutions and ionic equilibria

a. Acid–base equilibria

(1) According to the **Arrhenius dissociation theory**, an **acid** is a substance that liberates H^+ in aqueous solution. A **base** is a substance that liberates hydroxyl ions (OH^-) in aqueous solution. This definition applies only under aqueous conditions.

(2) The **Lowry–Brønsted theory** is a more powerful concept that applies to aqueous and nonaqueous systems. It is most commonly used for pharmaceutical and biologic systems because these systems are primarily aqueous.

(a) According to this definition, an **acid** is a substance (charged or uncharged) that is capable of donating a proton. A **base** is a substance (charged or uncharged) that is capable of accepting a proton from an acid. The dissociation of an acid (HA) always produces a base (A^-) according to the following formula:

$$HA \leftrightarrow H^+ + A^-$$

(b) HA and A^- are a **conjugate acid–base pair** (an acid and a base that exist in equilibrium and differ in structure by a proton). The proton of an acid does not exist free in solution, but combines with the solvent. In water, this **hydrated proton** is a **hydronium ion** (H_3O^+).

(c) The relative **strengths** of acids and bases are determined by their ability to donate or accept protons. For example, in water, HCl donates a proton more readily than does acetic acid. Thus HCl is a stronger acid. Acid strength is also determined by the affinity of the solvent for protons. For example, HCl may dissociate completely in liquid ammonia, but only very slightly in glacial acetic acid. Thus, HCl is a strong acid in liquid ammonia and a weak acid in glacial acetic acid.

(3) The **Lewis theory** extends the acid–base concept to reactions that do not involve protons. It defines an **acid** as a molecule or ion that accepts an electron pair from another atom and a **base** as a substance that donates an electron pair to be shared with another atom.

b. H^+ concentration values are very small. Therefore, they are expressed in **exponential notation as pH**. The pH is the logarithm of the reciprocal of the H^+ concentration

$$pH = \log\left(\frac{1}{[H^+]}\right)$$

where $[H^+]$ is the molar concentration of H^+. Because the logarithm of a reciprocal equals the **negative logarithm** of the number, this equation may be rewritten as

$$pH = -\log [H^+]$$

or

$$[H^+] = 10^{-pH}$$

Thus, the pH value may be defined as the negative logarithm of the $[H^+]$ value. For example, if the H^+ concentration of a solution is 5×10^{-6}, the pH value may be calculated as follows:

$$\begin{aligned} pH &= -\log (5 \times 10^{-6}) \\ \log 5 &= 0.699 \\ \log 10^{-6} &= -6.0 \\ pH &= -(-6 + 0.699) \\ &= -(-5.301) \\ &= 5.301 \end{aligned}$$

c. As pH decreases, **H^+ concentration increases exponentially**. When the pH decreases from 6 to 5, the H^+ concentration increases from 10^{-6} to 10^{-5}, or 10 times its original value. When the pH falls from 5 to 4.7, the H^+ concentration increases from 1×10^{-5} to 2×10^{-5}, or double its initial value.

d. **Dissociation constants. Ionization** is the complete separation of the ions in a crystal lattice when the salt is dissolved. **Dissociation** is the separation of ions in solution when the ions are associated by interionic attraction.

(1) For **weak electrolytes**, dissociation is a reversible process. The equilibrium of this process can be expressed by the law of mass action. This law states that the rate of the chemical reaction is proportional to the product of the concentration of the reacting substances, each raised to a power of the number of moles of the substance in solution.

(2) For **weak acids**, dissociation in water is expressed as

$$HA \leftrightarrow H^+ + A^-$$

The dynamic equilibrium between the simultaneous forward and reverse reactions is indicated by the arrows. By the law of mass action,

$$\begin{aligned} \text{rate of forward reaction} &= K_1[HA] \\ \text{rate of reverse reaction} &= K_2[H^+][A^-] \end{aligned}$$

At equilibrium, the forward and reverse rates are equal. Therefore,

$$K_1[HA] = K_2[H^+][A^-]$$

Thus, **the equilibrium expression for the dissociation of a weak acid** is written as

$$K_a = \frac{K_1}{K_2} = \frac{[H^+][A^-]}{[HA]}$$

where K_a represents the acid dissociation constant. For a weak acid, the **acid dissociation constant** is conventionally expressed as **pK_a**, which is $-\log K_a$. For example, the K_a of acetic acid at 25°C is 1.75×10^{-5}. The pK_a is calculated as follows:

$$\begin{aligned} pK_a &= -\log (1.75 \times 10^{-5}) \\ \log 1.75 &= 0.243 \\ \log 10^{-5} &= -5 \\ pH &= -(-5 + 0.243) \\ &= -(-4.757) \\ &= 4.76 \end{aligned}$$

(3) For **weak bases**, dissociation may also be expressed with the K_a expression for the **conjugate acid of the base**. This acid is formed when a proton reacts with the base. For a base that does not contain a hydroxyl group,

$$BH^+ \leftrightarrow H^+ + B$$

The **dissociation constant** for this reaction is expressed as

$$K_a = \frac{[H^+][B]}{[BH^+]}$$

However, a **base dissociation constant** is traditionally defined for a weak base with this expression:

$$B + H_2O \leftrightarrow OH^- + BH^+$$

$$K_b = \frac{[OH^-][BH^+]}{[B]}$$

where K_b represents the dissociation constant of a weak base. This **dissociation constant** can be expressed as **pK_b** as follows:

$$pK_b = -\log K_b$$

(4) **Certain compounds** (acids or bases) can accept or donate more than one proton. Consequently, they have **more than one dissociation constant**.

e. **Henderson–Hasselbalch equations** describe the relation between the ionized and the un-ionized species of a weak electrolyte.

(1) For **weak acids**, the Henderson–Hasselbalch equation is obtained from the equilibrium relation described in IV.A.3d.(2).

$$pH = pK_a + \log \frac{[salt]}{[acid]}$$

(2) Similarly, the Henderson–Hasselbalch equation for **weak bases** is as follows:

$$pH = pK_a + \log \frac{[B]}{[BH^+]}$$

where B is the un-ionized weak base and BH^+ is the protonated base.

f. The **degree of ionization (α)**, the fraction of a weak electrolyte that is ionized in solution, is calculated from the following equation:

$$\alpha = \frac{[I]}{[I] + [U]}$$

where [I] and [U] represent the concentrations of the ionized and un-ionized species, respectively. The degree of ionization depends solely on the pH of the solution and the pK_a of the weak electrolyte. **When pH = pK_a**, the Henderson–Hasselbalch equations are for a weak acid and a weak base, respectively:

$$pH - pK_a = 0 = \log \frac{[A^-]}{[HA]}$$

thus

$$\frac{[A^-]}{[HA]} = 1$$

$$pH - pK_a = 0 = \log \frac{[B]}{[BH^+]}$$

thus

$$\frac{[B]}{[BH^+]} = 1$$

In effect, when the pH of the solution is numerically equivalent to the pK_a of the weak electrolyte, whether a weak base or a weak acid, [I] = [U] and the degree of ionization $\alpha = 0.5$ (i.e., 50% of the solute is ionized).

g. **Solubility of a weak electrolyte** varies as a function of pH.

(1) For a **weak acid**, the total solubility C_s is given by the expression

$$C_s = [HA] + [A^-]$$

where [HA] is the intrinsic solubility of the un-ionized weak acid and is denoted as C_0, whereas $[A^-]$ is the concentration of its anion. Because $[A^-]$ can be expressed in terms of C_0 and the dissociation constant K_a,

$$C_s = C_0 + \frac{K_a\, C_0}{[H^+]}$$

Thus, the **solubility of a weak acid increases with increasing pH** (i.e., with an increasing degree of ionization, as the anion is more polar and therefore more water soluble than the un-ionized weak acid).

(2) Similarly, for **weak bases,**

$$C_s = C_0 + \frac{C_0[H^+]}{K_a}$$

Thus, the **solubility decreases with increasing pH** because more of the weak base is in the unprotonated form. This form is less polar and therefore less water soluble.

h. **Buffers and buffer capacity**

(1) A **buffer** is a mixture of salt with acid or base that resists changes in pH when small quantities of acid or base are added. A buffer can be a **combination** of a weak acid and its conjugate base (salt) or a combination of a weak base and its conjugate acid (salt). However, buffer solutions are more **commonly prepared** from weak acids and their salts. They are not ordinarily prepared from weak bases and their salts because weak bases are often unstable and volatile.

(a) For a **weak acid and its salt,** the following buffer equation is satisfactory for calculations with a pH of 4 to 10. It is important in the preparation of buffered pharmaceutical solutions:

$$pH = pK_a + \log \frac{[salt]}{[acid]}$$

(b) For a **weak base and its salt,** the buffer equation is similar but also depends on the dissociation constant of water (pK_w). The equation becomes

$$pH = pK_w - pK_b \log \frac{[base]}{[salt]}$$

(2) **Buffer action** is the resistance to a change in pH.

(3) **Buffer capacity** is the ability of a buffer solution to resist changes in pH. The **smaller the pH change** caused by addition of a given amount of acid or base, the **greater the buffer capacity** of the solution.

(a) Buffer capacity is the number of gram equivalents of an acid or base that changes the pH of 1 L of buffer solution by 1 U.

(b) Buffer capacity is affected by the concentration of the buffer constituents. A higher concentration provides a greater acid or base reserve. Buffer capacity (β) is related to total concentration (C) as follows:

$$\beta = \frac{2.3\, CK_a[H^+]}{(K_a + [H^+])^2}$$

where C represents the molar concentrations of the acid and the salt.

(c) Thus, buffer capacity depends on the value of the ratio of the salt to the acid form. It increases as the ratio approaches unity. Maximum buffer capacity occurs when $pH = pK_a$ and is represented by $\beta = 0.576C$.

B. Heterogeneous (disperse) systems

1. Introduction

a. A **suspension** is a two-phase system that is composed of a solid material dispersed in an oily or aqueous liquid. The particle size of the dispersed solid is usually > 0.5 μm.

b. An **emulsion** is a heterogeneous system that consists of at least one immiscible liquid that is intimately dispersed in another in the form of droplets. The droplet diameter usually exceeds 0.1 μm. Emulsions are **inherently unstable** because the droplets of the dispersed liquid tend to coalesce to form large droplets until all of the dispersed droplets have coalesced. The third component of the system is an **emulsifying agent**. This agent prevents coalescence and maintains the integrity of the individual droplets.

2. **Dispersion stability**. In an **ideal dispersion**, the dispersed particles do not interact. The particles are uniform in size and undergo no change in position other than the random movement that results from Brownian motion. In contrast, in a **real dispersion**, the particles are not uniformly sized (i.e., they are not **monodisperse**). The particles are subject to particulate aggregation, or clumping, and the dispersion becomes more heterogeneous with time. The **rate of settling (separating or creaming)** of the dispersed phase in the dispersion medium is a function of the particle size, dispersion phase viscosity, and difference in density between the dispersed phase and the dispersion medium, in accordance with **Stokes's law**:

$$\text{sedimentation rate} = \frac{d^2 g(\rho_1 - \rho_2)}{18\,\eta}$$

where d is the particle diameter, g is the acceleration owing to gravity, η is the viscosity of the dispersion medium, and $(\rho_1 - \rho_2)$ is the difference between the density of the particles (ρ_1) and the density of the dispersion medium (ρ_2). Although Stokes's law was derived to determine the settling, or sedimentation, of noninteracting spherical particles, it also provides guidance for determining the stabilization of dispersion:

a. **Particle size** should be as **small** as possible. Smaller particles yield slower sedimentation, or flotation, rates.

b. **High particulate (dispersed phase) concentrations** increase the rate of particle–particle collisions and interaction. As a result, particle aggregation occurs, and instability increases as the aggregates behave as larger particles. In the case of liquid–liquid dispersions, particle–particle collisions can lead to coalescence (i.e., larger particles) and decrease dispersion stability.

c. **Avoidance of particle–particle interactions**

(1) Aggregation can be prevented if the particles have a similar electrical charge. Particles in an aqueous system always have some electrical charge because of **ionization** of chemical groups on the particle surface or **adsorption** of charged molecules or ions at the interface. If the adsorbed species is an **ionic surfactant** (e.g., sodium lauryl sulfate), the charge associated with the surfactant ion (e.g., lauryl sulfate anion) will accumulate at the interface. However, if a relatively non–surface-active electrolyte is adsorbed, the sign of the charge of the adsorbed ion is less readily predicted.

(2) The **magnitude of the charge** is the difference in electrical potential between the charged surface of the particle and the bulk of the dispersion medium. This magnitude is approximated by the **electrokinetic**, or **zeta**, **potential** (**ζ**). The zeta potential is measured from the fixed, avidly bound layers of ions and solvent molecules on the particle surface. When ζ is high (e.g., ≥ 25 mV), interparticulate **repulsive forces** exceed the attractive forces. As a result, the dispersion is **deflocculated** and relatively stable to collision and subsequent aggregation (**flocculation**). When ζ is so low that interparticulate **attractive forces** predominate, loose particle aggregates, or **flocs**, form (i.e., **flocculation** occurs).

d. **Density** can be manipulated to decrease the rate of dispersion instability. The settling rate decreases as $(\rho_1 - \rho_2)$ approaches zero. However, the density of the dispersion medium usually cannot be altered sufficiently to halt the settling (or flotation) process. In the dispersed phase, the density of solid particles is not readily altered; altering the density of liquid particles would require the addition of a miscible liquid of higher (or lower) density. Altering the composition of suspensions is also problematic because most solid particles are denser than the dispersion medium. Additives of higher (or lower) density might alter the biopharmaceutical characteristics of the formulation (e.g., rate of drug release, residence time at the site of administration, or absorption).

e. The **sedimentation**, or **flotation**, **rate** is inversely proportional to the **viscosity**. An **increase** in the **viscosity of the dispersion medium** decreases the rate of settling, or flotation. However, although the rate of destabilization can be slowed by an increase in viscosity, it cannot be halted.

3. **Emulsion stability**. **Coalescence** occurs in emulsion systems when the liquid particles of the dispersed phase merge to form larger particles. Coalescence is largely prevented by the **interfacial film** of surfactant around the droplets. This film prevents direct contact of the liquid phase of the droplets. Coalescence of droplets in oil in water (o/w) emulsions is also inhibited by the **electrostatic repulsion** of similarly charged particles. **Creaming** is the **reversible** separation of a layer of emulsified particles. Because mixing or shaking may be sufficient to reconstitute the emulsion system, creaming is not necessarily unacceptable. However, **cracking**, or **irreversible phase separation**, is never acceptable. **Phase inversion**, or emulsion-type reversal, involves the reversion of an emulsion from an o/w to water in oil (w/o) form, or vice versa. Phase inversion can change the consistency or texture of the emulsion or cause further deterioration in its stability.

V. CHEMICAL KINETICS AND DRUG STABILITY

A. **Introduction**. The **stability** of the **active component** of a drug is a major criterion in the rational design and evaluation of drug dosage forms. Problems with **stability** can determine whether a given formulation is accepted or rejected.

1. Extensive chemical degradation of the active ingredient can cause **substantial loss** of active ingredient from the dosage form.
2. Chemical degradation can produce a **toxic product** that has undesirable side effects.
3. Instability of the drug product can cause **decreased bioavailability**. As a result, the therapeutic efficacy of the dosage form may be substantially reduced.

B. **Rates and orders of reactions**

1. The **rate of a reaction**, or degradation rate, is the velocity with which the reaction occurs. This rate is expressed as dC/dt (the change in concentration, or C, within a given time interval, or dt).
   a. Reaction rates depend on certain conditions (e.g., **reactant concentration**, **temperature**, **pH**, **presence of solvents or additives**). Radiation and catalytic agents (e.g., polyvalent cations) also have an effect.
   b. The effective study of reaction rates in the body requires application of **pharmacokinetic principles** (see Chapter 5).
2. The **order of a reaction** is the way in which the concentration of the drug or reactant in a chemical reaction affects the rate. The rate of a reaction, dC/dt, is proportional to the concentration to the nth power, where n is the order of the reaction—that is,

$$\frac{dC}{dt} \propto C^n$$

The study of reaction orders is a crucial aspect of pharmacokinetics (see Chapter 5). Usually, **pharmaceutical degradation** can be treated as a **zero-order**, **first-order**, or **higher order reaction**. The first two are summarized as follows:

   a. In a **zero-order reaction**, the **rate is independent of the concentration of the reactants** (i.e., $dC/dt \propto C^0$) (see Chapter 5). Other factors, such as absorption of light in certain photochemical reactions, determine the rate.
      (1) A **zero-order reaction** can be expressed as

$$C = -k_0t + C_0$$

where C is the drug concentration, k_0 is the zero-order rate constant in units of concentration/time, t is the time, and C_0 is the initial concentration.

      (2) When this equation is plotted with C on the vertical axis (ordinate) against t on the horizontal axis (abscissa), the **slope of the line is equal to $-k_0$** (*Figure 2-6*). The negative sign indicates that the slope is decreasing.

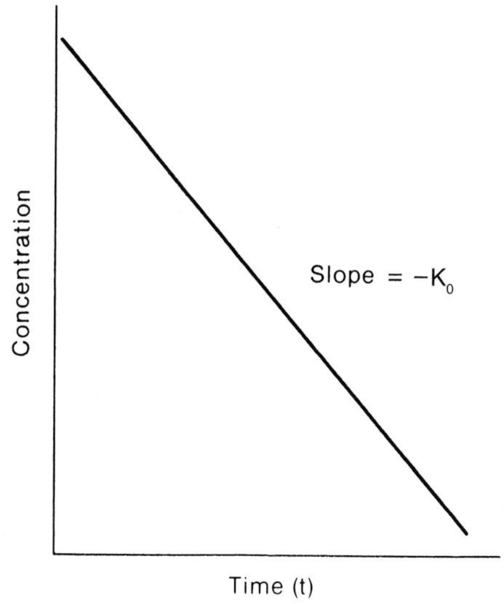

Figure 2-6. Concentration *(C)* versus time *(t)* for a zero-order reaction. The slope of the line equals $-k_0$. The slope of the line is not equal to the rate constant because it includes the minus sign.

b. In a **first-order reaction**, the **rate depends on the first power of the concentration of a single reactant** (i.e., $dC/dt \propto C^1$).

(1) In a first-order reaction, **drug concentration decreases exponentially with time**, in accordance with the equation

$$C = C_0 e^{-k_1 t}$$

where C is the concentration of the reacting material, C_0 is the initial concentration, k_1 is the first-order rate constant in units of reciprocal time, and t is time. A plot of the logarithm of concentration against time produces a straight line with a slope of $-k/2.303$ (*Figure 2-7*).

(2) The **half-life** ($t_{1/2}$) of a reaction is the time required for the concentration of a drug to decrease by one-half. For a first-order reaction, half-life is expressed by

$$t_{1/2} = \frac{0.693}{k_1}$$

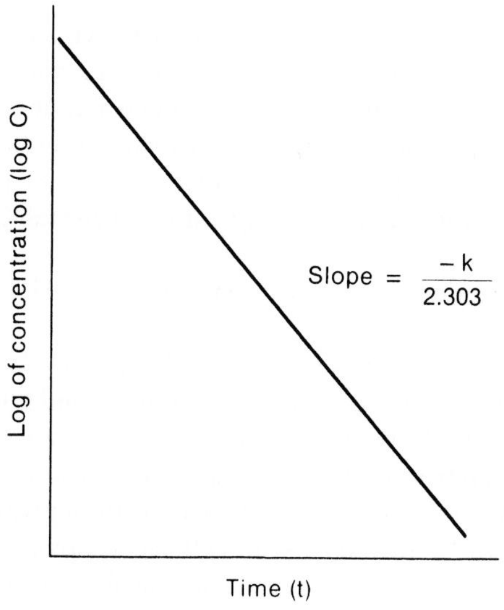

Figure 2-7. Logarithm of concentration (log *C*) versus time (*t*) for a first-order reaction. The slope of the line equals $-k/2.303$.

(3) The **time required for a drug to degrade** to 90% of its original concentration ($t_{90\%}$) is also important. This time represents a reasonable limit of degradation for the active ingredients. The $t_{90\%}$ can be calculated as

$$t_{90\%} = \frac{2.303}{k_1} \log \frac{100}{90} = \frac{0.105}{k_1}$$

(a) because

$$k_1 = 0.693 / t_{½}$$

(b) then

$$t_{90\%} = \frac{0.105}{0.693 / t_{½}} = 0.152 \times t_{½}$$

(4) Both $t_{½}$ and $t_{90\%}$ are **concentration independent**. Thus, for $t_{½}$, it takes the same amount of time to reduce the concentration of the drug from 100 to 50 mM as it does from 50 to 25 mM.

C. **Factors that affect reaction rates.** Factors other than concentration can affect the reaction rate and stability of a drug. These factors include temperature, the presence of a solvent, pH, and the presence of additives.

1. **Temperature.** An **increase in temperature** causes an increase in reaction rate, as expressed in the equation first suggested by Arrhenius:

$$k = A \cdot e - ^{Ea/RT}$$

or

$$\log k = \log A - \left(\frac{Ea}{2.303} \times \frac{1}{RT} \right)$$

where k is the specific reaction rate constant, A is a constant known as the frequency factor, Ea is the energy of activation, R is the molar gas constant (1.987 cal/degree × mole), and T is the absolute temperature.

a. The **constants *A* and *Ea*** are obtained by determining k at several temperatures and then plotting $\log k$ against $1/T$. The slope of the resulting line equals $-Ea/(2.303 \times R)$. The intercept on the vertical axis equals $\log A$.

b. The activation energy (Ea) is the amount of energy required to put the molecules in an **activated state**. Molecules must be activated to react. As **temperature increases**, more molecules are activated, and the **reaction rate increases**.

2. **Presence of solvent.** Many dosage forms require the incorporation of a water-miscible solvent—for example, low-molecular-weight alcohols, such as the polyethylene glycols (PEGs)—to stabilize the drug.

a. A change in the solvent system **alters** the transition state and the **activity coefficients** of the reactant molecules. It can also cause simultaneous changes in physicochemical parameters, such as pK_a, surface tension, and viscosity. These changes **indirectly affect the reaction rate.**

b. In some cases, **additional reaction pathways** are generated. For example, with an increasing concentration of ethanol in an aqueous solution, aspirin degrades by an extra route and forms the ethyl ester of acetylsalicylic acid. However, a **change in solvent can also stabilize the drug.**

3. **Change in pH.** The magnitude of the rate of a hydrolytic reaction catalyzed by H^+ and OH^- can vary considerably with pH.

a. **H^+ catalysis** predominates at **lower pH**, whereas **OH^- catalysis** operates at **higher pH.** At **intermediate pH**, the rate may be **pH independent** or may be catalyzed by **both H^+ and OH^-.** Rate constants in the intermediate pH range are typically less than those at higher or lower pH.

b. To determine the **effect of pH on degradation kinetics**, decomposition is measured at several H^+ concentrations. The **pH of optimum stability** can be determined by plotting the logarithm of the rate constant (k) as a function of pH (*Figure 2-8*). The **point of inflection** of the plot is the pH of optimum stability. This value is useful in the development of a stable drug formulation.

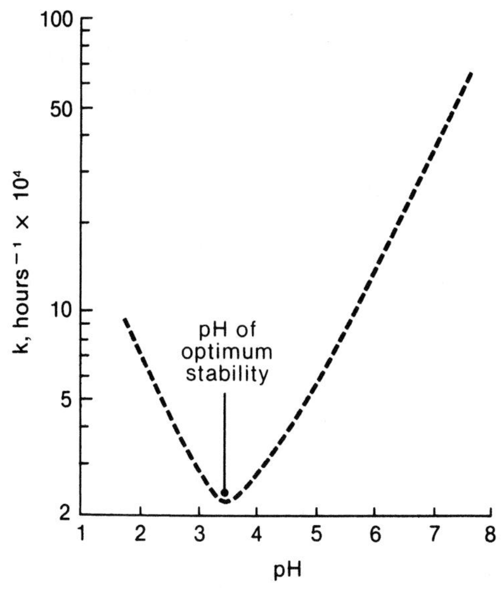

Figure 2-8. Semilogarithmic plot of the rate constant (*k*) versus pH. This plot is used to determine the pH of optimum stability.

4. **Presence of additives**
   a. **Buffer salts** must be added to many drug solutions to maintain the formulation at optimum pH. These salts **can affect the rate of degradation**, primarily as a result of salt increasing the ionic strength.
      (1) Increasing salt concentrations, particularly from polyelectrolytes (e.g., citrate, phosphate), can **substantially affect the magnitude of pK_a**. In this way, they change the rate constant.
      (2) Buffer salts can also **promote drug degradation** through general acid or base catalysis.
   b. The **addition of surfactants** may accelerate or decelerate drug degradation.
      (1) **Acceleration of degradation** is common and is caused by micellar catalysis.
      (2) **Stabilization of a drug** through the addition of a surfactant is less common.
   c. **Complexing agents** can improve drug stability. Aromatic esters (e.g., benzocaine, procaine, tetracaine) **increase in half-life** in the presence of caffeine. This increased stability appears to result from the formation of a less reactive complex between the aromatic ester and the caffeine.

D. **Modes of pharmaceutical degradation**. The decomposition of active ingredients in a dosage form occurs through several pathways (e.g., hydrolysis, oxidation, photolysis; see Chapter 8, II.A).
1. **Hydrolysis** is the most common type of degradation because many medicinal compounds are esters, amides, or lactams.
   a. **H^+ and OH^-** are the most common catalysts of hydrolytic degradation in solution.
   b. **Esters** usually undergo hydrolytic reactions that cause drug instability. Because esters are rapidly degraded in aqueous solution, formulators are reluctant to incorporate drugs that have ester functional groups into liquid dosage forms.
2. **Oxidation** is usually mediated through reaction with atmospheric oxygen under ambient conditions (auto-oxidation).
   a. Medicinal compounds that undergo auto-oxidation at room temperature are affected by **oxygen dissolved in the solvent** and in the head space of their packages. These compounds should be packed in an **inert atmosphere** (e.g., nitrogen) to exclude air from their containers.
   b. Most oxidation reactions involve a **free radical mechanism** and a **chain reaction**. Free radicals tend to take electrons from other compounds.
      (1) **Antioxidants** in the formulation react with the free radicals by providing electrons and easily available hydrogen atoms. In this way, they prevent the propagation of chain reactions.
      (2) **Commonly used antioxidants** include ascorbic acid, butylated hydroxyanisole (BHA), butylated hydroxytoluene (BHT), propyl gallate, sodium bisulfite, sodium sulfite, and the tocopherols.
3. **Photolysis** is the degradation of drug molecules by normal sunlight or room light.
   a. Molecules may absorb the proper wavelength of light and **acquire sufficient energy to undergo reaction**. Usually, photolytic degradation occurs on exposure to light of wavelengths < 400 nm.

b. An **amber glass bottle** or an **opaque container** acts as a barrier to this light, thereby preventing or retarding photolysis. For example, sodium nitroprusside in aqueous solution has a shelf life of only 4 hrs if exposed to normal room light. When protected from light, the solution is stable for at least 1 year.

E. **Determination of shelf life**. The shelf life of a drug preparation is the amount of time that the product can be stored before it becomes unfit for use, through either chemical decomposition or physical deterioration.

1. **Storage temperature** affects shelf life. It is generally understood to be ambient temperature unless special storage conditions are specified.
2. **In general, a preparation is considered fit for use if it varies from the nominal concentration or dose by no more than 10%**, provided that the decomposition products are not more toxic or harmful than the original material.
3. **Shelf life testing** aids in determining the standard shelf life of a formulation.
   a. Samples are stored at 3° to 5°C and at room temperature (20° to 25°C). The samples are then analyzed at various intervals to determine the **rate of decomposition**. Shelf life is calculated from this rate.
   b. Because storage time at these temperatures can result in an extended testing time, **accelerated testing** is conducted as well, with a range of higher temperatures. The **rate constants** obtained from these samples are used to predict shelf life at ambient or refrigeration temperatures. **Temperature-accelerated stability testing** is not useful if temperature changes are accompanied by changes in the reaction mechanism or by physical changes in the system (e.g., change from the solid to the liquid phase).
   c. **Stability at room temperature** can be predicted from accelerated testing data by the Arrhenius equation:

$$\log\left(\frac{k_{T_2}}{k_{T_1}}\right) = \frac{Ea(T_2 - T_1)}{2.303 \times R \times T_2 \times T_1}$$

   where k_{T_2} and k_{T_1} are the rate constants at the absolute temperatures T_2 and T_1, respectively; R is the molar gas constant; and Ea is the energy of activation.
   d. Alternatively, an expression of concentration can be plotted as a linear function of time. Rate constants (k) for degradation at several temperatures are obtained. The logarithm of the rate constant ($\log k$) is plotted against the reciprocal of absolute temperature ($1/T$) to obtain, by extrapolation, the rate constant for degradation at room temperature (*Figure 2-9*).

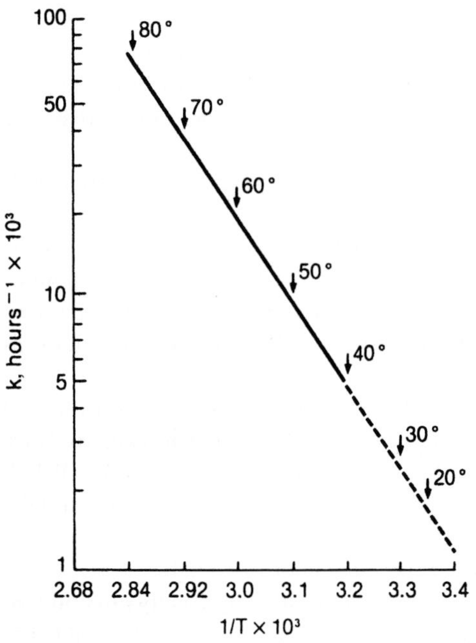

Figure 2-9. Semilogarithmic plot of the rate constant (k) versus the reciprocal of absolute temperature ($1/T$), showing the temperature dependency of degradation rates.

e. The **length of time that the drug will maintain its required potency** can also be predicted by calculation of the $t_{90\%}$ (see V.B.2.b.(3)). This method applies to chemical reactions with activation energies of 10 to 30 kcal/mol—the magnitude of the activation energy for many pharmaceutical degradations that occur in a solution.

VI. DRUG DOSAGE FORMS AND DELIVERY SYSTEMS

A. **Oral solutions**. The ***United States Pharmacopeia*** **(*USP*) 34/*National Formulary*** **(*NF*) 29** categorizes **oral solutions** as "liquid preparations, intended for oral administration, that contain one or more substances with or without flavoring, sweetening, or coloring agents dissolved in water or cosolvent-water mixtures." Oral solutions can contain certain polyols (e.g., sorbitol, glycerin) to inhibit crystallization and to modify solubility, taste, mouth feel, and other vehicle properties. They can be "formulated for direct oral administration to the patient or they may be dispensed in a more concentrated form that must be diluted prior to administration." **Drugs in solution** are more homogeneous and easier to swallow than drugs in solid form. For drugs that have a slow dissolution rate, onset of action and bioavailability are also improved. However, drugs in solution are bulkier dosage forms, degrade more rapidly, and are more likely to interact with constituents than those in solid form.

1. **Water** is the **most commonly used vehicle** for drug solutions. The ***USP*** recognizes seven types of water for the preparation of dosage forms:
   a. **Purified water *USP*** is water obtained by distillation, ion exchange, reverse osmosis, or other suitable treatment. It cannot contain more than 10 parts per million (ppm) of total solid and should have a pH between 5 and 7. Purified water is used in prescriptions and finished manufactured products except parenteral and ophthalmic products.
   b. **Water for injection *USP*** is water obtained by distillation or by reverse osmosis. It conforms to the standards of purified water but is also free of pyrogen. Water for injection is used as a solvent for the preparation of parenteral solutions.
   c. **Sterile water for injection *USP*** is water for injection that is sterilized and packaged in single-dose containers of type I and II glass. These containers do not exceed a capacity of 1 L. The limitations for total solids depend on the size of the container.
   d. **Bacteriostatic water for injection *USP*** is sterile water for injection that contains one or more suitable antimicrobial agents. It is also packaged in single- or multiple-dose containers of type I or II glass. These containers do not exceed the capacity of 30 mL.
   e. **Sterile water for inhalation *USP*** is water that is purified by distillation or by reverse osmosis (i.e., water for injection) and rendered sterile. It contains no antimicrobial agents, except when used in humidifiers or similar devices. This type of water should not be used for parenteral administration or for other sterile dosage forms.
   f. **Sterile water for irrigation *USP*** is water for injection that is sterilized and suitably packaged. It contains no antimicrobial agents or other added substance.
   g. **Sterile purified water *USP*** is purified water sterilized and suitably packaged. It contains no antimicrobial agent. It is not intended for use in parenterals.
2. **Oral drug solutions** include **syrups** and **elixirs** as well as other less widely prescribed classic (**galenical**) formulations, such as **aromatic waters**, **tinctures**, **fluid extracts**, and **spirits**.
   a. **Syrups** are traditionally per oral solutions that contain high concentrations of sucrose or other sugars. Through common usage, the term *syrup* has also come to include any other liquid dosage form prepared in a sweet, viscous vehicle, including per oral suspensions.
      (1) **Syrup *NF*** (**simple syrup**) is a concentrated or nearly saturated aqueous solution of sugar (85%; 65% w/w).
      (2) Syrups have a **low solvent capacity for water-soluble drugs** because the hydrogen bonding between sucrose and water is very strong. For this reason, it can be difficult or impossible to dissolve a drug in syrup. Often, the drug is best dissolved in a small quantity of water, and the flavoring syrup is added.
      (3) The **sucrose concentration** of syrup plays a crucial role in the control of microbial growth. Dilute sucrose solutions are excellent media for microorganisms. As the concentration of sucrose approaches saturation, the syrup becomes self-preserving (i.e., requires no additional preservative). However, a saturated solution is undesirable because temperature

fluctuations may cause crystallization. **Syrup *NF*** is a self-preserved solution with a minimal tendency to undergo crystallization.

b. **Elixirs** are traditionally per oral solutions that contain alcohol as a cosolvent. Many per oral solutions are not described as elixirs but contain alcohol.
   (1) To be considered an elixir, the solution **must contain alcohol**. Traditionally, the alcohol content of elixirs has varied from 5% to 40%. Most elixirs become turbid when moderately diluted by aqueous liquids. Elixirs are not the preferred vehicle for salts because alcohol accentuates saline taste. Salts also have limited solubility in alcohol. Therefore, the alcoholic content of salt-containing elixirs must be low.
   (2) **Aromatic elixir *NF***, prepared in part from syrup, contains approximately 22% alcohol. The limited usefulness of this elixir as a solvent for drugs was offset by the development of **iso-alcoholic elixir**. It is a combination of **low-alcoholic elixir**, an elixir with low alcoholic content (8% to 10% alcohol), and **high-alcoholic elixir**, an elixir with high alcoholic content (73% to 78% alcohol). Mixing appropriate volumes of the two elixirs provides an alcoholic content sufficient to dissolve the drugs.

B. Miscellaneous solutions

1. **Aromatic waters** are clear, **saturated aqueous solutions of volatile oils** or other aromatic or volatile substances. Aromatic waters may be used as pleasantly flavored vehicles for a water-soluble drug or as an aqueous phase in an emulsion or suspension. If a large amount of water-soluble drug is added to aromatic water, then an insoluble layer may form at the top. This **"salting out"** is a competitive process. The molecules of water-soluble drugs have more attraction for the solvent molecules of water than the "oil" molecules. The associated water molecules are pulled away from the oil molecules, which are no longer held in solution. Aromatic waters should be stored in tight, light-resistant bottles to reduce volatilization and degradation from sunlight. Aromatic waters are usually prepared by one of the following methods:
   a. **Distillation** is a universal method but is not practical or economical for most products. It is the only method, however, for preparing strong rose water and orange flower water.
   b. With the **solution method**, the volatile or aromatic substance is admixed with water, with or without the use of a dispersant (e.g., talc).
2. **Spirits**, or **essences**, are alcoholic or hydroalcoholic solutions of volatile substances that contain 50% to 90% alcohol. This **high alcoholic content** maintains the water-insoluble volatile oils in solution. If water is added to a spirit, the oils separate. Some spirits are **medicinal** (e.g., aromatic ammonia spirit). Many spirits (e.g., compound orange spirit, compound cardamom spirit) are used as flavoring agents. Spirits should be stored in tight containers to reduce loss by evaporation.
3. **Tinctures** are alcoholic or hydroalcoholic solutions of chemicals or soluble constituents of vegetable drugs. Although tinctures vary in drug concentration ($\leq$ 50%), those prepared from potent drugs are usually 10% in strength (i.e., 100 mL of the tincture has the activity of 10 g of the drug). Tinctures are usually considered stable. The alcohol content of the official tinctures varies from 17% to 21% for opium tincture *USP* and from 74% to 80% for compound benzoin tincture *USP*. Most tinctures are prepared by an **extraction process** of maceration or percolation. The selection of a **solvent**, or menstruum, is based on the solubility of the active and inert constituents of the crude drugs. Aging can cause precipitation of the inactive constituents of tinctures. Glycerin may be added to the hydroalcoholic solvent to increase the solubility of the active constituent and reduce precipitation on storage. Tinctures must be tightly stoppered and kept from excessive temperatures. Because many of their constituents undergo a photochemical change when exposed to light, tinctures must be stored in light-resistant containers.
4. **Fluid extracts** are liquid extracts of vegetable drugs that contain alcohol as a solvent, preservative, or both. Fluid extracts are prepared by percolation so that each milliliter contains the therapeutic constituents of 1 g of the standard drug. Because of their high drug content, fluid extracts are sometimes referred to as "100% tinctures." Fluid extracts of potent drugs are usually 10 times as concentrated, or potent, as the corresponding tincture. For example, the usual dose of tincture belladonna is 0.6 mL; the equivalent dose of the more potent fluid extract is 0.06 mL. Many fluid extracts are considered too potent for self-administration by patients, so they are almost never prescribed. In addition, many fluid extracts are simply too bitter. Today, most fluid extracts are modified by either flavoring or sweetening agents.

5. **Nasal**, **ophthalmic**, **otic**, and **parenteral solutions** are classified separately because of their specific use and method of preparation.
6. **Mouthwashes** are solutions that are used to cleanse the mouth or treat diseases of the oral mucous membrane. They often contain alcohol or glycerin to aid in dissolving the volatile ingredients. Mouthwashes are more often used cosmetically than therapeutically.
7. **Astringents** are locally applied solutions that precipitate protein. They reduce cell permeability without causing injury. Astringents cause **constriction**, with wrinkling and blanching of the skin. Because astringents **reduce secretions**, they can be used as antiperspirants.
   a. **Aluminum acetate** and **aluminum subacetate solutions** are used as wet dressings in contact dermatitis. The precipitation is minimized by the addition of boric acid.
   b. **Calcium hydroxide solution** is a mild stringent that is used in lotions as a reactant and an alkalizer.
8. **Antibacterial topical solutions** (e.g., benzalkonium chloride, strong iodine, povidone–iodine) kill bacteria when applied to the skin or mucous membrane in the proper strength and under appropriate conditions.

C. **Suspensions**

1. **Lotions**, **magmas** (i.e., suspensions of finely divided material in a small amount of water), and **mixtures** are all suspensions that have had official formulas for some time (e.g., calamine lotion *USP*, kaolin mixture with pectin *NF*). Official formulas are given in the *USP/NF*.
   a. A **complete formula** and a **detailed method of preparation** are available for some official suspensions. For others, only the **concentration** of the active ingredients is given, and the manufacturer has considerable latitude in the formulation.
   b. Some drugs are packaged in a **dry form** to circumvent the instability of aqueous dispersions. Water is added at the time of dispensing to reconstitute the suspension.
2. **Purposes of suspension**
   a. **Sustaining effect**. For a sustained-release preparation, a suspension necessitates drug dissolution before absorption.
   b. **Stability**. Drug degradation in suspension or solid dosage forms occurs much more slowly than degradation in solution form.
   c. **Taste**. A drug with an unpleasant taste can be converted into an insoluble form and then prepared as a suspension.
   d. **Basic solubility**. When suitable solvents are not available, the suspension provides an alternative. For example, only water can be used as a solvent for ophthalmic preparations because of the possibility of corneal damage. Ophthalmic suspensions provide an alternative to ophthalmic solutions.
3. **Suspending agents** include hydrophilic colloids, clays, and a few other agents. Some are also used as **emulsifying agents** (see VI.D.3).
   a. **Hydrophilic colloids** (i.e., **hydrocolloids**) increase the viscosity of water by binding water molecules, thus limiting their mobility, or fluidity. Viscosity is proportional to the concentration of the hydrocolloid. These agents **support the growth of microorganisms** and require a preservative. They are mostly **anionic**, with the exception of methyl cellulose (neutral) and chitosan (cationic). Thus, the anionic hydrocolloids are incompatible with quaternary antibacterial agents and other positively charged drugs. Chitosan is incompatible with negatively charged drugs and excipients. Most hydrocolloids are **insoluble in alcoholic solutions**.
      (1) **Acacia** is usually used as 35% dispersion in water (mucilage). Its viscosity is greatest between pH 5 and pH 9. Acacia is susceptible to microbial decomposition.
      (2) **Tragacanth** is usually used as 6% dispersion in water (mucilage). One advantage of tragacanth over acacia is that less is needed. Also, tragacanth does not contain the oxidase that is present in acacia. This oxidase catalyzes the decomposition of organic chemicals. The viscosity of tragacanth is greatest at pH 5.
      (3) **Methyl cellulose** is a polymer that is nonionic and stable to heat and light. It is available in several viscosity grades. Because it is soluble in cold water, but not in hot water, dispersions are prepared by adding methyl cellulose to boiling water and then cooling the preparation until the material dissolves.
      (4) **Carboxymethylcellulose** is an anionic material that is soluble in water. Prolonged exposure to heat causes loss of viscosity.

b. **Clays** (e.g., bentonite, Veegum) are silicates that are anionic in aqueous dispersions. They are strongly hydrated and exhibit **thixotropy** (the property of forming a gel-like structure on standing and becoming fluid on agitation).
   (1) The official form of **bentonite** is the 5% magma.
   (2) **Veegum** is hydrated to a greater degree than bentonite. Thus, it is more viscous at the same concentration.

c. **Other agents** include agar, chondrus (carrageenan), gelatin, pectin, and gelatinized starch. Their use is limited by their susceptibility to bacterial attack, their incompatibilities, and their cost. Xanthan gum is used in many modern suspension formulations because of its cosolvent compatibility, its stability, and its solution's high viscosity relative to concentration.

4. **Preparation**
   a. **Solids are wetted initially** to separate individual particles and coat them with a layer of dispersion medium. Wetting is accomplished by **levigation** (i.e., addition of a suitable nonsolvent, or **levigating agent**, to the solid material, followed by blending to form a paste), using a glass mortar and pestle or an ointment slab. A **surfactant** can also be used.
   b. **Suspending agents** are then added as dry powder along with the active ingredient. For best results, the suspending agent is added in the form of its **aqueous dispersion**.
      (1) The aqueous dispersion is added to the solid (or the levigated solid) by **geometric dilution**.
      (2) The preparation is brought to the desired volume by stirring in the appropriate vehicle.

D. Emulsions

1. **Purposes of emulsions**
   a. **Increased drug solubility**. Many drugs have limited aqueous solubility but have maximum solubility in the oil phase of an emulsion. Drug partitioning from the oil phase to the water phase can maintain or enhance activity.
   b. **Increased drug stability**. Many drugs are more stable when incorporated into an emulsion rather than an aqueous solution.
   c. **Prolonged drug action**. Incorporation of a drug into an emulsion can prolong bioavailability, as with certain intramuscular injection preparations.
   d. **Improved taste**. Drugs with an unpleasant taste are more palatable and thus more conveniently administered in emulsion form.
   e. **Improved appearance**. Oily materials intended for topical application are more appealing in an emulsified form.

2. **Phases of emulsions**. Most emulsions are considered **two-phase systems**.
   a. The **liquid droplet** is known as the **dispersed**, **internal**, or **discontinuous phase**. The other liquid is known as the **dispersion medium**, **external phase**, or **continuous phase**.
   b. In pharmaceutical applications, one phase is usually an **aqueous solution**. The other phase is usually **lipid** or **oily**. The lipids range from vegetable or hydrocarbon oils to semisolid hydrocarbons and waxes. Emulsions are usually described in terms of water and oil. Oil is the lipid, or nonaqueous, phase regardless of its composition.
      (1) If water is the **internal phase**, the emulsion is classified as **w/o**.
      (2) If water is the **external phase**, the emulsion is classified as **o/w**.
   c. The **type of emulsion** formed is primarily determined by the **relative phase volumes** and the **emulsifying agent** used.
      (1) For an ideal emulsion, the maximum concentration of internal phase is 74% (i.e., theoretically, an o/w emulsion can be prepared containing $\leq$ 74% oil).
      (2) The choice of an emulsifying agent is more important than the relative phase volumes in determining the final emulsion type. Most agents preferentially form one type of emulsion or the other if the phase volume permits.

3. **Emulsifying agents**. Any compound that lowers the interfacial tension and forms a film at the interface can potentially function as an emulsifying agent. The effectiveness of the emulsifying agent depends on its chemical structure, concentration, solubility, pH, physical properties, and electrostatic effect. **True emulsifying agents** (primary agents) can form and stabilize emulsions by themselves. **Stabilizers** (auxiliary agents) do not form acceptable emulsions when used alone,

but assist primary agents in stabilizing the product (e.g., increase viscosity). Emulsifying agents are either **natural** or **synthetic**.

a. **Natural emulsifying agents**
   (1) **Acacia** forms a good, stable emulsion of low viscosity. It tends to cream easily, is acidic, and is stable at a pH range of 2 to 10. Like other gums, it is negatively charged, dehydrates easily, and usually requires a preservative. It is incompatible with Peruvian balsam, bismuth salts, and carbonates.
   (2) **Tragacanth** forms a stable emulsion that is coarser than acacia emulsion. It is anionic, is difficult to hydrate, and is used mainly for its effects on viscosity. Less than 1/10 of the amount used for acacia is needed.
   (3) **Agar** is an anionic gum that is primarily used to increase viscosity. Its stability is affected by heating, dehydration, and destruction of charge. It is also susceptible to microbial degradation.
   (4) **Pectin** is a quasi-emulsifier that is used in the same proportion as tragacanth.
   (5) **Gelatin** provides good emulsion stabilization in a concentration of 0.5% to 1.0%. It may be anionic or cationic, depending on its isoelectric point. Type A gelatin (+), prepared from an acid-treated precursor, is used in acidic media. Type B gelatin (−), prepared from an alkali-treated precursor, is used in basic media.
   (6) **Methyl cellulose** is nonionic and induces viscosity. It is used as a primary emulsifier with mineral oil and cod liver oil, and yields an o/w emulsion. It is usually used in 2% concentration.
   (7) **Carboxymethylcellulose** is anionic and is usually used to increase viscosity. It tolerates alcohol up to 40%, forms a basic solution, and precipitates in the presence of free acids.

b. **Synthetic emulsifying agents** are anionic, cationic, or nonionic. Although these surfactants are amphiphilic molecules, their lipophilic and hydrophilic regions are seldom inverse equals of each other: Some surfactant molecules tend to be predominantly lipophilic, whereas others are predominantly hydrophilic. This imbalance is reflected in the hydrophilic–lipophilic balance (HLB) scale: The larger the HLB value, the more hydrophilic the molecule. *Table 2-1* lists HLB values for surfactants and their corresponding uses.
   (1) **Anionic** synthetic agents include **sulfuric acid esters** (e.g., sodium lauryl sulfate), **sulfonic acid derivatives** (e.g., dioctyl sodium sulfosuccinate), and **soaps**. Soaps are for external use. They have a high pH and are, therefore, sensitive to the addition of acids and electrolytes.
      (a) **Alkali soaps** are hydrophilic and form an o/w emulsion.
      (b) **Metallic soaps** are water insoluble and form a w/o emulsion.
      (c) **Monovalent soaps** form an o/w emulsion.
      (d) **Polyvalent soaps** form a w/o emulsion.
   (2) **Cationic** synthetic agents (e.g., benzalkonium chloride) are used as surface-active agents in 1% concentration. They are incompatible with soaps.
   (3) **Nonionic** synthetic agents are resistant to the addition of acids and electrolytes.
      (a) The **sorbitan esters** known as **Spans** are hydrophobic in nature and form w/o emulsions. They have low hydrophilic–lipophilic balance values (1–9) (*Table 2-2*).

Table 2-1 HYDROPHILIC–LIPOPHILIC BALANCE (HLB)

HLB Value Range	Surfactant Application
0–3	Antifoaming agents
4–6	Water-in-oil emulsifying agents
7–9	Wetting agents
8–18	Oil-in-water emulsifying agents
13–15	Detergents
10–18	Solubilizing agents

Table 2-2 COMMONLY USED SURFACTANTS AND THEIR HYDROPHILIC–LIPOPHILIC BALANCE (HLB) VALUES

Agent	HLB Value
Sorbitan trioleate (Span 85, Arlacel 85)	1.8
Sorbitan tristearate (Span 65)	2.1
Propylene glycol monostearate (pure)	3.4
Sorbitan sesquioleate (Arlacel C)	3.7
Sorbitan monooleate (Span 80y)	4.3
Sorbitan monostearate (Arlacel 60)	4.7
Sorbitan monopalmitate (Span 40, Arlacel 40)	6.7
Sorbitan monolaurate (Span 20, Arlacel 20)	8.6
Glyceryl monostearate (Aldo 28, Tegin)	5.5
Gelatin	9.8
Triethanolamine oleate (Trolamine)	12.0
Polyoxyethylene alkyl phenol (Igepal CA-630)	12.8
Tragacanth	13.2
Polyoxyethylene sorbitan monolaurate (Tween 21)	13.3
Polyoxyethylene castor oil (Atlas G-1794)	13.3
Polyoxyethylene sorbitan monooleate (Tween 80)	15.0
Polyoxyethylene sorbitan monopalmitate (Tween 40)	15.6
Polyoxyethylene sorbitan monolaurate (Tween 20)	16.7
Polyoxyethylene lauryl ether (Brij 35)	16.9
Sodium oleate	18.0
Sodium lauryl sulfate	40.0

(b) The **polysorbates** known as **Tweens** are hydrophilic and tend to form o/w emulsions. They may form complexes with phenolic compounds. They have high hydrophilic–lipophilic balance values (11–20).

4. **Preparation**. Various methods are used to prepare emulsions, depending on the type of emulsifying agent.
   a. Classical, acacia-stabilized emulsions are prepared by one of the following four methods:
      (1) **Wet gum (English) method**. A primary emulsion of fixed oil, water, and acacia (in a 4:2:1 ratio) is prepared as follows:
         (a) Two parts of water are added all at once to one part of acacia. The mixture is triturated until a smooth mucilage is formed.
         (b) Oil is added in small increments (1 to 5 mL), with continuous trituration, until the primary emulsion is formed.
         (c) The mixture (an o/w emulsion) is triturated for another 5 mins.
         (d) The o/w mixture can then be brought to volume with water and mixed to achieve homogeneity.
      (2) **Dry gum (continental) method**. A primary emulsion of the fixed oil, water, and acacia (in a 4:2:1 ratio) is prepared as follows:
         (a) Oil is added to the acacia, and the mixture is triturated until the powder is distributed uniformly throughout the oil. Water is added all at once, followed by rapid trituration to form the primary emulsion.
         (b) Any remaining water and other ingredients are added to finish the product.
            (i) **Electrolytes in high concentration** tend to crack an emulsion. They should be added last and in as dilute a form as possible.
            (ii) **Alcoholic solutions** tend to dehydrate and precipitate hydrocolloids. They should be added in as dilute a concentration as possible.

(3) **Bottle method** (a variation of the dry gum method used for volatile oils). Oil is added to the acacia in a bottle. The ratio of oil, water, and acacia should be 3:2:1 or 2:1:1. The low viscosity of the volatile oil requires a higher proportion of acacia.

(4) **Nascent soap method.** A soap is formed by mixing relatively equal volumes of an oil and an aqueous solution that contains a sufficient amount of alkali. The soap acts as an emulsifying agent.

(a) This method is used to form an o/w or a w/o emulsion, depending on the soap formed. For example, olive oil, which contains oleic acid, is mixed with lime water during the preparation of calamine lotion to calcium oleate, an emulsifying agent.

(b) A 50:50 ratio of oil to water ensures sufficient emulsion, provided that the oil contains an adequate amount of free fatty acid. Olive oil usually does. Cottonseed oil, peanut oil, and some other vegetable oils do not.

(c) The addition of an acid destroys the emulsifying soap and causes the emulsion to separate.

b. Emulsions stabilized by synthetic emulsifying agents are readily prepared by a two-phase procedure.

(1) Oil-miscible ingredients and water-miscible ingredients are separately admixed, using heat if necessary to ensure liquefaction and ease of mixing of each phase.

(a) High melting point oil-miscible ingredients (e.g., waxes) are melted before lower melting point ingredients (e.g., oils) are added.

(2) The two phases are heated to 70° to 80°C and then combined with stirring until the resultant emulsion has cooled.

(a) In general, heat-labile or volatile ingredients should not be incorporated in the separate phases but in the resultant emulsion after it has cooled to about 40°C or less.

(3) Further mechanical processing of the emulsion by a hand homogenizer, immersion blender, or other equipment may be warranted to improve the homogeneity and stability of the product.

5. Incorporation of medicinal agents. Medicinal agents can be incorporated into an emulsion either during or after its formation.

a. Addition of a drug during emulsion formation. It is best to incorporate a drug into a vehicle during emulsion formation, when it can be incorporated in molecular form. Soluble drugs should be dissolved in the appropriate phase (e.g., drugs that are soluble in the external phase of the emulsion should be added as a solution to the primary emulsion).

b. Addition of a drug to a preformed emulsion can present some difficulty, depending on the type of emulsion and the nature of the emulsifier (*Table 2-3*).

(1) **Addition of oleaginous materials to a w/o emulsion** presents no problem because of the miscibility of the additive with the external phase. However, **addition of oleaginous materials to an o/w emulsion** can be difficult after emulsion formation.

(a) Occasionally, a small amount of oily material is added if excess emulsifier was used in the original formation.

(b) A small amount of an oil-soluble drug can be added if it is dissolved in a very small quantity of oil with geometric dilution techniques.

(2) **Addition of water or an aqueous material to a w/o emulsion** is extremely difficult, unless enough emulsifier has been incorporated into the emulsion. However, **addition of aqueous materials to an o/w emulsion** usually presents no problems if the added material does not interact with the emulsifying agent. Potential interactions should be expected with cationic compounds and salts of weak bases.

(3) **Addition of small quantities of alcoholic solutions to an o/w emulsion** is possible if the solute is compatible or dispersible in the aqueous phase of the emulsion. If acacia or another gum is used as the emulsifying agent, the alcoholic solution should be diluted with water before it is added. *Table 2-3* lists some commercial emulsion bases and their general composition.

(4) **Addition of crystalline drugs to a w/o emulsion** occurs more easily if the drugs are dissolved or dispersed in a small quantity of oil before they are added.

Table 2-3 SELECTED COMMERCIAL EMULSION BASES: EMULSION TYPE AND EMULSIFIER USED

Commercial Base	Emulsion Type	Emulsifier Type
Allercreme skin lotion	o/w	Triethanolamine stearate
Almay emulsion base	o/w	Fatty acid glycol esters
Cetaphil	o/w	Sodium lauryl sulfate
Dermovan	o/w	Fatty acid amides
Eucerin	w/o	Wool wax alcohol
HEB base	o/w	Sodium lauryl sulfate
Keri lotion	o/w	Nonionic emulsifiers
Lubriderm	o/w	Triethanolamine stearate
Neobase	o/w	Polyhydric alcohol esters
Neutrogena lotion	o/w	Triethanolamine lactate
Nivea cream	w/o	Wool wax alcohols
pHorsix	o/w	Polyoxyethylene emulsifiers
Polysorb hydrate	w/o	Sodium sesquioleate
Velvachol	o/w	Sodium lauryl sulfate

o/w, oil in water; w/o, water in oil.

E. Ointments

1. **Introduction. Ointments** are **semisolid preparations intended for external use**. They are easily spread. Modifying the formulation controls their plastic viscosity. Ointments are typically used as
   a. **emollients** to make the skin more pliable,
   b. **protective barriers** to prevent harmful substances from coming in contact with the skin, and
   c. **vehicles** in which to incorporate medication.
2. **Ointment bases**
   a. **Oleaginous bases** are anhydrous and insoluble in water. They cannot absorb or contain water and are not washable in water.
      (1) **Petrolatum** is a good base for oil-insoluble ingredients. It forms an occlusive film on the skin, absorbs < 5% water under normal conditions, and does not become rancid. Wax can be incorporated to stiffen the base.
      (2) **Synthetic esters** are used as constituents of oleaginous bases. These esters include glyceryl monostearate, isopropyl myristate, isopropyl palmitate, butyl stearate, and butyl palmitate. Long-chain alcohols (e.g., cetyl alcohol, stearyl alcohol, PEG) can also be used.
      (3) **Lanolin derivatives** are often used in topical and cosmetic preparations. Examples are lanolin oil and hydrogenated lanolin.
   b. **Absorption bases** are anhydrous and water insoluble. Therefore, they are not washable in water, although they can absorb water. These bases permit water-soluble medicaments to be included through prior solution and uptake as the internal phase.
      (1) **Wool fat** (anhydrous lanolin) contains a high percentage of cholesterol as well as esters and alcohol that contain fatty acids. It absorbs twice its weight in water and melts between 36°C and 42°C.
      (2) **Hydrophilic petrolatum** is a white petrolatum combined with 8% beeswax, 3% stearyl alcohol, and 3% cholesterol. These components are added to a w/o emulsifier. Prepared forms include Aquaphor, which uses wool alcohol to render white petrolatum emulsifiable. Aquaphor is superior in its ability to absorb water.
   c. **Emulsion bases** may be w/o emulsions, which are water insoluble and are not washable in water. These emulsions can absorb water because of their aqueous internal phase. Emulsion bases may also be o/w emulsions, which are water insoluble but washable in water. They can absorb water in their aqueous external phase.
      (1) **Hydrous wool fat** (lanolin) is a w/o emulsion that contains approximately 25% water. It acts as an emollient and occlusive film on the skin, effectively preventing epidermal water loss.

(2) **Cold cream** is a w/o emulsion that is prepared by melting white wax, spermaceti, and expressed almond oil together; adding a hot aqueous solution of sodium borate; and stirring until the mixture is cool.

(a) The use of mineral oil rather than almond oil makes a more stable cold cream. However, cold cream prepared with almond oil makes a better emollient base.

(b) This ointment should be freshly prepared.

(3) **Hydrophilic ointment** is an o/w emulsion that uses sodium lauryl sulfate as an emulsifying agent. It absorbs 30% to 50% w/w without losing its consistency. It is readily miscible with water and is removed from the skin easily.

(4) **Vanishing cream** is an o/w emulsion that contains a large percentage of water as well as humectant (e.g., glycerin, propylene glycol) that retards moisture loss. An excess of stearic acid in the formula helps form a thin film when the water evaporates.

(5) **Other emulsion bases** include Dermovan, a hypoallergenic, greaseless emulsion base, and Unibase, a nongreasy emulsion base that absorbs approximately 30% of its weight in water and has a pH close to that of the skin.

d. **Water-soluble bases** may be anhydrous or may contain some water. They are washable in water and absorb water to the point of solubility.

(1) **PEG ointment** is a blend of water-soluble polyethylene glycols that form a semisolid base. This base can solubilize water-soluble drugs and some water-insoluble drugs. It is compatible with a wide range of drugs.

(a) This base contains 40% PEG 3350 and 60% PEG 400. It is prepared by the fusion method (see VI.E.3.b).

(b) Only a small amount of liquid ($< 5\%$) can be incorporated without loss of viscosity. This base can be made stiffer by increasing the amount of PEG 3350 to 60%.

(c) If 6% to 25% of an aqueous solution is to be incorporated, 5 g of the 40 g of PEG 3350 can be replaced with an equal amount of stearyl alcohol.

(2) **Propylene glycol** and **propylene glycol–ethanol** form a clear gel when mixed with 2% hydroxypropyl cellulose. This base is a popular dermatologic vehicle.

3. **Incorporation of medicinal agents**. Medicinal substances may be incorporated into an ointment base by **levigation** or by the **fusion method**. Insoluble substances should be reduced to the finest possible form and levigated before incorporation with a small amount of compatible levigating agent or with the base itself.

a. **Levigation**. The substance is incorporated into the ointment by levigation on an ointment slab.

(1) A stainless-steel spatula with a long, broad, flexible blade should be used. If the substance may interact with a metal spatula (e.g., when incorporating iodine and mercuric salts), then a hard rubber spatula can be used.

(2) Insoluble substances should be powdered finely in a mortar and mixed with an equal quantity of base until a smooth, grit-free mixture is obtained. The rest of the base is added in increments.

(3) Levigation of powders into a small portion of base is facilitated by the use of a melted base or a small quantity of compatible levigation aid (e.g., mineral oil, glycerin).

(4) Water-soluble salts are incorporated by dissolving them in the smallest possible amount of water and incorporating the aqueous solution directly into a compatible base.

(a) Usually, organic solvents (e.g., ether, chloroform, alcohol) are not used to dissolve the drug because the drug may crystallize as the solvent evaporates.

(b) Solvents are used as levigating aids only if the solid will become a fine powder after the solvent evaporates.

b. **Fusion method**. This method is used when the base contains solids that have higher melting points (e.g., waxes, cetyl alcohol, glyceryl monostearate). This method is also useful for solid medicaments, which are readily soluble in the melted base.

(1) The oil phase should be melted separately, starting with materials that have the highest melting point. All other oil-soluble ingredients are added in decreasing order of melting point.

(2) The ingredients in the water phase are combined and heated separately to a temperature that is equal to or several degrees above that of the melted oil phase.

(3) The two phases are combined. If a w/o system is desired, then the hot aqueous phase is incorporated into the hot oil phase with agitation. If an o/w system is preferred, then the hot oil phase is incorporated into the hot aqueous phase.

(4) Volatile materials (e.g., menthol, camphor, iodine, alcohol, perfumes) are added after the melted mixture cools to 40°C or less.

F. Suppositories

1. **Introduction**. A suppository is a **solid or semisolid mass intended to be inserted into a body orifice** (i.e., rectum, vagina, urethra). After it is inserted, a suppository either melts at body temperature or dissolves (or disperses) into the aqueous secretions of the body cavity.
   a. Suppositories are often used for local effects (e.g., relief of hemorrhoids or infection).
   b. When used rectally, suppositories can provide systemic medication. The absorption of a drug from a suppository through the rectal mucosa into the circulation involves two steps:
      (1) The drug is released from a vehicle and partitions/diffuses through the mucosa.
      (2) The drug is transported through the veins or lymph vessels into systemic fluids or tissues. The first-pass effect is avoided because the rectal veins "bypass" the liver.
   c. Rectal suppositories are useful when oral administration is inappropriate, as with infants, debilitated or comatose patients, and patients who have nausea, vomiting, or gastrointestinal disturbances. Some drugs can cause disturbances of the gastrointestinal tract.
2. **Types of suppositories**
   a. **Rectal suppositories** are usually cylindrical and tapered to a point, forming a bullet-like shape. As the rectum contracts, a suppository of this shape moves inward rather than outward. Suppositories for adults weigh approximately 2 g. Suppositories for infants and children are smaller.
   b. **Vaginal suppositories** are oval and typically weigh approximately 5 g. Drugs administered by this route are intended to have a local effect, but systemic absorption can occur. Antiseptics, contraceptive agents, and drugs used to treat trichomonal, monilial, or bacterial infections are often formulated as vaginal suppositories.
   c. **Urethral suppositories** are typically long and tapered. They are approximately 60 mm long and 4 to 5 mm in diameter. They are administered for a local effect and are most often used for anti-infective agents. Alprostadil, or prostaglandin E_1 (PGE_1), when used to treat erectile dysfunction, is available for urethral insertion in the form of a micropellet, or microsuppository, that is only 3 to 6 mm long and 1.4 mm in diameter.
3. **Suppository bases**
   a. **Criteria for satisfactory suppository bases**. Suppository bases should
      (1) Remain firm at room temperature to allow insertion. The suppository should not soften $< 30°C$ to avoid melting during storage.
      (2) Have a narrow, or sharp, melting range
      (3) Yield a clear melt just below body temperature or dissolve rapidly in the cavity fluid
      (4) Be inert and compatible with a variety of drugs
      (5) Be nonirritating and nonsensitizing
      (6) Have wetting and emulsifying properties
      (7) Have an acid value of < 0.2, a saponification value of 200 to 245, and an iodine value of < 7 if the base is fatty
   b. **Selecting a suppository base**. Lipid–water solubility must be considered because of its relation to the drug-release rate.
      (1) If an oil-soluble drug is incorporated into an oily base, then the rate of absorption is somewhat less than that achieved with a water-soluble base. The lipid-soluble drug tends to remain dissolved in the oily pool from the suppository. It is less likely to escape into the mucous secretions from which it is ultimately absorbed.
      (2) Conversely, a water-soluble drug tends to pass more rapidly from the oil phase to the aqueous phase. Therefore, if rapid onset of action is desired, the water-soluble drug should be incorporated into the oily base.
   c. **Bases that melt** include **cocoa butter**, other **combinations of fats and waxes**, **Witepsol bases**, and **Wecobee bases** (*Table 2-4*).
      (1) **Cocoa butter** (theobroma oil) is the most widely used suppository base. It is firm and solid up to a temperature of 32°C, at which point it begins to soften. At 34° to 35°C, it melts to produce a thin, bland, oily liquid.
         (a) Cocoa butter is a good base for a **rectal suppository**, but it is less than ideal for a vaginal or urethral suppository.

Table 2-4 COMPOSITION, MELTING RANGE, AND CONGEALING RANGE OF SELECTED BASES THAT MELT

Base	Composition	Melting Range (°C)	Congealing Range (°C)
Cocoa butter	Mixed triglycerides of oleic, palmitic, and stearic acids	34–35	28 or less
Cotmar	Partially hydrogenated cottonseed oil	34–75	—
Dehydag	Hydrogenated fatty alcohols		
Base I	and esters	33–36	32–33
Base II		37–39	36–37
Base III		9 ranges	9 ranges
Wecobee R	Glycerides of saturated fatty acids C_{12}–C_{18}	33–35	31–32
Wecobee SS	Triglycerides derived from coconut oil	40–43	33–35
Witepsol	Triglycerides of saturated fatty		
H12	acids C_{12}–C_{18}, with varied	32–33	29–32
H15	portions of the corresponding	33–35	32–34
H85	partial glycerides	42–44	36–38

(b) A mixture of triglycerides, cocoa butter exhibits polymorphism. Depending on the fusion temperature, it can crystallize into any one of four crystal forms.

(c) **Major limitations of cocoa butter**. Because of the following limitations, many combinations of fats and waxes are used as substitutes (*Table 2-4*):

(i) **An inability to absorb aqueous solutions**. The addition of nonionic surfactants to the base ameliorates this problem to some extent. However, the resultant suppositories have poor stability and may turn rancid rapidly.

(ii) **The lowering of the melting point produced by certain drugs** (e.g., chloral hydrate).

(2) **Witepsol** bases contain natural saturated fatty acid chains between C_{12} and C_{18}. Lauric acid is the major component. All 12 bases of this series are colorless and almost odorless. The drug-release characteristics of Witepsol H15 are similar to those of cocoa butter.

(a) Unlike cocoa butter, Witepsol bases do not exhibit polymorphism when heated and cooled.

(b) The interval between softening and melting temperatures is very small. Because Witepsol bases solidify rapidly in the mold, lubrication of the mold is not necessary.

(3) **Wecobee** bases are derived from coconut oil. Their action is similar to that of Witepsol bases. Incorporation of glyceryl monostearate and propylene glycol monostearate makes these bases emulsifiable.

d. **Bases that dissolve** include **PEG** polymers with a molecular weight of 400 to 6000.

(1) At room temperature, PEG 400 is a liquid, PEG 1000 is a semisolid, PEG 1500 and 1600 are fairly firm semisolids, and PEG 3350 and 6000 are firm waxlike solids.

(2) These bases are water soluble, but the dissolution process is very slow. In the rectum and vagina, where the amount of fluid is very small, they dissolve very slowly, but they soften and spread.

(3) PEGs complex with several drugs and affect drug release and absorption.

(4) Mixtures of PEG polymers in varying proportions provide a base of different properties (*Table 2-5*).

4. **Preparation**. Suppositories are prepared by the following three methods:

a. **Hand-rolling** involves molding the suppository with the fingers after a plastic mass is formed.

(1) A finely powdered drug is mixed with the grated base in a mortar and pestle, using levigation and geometric dilution techniques. A small quantity of fixed oil may be added to facilitate preparation.

Table 2-5 MIXTURES OF POLYETHYLENE GLYCOL (PEG) BASES PROVIDING SATISFACTORY ROOM TEMPERATURE STABILITY AND DISSOLUTION CHARACTERISTICS

Base	Comments	Components	Proportion (%)
1	Provides a good general-purpose, water-soluble suppository	PEG 6000	50
		PEG 1540	30
		PEG 400	20
2	Provides a good general-purpose base that is slightly softer than base 1 and dissolves more rapidly	PEG 4000	60
		PEG 1500	30
		PEG 400	10
3	Has a higher melting point than the other bases, which is usually sufficient to compensate for the melting point lowering effect of such drugs as chloral hydrate and camphor	PEG 6000	30
		PEG 1540	70

(2) The uniformly mixed semiplastic mass is kneaded further, rolled into a cylinder, and divided into the requisite number of suppositories. Each small cylinder is rolled by hand until a suppository shape is fashioned.

b. Compression is generally used when cocoa butter is used as a base.

(1) A uniform mixture of drug and base is prepared as for the hand-rolling method.

(2) The mixture is placed into a suppository compression device. Pressure is applied, and the mixture is forced into lubricated compression mold cavities. The mold is then cooled and the suppositories ejected.

(3) This procedure generally produces a 2-g suppository. However, a large volume of the active ingredients can affect the amount of cocoa butter required for an individual formula.

(a) The amount of cocoa butter needed is determined by calculating the total amount of active ingredient to be used, dividing this number by the cocoa butter density factor (*Table 2-6*), and subtracting the resulting number from the total amount of cocoa butter required for the desired number of suppositories.

(b) For example, suppose 12 suppositories, each containing 300 mg aspirin, are required. Each mold cavity has a 2-g capacity. For 13 suppositories (calculated to provide one

Table 2-6 COCOA BUTTER DENSITY FACTORS OF DRUGS COMMONLY USED IN SUPPOSITORIES

Drug	Cocoa Butter Density Factor	Drug	Cocoa Butter Density Factor
Aloin	1.3	Dimenhydrinate	1.3
Aminophylline	1.1	Diphenhydramine hydrochloride	1.3
Aminopyrine	1.3	Gallic acid	2.0
Aspirin	1.1	Morphine hydrochloride	1.6
Barbital sodium	1.2	Pentobarbital	1.2
Belladonna extract	1.3	Phenobarbital sodium	1.2
Bismuth subgallate	2.7	Salicylic acid	1.3
Chloral hydrate	1.3	Secobarbital sodium	1.2
Codeine phosphate	1.1	Tannic acid	1.6
Digitalis leaf	1.6		

extra), 3.9 g aspirin (13 × 0.3 g = 3.9 g) is required. This number is divided by the density factor of aspirin (1.1) (*Table 2-6*). Thus, 3.9 g of aspirin replaces 3.55 g of cocoa butter. The total amount of cocoa butter needed for 13 suppositories of 2 g each equals 26 g. The amount of cocoa butter required is 26 g − 3.55 g, or 22.45 g.

c. The **fusion method** is the principal way that suppositories are made commercially. This method is used primarily for suppositories that contain cocoa butter, PEG, and glycerin–gelatin bases. Molds made of aluminum, brass, or nickel–copper alloys are used and can make 6 to 50 suppositories at one time.
   (1) The **capacity of the molds** is determined by melting a sufficient quantity of base over a steam bath, pouring it into the molds, and allowing it to congeal. The "blank" suppositories are trimmed, removed, and weighed. Once the weight is known, the drug-containing suppositories are prepared.
      (a) To prepare suppositories, the drug is reduced to a fine powder. A small amount of grated cocoa butter is liquefied in a suitable container placed in a water bath at 33°C or less.
      (b) The finely powdered drug is mixed with melted cocoa butter with continuous stirring.
      (c) The remainder of the grated cocoa butter is added with stirring. The temperature is maintained at or below 33°C. The liquid should appear creamy rather than clear.
      (d) The mold is very lightly lubricated with mineral oil, and the creamy melt is poured into the mold at room temperature. The melt is poured continuously to avoid layering.
      (e) After the suppositories congeal, they are placed in a refrigerator to harden. After 30 mins, they are removed from the refrigerator, trimmed, and unmolded.
   (2) The fusion process should be used carefully with **thermolabile drugs** and **insoluble powders**.
      (a) Insoluble powders in the melt may settle or float during pouring, depending on their density. They may also collect at one end of the suppository before the melt congeals, and cause a nonuniform drug distribution.
      (b) Hard crystalline materials (e.g., iodine, merbromin) can be incorporated by dissolving the crystals in a minimum volume of suitable solvent before they are incorporated into the base.
      (c) Vegetable extracts can be incorporated by moistening with a few drops of alcohol and levigating with a small amount of melted cocoa butter.

G. **Powders**

1. **Introduction**. A pharmaceutical powder is a mixture of finely divided drugs or chemicals in dry form. The powder may be used internally or externally.
   a. **Advantages** of powders
      (1) Flexibility of compounding
      (2) Good chemical stability
      (3) Rapid dispersion of ingredients because of the small particle size
   b. **Disadvantages** of powders
      (1) Time-consuming preparation
      (2) Inaccuracy of dose
      (3) Unsuitability for many unpleasant-tasting, hygroscopic, and deliquescent drugs
   c. **Milling** is the mechanical process of reducing the particle size of solids (**comminution**) before mixing with other components, further processing, or incorporation into a final product (*Tables 2-7 and 2-8*). The particle size of a powder is related to the proportion of the powder that can pass through the opening of standard sieves of various dimensions in a specified amount of time. **Micromeritics** is the study of particles.
      (1) **Advantages** of milling
         (a) Increases the surface area, which may increase the dissolution rate as well as bioavailability (e.g., griseofulvin)
         (b) Increases extraction, or leaching, from animal glands (e.g., liver, pancreas) and from crude vegetable extracts
         (c) Facilitates drying of wet masses by increasing the surface area and reducing the distance that moisture must travel to reach the outer surface. Micronization and subsequent drying, in turn, increase stability as occluded solvent is removed.

Table 2-7 *UNITED STATES PHARMACOPEIA* STANDARDS FOR POWDERS OF ANIMAL AND VEGETABLE DRUGS

Type of Powder	Sieve Size All Particles Pass Through	Sieve Size Percentage of Particles Pass Through
Very coarse (#8)	#20 sieve	20% through a #60 sieve
Coarse (#20)	#20 sieve	40% through a #60 sieve
Moderately coarse (#40)	#40 sieve	40% through a #80 sieve
Fine (#60)	#60 sieve	40% through a #100 sieve
Very fine (#80)	#80 sieve	No limit

(d) Improves mixing, or blending, of several solid ingredients if they are reduced to approximately the same size; also minimizes segregation and provides greater dose uniformity

(e) Permits uniform distribution of coloring agents in artificially colored solid pharmaceuticals

(f) Improves the function of lubricants used to coat the surface of the granulation or powder in compressed tablets and capsules

(g) Improves the texture, appearance, and physical stability of ointments, creams, and pastes

(2) Disadvantages of milling

(a) Can change the polymorphic form of the active ingredient, rendering it less active

(b) Can degrade the drug as a result of heat buildup, oxidation, or adsorption of unwanted moisture because of increased surface area

(c) Decreases the bulk density of the active compound and excipients, causing flow problems and segregation.

(d) Decreases the particle size of the raw materials and may create problems with static charge, which may cause particle aggregation and decrease the dissolution rate

(e) Increases surface area, which may promote air adsorption and inhibit wettability

(3) Comminution techniques. On a large scale, various mills and pulverizers (e.g., rotary cutter, hammer, roller, fluid energy mill) are used during manufacturing. On a small scale, the pharmacist usually uses one of the following comminution techniques:

(a) Trituration. The substance is reduced to small particles by rubbing it in a mortar with a pestle. Trituration also describes the process by which fine powders are intimately mixed in a mortar.

(b) Pulverization by intervention. Substances are reduced and subdivided with an additional material (i.e., solvent) that is easily removed after pulverization. This technique is often used with gummy substances that reagglomerate or resist grinding. For example, camphor is readily reduced after a small amount of alcohol or other volatile solvent is added. The solvent is then permitted to evaporate.

Table 2-8 *UNITED STATES PHARMACOPEIA* STANDARDS FOR POWDERS OF CHEMICALS

Type of Powder	Sieve Size All Particles Pass Through	Sieve Size Percentage of Particles Pass Through
Coarse (#20)	#20 sieve	60% through a #40 sieve
Moderately coarse (#40)	#40 sieve	60% through a #60 sieve
Fine (#80)	#80 sieve	No limit
Very fine (#120)	#120 sieve	No limit

(c) **Levigation**. The particle size of the substance is reduced by adding a suitable nonsolvent (levigating agent) to form a paste. The paste is then rubbed in a mortar and pestle or using an ointment slab and spatula. This method is often used to prevent a gritty feel when solids are incorporated into dermatologic or ophthalmic ointments and suspensions. Mineral oil is a common levigating agent.

2. **Mixing powders**. Powders are mixed, or blended, by the following five methods:
   a. **Spatulation**. A spatula is used to blend small amounts of powders on a sheet of paper or a pill tile.
      (1) This method is not suitable for large quantities of powders or for powders that contain potent substances because homogeneous blending may not occur.
      (2) This method is particularly useful for solid substances that liquefy or form **eutectic mixtures** (i.e., mixtures that melt at a lower temperature than any of their ingredients) when in close, prolonged contact with one another because little compression or compaction results.
         (a) These substances include phenol, camphor, menthol, thymol, aspirin, phenylsalicylate, and phenacetin.
         (b) To diminish contact, powders prepared from these substances are commonly mixed with an inert diluent (e.g., light magnesium oxide or magnesium carbonate, kaolin, starch, bentonite).
         (c) Silicic acid (approximately 20%) prevents eutexia with aspirin, phenylsalicylate, and other troublesome compounds.
   b. **Trituration** is used both to comminute and to mix powders.
      (1) If comminution is desired, a porcelain or ceramic mortar with a rough inner surface is preferred to a glass mortar with a smooth working surface.
      (2) A glass mortar is preferable for chemicals that stain a porcelain or ceramic surface as well as for simple admixture of substances without special need for comminution. A glass mortar cleans more readily after use.
   c. **Geometric dilution** is used when potent substances must be mixed with a large amount of diluent.
      (1) The potent drug and an approximately equal volume of diluent are placed in a mortar and thoroughly mixed by trituration.
      (2) A second portion of diluent, equal in volume to the powder mixture in the mortar, is added, and trituration is repeated. The process is continued; equal volumes of diluent are added to the powder mixture in the mortar until all of the diluent is incorporated.
   d. **Sifting**. Powders are mixed by passing them through sifters similar to those used to sift flour. This process results in a light, fluffy product. Usually, it is not acceptable for incorporating potent drugs into a diluent base.
   e. **Tumbling** is the process of mixing powders in a large container rotated by a motorized process. These blenders are widely used in industry, as are large-volume powder mixers that use motorized blades to blend the powder in a large mixing vessel.
3. **Use and packaging of powders**. Depending on their intended use, powders are packaged and dispensed by pharmacists as bulk powders or divided powders.
   a. Bulk powders are dispensed by the pharmacist in bulk containers. A **perforated**, or **sifter**, **can** is used for external dusting, and an **aerosol container** is used for spraying on skin. A **wide-mouthed glass jar** permits easy removal of a spoonful of powder.
      (1) Powders commonly dispensed in bulk form
         (a) **Antacid and laxative powders** are used by mixing the directed amount of powder (usually approximately 1 teaspoon) in a portion of liquid, which the patient then drinks.
         (b) **Douche powders** are dissolved in warm water and applied vaginally.
         (c) **Medicated and nonmedicated powders for external use** are usually dispensed in a sifter for convenient application to the skin.
         (d) **Dentifrices**, or **dental cleansing powders**, are used for oral hygiene.
         (e) Powders for the **ear**, **nose**, **throat**, **tooth sockets**, or **vagina** are administered with an insufflator or powder blower.
      (2) **Nonpotent substances** are usually dispensed in bulk powder form. Those intended for external use should be clearly labeled.

(3) **Hygroscopic**, **deliquescent**, or **volatile** powders should be packed in glass jars rather than pasteboard containers. Amber or green glass should be used if needed to prevent decomposition of light-sensitive components. All powders should be stored in tightly closed containers.

b. **Divided powders** are dispensed in individual doses, usually in folded **papers** (i.e., chartulae). They may also be dispensed in metal foil, small heat-sealed or resealable **plastic bags**, or other containers.

(1) After the ingredients are weighed, comminuted, and mixed, the powders must be accurately **divided** into the prescribed number of doses.

(2) Depending on the potency of the drug substance, the pharmacist decides whether to **weigh** each portion separately before packaging or to approximate portions by the **block-and-divide method**.

(3) **Powder papers** can be of any convenient size that fits the required dose. Four basic types are used:

(a) **Vegetable parchment** is a thin, semiopaque, moisture-resistant paper.

(b) **White bond** is an opaque paper that has no moisture-resistant properties.

(c) **Glassine** is a glazed, transparent, moisture-resistant paper.

(d) **Waxed paper** is a transparent waterproof paper.

(4) Hygroscopic and volatile drugs are best protected with waxed paper that is double wrapped and covered with a bond paper to improve the appearance. Parchment and glassine papers are of limited use for these drugs.

4. **Special problems**. Volatile substances, eutectic mixtures, liquids, and hygroscopic or deliquescent substances present problems when they are mixed into powders that require special treatment.

a. **Volatile substances** (e.g., camphor, menthol, essential oils) can be lost by volatilization after they are incorporated into powders. This process is prevented or retarded by the use of heat-sealed plastic bags or by double wrapping with waxed or glassine paper inside white bond paper.

b. **Liquids** are incorporated into divided powders in small amounts.

(1) Magnesium carbonate, starch, or lactose can be added to increase the absorbability of the powders by increasing the surface area.

(2) When the liquid is a solvent for a nonvolatile heat-stable compound, it is evaporated gently in a water bath. Some fluid extracts and tinctures are treated in this way.

c. **Hygroscopic and deliquescent substances** that become moist because of an affinity for moisture in the air can be prepared as divided powders by adding inert diluents. Double wrapping is desirable for further protection.

d. **Eutectic mixtures**

H. Capsules

1. **Introduction**. Capsules are solid dosage forms in which one or more medicinal or inert substances (as powder, compact, beads, or granulation) are enclosed within a small gelatin shell. Gelatin capsules may be hard or soft. Most capsules are intended to be swallowed whole, but occasionally, the contents are removed from the gelatin shell and used as a premeasured dose.

2. **Hard gelatin capsules**

a. **Preparation of filled hard capsules** includes preparing the formulation, selecting the appropriate capsule, filling the capsule shells, and cleaning and polishing the filled capsules.

(1) Empty hard capsule shells are manufactured from a mixture of gelatin, colorants, and sometimes an opacifying agent (e.g., titanium dioxide). The *USP* also permits the addition of 0.15% sulfur dioxide to prevent decomposition of gelatin during manufacture.

(2) Gelatin *USP* is obtained by partial hydrolysis of collagen obtained from the skin, white connective tissue, and bones of animals. Types A and B are obtained by acid and alkali processing, respectively.

(3) Capsule shells are cast by dipping cold metallic molds or pins into gelatin solutions that are maintained at a uniform temperature and an exact degree of fluidity.

(a) Variation in the viscosity of the gelatin solution increases or decreases the thickness of the capsule wall.

(b) After the pins are withdrawn from the gelatin solution, they are rotated while being dried in kilns. A strong blast of filtered air with controlled humidity is forced through the kilns. Each capsule is then mechanically stripped, trimmed, and joined.

b. **Storage**. Hard capsules should be stored in tightly closed glass containers and protected from dust and extremes of humidity and temperature.
   (1) These capsules contain 12% to 16% water, varying with storage conditions. When humidity is low, the capsules become brittle. When humidity is high, the capsules become flaccid and shapeless.
   (2) Storage at high temperatures also affects the quality of hard gelatin capsules.

c. **Sizes**. Hard capsules are available in various sizes.
   (1) Empty capsules are **numbered** from 000, which is the largest size that can be swallowed, to 5, the smallest size. The approximate capacity of capsules ranges from 600 to 30 mg for capsules from 000 to 5, respectively. The capacity varies because of varying densities of powdered drug materials and the degree of pressure used to fill the capsules.
   (2) Large capsules are available for **veterinary medicine**.
   (3) **Selecting capsules**. Capsule size should be chosen carefully. A properly filled capsule should have its body filled with the drug mixture and its cap fully extended down the body. The cap is meant to enclose the powder, not to retain additional powder. Typically, hard gelatin capsules are used to encapsulate between 65 mg and 1 g of powdered material, including the drug and any diluents needed.
      (a) If the drug dose is inadequate to fill the capsule, a diluent (e.g., lactose) is added.
      (b) If the amount of drug needed for a usual dose is too large to place in a single capsule, two or more capsules may be required.
      (c) Lubricants such as magnesium stearate (frequently, 1%) are added to facilitate the flow of the powder when an automatic capsule-filling machine is used.
      (d) Wetting agents (e.g., sodium lauryl sulfate) may be added to capsule formulations to enhance drug dissolution.

d. **Filling capsules**. Whether on a large- or a small-production scale, the cap is first separated from the body of the capsule before filling the capsule body with the formulation and then reattaching the cap. Automated and semiautomated capsule-filling equipment fill the capsule bodies with the formulation by gravity fill, tamping, or a screw-feed (i.e., auger) mechanism. Extemporaneously compounded capsules are usually filled by the punch method.
   (1) The powder is placed on paper and flattened with a spatula so that the layer of powder is no more than approximately one-third the length of the capsule. The paper is held in the left hand. The body of the capsule is held in the right hand and repeatedly pressed into the powder until the capsule is filled. The cap is replaced and the capsule weighed.
   (2) **Granular** material that does not lend itself well to the punch method can be poured into each capsule from the powder paper on which it was weighed.
   (3) **Crystalline** materials, especially those that consist of a mass of filament-like crystals (e.g., quinine salts), will not fit into a capsule easily unless they are powdered.
   (4) After they are filled, capsules must be cleaned and polished.
      (a) On a **small scale**, capsules are cleaned individually or in small numbers by rubbing them on a clean gauze or cloth.
      (b) On a **large scale**, many capsule-filling machines have a cleaning vacuum that removes any extraneous material as the capsules leave the machine.

3. **Soft gelatin capsules**

a. **Preparation**
   (1) Soft gelatin capsules are prepared from gelatin shells. Glycerin or a polyhydric alcohol (e.g., sorbitol) is added to these shells to make them elastic or plastic-like.
   (2) These shells contain preservatives (e.g., methyl and propyl parabens, sorbic acid) to prevent the growth of fungi.

b. **Uses**. Soft gelatin shells are oblong, elliptical, or spherical. They are used to contain liquids, suspensions, pastes, dry powders, or pellets.
   (1) Drugs that are commercially prepared in soft capsules include demeclocycline hydrochloride (Declomycin, Lederle), chloral hydrate, digoxin (Lanoxicaps, GlaxoSmithKline), vitamin A, and vitamin E.
   (2) Soft gelatin capsules are usually prepared by the plate process or by the rotary or reciprocating die process.

(b) **Common disintegrants** include cornstarch and potato starch, starch derivatives (e.g., sodium starch glycolate), cellulose derivatives (e.g., sodium carboxymethylcellulose, croscarmellose sodium), clays (e.g., Veegum, bentonite), and cation exchange resins.

(c) The total **amount of disintegrant** is not always added to the drug–diluent mixture. A portion can be added, with the lubricant, to the prepared granulation of the drug. This approach causes double disintegration of the tablet. The portion of disintegrant that is added last causes the tablet to break into small pieces or chunks. The portion that is added first breaks the pieces of tablet into fine particles.

(4) **Lubricants**, **antiadherents**, and **glidants** have overlapping function.

(a) **Lubricants** reduce the friction that occurs between the walls of the tablet and the walls of the die cavity when the tablet is ejected. Talc, magnesium stearate, and calcium stearate are commonly used.

(b) **Antiadherents** reduce sticking, or adhesion, of the tablet granulation or powder to the faces of the punches or the die walls.

(c) **Glidants** promote the flow of the tablet granulation or powder by reducing friction among particles.

(5) **Colors and dyes** disguise off-color drugs, provide product identification, and produce a more aesthetically appealing product. **Food**, **drug**, and **cosmetic dyes** are applied as solutions. **Lakes** are dyes that have been absorbed on a hydrous oxide. Lakes are typically used as dry powders.

(6) **Flavoring agents** are usually limited to chewable tablets or tablets that are intended to dissolve in the mouth.

(a) Water-soluble flavors usually have poor stability. For this reason, flavor oils or dry powders are typically used.

(b) Flavor oils may be added to tablet granulations in solvents, dispersed on clays and other adsorbents, or emulsified in aqueous granulating agents. Usually, the maximum amount of oil that can be added to a granulation without affecting its tablet characteristics is 0.5% to 0.75%.

(7) **Artificial sweeteners**, like flavors, are typically used only with chewable tablets or tablets that are intended to dissolve in the mouth.

(a) Some **sweetness** may come from the diluent (e.g., mannitol, lactose). Other agents (e.g., saccharin, aspartame) may also be added.

(b) **Saccharin** has an unpleasant aftertaste.

(c) **Aspartame** is not stable in the presence of moisture and heat.

(8) **Adsorbents** (e.g., magnesium oxide, magnesium carbonate, bentonite, silicon dioxide) hold quantities of fluid in an apparently dry state.

3. **Tablet types and classes.** Tablets are classified according to their route of administration, drug delivery system, and form and method of manufacture (*Table 2-10*).

a. **Tablets for oral ingestion** are designed to be swallowed intact, with the exception of chewable tablets. Tablets may be coated for a number of reasons: to mask the taste, color, or odor of the drug; to control drug release; to protect the drug from the acid environment of the stomach; to incorporate another drug and provide sequential release or avoid incompatibility; or to improve appearance.

(1) **Compressed tablets** are formed by compression and have no special coating. They are made from powdered, crystalline, or granular materials, alone or in combination with excipients such as binders, disintegrants, diluents, and colorants.

(2) **Multiple compressed tablets** are layered or compression coated.

(a) **Layered tablets** are prepared by compressing a tablet granulation around a previously compressed granulation. The operation is repeated to produce multiple layers.

(b) **Compression-coated, or dry-coated, tablets** are prepared by feeding previously compressed tablets into a special tableting machine. This machine compresses an outer shell around the tablets. This process applies a thinner, more uniform coating than sugar coating, and it can be used safely with drugs that are sensitive to moisture.

Table 2-10 TABLET TYPES AND CLASSES

Tablets for oral ingestion	Tablets used in the oral cavity
Compressed	Buccal
Multiple compressed	Sublingual
Layered	Troches, lozenges, and dental cones
Compression coated	
Repeat-action	**Tablets used to prove solutions**
Delayed action and enteric coated	Effervescent
Sugar coated and chocolate coated	Dispensing
Film coated	Hypodermic
Air suspension coated	Triturates
Chewable	

This process can be used to separate incompatible materials, to produce repeat-action or prolonged-action products, or to produce tablets with a multilayered appearance.

(3) **Repeat-action tablets** are layered or compression-coated tablets in which the outer layer or shell rapidly disintegrates in the stomach (e.g., Repetabs, Schering, Extentabs, Wyeth). The components of the inner layer or inner tablet are insoluble in gastric media but soluble in intestinal media.

(4) **Delayed-action** and **enteric-coated tablets** delay the release of a drug from a dosage form. This delay is intended to prevent destruction of the drug by gastric juices, to prevent irritation of the stomach lining by the drug, or to promote absorption, which is better in the intestine than in the stomach.
   (a) **Enteric-coated** tablets are coated and remain intact in the stomach, but yield their ingredients in the intestines (e.g., Ecotrin, GlaxoSmithKline). Enteric-coated tablets are a form of delayed-action tablet. However, not all delayed-action tablets are enteric or are intended to produce an enteric effect.
   (b) Agents used to coat these tablets include fats, fatty acids, waxes, shellac, and cellulose acetate phthalate.

(5) **Sugar-coated** and **chocolate-coated tablets** are compressed tablets that are coated for various reasons. The coating may be added to protect the drug from air and humidity, to provide a barrier to a drug's objectionable taste or smell, or to improve the appearance of the tablet.
   (a) Tablets may be coated with a colored or an uncolored sugar. The process includes **seal coating** (waterproofing), **subcoating**, **syrup coating** (for smoothing and coloring), and **polishing**. These steps take place in a series of mechanically operated coating pans.
   (b) **Disadvantages** of sugar-coated tablets include the time and expertise required for the process and the increase in tablet size and weight. Sugar-coated tablets may be 50% larger and heavier than the original tablets.
   (c) Chocolate-coated tablets are rare today.

(6) **Film-coated tablets** are compressed tablets that are coated with a thin layer of a water-insoluble or water-soluble polymer (e.g., hydroxypropyl methylcellulose [hypromellose], ethylcellulose, povidone, PEG).
   (a) The film is usually colored. It is more durable, less bulky, and less time consuming to apply than sugar coating. Although the film typically increases tablet weight by only 2% to 3%, it increases formulation efficiency, resistance to chipping, and output.
   (b) Film-coating solutions usually contain a film former, an alloying substance, a plasticizer, a surfactant, opacifiers, sweeteners, flavors, colors, glossants, and a volatile solvent.
   (c) The volatile solvents used in these solutions are expensive and potentially toxic when released into the atmosphere. Specifically formulated **aqueous dispersions** of

polymers (e.g., ethylcellulose) are now available as alternatives to organic solvent-based coating solutions.

(7) **Air suspension–coated tablets** are fed into a vertical cylinder and supported by a column of air that enters from the bottom of the cylinder. As the coating solution enters the system, it is rapidly applied to the suspended, rotating solids (**Wurster process**). Rounding coats can be applied in < 1 hr when blasts of warm air are released in the chamber.

(8) **Chewable tablets** disintegrate smoothly and rapidly when chewed or allowed to dissolve in the mouth. These tablets contain specially colored and flavored mannitol and yield a creamy base.

(a) Chewable tablets are especially useful in formulations for children.

(b) They are commonly used for multivitamin tablets and are used for some antacids and antibiotics.

b. Tablets used in the oral cavity are allowed to dissolve in the mouth.

(1) **Buccal** and **sublingual** tablets allow absorption through the oral mucosa after they dissolve in the buccal pouch (buccal tablets) or below the tongue (sublingual tablets). These forms are useful for drugs that are destroyed by gastric juice or poorly absorbed from the intestinal tract. Examples include sublingual nitroglycerin tablets, which dissolve promptly to give rapid drug effects, and buccal progesterone tablets, which dissolve slowly.

(2) **Troches**, **lozenges**, and **dental cones** dissolve slowly in the mouth and provide primarily local effects.

c. Tablets used to prepare solutions are dissolved in water before administration.

(1) **Effervescent tablets** are prepared by compressing granular effervescent salts or other materials (e.g., citric acid, tartaric acid, sodium bicarbonate) that release carbon dioxide gas when they come into contact with water. Commercial alkalinizing analgesic tablets are often made to effervesce to encourage rapid dissolution and absorption (e.g., Alka-Seltzer, Bayer).

(2) Other tablets used to prepare solutions include **dispensing tablets**, **hypodermic tablets**, and **tablet triturates**.

4. Processing problems

a. **Capping** is the partial or complete separation of the top or bottom crown from the main body of the tablet. **Lamination** is separation of a tablet into two or more distinct layers. These problems are usually caused by entrapment of air during processing.

b. **Picking** is removal of the surface material of a tablet by a punch. Sticking is adhesion of tablet material to a die wall. These problems are caused by excessive moisture or the inclusion of substances with low melting temperatures in the formulation.

c. **Mottling** is unequal color distribution, with light or dark areas standing out on an otherwise uniform surface. This problem occurs when a drug has a different color than the tablet excipients or when a drug has colored degradation products. Colorants solve the problem but can create other problems.

5. Tablet evaluation and control

a. The general appearance of tablets is an important factor in consumer acceptance. It also allows monitoring of lot-to-lot uniformity, tablet-to-tablet uniformity, and elements of the manufacturing process. The appearance of the tablet includes visual identity and overall appearance. The appearance of the tablet is controlled by measurement of attributes such as size, shape, color, odor, taste, surface, texture, physical flaws, consistency, and legibility of markings.

b. Hardness and resistance to friability are necessary for tablets to withstand the mechanical shocks of manufacture, packaging, and shipping, and to ensure consumer acceptance. Hardness involves both tablet disintegration and drug dissolution. Certain tablets that are intended to dissolve slowly are made hard. Other tablets that are intended to dissolve rapidly are made soft. Friability is the tendency of the tablet to crumble.

(1) Tablet hardness testers measure the degree of force required to break a tablet.

(2) **Friabilators** determine **friability** by allowing the tablet to roll and fall within a rotating tumbling apparatus. The tablets are weighed before and after a specified number of rotations, and the weight loss is determined.

(a) Resistance to weight loss indicates the ability of the tablet to withstand abrasion during handling, packaging, and shipping. Compressed tablets that lose $< 0.5\%$ to 1% of their weight are usually considered acceptable.

(b) Some chewable tablets and most effervescent tablets are highly friable and require special unit packaging.

c. Tablets are routinely weighed to ensure that they contain the proper amount of drug.
(1) The *USP* defines a **weight variation standard** to which tablets must conform.
(2) These standards apply to tablets that contain 50 mg or more of drug substance when the drug substance is 50% or more (by weight) of the dosage form unit.

d. **Content uniformity** is evaluated to ensure that each tablet contains the desired amount of drug substance, with little variation among contents within a batch. The *USP* defines content uniformity tests for tablets that contain 50 mg or less of drug substance.

e. **Disintegration** is evaluated to ensure that the drug substance is fully available for dissolution and absorption from the gastrointestinal tract.
(1) All *USP* tablets must pass an official **disintegration test** that is conducted in vitro with special equipment.
(a) Disintegration times for uncoated *USP* tablets are as low as 2 mins (nitroglycerin) to 5 mins (aspirin). Most have a maximum disintegration time of less than 30 mins.
(b) Buccal tablets must disintegrate within 4 hrs.
(c) Enteric-coated tablets must show no evidence of disintegration after 1 hr in simulated gastric fluid. In simulated intestinal fluid, they should disintegrate in 2 hrs plus the time specified.
(2) **Dissolution requirements** in the *USP* have replaced earlier disintegration requirements for many drugs.

f. Dissolution characteristics are tested to determine drug absorption and physiologic availability.
(1) The *USP* gives standards for tablet dissolution.
(2) An increased emphasis on testing tablet dissolution and determining drug bioavailability has increased the use of sophisticated testing systems.

J. **Aerosol products**

1. Introduction. Aerosol products, or **aerosols**, are **pressurized dosage forms**. They are designed to deliver drug systemically or topically with the aid of a liquefied or propelled gas (propellant). Aerosol products consist of a pressurizable container (tin-plated steel, aluminum, glass, or plastic), a valve that allows the pressurized product to be expelled from the container (either continuously or intermittently) when the actuator is pressed, and a dip tube that conveys the formulation from the bottom of the container to the valve assembly. Aerosols are prepared by special methods (cold filling, pressure filling) because of the gaseous components.

2. Systemic or pulmonary drug delivery is provided by aerosol drug delivery systems, or **metered dose inhalers (MDIs)**. These devices allow a drug to be inhaled as a fine mist of drug or drug-containing particles. MDIs use special metering valves to regulate the amount of formulation and drug that is dispensed with each dose (i.e., each actuation of the container). Aerosol products are used for topical drug delivery. The formulations range from solutions to dispersions. Metering valves may also be used with topical aerosol products to regulate the amount of drug applied per application.

3. **Propellants** used in aerosol products

a. **Compressed gases** include carbon dioxide, nitrogen, and nitrous oxide. Aerosol products that contain compressed gas tend to lose pressure over time as the product is dispensed. The drop in pressure reflects the expansion of the head space in the container (i.e., increase in the volume that the gas can occupy) as formulation is withdrawn for use. For this reason, higher initial pressures are typically used with compressed gas-based systems than with liquefiable gas-based formulations.

b. **Liquefiable gases** include saturated hydrocarbons (n-butane, isobutane, propane); chlorofluorocarbons (CFCs), including tetrafluorodichloroethane (propellant 114), dichlorodifluoromethane (propellant 12), and trichlorofluoromethane (propellant 11); dimethyl ether; and hydrofluorocarbons, such as 1,1,1,2-fluoroethane (propellant 134a) and 1,1-difluoroethane (propellant 152a). The negative effect of older CFCs on atmospheric ozone and the potential for global warming led to the worldwide reduction in CFC production under the Montreal Protocol. This plan called for a general ban on CFC production in industrialized countries by January 1996. As a result, the use of CFCs in pharmaceutical products is being phased out. Temporary exemptions for CFCs in MDIs will eventually lapse (in 2008) as stable, safe, and effective alternative formulations are developed with more acceptable propellants (e.g., hydrofluorocarbons).

4. Advantages of aerosol products include the convenience of push-button dispensing of medication and the stability afforded by a closed, pressurized container that minimizes the likelihood of tampering and protects the contents from light, moisture, air (oxygen), and microbial contamination. Aerosol formulations and packaging components (valves, actuators) permit a wide range of products to be dispensed as sprays, foams, or semisolids.
5. The principal disadvantage of aerosol products is environmental (e.g., disposal of pressurized packages, venting of propellants to the atmosphere).

K. Controlled-release dosage forms

1. Introduction. Controlled-release dosage forms are also known as delayed-release, sustained-action, prolonged-action, sustained-release, prolonged-release, timed-release, slow-release, extended-action, and extended-release forms. They are designed to release drug substance slowly to provide prolonged action in the body.
2. Advantages of controlled-release forms:
   - a. Fewer problems with patient compliance
   - b. Use of less total drug
   - c. Fewer local or systemic side effects
   - d. Minimal drug accumulation with long-term dosage
   - e. Fewer problems with potentiation or loss of drug activity with long-term use
   - f. Improved treatment efficiency
   - g. More rapid control of the patient's condition
   - h. Less fluctuation in drug level
   - i. Improved bioavailability for some drugs
   - j. Improved ability to provide special effects (e.g., morning relief of arthritis by bedtime dose)
   - k. Reduced cost
3. Sustained-release forms can be grouped according to their pharmaceutical mechanism.
   - a. **Coated beads** or **granules** (e.g., Spansules, GlaxoSmithKline, Sequels, Wyeth) produce a blood level profile similar to that obtained with multiple dosing.
     - (1) A solution of the drug substance in a nonaqueous solvent (e.g., alcohol) is coated on small, inert beads, or granules, made of a combination of sugar and starch. When the drug dose is large, the starting granules may be composed of the drug itself.
     - (2) Some of the granules are left uncoated to provide immediate release of the drug.
     - (3) Coats of a lipid material (e.g., beeswax) or a cellulosic material (e.g., ethylcellulose) are applied to the remaining granules. Some granules receive few coats, and some receive many. The various coating thicknesses produce a sustained-release effect.
   - b. **Microencapsulation** is a process by which solids, liquids, or gases are encased in microscopic capsules. Thin coatings of a "wall" material are formed around the substance to be encapsulated.
     - (1) **Coacervation** is the most common method of microencapsulation. It occurs when a hydrophilic substance is added to colloidal drug dispersion and causes layering and the formation of microcapsules.
     - (2) Film-forming substances that are used as the coating material include a variety of natural and synthetic polymers. These materials include shellacs, waxes, gelatin, starches, cellulose acetate phthalate, and ethylcellulose. After the coating material dissolves, all of the drug inside the microcapsule is immediately available for dissolution and absorption. The thickness of the wall can vary from 1 to 200 mm, depending on the amount of coating material used (3% to 30% of total weight).
   - c. **Matrix tablets** use insoluble plastics (e.g., polyethylene, polyvinyl acetate, polymethacrylate), hydrophilic polymers (e.g., methylcellulose, hydroxypropyl methylcellulose), or fatty compounds (e.g., various waxes, glyceryl tristearate). Examples include Gradumet (Abbott) and Dospan (Aventis).
     - (1) The most common method of preparation is mixing of the drug with the matrix material followed by compression of the material into tablets.
     - (2) The primary dose, or the portion of the drug to be released immediately, is placed on the tablet as a layer, or coat. The rest of the dose is released slowly from the matrix.

d. **Osmotic systems** include the Oros system (Alza), which is an oral osmotic pump composed of a core tablet and a semipermeable coating that has a small hole (0.4 mm in diameter) for drug exit. The hole is produced by a laser beam. Examples include Glucotrol XL (glipizide extended-release tablets, Pfizer) and Procardia XL (nifedipine extended-release tablets, Pfizer).
   (1) This system requires only osmotic pressure to be effective. It is essentially independent of pH changes in the environment.
   (2) The drug-release rate can be changed by changing the tablet surface area, the nature of the membrane, or the diameter of the drug-release aperture.

e. **Ion-exchange resins** can be complexed with drugs by passage of a cationic drug solution through a column that contains the resin. The drug is complexed to the resin by replacement of hydrogen atoms. Examples include Ionamin capsules (Celltech; resin complexes of phentermine) and the Pennkinetic system (Celltech), which incorporates a polymer barrier coating and bead technology in addition to the ion-exchange mechanism.
   (1) After the components are complexed, the resin–drug complex is washed and tableted, encapsulated, or suspended in an aqueous vehicle.
   (2) Release of drug from the complex depends on the ionic environment within the gastrointestinal tract and on the properties of the resin. Usually, release is greater in the highly acidic stomach than in the less acidic small intestine.

f. **Complex formation** is used for certain drug substances that combine chemically with other agents. For example, hydroxypropyl-β-cyclodextrin forms a chemical complex that can be only slowly soluble from body fluids, depending on the pH of the environment. Tannic acid (i.e., tannates) complexes with the amino groups of weak bases dissolve at a slow rate in the gastrointestinal tract, thereby providing for a prolonged release of drug. Examples of the latter include brompheniramine tannate (Brovex, Athlon) and chlorpheniramine/phenylephrine tannates (Rynatan, Wallace).

Study Questions

Directions for questions 1–28: Each of the questions, statements, or incomplete statements in this section can be correctly answered or completed by one of the suggested answers or phrases. Choose the best answer.

1. Which substance is classified as a weak electrolyte?
   (A) glucose
   (B) urea
   (C) ephedrine
   (D) sodium chloride
   (E) sucrose

2. The pH value is calculated mathematically as the
   (A) log of the hydroxyl ion (OH^-) concentration.
   (B) negative log of the OH^- concentration.
   (C) log of the hydrogen ion (H^+) concentration.
   (D) negative log of the H^+ concentration.
   (E) ratio of H^+/OH^- concentration.

3. Which property is classified as colligative?
   (A) solubility of a solute
   (B) osmotic pressure
   (C) hydrogen ion (H^+) concentration
   (D) dissociation of a solute
   (E) miscibility of the liquids

4. The colligative properties of a solution are related to the
   (A) pH of the solution.
   (B) number of ions in the solution.
   (C) total number of solute particles in the solution.
   (D) number of un-ionized molecules in the solution.
   (E) pK_a of the solution.

5. The pH of a buffer system can be calculated with the
   (A) Noyes–Whitney equation.
   (B) Henderson–Hasselbalch equation.
   (C) Michaelis–Menten equation.
   (D) Young equation.
   (E) Stokes equation.

6. Which mechanism is most often responsible for chemical degradation?
(A) racemization
(B) photolysis
(C) hydrolysis
(D) decarboxylation
(E) oxidation

7. Which equation is used to predict the stability of a drug product at room temperature from experiments at accelerated temperatures?
(A) Stokes equation
(B) Young equation
(C) Arrhenius equation
(D) Michaelis–Menten equation
(E) Hixson–Crowell equation

8. Based on the relation between the degree of ionization and the solubility of a weak acid, the drug aspirin (pK_a = 3.49) will be most soluble at
(A) pH 1.0.
(B) pH 2.0.
(C) pH 3.0.
(D) pH 4.0.
(E) pH 6.0.

9. Which solution is used as an astringent?
(A) strong iodine solution *USP*
(B) aluminum acetate topical solution *USP*
(C) acetic acid *NF*
(D) aromatic ammonia spirit *USP*
(E) benzalkonium chloride solution *NF*

10. The particle size of the dispersed solid in a suspension is usually greater than
(A) 0.5 μm.
(B) 0.4 μm.
(C) 0.3 μm.
(D) 0.2 μm.
(E) 0.1 μm.

11. In the extemporaneous preparation of a suspension, levigation is used to
(A) reduce the zeta potential.
(B) avoid bacterial growth.
(C) reduce particle size.
(D) enhance viscosity.
(E) reduce viscosity.

12. Which compound is a natural emulsifying agent?
(A) acacia
(B) lactose
(C) polysorbate 20
(D) polysorbate 80
(E) sorbitan monopalmitate

13. Vanishing cream is an ointment that may be classified as
(A) a water-soluble base.
(B) an oleaginous base.
(C) an absorption base.
(D) an emulsion base.
(E) an oleic base.

14. Rectal suppositories intended for adult use usually weigh approximately
(A) 1 g.
(B) 2 g.
(C) 3 g.
(D) 4 g.
(E) 5 g.

15. In the fusion method of making cocoa butter suppositories, which substance is most likely to be used to lubricate the mold?
(A) mineral oil
(B) propylene glycol
(C) cetyl alcohol
(D) stearic acid
(E) magnesium silicate

16. A very fine powdered chemical is defined as one that
(A) completely passes through a #80 sieve.
(B) completely passes through a #120 sieve.
(C) completely passes through a #20 sieve.
(D) passes through a #60 sieve and not more than 40% through a #100 sieve.
(E) passes through a #40 sieve and not more than 60% through a #60 sieve.

17. Which technique is typically used to mill camphor?
(A) trituration
(B) levigation
(C) pulverization by intervention
(D) geometric dilution
(E) attrition

18. The dispensing pharmacist usually blends potent powders with a large amount of diluent by
(A) spatulation.
(B) sifting.
(C) trituration.
(D) geometric dilution.
(E) levigation.

19. Which type of paper best protects a divided hygroscopic powder?
(A) waxed paper
(B) glassine
(C) white bond
(D) blue bond
(E) vegetable parchment

20. Which capsule size has the smallest capacity?

(A) 5
(B) 4
(C) 1
(D) 0
(E) 000

21. The shells of soft gelatin capsules may be made elastic or plastic-like by the addition of

(A) sorbitol.
(B) povidone.
(C) polyethylene glycol (PEG).
(D) lactose.
(E) hydroxypropyl methylcellulose.

22. The *United States Pharmacopeia* (*USP*) content uniformity test for tablets is used to ensure which quality?

(A) bioequivalency
(B) dissolution
(C) potency
(D) purity
(E) toxicity

23. All of the following statements about chemical degradation are true *except*

(A) as temperature increases, degradation decreases.
(B) most drugs degrade by a first-order process.
(C) chemical degradation may produce a toxic product.
(D) chemical degradation may result in a loss of active ingredients.
(E) chemical degradation may affect the therapeutic activity of a drug.

24. All of the following statements concerning zero-order degradation are true *except*

(A) its rate is independent of the concentration.
(B) a plot of concentration versus time yields a straight line on rectilinear paper.
(C) its half-life is a changing parameter.
(D) its concentration remains unchanged with respect to time.
(E) the slope of a plot of concentration versus time yields a rate constant.

25. All of the following statements about first-order degradation are true *except*

(A) its rate is dependent on the concentration.
(B) its half-life is a changing parameter.
(C) a plot of the logarithm of concentration versus time yields a straight line.
(D) its $t_{90\%}$ is independent of the concentration.
(E) a plot of the logarithm of concentration versus time allows the rate constant to be determined.

26. A satisfactory suppository base must meet all of the following criteria *except*

(A) it should have a narrow melting range.
(B) it should be nonirritating and nonsensitizing.
(C) it should dissolve or disintegrate rapidly in the body cavity.
(D) it should melt $< 30°C$.
(E) it should be inert.

27. Cocoa butter (theobroma oil) exhibits all of the following properties *except*

(A) it melts at temperatures between 33°C and 35°C.
(B) it is a mixture of glycerides.
(C) it is a polymorph.
(D) it is useful in formulating rectal suppositories.
(E) it is soluble in water.

28. *United States Pharmacopeia* (*USP*) tests to ensure the quality of drug products in tablet form include all of the following *except*

(A) disintegration.
(B) dissolution.
(C) hardness and friability.
(D) content uniformity.
(E) weight variation.

Directions for questions 29–42: The questions and incomplete statements in this section can be correctly answered or completed by **one or more** of the suggested answers. Choose the answer, **A–E.**

A if **I only** is correct
B if **III only** is correct
C if **I** and **II** are correct
D if **II** and **III** are correct
E if **I**, **II**, and **III** are correct

29. Forms of water that are suitable for use in parenteral preparations include

I. purified water *USP*.
II. water for injection *USP*.
III. sterile water for injection *USP*.

30. The particles in an ideal suspension should satisfy which of the following criteria?

I. Their size should be uniform.
II. They should be stationary or move randomly.
III. They should remain discrete.

31. The sedimentation of particles in a suspension can be minimized by

I. adding sodium benzoate.
II. increasing the viscosity of the suspension.
III. reducing the particle size of the active ingredient.

32. Ingredients that may be used as suspending agents include

- **I.** methylcellulose.
- **II.** acacia.
- **III.** talc.

33. Mechanisms that are thought to provide stable emulsifications include the

- **I.** formation of interfacial film.
- **II.** lowering of interfacial tension.
- **III.** presence of charge on the ions.

34. Nonionic surface-active agents used as synthetic emulsifiers include

- **I.** tragacanth.
- **II.** sodium lauryl sulfate.
- **III.** sorbitan esters (Spans).

35. Advantages of systemic drug administration by rectal suppositories include

- **I.** avoidance of first-pass effects.
- **II.** suitability when the oral route is not feasible.
- **III.** predictable drug release and absorption.

36. True statements about the milling of powders include

- **I.** a fine particle size is essential if the lubricant is to function properly.
- **II.** an increased surface area may enhance the dissolution rate.
- **III.** milling may cause degradation of thermolabile drugs.

37. Substances used to insulate powder components that liquefy when mixed include

- **I.** talc.
- **II.** kaolin.
- **III.** light magnesium oxide.

38. A ceramic mortar may be preferable to a glass mortar when

- **I.** a volatile oil is added to a powder mixture.
- **II.** colored substances (dyes) are mixed into a powder.
- **III.** comminution is desired in addition to mixing.

39. Divided powders may be dispensed in

- **I.** individual-dose packets.
- **II.** a bulk container.
- **III.** a perforated, sifter-type container.

40. True statements about the function of excipients used in tablet formulations include

- **I.** binders promote granulation during the wet granulation process.
- **II.** glidants help promote the flow of the tablet granulation during manufacture.
- **III.** lubricants help the patient swallow the tablets.

41. Which manufacturing variables would be likely to affect the dissolution of a prednisone tablet in the body?

- **I.** the amount and type of binder added
- **II.** the amount and type of disintegrant added
- **III.** the force of compression used during tableting

42. Agents that may be used to coat enteric-coated tablets include

- **I.** hydroxypropyl methylcellulose.
- **II.** carboxymethylcellulose.
- **III.** cellulose acetate phthalate.

Directions for questions 43–46: Each of the following tablet-processing problems can be the result of one of the following reasons. The processing problems may be used more than once or not at all. Choose the **best** answer, **A–E**.

- **A** excessive moisture in the granulation
- **B** entrapment of air
- **C** tablet friability
- **D** degraded drug
- **E** tablet hardness

43. Picking

44. Mottling

45. Capping

46. Sticking

Directions for questions 47–49: Each of the following processes can be described by one of the following comminution procedures. The processes may be used more than once or not at all. Choose the **best** answer, **A–E**.

- **A** trituration
- **B** spatulation
- **C** levigation
- **D** pulverization by intervention
- **E** tumbling

47. Rubbing or grinding a substance in a mortar that has a rough inner surface

48. Reducing and subdividing a substance by adding an easily removed solvent

49. Adding a suitable agent to form a paste and then rubbing or grinding the paste in a mortar

Directions for questions 50–53: Each of the following controlled-release dosage forms is represented by one of the following drug products. The dosage forms may be used more than once or not at all. Choose the **best** answer, **A–E**.

A matrix formulations
B ion-exchange resin complex
C drug complexes
D osmotic system
E coated beads or granules

50. Ionamin capsules

51. Thorazine Spansule capsules

52. Rynatan pediatric suspension

53. Procardia XL

Answers and Explanations

1. The answer is C *[see IV.A.1.a; IV.A.3.d].*
Glucose, urea, and sucrose are nonelectrolytes. Sodium chloride is a strong electrolyte. Electrolytes are substances that form ions when dissolved in water. Thus, they can conduct an electric current through the solution. Ions are particles that bear electrical charges: Cations are positively charged, and anions are negatively charged. Strong electrolytes are completely ionized in water at all concentrations. Weak electrolytes (e.g., ephedrine) are only partially ionized at most concentrations. Because nonelectrolytes do not form ions when in solution, they are nonconductors.

2. The answer is D *[see IV.A.3.b].*
The pH is a measure of the acidity, or hydrogen ion concentration, of an aqueous solution. The pH is the logarithm of the reciprocal of the hydrogen ion (H^+) concentration expressed in moles per liter. Because the logarithm of a reciprocal equals the negative logarithm of the number, the pH is the negative logarithm of the H^+ concentration. A pH of 7.0 indicates neutrality. As the pH decreases, the acidity increases. The pH of arterial blood is 7.35 to 7.45; of urine, 4.8 to 7.5; of gastric juice, approximately 1.4; and of cerebrospinal fluid, 7.35 to 7.40. The concept of pH was introduced by Sörensen in the early 1900s. Alkalinity is the negative logarithm of $[OH^-]$ and is inversely related to acidity.

3. The answer is B *[see IV.A.2.d].*
Osmotic pressure is an example of a colligative property. The osmotic pressure is the magnitude of pressure needed to stop osmosis across a semipermeable membrane between a solution and a pure solvent. The colligative properties of a solution depend on the total number of dissociated and undissociated solute particles. These properties are independent of the size of the solute. Other colligative properties of solutes are reduction in the vapor pressure of the solution, elevation of its boiling point, and depression of its freezing point.

4. The answer is C *[see IV.A.1.b].*
The colligative properties of a solution are related to the total number of solute particles that it contains. Examples of colligative properties are the osmotic pressure, lowering of the vapor pressure, elevation of the boiling point, and depression of the freezing or melting point.

5. The answer is B *[see IV.A.3.e].*
The Henderson–Hasselbalch equation for a weak acid and its salt is as follows:

$$pH = pK_a + \log \frac{[salt]}{[acid]}$$

where pK_a is the negative log of the dissociation constant of a weak acid and [salt]/[acid] is the ratio of the molar concentration of salt and acid used to prepare a buffer.

6. The answer is C *[see V.D.1].*
Although all of the mechanisms listed can be responsible, the chemical degradation of medicinal compounds, particularly esters in liquid formulations, is usually caused by hydrolysis. For this reason, drugs that have ester functional groups are formulated in dry form whenever possible. Oxidation is another common mode of degradation and is minimized by including antioxidants (e.g., ascorbic acid) in drug formulations. Photolysis is reduced by packaging susceptible products in amber or opaque containers. Decarboxylation, which is the removal of COOH groups, affects compounds that include carboxylic acid. Racemization neutralizes the effects of an optically active compound by converting half of its molecules into their mirror-image configuration. As a result, the dextrorotatory and levorotatory forms cancel each other out. This type of degradation affects only drugs that are characterized by optical isomerism.

7. **The answer is C** *[see V.E.3.d].*
Testing of a drug formulation to determine its shelf life can be accelerated by applying the Arrhenius equation to data obtained at higher temperatures. The method involves determining the rate constant (k) values for the degradation of a drug at various elevated temperatures. The log of k is plotted against the reciprocal of the absolute temperature, and the k value for degradation at room temperature is obtained by extrapolation.

8. **The answer is E** *[see IV.A.3.g].*
The solubility of a weak acid varies as a function of pH. Because pH and pK_a (the dissociation constant) are related, solubility is also related to the degree of ionization. Aspirin is a weak acid that is completely ionized at a pH that is two units greater than its pK_a. Therefore, it is most soluble at pH 6.0.

9. **The answer is B** *[see VI.B.7].*
Aluminum acetate and aluminum subacetate solutions are astringents that are used as antiperspirants and as wet dressings for contact dermatitis. Strong iodine solution and benzalkonium chloride are topical antibacterial solutions. Acetic acid is added to products as an acidifier. Aromatic ammonia spirit is a respiratory stimulant.

10. **The answer is A** *[see IV.B.1.a].*
A suspension is a two-phase system that consists of a finely powdered solid dispersed in a liquid vehicle. The particle size of the suspended solid should be as small as possible to minimize sedimentation, but it is usually $> 0.5\ \mu m$.

11. **The answer is C** *[see VI.E.3.a].*
Levigation is the process of blending and grinding a substance to separate the particles, reduce their size, and form a paste. Levigation is performed by adding a small amount of suitable levigating agent (e.g., glycerin) to the solid and blending the mixture with a mortar and pestle.

12. **The answer is A** *[see VI.D.3].*
Acacia, or gum arabic, is the exudate obtained from the stems and branches of various species of *Acacia*, a woody plant native to Africa. Acacia is a natural emulsifying agent that provides a stable emulsion of low viscosity. Emulsions are droplets of one or more immiscible liquids dispersed in another liquid. Emulsions are inherently unstable: The droplets tend to coalesce into larger and larger drops. The purpose of an emulsifying agent is to keep the droplets dispersed and prevent them from coalescing. Polysorbate 20, polysorbate 80, and sorbitan monopalmitate are also emulsifiers, but are synthetic, not natural, substances.

13. **The answer is D** *[see VI.E.2].*
Ointments are typically used as emollients to soften the skin, as protective barriers, or as vehicles for medication. A variety of ointment bases are available. Vanishing cream, an emulsion type of ointment base, is an oil-in-water emulsion that contains a high percentage of water. Stearic acid is used to create a thin film on the skin when the water evaporates.

14. **The answer is B** *[see VI.F.2.a].*
By convention, a rectal suppository for an adult weighs approximately 2 g. Suppositories for infants and children are smaller. Vaginal suppositories typically weigh approximately 5 g. Rectal suppositories are usually shaped like an elongated bullet (cylindrical and tapered at one end). Vaginal suppositories are usually ovoid.

15. **The answer is A** *[see VI.F.4.c].*
In the fusion method of making suppositories, molds made of aluminum, brass, or nickel–copper alloys are used. Finely powdered drug mixed with melted cocoa butter is poured into a mold that is lubricated very lightly with mineral oil.

16. **The answer is B** *[see VI.G; Table 2-8].*
The *USP* defines a very fine chemical powder as one that completely passes through a standard #120 sieve, which has 125-μm openings. The *USP* classification for powdered vegetable and animal drugs differs from that for powdered chemicals. To be classified as very fine, powdered vegetable and animal drugs must pass completely through a #80 sieve, which has 180-μm openings.

17. **The answer is C** *[see VI.G.1.c.(3.(b)].*
Pulverization by intervention is the milling technique that is used for drug substances that are gummy and tend to reagglomerate or resist grinding (e.g., camphor, iodine). In this sense, intervention is the addition of a small amount of material that aids milling and can be removed easily after pulverization is complete. For example, camphor can be reduced readily if a small amount of volatile solvent (e.g., alcohol) is added. The solvent is then allowed to evaporate.

18. **The answer is D** *[see VI.G.2.c].*
The pharmacist uses geometric dilution to mix potent substances with a large amount of diluent. The potent drug and an equal amount of diluent are first mixed in a mortar by trituration. A volume of diluent equal to the mixture in the mortar is added, and the mix is again triturated. The procedure is repeated, and each time, diluent equal in volume to the mixture then in the mortar is added, until all of the diluent is incorporated.

19. The answer is A *[see VI.G.3.b.(4)].*
Hygroscopic and volatile drugs are best protected by waxed paper, which is waterproof. The packet may be double-wrapped with a bond paper to improve the appearance of the completed powder.

20. The answer is A *[see VI.H.2.c.(1)].*
Hard capsules are numbered from 000 (largest) to 5 (smallest). Their approximate capacity ranges from 600 to 30 mg; however, the capacity of the capsule depends on the density of the contents.

21. The answer is A *[see VI.H.3.a–b].*
The shells of soft gelatin capsules are plasticized by the addition of a polyhydric alcohol (polyol), such as glycerin or sorbitol. An antifungal preservative can also be added. Both hard and soft gelatin capsules can be filled with a powder or another dry substance. Soft gelatin capsules are also useful dosage forms for fluids or semisolids.

22. The answer is C *[see VI.H.4.a].*
A content uniformity test is a test of potency. To ensure that each tablet or capsule contains the intended amount of drug substance, the *USP* provides two tests: weight variation and content uniformity. The content uniformity test can be used for any dosage unit but is required for coated tablets, for tablets in which the active ingredient makes up < 50% of the tablet, for suspensions in single-unit containers or in soft capsules, and for many solids that contain added substances. The weight variation test can be used for liquid-filled soft capsules, for any dosage form unit that contains at least 50 mg of a single drug if the drug makes up at least 50% of the bulk, for solids that do not contain added substances, and for freeze-dried solutions.

23. The answer is A *[see V.A and V.B].*
The reaction velocity, or degradation rate, of a pharmaceutical product is affected by several factors, including temperature, solvents, and light. The degradation rate increases two to three times with each 10°C increase in temperature. The effect of temperature on reaction rate is given by the Arrhenius equation:

$$k = Ae^{-Ea/RT}$$

where k is the reaction rate constant, A is the frequency factor, Ea is the energy of activation, R is the gas constant, and T is the absolute temperature.

24. The answer is D *[see V.B.2.a].*
In zero-order degradation, the concentration of a drug decreases over time. However, the change of concentration with respect to time is unchanged. In the equation

$$-\frac{dC}{dt} = k$$

the fact that dC/dt is negative signifies that the concentration is decreasing. However, the velocity of the concentration change is constant.

25. The answer is B *[see V.B.2.b.(2)].*
The half-life ($t_{1/2}$) is the time required for the concentration of a drug to decrease by one-half. For a first-order degradation:

$$t_{1/2} = \frac{0.693}{k}$$

Because both k and 0.693 are constants, $t_{1/2}$ is a constant.

26. The answer is D *[see VI.F.3].*
A satisfactory suppository base should remain firm at room temperature. Preferably, it should not melt < 30°C to avoid premature softening during storage and insertion. It should also be inert, nonsensitizing, nonirritating, and compatible with a variety of drugs. Moreover, it should melt just below body temperature and should dissolve or disintegrate rapidly in the fluid of the body cavity into which it is inserted.

27. The answer is E *[see VI.F.3.c.(1)].*
Cocoa butter is a fat that is obtained from the seed of *Theobroma cacao*. Chemically, it is a mixture of stearin, palmitin, and other glycerides that are insoluble in water and freely soluble in ether and chloroform. Depending on the fusion temperature, cocoa butter can crystallize into any one of four crystal forms. Cocoa butter is a good base for rectal suppositories, although it is less than ideal for vaginal or urethral suppositories.

28. The answer is C *[see VI.I.5].*
To satisfy the *USP* standards, tablets are required to pass one of two tests. A weight variation test is used if the active ingredient makes up the bulk of the tablet. A content uniformity test is used if the tablet is coated or if the active ingredient makes up < 50% of the bulk of the tablet. Many tablets for oral administration are required to meet a disintegration test. Disintegration times are specified in the individual monographs. A dissolution test may be required instead if the active component of the tablet has limited water solubility. Hardness and friability would affect the disintegration and dissolution rates, but hardness and friability tests are in-house quality control tests, not official *USP* tests.

29. **The answer is D (II, III)** *[see VI.A.1].*
Water for injection *USP* is water that has been purified by distillation or by reverse osmosis. This water is used to prepare parenteral solutions that are subject to final sterilization. For parenteral solutions that are prepared aseptically and not subsequently sterilized, sterile water for injection *USP* is used. Sterile water for injection *USP* is water for injection *USP* that has been sterilized and suitably packaged. This water meets the *USP* requirements for sterility. Bacteriostatic water for injection *USP* is sterile water for injection *USP* that contains one or more antimicrobial agents. It can be used in parenteral solutions if the antimicrobial additives are compatible with the other ingredients in the solution, but it cannot be used in newborns. Purified water *USP* is not used in parenteral preparations.

30. **The answer is E (I, II, III)** *[see IV.B.2].*
An ideal suspension would have particles of uniform size, minimal sedimentation, and no interaction between particles. Although these ideal criteria are rarely met, they can be approximated by keeping the particle size as small as possible, the densities of the solid and the dispersion medium as similar as possible, and the dispersion medium as viscous as possible.

31. **The answer is D (II, III)** *[see IV.B.2].*
As Stokes's law indicates, the sedimentation rate of a suspension is slowed by reducing its density, reducing the size of the suspended particles, or increasing its viscosity by incorporating a thickening agent. Sodium benzoate is an antifungal agent and would not reduce the sedimentation rate of a suspension.

32. **The answer is C (I, II)** *[see VI.C.3].*
Acacia and methylcellulose are common suspending agents. Acacia is a natural product, and methylcellulose is a synthetic polymer. By increasing the viscosity of the liquid, these agents enable particles to remain suspended for a longer period.

33. **The answer is E (I, II, III)** *[see VI.D.3].*
Emulsifying agents provide a mechanical barrier to coalescence. They also reduce the natural tendency of the droplets in the internal phase (oil or water) of the emulsion to coalesce. Three mechanisms appear to be involved. Some emulsifiers promote stability by forming strong, pliable interfacial films around the droplets. Emulsifying agents also reduce interfacial tension. Finally, ions (from the emulsifier) in the interfacial film can lead to charge repulsion that causes droplets to repel one another, thereby preventing coalescence.

34. **The answer is B (III)** *[see VI.D.3].*
All of the substances listed are emulsifying agents, but only sorbitan esters are nonionic synthetic agents. Tragacanth, like acacia, is a natural emulsifying agent. Sodium lauryl sulfate is an anionic surfactant. Sorbitan esters (known colloquially as Spans because of their trade names) are hydrophobic and form water-in-oil emulsions. The polysorbates (known colloquially as Tweens) are also nonionic, synthetic sorbitan derivatives. However, they are hydrophilic and therefore form oil-in-water emulsions. Sodium lauryl sulfate, as alkali soap, is also hydrophilic and thus forms oil-in-water emulsions.

35. **The answer is C (I, II)** *[see VI.F.1–2].*
Rectal suppositories are useful for delivering systemic medication under certain circumstances. Absorption of a drug from a rectal suppository involves release of the drug from the suppository vehicle, diffusion through the rectal mucosa, and transport to the circulation through the rectal veins. The rectal veins bypass the liver, so this route avoids rapid hepatic degradation of certain drugs (first-pass effect). The rectal route is also useful when a drug cannot be given orally (e.g., because of vomiting). However, the extent of drug release and absorption is variable. It depends on the properties of the drug, the suppository base, and the environment in the rectum.

36. **The answer is E (I, II, III)** *[see VI.G.1.c].*
Milling is the process of mechanically reducing the particle size of solids before they are formulated into a final product. To work effectively, a lubricant must coat the surface of the granulation or powder. Hence, fine particle size is essential. Decreasing the particle size increases the surface area and can enhance the dissolution rate. Thermolabile drugs may undergo degradation because of the buildup of heat during milling.

37. **The answer is D (II, III)** *[see VI.G.2.a.(2)].*
Some solid substances (e.g., aspirin, phenylsalicylate, phenacetin, thymol, camphor) liquefy or form eutectic mixtures when in close, prolonged contact with one another. These substances are best insulated by the addition of light magnesium oxide or magnesium carbonate. Other inert diluents that can be used are kaolin, starch, and bentonite.

38. **The answer is B (III)** *[see VI.G.2.b].*
When powders are mixed, if comminution is especially important, a porcelain or ceramic mortar that has a rough inner surface is preferred over the smooth working surface of a glass mortar. Because a glass mortar cleans more easily after use, it is preferred for chemicals that may stain a porcelain or ceramic mortar as well as for simple mixing of substances that do not require comminution.

39. **The answer is A (I)** *[see VI.G.3.a–b].*
Powders for oral use can be dispensed by the pharmacist in bulk form or divided into premeasured doses (divided powders). Divided powders are traditionally dispensed in folded paper packets (chartulae) made of parchment, bond paper, glassine, or waxed paper. However, individual doses can be packaged in metal foil or small plastic bags if the powder needs greater protection from humidity or evaporation.

40. **The answer is C (I, II)** *[see VI.I.2.b].*
Tablets for oral ingestion usually contain excipients that are added to the formulation for their special functions. Binders and adhesives are added to promote granulation or compaction. Diluents are fillers that are added to make up the required tablet bulk. They can also aid in the manufacturing process. Disintegrants aid in tablet disintegration in gastrointestinal fluids. Lubricants, antiadherents, and glidants aid in reducing friction or adhesion between particles or between tablet and die. For example, lubricants are used in the manufacture of tablets to reduce friction when the tablet is ejected from the die cavity. Lubricants are usually hydrophobic substances that can affect the dissolution rate of the active ingredient.

41. **The answer is E (I, II, III)** *[see VI.2.b.(3)].*
Disintegrants are added to tablet formulations to facilitate disintegration in gastrointestinal fluids. Disintegration of the tablet in the body is critical to its dissolution and subsequent absorption and bioavailability. The binder and the compression force used during tablet manufacturing affect the hardness of the tablet as well as tablet disintegration and drug dissolution.

42. **The answer is B (III)** *[see VI.I.3.a.(4)].*
An enteric-coated tablet has a coating that remains intact in the stomach, but dissolves in the intestines to yield the tablet ingredients there. Enteric coatings include various fats, fatty acids, waxes, and shellacs. Cellulose acetate phthalate remains intact in the stomach because it dissolves only when the $pH > 6$. Other enteric-coating materials include povidone (polyvinylpyrrolidone), polyvinyl acetate phthalate, and hydroxypropyl methylcellulose phthalate.

43. **The answer is A** *[see VI.I.4].*

44. **The answer is D** *[see VI.I.4].*

45. **The answer is B** *[see VI.I.4].*

46. **The answer is A** *[see VI.I.4].*
Sticking is adhesion of tablet material to a die wall. It may be caused by excessive moisture or by the use of ingredients that have low melting temperatures. Mottling is uneven color distribution. It is most often caused by poor mixing of the tablet granulation but may also occur when a degraded drug produces a colored metabolite. Capping is separation of the top or bottom crown of a tablet from the main body. Capping implies that compressed powder is not cohesive. Reasons for capping include excessive force of compression, use of insufficient binder, worn tablet tooling equipment, and entrapment of air during processing. Picking is adherence of tablet surface material to a punch. It can be caused by a granulation that is too damp, by a scratched punch, by static charges on the powder, and particularly by the use of a punch tip that is engraved or embossed.

47. **The answer is A** *[see VI.G.1.c; VI.G.2].*

48. **The answer is D** *[see VI.G.1.c; VI.G.2].*

49. **The answer is C** *[see VI.G.1.c; VI.G.2].*
Comminution is the process of reducing the particle size of a powder to increase its fineness. Several comminution techniques are suitable for small-scale use in a pharmacy. Trituration is used both to comminute and to mix dry powders. If comminution is desired, the substance is rubbed in a mortar that has a rough inner surface. Pulverization by intervention is often used for substances that tend to agglomerate or resist grinding. A small amount of easily removed (e.g., volatile) solvent is added. After the substance is pulverized, the solvent is allowed to evaporate or is otherwise removed. Levigation is often used to prepare pastes or ointments. The powder is reduced by adding a suitable nonsolvent (levigating agent) to form a paste and then either rubbing the paste in a mortar with a pestle or rubbing it on an ointment slab with a spatula. Spatulation and tumbling are techniques that are used to mix or blend powders, not to reduce them. Spatulation is blending small amounts of powders by stirring them with a spatula on a sheet of paper or a pill tile. Tumbling is blending large amounts of powder in a large rotating container.

50. **The answer is B** *[see VI.K.3.e].*

51. **The answer is E** *[see VI.K.3.a].*

52. **The answer is C** *[see VI.K.3.f].*

53. **The answer is D** *[see VI.K.3.d].*
Controlled-release dosage forms are designed to release a drug slowly for prolonged action in the body. A variety of pharmaceutical mechanisms are used to provide the controlled release. Ion-exchange resins may be complexed to drugs by passing a cationic drug solution through a column that contains the resin. The drug is complexed to the resin by replacement of hydrogen atoms. Release of drug from the complex depends on the ionic environment within the gastrointestinal tract and on the properties of the resin. Coated beads (e.g., Thorazine Spansule capsules) or granules produce blood levels similar to those obtained with multiple dosing. The various coating thicknesses produce a sustained-release effect.
Matrix devices may use insoluble plastics, hydrophilic polymers, or fatty compounds. These components are mixed with the drug and compressed into a tablet. The primary dose, or the portion of the drug to be released immediately, is placed on the tablet as a layer or coat. The remainder of the dose is released slowly from the matrix. Relatively insoluble tannate–amine complexes provide for a prolonged gastrointestinal absorption phase and sustained systemic concentrations of the weak bases. Osmotic systems employ osmotic pressure to control the release of the active ingredient from the formulation. Osmotic tablet formulations provide a semipermeable membrane as a coating that surrounds the osmotically active core. The coating allows water to diffuse into the core but does not allow drug to diffuse out. As water flows into the tablet, the drug dissolves. The laser-drilled hole in the coating allows the drug solution within the tablet to flow to the outside at a rate that is equivalent to the rate of water flow into the tablet. The osmotic pressure gradient and a zero-order drug-release rate will be maintained as long as excess osmotically active solute (e.g., electrolyte) remains in the tablet core.

Biopharmaceutics and Drug Delivery Systems

3

LAWRENCE H. BLOCK

I. INTRODUCTION

A. Biopharmaceutics is the study of the relation of the physical and chemical properties of a drug to its bioavailability, pharmacokinetics, and pharmacodynamic and toxicologic effects.

1. A **drug product** is the finished dosage form (e.g., tablet, capsule, solution) that contains the active drug ingredient in association with nondrug (usually inactive) ingredients (**excipients**) that make up the **vehicle** or **formulation matrix**.
2. The phrase *drug delivery system* is often used interchangeably with the terms *drug product* or *dosage form*. However, a **drug delivery system** is a more comprehensive concept, which includes the drug formulation and the dynamic interactions among the drug, its formulation matrix, its container, and the patient.
3. **Bioavailability** is a measurement of the rate and extent (amount) of systemic absorption of the therapeutically active drug.

B. Pharmacokinetics is the study of the time course of drug movement in the body during absorption, distribution, and elimination (excretion and biotransformation).

C. Pharmacodynamics is the study of the relation of the drug concentration or amount at the site of action (receptor) and its pharmacologic response as a function of time.

II. DRUG TRANSPORT AND ABSORPTION

A. Transport of drug molecules *across* cell membranes. Drug absorption requires the drug to be transported across various cell membranes. Drug molecules may enter the bloodstream and be transported to the tissues and organs of the body. Drug molecules may cross additional membranes to enter cells. Drug molecules may also cross an intracellular membrane, such as the nuclear membrane or endoplasmic reticulum, to reach the site of action. *Figure 3-1* demonstrates some of the key transport processes involved in drug absorption.

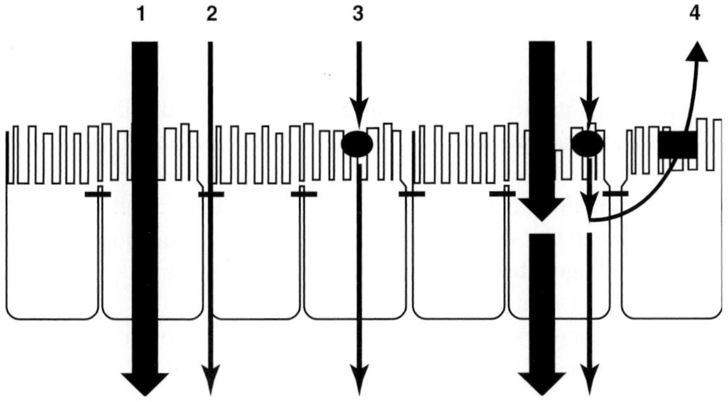

Figure 3-1. The key drug transport processes in intestinal epithelial cells. *1*, Transcellular passive (diffusion and partitioning); *2*, paracellular transport (diffusion and convection); *3*, carrier-mediated transport; *4*, P-glycoprotein–mediated efflux. Modified from Brayden DJ. Human intestinal epithelial cell monolayers as prescreens for oral drug delivery. *Pharm News.* 1997;4(1):11–15.

1. **General principles**
   a. A **cell membrane** is a semipermeable structure composed primarily of lipids and proteins.
   b. Drugs may be transported by **passive diffusion**, **partitioning**, **carrier-mediated transport**, **paracellular transport**, or **vesicular transport**.
   c. Usually, **proteins**, **drugs bound to proteins**, and **macromolecules** do not easily cross cell membranes.
   d. **Nonpolar lipid-soluble drugs** traverse cell membranes more easily than do **ionic** or **polar water-soluble drugs**.
   e. **Low-molecular-weight drugs** diffuse across a cell membrane more easily than do **high-molecular-weight drugs**.
2. **Passive diffusion and partitioning**
   a. ***Within* the cytoplasm** or in **interstitial fluid**, most drugs undergo transport by simple diffusion.
   b. **Fick's law of diffusion. Simple passive diffusion** involves the transfer of drugs from an area of high concentration (C_1) to an area of lower concentration (C_2) according to Fick's law of diffusion:

$$\frac{dQ}{dt} = \frac{DA}{h}(C_1 - C_2)$$

   where dQ/dt is the rate of drug diffusion, D is the diffusion coefficient for the drug, A is the surface area of the plane across which transfer occurs, h is the thickness of the region through which diffusion occurs, and $(C_1 - C_2)$ is the difference between the drug concentration in area 1 and area 2, respectively.
   c. Passive drug transport *across* cell membranes involves the successive **partitioning** of a solute between aqueous and lipid phases as well as **diffusion** within the respective phases. Modifying Fick's law of diffusion to accommodate the partitioning of drug gives the following:

$$\frac{dQ}{dt} = \frac{DAK}{h}(C_1 - C_2)$$

   The rate of drug diffusion, dQ/dt, now reflects its direct dependence on K, the oil to water partition coefficient of the drug, as well as on A and $(C_1 - C_2)$.
   d. **Ionization of a weak electrolyte** is affected by the pH of the medium in which the drug is dissolved as well as by the pK_a of the drug. The nonionized species is more lipid soluble than the ionized species, and it partitions more readily across cell membranes.
3. **Carrier-mediated transport**
   a. **Active transport** of the drug across a membrane is a carrier-mediated process that has the following characteristics:
      (1) The drug moves against a concentration gradient.
      (2) The process requires energy.
      (3) The carrier may be selective for certain types of drugs that resemble natural substrates or metabolites that are normally actively transported.
      (4) The carrier system may be saturated at a high drug concentration.
      (5) The process may be competitive (i.e., drugs with similar structures may compete for the same carrier).
   b. **Facilitated diffusion** is also a carrier-mediated transport system. However, facilitated diffusion occurs with (i.e., in the direction of) a concentration gradient and does not require energy.
4. **Paracellular transport.** Drug transport across tight (narrow) junctions between cells or transendothelial channels of cells is known as **paracellular transport**. It involves both diffusion and the **convective** (bulk) flow of water and accompanying water-soluble drug molecules through the paracellular channels.
5. **Vesicular transport** is the process of engulfing particles or dissolved materials by a cell. Vesicular transport is the only transport mechanism that does not require a drug to be in an aqueous solution to be absorbed. **Pinocytosis** and **phagocytosis** are forms of vesicular transport.
   a. **Pinocytosis** is the engulfment of small solute or fluid volumes.
   b. **Phagocytosis** is the engulfment of larger particles, or macromolecules, generally by macrophages.
   c. **Endocytosis** and **exocytosis** are the movement of macromolecules into and out of the cell, respectively.

6. **Other transport mechanisms: transporter proteins.** Various **transporter proteins** (e.g., **P-glycoprotein**) are embedded in the lipid bilayer of cell membranes in tandem in α-helical transmembrane regions or domains. These proteins are adenosine triphosphate (ATP; energy) dependent "pumps," which can facilitate the efflux of drug molecules from the cell. Because these transmembrane efflux pumps are often found in conjunction with metabolizing enzymes such as **cytochrome P450 3A4**, their net effect is to substantially reduce intracellular drug concentrations. Thus they determine, to a large extent, the pharmacokinetic disposition and circulating plasma concentrations of drugs (e.g., cyclosporine, nifedipine, digoxin) that are substrates for these proteins.

B. Routes of drug administration

1. **Parenteral administration**
   a. **Intravenous bolus injection.** The drug is injected directly into the bloodstream, distributes throughout the body, and acts rapidly. Any side effects, including an intense pharmacologic response, anaphylaxis, or overt toxicity, also occur rapidly.
   b. **Intra-arterial injection.** The drug is injected into a specific artery to achieve a high drug concentration in a specific tissue before drug distribution occurs throughout the body. Intra-arterial injection is used for diagnostic agents and occasionally for chemotherapy.
   c. **Intravenous infusion.** The drug is given intravenously at a constant input rate. Constant-rate intravenous infusion maintains a relatively constant plasma drug concentration once the infusion rate is approximately equal to the drug's elimination rate from the body (i.e., once steady state is reached).
   d. **Intramuscular injection.** The drug is injected deep into a skeletal muscle. The rate of absorption depends on the vascularity of the muscle site, the lipid solubility of the drug, and the formulation matrix.
   e. **Subcutaneous injection.** The drug is injected beneath the skin. Because the subcutaneous region is less vascular than muscle tissues, drug absorption is less rapid. The factors that affect absorption from intramuscular depots also affect subcutaneous absorption.
   f. **Miscellaneous parenteral routes**
      (1) **Intra-articular injection.** The drug is injected into a joint.
      (2) **Intradermal (intracutaneous) injection.** The drug is injected into the dermis (i.e., the vascular region of the skin below the epidermis).
      (3) **Intrathecal injection.** The drug is injected into the spinal fluid.
2. **Enteral administration**
   a. **Buccal and sublingual administration.** A tablet or lozenge is placed under the tongue (**sublingual**) or in contact with the mucosal (**buccal**) surface of the cheek. This type of administration allows a nonpolar, lipid-soluble drug to be absorbed across the epithelial lining of the mouth. After buccal or sublingual administration, the drug is absorbed directly into the systemic circulation, bypassing the liver and any first-pass effects.
   b. **Peroral (oral) drug administration.** The drug is administered orally, is swallowed, and undergoes absorption from the gastrointestinal tract through the mesenteric circulation to the hepatic portal vein into the liver and then to the systemic circulation. The peroral route is the most common route of administration.
      (1) The peroral route is the most convenient and the safest route.
      (2) Disadvantages of this route include the following:
         (a) The drug may not be absorbed from the gastrointestinal tract consistently or completely.
         (b) The drug may be digested by gastrointestinal enzymes or decomposed by the acid pH of the stomach.
         (c) The drug may irritate mucosal epithelial cells or complex with the contents of the gastrointestinal tract.
         (d) Some drugs may be incompletely absorbed because of first-pass effects or presystemic elimination (e.g., the drug is metabolized by the liver before systemic absorption occurs).
         (e) The absorption rate may be erratic because of delayed gastric emptying or changes in intestinal motility.
      (3) Most drugs are **xenobiotics** or **exogenous** molecules and, consequently, are absorbed from the gastrointestinal tract by **passive diffusion** and **partitioning**. **Carrier-mediated transport**, **paracellular transport**, and **vesicular transport** play smaller—but critical—roles, particularly for endogenous molecules.

(4) Drug molecules are absorbed throughout the gastrointestinal tract; but the **duodenal region**, which has a large surface area because of the villi and microvilli, is the primary absorption site. The large blood supply provided by the mesenteric vessels allows the drug to be absorbed more efficiently (see II.A.2).

(5) **Altered gastric emptying** affects arrival of the drug in the duodenum for systemic absorption. **Gastric emptying time** is affected by food content, food composition (fats, acids delay gastric emptying), emotional state, circadian effects (gastric emptying tends to be more rapid in the morning than in the evening), and drugs that alter gastrointestinal tract motility (e.g., anticholinergics, narcotic analgesics, prokinetic agents). In general, the T_{max} (**time** of peak systemic drug concentration) occurs earlier, when gastric emptying is faster than normal, and later, when gastric emptying is slower than normal. The effect of gastric emptying on C_{max} (**peak** systemic drug concentration) varies, depending on the absorption mechanism, pH dependence of dissolution, extent of presystemic elimination, etc.

(6) Normal intestinal motility from **peristalsis** brings the drug in contact with the intestinal epithelial cells. A sufficient period of contact (residence time) is needed to permit drug absorption across the cell membranes from the mucosal to the serosal surface.

(7) Some drugs, such as **cimetidine** and **acetaminophen**, when given in an immediate-release peroral dosage form to fasted subjects produce a systemic drug concentration time with two peaks. This **double-peak phenomenon** is attributed to variability in stomach emptying, variable intestinal motility, and enterohepatic cycling.

c. **Rectal administration.** The drug in solution (enema) or suppository form is placed in the rectum. Drug diffusion from the solution or release from the suppository leads to absorption across the mucosal surface of the rectum. Drug absorbed in the lower two-thirds of the rectum enters the systemic circulation directly, bypassing the liver and any first-pass effects.

3. **Respiratory tract administration**

a. **Intranasal administration.** The drug contained in a solution or suspension is administered to the nasal mucosa, either as a spray or as drops. The medication may be used for local (e.g., nasal decongestants, intranasal steroids) or systemic effects.

b. **Pulmonary inhalation.** The drug, as liquid or solid particles, is inhaled perorally (with a nebulizer or a metered-dose aerosol) into the pulmonary tree. In general, **particles > 60 μm** are primarily deposited in the **trachea**. **Particles > 20 μm** do not reach the bronchioles, and **particles < 0.6 μm** are not deposited and are **exhaled**. Particles between **2 and 6 μm** can reach the **alveolar ducts**, although only particles of **1 to 2 μm are retained in the alveoli**.

4. **Transdermal and topical administration**

a. **Transdermal (percutaneous)** drug absorption is the placement of the drug (in a lotion, ointment, cream, paste, or patch) on the skin surface for systemic absorption. An occlusive dressing or film improves systemic drug absorption from the skin. Small lipid-soluble molecules, such as nitroglycerin, nicotine, scopolamine, clonidine, fentanyl, and steroids (e.g., 17-β-estradiol, testosterone), are readily absorbed from the skin.

b. Drugs (e.g., antibacterials, local anesthetic agents) are applied **topically** to the skin for a local effect.

5. Miscellaneous routes of drug administration include **ophthalmic**, **otic**, **urethral**, and **vaginal** administration. These routes of administration are generally used for local therapeutic activity. However, some systemic drug absorption may occur.

C. **Local drug activity** versus **systemic drug absorption.** The route of administration, absorption site, and bioavailability of the drug from the dosage form are major factors in the design of a drug product.

1. Drugs intended for **local activity** such as topical antibiotics, anti-infectives, antifungal agents, and local anesthetics are formulated in dosage forms that minimize systemic absorption. The concentration of these drugs at the application site affects their activity.

2. When **systemic absorption** is desired, the bioavailability of the drug from the dosage form at the absorption site must be considered (e.g., a drug given intravenously is 100% bioavailable because all of the drug is placed directly into the systemic circulation). The amount, or dose, of drug in the dosage form is based on the extent of drug absorption and the desired systemic drug concentration. The type of dosage form (e.g., immediate release, controlled release) affects the rate of drug absorption.

III. BIOPHARMACEUTIC PRINCIPLES

A. Physicochemical properties

1. **Drug dissolution.** For most drugs with limited water solubility, the rate at which the solid drug enters into solution (i.e., the rate of dissolution) is often the rate-limiting step in bioavailability. The **Noyes–Whitney** equation describes the diffusion-controlled rate of drug dissolution (dm/dt; i.e., the change in the amount of drug in solution with respect to time):

$$\frac{dm}{dt} = \frac{DA}{\delta}(C_s - C_b)$$

where D is the diffusion coefficient of the solute, A is the surface area of the solid undergoing dissolution, δ is the thickness of the diffusion layer, C_s is the concentration of the solvate at saturation, and C_b is the concentration of the drug in the bulk solution phase at time t.

2. **Drug solubility** in a saturated solution (see Chapter 2, IV) is a static (equilibrium) property. The dissolution rate of a drug is a dynamic property related to the rate of absorption.
3. **Particle size** and **surface area** are inversely related. As solid drug particle size decreases, particle surface area increases.
   - a. As described by the Noyes–Whitney equation, the dissolution rate is directly proportional to the surface area. An increase in surface area allows for more contact between the solid drug particles and the solvent, resulting in a faster dissolution rate (see III.A.1).
   - b. With certain **hydrophobic drugs**, excessive particle size reduction does not always increase the dissolution rate. Small particles tend to reaggregate into larger particles to reduce the high surface free energy produced by particle size reduction.
   - c. To prevent the formation of aggregates, small drug particles are molecularly dispersed in polyethylene glycol (PEG), polyvinylpyrrolidone (PVP; povidone), dextrose, or other agents. For example, a molecular dispersion of griseofulvin in a water-soluble carrier such as PEG 4000 (e.g., Gris–PEG) enhances its dissolution and bioavailability.
4. **Partition coefficient and extent of ionization**
   - a. The **partition coefficient** of a drug is the ratio of the solubility of the drug, at equilibrium, in a nonaqueous solvent (e.g., *n*-octanol) to that in an aqueous solvent (e.g., water; pH 7.4 buffer solution). Hydrophilic drugs with higher water solubility have a faster dissolution rate than do hydrophobic or lipophilic drugs, which have poor water solubility.
   - b. **Extent of ionization.** Drugs that are weak electrolytes (acids or bases) exist in both an ionized form and a nonionized form in solution. The extent of ionization depends on the pK_a of the weak electrolyte and the pH of the solution. The ionized form is more polar, and therefore more water soluble, than the nonionized form. The **Henderson–Hasselbalch equation** describes the relation between the ionized and the nonionized forms of a drug as a function of pH and pK_a. When the pH of the medium equals the pK_a of the drug, 50% of the drug in solution is nonionized and 50% is ionized, as can be shown from the following equations:
     - (1) **For weak acids:**

$$pH = pK_a + \log\left(\frac{\text{salt}}{\text{nonionized acid}}\right)$$

     - (2) **For weak bases:**

$$pH = pK_a + \log\left(\frac{\text{nonionized base}}{\text{salt}}\right)$$

5. **Salt formation**
   - a. The choice of salt form for a drug depends on the desired physical, chemical, or pharmacologic properties. Certain salts are designed to provide slower dissolution, slower bioavailability, and longer duration of action. Other salts are selected for greater stability, less local irritation at the absorption site, or less systemic toxicity.
     - (1) Some soluble salt forms are less stable than the nonionized form. For example, sodium aspirin is less stable than aspirin in the acid form.
     - (2) A solid dosage form containing buffering agents may be formulated with the free acid form of the drug (e.g., buffered aspirin).

(a) The buffering agent forms an alkaline medium in the gastrointestinal tract, and the drug dissolves in situ.
(b) The dissolved salt form of the drug diffuses into the bulk fluid of the gastrointestinal tract, forms a fine precipitate that redissolves rapidly, and becomes available for absorption.

b. **Effervescent granules** or **tablets** containing the acid drug in addition to sodium bicarbonate, tartaric acid, citric acid, or other ingredients are added to water just before oral administration. The excess sodium bicarbonate forms an alkaline solution in which the drug dissolves. Carbon dioxide is also formed by the decomposition of carbonic acid.

c. For weakly acidic drugs, potassium and sodium salts are more soluble than divalent cation salts (e.g., calcium, magnesium) or trivalent cation salts (e.g., aluminum).

d. For weak bases, common water-soluble salts include the hydrochloride, sulfate, citrate, and gluconate salts. The estolate, napsylate, and stearate salts are less water soluble.

6. Polymorphism is the ability of a drug to exist in more than one crystalline form.

a. Different polymorphs have different physical properties, including melting point and dissolution rate.

b. **Amorphous**, or **noncrystalline, forms** of a drug have faster dissolution rates than do crystalline forms.

7. Chirality is the ability of a drug to exist as **optically active stereoisomers** or **enantiomers**. Individual enantiomers may not have the same pharmacokinetic and pharmacodynamic activity. Because most chiral drugs are used as racemic mixtures, the results of studies with such mixtures may be misleading because the drug is assumed to behave as a single entity. For example, ibuprofen exists as the *R*- and *S*-enantiomers; only the *S*-enantiomer is pharmacologically active. When the racemic mixture of ibuprofen is taken orally, the *R*-enantiomer undergoes presystemic inversion in the gut to the *S*-enantiomer. Because the rate and extent of inversion are site specific and formulation dependent, ibuprofen activity may vary considerably.

8. Hydrates. Drugs may exist in a **hydrated**, or **solvated, form** or as an **anhydrous molecule**. Dissolution rates differ for hydrated and anhydrous forms. For example, the anhydrous form of ampicillin dissolves faster and is more rapidly absorbed than the hydrated form.

9. Complex formation. A **complex** is a species formed by the reversible or irreversible association of two or more interacting molecules or ions. **Chelates** are complexes that typically involve a ringlike structure formed by the interaction between a partial ring of atoms and a metal. Many biologically important molecules (e.g., hemoglobin, insulin, cyanocobalamin) are chelates. Drugs such as tetracycline form chelates with divalent (e.g., Ca^{++}, Mg^{++}) and trivalent (e.g., Al^{+++}, Bi^{+++}) metal ions. Many drugs adsorb strongly on charcoal or clay (e.g., kaolin, bentonite) particles by forming complexes. Drug complexes with proteins, such as albumin or α_1-acid glycoprotein, often occur.

a. Complex formation usually alters the physical and chemical characteristics of the drug. For example:
(1) The chelate of tetracycline with calcium is less water soluble and is poorly absorbed.
(2) Theophylline complexed with ethylenediamine to form aminophylline is more water soluble and is used for parenteral and rectal administration.
(3) Cyclodextrins are used to form complexes with many drugs to increase their water solubility.

b. Large drug complexes, such as drug–protein complexes, do not cross cell membranes easily. These complexes must dissociate to free the drug for absorption at the absorption site or to permit transport across cell membranes or glomerular filtration before the drug is excreted into the urine.

B. Drug product and delivery system formulation

1. General considerations

a. **Design of the appropriate dosage form** or **delivery system** depends on the
(1) physical and chemical properties of the drug,
(2) dose of the drug,
(3) route of administration,
(4) type of drug delivery system desired,
(5) desired therapeutic effect,
(6) physiologic release of the drug from the delivery system,

(7) bioavailability of the drug at the absorption site, and
(8) pharmacokinetics and pharmacodynamics of the drug.

b. **Bioavailability.** The more complicated the formulation of the finished drug product (e.g., controlled-release tablet, enteric-coated tablet, transdermal patch), the greater the potential for a bioavailability problem. For example, the **release** of a drug from a peroral dosage form and its subsequent bioavailability depend on a succession of rate processes (*Figure 3-2*). These processes may include the following:
(1) **Attrition**, **disintegration**, or **disaggregation** of the drug product
(2) **Dissolution** of the drug in an aqueous environment
(3) **Convection** and **diffusion** of the drug molecules to the absorbing surface
(4) **Absorption** of the drug across cell membranes into the systemic circulation

c. The **rate-limiting step** in the bioavailability of a drug from a drug product is the slowest step in a series of kinetic processes.
(1) For most conventional solid drug products (e.g., capsules, tablets), the dissolution rate is the slowest, or rate-limiting, step for bioavailability.
(2) For a controlled- or sustained-release drug product, the release of the drug from the delivery system is the rate-limiting step.

2. **Solutions** are homogeneous mixtures of one or more solutes dispersed molecularly in a dissolving medium (solvent).

a. Compared with other oral and peroral drug formulations, a drug dissolved in an aqueous solution is in the most bioavailable and consistent form. Because the drug is already in solution,

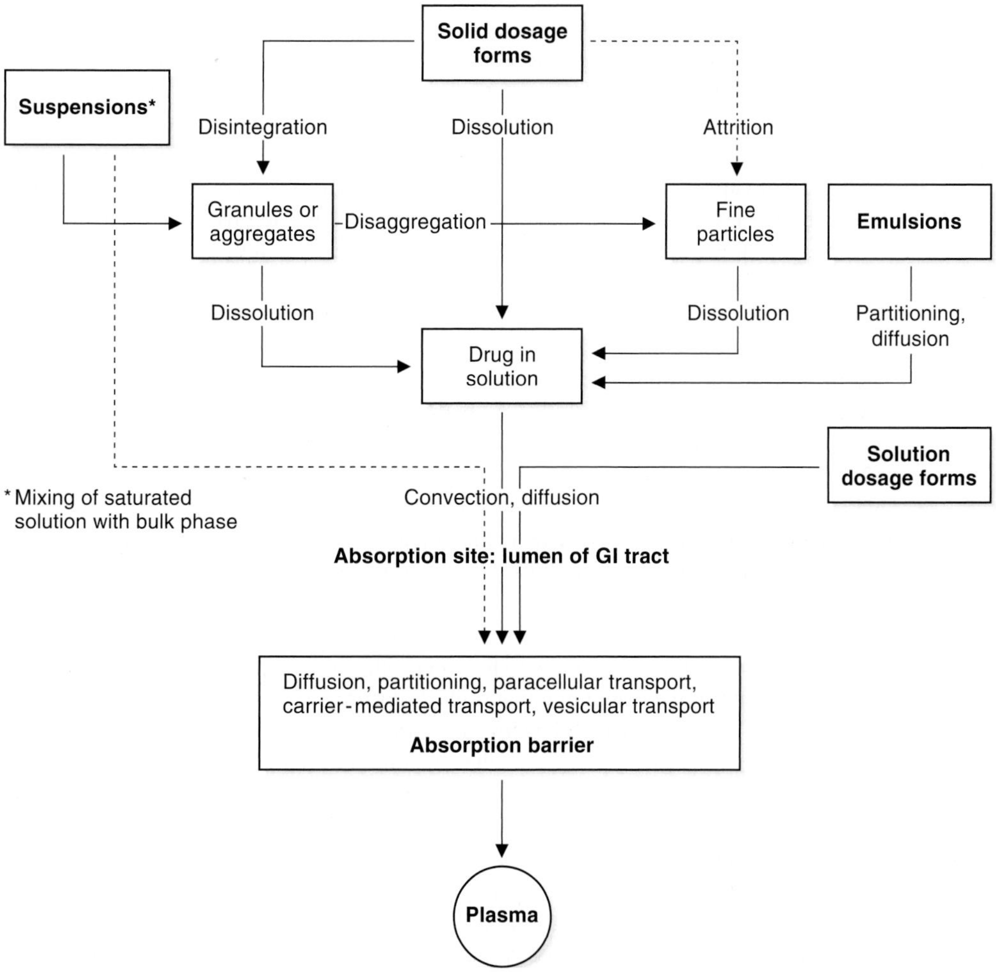

Figure 3-2. The processes involved in drug release from peroral dosage forms. *GI*, gastrointestinal.

no dissolution step is necessary before systemic absorption occurs. Peroral drug solutions are often used as the reference preparation for solid peroral formulations.

b. A drug dissolved in a hydroalcoholic solution (e.g., elixir) also has good bioavailability. Alcohol aids drug solubility. However, when the drug is diluted by gastrointestinal tract fluid and other gut contents (e.g., food), it may form a finely divided precipitate in the lumen of the gastrointestinal tract. Because of the extensive dispersion and large surface area of such finely divided precipitates, redissolution and subsequent absorption occur rapidly.

c. A viscous drug solution (e.g., syrup) may interfere with dilution and mixing with gastrointestinal tract contents. The solution decreases the gastric emptying rate and the rate of transfer of drug solution to the duodenal region, where absorption is most efficient.

3. Suspensions are dispersions of finely divided solid particles of a drug in a liquid medium in which the drug is not readily soluble. The liquid medium of a suspension comprises a saturated solution of the drug in equilibrium with the solid drug.

a. The bioavailability of the drug from suspensions may be similar to that of a solution because the finely divided particles are dispersed and provide a large surface area for rapid dissolution. On the other hand, a slow dissolution rate decreases the absorption rate.

b. Suspending agents are often hydrophilic colloids (e.g., cellulose derivatives, acacia, xanthan gum) added to suspensions to increase viscosity, inhibit agglomeration, and decrease the rate at which particles settle. Highly viscous suspensions may prolong gastric emptying time, slow drug dissolution, and decrease the absorption rate.

4. Capsules are solid dosage forms with hard or soft gelatin shells that contain drugs, usually admixed with excipients. **Coating** the capsule shell or the drug particles within the capsule can affect bioavailability.

a. Hard gelatin capsules are usually filled with a powder blend that contains the drug. Typically, the powder blend is simpler and less compacted than the blend in a compressed tablet. After ingestion, the gelatin softens, swells, and begins to dissolve in the gastrointestinal tract. Encapsulated drugs are released rapidly and dispersed easily, and bioavailability is good. Hard gelatin capsules are the preferred dosage form for early clinical trials of new drugs.

b. Soft gelatin capsules may contain a nonaqueous solution, a powder, or a drug suspension. The vehicle may be water miscible (e.g., PEG). The cardiac glycoside digoxin, dispersed in a water-miscible vehicle (Lanoxicaps), has better bioavailability than a compressed tablet formulation (Lanoxin). However, a soft gelatin capsule that contains the drug dissolved in a **hydrophobic** vehicle (e.g., vegetable oil) may have poorer bioavailability than a compressed tablet formulation of the drug.

c. Aging and **storage conditions** can affect the moisture content of the gelatin component of the capsule shell and the bioavailability of the drug.

(1) At low moisture levels, the capsule shell becomes brittle and is easily ruptured.

(2) At high moisture levels, the capsule shell becomes moist, soft, and distorted. Moisture may be transferred to the capsule contents, particularly if the contents are hygroscopic.

5. Compressed tablets are solid dosage forms in which high pressure is used to compress a powder blend or granulation that contains the drug and other ingredients, or excipients, into a solid mass.

a. Excipients, including diluents (fillers), binders, disintegrants, lubricants, glidants, surfactants, dye, and flavoring agents, have the following properties:

(1) They permit the efficient manufacture of compressed tablets.

(2) They affect the physical and chemical characteristics of the drug.

(3) They affect bioavailability. The higher the ratio of excipient to active drug, the greater the likelihood that the excipients affect bioavailability.

b. Examples

(1) Disintegrants (e.g., starch, croscarmellose, sodium starch glycolate) vary in action, depending on their concentration; the method by which they are mixed with the powder formulation or granulation; and the degree of tablet compaction. Although tablet disintegration is usually not a problem because it often occurs more rapidly than drug dissolution, it is necessary for dissolution in immediate-release formulations. Inability to disintegrate may interfere with bioavailability.

(2) **Lubricants** are usually hydrophobic, water-insoluble substances such as stearic acid, magnesium stearate, hydrogenated vegetable oil, and talc. They may reduce wetting of the surface of the solid drug particles, slowing the dissolution and bioavailability rates of the drug. Water-soluble lubricants, such as L-leucine, do not interfere with dissolution or bioavailability.
(3) **Glidants** (e.g., colloidal silicon dioxide) improve the flow properties of a dry powder blend before it is compressed. Rather than posing a potential problem with bioavailability, glidants may reduce tablet-to-tablet variability and improve product efficacy.
(4) **Surfactants** enhance drug dissolution rates and bioavailability by reducing interfacial tension at the boundary between solid drug and liquid and by improving the wettability (contact) of solid drug particles by the solvent.

c. **Coated compressed tablets** have a sugar coat, a film coat, or an enteric coat with the following properties:
(1) It protects the drug from moisture, light, and air.
(2) It masks the taste or odor of the drug.
(3) It improves the appearance of the tablet.
(4) It may affect the release rate of the drug.

d. In addition, **enteric coatings** minimize contact between the drug and the gastric region by resisting dissolution or attrition and preventing contact between the underlying drug and the gastric contents or gastric mucosa. Some enteric coatings minimize gastric contact because they are insoluble at acidic pHs. Other coatings resist attrition and remain whole long enough for the tablet to leave the gastric area. By resisting dissolution or attrition, enteric coatings may decrease bioavailability. Enteric coatings are used to
(1) minimize irritation of the gastric mucosa by the drug;
(2) prevent inactivation or degradation of the drug in the stomach; and
(3) delay the release of drug until the tablet reaches the small intestine, where conditions for absorption may be optimal.

6. **Modified-release dosage forms** are drug products that alter the rate or timing of drug release. Because modified-release dosage forms are more complex than conventional immediate-release dosage forms, more stringent quality control and bioavailability tests are required. **Dose dumping** or the abrupt, uncontrolled release of a large amount of drug is a problem.
   a. **Extended-release dosage forms** include **controlled-release**, **sustained-action**, and **long-acting drug delivery systems.** These delivery systems allow at least a twofold reduction in dosing frequency compared with conventional immediate-release formulations.
   (1) The extended, slow release of controlled-release drug products produces a relatively flat, sustained plasma drug concentration that avoids toxicity (from high drug concentrations) or lack of efficacy (from low drug concentrations).
   (2) Extended-release dosage forms provide an immediate (initial) release of the drug, followed by a slower sustained release.
   b. **Delayed-release dosage forms** release active drug at a time other than immediately after administration at a desired site in the gastrointestinal tract. For example, an enteric-coated drug product does not allow for dissolution in the acid environment of the stomach but, rather, in the less acidic environment of the small intestine.

7. **Transdermal drug delivery systems**, or **patches**, are controlled-release devices that contain the drug for systemic absorption after topical application to the skin surface. Transdermal drug delivery systems are available for a number of drugs (nitroglycerin, nicotine, scopolamine, clonidine, fentanyl, 17-β-estradiol, and testosterone). Although the formulation matrices of these delivery systems differ somewhat, they all differ from conventional topical formulations in the following ways:
   a. They have an impermeable **occlusive backing film** that prevents insensible water loss from the skin beneath the patch. This film causes increased hydration and skin temperature under the patch and enhanced permeation of the skin by the drug.
   b. The formulation matrix of the patch maintains the drug concentration gradient within the device after application so that drug delivery to the interface between the patch and the skin is sustained. As a result, drug partitioning and diffusion into the skin persist, and systemic absorption is maintained throughout the dosing interval.
   c. Transdermal drug delivery systems are kept in place on the skin surface by an **adhesive layer**, ensuring drug contact with the skin and continued drug delivery.

8. **Targeted (site-specific) drug delivery systems** are drug carrier systems that place the drug at or near the receptor site. Examples include macromolecular drug carriers (protein drug carriers), particulate drug delivery systems (e.g., liposomes, nanoparticles), and monoclonal antibodies. With targeted drug delivery, the drug may be delivered to
   a. the capillary bed of the active site,
   b. a special type of cell (e.g., tumor cells) but not to normal cells, and
   c. a specific organ or tissue by complexing with a carrier that recognizes the target.
9. **Inserts, implants**, and **devices** are used to control drug delivery for localized or systemic drug effects. The drug is impregnated into a biodegradable or nonbiodegradable material and is released slowly. The inserts, implants, and devices are inserted into a variety of cavities (e.g., vagina, buccal cavity) or tissues (e.g., skin). For example, the leuprolide acetate implant, Viadur, is inserted beneath the skin of the upper arm. It provides palliative treatment of advanced prostate cancer for 1 year.

Study Questions

Directions: Each question, statement, or incomplete statement in this section can be correctly answered or completed by **one** of the suggested answers or phrases. Choose the **best** answer.

1. Which statement best describes bioavailability?
   (A) relation between the physical and the chemical properties of a drug and its systemic absorption
   (B) measurement of the rate and amount of therapeutically active drug that reaches the systemic circulation
   (C) movement of the drug into body tissues over time
   (D) dissolution of the drug in the gastrointestinal tract
   (E) amount of drug destroyed by the liver before systemic absorption from the gastrointestinal tract occurs

2. The route of drug administration that gives the most rapid onset of the pharmacologic effect is
   (A) intramuscular injection.
   (B) intravenous injection.
   (C) intradermal injection.
   (D) peroral administration.
   (E) subcutaneous injection.

3. The route of drug administration that provides complete (100%) bioavailability is
   (A) intramuscular injection.
   (B) intravenous injection.
   (C) intradermal injection.
   (D) peroral administration.
   (E) subcutaneous injection.

4. After peroral administration, drugs generally are absorbed best from the
   (A) buccal cavity.
   (B) stomach.
   (C) duodenum.
   (D) ileum.
   (E) rectum.

5. The characteristics of an active transport process include all of the following *except* for which one?
   (A) Active transport moves drug molecules against a concentration gradient.
   (B) Active transport follows Fick's law of diffusion.
   (C) Active transport is a carrier-mediated transport system.
   (D) Active transport requires energy.
   (E) Active transport of drug molecules may be saturated at high drug concentrations.

6. The passage of drug molecules from a region of high drug concentration to a region of low drug concentration is known as
   (A) active transport.
   (B) bioavailability.
   (C) biopharmaceutics.
   (D) simple diffusion.
   (E) pinocytosis.

7. Which equation describes the rate of drug dissolution from a tablet?
   (A) Fick's law
   (B) Henderson–Hasselbalch equation
   (C) Law of mass action
   (D) Michaelis–Menten equation
   (E) Noyes–Whitney equation

8. Which condition usually increases the rate of drug dissolution from a tablet?
   (A) increase in the particle size of the drug
   (B) decrease in the surface area of the drug
   (C) use of the free acid or free base form of the drug
   (D) use of the ionized, or salt, form of the drug
   (E) use of sugar coating around the tablet

9. Dose dumping is a problem in the formulation of
   (A) compressed tablets.
   (B) modified-release drug products.
   (C) hard gelatin capsules.
   (D) soft gelatin capsules.
   (E) suppositories.

10. The rate-limiting step in the bioavailability of a lipid-soluble drug formulated as an immediate-release compressed tablet is the rate of
    (A) disintegration of the tablet and release of the drug.
    (B) dissolution of the drug.
    (C) transport of the drug molecules across the intestinal mucosal cells.
    (D) blood flow to the gastrointestinal tract.
    (E) biotransformation, or metabolism, of the drug by the liver before systemic absorption occurs.

11. The extent of ionization of a weak electrolyte drug depends on the
    (A) pH of the media and pK_a of the drug.
    (B) oil to water partition coefficient of the drug.
    (C) particle size and surface area of the drug.
    (D) Noyes–Whitney equation for the drug.
    (E) polymorphic form of the drug.

12. The rate of drug bioavailability is most rapid when the drug is formulated as a
    (A) controlled-release product.
    (B) hard gelatin capsule.
    (C) compressed tablet.
    (D) solution.
    (E) suspension.

13. The amount of drug that a transdermal patch (i.e., transdermal drug delivery system) delivers within a 24-hrs period depends on the
    (A) patch composition, which includes an occlusive backing and an adhesive film in contact with the skin.
    (B) affinity of the drug for the formulation matrix relative to its affinity for the stratum corneum.
    (C) rate of drug partitioning and/or diffusion through the patch to the skin surface.
    (D) surface area of the patch.
    (E) All of the above

Answers and Explanations

1. **The answer is B** *[see I.A.3]*.
   Bioavailability is the measurement of the rate and extent (amount) of therapeutically active drug that reaches the systemic circulation. The relation of the physical and the chemical properties of a drug to its systemic absorption (i.e., bioavailability) is known as its biopharmaceutics. The movement of a drug into body tissues is an aspect of pharmacokinetics, which is the study of drug movement in the body over time. The dissolution of a drug in the gastrointestinal tract is a physicochemical process that affects bioavailability. Significant destruction of a drug by the liver before it is systemically absorbed (known as the first-pass effect because it occurs during the first passage of the drug through the liver) decreases bioavailability.

2. **The answer is B** *[see II.B.1.a]*.
   When the active form of the drug is given intravenously, it enters the systemic circulation directly. The drug is delivered rapidly to all tissues, including the drug receptor sites. For all other routes of drug administration, except intra-arterial injection, the drug must be systemically absorbed before it is distributed to the drug receptor sites. For this reason, the onset of pharmacologic effects is slower. If the drug is a prodrug that must be converted to an active drug, oral administration, not intravenous injection, may not provide the most rapid onset of activity if conversion to the active form takes place in the gastrointestinal tract or liver.

3. **The answer is B** *[see II.C.2]*.
   When a drug is given by intravenous injection, the entire dose enters the systemic circulation. With other routes of administration, the drug may be lost before it reaches the systemic circulation. For example, with first-pass effects, a portion of an orally administered drug is eliminated, usually through degradation by liver enzymes, before the drug reaches its receptor sites.

4. **The answer is C** *[see II.B.2.b.(4)]*.
   Drugs given orally are well absorbed from the duodenum. The duodenum has a large surface area because of the presence of villi and microvilli. In addition, because the duodenum is well perfused by the mesenteric blood vessels, a concentration gradient is maintained between the lumen of the duodenum and the blood.

5. **The answer is B** *[see II.A.2–3].*
Fick's law of diffusion describes passive diffusion of drug molecules moving from a high concentration to a low concentration. This process is not saturable and does not require energy.

6. **The answer is D** *[see II.A.2].*
The transport of a drug across a cell membrane by passive diffusion follows Fick's law of diffusion: The drug moves with a concentration gradient (i.e., from an area of high concentration to an area of low concentration). In contrast, drugs that are actively transported move against a concentration gradient.

7. **The answer is E** *[see III.A.1].*
The Noyes–Whitney equation describes the rate at which a solid drug dissolves. Fick's law is similar to the Noyes–Whitney equation in that both equations describe drug movement caused by a concentration gradient. Fick's law generally refers to passive diffusion, or passive transport, of drugs. The law of mass action describes the rate of a chemical reaction, the Michaelis–Menten equation involves enzyme kinetics, and the Henderson–Hasselbalch equation gives the pH of a buffer solution.

8. **The answer is D** *[see III.A.1–3].*
The ionized, or salt, form of a drug has a charge and is generally more water soluble and therefore dissolves more rapidly than the nonionized (free acid or free base) form of the drug. The dissolution rate is directly proportional to the surface area and inversely proportional to the particle size. An increase in the particle size or a decrease in the surface area slows the dissolution rate.

9. **The answer is B** *[see III.B.6].*
A modified-release, or controlled-release, drug product contains two or more conventional doses of the drug. An abrupt release of the drug, known as dose dumping, may cause intoxication.

10. **The answer is B** *[see III.B.1.c].*
For lipid-soluble drugs, the rate of dissolution is the slowest (i.e., rate-limiting) step in drug absorption and thus in bioavailability. The disintegration rate of an immediate-release or conventional compressed tablet is usually more rapid than the rate of drug dissolution. Because the cell membrane is a lipoprotein structure, transport of a lipid-soluble drug across the cell membrane is usually rapid.

11. **The answer is A** *[see III.A.4.b].*
The extent of ionization of a weak electrolyte is described by the Henderson–Hasselbalch equation, which relates the pH of the solution to the pK_a of the drug.

12. **The answer is D** *[see III.B.2.a].*
Because a drug in solution is already dissolved, no dissolution is needed before absorption. Consequently, compared with other drug formulations, a drug in solution has a high rate of bioavailability. A drug in aqueous solution has the highest bioavailability rate and is often used as the reference preparation for other formulations. Drugs in hydroalcoholic solution (e.g., elixirs) also have good bioavailability. The rate of drug bioavailability from a hard gelatin capsule, compressed tablet, or suspension may be equal to that of a solution if an optimal formulation is manufactured and the drug is inherently rapidly absorbed.

13. **The answer is E** *[see III.B.7].*
Drug delivery from a transdermal drug delivery system depends on all of the factors cited—that is, on the presence of an occlusive backing (to maintain skin hydration and elevate skin temperature slightly) and an adhesive film to maintain contact of the formulation matrix with the skin to enable drug transfer from the patch into the skin. If the drug's affinity for the formulation matrix is greater than its affinity for the stratum corneum, the drug's escaping tendency from the patch will be reduced, minimizing the gradient for drug transfer into the skin. The microviscosity of the formulation matrix, the presence of a membrane between the drug reservoir in the patch and the skin surface, and the interaction of the drug with the formulation matrix affect the rate and extent of diffusion and/or partitioning of the drug through the patch to the skin surface. Finally, the extent of drug delivery from the patch is directly proportional to the surface area of the patch in contact with the skin surface.

4

Extemporaneous Prescription Compounding

LOYD V. ALLEN JR.

I. INTRODUCTION

A. **Definitions**

1. **Compounding versus manufacturing**
2. It is important, but oftentimes difficult, to distinguish between compounding and manufacturing.
3. **Compounding** is defined by the *United States Pharmacopeia* (*USP*) as the preparation, mixing, assembling, altering, packaging, and labeling of a drug, drug delivery device, or device in accordance with a licensed practitioner's prescription, medication order, or initiative based on the practitioner/patient/pharmacist/compounder relationship in the course of professional practice. Compounding includes the following:
   - Preparation of drug dosage forms for both human and animal patients
   - Preparation of drugs or devices in anticipation of prescription drug orders based on routine, regularly observed prescribing patterns
   - Reconstitution or manipulation of commercial products that may require the addition of one or more ingredients
   - Preparation of drugs or devices for the purposes of, or as an incident to, research (clinical or academic), teaching, or chemical analysis
   - Preparation of drugs and devices for prescriber's office use where permitted by federal and state law
4. **Manufacturing** has been defined as the production, preparation, propagation, conversion, or processing of a drug or device, either directly or indirectly, by extraction of the drug from substances of natural origin or by means of chemical or biological synthesis. Manufacturing may also include any packaging or repackaging of the substance(s) or labeling or relabeling of container for resale by pharmacies, practitioners, or other persons.
5. The purpose of pharmaceutical compounding is to prepare an individualized drug treatment for a patient based on an order from a duly licensed prescriber. The fundamental difference between compounding and manufacturing is the existence of a pharmacist/prescriber/patient relationship that controls the compounding of the drug preparation. Compounded drugs are not for resale but rather are personal and responsive to the patient's immediate needs. They are prepared and administered by the patient, caregiver, or patient's health care professionals, which allows for the monitoring of patient outcomes. On the other hand, drug manufacturers produce batches consisting of tens or hundreds of thousands of dosage units, such as tablets or capsules, for resale, using many personnel and large-scale manufacturing equipment. These products are distributed through the normal channels of interstate commerce to individuals unknown to the company. Manufacturers are not required to, and do not, provide oversight of individual patients. It is also acceptable and routine practice for pharmacists to compound for "office use" those preparations that are not commercially available. These preparations are "for office use only" and are not for resale or to be given to the patients to take home; they are to be administered at the office.

6. The *USP* uses the term *preparation* to refer to compounded prescriptions and the term *products* to refer to manufactured pharmaceuticals. Also, for stability purposes, compounded preparations are assigned a "beyond-use" date, and manufactured products are assigned an "expiration date."

B. **Regulation**

1. **Current good manufacturing practices (cGMPs)** are the standards of practice used in the pharmaceutical industry and are regulated by the U.S. Food and Drug Administration (FDA).
2. **Good compounding practices (GCPs)** are the standards of practice detailed in the *USP*, Chapter [795]. Community pharmacists must comply with state board of pharmacy laws, regulations, and guidelines to ensure a quality preparation, which includes using proper materials, weighing equipment, documented techniques, and dispensing and storage instructions.
3. **Legal considerations**
   a. Extemporaneous compounding by the pharmacist or a prescription order from a licensed practitioner, as with the dispensing of any other prescription, is controlled by the state boards of pharmacy.
   b. The legal risk (liability) of compounding is no greater than the risk of filling a prescription for a manufactured product because the pharmacist must ensure that the correct drug, dose, and directions are provided. The pharmacist is also responsible for preparing a quality pharmaceutical preparation, providing proper instructions regarding its storage, and advising the patient of any adverse effects.
4. **U.S. Food and Drug Administration.** The FDA has developed a list of preparations that should not be extemporaneously compounded. This list was developed primarily from commercial products that have been removed from the market owing to safety and/or efficacy concerns. This is a lengthy list and must be read carefully because, in some cases, only certain dosage forms of a specific drug are included on the list and others are not. The list is too extensive to include here but can be accessed at http://www.gpo.gov/fdsys/pkg/FR-1999-03-08/html/99-5517.htm.

C. **Stability and quality control of compounded preparations**

1. **Beyond-use dates.** The assignment of a beyond-use date is one of the most difficult tasks required of a compounding pharmacist. Chapters [795] and [797] of the *USP* provide guidelines for this task. Chapter [795] involves nonsterile preparations, and Chapter [797] involves sterile preparations. For nonsterile preparations, the current *USP* criteria are applicable in the absence of stability information to a specific drug and preparation. For nonaqueous liquids and solid formulations (for which a manufactured drug product is the source of active ingredients), include a beyond-use date not later than 25% of the time remaining until the product's expiration date or 6 months, whichever is earlier. When a *USP* or *National Formulary* (*NF*) substance is the source of active ingredient, the beyond-use date is not later than 6 months. For water-containing oral formulations, the beyond-use date is not later than 14 days when stored at cold temperatures; for water-containing topical/dermal and mucosal liquid and semisolid formulations, the beyond-use date is not later than the intended duration of therapy or 30 days. These beyond-use dates may be exceeded when there is supporting valid scientific stability information that is directly applicable to the specific preparation.

   For sterile preparations and if not sterility tested, the following can be used provided that the preparation is properly packaged and stored. If the preparation is sterility tested, the beyond-use dates for nonsterile preparations apply.

   Low-risk level compounded sterile preparations: Not more than 48 hrs at controlled room temperature, not more than 14 days at a cold temperature (refrigerator), and for 45 days frozen at −20°C or colder.

   Medium-risk level compounded sterile preparations: Not more than 30 hrs at controlled room temperature, not more than 9 days at cold temperature (refrigerator), and for 45 days frozen at −20°C or colder.

   High-risk level compounded sterile preparations: Not more than 24 hrs at controlled room temperature, not more than 3 days at cold temperature (refrigerator), and for 45 days frozen at −20°C or colder.

   As in nonsterile compounding, these beyond-use dates for sterile compounding may be exceeded when there is supporting valid scientific stability information that is directly applicable to the specific preparation.

2. **Quality control.** Quality control is becoming one of the fastest growing aspects of pharmacy compounding. Guidelines for establishing a quality control program are detailed in *USP* [1163] Quality Assurance in Pharmaceutical Compounding. Pharmacists are becoming more involved in the final testing of compounded preparations or are sending them to contract laboratories for testing. For example, the following quality control tests can be considered for the respective compounded dosage forms:
   a. **Ointments, creams, and gels.** Theoretical weight compared to actual weight, pH, specific gravity, active drug assay, physical observations (color, clarity, texture–surface, texture–spatula spread, appearance, feel), and rheological properties
   b. **Hard gelatin capsules.** Weight overall, average weight, individual weight variation, dissolution of capsule shell, disintegration of capsule contents, active drug assay, physical appearance (color, uniformity, extent of fill, locked), and physical stability (discoloration, changes in appearance)
   c. **Special hard gelatin capsules.** Weight overall, average weight, individual weight variation, dissolution of capsule shell, disintegration of capsule contents, active drug assay, physical appearance (color, uniformity of appearance, uniformity of extent of fill, closures), and physical stability (discoloration or other changes)
   d. **Suppositories, troches, lollipops, and sticks.** Weight, specific gravity, active drug assay, physical observations (color, clarity, texture of surface, appearance, feel), melting test, dissolution test, and physical stability
   e. **Oral and topical liquids.** Weight to volume, pH, specific gravity, active drug assay, globule size range, rheological properties/pourability, physical observations (color, clarity), and physical stability (discoloration, foreign materials, gas formation, mold growth)
   f. **Parenteral preparations.** Weight or volume, pH, specific gravity, osmolality, assay, physical observations (color, clarity), particulate matter, sterility, and pyrogenicity
3. **Quality control testing.** Pharmacists have the option of doing testing in-house or outsourcing it to laboratories.
   a. **In-house testing** can include measurements such as weight, volume, pH, specific gravity, osmolality, physical observations, sterility, and endotoxins.
   b. **Out-sourced testing** can include sterility, endotoxins, potency, and dissolution.
   c. **Test results** should be kept on file with the compounding records for the individual compounded preparations.

II. REQUIREMENTS FOR COMPOUNDING

A. **Sources for chemicals and drugs.** Pharmacists can obtain small quantities of the appropriate chemicals or drugs from wholesalers or chemical supply houses. These suppliers then may also serve as compounding consultants to the pharmacists to aid in ensuring their product's purity and quality.

B. **Equipment.** The correct equipment is important in a compounding pharmacy. Many state boards of pharmacy have a required minimum list of equipment for compounding prescriptions. Equipment appropriate for the type and extent of compounding being conducted is vital. Appropriate standard operating procedures must be in place and followed for the maintenance, operation, and calibration of the equipment.

C. **Location of compounding area.** Many pharmacies actively involved in compounding have dedicated a separate area in the pharmacy to this process. The ideal location is away from heavy foot traffic and is near a sink where there is sufficient space to work and store all chemicals and equipment. For compounding of sterile preparations, a laminar airflow hood and a clean room are current practice, or isolation barrier technology equipment appropriately positioned.

D. **Sources of information**
   1. Library at a college of pharmacy
   2. **References**
      a. Allen LV Jr. *The Art, Science and Technology of Pharmaceutical Compounding.* 4th ed. Washington, DC: American Pharmaceutical Association; 2012.
      b. Allen LV Jr, ed. *Remington: The Science and Practice of Pharmacy.* 22nd ed. Baltimore, MD: Pharmaceutical Press; 2012.
      c. O'Neil MJ, ed. *Merck Index.* 14th ed. Whitehouse Station, NJ: Merck & Co; 2006.

d. *The USP Pharmacists' Pharmacopeia*. 2nd ed. Rockville, MD: U.S. Pharmacopeial Convention, Inc.; 2008.
e. Allen LV Jr, Popovich NG, Ansel HC. *Ansel's Pharmaceutical Dosage Forms and Drug Delivery Systems*. 9th ed. Philadelphia, PA: Lippincott Williams & Wilkins; 2008.

3. **Journals**
   a. *International Journal of Pharmaceutical Compounding*
   b. *U.S. Pharmacist*
   c. *Pharmacy Times*
   d. *Lippincott's Hospital Pharmacy*
4. Manufacturers' drug product information inserts; compounding specialty suppliers
5. **Web sites**
   a. Compounding Today: http://www.CompoundingToday.com
   b. *International Journal of Pharmaceutical Compounding*: http://www.ijpc.com
   c. Paddock Laboratories, Inc.: http://www.paddocklabs.com

III. COMPOUNDING OF SOLUTIONS

A. **Definition.** *USP* 34 defines **solutions** as liquid preparations that contain one or more chemical substances dissolved (i.e., molecularly dispersed) in a suitable solvent or mixture of mutually miscible solvents. Although the uniformity of the dosage in a solution can be assumed, the stability, pH, solubility of the drug or chemicals, taste (for oral solutions), and packaging need to be considered.

B. **Types of solutions**
   1. **Sterile parenteral and ophthalmic solutions** require special consideration for their preparation (see XI).
   2. **Nonsterile solutions** include oral, topical, and otic solutions.

C. **Preparation of solutions.** Solutions are the easiest of the dosage forms to compound extemporaneously, as long as a few general rules are followed.
   1. Each drug or chemical is dissolved in the solvent in which it is most soluble. Thus, the solubility characteristics of each drug or chemical must be known.
   2. If an alcoholic solution of a poorly water-soluble drug is used, the aqueous solution is added to the alcoholic solution to maintain as high an alcohol concentration as possible.
   3. The salt form of the drug—not the free acid or base form, which both have poor solubility—is used.
   4. Flavoring or sweetening agents are prepared ahead of time.
   5. When adding a salt to a syrup, dissolve the salt in a few milliliters of water first; then add the syrup to volume.
   6. The proper vehicle (e.g., syrup, elixir, aromatic water, purified water) must be selected.

D. **Examples**
   1. **Example 1**
      a. **Medication order**

Triamcinolone acetonide	100 mg
Menthol	50 mg
Ethanol	10 mL
Propylene glycol	30 mL
Glycerin	20 mL
Sorbitol 70% solution, q.s.	100 mL
Sodium saccharin	100 mg
Sodium metabisulfite	20 mg
Disodium EDTA	100 mg
Purified water	5 mL

      b. **Compounding procedure.** Triamcinolone acetonide 0.1% mouthwash solution is prepared by dissolving the triamcinolone acetonide and menthol in the ethanol. Add the propylene glycol, glycerin, and about 10 mL of the 70% sorbitol and mix well. Dissolve the sodium saccharin, sodium metabisulfite, and disodium EDTA in the purified water. Add the aqueous solution to the drug mixture and mix well. Add sufficient 70% sorbitol solution to volume and mix well.

How much of the triamcinolone base is present in this prescription? The molecular weight of triamcinolone is 394.4 and that of triamcinolone acetonide is 434.5.

$$\frac{394.4}{434.5} \times 100 \text{ mg} = 91 \text{ mg of triamcinolone base}$$

2. **Example 2**
   a. **Medication order**

Potassium chloride	1 mEq/mL
Preserved flavored, oral vehicle, q.s.	100 mL

   b. **Calculations.** The molecular weight of potassium chloride is 74.5 (K = 39; Cl = 35.5). One milliequivalent (mEq) weighs 74.5 mg.

$$100 \text{ mL} \times 74.5 \text{ mg/mL} = 7450 \text{ mg or } 7.45 \text{ g of KCl required}$$

   What is the molar concentration of this prescription?
   7.45 g per 100 mL or 74.5 g per 1000 mL
   1 mole of KCl weighs 74.5 g
   It is a 1 molar solution.

   c. **Compounding procedure.** The solubility of potassium chloride is 1 g in 2.8 mL water. Therefore, dissolve the 7.45 g KCl in 21 mL of purified water. Add sufficient preserved flavored oral vehicle to volume and mix well.

3. **Example 3**
   a. **Medication order**

Salicylic acid	2%
Lactic acid	6 mL
Flexible collodion, a.d.	30 mL

   b. **Compounding procedure.** Pharmacists must use caution when preparing this prescription because flexible collodion is extremely flammable. A 1-oz applicator-tip bottle is calibrated, using ethanol, which is poured out and any remaining alcohol is allowed to evaporate, resulting in a dry bottle. Salicylic acid (0.6 g) is added directly into the bottle, to which is added the 6 mL of lactic acid. The bottle is agitated or a glass stirring rod is used to dissolve the salicylic acid. Flexible collodion is added up to the calibrated 30-mL mark on the applicator-tip bottle.

4. **Example 4**
   a. **Medication order**

Iodine	2%
Sodium iodide	2.4%
Alcohol, q.s.	30 mL

   b. **Compounding procedure.** Iodine (0.6 g) and sodium iodide (0.72 g) are dissolved in the alcohol, and the final solution is placed in an amber bottle. A rubber or plastic spatula is used because iodine is corrosive.

IV. COMPOUNDING OF SUSPENSIONS

A. **Definition. Suspensions** are defined by *USP* 34 as liquid preparations that consist of solid particles dispersed throughout a liquid phase in which the particles are not soluble.

B. **General characteristics**
   1. Some suspensions should contain an antimicrobial agent as a preservative.
   2. Particles settle in suspensions even when a suspending agent is added; thus, suspensions must be well shaken before use to ensure the distribution of particles for a uniform dose.
   3. Tight containers are necessary to ensure the stability of the final preparation.
   4. Principles to keep in mind when compounding include the following:
      a. Insoluble powders should be small and uniform in size to decrease settling.
      b. The suspension should be viscous.
      c. Topical suspensions should have a smooth, impalpable texture.
      d. Oral suspensions should have a pleasant odor and taste.

C. **Formation of suspensions.** Suspensions are easy to compound; however, physical stability after compounding the final preparation is problematic. The following steps may minimize stability problems.
   1. The particle size of all powders used in the formulation should be reduced.
   2. A thickening (suspending) agent may be used to increase viscosity. Common thickening agents include alginic acid, bentonite, VEEGUM, methylcellulose, and tragacanth.
   3. A levigating agent may aid in the initial dispersion of insoluble particles. Common levigating agents include glycerin, propylene glycol, alcohol, syrups, and water.
   4. Flavoring agents and preservatives should be selected and added if the preparation is intended for oral use. Common preservatives include methylparaben, propylparaben, benzoic acid, and sodium benzoate. Flavoring agents may be any flavored syrup or flavored concentrate (*Table 4-1*).
   5. The source of the active ingredients (e.g., bulk powders vs. tablets or capsules) must be considered; if commercial dosage forms are used, the inactive ingredients must be considered and only immediate-release tablets or capsules should be used and not modified release, unless necessary and they can be used appropriately.

D. **Preparation of suspensions**
   1. The insoluble powders are triturated to a fine powder.
   2. A small portion of liquid is used as a levigating agent, and the powders are triturated until a smooth paste is formed.
   3. The vehicle containing the suspending agent is added in divided portions. A high-speed mixer greatly increases the dispersion.
   4. The preparation is brought to the required volume using the vehicle.
   5. The final mixture is transferred to a "tight" bottle for dispensing to the patient.
   6. All suspensions are dispensed with a "shake well" label.
   7. Suspensions are not filtered.
   8. The water-soluble ingredients, including flavoring agents, are mixed in the vehicle before mixing with the insoluble ingredients.

E. **Examples**
   1. **Example 1**
      a. **Medication order**

Propranolol HCl	4 mg/mL
Disp	30 mL
Sig:	1 mL p.o. t.i.d.

      b. **Calculations.** Propranolol HCl: 4 mg/mL × 30 mL = 120 mg. Propranolol HCl is available as a powder or in immediate-release and extended-release (long-acting) dosage forms. Only the powder or the immediate-release tablets are used for compounding prescriptions; therefore, some combination of propranolol HCl tablets that yields 120-mg active drug (e.g., 3 × 40-mg tablets) may be used.
      c. **Compounding procedure.** The propranolol tablets are reduced to a fine powder in a mortar. The powder or the comminuted tablets are levigated to a smooth paste, using a 2% methylcellulose

Table 4-1 SELECTED FLAVOR APPLICATIONS

Drug Category	Preferred Flavors
Antibiotics	Cherry, maple, pineapple, orange, raspberry, banana-pineapple, banana-vanilla, butterscotch-maple, coconut custard, strawberry, vanilla, lemon custard, cherry custard, fruit-cinnamon
Antihistamines	Apricot, black currant, cherry, cinnamon, custard, grape, honey, lime, loganberry, peach-orange, peach-rum, raspberry, root beer, wild cherry
Barbiturates	Banana-pineapple, banana-vanilla, black currant, cinnamon-peppermint, grenadine-strawberry, lime, orange, peach-orange, root beer
Decongestants and expectorants	Anise, apricot, black currant, butterscotch, cherry, coconut custard, custard mint-strawberry, grenadine-peach, strawberry, lemon, coriander, orange-peach, pineapple, raspberry, strawberry, tangerine
Electrolyte solutions	Cherry, grape, lemon-lime, raspberry, wild cherry, black currant, grenadine-strawberry, lime, Port wine, Sherry wine, root beer, wild strawberry

solution. To this mixture, about 10 mL of a suitable flavoring agent is added. The mixture is transferred to a calibrated container and brought to the final volume with purified water or suitable suspending vehicle. A "shake well" label is attached to the prescription container.

2. **Example 2**
   a. Medication order

Zinc oxide	10 g
Ppt sulfur	10 g
Bentonite	3.6 g
Purified water, a.d.	90 mL
Sig:	Apply t.i.d.

   b. **Compounding procedure.** The powders are reduced to a fine uniform mixture in a mortar. The powders are mixed to form a smooth paste using water and transferred to a calibrated bottle. The final volume is attained with purified water. A "shake well" label is attached to the prescription container.

3. **Example 3**
   a. **Medication order**

Rifampin suspension	20 mg/mL
Disp	120 mL
Sig:	u.d.

   b. **Calculations.** Rifampin: 20 mg/mL × 120 mL = 2400 mg. Rifampin is available in 150-mg and 300-mg capsules. Hence, 8 capsules containing 300 mg of rifampin in each capsule or 16 capsules containing 150 mg of rifampin per capsule are needed.
   c. **Compounding procedure.** The contents of the appropriate number of rifampin capsules are emptied into a mortar and comminuted with a pestle. This powder is levigated with a small amount of 1% methylcellulose solution. Then 20 mL of simple syrup are added and mixed. The mixture is brought to the final volume with simple syrup. "Shake well" and "refrigerate" labels are attached to the prescription container.

V. EMULSIONS

A. **Definition.** Emulsions are **two-phase systems** in which one liquid is dispersed throughout another liquid in the form of small droplets.

B. **General characteristics.** Emulsions can be used externally as lotions and creams or internally to mask the taste of medications.
   1. The two liquids in an emulsion are immiscible and require the use of an emulsifying agent.
   2. Emulsions are classified as either **oil-in-water (o/w)** or **water-in-oil (w/o)**; there can also be multiple emulsions, such as **oil-in-water-in-oil (o/w/o)** and **water-in-oil-in-water (w/o/w)**, as well as emulsion gels, in which the external phase of an oil in water emulsion is thickened with a gelling agent.
   3. Emulsions are **unstable** by nature, and the following steps should be taken to prevent the two phases of an emulsion from separating into two layers after preparation.
      a. The correct **proportions** of oil and water should be used during preparation. The internal phase should represent 40% to 60% of the total volume.
      b. An emulsifying **agent** is needed for emulsion formation.
      c. A **hand homogenizer**, which reduces the size of globules of the internal phase, may be used; if small quantities are compounded, two 60-mL syringes attached with a Luer-Lock adapter can be used and the materials pushed back and forth between the two syringes.
      d. **Preservatives** should be added if the preparation is intended to last longer than a few days. Generally, a combination of methylparaben (0.2%) and propylparaben (0.02%) may be used.
      e. A **"shake well"** label should be placed on the final preparation.
      f. The preparation should be **protected** from light and extreme temperature. Both freezing and heat may have an effect on stability.

C. **Emulsifying agents**
   1. **Gums**, such as acacia or tragacanth, are used to form o/w emulsions. These emulsifying agents are for general use, especially for emulsions intended for internal administration (*Table 4-2*).
      a. Use 1 g of acacia powder for every 4 mL of fixed oil or 1 g to 2 mL for a volatile oil.
      b. If using tragacanth in place of acacia, 0.1 g of tragacanth is used for every 1 g of acacia.

Table 4-2 AGENTS USED IN PRESCRIPTION COMPOUNDING

Ointments	
Oleaginous or hydrocarbon bases	Hydrous emulsion bases (w/o)
Anhydrous	Hydrous
Nonhydrophilic	Will absorb water
Insoluble in water	Insoluble in water
Not water removable (occlusive)	Not water removable (occlusive)
Good vehicles for antibiotics	Examples
Example	Cold cream
Petrolatum	Hydrous lanolin
Absorption bases	Emulsion bases (o/w)
Anhydrous	Hydrous
Will absorb water	Hydrophilic
Insoluble in water	Insoluble in water
Not water removable (occlusive)	Water removable
Examples	Can absorb 30%–50% of weight
Hydrophilic petrolatum	Examples
Lanolin *USP* (anhydrous)	Hydrophilic ointment *USP*
	Acid mantle cream
	Water soluble
	Anhydrous or hydrous
	Soluble in water
	Water removable
	Hydrophilic
	Example
	Polyethylene glycol ointment
Suspending Agents	
Acacia 10%	Methylcellulose 1%–7%
Alginic acid 1%–2%	Sodium alginate 1%–2%
Bentonite 6%	Tragacanth 1%–3%
Carboxymethylcellulose 1%–5%	VEEGUM 6%
Preservatives	
Methylparaben 0.02%–0.2%	Propylparaben 0.01%–0.04%
Emulsifying Agents	
Hydrophilic colloids	Surfactants, nonionic
Acacia	Concentrations used (1%–30%)
Tragacanth	Tweens (e.g., polysorbate 80)
Pectin; favor o/w	Spans
Carboxymethylcellulose	
Methylcellulose	
Proteins	Soaps
Gelatin	Triethanolamine
Egg whites; favor o/w	Stearic acid
Inorganic gels and magmas	Others
Milk of magnesia	Sodium lauryl sulfate
Bentonite; favor o/w	Dioctyl sodium sulfosuccinate
	Cetylpyridinium chloride

o/w, oil-in-water; *w/o*, water-in-oil.

2. **Methylcellulose and carboxymethylcellulose** are used for o/w emulsions. The concentrations of these agents vary, depending on the grade that is used. Methylcellulose is available in several viscosity grades, ranging from 15 to 4000 and designated by a centipoise number, which is a unit of viscosity.
3. **Soaps** can be used to prepare o/w or w/o emulsions for external preparations.
4. **Nonionic emulsifying agents** can be used for o/w and w/o emulsions.

D. **Formation and preparation of emulsions.** The procedure for preparing an emulsion depends on the desired emulsifying agent in the formulation.

1. A **mortar** and **pestle** are frequently all the equipment that is needed.
   a. A mortar with a **rough surface** (e.g., Wedgwood) should be used. This rough surface allows maximal dispersion of globules to produce a fine particle size.
   b. A **rapid motion** is essential when triturating an emulsion using a mortar and pestle.
   c. The mortar should be able to hold at least three times the **quantity** being made. Trituration seldom requires more than 5 mins to create the emulsion.
2. **Electric mixers** and hand homogenizers are useful for producing emulsions after the coarse emulsion is formed in the mortar.
3. The **order** of mixing of ingredients in an emulsion depends on the type of emulsion being prepared (i.e., o/w or w/o) as well as the emulsifying agent chosen. Methods used for compounding include the following:
   a. **Dry gum** (continental) method is used for forming emulsions using natural emulsifying agents and requires a specific order of mixing.
   b. **Wet gum** (English) method is used for forming emulsions using natural emulsifying agents and requires a specific order of mixing.
   c. **Bottle method** is used for forming emulsions using natural emulsifying agents and requires a specific order of mixing.
   d. **Beaker method** is used to prepare emulsions using synthetic emulsifying agents and produces a satisfactory preparation regardless of the order of mixing.
4. **Preservatives.** If the emulsion is kept for an extended period, refrigeration is usually sufficient. The preparation should not be frozen. If a preservative is used, it must be soluble in the water phase to be effective.
5. **Flavoring agents.** If the addition of a flavor is needed to mask the taste of the oil phase, the flavor should be added to the external phase before emulsification (*Table 4-3*).

E. **Examples**

1. **Example 1**
   a. **Medication order**

Mineral oil	18 mL
Acacia	q.s.
Distilled water, q.s. a.d.	90 mL
Sig:	1 tablespoon q.d.

   b. **Compounding procedure.** With the dry gum method, an initial emulsion (primary emulsion) is formed, using four parts (18 mL) of oil, two parts (9 mL) of water, and one part (4.5 g) of powdered acacia. The mineral oil is triturated with the acacia in a Wedgwood mortar. The 9 mL of water is added all at once and, with rapid trituration, form the primary emulsion, which is triturated for about 5 mins. The remaining water is incorporated in small amounts

Table 4-3 FLAVOR SELECTION GUIDE

Taste	Masking Flavor
Salt	Butterscotch, maple
Bitter	Wild cherry, walnut, chocolate mint, licorice
Sweet	Fruit, berry, vanilla
Acid	Citrus

Table 4-4 APPROXIMATE AMOUNT OF POWDER CONTAINED IN CAPSULES

Capsule Size	Range of Powder Capacity (mg)
No. 5	60–130
No. 4	95–260
No. 3	130–390
No. 2	195–520
No. 1	225–650
No. 0	325–910
No. 00	390–1300
No. 000	650–2000

4. Capsules for veterinarians are available in no. 10, no. 11, and no. 12, containing approximately 30, 15, and 7.5 g, respectively.

C. **Preparation of hard and soft capsules**
1. As with the bulk powders, all ingredients are triturated and blended, using geometric dilution.
2. The correct size capsule must be determined by trying different capsule sizes, weighing them, and then choosing the appropriate size.
3. Before filling capsules with the medication, the body and cap of the capsule are separated. Filling is accomplished by using the "punch" method (Alternatively, small capsule machines are commonly used to prepare up to 300 capsules at a time, extemporaneously).
   a. The powder formulation is compressed with a spatula on a pill tile or paper sheet with a uniform depth of approximately half the length of the capsule body.
   b. The empty capsule body is repeatedly pressed into the powder until full.
   c. The capsule is then weighed to ensure an accurate dose. An empty tare capsule of the same size is placed on the pan containing the weights.
4. For a large number of capsules, capsule-filling machines can be used for small-scale use to save time. Most commonly, capsule machines used are capable of preparing 100 to 300 capsules at a time.
5. The capsule is wiped clean of any powder or oil and dispensed in a suitable prescription vial.

D. **Examples**
1. **Example 1**
   a. **Medication order**

      Rifampin 100 mg
      dtd #50
      Sig: 1 cap p.o. q.d.

   b. **Calculations.** Compound this prescription using the commercially available 300-mg capsules as the drug source. Calculate for at least one extra capsule.

$$51 \text{ caps} \times 100 \text{ mg/cap} = 5100 \text{ mg rifampin}$$

$$5100 \text{ mg rifampin} \div 300 \text{ mg/cap} = 17 \text{ caps}$$

   c. **Compounding procedure.** Use 17 rifampin capsules, each containing 300 mg rifampin. The content of each capsule is emptied, and the powder is weighed. The powder equivalent to 100 mg rifampin is placed in a capsule (e.g., if the total contents of one capsule weigh 360 mg; then $100/300 = x/360$; $x = 120$ mg of active drug powder required from the capsule contents to provide 100 mg active drug) and sufficient lactose added to fill the capsule. The total filled capsule contents weigh 200 mg. The weight of the active drug powder is subtracted from 200 mg to obtain the amount of lactose required per capsule, which is 200 mg − 120 mg = 80 mg. This is multiplied by 51 capsules. Enough lactose (51 capsules × 80 mg/

cap = 4.08 g) is added to make a total of 10.2 g of powder. The powders are combined, using geometric dilution, and 50 capsules can be punched out. Each capsule should weigh 200 mg (10.2 g/51 caps).

2. **Example 2**
   a. **Medication order.** This order is for veterinary use only.

Castor oil	8 mL
Disp	12 caps
Sig:	2 caps p.o. h.s.

   b. **Calculations.** No calculations are necessary.
   c. **Compounding procedure.** A no. 11 veterinary capsule is used. Using a calibrated dropper or a pipette, 8 mL of the oil is carefully added to the inside of each capsule body. Next, the lower inside portion of the cap is moistened, using a glass rod or brush. The cap and body are joined together, using a twisting motion, to form a tight seal. The capsules are placed on a piece of filter paper and checked for signs of leakage. The capsules are dispensed in the appropriate size and type of prescription vial. They can be stored in a refrigerator if desired.

VIII. MOLDED TABLETS (TABLET TRITURATES)

A. **Definition.** Tablet triturates are small, usually cylindrical molded or compressed tablets. They are made of powders created by moistening the powder mixture with alcohol and water or by the process of sintering. They can be used for compounding potent drugs in small doses and for preparation of a rapidly disintegrating/dissolving dosage form.

B. **Formulation and preparation of tablet triturates using moistened powders**
   1. Tablet triturates are made in special molds consisting of a pegboard and a corresponding perforated plate.
   2. In addition to the mold, a diluent, usually a mixture of lactose and sucrose (80:20), and a moistening agent, usually a mixture of ethyl alcohol and water (60:40), are required.
   3. The diluent is triturated with the active ingredients.
   4. A paste is then made, using the alcohol and water mixture.
   5. This paste is spread into the mold; the tablets are punched out and remain on the pegs until dry.

C. **Example**
   1. **Medication order**

Atropine sulfate	0.4 mg
Disp	#500 TT
Sig:	u.d.

   2. **Calculations.** For 500 TT: 500×0.4 mg = 200 mg atropine sulfate
   3. **Compounding procedure.** The mold prepares 70-mg tablets. The 200 mg of atropine sulfate, 6.8 g of sucrose, and 28 g of lactose are weighed and mixed by geometric dilution. The powder is wet with a mixture of 40% purified water and 60% ethyl alcohol (95%). The paste that is formed is spread onto the tablet triturate mold; the tablets are then punched out of the mold and allowed to dry on the pegs. This procedure is repeated until the required number of tablet triturates has been prepared.

D. **Formulation and preparation of tablet triturates using sintering**
   1. These tablet triturates are made in special molds consisting of materials that can tolerate heat to about 100°C.
   2. In addition to the mold, a diluent, usually a mixture of active drug and diluent, which make up approximately 65% of the tablet weight, are blended together. Mannitol is good to use in combination with lactose for particle sizes of 60 to 80 mesh fraction.
   3. The mixture is triturated with polyethylene glycol 3350 with a particle size of 80 to 100 mesh fraction.
   4. The powder mixture is placed into appropriate molds and lightly tamped.
   5. The molds containing the powder are placed in an oven at about 90°C for 10 to 20 mins, removed, and allowed to cool. Depending on the molds used, the tablets can be dispensed in the molds or removed from the molds and packaged and labeled.

E. **Example**

1. **Medication order**

Homatropine hydrobromide	300 mg
Mannitol	3.5 g
Lactose	3.47 g
Flavor (dry powder type)	q.s.
Polyethylene glycol 3350	3.5 g

2. **Calculations.** As presented, this formula is for 100 rapid-dissolving tablet triturates.
3. **Compounding procedure.** Blend the homatropine hydrobromide, mannitol, lactose, and dry flavor together until fine and uniformly mixed. Separately, reduce the particle size of the polyethylene glycol 3350 to 100 to 200 mesh fraction. Lightly blend in the polyethylene glycol 3350 into the previously blended powders. Place 100 mg of the powder into the cavities of a mold (some blister packs work well; otherwise, obtain a tablet triturate mold or a special mold for preparing these tablets). Place the mold containing the powder in an oven at 80° to 90°C for 15 to 20 mins. The time depends on the mold, formulation, oven, etc. Remove from the oven and place in a refrigerator for approximately 5 mins. Remove from the refrigerator and let set at room temperature. Package and label.

IX. OINTMENTS, CREAMS, PASTES, AND GELS

A. **Definitions**

1. **Ointments**, **creams**, and **pastes** are semisolid dosage forms intended for topical application to the skin or mucous membranes. **Ointments** are characterized as being oleaginous in nature; **creams** are generally o/w or w/o emulsions, and **pastes** are characterized by their high content of solids (about 25%).
2. Gels (sometimes called jellies) are semisolid systems consisting of suspensions made up of either small inorganic particles or large organic molecules interpenetrated by a liquid.

B. **General characteristics.** These dosage forms are semisolid preparations generally applied externally. Semisolid dosage forms may contain active drugs intended to

1. act solely on the surface of the skin to produce a local effect (e.g., antifungal agent, topicals);
2. release the medication, which, in turn, penetrates into the skin (e.g., hydrocortisone cream); and
3. release medication for systemic absorption through the skin (e.g., nitroglycerin, transdermals).

C. **Types of ointment bases**

1. Hydrophobic bases feel greasy and contain mixtures of fats, oils, and waxes. Hydrophobic bases cannot be washed off using water.
2. Hydrophilic bases are usually emulsion bases. The o/w-type emulsion bases can be easily washed off with water, but the w/o type is slightly more difficult to remove.

D. **Preparation of ointments, creams, pastes, and gels**

1. Mixing can be done in a mortar or on an ointment slab or tile or using an ointment mill.
2. Liquids are incorporated by gradually adding them to an absorption-type base and mixing.
3. Insoluble powders are reduced to a fine powder and then added to the base, using geometric dilution.
4. Water-soluble substances are dissolved with water and then incorporated into the base.
5. The final preparation should be smooth (impalpable) and free of any abrasive particles.

E. **Examples**

1. **Example 1**

a. **Medication order**

Sulfur	
Salicylic acid, a.a.	600 mg
White petrolatum, a.d.	30 g
Sig:	Apply t.i.d.

b. **Compounding procedure.** The particle sizes of the sulfur and salicylic acid are reduced separately in a Wedgwood mortar and then blended together. Using a pill tile, the powder mixture is levigated with the base. Using geometric dilution, the base and powders are blended to the final weight. An ointment jar or plastic tube is used for dispensing, and an "external use only" label is placed on the container.

c. **Alternate method.** Suppose you have sulfur 5% in white petrolatum ointment and a salicylic acid 5% ointment. **How can you prepare the prescription using these and diluting with white petrolatum?**

However, since we are using two different 5% ointments, two parts of each, this leaves one part for the white petrolatum. A total of five parts is to be used to make 30 g (6 g per part): two parts (12 g) of the sulfur 5%, two parts (12 g) of the salicylic acid 5%, and one part (6 g) of the white petrolatum could be used. To check:

$$12\text{ g} \times 0.05 = 600\text{ mg of sulfur}$$

$$12\text{ g} \times 0.05 = 600\text{ mg of salicylic acid}$$

$$12\text{ g} + 12\text{ g} + 6\text{ g} = 30\text{ g}$$

2. **Example 2**

a. **Medication order**

Methylparaben	0.25 g
Propylparaben	0.15 g
Sodium lauryl sulfate	10 g
Propylene glycol	120 g
Stearyl alcohol	250 g
White petrolatum	250 g
Purified water	370 g
Disp	60 g
Sig:	Apply u.d.

b. **Calculations.** The quantity of each ingredient required to prepare 60 g is obtained as follows. The medication order is for 1000 g; therefore, the multiplication factor is 60/1000 = 0.06.

$$0.25\text{ g} \times 0.06 = 0.15\text{ g methylparaben}$$
$$0.15\text{ g} \times 0.06 = 0.009\text{ g propylparaben}$$
$$10\text{ g} \times 0.06 = 0.6\text{ g sodium lauryl sulfate}$$
$$120\text{ g} \times 0.06 = 7.2\text{ g propylene glycol}$$
$$250\text{ g} \times 0.06 = 15\text{ g stearyl alcohol}$$
$$250\text{ g} \times 0.06 = 15\text{ g white petrolatum}$$
$$370\text{ g} \times 0.06 = 22.2\text{ g purified water}$$

Since the 0.009 g of propylparaben is too small to accurately weigh, a dilution can be prepared as follows, assuming a minimum weighable quantity of 120 mg. Weigh 120 mg of propylparaben and add to 40 mL of propylene glycol, resulting in a propylparaben concentration of 3 mg/mL. Take 3 mL of this solution to obtain the propylparaben and subtract the 3 mL from the quantity of propylene glycol required in the formula.

c. **Compounding procedure.** The stearyl alcohol and the white petrolatum are melted on a steam bath and heated to about 75°C. The other ingredients, previously dissolved in purified water at about 78°C, are added. The mixture is stirred until it congeals. An ointment jar is used for dispensing, and an "external use only" label is placed on the jar.

3. **Example 3**

a. **Medication order**

Scopolamine hydrobromide	0.25%
Soy lecithin	12 g
Isopropyl palmitate	12 g
Pluronic F-127 20% gel, q.s.	100 mL
Sig:	Apply 0.1 mL t.i.d.

b. **Calculations.** The quantity of scopolamine hydrobromide required for the prescription will be

$$0.0025 \times 100\text{ mL} = 0.25\text{ g or }250\text{ mg}$$

c. **Compounding procedure.** Mix the soy lecithin with the isopropyl palmitate. Dissolve the scopolamine hydrobromide in about 3 mL of purified water and add to about 70 mL of the Pluronic F-127 gel. Add the soy lecithin–isopropyl palmitate mixture, and mix well. Add sufficient Pluronic F-127 gel to volume and mix well using a shearing technique. Package and label.

X. SUPPOSITORIES

A. **General characteristics**

1. Suppositories are **solid bodies** of various weights and shapes, adapted for introduction into the rectal, vaginal, or urethral orifices of the human body. They are used to deliver drugs for their local or systemic effects.
2. Suppositories differ in **size** and **shape** and include
   a. rectal,
   b. vaginal, and
   c. urethral.

B. **Common suppository bases**

1. **Cocoa butter** (theobroma oil), which melts at body temperature, is a fat-soluble mixture of triglycerides that is most often used for rectal suppositories. Witepsol is a synthetic triglyceride. Fatty acid bases include Fattibase.
2. **Polyethylene glycol** (PEG, carbowax) derivatives are water-soluble bases suitable for vaginal and rectal suppositories. Polybase is an example.
3. **Glycerinated gelatin** is a water-miscible base often used in vaginal and rectal suppositories.

C. **Suppository molds**

1. Suppository molds can be made of rubber, plastic, brass, stainless steel, or other suitable material.
2. The formulation and volume of the base depend on the size of the mold used, less the displacement caused by the active ingredient.

D. **Methods of preparing and dispensing suppositories**

1. **Molded suppositories** are prepared by first melting the base and then incorporating the medications uniformly into the base. This mixture is then poured into the suppository mold (fusion method).
2. **Hand-rolled suppositories** require a special technique. With proper technique, it is possible to make a preparation equal in quality to the molded suppositories.
3. **Containers for the suppositories** are determined by the method and base used in preparation. Hand-rolled and molded suppositories should be dispensed in special boxes that prevent the suppositories from coming in contact with each other. Suppositories made using plastic strip molds are easily dispensed in various types of packages.
4. **Storage conditions.** If appropriate, a "refrigerate" label should appear on the container. Regardless of the base or medication used in the formulation, the patient should be instructed to store the suppositories in a cool, dry place.

E. **Examples**

1. **Example 1**
   a. **Medication order**

Naproxen suppository	500 mg
Disp	#12
Sig:	Insert u.d. into rectum

   b. **Calculations.** Each standard adult suppository should weigh 2 g, but it depends on the mold used and should be calibrated before compounding. Also, the displacement must be determined for the added powder.

2 g (total weight) − 0.540 g (weight of base displaced by the 500-mg tablet) per suppository

= 1.46 g cocoa butter per suppository × 13 suppositories
= 18.98 g cocoa butter

   c. **Compounding procedure.** The 13 naproxen 500-mg tablets are triturated to a fine powder, using a Wedgwood or porcelain mortar. The 18.98 g cocoa butter base is melted in a beaker, using a water bath. The temperature of the water bath should not exceed 36°C. The powder is then added and stirred until mixed. The mixture is poured into an appropriate rectal suppository mold (about 2 g per suppository) and placed into a refrigerator until the suppositories congeal. Any excess is scraped from the top of the mold, and a suppository box is used for dispensing. A "refrigerate" label is placed on the box.

2. **Example 2**
   a. **Medication order**

Progesterone	50 mg
Disp	#14
Sig:	1 per vagina once daily on days 14 to 28 of cycle

   b. **Calculations.** Total weight of each vaginal suppository is 1.9 g. Assuming 50 mg progesterone displaces 50 mg PEG base:
      50 mg progesterone/suppository × 15 = 750 mg progesterone
      1.9 g (total weight) − 0.050 g progesterone
      = 1.85 g PEG × 15 suppositories
      = 27.75 g PEG total
   c. **Compounding procedure.** The PEG is melted to 55° to 57°C, and 750 mg progesterone is added. This mixture is poured into a vaginal suppository mold, allowed to cool, cleaned, and dispensed.

XI. STERILE PREPARATIONS

A. **General requirements.** The extemporaneous compounding of sterile preparations occurs in many pharmacy environments, including community, home health care, hospital, and nuclear. Minimum requirements include
   1. proper equipment and supplies;
   2. proper facilities, including a laminar-flow clean bench and a clean room or isolation barrier technology equipment;
   3. proper documentation of all preparations made;
   4. quality control, including batch sterility testing;
   5. proper storage both at the facility and in transport to the patient's home;
   6. proper labeling of the prescription preparation;
   7. knowledge of product's/preparation's stability and incompatibilities; and
   8. knowledge of all ancillary equipment involved in compounding or delivery of the medications.

B. **Compounding of parenteral preparations**
   1. Compounding of sterile preparations, including intravenous admixtures, requires special skills and training. Compounding parenteral preparations or providing this service without proper training should not be attempted.
   2. These preparations must be compounded in a clean environment, using aseptic technique (i.e., working under controlled conditions to minimize contamination).
   3. Dry powders of parenteral drugs for reconstitution are used for drug products or preparations that are unstable as solutions. It is important to know the correct diluents that can be used to yield a solution.
   4. Solutions of drugs for parenteral administration may also be further diluted before administration. If further dilution is required, then the pharmacist must know the stability and compatibility of the drug in the diluent.

C. **Reconstitution of a dry powder from a vial**
   1. Work takes place in a clean-air environment, observing aseptic technique.
   2. The manufacturer's instructions should be checked to determine the required volume of diluent.
   3. The appropriate needle size and syringe are chosen, keeping in mind that the capacity of the syringe should be slightly larger than the volume required for reconstitution.
   4. Using the correct diluent, the surface of the container is cleaned, using an alcohol prep pad, after which the alcohol is permitted to evaporate.
   5. The syringe is filled with the diluent to the proper volume.
   6. The surface of the vial containing the sterile powder is cleaned, using an alcohol prep pad, after which it is permitted to dry. The diluent is injected into the vial containing the dry powder.
   7. The vial is gently shaken or rolled, and the powder is allowed to dissolve.
   8. After the powder has dissolved, the vial is inverted, and the desired volume is withdrawn.

Study Questions

Directions for questions 1–3: Each question or incomplete statement in this section can be correctly answered or completed by **one** of the suggested answers or phrases. Choose the **best** answer.

The following medication order is given to the pharmacist by the physician.

Olive oil	60 mL
Vitamin A	60,000 U
Water	120 mL
Sig:	15 mL t.i.d.

1. The final dosage form of this prescription will be

(A) a solution.
(B) an elixir.
(C) an emulsion.
(D) a suspension.
(E) a lotion.

2. When preparing this prescription, the pharmacist needs to add

(A) Tween 80.
(B) acacia.
(C) glycerin.
(D) alcohol.
(E) propylene glycol.

3. Which of the following caution labels should the pharmacist affix to the container when dispensing this preparation?

(A) Do not refrigerate.
(B) Shake well.
(C) For external use only.
(D) No preservatives added.

Directions for questions 4–9: Each question or statement in this section can be correctly answered or completed by one or more of the suggested answers or phrases. Choose the correct answer, A–E:

A if **I** only is correct
B if **III** only is correct
C if **I** and **II** are correct
D if **II** and **III** are correct
E if **I, II,** and **III** are correct

4. Which statements about the following prescription are correct?

Morphine	1 mg/mL
Flavored vehicle, q.s. a.d.	120 mL
Sig:	5 to 20 mg p.o. q 3 to 4 hrs p.r.n. pain

I. The amount of morphine needed is 240 mg.
II. Powdered morphine alkaloid should be used when compounding this prescription.
III. The final dosage form of this prescription is a solution.

5. When preparing the following prescription, the pharmacist should

Podophyllum	5%
Salicylic acid	10%
Acetone	20%
Flexible collodion, a.d.	30 mL
Sig:	Apply q h.s.

I. triturate 1.5 g of podophyllum with the 8 mL of acetone.
II. add 3 g of salicylic acid to the collodion with trituration.
III. affix an "external use only" label to the container.

6. Which statements about the following prescription are correct?

Sulfur	6 g
Purified water	
Camphor water, a.a. q.s. a.d.	60

I. Precipitated sulfur can be used to prepare this prescription.
II. The sulfur can be triturated with glycerin before mixing with other ingredients.
III. A "shake well" label should be affixed to the bottle.

7. Which statements about the following prescription are correct?

Starch	10%
Menthol	1%
Camphor	2%
Calamine, q.s. a.d.	120

I. The powders should be blended together in a mortar, using geometric dilution.
II. The prescription should be prepared by dissolving the camphor in a sufficient amount of 90% alcohol.
III. A eutectic mixture should be avoided.

8. When preparing the following prescription, the pharmacist should

Salicylic acid	3 g
Sulfur ppt	7 g
Lanolin	10 g
White petrolatum	10 g

I. reduce the particle size of the powders, using a mortar and pestle or using the pill tile with a spatula.

II. place on an ointment tile and levigate the ingredients, using geometric dilution.

III. package the ointment in an ointment jar or tube.

9. An equal volume of air is injected when removing drug solutions from

I. vials.
II. ampules.
III. syringes.

Answers and Explanations

1. The answer is C *[see V.B.1.]*.

2. The answer is B *[see V.B.2; V.C.1]*.

3. The answer is B *[see V.B.3]*.
For 1–3: Because olive oil and water are two immiscible liquids, their incorporation requires a two-phase system in which one liquid is dispersed throughout another liquid in the form of small droplets. To accomplish this, an emulsifying agent is necessary. Acacia is the most suitable emulsifying agent when forming an oil-in-water emulsion that is intended for internal use. Emulsions are physically unstable, and they must be protected against the effects of microbial contamination and physical separation. Shaking before use redistributes the two layers of emulsion. Because light, air, and microorganisms also affect the stability of an emulsion, preservatives can be added.

4. The answer is B (III) *[see III.C.3]*.
The concentration of morphine needed for the prescription described in the question is 1 mg/mL, and because 120 mL is the final volume, 120 mg of morphine is needed to compound this prescription. Morphine alkaloid has poor solubility; therefore, one of the salt forms should be used. Because morphine is dissolved in the vehicle, resulting in a liquid preparation, the final dosage form is a solution.

5. The answer is B (III) *[see III.C.1; III.C.5; III.D.3]*.
Calculating for the amount of each ingredient of the prescription in the question requires 1.5 g of podophyllum, 3 g of salicylic acid, and 6 mL of acetone. The correct procedure would be to triturate the podophyllum with the acetone, then add the triturated salicylic acid to a calibrated bottle containing the podophyllum and acetone. Flexible collodion is then added up to the 30-mL calibration. An "external use only" label should be affixed to the container.

6. The answer is E (I, II, and III) *[see IV.B.2; IV.C.5; IV.D.1–2]*.
Although precipitated sulfur can be used to prepare the prescription described in the question, it is difficult to triturate; therefore, it must first be levigated with a suitable levigating agent (e.g., glycerin). All suspensions, owing to their instability, require shaking before use to redistribute the insoluble ingredients.

7. The answer is A (I) *[see VI.C.3; VI.D.1]*.
The proper procedure for compounding the prescription described in the question is to first form a liquid eutectic. This is done by triturating the menthol and camphor together in a mortar. This eutectic is then blended with the powdered starch and calamine, using geometric dilution.

8. The answer is E (I, II, and III) *[see IX.D.1–3; IX.E.1]*.
The proper procedure for preparing the prescription given in the question is to reduce the particle size of each powder and mix them together, using geometric dilution. This ensures the proper blending of the powders. Next, this powdered mixture is incorporated, geometrically, with the petrolatum. Then, the lanolin is added geometrically.

9. The answer is A (I) *[see XI.E.2]*.
An equal volume of air must be injected when removing a drug solution from a vial. This is done to prevent the formation of a vacuum within the vial. This problem does not occur with ampules and syringes containing drug solutions; therefore, it is unnecessary to inject any air when removing them.

5 Basic Pharmacokinetics

ELISE DUNZO, LEON SHARGEL

I. PHARMACOKINETICS

A. **Introduction**

1. **Pharmacokinetics** is the quantitative measurement of drug absorption, distribution, and elimination (i.e., excretion and metabolism) and includes the rate processes for drug movement into the body, within the body, and out of the body.
2. Commonly used units in pharmacokinetics are tabulated in *Table 5-1*.
3. **Rates and orders of reactions.** The **rate** of a chemical reaction or pharmacokinetic process is the velocity with which it occurs. **The order** of a reaction is the way in which the concentration of a drug or reactant in a chemical reaction affects the rate.
   a. **Zero-order reaction.** The drug concentration changes with respect to time at a constant rate, according to the following equation:

$$\frac{dC}{dt} = -k_0$$

Table 5-1 COMMON UNITS IN PHARMACOKINETICS

Pharmacokinetic Parameter	Abbreviation	Fundamental Units	Units Example
Area under the curve	AUC	Concentration × time	μg × hr/mL
Total body clearance	Cl_T	Volume/time	L/hr
Renal clearance	Cl_R	Volume/time	L/hr
Hepatic clearance	Cl_H	Volume/time	L/hr
Apparent volume of distribution	V_D	Volume	L
Volume of distribution at steady state	V_{ss}	Volume	L
Peak plasma drug concentration	C_{max}	Concentration	mg/L
Plasma drug concentration	C_p	Concentration	mg/L
Steady-state drug concentration	C_{ss} or C_{av}	Concentration	mg/L
Time for peak drug concentration	T_{max}	Time	hr
Dose	D_0	Mass	mg
Loading dose	D_L	Mass	mg
Maintenance dose	D_M	Mass	mg
Amount of drug in the body	D_B	Mass	mg
Rate of drug infusion	R	Mass/time	mg/hr
First-order rate constant for drug absorption	k_A	1/time	1/hr or hr^{-1}
Zero-order rate constant for drug absorption	k_0	Mass/time	mg/hr
First-order rate constant for drug elimination	k (sometimes referred to as kel)	1/time	1/hr or hr^{-1}
Elimination half-life	$t_{1/2}$	Time	hr
Fraction of drug absorbed	F	(no units)	Ranges from 0 to 1 (0%–100%)

where C is the drug concentration and k_0 is the **zero-order rate constant** expressed in units of concentration per time (e.g., milligrams per milliliter per hour). Integration of this equation yields the linear (straight-line) equation:

$$C = -k_0 t + C_0$$

where k_0 is the slope of the line (see *Figure 2-6*) and C_0 is the y intercept, or drug concentration, when time (t) equals zero. The negative sign indicates that the slope is decreasing.

b. **First-order reaction.** The change in drug concentration with respect to time equals the product of the rate constant and the concentration of drug remaining, according to the following equation:

$$\frac{dC}{dt} = -kC$$

where k is the first-order rate constant, expressed in units of reciprocal time, or time^{-1} (e.g., 1/hr or hr^{-1}).

(1) Integration and subsequent transformation of this equation yields the following mathematically equivalent equations:

$$C = C_0 e^{-kt}$$

$$\ln C = -kt + \ln C_0$$

$$\log C = \frac{-kt}{2.3} + \log C_0$$

(2) A graph of the equation in *Figure 5-1* shows the linear relation of the log of the concentration versus time. In *Figure 5-1*, the slope of the line is equal to $-k/2.3$, and the y intercept is C_0. The values for C are plotted on logarithmic coordinates, and the values for t are shown on linear coordinates.

(3) The **half-life** ($t_{1/2}$) of a reaction or process is the time required for the concentration of a drug to decrease by one-half. For a first-order reaction or process, the half-life is a constant and is related to the first-order rate constant, according to the following equation:

$$t_{1/2} = \frac{0.693}{k}$$

4. **Models and compartments**
   a. A **model** is a mathematic description of a biologic system and is used to express quantitative relationships.
   b. A **compartment** is a group of tissues with similar blood flow and drug affinity. A compartment is not a real physiologic or anatomic region.
5. **Drug distribution**
   a. Drugs distribute rapidly to tissues with high blood flow (e.g., liver) and more slowly to tissues with low blood flow (e.g., adipose).
   b. Drugs rapidly cross capillary membranes into tissues because of **passive diffusion** and **hydrostatic pressure. Drug permeability** across capillary membranes varies.
      (1) Drugs easily cross the capillaries of the glomerulus of the kidney and the sinusoids of the liver.
      (2) The capillaries of the brain are surrounded by glial cells that create a **blood–brain barrier**, which acts as a thick lipid membrane. Polar and ionic hydrophilic drugs cross this barrier slowly.
      (3) In disease states, membranes may become more permeable to drugs. For example, in meningitis, the blood–brain barrier becomes more permeable to the penetration of drugs into the brain.
   c. **Drugs may accumulate in tissues** as a result of their physicochemical characteristics or special affinity of the tissue for the drug.
      (1) Lipid-soluble drugs may accumulate in adipose (fat) tissue because of partitioning of the drug.
      (2) Tetracycline may accumulate in bone because complexes are formed with calcium.

d. Plasma protein binding of drugs affects drug distribution.

(1) A drug bound to a protein forms a complex that is too large to cross cell membranes.

(2) **Albumin** is the major plasma protein involved in drug protein binding. **α_1-Glycoprotein,** also found in plasma, is important for the binding of such basic drugs as propranolol.

(3) Potent drugs, such as phenytoin, that are highly bound (> 95%) to plasma proteins may be displaced by other highly bound drugs. The displacement of the bound drug results in more free (nonbound) drug, which rapidly reaches the drug receptors and may cause a more intense pharmacologic response.

(4) A few hormonal drugs bind to specific plasma proteins. For example, prednisone binding to transcortin (and albumin) results in dose-dependent pharmacokinetics of prednisone. This nonlinear pharmacokinetics is due to saturable protein binding. Transcortin has high affinity and low capacity, whereas albumin has low affinity and high capacity.

B. One-compartment model

1. Intravenous bolus injection. The entire drug dose enters the body instantaneously, and the rate of absorption is therefore assumed to be negligible in calculations (*Figure 5-1*). The entire body acts as a single compartment, and the drug rapidly equilibrates with all of the tissues in the body.

a. Drug elimination is generally a first-order kinetic process according to the equations in I.A.3.b.

(1) The first-order elimination rate constant (k or k_{el}) is the sum of the rate constants for removal of drug from the body, including the rate constants for renal excretion and metabolism (**biotransformation**) as described by the following equation:

$$k = k_e + k_m$$

where k_e is the rate constant for renal excretion and k_m is the rate constant for metabolism. This equation assumes that all rates are first-order processes.

(2) The **elimination half-life ($t_{1/2}$)** is given by the following equation:

$$t_{1/2} = \frac{0.693}{k}$$

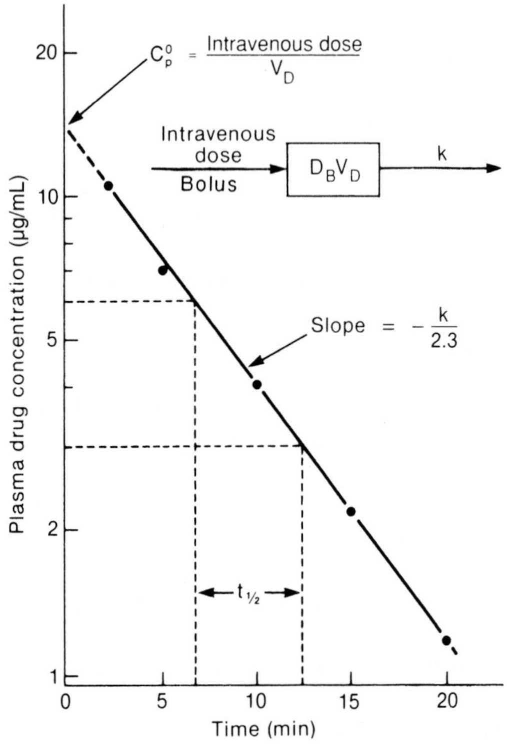

Figure 5-1. Generalized pharmacokinetic model for a drug administered by rapid intravenous bolus injection. C_p^0, extrapolated drug concentration; V_D, apparent volume of distribution; D_B, amount of drug in the body; k, elimination rate constant; $t_{1/2}$, elimination half-life. Adapted with permission from Gibaldi M, Perrier D. *Pharmacokinetics*. 2nd ed. New York, NY: Marcel Dekker, Inc.; 1982. Copyright © 1982 Routledge/Taylor & Francis Group, LLC.

b. **Apparent volume of distribution** (V_D) is the hypothetical volume of body fluid in which the drug is dissolved. This value is not a true anatomic or physical volume.

(1) V_D is needed to estimate the amount of drug in the body relative to the concentration of drug in the plasma, as shown in the following:

$$V_D \times C_p = D_B$$

where V_D (liters) is the apparent volume of distribution, C_p (milligrams per liter) is the plasma drug concentration, and D_B (milligram) is the amount of drug in the body.

(2) To calculate the V_D after an intravenous bolus injection, the equation is rearranged to give:

$$V_D = \frac{D_B^0}{C_P^0}$$

where D_B^0 is the dose (D_B) of drug given by intravenous bolus and C_P^0 is the extrapolated drug concentration at zero time on the *y* axis, after the drug equilibrates (*Figure 5-1*).

(3) According to the equation, V_D is increased and C_P^0 is decreased when the drug is distributed more extravascularly into the tissues. When more drug is contained in the vascular space or plasma, C_P^0 is increased and V_D is decreased.

2. **Single oral dose.** If the drug is given in an oral dosage form (e.g., tablet, capsule), the drug is generally absorbed by first-order kinetics. Elimination of the drug also follows the principles of first-order kinetics (*Figure 5-2*).

a. The following equation describes the pharmacokinetics of **first-order absorption and elimination**:

$$C_P = \frac{FD_0k_A}{V_D(k_A - k)}(e^{-kt} - e^{-K_At})$$

where k_A is the first-order absorption rate constant and *F* is the fraction of drug bioavailable. Changes in *F*, D_0, V_D, k_A, and *k* affect the plasma drug concentration.

b. The time for maximum, or **peak, drug absorption** is given by the following equations:

$$t_{max} = \frac{2.3 \log (k_A/k)}{k_A - k}$$

where t_{max} depends only on the rate constants k_A and *k*, not on *F*, D_0, or V_D.

c. After t_{max} is obtained, the peak drug concentration (C_{max}) is calculated, using the equation in I.B.2.a and substituting t_{max} for *t*.

d. The area under the curve (AUC) may be determined by integration of $\int_0^t C_P \, dt$ using the trapezoidal rule or by the following equation:

$$[AUC]_0^\infty = \int_0^\infty C_P \, dt = \frac{FD_0}{V_Dk}$$

changes in *F*, D_0, *k*, and V_D affect the AUC. Minor changes in k_A do not affect the AUC.

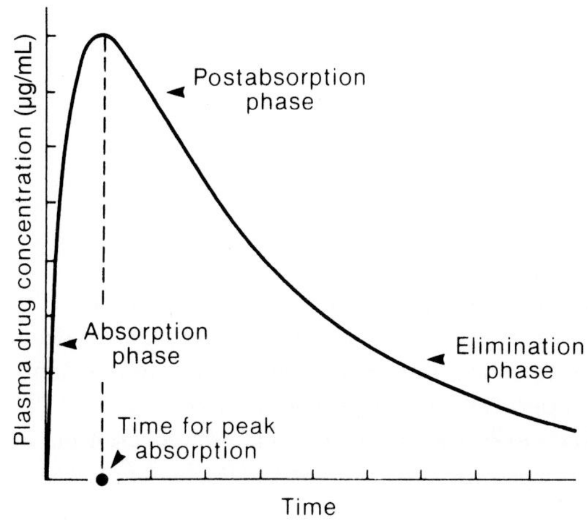

Figure 5-2. Generalized plot for a one-compartment model showing first-order drug absorption and first-order drug elimination. Adapted with permission from Shargel L, Wu-Pong S, Yu ABC. *Applied Biopharmaceutics and Pharmacokinetics*. 5th ed. New York, NY: McGraw-Hill; 2005.

e. To obtain $[AUC]_0^\infty$, obtain the [AUC] from 0 to t by the trapezoidal rule and add on the extrapolated section of AUC, which is the last measurable drug concentration at time, t, divided by the slope of the terminal elimination curve, as shown in the following equation:

$$[AUC]_0^\infty = [AUC]_0^t + \frac{C_{P,t}}{k}$$

f. **Lag time** occurs at the beginning of systemic drug absorption. For some individuals, systemic drug absorption is delayed after oral drug administration because of delayed stomach emptying or other factors.

3. Intravenous infusion

a. Intravenous infusion is an example of zero-order absorption and first-order elimination (*Figure 5-3*).

b. A few oral controlled-release drug products release the drug by zero-order kinetics and have **zero-order systemic absorption.**

c. The plasma drug concentration at any time after the start of an intravenous infusion is given by the following equation:

$$C_P = \frac{R}{V_D k}(1 - e^{-kt})$$

where R is the zero-order rate of infusion given in units as milligrams per hour or milligrams per minute.

d. If the intravenous infusion is discontinued, the plasma drug concentration declines by a first-order process. The elimination half-life or elimination rate constant, k, may be obtained from the declining plasma drug concentration versus time curve.

e. As the drug is infused, the plasma drug concentration increases to a plateau, or **steady-state concentration** (**C_{SS}**).

(1) Under steady-state conditions, the fraction of drug absorbed equals the fraction of drug eliminated from the body.

(2) The plasma concentration at steady state (C_{ss}) is given by the following equation:

$$C_{ss} = \frac{R}{V_D k} = \frac{R}{Cl_T}$$

where Cl_T is total body clearance (see section I.E.).

(3) The rate of drug infusion (R) may be calculated from a rearrangement of the equation if the desired C_{ss}, the V_D, and the k are known. These values can often be obtained from the drug literature. To calculate the rate of infusion, the following equation is used:

$$R = C_{ss} V_D k = C_{ss} Cl_T$$

where C_{ss} is the desired (target) plasma drug concentration and Cl_T is total body clearance.

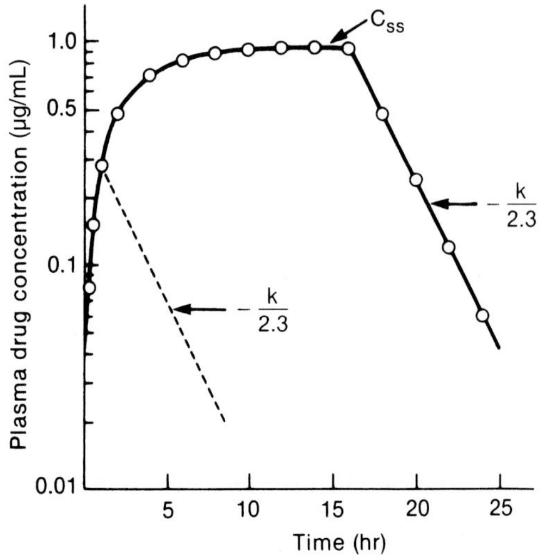

Figure 5-3. Generalized semilogarithmic plot for a drug showing zero-order absorption and first-order elimination. C_{ss}, steady-state concentration; k, elimination rate constant. Adapted with permission from Gibaldi M, Perrier D. *Pharmacokinetics*. 2nd ed. New York, NY: Marcel Dekker, Inc.; 1982. Copyright © 1982 Routledge/Taylor & Francis Group, LLC.

f. A **loading dose (D_L)** is given as an initial intravenous bolus dose to produce the C_{ss} as rapidly as possible. The intravenous infusion is started at the same time as the D_L.

(1) The time to reach C_{ss} depends on the elimination half-life of the drug. Reaching 90%, 95%, or 99% of the C_{ss} without a D_L takes 3.32, 4.32, or 6.65 half-lives, respectively. Thus, for a drug with an elimination $t_{½}$ of 8 hrs, it will take 3.32 × 8 hrs, or 26.56 hrs, to reach 90% of C_{ss} if no loading dose is given.

(2) The D_L is the amount of drug that, when dissolved in the apparent V_D, produces the desired C_{ss}. Thus, D_L is calculated by the following equation:

$$D_L = C_{ss} V_D \text{ and } D_L = \frac{R}{k}$$

g. An intravenous infusion provides a relatively constant plasma drug concentration and is particularly useful for drugs that have a narrow therapeutic range. The IV infusion keeps the plasma drug concentration between the *minimum toxic concentration* (MTC) and the *minimum effective concentration* (MEC).

4. **Intermittent intravenous infusions**

a. Intermittent intravenous infusions are infusions in which the drug is infused for short periods to prevent accumulation and toxicity.

b. Intermittent intravenous infusions are used for a few drugs, such as the aminoglycosides. For example, gentamicin may be given as a 1-hr infusion every 12 hrs. In this case, steady-state drug concentrations are not achieved.

c. The peak drug concentration in the plasma for a drug given by intermittent intravenous infusion may be calculated by the following equation:

$$C_{p,\,n} = \frac{R(1 - e^{-kt})(1 - e^{-nk\tau})}{Cl(1 - e^{-k\tau})}$$

where $C_{p,n}$ is the peak drug concentration, R is the rate of drug infusion, Cl is total body clearance, k is the dosage interval, n is the number of infusions, t is the time for the infusion, and τ is the dosage interval.

5. **Multiple doses**. Many drugs are given intermittently in a multiple-dose regimen for continuous or prolonged therapeutic activity. This regimen is often used to treat chronic disease.

a. If drug doses are given frequently before the previous dose is completely eliminated, then plasma drug concentrations accumulate and increase to a steady-state level.

b. At **steady state**, plasma drug concentration fluctuates between a maximum $(C^{\infty}_{\min})$ and a minimum $(C^{\infty}_{\min})$ value (*Figure 5-4*).

c. When a multiple-dose regimen is calculated, the **superposition principle** assumes that previous drug doses have no effect on subsequent doses. Thus, the predicted plasma drug

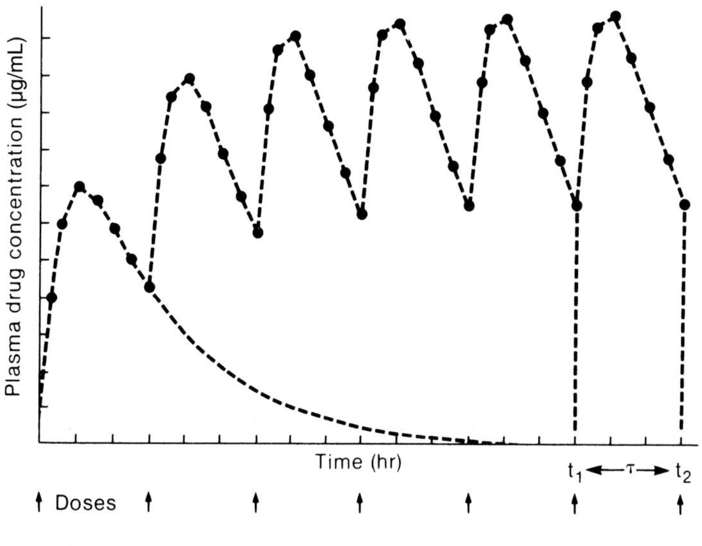

Figure 5-4. Generalized plot showing plasma drug concentration levels after administration of multiple doses and levels of accumulation when equal doses are given at equal time intervals. τ, time interval between doses (*t*), or the frequency of dosing. Adapted with permission from Shargel L, Wu-Pong S, Yu ABC. *Applied Biopharmaceutics and Pharmacokinetics*. 5th ed. New York, NY: McGraw-Hill; 2005.

concentration is the total plasma drug concentration obtained by adding the residual drug concentrations found after each previous dose.

d. When a multiple-dose regimen is designed, only the **dosing rate** (D_0/τ) can be adjusted easily.

(1) The dosing rate is based on the **size of the dose** (D_0) and the **interval** (τ) **between doses**, or the **frequency of dosing**.

(2) The dosing rate is given by the following equation:

$$\text{Dosing rate} = \frac{D_0}{\tau}$$

(3) As long as the dosing rate is the same, the expected **average drug concentration at steady state** $\left(C^{\infty}_{min}\right)$ is the same (*Figure 5-4*).

(a) For example, if a 600-mg dose is given every 12 hrs, the dosing rate is 600 mg/12 hrs, or 50 mg/hr.

(b) A dose of 300 mg every 6 hrs or 200 mg every 4 hrs also gives the same dosing rate (50 mg/hr), with the same expected C^{∞}_{Av}. However, the C^{∞}_{max} and C^{∞}_{min} values will be different.

(c) For a larger dose given over a longer interval (e.g., 600 mg every 12 hrs), the C^{∞}_{max} is higher and the C^{∞}_{min} is lower compared with a smaller dose given more frequently (e.g., 200 mg every 4 hrs).

e. Certain antibiotics are given by **multiple rapid intravenous bolus injections.**

(1) The peak, or **maximum, serum drug concentration** at steady state may be estimated by the following equation:

$$C^{\infty}_{max} = \frac{\dfrac{D_0}{V_D}}{1 - e^{-k\tau}}$$

(2) The **minimum serum drug concentration** $\left(C^{\infty}_{min}\right)$ at steady state is the drug concentration after the drug declines one dosage interval. Thus, C^{∞}_{min} is determined by the following equation:

$$C^{\infty}_{min} = C^{\infty}_{min}\, e^{-k\tau}$$

(3) The **average drug concentration** $\left(C^{\infty}_{Av}\right)$ at steady state is estimated with the equation used for multiple oral doses:

$$C^{\infty}_{Av} = \frac{FD_0}{kV_D\tau}$$

For intravenous bolus injections, $F = 1$.

f. Orally administered drugs given in **immediate-release dosage forms** (e.g., solutions, conventional tablets, capsules) by multiple oral doses are usually rapidly absorbed ($k_A \geq k$) and slowly eliminated. C^{∞}_{max} and C^{∞}_{min} for these drugs are approximated by the equations shown in I.B.5.e.(1)–(2).

(1) For more exact calculations of C^{∞}_{min} and C^{∞}_{max} after multiple oral doses, the following equations are used:

$$C^{\infty}_{max} = \frac{FD_0k_A}{V_D(k_A - k)}\left(\frac{1}{1 - e^{-k\tau}}\right) \text{ and}$$

$$C^{\infty}_{min} = \frac{FD_0k_A}{V_D(k_A - k)}\left(\frac{1}{1 - e^{-k\tau}}\right) e^{-k\tau}$$

(2) The calculation of C^{∞}_{Av} is the same as for multiple intravenous bolus injections, using the equation shown in I.B.5.e.(3).

(3) The term $1/(1 - e^{-k\tau})$ is known as the **accumulation rate.**

(4) The fraction of drug remaining in the body (f) after a dosage interval is given by the following equation:

$$f = e^{-k\tau}$$

g. Loading dose. An initial loading dose (D_L) is given to obtain a therapeutic steady-state drug level quickly.

(1) For multiple oral doses, D_L is calculated by:

$$D_L = D_M \frac{1}{1 - e^{-k\tau}}$$

where D_M is the maintenance dose.

(2) If D_M is given at a dosage interval equal to the elimination half-life of the drug, then D_L equals twice the maintenance dose.

C. Multicompartment models

1. Drugs that exhibit multicompartment pharmacokinetics distribute into different tissue groups at different rates. Tissues with high blood flow equilibrate with a drug more rapidly than tissues with low blood flow. Drug concentration in various tissues depends on the physical and chemical characteristics of the drug and the nature of the tissue. For example, highly lipid-soluble drugs accumulate slowly in fat (lipid) tissue.

2. Two-compartment model (intravenous bolus injection)

a. After an intravenous bolus injection, the drug distributes and equilibrates rapidly into highly perfused tissues (**central compartment**) and more slowly into peripheral tissues (**tissue compartment**).

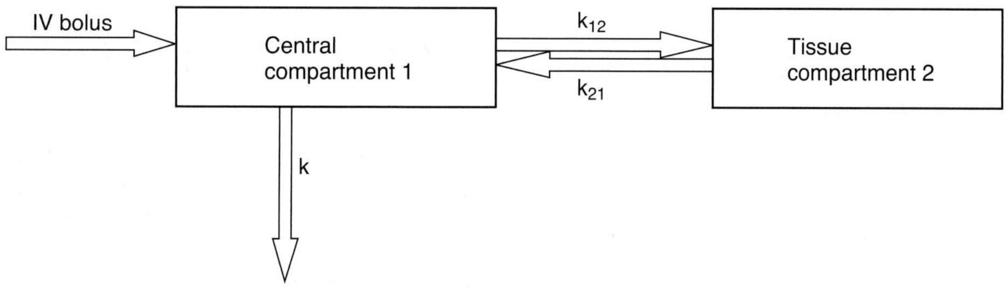

b. The initial rapid decline in plasma drug concentration is known as the **distribution phase.** The slower rate of decline in drug concentration after complete equilibration is achieved is known as the **elimination phase** (*Figure 5-5*).

c. The **plasma drug concentration** at any time is the sum of two first-order processes, as given in the following equation:

$$C_p = Ae^{-at} + Be^{-bt}$$

where a and b are hybrid first-order rate constants and A and B are y intercepts.

(1) The **hybrid first-order rate constant *b*** is obtained from the slope of the elimination phase of the curve (*Figure 5-5*) and represents the first-order elimination of drug from the body after the drug equilibrates with all tissues.

(2) The **hybrid first-order rate constant *a*** is obtained from the slope of the residual line of the distribution phase after the elimination phase is subtracted.

d. The **apparent volume of distribution** depends on the type of pharmacokinetic calculation. Volumes of distribution include the volume of the central compartment (V_p), the volume of distribution at steady state (V_{ss}), and the volume of the tissue compartment (V_t).

3. Two-compartment model (oral drug administration)

a. A drug with a rapid distribution phase may not show two-compartment characteristics after oral administration. As the drug is absorbed, it equilibrates with the tissues so that the elimination half-life of the elimination portion of the curve equals $0.693/b$.

b. Two-compartment characteristics are seen if the drug is absorbed rapidly and the distribution phase is slower.

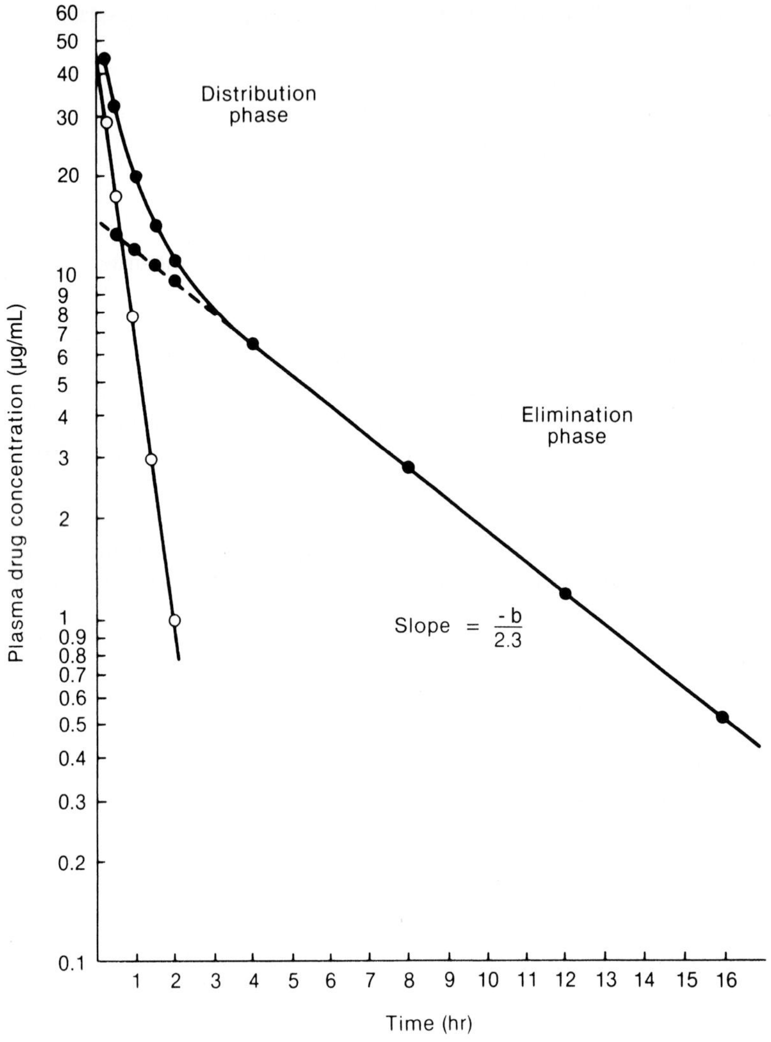

Figure 5-5. Generalized plot showing drug distribution and equilibration for a two-compartment model (intravenous bolus injection). The distribution phase is the initial rapid decline in plasma drug concentration. The elimination phase is the slower rate of decline after complete equilibration of the drug is achieved. Adapted with permission from Shargel L, Wu-Pong S, Yu ABC. *Applied Biopharmaceutics and Pharmacokinetics.* 5th ed. New York, NY: McGraw-Hill; 2005.

4. **Models with additional compartments**
   a. The addition of each new compartment to the model requires an additional first-order plot.
   b. The addition of a third compartment suggests that the drug slowly equilibrates into a deep tissue space. If the drug is given at frequent intervals, the drug begins to accumulate into the third compartment.
   c. The terminal linear phase generally represents the elimination of the drug from the body after equilibration occurs. The rate constant from the elimination phase is used to calculate dosage regimens.
   d. Adequate pharmacokinetic description of multicompartment models is often difficult and depends on proper plasma sampling and determination of drug concentrations.
5. **Elimination rate constants**
   a. The elimination rate constant, *k*, represents drug elimination from the central compartment.
   b. The terminal elimination rate constant (λ or *b* in the two-compartment model) represents drug elimination after drug distribution is mostly completed.

D. **Nonlinear pharmacokinetics** is also known as capacity-limited, dose-dependent, or saturation pharmacokinetics. Nonlinear pharmacokinetics do not follow first-order kinetics as the dose increases (*Figure 5-6*). Nonlinear pharmacokinetics may result from the saturation of an enzyme- or carrier-mediated system.

1. **Characteristics of nonlinear pharmacokinetics** include the following:
   a. The AUC is not proportional to the dose.
   b. The amount of drug excreted in the urine is not proportional to the dose.
   c. The elimination half-life may increase at high doses.
   d. The ratio of metabolites formed changes with increased dose.

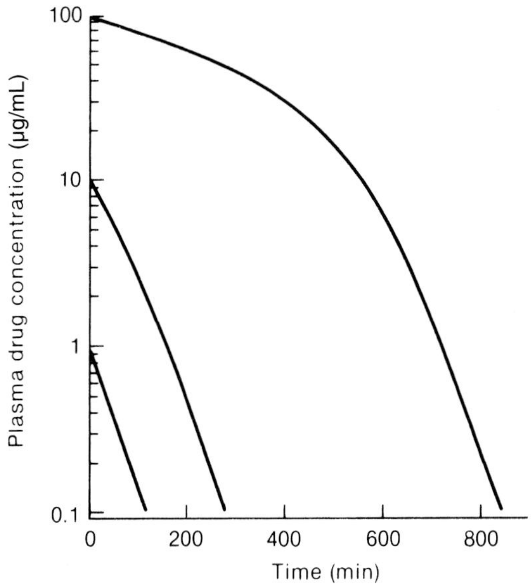

Figure 5-6. Generalized plot showing plasma drug concentration versus time for a drug with Michaelis–Menten (nonlinear) elimination kinetics. For this one-compartment model (intravenous injection), the doses are 1 mg, 10 mg, and 100 mg, and the apparent in vivo rate constant (k_M) is 10 mg. The maximum velocity of the reaction (V_{max}) is 0.2 mg/min. Adapted with permission from Gibaldi M, Perrier D. *Pharmacokinetics*. 2nd ed. New York, NY: Marcel Dekker, Inc.; 1982. Copyright © 1982 Routledge/Taylor & Francis Group, LLC.

2. **Michaelis–Menten kinetics** describes the velocity of enzyme reactions. Michaelis–Menten kinetics is used to describe nonlinear pharmacokinetics.
   a. The **Michaelis–Menten equation** describes the rate of change (velocity) of plasma drug concentration after an intravenous bolus injection as follows:

$$\frac{dC_p}{dt} = \frac{-V_{max}C_p}{k_M + Cp}$$

   where V_{max} is the maximum velocity of the reaction, C_p is the substrate or plasma drug concentration, and k_M is the Michaelis constant equal to the C_p at 0.5 V_{max}.
   b. At low C_p values, where $C_p << k_M$, this equation reduces to a first-order rate equation because both k_M and V_{max} are constants.

$$\frac{dC_p}{dt} = \frac{-V_{max}C_p}{k_M} = -k'C_p$$

   c. At high C_p values, where $C_p >> k_M$, the Michaelis–Menten equation is a zero-order rate equation as follows:

$$\frac{dC_p}{dt} = -V_{max}$$

3. Drugs that follow nonlinear pharmacokinetics may show zero-order elimination rates at high drug concentrations, fractional-order elimination rates at intermediate drug concentrations, and first-order elimination rates at low drug concentrations (*Figure 5-6*).

E. **Clearance** is a measurement of drug elimination from the body. Units for clearance are volume per time (e.g., liters per hour).
   1. **Total body clearance (Cl_T)** is the drug elimination rate divided by the plasma drug concentration. According to the concept of clearance, the body contains an apparent volume of distribution in which the drug is dissolved. A constant portion of this volume is cleared, or removed, from the body per unit time.
      a. The following equations express the measurement of total body clearance:

$$Cl_T = \frac{\text{drug elimination}}{\text{plasma drug concentration}} = \frac{(dDe/dt)}{Cp}$$

$$Cl_T = V_D k$$

$$Cl_T = \frac{FD_0}{\text{AUC}}$$

b. For drugs that follow first-order (linear) pharmacokinetics, total body clearance is the sum of all the clearances in the body, as shown in the following equation:

$$Cl_T = Cl_R + Cl_{NR}$$

where Cl_R is renal clearance and Cl_{NR} is nonrenal clearance. Nonrenal clearance, Cl_{NR}, is often equated with hepatic clearance, Cl_H.

c. The relation between Cl_T and $t_{½}$ is obtained by substituting $0.693/t_{½}$ for k in the equation in I.E.1 a to obtain the following expression:

$$t_{½} = \frac{0.693\,V_D}{Cl_T}$$

where V_D and Cl_T are considered independent variables, and $t_{½}$ is considered a dependent variable.

d. As clearance decreases (e.g., in renal disease), $t_{½}$ increases. Changes in V_D also cause proportional changes in $t_{½}$.

2. Renal drug excretion is the major route of drug elimination for polar drugs, water-soluble drugs, drugs with low molecular weight ($<$ 500 g/mol), and drugs that are biotransformed slowly. The relation between the drug excretion rate and the plasma drug concentration is shown in *Figure 5-7.* Drugs are excreted through the kidney into the urine by glomerular filtration, tubular reabsorption, and active tubular secretion.

a. Glomerular filtration is a passive process by which small molecules and drugs are filtered through the glomerulus of the nephron.

(1) Drugs bound to plasma proteins are too large to be filtered at the glomerulus.

(2) Drugs such as **creatinine and inulin** are not actively secreted or reabsorbed. They are used to measure the **glomerular filtration rate (GFR)**.

b. Tubular reabsorption is a passive process that follows Fick's law of diffusion.

(1) Lipid-soluble drugs are reabsorbed from the lumen of the nephron back into the systemic circulation.

(2) For weak electrolyte drugs, urine pH affects the ratio of nonionized and ionized drug.

(a) If the drug exists primarily in the nonionized or lipid-soluble form, then it is reabsorbed more easily from the lumen of the nephron.

(b) If the drug exists primarily in the ionized or water-soluble form, then it is excreted more easily in the urine.

(c) Depending on the pK_a of the drug, alteration of urine pH alters the ratio of ionized to nonionized drug and affects the rate of drug excretion. For example, alkalinization of the urine by the administration of sodium bicarbonate increases the excretion of salicylates (weak acids) into the urine.

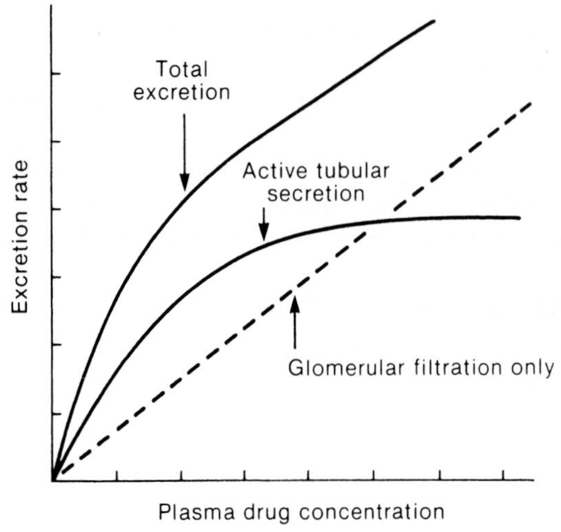

Figure 5-7. Generalized plot showing the excretion rate versus plasma drug concentration for a drug with active tubular secretion and for a drug secreted by glomerular filtration only. Adapted with permission from Shargel L, Wu-Pong S, Yu ABC. *Applied Biopharmaceutics and Pharmacokinetics.* 5th ed. New York, NY: McGraw-Hill; 2005.

(3) An increase in urine flow caused by simultaneous administration of a diuretic decreases the time for drug reabsorption. Consequently, more drug is excreted if given with a diuretic.

c. **Active tubular secretion** is a carrier-mediated active transport system that requires energy.

(1) Two active tubular secretion pathways exist in the kidney: one system for weak acids and one system for weak bases.

(2) The active tubular secretion system shows competition effects. For example, **probenecid** (a weak acid) competes for the same system as penicillin, decreasing the rate of penicillin excretion, resulting in a longer penicillin $t_{1/2}$.

(3) The renal clearance of drugs that are actively secreted, such as ***p*-aminohippurate (PAH)**, is used to measure **effective renal blood flow (ERBF).**

3. **Renal clearance** is the volume of drug contained in the plasma that is removed by the kidney per unit time. **Units for renal clearance** are expressed in volume per time (e.g., milliliters per minute or liters per hour).

a. Renal clearance may be measured by dividing the rate of drug excretion by the plasma drug concentration, as shown in the following equation:

$$Cl_R = \frac{\text{rate of drug excretion}}{C_p} = \frac{\frac{dD_u}{dt}}{C_p}$$

b. Measurement of renal clearance may also be expressed by the following equation:

$$Cl_R = k_e V_D$$

where k_e is the first-order renal excretion rate constant, and

$$Cl_R = \frac{D_u^\infty}{\text{AUC}}$$

where D_u^∞ is the total amount of parent (unchanged) drug excreted in the urine.

c. Renal clearance is measured without regard to the physiologic mechanism of renal drug excretion. The probable mechanism for renal clearance is obtained with a **clearance ratio**, which relates drug clearance to inulin clearance (a measure of GFR).

(1) If the clearance ratio is < 1.0, the mechanism for drug clearance may result from filtration plus reabsorption.

(2) If the ratio is 1.0, the mechanism may be filtration only.

(3) If the ratio is > 1.0, the mechanism may be filtration plus active tubular secretion.

4. **Hepatic clearance** is the volume of plasma-containing drug that is cleared by the liver per unit time.

a. **Measurement of hepatic clearance**. Hepatic clearance is usually measured indirectly, as the difference between total body clearance and renal clearance, as shown in the following equation:

$$Cl_H = Cl_T - Cl_R$$

where Cl_H is the hepatic clearance. Hepatic clearance is generally considered to be equivalent to Cl_{NR}, or nonrenal drug clearance. Hepatic clearance can also be calculated as the **product of the liver blood flow (*Q*)** and the **extraction ratio (ER)**, as shown in the following equation:

$$Cl_H = Q(\text{ER})$$

(1) The **extraction ratio** is the fraction of drug that is irreversibly removed by an organ or tissue as the plasma-containing drug perfuses that tissue.

(2) The extraction ratio is obtained by measuring the plasma drug concentration entering the liver and the plasma drug concentration exiting the liver:

$$\text{ER} = \frac{C_a - C_v}{C_a}$$

where C_a is the arterial plasma drug concentration entering the liver and C_v is the venous plasma drug concentration exiting the liver.

(3) Values for the ER range from 0 to 1. For example, if the ER is 0.9, then 90% of the incoming drug is removed as the plasma perfuses the liver. If the ER is 0, then no drug is removed by the liver.

b. **Blood flow**, **intrinsic clearance**, and **protein binding** affect hepatic clearance.
   (1) **Blood flow** to the liver is approximately 1.5 L/min and may be altered by exercise, food, disease, or drugs.
      (a) Blood enters the liver through the hepatic portal vein and hepatic artery and leaves through the hepatic vein.
      (b) After oral drug administration, the drug is absorbed from the gastrointestinal tract into the mesenteric vessels and proceeds to the hepatic portal vein, liver, and systemic circulation.
   (2) **Intrinsic clearance, Cl_{int},** describes the ability of the liver to remove the drug independently of blood flow.
      (a) Intrinsic drug clearance primarily occurs because of the inherent ability of the **biotransformation enzymes** (mixed-function oxidases) to metabolize the drug as it enters the liver.
      (b) Normally, basal level mixed-function oxidase enzymes biotransform drugs. Levels of these enzymes may be increased by various drugs (e.g., phenobarbital) and environmental agents (e.g., tobacco smoke). These enzymes may be inhibited by other drugs and environmental agents (e.g., cimetidine, acute lead poisoning).
   (3) **Protein binding.** Drugs that are bound to protein are not easily cleared by the liver or kidney because only the free, or nonplasma protein-bound, drug crosses the cell membrane into the tissue.
      (a) **The free drug** is available to drug-metabolizing enzymes for biotransformation.
      (b) A sudden increase in free-drug plasma concentration results in more available drug at pharmacologic receptors, producing a more intense effect in the organs (e.g., kidney, liver) involved in drug removal.
      (c) **Blood flow (Q), intrinsic clearance (Cl_{int}),** and fraction of free drug in plasma (f) are related to hepatic clearance as shown in the following equation:

$$Cl_H = Q\left(\frac{fCl_{int}}{Q + fCl_{int}}\right)$$

   (4) The hepatic clearance of drugs that have high extraction ratios and high Cl_{int} values (e.g., propranolol) is most affected by changes in blood flow and inhibitors of the drug metabolism enzymes.
   (5) The hepatic clearance of drugs that have low extraction ratios and low Cl_{int} values (e.g., theophylline) is most affected by changes in Cl_{int} and is affected only slightly by changes in hepatic blood flow.
   (6) Only drugs that are highly plasma protein bound (i.e., $> 95\%$) and have a low intrinsic clearance (e.g., phenytoin) are affected by a sudden shift in protein binding. This shift causes an increase in free drug plasma concentration.
c. **Biliary drug excretion**, an active transport process, is also included in hepatic clearance. Separate active secretion systems exist for weak acids and weak bases.
   (1) Drugs that are excreted in bile are usually high-molecular-weight compounds (i.e., > 500 g/mol) or polar drugs, such as reserpine, digoxin, and various glucuronide conjugates.
   (2) Drugs may be recycled by the **enterohepatic circulation**.
      (a) Some drugs are absorbed from the gastrointestinal tract through the mesenteric and hepatic portal veins, proceeding to the liver. The liver may secrete some of the drug (unchanged or as a glucuronide metabolite) into the bile.
      (b) The bile and drug are stored in the gallbladder and will empty into the gastrointestinal tract through the bile duct and then may be reabsorbed.
      (c) If the drug is a **glucuronide metabolite**, bacteria in the gastrointestinal tract may hydrolyze the glucuronide moiety, allowing the released drug to be reabsorbed.
d. **First-pass effects (presystemic elimination)** occur with drugs given orally. A portion of the drug is eliminated before systemic absorption occurs.
   (1) First-pass effects generally result from rapid drug biotransformation by liver enzymes. Other mechanisms include metabolism of the drug by gastrointestinal mucosal cells, intestinal flora, and biliary secretion.

(2) First-pass effects are usually observed by measuring the **absolute bioavailability** (F) of the drug (see Chapter 6). If $F < 1$, then some of the drug was eliminated before systemic drug absorption occurred.

(3) Drugs that have a **high hepatic extraction ratio**, such as propranolol and morphine, show first-pass effects.

(4) To obtain better systemic absorption of a drug that demonstrates high first-pass effects, then either

(a) the drug dose could be increased (e.g., propranolol, penicillin);

(b) the drug could be given by an alternate route of administration (e.g., nitroglycerin sublingual, insulin subcutaneous, estradiol transdermal); or

(c) the dosage form could be modified as a delayed-release drug product (e.g., enteric-coated aspirin, mesalamine), so that the drug may be absorbed more distally in the gastrointestinal (GI) tract.

F. **Noncompartment methods**. Some pharmacokinetic parameters for absorption, distribution, and elimination may be estimated with noncompartment methods. These methods usually require comparison of the areas under the curve.

1. **Mean residence time**

a. **Mean residence time (MRT)** is the average time for the drug molecules to reside in the body. MRT is also known as the *mean transit time* and *mean sojourn time*.

b. The MRT depends on the route of administration and assumes that the drug is eliminated from the central compartment.

c. The MRT is the total residence time for all molecules in the body divided by the total number of molecules in the body, as shown in the following equation:

$$\text{MRT} = \frac{\text{total residence time for all drug molecules in the body}}{\text{total number of drug molecules}}$$

d. **MRT after IV bolus injection**

(1) The MRT after a bolus intravenous injection is calculated by the following equation:

$$\text{MRT}_{\text{IV}} = \frac{\text{AUMC}}{\text{AUC}_{0-\infty}}$$

where AUMC is the area under the first moment versus time curve from $t = 0$ to $t =$ infinity and $\text{AUC}_{0-\infty}$ is the area under the plasma drug concentration versus time curve from $t = 0$ to $t =$ infinity. $\text{AUC}_{0-\infty}$ is also known as the *zero-moment curve*.

(2) The MRT_{IV} is related to the elimination rate constant by the following expression:

$$\text{MRT}_{\text{IV}} = 1/k$$

(3) During MRT_{IV}, 62.3% of the intravenous bolus dose is eliminated.

(4) The MRT for a drug given by a noninstantaneous input is longer than the MRT_{IV}.

2. **Mean absorption time (MAT)** is the difference between MRT and MRT_{IV} after an extravascular route is used.

$$\text{MAT} = \text{MRT}_{\text{ev}} - \text{MRT}_{\text{IV}}$$

When first-order absorption occurs, $\text{MAT} = 1/ka$.

3. **Clearance** is the volume of plasma cleared of drug per unit time and may be calculated without consideration of the compartment model.

$$Cl = \frac{FD_0}{\text{AUC}_{0-\infty}}$$

After an IV dose, $F = 1$.

4. **Steady-state volume of distribution (V_{ss})**

a. The steady-state volume of distribution is the ratio of the amount of drug in the body at steady state and the average steady-state drug concentration.

b. After an intravenous bolus injection, V_{ss} is calculated by the following equation:

$$V_{ss} = \frac{\text{dose}_{\text{IV}}\,(\text{AUMC})}{\text{AUC}^2}$$

II. CLINICAL PHARMACOKINETICS

A. **Definition**

1. Clinical pharmacokinetics is the application of pharmacokinetic principles for the rational design of an individualized dosage regimen. The two main objectives are **maintenance of an optimum drug concentration at the receptor site** to produce the desired therapeutic response for a specific period and **minimization of any adverse or toxic effects** of the drug.

III. TOXICOKINETICS

A. **Definitions**

1. Toxicokinetics is the application of pharmacokinetic principles to the design, conduct, and interpretation of drug safety evaluation studies.
2. **Toxicokinetics** is also used to validate dose-related exposure in animals. Toxicokinetic studies are performed in animals during preclinical drug development to aid in prediction of human drug toxicity. Toxicokinetic (nonclinical) studies may continue after the drug has been tested in humans.
3. **Clinical toxicology** is the study of adverse effects of drugs and toxic substances (poisons) in the human body. The pharmacokinetics of a drug in an overmedicated (intoxicated) patient may be very different from the pharmacokinetics of the same drug given in therapeutic doses. For example, a very high toxic dose may show nonlinear pharmacokinetics due to saturation kinetics compared to the drug given at lower therapeutic doses in which the drug levels follow linear pharmacokinetics.

IV. POPULATION PHARMACOKINETICS

A. **Definition**

1. Population pharmacokinetics is the study of sources and correlates of variability in drug concentrations among individuals who are the target patient population. Population pharmacokinetics is most often applied to the clinical patient who is receiving relevant doses of a drug of interest. Both pharmacokinetic and nonpharmacokinetic data may be considered, including gender, age, weight, creatinine clearance, and concomitant disease. Population pharmacokinetics can be used to assist with therapeutic drug monitoring and the principles of dosage adjustments (see Chapter 26).

Study Questions

Directions: Each question, statement, or incomplete statement in this section can be correctly answered or completed by **one** of the suggested answers or phrases. Choose the **best** answer.

1. Creatinine clearance is used as a measurement of
   - (A) renal excretion rate.
   - (B) glomerular filtration rate (GFR).
   - (C) active renal secretion.
   - (D) passive renal absorption.
   - (E) drug metabolism rate.

For questions 2–5: A new cephalosporin antibiotic was given at a dose of 5 mg/kg by a single intravenous bolus injection to a 58-year-old man who weighed 75 kg. The antibiotic follows the pharmacokinetics of a one-compartment model and has an elimination half-life of 2 hrs. The apparent volume of distribution is 0.28 L/kg, and the drug is 35% bound to plasma proteins.

2. What is the initial plasma drug concentration (C_p^0) in this patient?
   - (A) 0.24 mg/L
   - (B) 1.80 mg/L
   - (C) 17.9 mg/L
   - (D) 56.0 mg/L
   - (E) 1339 mg/L

3. What is the predicted plasma drug concentration (C_p) at 8 hr after the dose?
   (A) 0.73 mg/L
   (B) 1.11 mg/L
   (C) 2.64 mg/L
   (D) 4.02 mg/L
   (E) 15.10 mg/L

4. How much drug remains in the patient's body (D_B) 8 hrs after the dose?
   (A) 15.3 mg
   (B) 23.3 mg
   (C) 84.4 mg
   (D) 100.0 mg
   (E) 112.0 mg

5. How long after the dose is exactly 75% of the drug eliminated from the patient's body?
   (A) 2 hrs
   (B) 4 hrs
   (C) 6 hrs
   (D) 8 hrs
   (E) 10 hrs

For questions 6–11: A 35-year-old man who weighs 70 kg and has normal renal function needs an intravenous infusion of the antibiotic carbenicillin. The desired steady-state plasma drug concentration is 15 mg/dL. The physician wants the antibiotic to be infused into the patient for 10 hrs. Carbenicillin has an elimination half-life ($t_{½}$) of 1 hr and an apparent volume distribution (V_D) of 9 L in this patient.

6. Assuming that no loading dose was given, what rate of intravenous infusion is recommended for this patient?
   (A) 93.6 mg/hr
   (B) 135.0 mg/hr
   (C) 468.0 mg/hr
   (D) 936.0 mg/hr
   (E) 1350.0 mg/hr

7. Assuming that no loading intravenous dose was given, how long after the initiation of the intravenous infusion would the plasma drug concentration reach 95% of the theoretic steady-state drug concentration?
   (A) 1.0 hrs
   (B) 3.3 hrs
   (C) 4.3 hrs
   (D) 6.6 hrs
   (E) 10.0 hrs

8. What is the recommended loading dose?
   (A) 93.6 mg
   (B) 135.0 mg
   (C) 468.0 mg
   (D) 936.0 mg
   (E) 1350.0 mg

9. To infuse the antibiotic as a solution containing 10-g drug in 500 mL 5% dextrose, how many milliliters per hour of the solution would be infused into the patient?
   (A) 10.0 mL/hr
   (B) 46.8 mL/hr
   (C) 100.0 mL/hr
   (D) 936.0 mL/hr
   (E) 1141.0 mL/hr

10. What is the total body clearance rate for carbenicillin in this patient?
    (A) 100 mL/hr
    (B) 936 mL/hr
    (C) 4862 mL/hr
    (D) 6237 mL/hr
    (E) 9000 mL/hr

11. If the patient's renal clearance for carbenicillin is 86 mL/min, what is the hepatic clearance for carbenicillin?
    (A) 108 mL/hr
    (B) 1077 mL/hr
    (C) 3840 mL/hr
    (D) 5160 mL/hr
    (E) 6844 mL/hr

12. The earliest evidence that a drug is stored in tissue is
    (A) an increase in plasma protein binding.
    (B) a large apparent volume of distribution (V_D).
    (C) a decrease in the rate of formation of metabolites by the liver.
    (D) an increase in the number of side effects produced by the drug.
    (E) a decrease in the amount of free drug excreted in the urine.

13. The intensity of the pharmacologic action of a drug is most dependent on the
    (A) concentration of the drug at the receptor site.
    (B) elimination half-life ($t_{½}$) of the drug.
    (C) onset time of the drug after oral administration.
    (D) minimum toxic concentration (MTC) of the drug in plasma.
    (E) minimum effective concentration (MEC) of the drug in the body.

14. Drugs that show nonlinear pharmacokinetics have which property?
    (A) A constant ratio of drug metabolites is formed as the administered dose increases.
    (B) The elimination half-life ($t_{½}$) increases as the administered dose increases.
    (C) The area under the plasma drug concentration versus time curve (AUC) increases in direct proportion to an increase in the administered dose.
    (D) Both low and high doses follow first-order elimination kinetics.
    (E) The steady-state drug concentration increases in direct proportion to the dosing rate.

The patient's total body clearance (Cl_T) is calculated as follows:

$$Cl_T = kV_D$$

$$Cl_T = \frac{0.693}{1} \times 9000 \text{ mL} = 6237 \text{ mL/hr}$$

The hepatic clearance (Cl_H) is the difference between total clearance (Cl_T) and renal clearance (Cl_R):

$$Cl_H = Cl_T - Cl_R$$

$$Cl_H = 6237 - (86 \text{ mL/min} \times 60 \text{ min/hr}) = 1077 \text{ mL/hr}$$

12. **The answer is B** *[see I.B.1.b.(1)].*
A large apparent volume of distribution (V_D) is an early sign that a drug is not concentrated in the plasma but is distributed widely in tissue. An increase in plasma protein binding suggests that the drug is located in the plasma rather than in tissue. A decrease in hepatic metabolism, an increase in side effects, or a decrease in urinary excretion of free drug is caused by a decrease in drug elimination.

13. **The answer is A** *[see I.A.5.d.(3)].*
As more drug is concentrated at the receptor site, more receptors interact with the drug to produce a pharmacologic effect. The intensity of the response increases until it reaches a maximum. When all of the available receptors are occupied by drug molecules, additional drug does not produce a more intense response.

14. **The answer is B** *[see I.D].*
Nonlinear pharmacokinetics is a term used to indicate that first-order elimination of a drug does not occur at all drug concentrations. With some drugs, such as phenytoin, as the plasma drug concentration increases, the elimination pathway for metabolism of the drug becomes saturated and the half-life increases. The area under the plasma drug concentration versus time curve (AUC) of the drug is not proportional to the dose, neither is the rate of metabolite formation. The metabolic rate is related to the effects of the drug.

15. **The answer is D** *[see I.B.1.b.(2); I.B.5.g.(1)].*
A loading dose (D_L) of a drug is given to obtain a therapeutic plasma drug level as rapidly as possible. The D_L is calculated based on the apparent volume of distribution (V_D) and the desired plasma level of the drug.

16. **The answer is E** *[see I.E.3.c].*
Inulin is neither reabsorbed nor actively secreted. Therefore, it is excreted by glomerular filtration only. The inulin clearance rate is used as a standard measure of the GFR, a test that is useful both in a clinical situation and in the development of new drugs.

17. **The answer is E** *[see I.A.5.d].*
Drugs that are highly bound to plasma proteins diffuse poorly into tissue and have a low apparent volume of distribution (V_D).

18. **The answer is B** *[see I.B.3.g].*
The onset time is the time from the administration of the drug to the time when absorbed drug reaches the MEC. The MEC is the drug concentration in the plasma that is proportional, but not necessarily equal, to the minimum drug concentration at the receptor site that elicits a pharmacologic response.

19. **The answer is A** *[see I.A.5.a].*
The initial distribution of a drug is chiefly determined by blood flow, whereas the affinity of the drug for tissue determines whether the drug concentrates at that site. The GFR affects the renal clearance of a drug, not its initial distribution. The gastric emptying time and degree of plasma protein binding affect drug distribution but are less important than the rate of blood flow to tissue.

20. **The answer is C** *[see I.E.4.b.(2)].*
The kidney, lung, skin, and intestine all have some capacity to biotransform, or metabolize, drugs; but the brain has little capacity for drug metabolism. The liver has the highest capacity for drug metabolism.

21. **The answer is D** *[see I.B.5.c].*
The superposition principle, which underlies the design of multiple-dose regimens, assumes that earlier drug doses do not affect subsequent doses. If the elimination rate constant or total body clearance of the drug changes during multiple dosing, then the superposition principle is no longer valid. Changes in the total body clearance (Cl_T) may be caused by enzyme induction, enzyme inhibition, or saturation of an elimination pathway. Any of these changes would cause nonlinear pharmacokinetics.

22. **The answer is D** *[see I.B.5.e.(3)].*

23. **The answer is E** *[see I.B.5.g.(1)].*

24. **The answer is A** *[see I.B.5.d.(2); I.B.5.e.(3)].*
The oral maintenance dose (D_0) should maintain the patient's average drug concentration at the effective drug concentration. The bioavailability of the drug (F), the apparent volume of distribution (V_D), the dosage interval (τ), and the excretion rate constant (k) must be considered in calculating the dose. The equation used is

$$C_{Av}^{\infty} = FD_0 / kV_D\tau$$

For this drug, $F = 0.75$, $k = 0.693/24$ hrs, $V_D = 3$ L/kg $\times$ 65 kg, $\tau = 24$ hrs, and $C^{\infty}_{Av} = 1.5$ ng/mL, or 1.5 μg/L. Therefore, by substitution, $D_0 = 270$ μg, or 0.270 mg. When the maintenance dose is given at a dosage frequency equal to the half-life, then the loading dose is equal to twice the maintenance dose, in this case 540 μg, or 0.540 mg. To determine the plasma drug concentration for a dosage regimen of 0.125 mg every 12 hrs, the C^{∞}_{Av} formula is used. This time, $F = 0.75$, $D_0 = 0.125$ mg, $k = 0.693/24$ hrs, $V_D = 3$ L/kg $\times$ 65 kg, and $\tau = 12$ hrs. Therefore, $C^{\infty}_{Av} = 1.39$ ng/mL. For cardiac glycosides, the peak (C_{max}) and trough (C_{min}) concentrations are calculated, and plasma drug concentrations are monitored after dosing. The loading dose (D_L) may be given in small increments over a specified period, according to the dosage regimen suggested by the manufacturer.

25. **The answer is C** *[see I.A.3.b]*.
For first-order elimination, it takes two half-lives for plasma drug concentration of 8 ng/mL to decline to 2 ng/mL. The first half-life, the plasma drug concentration declines to 4 ng/mL, and the next half-life, the plasma drug concentration declines to 2 ng/mL.

26. **The answer is A (I)** *[see I.A.3.a]*.
The first equation in the question describes a zero-order reaction (dA/dt) in which the reaction rate increases or decreases at a constant rate (k). A zero-order reaction produces a graph of a straight line with the equation of $A = -kt + A_o$ when A is plotted against time (t). The other equations in the question represent first-order reactions.

6 Bioavailability and Bioequivalence

MANISH ISSAR, LEON SHARGEL

I. DEFINITIONS[1]

A. **Bioavailability** is a measurement of the rate and extent (amount) to which the active ingredient or active moiety becomes available at the site of action. Bioavailability is also considered a measure of the rate and extent of therapeutically active drug that is systemically absorbed. For drug products that are not intended to be absorbed into the bloodstream, bioavailability may be assessed by measurements intended to reflect the rate and extent to which the active ingredient or active moiety becomes available at the site of action.

B. **Bioequivalent drug products**. A generic drug product is considered bioequivalent to the **reference listed drug** (**RLD**) **product** if both products are pharmaceutical equivalents and the generic drug product's rate and extent of systemic drug absorption (bioavailability) do not show a statistically significant difference when administered in the same molar dose of the active ingredient, in the same chemical form, in a similar dosage form, by the same route of administration, and under the same experimental conditions. The RLD is generally the brand product.

C. **Generic drug product**
   1. The generic drug product requires an **abbreviated new drug application** (ANDA) for approval by the U.S. Food and Drug Administration (FDA) and may be marketed after patent expiration of the reference drug product.
   2. The generic drug product must be a **therapeutic equivalent** to the reference drug product but may differ in certain characteristics, including shape, scoring configuration, packaging, and excipients (such as colors, flavors, preservatives, expiration date, and minor aspects of labeling).
   3. FDA believes that products classified as therapeutically equivalent can be substituted with the full expectation that the substituted product will produce the same clinical effect and safety profile as the prescribed product.

D. **Pharmaceutical equivalents** are drug products that contain the same therapeutically active drug ingredient(s); contain the same salt, ester, or chemical form; are of the same dosage form; and are identical in strength, concentration, and route of administration. Pharmaceutical equivalents may differ in characteristics such as shape, scoring configuration, release mechanisms, packaging, and excipients (including colors, flavoring, and preservatives).

E. **The reference listed drug product** is usually the currently marketed, brand-name product with a full **new drug application** (**NDA**) approved by the FDA. The RLD is the reference drug product identified by FDA (see *Electronic Orange Book* at http://www.accessdata.fda.gov/scripts/cder/ob/default.cfm).

[1]The U.S. Food and Drug Administration (FDA) annually publishes the book *Approved Drug Products with Therapeutic Equivalence Evaluation* also known as the *Electronic Orange Book* (available online at http://www.accessdata.fda.gov/scripts/cder/ob/default.cfm). This source should be consulted for the latest definitions of therapeutic equivalence–related terms.

F. **Therapeutic equivalent drug products** are pharmaceutical equivalents that can be expected to have the same clinical effect and safety profile when administered to patients under the same conditions specified in the labeling. Therapeutic equivalent drug products have the following criteria:
   1. The products are safe and effective.
   2. The products are pharmaceutical equivalents that contain the same active drug ingredient in the same dosage form, given by the same route of administration; meet compendial or other applicable standards of strength, quality, purity, and identity; and meet an acceptable in vitro standard.
   3. The drug products are bioequivalent in that they do not present a known potential problem and are shown to meet an appropriate bioequivalence standard.
   4. The drug products are adequately labeled.
   5. The drug products are manufactured in compliance with current good manufacturing practice regulations.

G. **Pharmaceutical alternatives** are drug products that contain the same therapeutic moiety but are different salts, esters, or complexes of that moiety (e.g., tetracycline hydrochloride vs. tetracycline phosphate) or are different dosage forms (e.g., tablet versus capsule; immediate-release dosage form versus controlled-release dosage form) or strengths.

II. DRUG PRODUCT PERFORMANCE

A. **Drug product performance**, in vivo, may be defined as the release of the drug substance from the drug product leading to bioavailability of the drug substance. Performance tests relate the quality of the drug product to its clinical safety and efficacy.

B. **Bioavailability studies** are used for establishing dosage regimens of new drug products. Bioavailability is one attribute to product quality that links in vivo performance of the drug product used to original formulation that was used in the clinical safety and efficacy studies.

C. **Bioequivalence studies** can be useful during the investigational new drug (IND) development or NDA development period to establish links between
   1. early and late clinical trial formulations;
   2. formulations used in clinical trial and stability studies, if different; and
   3. clinical trial formulations and to-be-marketed drug product.

D. **Bioequivalence studies** are a critical component of ANDA submissions.
   1. The purpose of these studies is to demonstrate bioequivalence between a pharmaceutically equivalent generic drug product and the corresponding reference listed drug (usually the brand drug product).
   2. Together with the determination of pharmaceutical equivalence, establishing bioequivalence allows a regulatory conclusion of therapeutic equivalence.

E. **Scale-up and post-approval changes (SUPACs)**. After market approval, a drug product may undergo a manufacturing change. A bioequivalence study may be needed to show that the new formulation or the new method of manufacture (test product) and the prior formulation or method of manufacture (reference product) are equivalent.

III. BIOAVAILABILITY AND BIOEQUIVALENCE.

These may be determined directly using pharmacokinetic studies (e.g., plasma drug concentration versus time profiles, urinary drug excretion studies), measurements of an acute pharmacodynamic effect, comparative clinical studies, or in vitro studies. The choice of study used is based on the site of action of the drug and the ability of the study design to compare drug delivered to that site by the two products.

A. **Acute pharmacodynamic effects**, such as changes in heart rate, blood pressure, electrocardiogram (ECG), clotting time, or forced expiratory volume in 1 sec (FEV_1) can be used to measure bioavailability when no assay for plasma drug concentration is available or when the plasma drug concentration does not relate to the pharmacological response (e.g., a bronchodilator such as albuterol given by inhalation). Quantitation of the pharmacological effect versus time profile can be used as a measure of bioavailability and/or bioequivalence (*Figure 6-1*).
   1. **Onset time**. As the drug is systemically absorbed, the drug concentration at the receptor rises to a **minimum effective concentration** (MEC), and a pharmacological response is initiated. The time from drug administration to the MEC is known as the onset time.

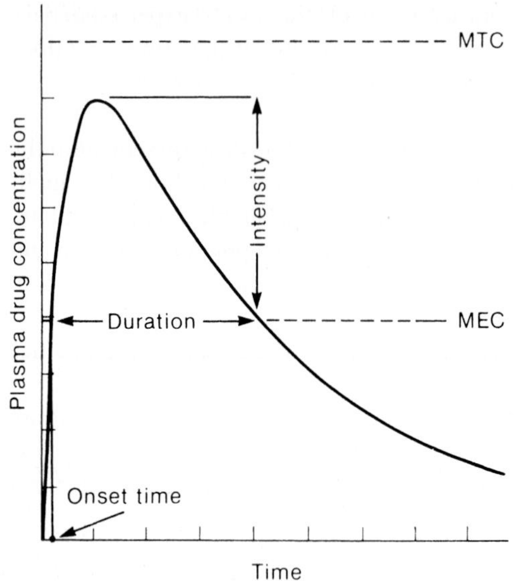

Figure 6-1. Generalized plasma drug concentration versus time curve after oral drug administration. *MEC*, minimum effective concentration; *MTC*, minimum toxic concentration. Adapted with permission from Shargel L, Wu-Pong S, Yu ABC. *Applied Biopharmaceutics and Pharmacokinetics*. 5th ed. New York, NY: McGraw-Hill; 2005:6.

2. **Intensity**. The intensity of the pharmacological effect is proportional to the number of receptors occupied by the drug up to a *maximum* pharmacological effect. The maximum pharmacological effect may occur before, after, or at peak drug absorption.
3. **Duration of action**. As long as the drug concentration remains above the MEC, pharmacological activity is observed. The duration of action is the time for which the drug concentration remains above the MEC.
4. **Therapeutic window**. As the drug concentration increases, other receptors may combine with the drug to exert a toxic or adverse response. This drug concentration is the **minimum toxic concentration** (MTC). The drug concentration range between the MEC and the MTC is known as the *therapeutic window*.

B. **Plasma drug concentration**. The plasma drug concentration versus time curve is most often used to measure the systemic bioavailability of a drug from a drug product (*Figure 6-2*).

1. **Time for peak plasma drug concentration** (T_{max}) relates to the rate constants for systemic drug absorption and elimination. If two oral drug products contain the same amount of active drug but different excipients, the dosage form that yields the faster rate of drug absorption has the shorter T_{max}.

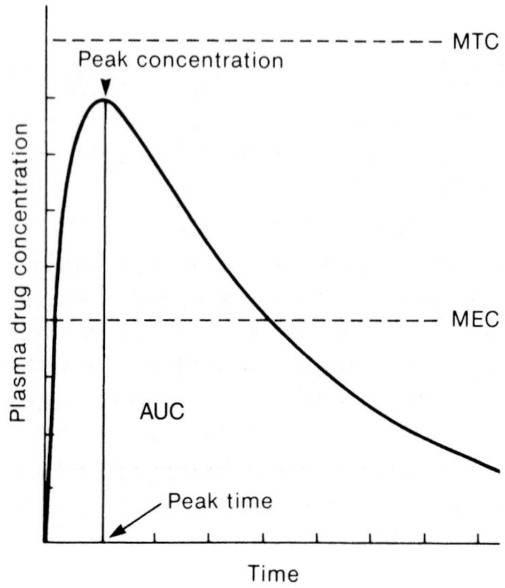

Figure 6-2. Generalized plasma drug concentration versus time curve, showing peak time and peak concentration. *AUC*, area under the curve; *MEC*, minimum effective concentration; *MTC*, minimum toxic concentration. Adapted with permission from Shargel L, Wu-Pong S, Yu ABC. *Applied Biopharmaceutics and Pharmacokinetics*. 5th ed. New York, NY: McGraw-Hill; 2005:7.

2. **Peak plasma drug concentration** (C_{max}). The plasma drug concentration at T_{max} relates to the intensity of the pharmacological response. Ideally, C_{max} should be within the therapeutic window.
3. **Area under the plasma drug concentration versus time curve** (AUC) relates to the amount or extent of drug absorption. The amount of systemic drug absorption is directly related to the AUC. The AUC is usually calculated by the **trapezoidal rule** and is expressed in units of concentration multiplied by time (e.g., μg/mL × hr).

C. **Urinary drug excretion**. Measurement of urinary drug excretion can determine bioavailability from a drug product. This method is most accurate if the active therapeutic moiety is excreted unchanged in significant quantity in the urine (*Figure 6-3*).
1. **The cumulative amount of active drug excreted in the urine** $\left(D_U^\infty\right)$ is directly related to the extent of systemic drug absorption.
2. **The rate of drug excretion in the urine** (dD_U/dt) is directly related to the rate of systemic drug absorption.
3. **The time for the drug to be completely excreted** (t^∞) corresponds to the total time for the drug to be systemically absorbed and completely excreted after administration.

D. **Comparative clinical trials** to a drug can be used to measure bioavailability quantitatively. Clinical studies are highly variable and less precise than other methods because of individual differences in drug pharmacodynamics and subjective measurements.

E. **In vitro measurements of bioequivalence**. Bioequivalence may sometimes be demonstrated using an in vitro bioequivalence standard, especially when such an in vitro test has been correlated with human in vivo bioavailability data. For example, the rate of drug dissolution in vitro for certain drug products correlates with drug bioavailability in vivo. If the dissolution test in vitro is considered statistically adequate to predict drug bioavailability, then, in some cases, dissolution may be used in place of an in vivo bioavailability study. This relationship between in vitro dissolution and in vivo bioavailability is also known as in vitro–in vivo correlation (IVIVC).

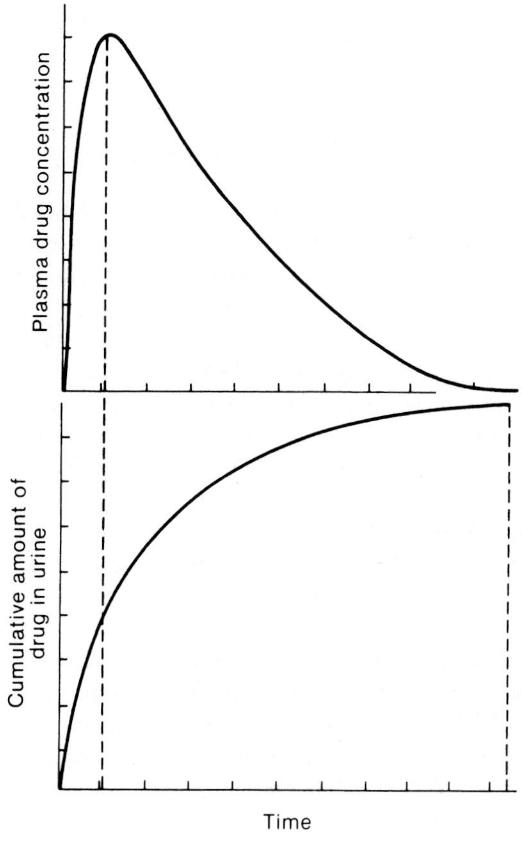

Figure 6-3. These corresponding plots show the relationship of the plasma drug concentration versus time curve to the cumulative amount of drug in the urine versus time curve. Adapted with permission from Shargel L, Wu-Pong S, Yu ABC. *Applied Biopharmaceutics and Pharmacokinetics*. 5th ed. New York, NY: McGraw-Hill; 2005:463.

IV. RELATIVE AND ABSOLUTE BIOAVAILABILITY

A. Relative bioavailability (RBA) is the systemic availability of the drug from a dosage form as compared to a reference standard given by the same route of administration. Relative bioavailability is calculated as the ratio of the AUC for the dosage form to the AUC for the reference dosage form given in the same dose. A relative bioavailability of 1 (or 100%) implies that drug bioavailability from both dosage forms is the same but does not indicate the completeness of systemic drug absorption. The determination of relative bioavailability is important in generic drug studies (e.g., bioequivalence studies). Bioequivalence is a relative bioavailability study.

$$RBA = \frac{[AUC]_{0\,oralTEST}^{\infty}/Dose_{oralTEST}}{[AUC]_{0\,REF.}^{\infty}/Dose_{REF.}}$$

B. Absolute bioavailability (F) is the fraction of drug systemically absorbed from the dosage form. F is calculated as the ratio of the AUC for the dosage form given orally to the AUC obtained after intravenous (IV) drug administration (adjusted for dose). A parenteral drug solution given by IV administration is considered to have 100% systemic absorption (i.e., $F = 1$). An F value of 0.80 (or 80%) indicates that only 80% of the drug was systemically available from the oral dosage form.

$$F = \frac{[AUC]_{0\,oral}^{\infty}/Dose_{oral}}{[AUC]_{0\,i.v.}^{\infty}/Dose_{i.v.}}$$

V. BIOEQUIVALENCE STUDIES FOR SOLID ORAL DRUG PRODUCTS

A. Objective of bioequivalence studies. The objective of a bioequivalence study is to measure and compare formulation performance between two or more pharmaceutically equivalent drug products.

B. Design of bioequivalence studies

1. The FDA's Division of Bioequivalence, Office of Generic Drugs provides guidance for the performance of in vitro dissolution and in vivo bioequivalence studies. These guidances are available at http://www.fda.gov/Drugs/GuidanceComplianceRegulatoryInformation/Guidances/default.htm.
2. **Fasting study**. Bioequivalence studies are usually evaluated by a single-dose, two-period, two-treatment, two-sequence, open-label, randomized crossover design, comparing equal doses of the test (generic) and reference (brand) products in fasted, adult, healthy subjects.
   - **a.** Both men and women may be used in the study.
   - **b.** Blood sampling is performed just before the dose (zero time) and at appropriate intervals after the dose to obtain an adequate description of the plasma drug concentration versus time profile.
3. **Food intervention study**. If the bioavailability of the active drug ingredient is known to be affected by food, the generic drug manufacturer must include a single-dose, randomized, crossover, food effects study comparing equal doses of the test product and reference products given immediately after a standard high-fat–content breakfast.
4. **Other study designs**. Crossover studies may not be practical in drugs with a long half-life in the body, and a parallel study design may be used instead. Alternate study methods, such as in vitro studies or equivalence studies with clinical or pharmacodynamic end points, are used for drug products where plasma concentrations are not useful to determine delivery of the drug substance to the site of activity (such as inhalers, nasal sprays, and topical products applied to the skin).
5. **Waiver of an in vivo bioequivalence study (biowaiver)**
   - **a.** A comparative in vitro dissolution (drug-release) study between the test and the reference products may be used in lieu of an in vivo bioequivalence study for some immediate-release (conventional) oral drug products.
   - **b.** No bioequivalence study is required for certain drug products given as a solution such as oral, parenteral, ophthalmic, or other solutions because bioequivalence is self-evident. In this case, the drug is in a pure aqueous solution, and there is no drug dissolution rate consideration.
   - **c.** Immediate-release (IR) solid oral drug products that meet biopharmaceutics classification system (BCS) class 1 drugs—that is, highly water soluble, rapidly dissolving, and rapid permeation of cellular membranes—may obtain a biowaiver.

d. Drug products containing a lower dose strength (e.g., 200 mg, 100 mg, and 50 mg IR tablets). The drug product must be in the same dosage form, lower strength, and is proportionately similar in its active and inactive ingredients.

C. **Pharmacokinetic evaluation of the data**. Pharmacokinetic analysis includes calculation for each subject of the AUC to the last quantifiable concentration (AUC_{0-t}) and to infinity ($AUC_{0-\infty}$), T_{max}, and C_{max}. In addition, the elimination rate constant (k), the elimination half-life ($t_{1/2}$), and other parameters may be estimated.

D. **Statistical evaluation of the data**

1. The statistical methodology for analyzing bioequivalence studies is called the *two one-sided test procedures*. Two situations are tested with this statistical methodology.
   a. The first of the two one-sided tests determines whether a generic product (test), when substituted for a brand-name product (reference), is significantly less bioavailable.
   b. The second of the two one-sided tests determines whether a brand-name product (reference), when substituted for a generic product (test), is significantly less bioavailable.
   c. Based on the opinions of FDA medical experts, a difference of $> 20\%$ for each of the aforementioned tests was determined to be significant and, therefore, undesirable for all drug products.
2. An analysis of variance (ANOVA) should be performed on the log transformed AUC and C_{max} values obtained from each subject. The 90% confidence intervals for both pharmacokinetic parameters, AUC and C_{max}, must be entirely within the 80% to 125% boundaries based on log transformation of the data. The ratio of the means of the study data (test to reference) should lie in the center of the 90% confidence interval, or close to 100% (equivalent to a test to reference ratio of 1) (*Table 6-1*).
3. Different statistical criteria are sometimes used when bioequivalence is demonstrated through comparative clinical trials, pharmacodynamic studies, or comparative in vitro methodology.
4. The bioequivalence methodology and criteria described earlier simultaneously control for both differences in the average response between test and reference products as well as the precision with which the average response in the population is estimated. This precision depends on the within-subject (normal volunteer or patient) variability in the pharmacokinetic parameters (AUC and C_{max}) of the two products and on the number of subjects in the study. The width of the 90% confidence interval is a reflection in part of the within-subject variability of the test and reference products in the bioequivalence study.

VI. BIOEQUIVALENCE ISSUES

A. **Problems in determining bioequivalence** include lack of an adequate study design; inability to accurately measure the drug analytes, including metabolites and enantiomers (chiral drugs); and lack of systemic drug absorption (*Table 6-2*).

B. **Bioequivalence studies** for which objective blood drug concentrations cannot be obtained require either a pharmacodynamic study, a clinical trial, or an in vitro study that has been correlated with human in vivo bioavailability data.

1. Pharmacodynamic measurements are more difficult to obtain, and the data tend to be variable, requiring a larger number of subjects compared to the bioequivalence studies for systemically absorbed drugs.
   a. A bioequivalence study using pharmacodynamic measurements tries to obtain a pharmacodynamic effect versus time profile for the drug in each subject.
   b. The area under the effect versus time profile, peak effect, and time for peak effect are obtained for the test and reference products and are then statistically analyzed.
2. Comparative clinical trials are more difficult to run, do not have easily quantifiable observations, and are quite costly.
3. In vitro studies may require the development of a reliable surrogate marker that may be correlated with human in vivo bioavailability data. Examples include the following:
   a. Comparative in vitro drug release/dissolution studies in which the dissolution profile of the test and reference drug products under different conditions of pH and media are performed.
   b. Comparison of binding of bile acids to cholestyramine (Questran®) and the test product.

Table 6-1 BIOAVAILABILITY COMPARISON OF A GENERIC (TEST) AND BRAND (REFERENCE) DRUG PRODUCT

		LN-Transformed Data						
		Geometric Mean			90% Confidence Interval			
PK Variable	Units	Test	Reference	% Ratio T/R	(Lower Limit, Upper Limit)	*P* Values for Product Effects	Power of ANOVA	ANOVA % CV
C_{max}	ng/mL	344.79	356.81	96.6	(89.5, 112)	.3586	0.8791	17.90%
AUC_{0-t}	ng hr/mL	2659.12	2674.92	99.4	(95.1, 104)	.8172	1.0000	12.60%
AUC_{inf}	ng hr/mL	2708.63	2718.52	99.6	(95.4, 103)	.8865	1.0000	12.20%
T_{max}	hr	4.29	4.24	101				
k_{elim}	1/hr	0.0961	0.0980	98.1				
$t_{½}$	hr	8.47	8.33	101.7				

AUC, area under the curve; C_{max}, peak plasma drug concentration; T_{max}, time for peak plasma drug concentration.
The results were obtained from a two-way crossover, single-dose, fasting study in 36 healthy adult volunteers. Mean values are reported. No statistical differences were observed between AUC and C_{max} values for the test and reference products.

Table 6-2 PROBLEM ISSUES IN THE DETERMINATION OF BIOEQUIVALENCE

Problem Issues	Example
Drugs with highly variable bioavailability[a]	Propranolol, verapamil
Drugs with active metabolites	Selegiline
Chiral drugs	Ibuprofen, albuterol
Drugs with nonlinear pharmacokinetics	Phenytoin
Orally administered drugs that are not systemically absorbed	Cholestyramine resin, sucralfate
Drugs with long elimination half-lives	Probucol
Variable-dosage forms	Dyazide, conjugated estrogens
Nonoral drug delivery	
Topical drugs	Steroids, antifungals
Transdermal delivery systems	Estrogen patch
Drugs given by inhalation aerosols	Bronchodilators, steroids
Intranasal drugs	Intranasal steroids
Biotechnology-derived drugs	Erythropoietin, interferon
Bioavailable drugs that should not reach peak drug levels	Potassium supplements, hormone replacement therapy
Target population used in the bioequivalence studies	Pediatric patients; renal disease

[a]These drugs have high intrasubject variability.

VII. DRUG PRODUCTION SELECTION

A. Generic drug substitution

1. **Generic drug substitution** is the process of dispensing a generic drug product in place of the prescribed drug product (e.g., generic product for brand-name product, generic product for another generic product, brand-name product for generic product). The substituted product must be a therapeutic equivalent to the prescribed product.
2. Generic drug products that are classified as therapeutic equivalents by the FDA are expected to produce the same clinical effect and safety profile as the prescribed drug.

B. Therapeutic substitution

1. Therapeutic substitution is the process of dispensing a therapeutic alternative in place of the prescribed drug product. For example, amoxicillin is dispensed for ampicillin.
2. The substituted drug product is usually in the same therapeutic class (e.g., calcium channel blocker) and is expected to have a similar clinical profile.

C. Formulary issues

1. A **formulary** is a list of drugs. A **positive** formulary lists all the drugs that may be substituted, whereas a **negative** formulary lists drugs for which the pharmacist may not substitute. A **restrictive** formulary lists only those drugs that may be reimbursed without justification by the prescriber; for drugs not listed in the restrictive formulary, the prescriber must justify the need for the nonlisted drug.
2. Many states have legal requirements that address the issue of drug product selection. States may provide information and guidance in drug product selection through positive, negative, or restrictive formularies.
3. The FDA annually publishes *Approved Drug Products with Therapeutic Equivalence Evaluations* (the *Orange Book*). This publication is also reproduced in the *United States Pharmacopeia* (*USP*), DI Vol. III, *Approved Drug Products and Legal Requirements*, published annually by the *USP* Convention. The *Electronic Orange Book* may be found at http://www.accessdata.fda.gov/scripts/cder/ob/default.cfm.
   a. The *Orange Book* provides therapeutic evaluation codes for drug products (*Table 6-3*).
      (1) "A-rated" drug products are drug products that contain active ingredients and dosage forms that are not regarded as presenting either actual or potential bioequivalence problems or drug quality standards issues. However, all oral dosage forms must meet an appropriate in vitro bioequivalence standard that is acceptable to the FDA to be approved as therapeutically equivalent and may be interchanged.

Directions for questions 4–6: The questions and incomplete statements in this section can be correctly answered or completed by **one or more** of the suggested answers. Choose the answer, A–E.

A if **I only** is correct
B if **III only** is correct
C if **I and II** are correct
D if **II and III** are correct
E if **I, II, and III** are correct

4. For two drug products, generic (test) and brand (reference), to be considered bioequivalent,
   I. there should be no statistical difference between the extent of bioavailability of the drug from the test product compared to the reference product.
   II. the 90% confidence interval about the ratio of the means of the C_{max} and AUC values for the test product to reference product must be within 80% to 125% of the reference product.
   III. there should be no statistical differences between the mean C_{max} and AUC values for the test product compared to the reference product.

5. For which of the following products is measuring plasma drug concentrations not appropriate for estimating bioequivalence?
   I. metered-dose inhaler containing a bronchodilator
   II. antifungal agent for the treatment of a vaginal infection
   III. enteric-coated tablet containing a nonsteroidal anti-inflammatory agent

6. Bioequivalence studies compare the bioavailability
   I. of the generic drug product to the brand drug product.
   II. of a reformulated brand drug product to the original formulation of the brand product.
   III. of a to-be-marketed brand product to the drug product used in the clinical trials.

Answers and Explanations

1. The answer is B *[see III.B]*.
AUC relates to the extent of drug absorption. C_{max} and T_{max} relate to the rate of drug absorption. The elimination $t_{½}$ of the drug is usually independent of the route of drug administration and is not used as a measure of bioavailability. For the FDA, only the C_{max} and AUC parameters must meet 90% confidence intervals of 80% to 125% of the reference (brand) product (*Table 6-1*).

2. The answer is C *[see IV.B]*.
After an IV bolus injection or IV infusion, the entire dose is absorbed into the body. The ratio of the AUC of the drug given orally to the AUC of the drug given by IV injection is used to obtain the absolute bioavailability (F) of the drug.

3. The answer is E *[see IV.A]*.
The relative bioavailability is determined from the ratio of the AUC of the generic (test) product to the AUC of the reference standard. Thus, the relative bioavailability can exceed 100%, whereas the absolute bioavailability cannot exceed 100%. $AUC_{generic}/AUC_{reference} = 2822/2715 = 1.039$ or 103.9%.

4. The answer is E (I, II, III) *[see V.C]*.
Although T_{max} is an indication of rate of drug absorption, it is a discrete measurement and usually too variable to use for statistical comparisons in bioequivalence studies. Statistical comparisons use AUC and C_{max} values from test and reference drug products as the basis of bioequivalence.

5. The answer is C (I, II) *[see V.A]*.
Although some systemic absorption may be demonstrated after administering a metered dose inhaler containing a bronchodilator or a vaginal antifungal agent, bioequivalence can be determined only by using a clinical response measurement.

6. The answer is E (I, II, III) *[see I.A–E]*.
Bioequivalence studies compare the bioavailability of a drug from one drug product to another drug product containing the same active ingredient. Drug products such as capsules that are used in clinical trials should be bioequivalent to the marketed drug product, which may be a tablet. Generic drug products and the corresponding brand drug product must be bioequivalent. For any change in a formulation, the manufacturer (brand or generic) must demonstrate that the formulation change does not affect the bioavailability compared to the original product.

7

Biotechnology Drug Products

SUSANNA WU-PONG

I. INTRODUCTION.

Pharmaceutical biotechnology has enabled the creation, modification, and manufacture of recombinant biological products for therapeutic use. Cell lines, recombinant DNA, and highly sensitive and specific analytical methods are now routinely used to design, discover, and evaluate highly specific new drugs, imaging agents, and diagnostics.

A. Currently available biological drugs primarily fall into two categories: nucleic acid or protein/peptide drugs.
   1. **Nucleic acid drugs.** Macromolecular nucleic acid drugs include oligonucleotides and other compounds still in clinical trials, such as gene therapy or microRNAs.
   2. **Protein drugs.** Protein and peptide drugs include **monoclonal antibodies** (mAbs) and recombinant proteins. mAbs are also used as imaging and targeting agents.

B. Biological drugs are manufactured usually using engineered cells or recombinant methods in vitro, although smaller molecules may be chemically synthesized. Such cell- and gene-based methods are distinctly different from chemical synthetic techniques used to manufacture most small-molecule drugs; the manufacturing process and materials used for biologic products are intricately linked to the quality and properties of the product, even when identical gene sequences are being expressed. Several examples of differences in adverse reactions have been reported for the same recombinant proteins (erythropoietin, interferon-β1a, and botulism A toxin) made by different manufacturers or using slightly different processes or materials.

C. Recombinant DNA techniques are used to design and produce protein drugs and many of the emerging nucleic acid drugs. Therefore, these biologic products can be engineered to a specific sequence and/or structure.

D. Biologic drugs are biological products, so they have unique challenges in the areas of stability, delivery, formulation, and analysis. Protein drugs and products are dependent on having correct protein structure for activity and are often active in very low concentrations. Thus, formulation, storage, and analysis must be able to differentiate, preserve, and measure the active protein in low concentrations.

E. Most biologic products should be refrigerated at 2° to 8°C and should not be frozen, shaken, or exposed to light. Products must be used within a specified time after dilution. Specific product information should always be consulted before storage or use.

II. BASIC TERMINOLOGY

A. An **antigen** is a substance or molecule that stimulates the production of antibodies by the immune system.

B. An **antibody** is an immunoglobulin molecule that is produced by the immune system after stimulation from an antigen. The plasma contains a mixture of antibodies synthesized to bind many different antigens (**polyclonal** antibodies). **Monoclonal antibodies** are produced in vitro and consist of copies of a single antibody that binds a single epitope. Antibodies are part of the body's immune system, which identifies and neutralizes foreign molecules.

Table 7-1 THERAPEUTIC mAbs

Antibody	Brand Name	Type	Target	Warnings	Indication
Abciximab	ReoPro®	Chimeric	Glycoprotein IIb/IIIa	—	Cardiovascular disease
Adalimumab	Humira®	Human	TNF-α	Risk for fatal infections, malignancies especially in children, adolescents, and young adult males	Autoimmune disorders
Alefacept	Amevive®		CD2	—	Psoriasis
Alemtuzumab	Campath®	Humanized	CD52	Risk for hematologic toxicity, infection, infusion reactions	Chronic lymphocytic leukemia
Basiliximab	Simulect®	Chimeric	IL-2Rα receptor (CD25)	Should be administered by transplant physician	Transplant rejection
Bevacizumab	Avastin®	Humanized	VEGF	Risk for GI perforation, hemorrhage, wound-healing complications	Colorectal cancer
Cetuximab	Erbitux®	Chimeric	EGF receptor	Risk for cardiopulmonary arrest in patients also receiving radiation therapy, infusion reactions	Colorectal cancer, head and neck cancer
Certolizumab pegol	Cimzia®	Pegylated humanized	TNF-α	Risk for T-cell lymphoma, infection risk, evaluate for tuberculosis	Crohn's disease
Daclizumab	Zenapax®	Chimeric humanized	IL-2Rα receptor (CD25)	Should be administered by transplant physician	Transplant rejection
Eculizumab	Soliris®	Humanized	Complement system protein C5	Risk for meningococcal infection	Paroxysmal nocturnal hemoglobinuria
Gemtuzumab ozogamicin	Mylotarg®	Humanized	CD33	—	Acute myeloid and promyelocytic leukemia
Ibritumomab tiuxetan	Zevalin®	Murine (with ^{90}Y or ^{111}In)	CD20	Risk for cutaneous and mucocutaneous reactions, cytopenia, infusion reaction	Non-Hodgkin lymphoma
Infliximab	Remicade®	Chimeric	TNF-α	Risk for fatal infections, malignancies especially in children, adolescents, and young adult males	Autoimmune disorders
Muromonab-CD3	Orthoclone OKT3®	Murine	T-cell CD3 receptor	Risk for anaphylaxis, should be administered by transplant physician	Transplant rejection
Natalizumab	Tysabri®	Humanized	α4-Integrin	Risk for progressive multifocal leukoencephalopathy (PML)	Multiple sclerosis and Crohn's disease
Omalizumab	Xolair®	Humanized	IgE on mast cells and basophils	Risk for anaphylaxis	Allergic asthma
Palivizumab	Synagis®	Humanized	RSV	—	Respiratory syncytial virus
Panitumumab	Vectibix®	Human	EGF receptor	Risk for dermatologic toxicity (90% of patients), infusion reaction	Refractory metastatic colorectal cancer
Ranibizumab	Lucentis®	Humanized	VEGF-A	—	Macular degeneration
Rituximab	Rituxan® MabThera®	Chimeric	CD20	Risk for infusion reactions, mucocutaneous reactions, PML	Chronic lymphocytic leukemia
Tositumomab and ^{131}I tositumomab	Bexxar®	Murine	CD20	Radioisotope; risk for anaphylaxis, bone marrow suppression, and fetal toxicity	Non-Hodgkin lymphoma
Trastuzumab	Herceptin®	Humanized	Human EGFR	Risk for cardiotoxicity, pulmonary toxicity, infusion reactions, and fetal toxicity	HER-2 positive breast cancer and gastric adenocarcinoma

TNF, tumor necrosis factor; *IL*, interleukin; *GI*, gastrointestinal; *Ig*, immunoglobulin; *VEGF*, vascular endothelial growth factor; *EGF*, epidermal growth factor; *EGFR*, epidermal growth factor receptor; *RSV*, respiratory syncytial virus.

6. **Infliximab** (Remicade®) is a chimeric mAb that binds and inhibits TNF-α. Infliximab is used to treat Crohn's disease and has an onset of action of about 2 weeks and elimination half-life of 7 to 12 days. The drug is infused over 2 or more hrs at 3 to 5 mg/kg starting at 0, 2, and 6 weeks, then every 8 weeks thereafter. The drug is also used to treat other autoimmune diseases such as rheumatoid arthritis.
7. **Rituximab** (Rituxan®) is an mAb targeted to the CD20 major histocompatibility protein on B lymphocytes. It is used to treat cancers such as **CD20-positive non-Hodgkin lymphoma** and also **rheumatoid arthritis.** The elimination half-life is 18 to 78 days depending on the disease and the patient.

V. CYTOKINE IMMUNOMODULATORS

A. **Overview**

1. Cytokine immunomodulators include **colony-stimulating factors**, **interleukins**, **interferons**, **chemokines**, and **thymic hormones**.
2. CSFs are **glycoprotein** cytokines that regulate the production, differentiation, and activation of hematopoietic cells in the body. These include **macrophages**, **megakaryocytes**, **eosinophils**, **neutrophils**, **basophils**, and **platelets. Erythropoietin** stimulates red cell production and is in the CSF class. Natural and modified CSFs are used to treat several **congenital disorders** and several forms of cancer.
3. **Interleukins** are proteins secreted by leukocytes that mediate communication between leukocytes. IL actions are similar to TNF but without the ability to produce septic shock symptoms.
4. **Interferons** are secreted in response to infection. In combination with other cytokines, IFNs participate in the immune response to infection. IFN-α and IFN-β are produced by leukocytes and fibroblasts and act in the antiviral immune response, whereas IFN-γ is secreted by T lymphocytes to stimulate macrophages and innate immunity.
5. **Tumor necrosis factor** is secreted in response to bacterial lipopolysaccharide and then recruits neutrophils and monocytes to the site of infection. TNF also mediates the symptoms of **septic shock**, characterized by intravascular collapse and disseminated intravascular coagulation.

B. **Examples**

1. **Darbepoetin alfa** (Aranesp®) and **epoetin alfa** (Epogen® and Procrit®) are recombinant human erythropoietin used for the treatment of **anemia** associated with **chronic renal failure** (darbepoetin or epoetin) or HIV (epoetin). Erythropoiesis-stimulating agents should be used as hemoglobin falls below 10 g/dL. Some recombinant human erythropoietin's in vivo properties are product dependent. Darbepoetin's half-life (21 hrs) is approximately three times longer than epoetin (4 to 13 hrs) when administered IV.
2. **Filgrastim** (Neupogen®) is recombinant hG-CSF (human granulocyte colony-stimulating factor) used for severe, chronic **neutropenia,** neutropenia associated with chemotherapy and for **bone marrow transplant**. hG-CSF and filgrastim both promote the proliferation, differentiation, maturation, and activation of neutrophils. Onset of action is within 24 hrs, levels return to baseline within 4 days. **Pegfilgrastim** (Neulasta®) is **pegylated** filgrastim with a half-life of 15 to 80 hrs compared to 3.5 hrs for the unpegylated filgrastim.
3. **Aldesleukin** (Proleukin®), a lymphokine, is a human recombinant IL-2 product that is used to treat **metastatic renal cell carcinoma** and **metastatic melanoma**. The starting dose is 600,000 IU/kg every 8 hrs by a 15-mins intravenous infusion for no more than 14 doses, then repeated after 9 days. Aldesleukin follows two-compartment pharmacokinetics, with an α-half-life of 6 to 13 mins and a β-half-life of 80 to 120 mins, and is excreted renally. The drug has several black box warnings including risk for capillary leak syndrome, severe central nervous system (CNS) effects, and infection, and should not be used in patients with cardiopulmonary disease.
4. **Etanercept** (Enbrel®) is a dimeric soluble form of the TNF receptor that binds both TNF-α and TNF-β. Like Humira®, Enbrel® is used for autoimmune disorders such as Crohn's disease and rheumatoid arthritis, given as 50-mg weekly injections, either as a single or divided dose. Patients taking Enbrel® are at increased risk for infection.
5. **Interferon-β** (Betaseron®, Extavia®) differs from naturally occurring IFN-β in its lack of carbohydrate side chains and a single amino acid substitution. Many of its effects are similar to those of IFN-α. Betaseron® is used to treat **multiple sclerosis (MS)**, dosed at 0.0625 mg SQ every other day for relapsing MS (0.125 mg for secondary progressive MS), slowly increasing to a target dose of 0.25 mg every other day. Common side effects include lymphopenia (88%), injection site reaction (85%), headache (5%), muscle weakness (61%), and flulike syndrome (60%).

6. **Interferon β-1a** (Avonex®, Rebif®) is human recombinant IFN β-1a and used for relapsing multiple sclerosis. Avonex is dosed 30 mcg IM once weekly; Rebif® is dosed SQ three times weekly titrating up to 44 or 22 mcg/week.
7. **Interferon-γ** (Actimmune®) is human recombinant IFN-γ and plays a role in macrophage-induced killing. Recombinant IFN-γ is used to treat **chronic granulomatous disease**. Actimmune® has a half-life of 38 mins when given IV, 4 hrs when given IM, and 7 hrs when given SQ.
8. **Sargramostim** (Leukine®) is a GM-CSF used for myeloid reconstitution after **bone marrow transplant or chemotherapy**. Nausea (58% to 70%), diarrhea ($<$ 89%), vomiting (46% to 70%), and fever (81%) are the most common side effects. The onset of action is 7 to 14 days before changes in white blood cell (WBC) levels are measurable.

VI. PLASMA PROTEINS, COAGULATION, FIBRINOLYSIS

A. **Overview**. The human plasma is rich in proteins such as **albumin** that are designed to maintain osmotic balance, acid–base balance, viscosity of the plasma, act as a protein reserve for the body, and transport insoluble molecules such as vitamins and hormones via plasma protein binding. In addition, immune globulins are present in high concentration in the plasma as part of immune surveillance (see antibodies, discussed earlier). Also, **fibrinogen** is an important plasma protein involved in blood clotting. Several key proteins have been made available by recombinant methods for either replacement therapy or given in therapeutic doses for their pharmacologic activity.

B. **Proteins providing pharmacologic activity**

1. **Alteplase** (Activase®, Cathflo®) is a **thrombolytic** agent also known as **tissue plasminogen activator**. Intravenous alteplase lyses thrombi in coronary arteries after ST-elevation **myocardial infarction**, **acute ischemic stroke** (within 3 hrs of onset of symptoms), or **pulmonary embolism**. An unlabeled use is for **acute ischemic stroke** presenting 3 to 4.5 hrs after onset of symptoms. The drug is given as a bolus dose over 1 to 2 mins or over 2 hrs for pulmonary embolism. Practitioners should avoid agitation during dilution. **Bleeding complications** and **reperfusion arrhythmias** are the primary adverse events associated with this therapy. Other examples of thrombolytics include **reteplase** (Retavase®) and **tenecteplase** (TNKase®).
2. **Desirudin** (Iprivask®) inhibits thrombin and is used as an **anticoagulant**. Specifically, it is used for **DVT** prophylaxis and is dosed 15 mg SQ every 12 hrs. Bleeding is the most common adverse reaction with anticoagulants. Other thrombin inhibitors include **lepirudin** (Refludan®) and **bivalirudin** (Angiomax®).

C. **Proteins for replacement therapy**. **Protein C** is available in recombinant form as an anticoagulant for congenital protein C deficiency. **Antihemophilic factors VIIA, VIII, and IX** are also available in recombinant forms in the treatment of patients with hemophilia.

VII. MISCELLANEOUS OTHER PROTEIN DRUGS

A. **Enzymes**. Many congenital disorders result in insufficient or inactive enzyme expression. As a result, recombinant technology is perfectly suited to design drugs for replacement therapy. Examples of these types of drugs include **alglucosidase** for **Pompe disease**, **Pulmozyme** for **cystic fibrosis**, **galsulfase** for **Maroteaux–Lamy syndrome**, **imiglucerase** for **Gaucher disease**, **laronidase** for **Hurler syndrome**, **PEG-ADA** (pegylated adenosine deaminase) for **ADA deficiency**, and **idursulfase** for **Hunter syndrome**. Some enzyme drugs are used for their pharmacologic properties, such as **glucarpidase** for **methotrexate overdose**, **pegloticase** (pegylated uricase; half-life: 10 to 12 days) for **gout**, and **rasburicase** (uricase; half-life: 8 hrs) to manage uric acid levels in some malignancies.

B. **Hormones**. Congenital defects also can result in insufficient or inactive hormone synthesis or be administered in therapeutic doses to elicit a pharmacologic effect. **Parathyroid hormone** (**teriparatide**), **insulin-like growth factor** (**mecasermin**), and **platelet-derived growth factor** (**becaplermin**) are available in recombinant forms for hormone supplement. **Gonadotropin** (**follitropin-α, follitropin-β, leutropin, urofollitropin**) is also used to stimulate ovulation.

1. **Somatropin** (Genotropin®, Humatrope®, Norditropin®, Nutropin®, Omnitrope®, Saizen®, Serostim®, Tev-Tropin®, Zorbtive®) is recombinant human growth hormone. The most common side effect of somatropin is edema, arthralgias, and myalgias. Many manufacturers produce this protein, and each is dosed differently because of their different SQ bioavailabilities (product dependent, ranging from 70% to 90%) and formulations (*Table 7-2*). A now-discontinued growth hormone

Table 7-2 SOMATROPIN COMPARISONS

Trade (Manufacturer) Cell Line	Adult GH Deficiency	Pediatric GH Deficiency	Other Indications	Formulation
Genotropin® (Pfizer) *Escherichia coli*	0.15–0.3 mg/d SQ; increase by 0.1–0.2 mg/d every 1–2 mo	*GH deficiency:* 0.16–0.24 mg/kg/wk SQ × 6–7 doses/wk	*Turner syndrome*: 0.33 mg/kg divided into equal doses 6–7 d/wk *Decreased body growth*: 0.24 mg/kg/wk SQ × 6–7 d/wk	*Miniquick* (disposable premeasured syringe): no refrigeration Pen (reusable pen): refrigerate Mixer (reusable, automatic mixer): refrigerate
Humatrope® (Lilly) *E. coli*	0.15–0.3 mg/d SQ; increase by 0.1–0.2 mg/d every 1–2 mo	0.18–0.3 mg/kg/wk SQ	*Turner syndrome*: 0.375 mg/kg divided into equal doses 6–7 d/wk *SHOX deficiency*: 0.35 mg/kg divided into equal doses 6–7 d/wk	Injection powder for solution; SQ powder for solution
Norditropin® (Novo Nordisk) *E. coli*	0.15–0.3 mg/d SQ; increase by 0.1–0.2 mg/d every 1–2 mo	0.024–0.34 mg/kg/d SQ × 6–7 d/wk	*Turner syndrome*: up to 0.067 mg/kg/d	*FlexPro*: SQ solution *Nordiflex* (prefilled): no refrigeration after initial use *PenMate* (needle-free): SQ solution
Nutropin®; Nutropin AQ® (Genentech) *E. coli*	0.15–0.3 mg/d SQ; increase by 0.1–0.2 mg/d every 1–2 mo	0.3 mg/kg/wk SQ × 6–7 d/wk up to 0.7 mg/kg/wk for pubertal patients	*Turner* syndrome: ≤ 0.375 mg/kg divided into equal doses 3–7 d/wk	*AQ NuSpin 5* (prefilled automatic): SQ solution *AQ Pen cartridge*: SQ solution Nutropin: powder *Nutropin AQ*: SQ solution
Omnitrope® (Sandoz) *E. coli*	< 0.04 mg/kg/wk SQ in divided dose; may increase to < 0.08 mg/kg/wk	0.16–0.24 mg/kg/wk SQ × 6–7 d	*Decreased body growth*: 0.24 mg/kg/wk SQ × 6–7 d/wk	SQ powder; SQ solution
Serostim® (EMD Serono) mammalian cell			*AIDS-associated cachexia*: body weight < 35 kg, 0.1 mg/kg SQ; otherwise 4–6 mg SQ	SQ powder store at room temperature prior to reconstitution; discard after reconstitution
Saizen® (EMD Serono) mammalian cell	0.005 mg/kg/d SQ or IM; after 4 wks, may adjust to ≤ 0.01 mg/kg/d	0.6 mg/kg SQ or IM 3 × per wk		*Cool Click* (needle-free) *Easypod* (automated device) Store powder at room temperature; refrigerate after reconstitution
Tev-Tropin®		0.1 mg/kg SQ, 3 × per wk		Store powder at room temperature; refrigerate after reconstitution
Zorbtive® (EMD Serono) *E. coli*			*Short bowel syndrome*: 0.1 mg/kg SQ daily for 4 wks; increase to ≤ 8 mg/d	SQ powder

From Page AV, Caplan ES. Immunomodulators. In: Mandell GL, Bennett JE, Dolin R, eds. *Mandell, Douglas, and Bennett's Principles and Practice of Infectious Diseases*. 7th ed. Philadelphia, PA: Churchill Livingstone; 2010:611–624.

product contained an extra methionine amino acid at the N-terminus (Protropin®). **Growth hormone** antagonist (**pegvisomant**) is a pegylated growth hormone analog used in the treatment of **acromegaly** where growth hormone is overproduced.

2. **Insulin** (Humulin® R, Humulin® R U-500, Novolin®) is regular, short-acting human recombinant insulin used to treat diabetes mellitus. Insulin is either given as regular insulin SQ boluses (baseline plus bolus dosing) or via dosing two to three times per day using a mixture of regular and intermediate-acting isophane insulin, also known as NPH insulin (Humulin® N, Iletin® I NPH, Iletin® II NPH, Novolin®, Novolin® N Innolet®, ReliOn N, ReliOn N Innolet®). **NPH insulin** is insulin modified with zinc and protamine to promote dimer and hexamer formation, resulting in prolonged absorption and action. The disadvantage of NPH insulin is variable absorption but it does have a long clinical history compared to other types of insulin. Lente insulin is another type of intermediate-acting insulin product. Other insulin forms, such as rapid acting (semilente insulin, insulin aspart, insulin glulisine, and insulin lispro) or long acting (ultralente insulin insulin detemir, insulin glargine, protamine-zinc insulin), are also used in various combinations to individualize glucose control. **Insulin pumps** are also used for continuous infusion of basal insulin and also boluses at meals but must be changed every 3 days. **Inhaled insulin** (Exubera®) is no longer on the market.

VIII. MACROMOLECULAR NUCLEIC ACID DRUGS

A. Background

1. **DNA** (deoxyribonucleic acid) is a polymeric, double-stranded helix that comprises the genetic material of all organisms. DNA is transcribed into **RNA** (ribonucleic acid), which is translated into protein. DNA sequences can be modified with high accuracy using recombinant DNA technology. **Restriction endonucleases** are key tools for sequence-specific modification and recombination of DNA.
2. **Viruses**' genetic material may consist of either RNA or double-stranded or single-stranded DNA. RNA viruses, or retroviruses, use reverse transcriptase to transcribe their genome into DNA.
3. The **Human Genome Project** was designed to sequence the human genome. Other technologies using high-throughput sequencing have also been useful to sequence individual genes and their variants. Knowledge of the role of these genetic variants, or **polymorphisms**, are useful for better understanding disease etiology and for the development of new, more specific drugs.

B. Oligonucleotide drugs

1. **Background**. Oligonucleotide drugs are single-stranded DNA or RNA molecules that are usually chemically modified to improve in vivo stability and cellular uptake. They are used to block gene expression or act as substrate inhibitors. **Antisense** drugs bind to or "hybridize to" mRNA complementary sequences to inhibit translation. The primary applications for antisense therapy are cancer or antiviral therapies, but any disease or disorder where inhibition of a specific gene is desired has a potential application. An **aptamer** is an oligonucleotide with secondary structure that binds with high affinity to a substrate in the same manner that a DNA-binding protein binds DNA.
2. **Examples**. **Pegaptanib** (Macugen®) is a 2′-fluoro, PEG-conjugated, oligoribonucleotide aptamer, which binds to and inhibits VEGF. It is used in the treatment of **age-related macular degeneration**. The drug is administered 0.3 mg intravitreally every 6 weeks and has a plasma half-life of 6 to 14 days. Pegaptanib may cause hypertension or ocular side effects such as conjunctivitis. **Fomivirsen** (Vitravene®) is an antisense phosphorothioate oligonucleotide used to treat HIV patients with **cytomegaloviral** infections in the eye. It is dosed 330 mcg intravitreally every 2 weeks for two doses, then every 4 weeks thereafter. Onset and duration of action is 8 and 10 days, respectively.

C. Gene therapy

Gene therapy. Despite decades of research and development, and currently more than 1500 clinical trials worldwide, gene therapy therapeutics have not yet been approved by the U.S. Food and Drug Administration (FDA). Scores of gene therapy formulations are in advanced clinical trials, but the technology continues to be plagued by insufficient expression of the therapeutic gene and safety questions. Should this technology finally resolve its development hurdles, the ability to provide therapeutic genes to somatic cells has incredible potential, especially in the areas of cancer, cardiovascular disease, and genetic disorders.

Study Questions

Directions: Choose the **best** answer to each of the following questions.

1. Most biologic drugs are sensitive to all of the following **except**
   (A) heat.
   (B) shaking.
   (C) stainless steel.
   (D) light.

2. Recombinant protein drugs are designed to replicate which of the following types of molecules?
   (A) Antibodies
   (B) Enzymes
   (C) Proteins in the plasma
   (D) All of the above
   (E) None of the above

3. Nucleic acid drugs or drug candidates include which of the following?
   (A) Gene therapy
   (B) Oligonucleotides
   (C) A and B
   (D) None of the above

4. Glycoprotein is a protein linked to _____.
   (A) a carbohydrate
   (B) a nucleotide
   (C) an amino acid
   (D) a lipid molecule
   (E) None of the above

5. Examples of monoclonal antibody drugs include all of the following **except**
   (A) infliximab.
   (B) Herceptin.
   (C) trypsin.
   (D) rituximab.

6. An example of a recombinant cytokine is _____.
   (A) muromonab
   (B) albumin
   (C) oligonucleotide
   (D) interferon
   (E) growth hormone

7. A recombinant protein will have the same in vivo properties if the genetic sequence is the same. This statement is _____.
   (A) always true
   (B) not necessarily true
   (C) always false

8. Monoclonal antibodies are most often used for what type of clinical indications?
   (A) Cancer
   (B) Correcting congenital deficiencies
   (C) Replacement therapy
   (D) Psychiatric disorders
   (E) None of the above

9. Gene therapy _____.
   (A) is a technology that is widely used in patient care
   (B) involves short nucleic acid sequences to inhibit gene expression
   (C) has not been tested in clinical trials
   (D) All of the above
   (E) None of the above

10. Which of the following statements is true for polyethylene glycol (PEG)?
    (A) It is a carbohydrate used to increase clearance of drugs.
    (B) It is conjugated only to recombinant hormones.
    (C) It blocks the renal filtration of drugs.
    (D) It is naturally occurring on many biologic molecules.

Answers and Explanations

1. **The answer is C** *[see I.E.]*.
   Biologic drugs are sensitive to high (and very low) temperatures, agitation, and light.

2. **The answer is D** *[see IV; VI; VII.A.]*.
   Protein drugs are used for protein replacement or for providing pharmacologic activity when used in therapeutic doses. Besides enzymes, plasma proteins, mAbs, and cytokines, hormones are also classes of proteins that have been made into recombinant drugs.

3. **The answer is C** *[see VIII]*.
   Many macromolecular nucleic acid drugs are in clinical trials and preclinical development, such as miRNA, ribozymes, siRNA, and gene therapy, but only oligonucleotides have become approved drugs at this time. Nucleoside

drugs are small nucleic acid drug molecules and many are in use, especially for antiviral therapy.

4. **The answer is A** *[see II.K]*.
Glycoproteins are made of a carbohydrate linked to a protein.

5. **The answer is C** *[see IV.B; Table 7-1]*.
Trypsin is an enzyme that digests proteins. The other drugs listed are examples of mAbs.

6. **The answer is D** *[see V]*.
Muromonab is an mAb, albumin is a plasma protein, oligonucleotides are nucleic acid drugs, and growth hormone is a hormone. Only interferon is considered a cytokine of this list.

7. **The answer is B** *[see I.B; VII.B.1; Table 7-2]*.
Because product quality and even structure are dependent on the manufacturing process (including cell line, equipment, chemicals and their impurities, material handling, etc.), each biologic product is unique even if the original gene sequence used is identical. Therefore, generic versions of biologics are not available; rather, similar products that follow the innovator are called **biosimilars**.

8. **The answer is A** *[see IV.B; Table 7-1]*.
mAbs bind to unique epitopes on specific antigens, which either act as an antagonist to the antigen or employ the immune system to elicit an immune response against the target. Congenital defects in the immune system would result in an overall lack of antibody defense instead of lacking a single antibody type.

9. **The answer is E** *[see VIII.C]*.
Gene therapies are in clinical trials but have not yet been FDA approved. Gene therapy involves delivery of a gene (usually thousands of double-stranded nucleotides in size) compared to an oligonucleotide (15–30 single-stranded nucleotides).

10. **The answer is C** *[see Table 7-1; II.S; V.B.2; VII.A; VII.B.2; VIII.B.2]*.
Polyethylene glycol (PEG) is a synthetic polymer that is conjugated to protein and nucleic acid drugs to increase the half-life and decrease the renal clearance of a drug by glomerular filtration. Many different protein drugs have employed this method to improve the pharmacokinetic properties of the compound, including filgrastim, adenosine deamidase, and anti-TNF antibody.

8

Drug Metabolism, Prodrugs, and Pharmacogenetics

MICHAEL L. ADAMS, S. THOMAS ABRAHAM

I. INTRODUCTION TO DRUG METABOLISM.

Xenobiotic metabolism is a general term used to describe the protective biochemical process by which a living organism either enzymatically or nonenzymatically alters a xenobiotic (foreign substance) to a metabolite that is inactive or quickly eliminated from the organism. *Drug metabolism* is a more specific term that applies the concept of xenobiotic metabolism to pharmaceutical agents. In general, drug metabolism begins with a lipophilic drug or substrate and converts it to a more hydrophilic metabolite to facilitate its elimination. There are multiple enzymes and paths that are possible for a single xenobiotic, so it is common for multiple metabolites with varying properties to be observed. An understanding of the drug metabolism process and the potential outcomes is critical for developing safe and useful pharmaceuticals.

II. CONSEQUENCES OF DRUG METABOLISM.

In the process of converting a drug to a metabolite, the pharmacological activity of the drug may be changed. Metabolites can be broadly classified as either inactive or active metabolites.

A. **Inactive metabolites** of drugs are devoid of pharmacological activity that was characteristic of the drug or toxicant. This metabolic change may be considered an **inactivation** or **detoxification**. There may be a disruption in the pharmacophore, the chemical functional groups, and their orientation relative to each other that is required for proper receptor binding or activity, or a change in the distribution of the drug because of the change in the physicochemical properties of the drug that facilitates elimination.
   1. The hydrolysis of procaine (Novocain) to *p*-aminobenzoic acid and diethylethanolamine results in a loss of anesthetic activity (*Figure 8-1A*).
   2. Acetaminophen is glucuronidated on its phenolic hydroxyl group to an inactive metabolite that is rapidly eliminated (*Figure 8-1B*).

B. **Active metabolites** of drugs have pharmacological activity, which can either be similar to the desired pharmacological activity or a new activity that is absent from the parent drug.
   1. Metabolites with similar pharmacological activity retain the desired biological activity that is inherent in the parent compound.
      a. Codeine is demethylated to the more active analgesic, morphine (*Figure 8-2A*).
      b. Imipramine (Tofranil) is demethylated to the essentially equiactive antidepressant, desipramine (Norpramin) (*Figure 8-2B*).
   2. In the case that the metabolite has the **desired pharmacological activity** although the parent is inactive, the metabolism is called **bioactivation**. The parent compound devoid of pharmacological activity before metabolism is called a prodrug.
      a. The prodrug enalapril (Vasotec) is hydrolyzed to enalaprilat, a potent antihypertensive (*Figure 8-3A*).

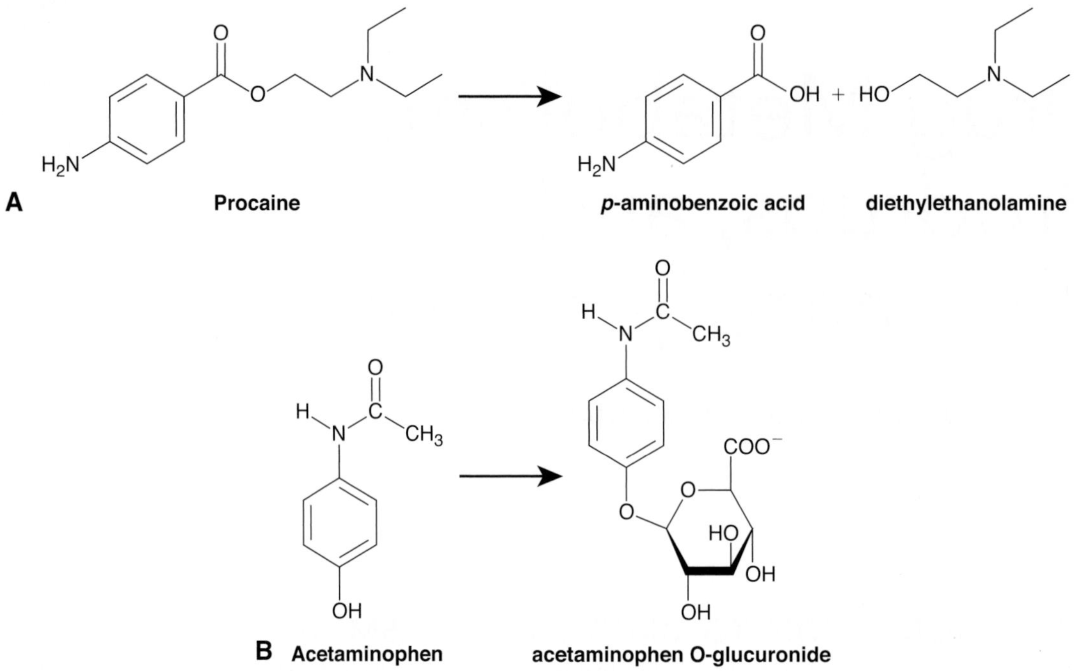

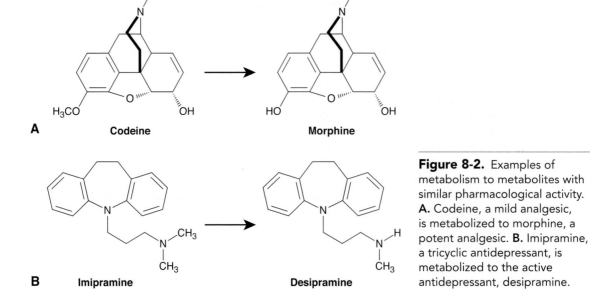

Figure 8-1. Examples of metabolism to inactive metabolites. **A.** Ester hydrolysis of the local anesthetic procaine to produce two inactive metabolites. **B.** Glucuronidation of acetaminophen to an inactive metabolite.

b. Nabumetone (Relafen) is a prodrug that is oxidized in the body to an active nonsteroidal anti-inflammatory drug (NSAID) (*Figure 8-3B*).

3. **Bioactivation** of a drug can also result in a **toxic metabolite**. The parent activated is called a protoxicant.
   a. Halothane (Fluothane) is a general anesthetic that is oxidized to a reactive metabolite that is associated with hepatotoxicity (*Figure 8-4A*).
   b. Acetaminophen (Tylenol) can be oxidized into a reactive metabolite, *N*-acetyl-*p*-benzoquinone imine (NAPQI), that can lead to hepatotoxicity (*Figure 8-4B*; Chapter 11, section IV.D.4).

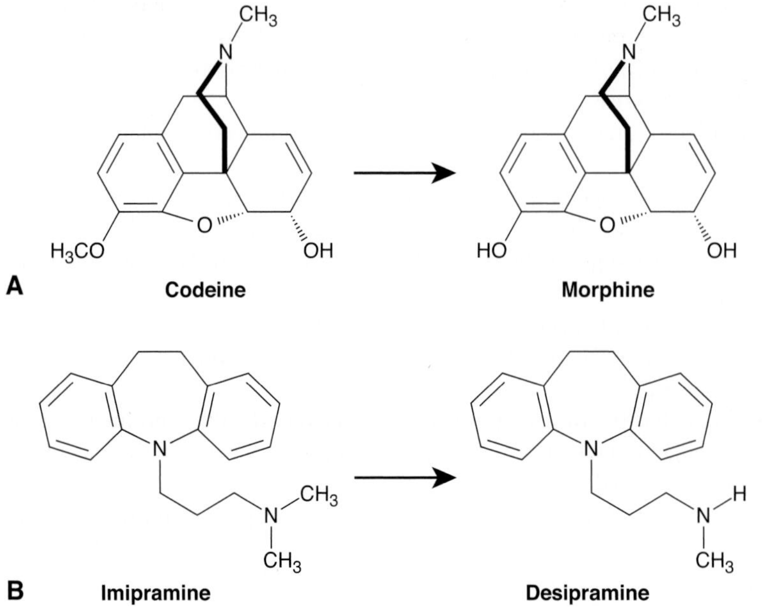

Figure 8-2. Examples of metabolism to metabolites with similar pharmacological activity. **A.** Codeine, a mild analgesic, is metabolized to morphine, a potent analgesic. **B.** Imipramine, a tricyclic antidepressant, is metabolized to the active antidepressant, desipramine.

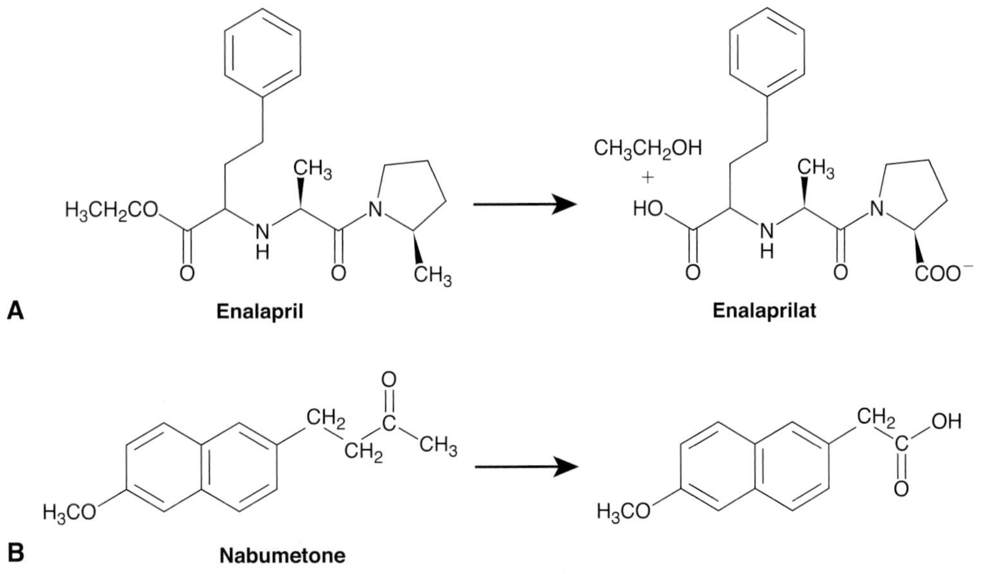

Figure 8-3. Examples of metabolism of an inactive prodrug to the desired pharmacological activity. **A.** Ester hydrolysis of the prodrug enalapril to the active enalaprilat. **B.** Oxidation of the ketone on the prodrug nabumetone to the active nonsteroidal anti-inflammatory carboxylic acid.

III. METABOLIC PATHWAYS.

Drug metabolism is performed by a large number of different enzymes and even by some nonenzymatic processes. The liver is the organ with the highest concentration of drug-metabolizing enzymes because of its localization between the gastrointestinal (GI) tract, where the body has the highest exposure to foreign substances, and the systemic circulation. The enzymes involved in drug metabolism can be classified by several different categories. The enzymes can either be localized in the cytosol (cytosolic) or the endoplasmic reticulum (ER) membrane (microsomal) portion of the cell. A general classification of enzymatic processes based on the type of reactions involved includes **phase I** and **phase II**.

A. **Phase I metabolism** is characterized as a **functionalization reaction**. Phase I reactions add or reveal a polar functional group on a substrate by oxidation, reduction, or hydrolysis. The addition of the polar group **increases** the overall **polarity** of the metabolites to increase water solubility and facilitate excretion in the urine. Many phase I metabolites are substrates for phase II reactions (see II.B).

1. **Oxidation** is the most common phase I reaction. Several phase I oxidation reactions are further described later and illustrated in *Table 8-1*.

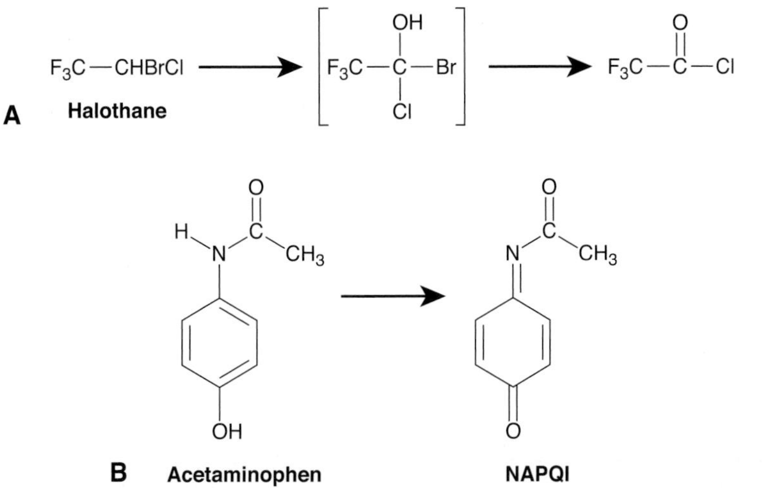

Figure 8-4. Examples of metabolism of active drugs to toxic metabolites. **A.** Halothane, a general anesthetic, is metabolized to a reactive metabolite associated with hepatotoxicity. **B.** Acetaminophen, an antipyretic, is metabolized to the reactive metabolite, NAPQI, associated with hepatotoxicity.

Table 8-1 COMMON OXIDATION REACTIONS

Reaction (Enzyme)	Examples
Aliphatic hydroxylation (CYP450)	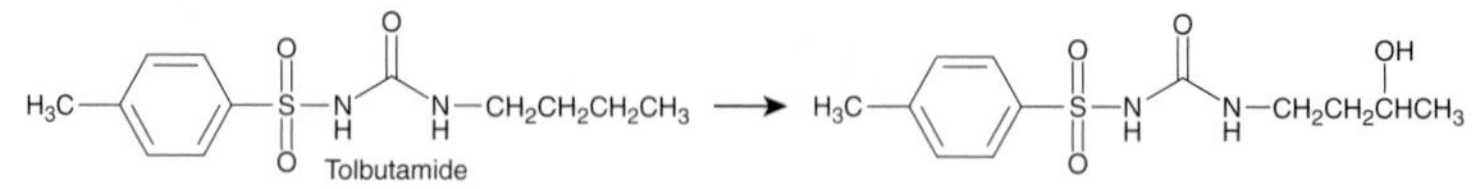
Allylic hydroxylation (CYP450)	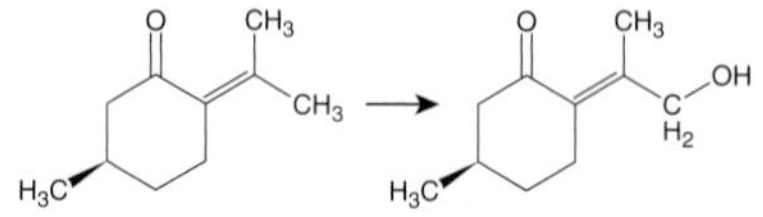
Benzylic hydroxylation (CYP450)	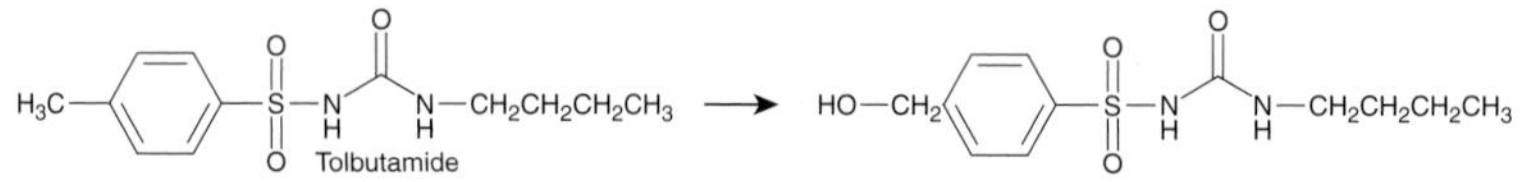
Aromatic hydroxylation (CYP450)	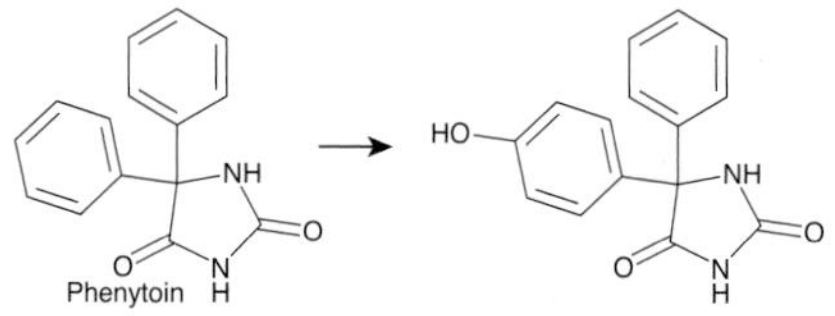
Epoxidation (CYP450)	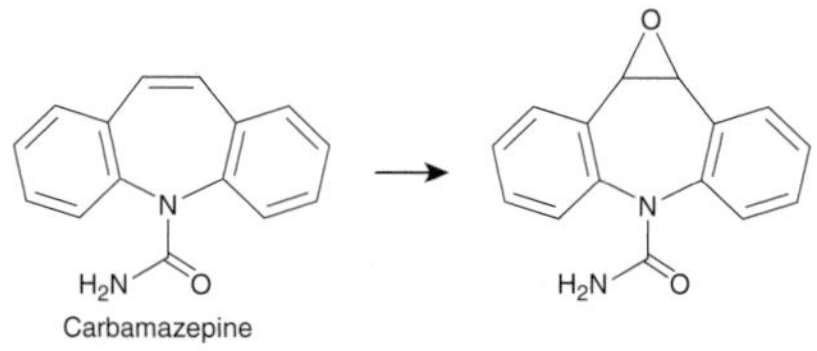
O-Dealkylation (CYP450)	Codeine to morphine (see *Figure 8-2A*)
S-Dealkylation (CYP450)	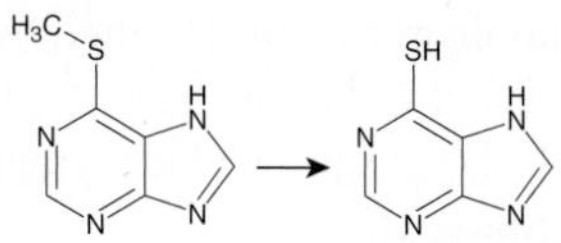
S-Oxidation (CYP450 or FMO)	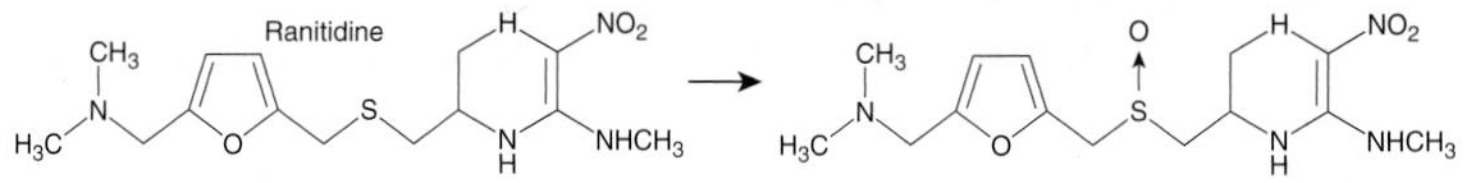
N-Dealkylation (CYP450)	Imipramine to desipramine (see *Figure 8-2B*)
N-Oxidation (FMO or CYP450)	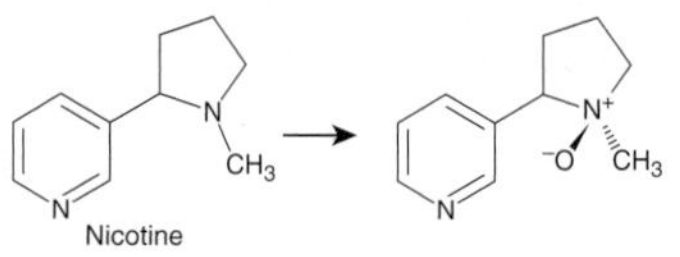
Deamination (CYP450 or monoamine oxidase)	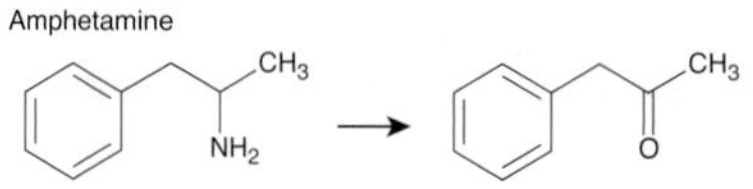
Dehalogenation (CYP450)	Halothane (see *Figure 8-4A*)
Alcohol oxidation (*1*) (alcohol dehydrogenase) Aldehyde oxidation (*2*) (aldehyde dehydrogenase)	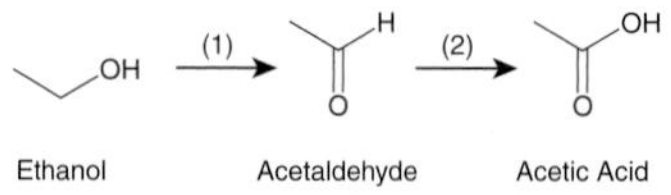
Oxidation (xanthine oxidase)	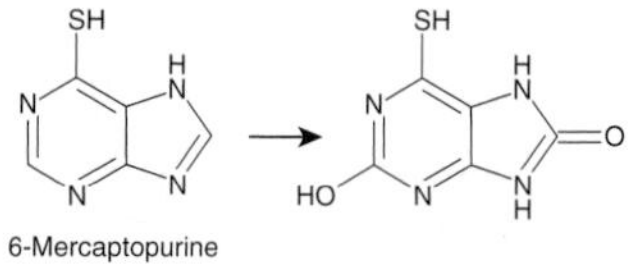

FMO, Flavin-containing monooxygenase; *CYP450*, Cytochrome P450s.

2. **Cytochrome P450** (CYP450) is a superfamily of mixed function oxidases that are responsible for the majority of oxidation reactions.
   a. CYP450 is classified as a **microsomal enzyme** and in the cell is bound to the ER. CYP450 is found in very **high concentrations in the liver** and to a lesser extent in the intestinal mucosa, lungs, and kidneys. CYP450 is dependent on the porphyrin prosthetic group, commonly called the heme group, and NADPH to metabolize a wide array of substrates to numerous metabolites. Common CYP450 reactions are illustrated in *Table 8-1*.
   b. There are **several isoforms of CYP450** responsible for drug metabolism, which gives wide substrate specificity to the family of CYP450 enzymes. Each isoform has different substrate specificities based on the size and amino acid composition of the CYP450 active site. The **nomenclature** for the CYP450 enzymes is based on **amino acid homology** and divides the CYP450's into **families** designated by an Arabic number, **subfamilies** designated by a letter, and individual genes designated by an Arabic number preceded by "CYP." For example, CYP3A4 is an example where the family is 3, the subfamily is A, and the individual gene is 4. The CYP450 families most responsible for drug metabolism include CYP1, CYP2, CYP3, and CYP4 with subfamilies CYP2C, CYP2D, and CYP3A metabolizing most drugs. CYP families CYP7, CYP11, CYP17, CYP19, CYP21, and CYP27 contribute to steroid and bile acid synthesis and metabolism required for homeostasis.
3. **Flavin-containing monooxygenase** (FMO) is a family of **microsomal phase I** drug-metabolizing enzymes responsible for the oxidation of N- and S-containing soft nucleophile substrates with metabolites similar to CYP450 metabolites (see *Table 8-1*).
4. **Alcohol dehydrogenase** is a **cytosolic** enzyme that oxidizes alcohols into aldehydes (from primary alcohols) or ketones (from secondary alcohols). This oxidation is reversible and is frequently observed in primary alcohols where the aldehyde can be further oxidized to a carboxylic acid (see Aldehyde Dehydrogenase, III.A.5).
5. **Aldehyde dehydrogenase** is a general name for a group of enzymes expressed both in the mitochondria and the cytosol that is responsible for oxidizing an aldehyde to a carboxylic acid. A common reaction performed by an aldehyde dehydrogenase and aldehyde oxidase is the conversion of acetaldehyde to acetic acid in the metabolism of ethanol.
6. **Xanthine oxidase** and **xanthine dehydrogenase** are the two forms of the same gene product that are responsible for the breakdown of **endogenous purines**. Xanthine oxidase is a cytosolic enzyme that contributes to the metabolism of the purine anticancer drugs (i.e., 6-mercaptopurine) and other xanthines including caffeine and theophylline. Xanthine oxidase is also inhibited by antigout drugs like allopurinol (Zyloprim) to slow the production of uric acid from purines.
7. **Monoamine** and **diamine oxidase** are mitochondrial enzymes that metabolize amines to aldehydes through an **oxidative deamination** process. Monoamine oxidase is responsible for the metabolic inactivation of catecholamines in neurons and the hepatic inactivation of biogenic amines absorbed from the GI tract. Monoamine oxidase is also a target for inhibition in the treatment of depression (i.e., monoamine oxidase inhibitors including phenelzine [Nardil]).
8. **Reduction reactions** are less common than oxidation but are still **phase I** reactions that add or reveal a functional group to increase the water solubility of the molecule to facilitate elimination. There are several reductase enzymes and even CYP450 may have reductase activity. Common reduction reactions include the reduction of disulfide bonds, carbonyls, and nitro or azo functional groups.
   a. A common reduction reaction is the **reduction of disulfide bonds** commonly found between cysteine residues in proteins. Other sulfhydryl-containing molecules can form disulfides that may be reduced back to the free sulfhydryls, or disulfide-containing drugs can be reduced like disulfiram (*Table 8-2*).
   b. **Aldo-keto reductases** reduce a carbonyl-containing compound back to an alcohol in a process opposite the oxidation performed by the alcohol dehydrogenases (*Table 8-2*; see also III.A.4).
   c. **Reduction** of the **aromatic nitro** (NO_2) group and the **azo** (N=N) group is performed by a class of enzymes generically called nitroreductases and azoreductases, respectively, to produce free aromatic amines. Example reactions are included in *Table 8-2*. The liver contains these reductases both in the cytosol and the microsomal cellular fraction. Additionally, gut bacteria have significant reductase activity for both nitro and azo groups.

Table 8-2 COMMON REDUCTION REACTIONS

Reaction (Enzyme)	Examples
Reduction of disulfide bond	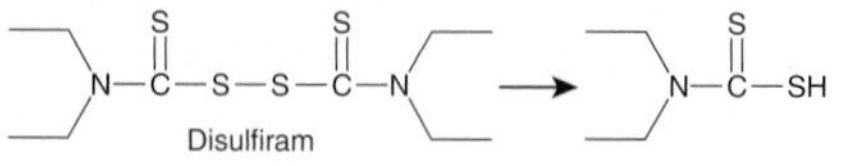 Disulfiram
Aldehyde and/or keto reduction	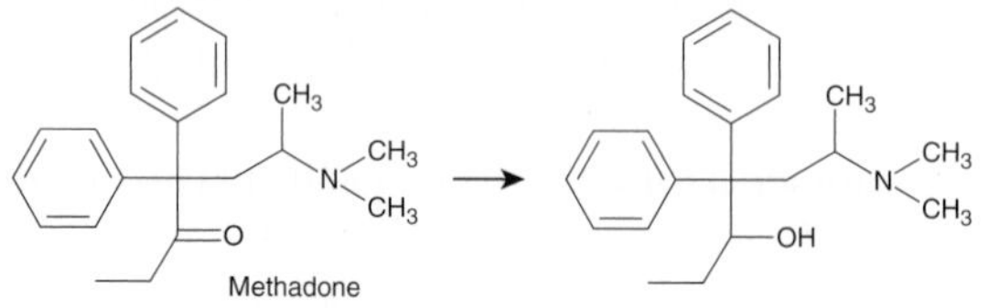 Methadone
Nitro (—NO_2) reductions	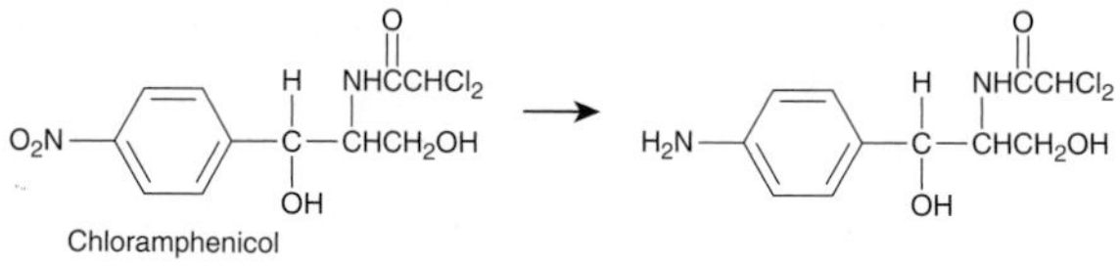 Chloramphenicol
Azo reductions (—N=N—)	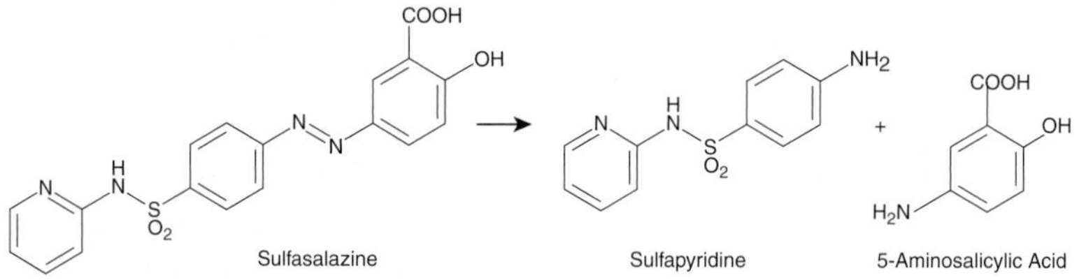 Sulfasalazine Sulfapyridine 5-Aminosalicylic Acid

9. **Hydrolysis** reactions add water across a bond to produce a more water-soluble metabolite. Common hydrolysis reactions include ester hydrolysis, amide hydrolysis, and epoxide hydrolysis.
   a. **Ester hydrolysis** is commonly performed by the ubiquitous **esterase** enzymes found throughout the body. There is a significant esterase activity in the plasma that is responsible for the hydrolysis of an ester into a more water-soluble alcohol and carboxylic acid. This metabolic process can be an inactivating or activating (see Prodrugs, V) reaction. A **lactone**, like found in erythromycin, is a cyclic ester that can also be metabolized by esterase enzymes.
   b. **Amide hydrolysis** is performed by **amidase** enzymes that are generally expressed in the liver. Analogous to the ester hydrolysis reaction, the products of amide hydrolysis are an amine and a carboxylic acid (*Table 8-3*). A cyclic amide is called a **lactam** and is the key structural feature for the β-lactam antibiotics.
   c. **Epoxide hydrolase** converts epoxides into diols, which can be targets for conjugation reactions to facilitate elimination of xenobiotics (*Table 8-3*). There is both a microsomal and cytosolic form of epoxide hydrolase.

B. **Phase II reactions** are commonly called **conjugation reactions** because they use a functional group on the xenobiotic (either from phase I metabolism or part of the xenobiotic itself) to add or conjugate a biomolecule that usually increases the polarity of the xenobiotic and facilitates elimination from the body. These conjugation reactions require an enzyme generally termed as **transferase** that transfers a high-energy molecule called the **cofactor** or **cosubstrate** to the xenobiotic. The transferred cofactor is usually large and very polar-forming inactive metabolites. There are exceptions like methylation (see later discussion) that do not increase polarity but do generally form inactive metabolites. Common phase II reactions are discussed later and examples are included in *Table 8-4*.

1. **Glucuronidation** is the most common phase II reaction. **Glucuronosyltransferase** is the microsomal enzyme that uses uridine diphosphate glucuronic acid (UDP-GA) as the cofactor to transfer the glucuronic acid to several different functional groups, including hydroxyl groups, carboxylic acid groups, hydroxylamines, and sulfonamides. The glucuronic acid adds a significant amount of hydrophilicity to the molecule and facilities its elimination in the urine. High-molecular-weight glucuronides (MW > 500 Da) are secreted into the bile, which ends up in the intestines.

Table 8-3 COMMON HYDROLYSIS REACTIONS

Reaction	Examples
Ester hydrolysis (esterase)	See *Figure 8-3A*
Amide hydrolysis (amidase; peptidase)	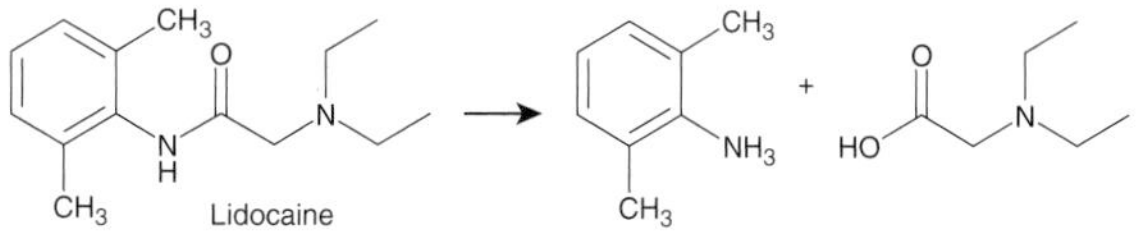
Epoxide hydrolysis (epoxide hydrolase)	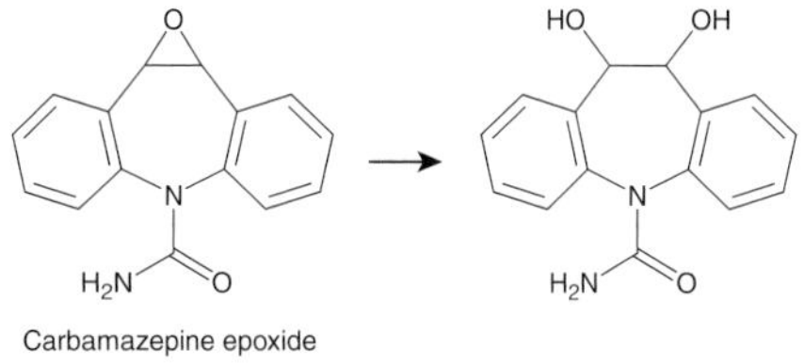

Table 8-4 COMMON PHASE II REACTIONS

Reaction	Enzyme	Cofactor	Examples
Glucuronidation	Glucuronosyltransferase	UDP-GA	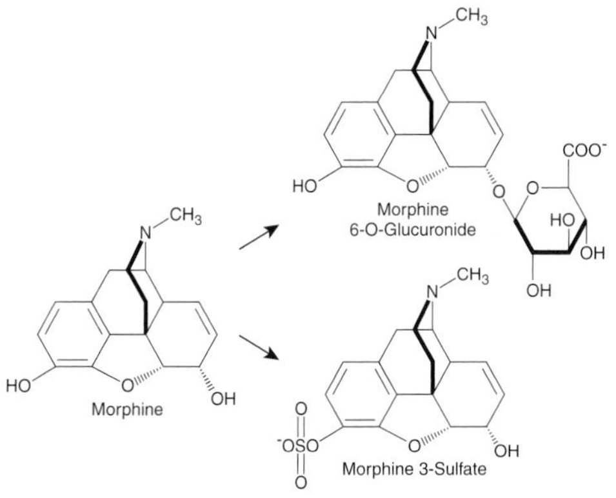
Sulfation	Sulfotransferase	PAPS	
Amino acid conjugation	*N*-Acyltransferase	Glycine and/ or glutamine	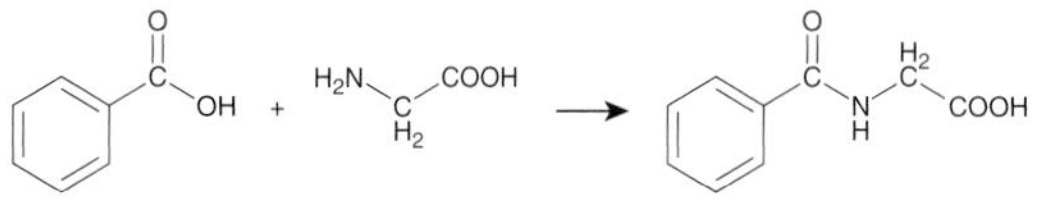
Glutathione conjugation	Glutathione-S-transferase	Glutathione	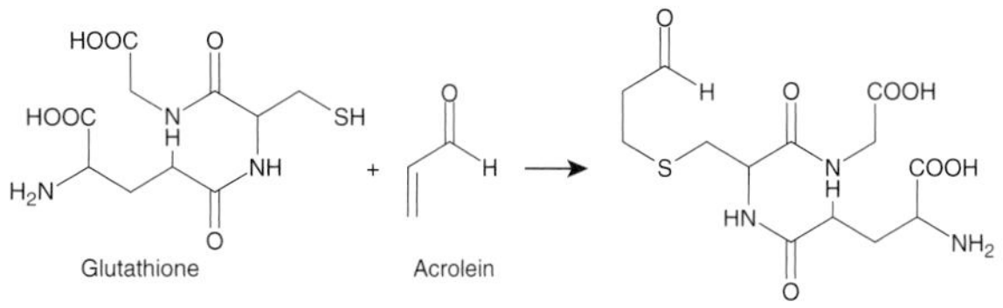
Methylation	Methyltransferase	SAM	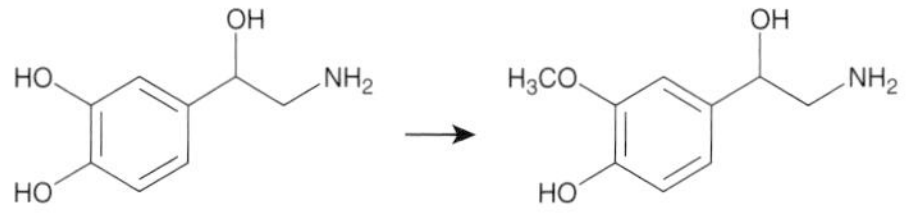
Acetylation	*N*-Acetyltransferase	Acetyl-CoA	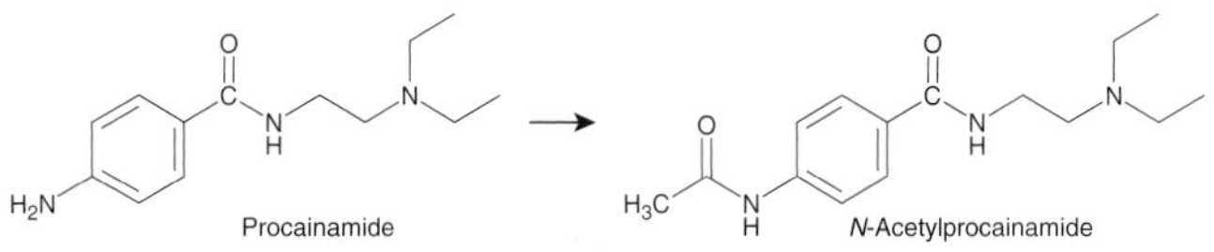

UDP-GA, uridine diphosphate glucuronic acid; *PAPS*, 3′-phosphoadenosine-5′-phosphosulfate; *SAM*, *S*-adenosylmethionine; *Acetyl-CoA*, acetyl coenzyme A.

polymorphic enzyme that results in the division of individuals into ultrarapid, intermediate, or poor metabolizers of substrates like debrisoquine and dextromethorphan.

C. **Gender**. Metabolic differences between the sexes have been observed for a number of compounds, suggesting that androgen, estrogen, and/or adrenocorticoid activity might affect the activity of certain CYP450 enzyme isozymes.
   1. Metabolism of diazepam (Valium), prednisolone (Orapred), caffeine, and acetaminophen (Tylenol) is slightly faster in women.
   2. Metabolism of propranolol (Inderal), chlordiazepoxide (Librium), lidocaine (Xylocaine), and some steroids is faster in men than in women.

D. **Age**
   1. The **fetus** and the **neonate** do not have fully developed drug-metabolizing enzymes, particularly phase II glucuronidation. As a result, smaller doses are often required to avoid drug accumulation and adverse effects during the first 6 to 8 weeks of life.
   2. The **elderly patient** shows a **decrease in the drug-metabolizing capacity** compared to young adults. This may be related to changes in hepatic blood flow, body mass, and/or other disease states. Drug clearance is therefore generally slower and blood concentrations are higher, increasing the potential for toxicity.

E. **Circadian rhythms**. The nocturnal plasma levels of drugs, such as theophylline (Theochron, Uniphyl) and diazepam (Valium), are lower than the diurnal plasma levels.

F. Various **disease states** that influence the function of the liver, the major site of drug metabolism, can affect a drug's hepatic clearance. Alterations in liver blood flow, loss of functional hepatocytes, and changes in albumin production can influence the extent of drug metabolism and toxicity and therefore require caution when administering a drug that requires hepatic biotransformation for detoxification or elimination.

G. The **nutritional status** of an individual can also influence the activity of drug-metabolizing enzymes by altering the amount of conjugating agents, protein, essential fatty acids, minerals, and/or vitamins available for use. Various alterations in drug-metabolizing activity have been identified for each category listed previously.

H. **Interacting substances**. Xenobiotics, whether they are drugs or not, can influence the activity of drug-metabolizing enzymes in a variety of ways.
   1. **Inducers** are xenobiotics that cause an increase in the drug-metabolizing activity of a target enzyme, usually by increasing the concentration of the enzyme in the liver or other tissue. Several **CYP450 enzymes** and **glucuronosyltransferases** are known to be inducible. In the case of drug–drug interactions, the compound causing the induction is called the **precipitant drug**, whereas the drug that is being affected is called the **object drug**. The consequence of induction is dependent on the extent of induction by the precipitant drug and the pharmacological characteristics of the object drug. For example, if the object drug is metabolized to a toxic metabolite, then induction by the precipitant drug may result in greater toxicity as a result of the increased drug-metabolizing activity.
   2. **Inhibitors** are opposite of inducers in that they **decrease** the metabolizing activity of a target enzyme, usually by competing with the object drug for the enzyme and preventing its metabolism. The extent of inhibition is dependent on the affinity of the inhibitor, the availability of **alternate metabolic pathways** of the object, and the **pharmacologic characteristics** of the object drug. For example, if the object drug has a narrow margin of safety and one metabolic route of elimination, the addition of an inhibitor to that pathway could result in accumulation of the object drug and ultimately toxicity.
   3. The extent of **protein binding** can be altered by the administration of another compound that is also highly protein bound. Two drugs that compete for similar binding sites on plasma proteins can result in the displacement of (usually) the agent with the lower affinity. As a result, there is an **increase in the free fraction** of one or both drugs that can lead to increased receptor interactions, metabolism, or toxicity of the displaced drug.
   4. **Antibiotic therapy** may also influence the metabolic rate of a drug that is dependent on the gut microflora for its metabolism or **enterohepatic circulation** (see III.C.2.b).

I. **Route of administration** can dramatically influence the metabolic rate of a drug.
   1. **Orally administered drugs** are subject to **first-pass metabolism in the liver** through the portal circulation or **presystemic metabolism in the gut**. This first-pass or presystemic metabolism can

significantly reduce the amount of drug that enters the systemic circulation. Often, this problem can be overcome by administering more drug orally so that the systemic concentration is sufficient for pharmacologic activity.

2. **Intravenous administration (IV) bypasses any barriers to GI absorption and first-pass metabolism** and generally requires a smaller dose for the same effect. For example, oral morphine undergoes significant first-pass metabolism so an equivalent IV dose is approximately one-sixth that of an oral dose. **Sublingual** and **buccal administrations** also bypass the first-pass metabolism because they are not part of the portal circulation. **Rectal administration** is more variable but also bypasses first-pass metabolism to a significant extent.

J. The **dose** can also influence the extent of metabolism. There is a finite amount of drug-metabolizing enzymes, so higher doses can result in **saturation** of a particular metabolic pathway. When this occurs, an alternate pathway may contribute to the metabolism of the drug. For example, acetaminophen (Tylenol) given at therapeutic doses is metabolized almost exclusively by glucuronidation and sulfation but toxic doses saturate these processes, leading to increased metabolism by CYP2E1 to the proposed toxic metabolite NAPQI causing hepatotoxicity.

V. PRODRUGS.

These drugs are molecules that are either inactive or very weakly active and require in vivo **biotransformation** to produce the pharmacologically active drug. The phase I metabolic processes discussed previously activate prodrugs. There are a variety of advantages to using a prodrug instead of the active form of the drug.

A. An **increase in water solubility** is useful for the preparation of ophthalmic and parenteral formulations. Sodium succinate esters and sodium phosphate esters have been used to make a number of water-soluble steroid prodrugs.

B. An **increase in lipid solubility** is useful for a variety of reasons.

1. **Increased oral absorption** is obtained by converting carboxylic acid groups to esters. These esters can then be rapidly converted to the active acids by plasma esterases. Enalaprilat is a potent angiotensin-converting enzyme (ACE) inhibitor that is used for parenteral administration, but, due to its high polarity, it is orally inactive. Its monoethyl ester, enalapril (Vasotec), is considerably more lipophilic and, thus, provides good oral absorption. This strategy has been successfully used for a variety of other compounds, including additional ACE inhibitors, fibric acid derivatives, ampicillin, and several cephalosporins.
2. **Increased duration of action**. Lipid-soluble esters of estradiol, such as benzoate, valerate, and cypionate, are used to prolong estrogenic activity. IM injections of these esters in oil result in a deposit of drug that is slowly released and hydrolyzed to free estradiol over a prolonged period (see section VI.A.3).
3. **Increased topical absorption** of steroids is obtained by masking hydroxyl groups with less polar functional groups such as esters or acetonides. This decrease in polarity allows for increased dermal permeability to treat inflammatory, allergic, and pruritic skin conditions. Examples include triamcinolone acetonide (Kenalog), diflorasone diacetate (ApexiCon), and betamethasone valerate (Betaderm).
4. **Increased palatability**. Antibiotics such as sulfisoxazole have a bitter taste and are not suitable for administration to children who are unable to swallow tablets or capsules. Esterification to produce sulfisoxazole acetyl decreases the water solubility of the antibiotic and, thus, decreases its interaction with bitter taste receptors on the tongue. This compound is marketed as a flavored suspension with erythromycin ethylsuccinate. Similar strategies have been used to mask the bitter taste of chloramphenicol and other antibiotics.

C. A **decrease in GI irritation**. NSAIDs produce gastric irritation and ulceration via two mechanisms: a direct irritant effect of the acidic molecule and inhibition of gastroprotective prostaglandin production. The prodrugs sulindac (Clinoril) and nabumetone (Relafen) produce less GI irritation because the gastric and intestinal mucosa are not exposed to high concentrations of active drug during oral administration. Additionally, nabumetone is a ketone, not an acid, and lacks any direct irritant effects.

D. **Site specificity** is useful for increasing the concentration of the drug at the active site and for decreasing side effects.

1. Methyldopa (Aldomet) is a prodrug that is structurally similar to L-dopa. As a result, methyldopa is transported into the central nervous system (CNS) and metabolized to the active

not subject to rapid first-pass metabolism and can be used orally. A similar strategy has been used to make orally active estradiol analogues.

2. **Tolbutamide** is an oral hypoglycemic with a short duration of action. This sulfonylurea rapidly undergoes oxidation of its para-methyl group. A structurally similar compound, **chlorpropamide**, has a nonmetabolizable para-chloro group and, as a result, has a much longer duration of action.
3. **Isoproterenol** is a potent β-adrenergic agonist used for the relief of bronchospasm associated with bronchial asthma. Because it is a catechol (i.e., 3,4-dihydroxy–substituted benzene ring), isoproterenol is subject to rapid metabolism by catechol-*O*-methyltransferase (COMT) and, thus, has poor oral activity. Alteration of the 3,4-dihydroxy substitution to a 3,5-dihydroxy substitution produces **metaproterenol**, a bronchodilator that is not susceptible to COMT, is orally active, and has a longer duration of action than isoproterenol.
4. **Octreotide** is a synthetic octapeptide used to suppress or inhibit severe diarrhea associated with certain tumors. Octreotide mimics the actions of **somatostatin**, a naturally occurring, 14–amino acid peptide. Somatostatin undergoes rapid proteolysis, has a half-life of 1 to 3 mins, and must be administered as a continuous intravenous infusion. Octreotide contains the amino acids essential for clinical efficacy but replaces two of the amino acids with their D-enantiomers. These unnatural D–amino acids are more resistant to hydrolysis. As a result, octreotide has an increased half-life and can be administered as a subcutaneous injection.

VII. PHARMACOGENETICS

VII. PHARMACOGENETICS is the study of the **genetic basis for variation in drug response**. Because genes code for the proteins involved in drug absorption, distribution, metabolism, elimination, and receptors, it is clear that gene changes will alter the response to drugs. In this chapter, we will focus on the genetic basis for variation in drug response with some emphasis on drug metabolism.

A. **Phenotypic description of variability**. Historically, genetic variation related to drug metabolism has been described in terms of phenotypic observations such as fast or slow metabolizers of a particular compound. Now that the genetics behind the phenotype is often understood, an observed effect or a phenotype can be connected to the gene sequence or **genotype**. With this knowledge, the phenotype can be predicted regardless of the medication in question. The ability to predict drug response as it relates to drug metabolism or other factors is critical in providing truly personalized medicine, the ultimate goal of pharmacogenetics.

B. **Genetics review**. A review of the vocabulary of genetics will help with the understanding of the genetic basis of variation in drug response and metabolism.

1. **Genes** are defined as a **segment of DNA** that can be replicated for cell division and direct the biosynthesis of specific proteins that include receptors, enzymes, and structural proteins.
2. An **allele** is **one of several variants of a gene**. An individual has two alleles, one allele from each parent, of each gene. In polymorphic genes, the wild-type or most common allele is indicated as the *1 allele and the variant alleles are numbered based on discovery. For example, CYP2D6*1 is the most common allele of cytochrome P450 2D6 but other variants include CYP2D6*3 and CYP2D6*4, both of which lack drug-metabolizing activity.
3. **Promoters** are segments of DNA that aid or direct the transcription of a particular gene.
4. **Transcription** is the process of **copying genes from DNA into complementary RNA called messenger RNA (mRNA)**. This is the first step in the process of expressing a gene as a protein.
5. **Splicing** is the **processing of mRNA** to remove the **introns** (noncoding RNA) and join together **exons** (coding mRNA) to make mature mRNA that encodes for the desired protein.
6. **Translation** is the process of converting the processed or mature **mRNA into protein**. Translation occurs on the **ribosomes** using transfer RNA (tRNA) to read the mRNA and produce a chain of amino acids. The amino acids are connected by peptide, or amide, bonds to make a protein.
7. **Polymorphism** is defined as the existence of two or more variants of a gene that occur in the population with a population frequency of at least 1% for the less common variant.

C. **Genetic variation** in the DNA sequence can cause certain populations of individuals to be more likely to develop specific disease states, to be more likely to follow a specific path of disease progression, to be more likely to respond to specific drug therapy, and/or to be more likely to develop certain adverse drug effects. It is estimated that individuals differ from one another by one nucleotide, or SNP, every 300–1000 nucleotides in the genome.

1. The most common type of genetic variation is the **single nucleotide polymorphism** (SNP). The consequence of a SNP depends on its location and the change itself.
   a. SNP, pronounced "snip," is a single base pair change in the DNA sequence at a particular point compared with the "common" or "wild-type" gene sequence.
   b. A **synonymous SNP** in the coding region does not result in a change in the amino acid sequence compared to the common or wild-type sequence and therefore generally has no discernible effects.
   c. A **nonsynonymous SNP** in the coding region results in a change in the amino acid sequence compared to the common or wild-type gene. This change can have negligible effects if the new amino acid has similar properties as compared to the original amino acid (e.g., aspartic acid replaced with a glutamic acid) or can have significant effects if the properties change sufficiently (e.g., aspartic acid replaced with lysine). As an example of a significant, nonsynonymous SNP, a mutation from A to C at position 3023 of the CYP2D6 gene results in histidine 324 in the native protein being replaced by a proline ($H_{324}P$). This change produces the allele identified as CYP2D6*7, which has no drug-metabolizing activity.
   d. SNPs outside of the coding region may not influence the amino acid composition of the protein but can have significant effects on the expression of a protein. SNPs in a **promoter** can alter the transcription rate of the target protein, resulting in either more or less of the protein being expressed. SNPs in a **splicing control** region may result in alternative splicing, creating either a novel protein or a nonsense codon that terminates that translation of the protein. In each of these examples, expression and activity of the gene is altered. Vitamin K epoxide reductase complex 1 (VKORC1) is an example of a protein where SNPs in the promoter region result in various levels of protein expression. This is important because VKORC1 is the molecular target for the anticoagulant warfarin. The efficacy of warfarin varies widely across the population and about 25% of this dose variation can be explained by variability in the expression of VKORC1.
2. Other common genetic variations, which may be SNPs, are **insertions** and **deletions**. Just as the name sounds, nucleotides are either inserted or deleted from the sequence of the gene. Recall that nucleotides are translated into amino acids using a three-nucleotide codon, so adding or deleting one nucleotide can result in the significant changes to the gene. The CYP2D6*3 allele is the result of a deletion of one nucleotide (A_{2637}), which causes a reading frameshift in translation. This change results in CYP2D6 with no activity.
3. **Copy number variations** are also a possible genetic variation. In this case, large segments of DNA are duplicated, deleted, or inverted. In duplications, the gene of interest is repeated in the genome multiple times. A deletion is a complete absence of the functional gene, and inversions may disrupt gene function by changing the location of the gene and its promoters. CYP2D6 is one drug-metabolizing enzyme identified to have multiple copies (CYP2D6xN where N is between 2 and 12 copies) of the functional CYP2D6 gene. These multiple copies result in a very high expression of functional CYP2D6. These patients are ultrarapid metabolizers of CYP2D6 substrates.

D. Clinical pharmacogenetic assays

1. The goal of a clinical pharmacogenetic assay is to provide the best patient care possible to prevent adverse effects while gaining the best response possible. Ideally, a useful clinical pharmacogenetic assay will place patients into one of four categories.
   a. Individuals who are most likely to respond and are at a low risk for adverse effects.
   b. Individuals who are most likely to respond and are at a high risk for adverse effects.
   c. Individuals who are less likely to respond and are at low risk for adverse effects.
   d. Individuals who are less likely to respond and are at a high risk for adverse effects.
2. There are several known genetic variations that affect specific drug efficacy and safety. These variations are related to alterations in drug-metabolizing enzymes, targets, or side effects.
   a. **Warfarin** (Coumadin). Patients demonstrate significant variation in the effective dose of warfarin, which requires careful monitoring and a personalized dose. Part of this variability can be explained by the variation in the drug-metabolizing enzyme CYP2C9. Polymorphisms in

CYP2C9 result in slower clearance of warfarin that translates into drug accumulation and increased risk for bleeding at average doses. Of particular concern are the patients that carry the CYP2C9*2 or CYP2C9*3 allele, which encode for CYP2C9 protein with greatly reduced enzymatic activity. As a result, the metabolism of warfarin is dramatically diminished and the risk for drug accumulation and bleeding is significant. More of the variation can be explained by the variable expression of vitamin K epoxidase (VKORC1), the molecular target for warfarin. This variation is dependent on a SNP in the promoter region of VKORC1. Genetic tests for both CYP2C9 and VKORC1 are recommended in the warfarin labeling as tests that will provide guidance in induction and final therapeutic dose for individuals with specific CYP2C9 and VKORC1 alleles.

b. **6-Mercaptopurine** (Purinethol) and **azathioprine** (Imuran), which is initially bioactivated to 6-mercaptopurine, are inactivated by the drug-metabolizing enzyme **thiopurine methyltransferase** (TPMT). Genetic variations in TPMT, including the TPMT*2, TPMT*3A, and TPMT*3C alleles, are known to result in decreased metabolizing capacity and increased bone marrow toxicity as 6-mercaptopurine accumulates in the body. Although the genotypes for TPMT are known, phenotyping of red blood cells is more commonly used to evaluate TPMT activity.

c. **Procainamide** (Pronestyl), **hydralazine** (Apresoline), and **isoniazid** (Stanozide) are metabolized by ***N*-acetyltransferase**, a polymorphic drug-metabolizing enzyme. Each of these drugs listed here has a different adverse effect profile based on the ability of variants of *N*-acetyltransferase to metabolize the targets. A slow acetylator taking these drugs is likely to accumulate the drug and develop symptoms of overdose, including hypotension and lupus-like syndrome for procainamide and hydralazine and peripheral neuropathy for isoniazid. Although genetic tests are commercially available, there is currently no recommendation for testing.

d. **Salmeterol** (Serevent Diskus) and **albuterol** (Proventil or Ventolin) are **β_2-adrenergic receptor agonists** used to treat **asthma**. Genetic variations in the β_2-adrenergic receptor yield different responses to these agonists, which results in differences in efficacy in the treatment of asthma. Currently, the labeling for the β_2-agonists does not include a recommendation for genetic testing.

e. **Maraviroc** (Selzentry) is an HIV drug that is only active against HIV infections that require the **CCR5 coreceptor** to penetrate cells. Maraviroc works by antagonizing the CCR5 receptor, but if the HIV does not require CCR5 to penetrate the cell, it will not be effective in the treatment of HIV infections. To determine the HIV-1 tropism, a DNA test of the virus in a patient's blood, called a Trofile DNA, can be performed. A phenotypic assay can also be performed if there is a significant viral load detected called Trofile.

f. **Abacavir** (Ziagen) is an HIV drug that is associated with a serious **hypersensitivity reaction** associated with a particular variation in the major histocompatibility complex, class I, B allele (i.e., HLA-B*5701). Patients with the HLA-B*5701 allele are about 15 times more likely to develop abacavir hypersensitivity when compared to patients without the HLA-B*5701 allele. Genetic screening for the HLA-B*5701 allele is recommended prior to abacavir treatment but does not eliminate the risk for serious abacavir hypersensitivity.

g. **Codeine** is a mild analgesic that is **metabolized by CYP2D6** to morphine, a much more potent analgesic. **CYP2D6 is highly polymorphic**, including a potential for multiple copies of the gene resulting in an ultrametabolizer phenotype. This can lead to increased metabolism to morphine and increases in morphine-related toxicity, including constipation and respiratory depression. CYP2D6 also contributes to the metabolism of several selective serotonin reuptake inhibitors (i.e., fluoxetine [Prozac]), tricyclic antidepressants (i.e., amitriptyline [Elavil]), antipsychotics (i.e., clozapine [Clozaril]), and beta-blockers (i.e., propranolol [Inderal]). In these cases, the CYP2D6 alleles, CYP2D6*3, *4, *5, or *6, that are associated with poor metabolizers result in drug accumulation and toxicity. Genetic testing for CYP2D6 is commercially available, and the consequences of polymorphisms are mentioned in the drug labeling of several agents, but genetic testing is not widely recommended.

Study Questions

Directions: Each of the numbered items or incomplete statements in this section is followed by answers or by completions of the statement. Select the one lettered answer or completion that is **best** in each case.

1. Which of the following statements concerning drug metabolism is true?

(A) Generally, a single metabolite is excreted for each drug administered.
(B) Often, a drug may undergo a phase II reaction followed by a phase I reaction.
(C) Drug-metabolizing enzymes are found only in the liver.
(D) All metabolites are less active pharmacologically than their parent drugs.
(E) Phase I metabolites more likely are able to cross cellular membranes than phase II metabolites.

2. Which of the following metabolites would be the least likely excretion product of orally administered aspirin (see structure below)?

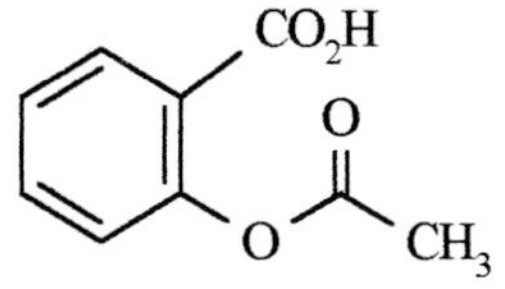

(A) Glycine conjugate
(B) Ester glucuronide
(C) Unchanged drug
(D) Ether glucuronide
(E) Hydroxylated metabolite

3. Sulfasalazine (see structure below) is a prodrug that is activated in the intestine by bacterial enzymes. The enzyme most likely responsible is

(A) azoreductase.
(B) pseudocholinesterase.
(C) *N*-acetyltransferase.
(D) β-glucuronidase.
(E) methyltransferase.

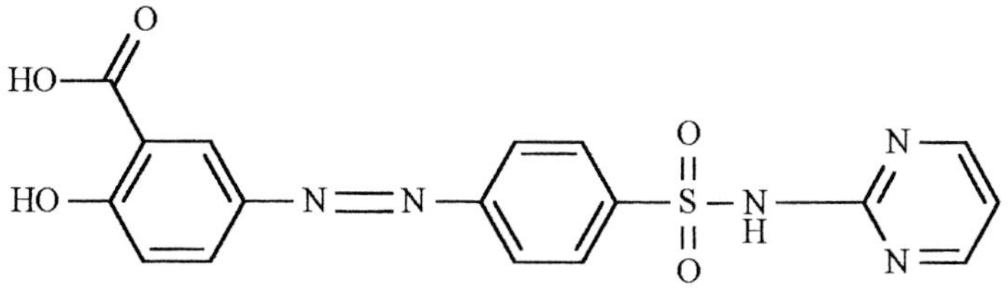

4. Chloramphenicol (see structure below) is considered to be toxic in infants (gray baby syndrome). This is due to tissue accumulation of unchanged chloramphenicol, resulting from an immature metabolic pathway. Which of the following enzymes would most likely be deficient?

(A) Pseudocholinesterase
(B) Glucuronyltransferase
(C) *N*-Acetyltransferase
(D) Azoreductase
(E) Methyltransferase

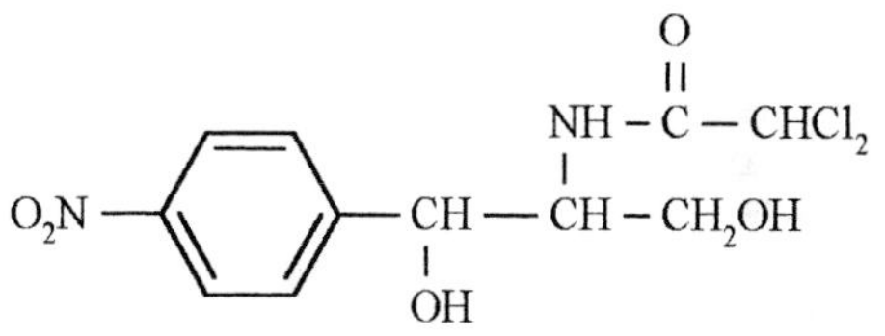

5. Which of the following therapeutic advantages cannot be obtained by the use of prodrugs?

(A) oral absorption
(B) water solubility
(C) duration of action
(D) potency
(E) palatability

6. Which of the following routes of administration would be subject to first-pass metabolism in the liver?

(A) IV (intravenous)
(B) Inhalation
(C) Sublingual
(D) IM (intramuscular)
(E) Oral

7. A compound that slows the metabolism of a xenobiotic is called a(n)

(A) inducer.
(B) epimer.
(C) reductase.
(D) inhibitor.
(E) object.

8. Which family of drug-metabolizing enzymes is characterized as a microsomal enzyme that contains a porphyrin prosthetic group?

(A) Glucuronosyltransferases
(B) Cytochrome P450s
(C) Flavin-containing monooxygenases
(D) Esterases
(E) *N*-Acetyltransferases

9. The most common type of genetic variation is a(n)

(A) copy number variation.
(B) insertion.
(C) deletion.
(D) frameshift.
(E) single nucleotide polymorphism.

10. Which polymorphic enzyme is responsible for the conversion of codeine to morphine?

(A) TPMT
(B) *N*-Acetyltransferase
(C) CYP2D6
(D) CYP2C9
(E) CCR5 coreceptor

Directions: Each question in this section contains three suggested answers, of which **one or more** is correct. Choose the answer.

A if **I only** is correct
B if **III only** is correct
C if **I and II** are correct
D if **II and III** are correct
E if **I, II, and III** are correct

11. Terms that may be used to describe the following metabolic reaction include

I. *N*-oxidation.
II. oxidative deamination.
III. phase I metabolism.

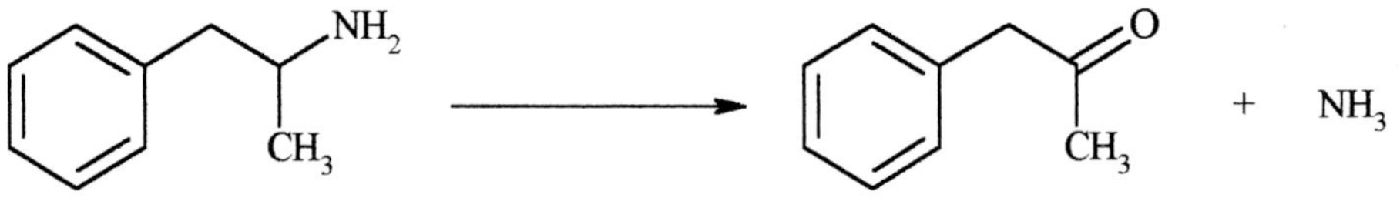

12. Which of the following reactions can be classified as phase II metabolism?

I.

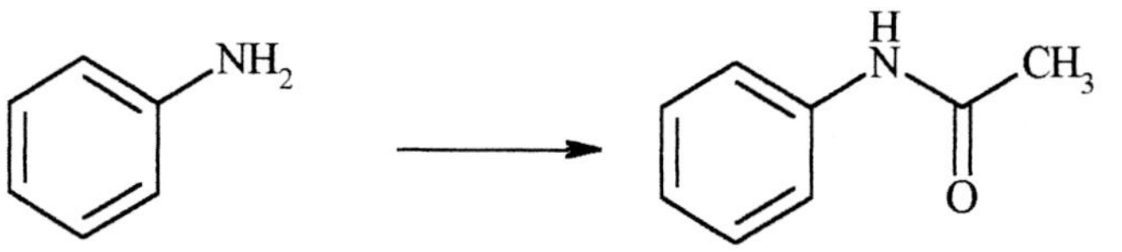

II.

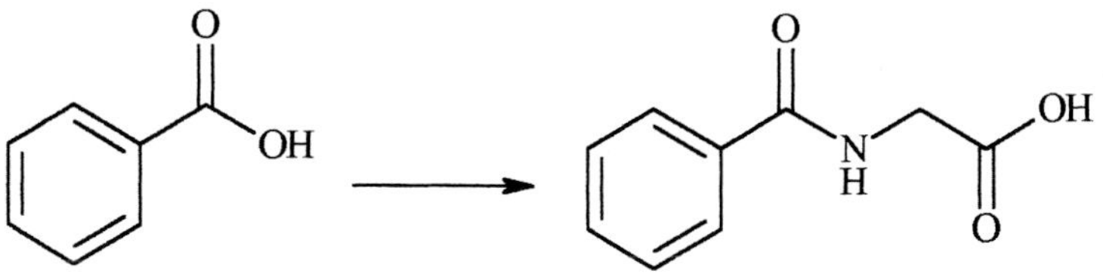

III.

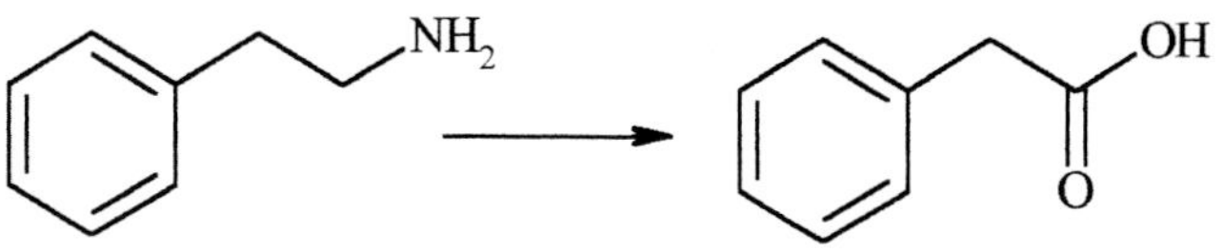

13. Conditions that tend to increase the action of an orally administered drug that undergoes phase II metabolism include

I. enterohepatic circulation.
II. enzyme saturation.
III. first-pass effect.

14. Which of the following statements concerning CYP450 are correct?

I. The CYP7, CYP11, and CYP27 subfamilies are involved in steroid and bile acid synthesis and metabolism.
II. A single drug may be metabolized by multiple isoforms of CYP450.
III. The majority of xenobiotics, or drugs, are metabolized by the CYP4B and CYP1A subfamilies.

15. Which of the following are genetic contributors to variation in the therapeutic dose of warfarin among patients?

I. CYP2C9
II. VKORC1
III. CYP2D6

16. Examples of phase II enzymes include

I. CYP450.
II. *N*-acetyltransferase.
III. sulfotransferase.

Directions: The group of items in this section consists of lettered options followed by a set of numbered items. For each item, select the **one** lettered option that is most closely associated with it. Each lettered option may be selected once, more than once, or not at all.

Questions 17–20

For each drug, select its most likely metabolic pathway.

(**A**) Ether glucuronidation
(**B**) Ester glucuronidation
(**C**) Nitroreduction
(**D**) Oxidative deamination
(**E**) Ester hydrolysis

17. Benzoic acid

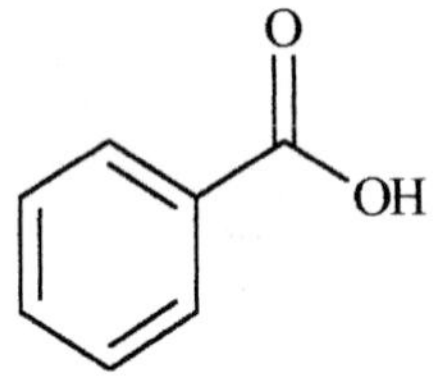

18. Procaine

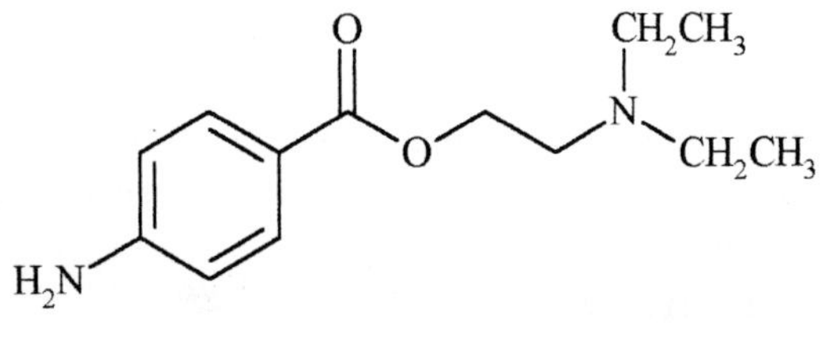

19. Acetaminophen

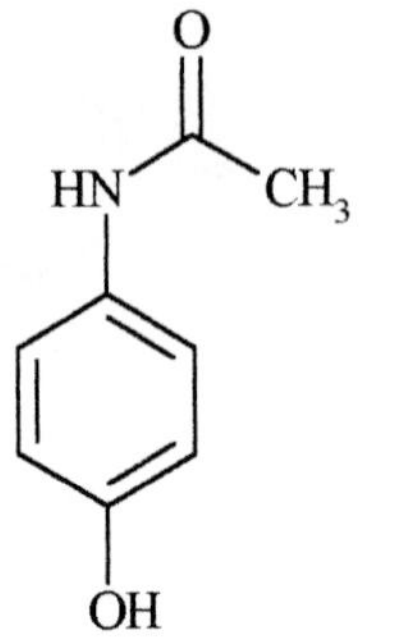

20. Amphetamine

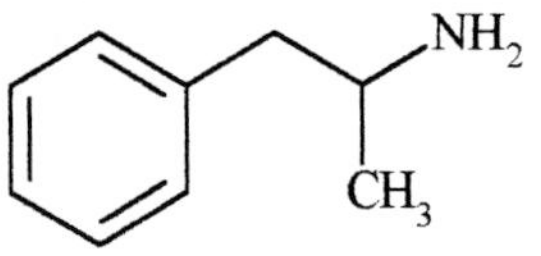

Answers and Explanations

1. **The answer is E** *[see III.A; III.B]*.
Phase I metabolites are often somewhat more polar than their parents. With the exception of acetylated and methylated metabolites, phase II metabolites are much more polar than their parents. Thus, phase I metabolites are more likely to retain some lipid solubility and are more likely to cross cellular membranes.

It is unusual for a single metabolite to be excreted for a given drug. Most drugs yield a mixture of metabolites. Because of the high polarity and subsequent high excretion of phase II metabolites, they are not likely to undergo further metabolism. Phase I metabolites, on the other hand, are less polar and are very likely to undergo further phase II metabolic reactions.

Whereas the major site of metabolism is the liver, there are many extrahepatic sites that secrete drug-metabolizing enzymes. Although many metabolites are less pharmacologically active than their parents, there are many drugs whose metabolites have equal or greater pharmacological activity and sometimes greater toxicity as well. Prodrugs (i.e., drugs inactive in the form administered) always form at least one active metabolite.

2. **The answer is C** *[see III.B.1; III.B.3; Table 8-1]*.
Because of the types of functional groups present, aspirin may undergo a number of different metabolic reactions. These include hydroxylation of the aromatic nucleus, conjugation of the carboxyl group with glycine,

conjugation of the carboxyl group with glucuronic acid with the formation of an ester glucuronide, hydrolysis of the acetate ester, and conjugation of the phenol group (resulting from hydrolysis of the acetate ester) with glucuronic acid to form an ether glucuronide.

Because the acetate ester is a simple ester, aspirin is susceptible to hydrolysis in the acid media of the stomach before absorption takes place. In addition, any acetylated molecules that are absorbed are subjected to hydrolysis and are catalyzed by the many esterases present in the circulation. Any acetylated molecules not hydrolyzed in the circulation are subject to hydrolysis in the liver. All of these processes occur before the drug reaches the glomerular filtrate; therefore, excretion of the unchanged acetylated drug is highly unlikely.

3. **The answer is A** *[see III.A.8.c; Table 8-2]*.
Sulfasalazine has both anti-inflammatory and antibacterial activity when converted to aminosalicylic acid and sulfapyridine in the body. This reaction occurs by reductive cleavage of the "azo" linkage contained in the sulfasalazine molecule and is catalyzed in the intestine by bacterial azoreductase. This is a form of site-specific delivery because the intact drug is not absorbed from the stomach or upper intestine and reaches the colon, where it is metabolized. Sulfasalazine is one of a few drugs that are effective for the treatment of ulcerative colitis.

4. **The answer is B** *[see IV.D.1; Table 8-4]*.
The chloramphenicol molecule contains an aromatic nucleus, which would be subject to hydroxylation; a nitro group that is subject to reduction; an amide group that is subject to liver hydrolysis; and alcohol groups that are subject to glucuronidation. Of all the enzyme systems responsible for these reactions, the system responsible for glucuronidation is developed poorly in premature infants and infants up to approximately 6 to 8 weeks of age.

5. **The answer is D** *[see V]*.
By definition, prodrugs are inactive or very weakly active molecules that require in vivo activation to the parent molecule. Thus, conversion of a drug molecule to a prodrug does not increase potency because the original molecule, with whatever potency it contains, is produced after administration. A variety of advantages, including increased water solubility, duration of action, oral absorption, and palatability, can be obtained through the use of prodrugs, but none of these advantages results in an increase in potency of the parent molecule.

6. **The answer is E** *[see IV.I.1–2]*.
First-pass metabolism in the liver refers to biotransformation of a xenobiotic after absorption from the GI tract before it reaches the systemic circulation. Orally administered drugs that are absorbed from the GI tract enter the portal circulation and pass through the liver where they are metabolized. Routes of administration that bypass the first-pass metabolism in the liver include IV, IM, sublingual, buccal, rectal, and inhalation. These routes of administration allow for absorption either outside of the GI tract or in regions of the GI tract that are not part of portal circulation.

7. **The answer is D** *[see IV.H.2]*.
An inhibitor, also called the precipitant drug, is a substance that blocks the metabolism of another drug called the *object drug*. An inducer is a compound that increases the expression of drug-metabolizing enzymes. Both inhibitors and inducers alter drug metabolism that may cause toxicity or lack of efficacy depending on the metabolic consequence of the object drug.

8. **The answer is B** *[see II.A.2.a]*.
The family of cytochrome P450 enzymes are microsomal proteins that contain a porphyrin prosthetic group. Glucuronosyltransferases and flavin-containing monooxygenases are both microsomal enzymes, but they do not contain the porphyrin group.

9. **The answer is E** *[see VII.C.1–3]*.
The most common genetic variation is a single nucleotide polymorphism (SNP), which may be an insertion or deletion that causes a frameshift. These polymorphisms can be called a synonymous SNP if the amino acid expressed is not changed or a nonsynonymous SNP if the amino acid expressed is different. These polymorphisms may also influence the promoter region or the splicing sites for proteins that would not result differences in the amino acids expressed. Multiple copies of a gene, as reported with CYP2D6, are called copy number variations.

10. **The answer is C** *[see VII.D.2.a–c, e, & g]*.
CYP2D6 is a highly polymorphic drug-metabolizing enzyme that is responsible for the conversion of codeine to morphine. TPMT, *N*-acetyltransferase, and CYP2C9 are polymorphic drug-metabolizing enzymes but are not responsible for the conversion codeine to morphine. The CCR5 coreceptor is not a drug-metabolizing enzyme but is involved in the cellular penetration of HIV.

11. The answer is D (II, III) *[see III.A; Table 8-1].*
The reaction shown in the question involves the conversion of one functional group to another (amine to carbonyl); thus, it is classified as a phase I reaction. The introduction of oxygen into the molecule indicates oxidation, and the loss of the amino group signifies deamination; thus, the reaction also can be classified as oxidative deamination. *N*-Oxidation reactions by CYP450 or FMO are observed but result in the addition of an oxygen to the nitrogen. In this case, no oxygen has been added to the nitrogen; therefore, this is not an *N*-oxidation reaction.

12. The answer is C (I, II) *[see III.A–B; Table 8-4].*
Phase II metabolic reactions involve masking an existing functional group with a natural endogenous constituent. The formulas shown in choices I and II represent this type of reaction, with choice I being an acetylation reaction and choice II a glycine conjugation reaction. Choice III represents a change in an existing functional group and, thus, represents a phase I reaction. It is an oxidative deamination reaction.

13. The answer is C (I, II) *[see III.C.2.b; IV.I.1; IV.J].*
Enterohepatic circulation refers to the process by which glucuronides, which are secreted into the intestine with the bile, are hydrolyzed by intestinal bacterial β-glucuronidase. The hydrolyzed free drug, which is no longer polar, becomes available for intestinal reabsorption into the system and subsequent penetration to its active site.

If an enzyme system becomes saturated, then the active drug cannot be inactivated by that pathway. If the drug cannot undergo an alternative pathway, the increased plasma levels of an unchanged active drug can result in increased activity or toxicity.

The first-pass effect results in metabolism of a drug by the liver before the drug reaches its site of action, resulting in an overall decrease in its activity. Drugs that undergo first-pass metabolism generally are effective in much smaller intravenous doses as compared to oral doses.

14. The answer is C (I, II) *[see I; III.A.2.b].*
There are six mammalian families involved in steroid and bile acid metabolism. These are CYP7, CYP11, CYP17, CYP19, CYP21, and CYP27. Because cholesterol is the common intermediate for the biosynthesis of all endogenous steroids, some of these enzymes are directly involved in cholesterol metabolism. The families listed, CYP7, CYP11, and CYP27, all metabolize cholesterol, whereas the other three families catalyze additional oxidations of the initial metabolites.

There are multiple enzymes and paths that are possible for a single xenobiotic, so it is common that multiple metabolites with varying properties are possible and observed. The cytochrome P450 subfamilies responsible for the majority of the biotransformations are CYP2C, CYP2D, and CYP3A.

15. The answer is C (I, II) *[see VII.D.2.a].*
Some of the individual variability in dosing is related to the metabolism of warfarin by CYP2C9 and by the level of expression of the warfarin target, VKORC1. With CYP2C9, the variability is related to differences in the metabolic efficiency of the different alleles, whereas differences in the promoter region of VKORC1 result in different levels of expression of the enzyme inhibited by warfarin. CYP2D6, although highly polymorphic, does not contribute to the variability of warfarin dosing.

16. The answer is D (II, III) *[see III.A.2; III.B.2 & 5].*
Phase II drug-metabolizing enzymes are commonly called transferase enzymes because they transfer a biomolecule from an activated cofactor to a target functional group. Phase II enzymes include glucuronosyltransferase, sulfotransferase, *N*-acyltransferase, glutathione-S-transferase, *N*-acetyltransferase, and methyltransferase. CYP450 is the most common phase I enzyme.

17–20. The answers are 17-B *[see III.B.1]*, **18-E** *[see III.A.9.a]*, **19-A** *[see III.B.1]*, **20-D** *[see Table 8-1].*
Benzoic acid contains a carboxylic acid, a functional group that commonly undergoes conjugation with glucuronic acid. The resulting conjugation produces an ester. Carboxylic acids can also undergo conjugation with the amino acids glycine and glutamine. Additionally, benzoic acid can undergo aromatic hydroxylation, a common phase I pathway for drugs containing unsubstituted aromatic rings. Of these options, ester glucuronidation is the only answer available here.

Procaine is an ester-containing local anesthetic. Due to the wide physiological distribution of esterase enzymes, it is extremely susceptible to in vivo hydrolysis. This susceptibility to hydrolysis is the major reason why ester-containing local anesthetics have shorter durations of action as compared to those in other chemical classes.

One of the principal functional groups in acetaminophen is the phenol group. Similar to the carboxylic acid in benzoic acid, the phenol commonly undergoes glucuronide conjugation. The one difference is that a phenol (or an alcohol) produces an **ether** glucuronide, whereas a carboxylic acid produces an **ester** glucuronide. Phenols also commonly undergo sulfate conjugation reactions and occasionally undergo O-methylation reactions.

The principal functional group in amphetamine is its primary amine. Oxidative deamination is a very common metabolic path for primary amines. Occasionally, primary amines undergo phase II acetylation; however, this is a less common pathway. Aromatic hydroxylation, similar to that discussed previously for benzoic acid, is also possible for amphetamine.

9

Pharmacology and Medicinal Chemistry of Drugs Affecting the Nervous System

S. THOMAS ABRAHAM, MICHAEL L. ADAMS

I. INTRODUCTION. Drugs affecting the nervous system can modulate neurotransmission in the **central nervous system (CNS) or peripheral nervous system (PNS)**. The CNS consists of the brain and the spinal cord, whereas the PNS is further divided into the **autonomic nervous system (ANS)** and the **somatic nervous system**. The ANS is composed of **sympathetic** and **parasympathetic** divisions that regulate several involuntary actions of the body, whereas the somatic nervous system innervates the skeletal muscles. Agents acting in the ANS include adrenergic agonists and antagonists, cholinergic agonists and antagonists, and indirectly acting agents that could affect one or the other system. These drugs are useful for treating various ailments, including blood pressure disturbances, bronchial asthma, cardiac dysfunctions, anaphylactic reactions, nasal congestion, and skeletal muscle spasticity. Drugs affecting the CNS produce anesthesia and sedation, relieve pain and anxiety, suppress movement disorders and epileptic seizures, and treat psychotic and affective disorders. Drugs acting on the nervous system achieve their pharmacologic effects by modifying the synaptic concentrations or receptor actions of neurotransmitters. Other drugs modulate the intracellular pathways by which neurotransmitter actions are conveyed to yield the ultimate physiological response.

II. DRUGS AFFECTING THE PERIPHERAL NERVOUS SYSTEM

A. **The sympathetic nervous system** produces global changes in multiple organs such as the heart, liver, kidneys, lungs, etc., to deal with a stressful (fight or flight) situation.

1. Activation of the sympathetic system is accomplished by the stimulation of preganglionic sympathetic nerves in the thoracic and lumbar portions of the spinal cord by input from higher brain centers (e.g., solitary tract nucleus, hypothalamus, the limbic/neostriatal/cortical axis).
2. Most preganglionic fibers synapse with postsynaptic sympathetic fibers in structures known as the paravertebral or chain ganglia. Postganglionic fibers innervate specific organs such as the heart, lungs, and liver, and alter their function by releasing the adrenergic neurotransmitter **norepinephrine (NE)**.
3. Preganglionic sympathetic nerves also stimulate the adrenal medulla to release **epinephrine (Epi)**, which is transported via the blood to the organs of the body. These catecholamines (NE, Epi) activate either **α**- or **β-adrenergic receptors** on various tissues to initiate specific biochemical signaling events (see Chapter 58), and thereby alter organ function.
4. *Table 9-1* lists the effects of the sympathetic nervous system on various organs as well as the predominant receptors that mediate these effects.

Table 9-1 ADRENERGIC RECEPTORS AND THEIR PREDOMINANT PHYSIOLOGICAL EFFECTS

Organ/Tissue	Adrenergic Receptor	Major Effect
Eye		
Iris radial muscle	α1	Pupillary dilation
Ciliary muscle	β_2	Relaxation for far vision
Heart		
Sinoatrial, atrioventricular nodes	β_1, β_2	Increased spontaneous depolarization
His-Purkinje system	β_1, β_2	Increased conduction velocity
Atria, ventricles	β_1, β_2	Increased contractility
Blood vessels		
Arteries, arterioles	α_1, α_2, β_2	Constriction via α_1, α_2; dilation via β_2
Veins, venules	α_1, α_2, β_2	Constriction via α_1, α_2; dilation via β_2
Lungs		
Tracheal, bronchial muscle	β_2	Relaxation of smooth muscle
Bronchial glands	α_1, β_2	Decreased secretions
GI tract		
Salivary glands	α_1	Decreased secretions
Stomach	α_1, α_2, β_2	Decreased motility; decreased secretions
Intestines	α_1, β_2	Decreased motility
Urinary bladder		
Detrusor	β_2	Relaxation, increased capacity
Trigone, sphincter	α_1	Contraction
Sex organs	α_1	Ejaculation
Skeletal muscle	β_2	Increased contractility; glycogenolysis
Liver	α_1, β_2	Increased glycogenolysis
Pancreas	β_2	Increased insulin release
Fat cells	β_1, β_2, β_3	Lipolysis
Kidneys	α_1, β_1	Increased renin release

5. The release of NE by postganglionic sympathetic nerves is regulated by the rate of action potentials reaching the nerve ending and also by several receptors on the nerve terminal membranes. The presynaptic α_2, adenosine, neuropeptide Y, and muscarinic M_2-receptors reduce neurotransmitter released by the nerve, whereas nicotinic-N_N, angiotensin AT1, and β_2-receptors enhance NE release.
6. The actions of NE and Epi on adrenergic receptors are terminated by uptake into postganglionic nerve endings via a **norepinephrine transporter (NET)** or the postsynaptic tissue by the extraneuronal transporter. Tricyclic antidepressants (e.g., imipramine) and cocaine are efficient inhibitors of NET function and thereby prolong NE actions at the receptor.
7. NE uptake into the nerve terminal may result in uptake into synaptic vesicles or metabolism by **monoamine oxidases (MAO)** and catechol-*O*-methyltransferases (COMT).

B. Pharmacology and medicinal chemistry of sympathomimetics

1. **Nonselective adrenergic agonists**, such as norepinephrine and epinephrine, interact directly with adrenergic receptors to elicit a response. Thus, pharmacological application of these agents results in the activation of α- and β-adrenoceptors throughout the body, resulting in the diverse actions listed in *Table 9-1*.
   a. The ethylamine chain common to these agonists is essential to their adrenergic activity, and the general pharmacophore is a primary or secondary amine two carbon atoms away from a substituted benzene ring (*Figure 9-1*).
   b. Intravenous epinephrine is used to treat cardiac arrest and hypotensive crisis (e.g., during anaphylactic reactions) due to its vasoconstrictor and positive ionotropic/chronotropic effects. Epinephrine is also mixed with local anesthetics, such as lidocaine, to produce localized vasoconstriction to prolong the duration of action and minimize the systemic effects of the latter.

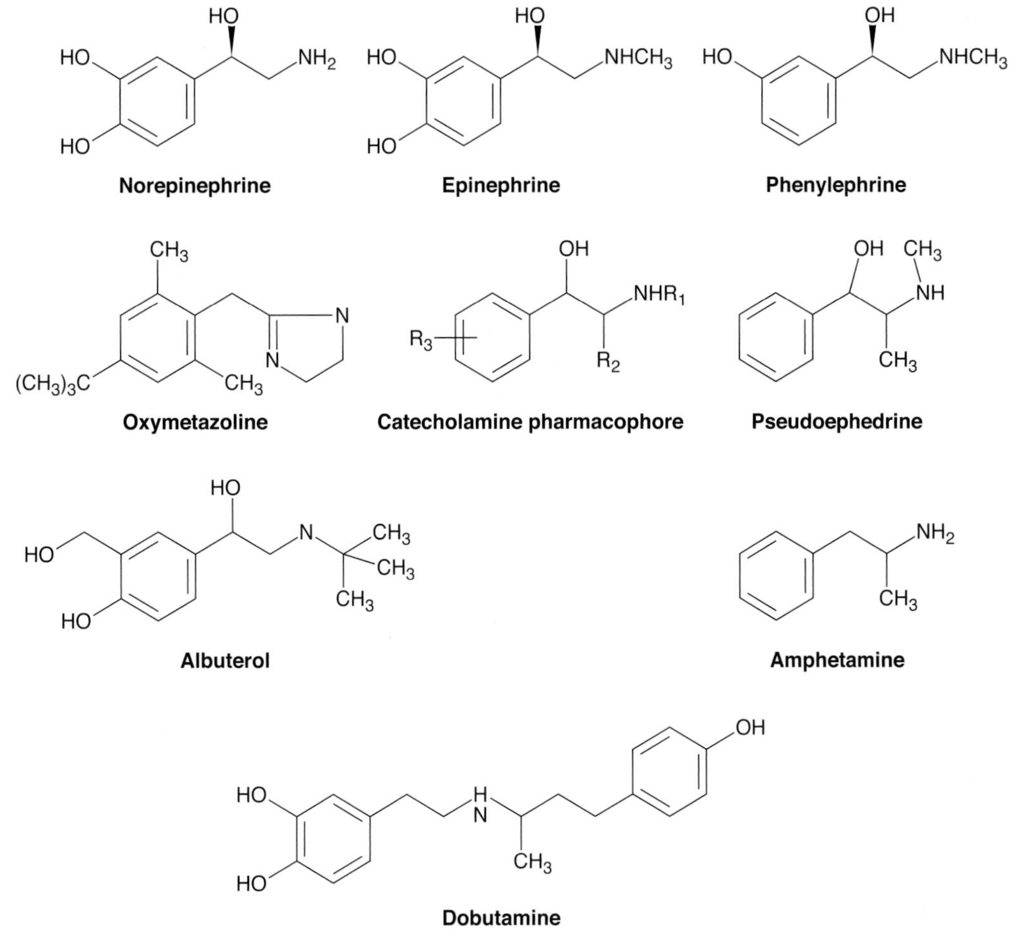

Figure 9-1. Structural formulas of the catecholamine pharmacophore with nonselective (epinephrine, norepinephrine), α_1-selective (phenylephrine), α-nonselective (oxymetazoline), β_1-selective (dobutamine), and β_2-selective (albuterol) agonists. Pseudoephedrine is a mixed α-agonist and indirect (NE releasing) agent, whereas amphetamine only releases catecholamines from sympathetic nerves (indirect action).

c. Dipivefrin (Propine®), the catechol diester prodrug of epinephrine, is used to treat open-angle glaucoma. Tissue esterases presumably cleave the ester bonds to regenerate epinephrine, which activates α_2-receptors on the ciliary body to decrease aqueous humor production.

2. **Selective α-adrenergic agonists.** To date, α_{1A}-, α_{1B}-, α_{1D}-, α_{2A}-, α_{2B}-, and α_{2C}-adrenergic receptors have been identified via pharmacological and molecular cloning methods.
   a. Methoxamine, phenylephrine, and clonidine, in general, have increased selectivity for α- versus β-receptors. Removal of the *para* hydroxyl group or substitution of the *meta* hydroxyl of Epi with a methoxy group increases α_1-receptor activity, as seen with phenylephrine (*Figure 9-1*) or methoxamine.
   b. Phenylephrine is useful as a topical (Neo-Synephrine®) or systemic (Sudafed-PE®) nasal decongestant. Intravenous administration of phenylephrine and methoxamine can be used to maintain systemic blood pressure in hypotensive conditions.
   c. Imidazoline derivatives such as oxymetazoline and clonidine have both α_1- and α_2-agonist activities with bulky *para* or *meta* substitutions on the benzene ring, generally increasing α1-selectivity (oxymetazoline; *Figure 9-1*). Oxymetazoline (Afrin®) is used as a topical nasal decongestant due to its direct vasoconstrictor action in the nasal mucosa. Clonidine (Catapres®) reduces tonic sympathetic output from the CNS by activating central α_2-adrenoceptors and is an effective antihypertensive agent.
   d. Derivatives of clonidine such as apraclonidine (Iopidine®)and brimonidine (Alphagan-P®) are used topically to selectively activate α_2-receptors in the eye to treat open-angle glaucoma.

e. The predominant adverse effect of imidazoline nasal decongestants is rebound congestion, whereas topical phenylephrine is less likely to produce this effect. Systemic clonidine administration can be associated with bradycardia, hypotension, sedation, and dry mouth. Sudden withdrawal of clonidine can result in enhanced central sympathetic outflow characterized by hypertension, sweating, tachycardia, and tremors.

3. **Selective β-adrenergic agonists.** To date, three distinct β-adrenergic receptors with unique functions (*Table 9-1*) have been identified; however, β_1- and β_2-receptors are the primary targets of pharmacological intervention.
   a. N-Substitutions of the catecholamine pharmacophore with isopropyl groups or aryl-alkyl groups, as in the case of albuterol (Ventolin®) or dobutamine (Dobutrex®; *Figure 9-1*), respectively, improve β-receptor selectivity over α-receptors. The bulky N-substitution of dobutamine confers some increased selectivity of the drug for β_1- relative to β_2-receptors.
   b. On the other hand, alteration of the *meta* hydroxyl on the benzene ring to a methoxy group (albuterol) or the catechol ring to a resorcinol (e.g., terbutaline) increases the selectivity of these agents for β_2- versus β_1-receptors.
   c. β_2-Selective agonists (albuterol, terbutaline, metaproterenol) are used as rescue bronchodilators in asthma or obstructive pulmonary disease and are often administered via metered-dose inhalers. By activating β_2-receptors, these agents elevate bronchial smooth muscle cAMP leading to decreased intracellular calcium and prompt bronchodilation.
   d. Terbutaline and ritodrine administered systemically have found use in slowing down premature labor.
   e. Dobutamine is used in acute heart failure for its positive ionotropic actions on the myocardium via β_1-receptor stimulation. Receptor stimulation leads to increased myocardial cAMP; however, in this case, the consequence is increased opening of L-type calcium channels and intracellular calcium, followed by enhanced contractility.
   f. Adverse effects such as tachycardia, muscle tremors, and insomnia with β_2-agonist use are generally due to their actions at cardiac and other β-receptors because their selectivity is not absolute. Dobutamine has been associated with tachyarrhythmias and ischemia during use.

4. **Indirect acting sympathomimetics**
   a. Removal of the hydroxyls on the catechol ring and addition of a α-methyl group partially reduce direct receptor agonist activity but increase indirect activity. Thus, ephedrine and pseudoephedrine (*Figure 9-1*) have the ability to activate α-adrenergic receptors and be taken up into the nerve terminal (via NET) and cause NE release from neurotransmitter vesicles.
   b. The lack of catechol hydroxyls also reduces metabolism by COMT and increases CNS penetration of these phenylethanolamines.
   c. Ephedrine and pseudoephedrine are used systemically to reduce nasal congestion, and their predominant adverse effects are insomnia, appetite suppression, and hypertension.
   d. Amphetamine (Adderall®; *Figure 9-1*), methamphetamine (Desoxyn®), and methylphenidate (Ritalin®) have little or no direct receptor action but enhance catecholamine release in the CNS.
   e. They are primarily used to treat attention deficit hyperactivity disorders, narcolepsy, and to suppress appetite. Adverse events related to their use are multiple and include dizziness, tremors, euphoria, confusion, aggressiveness, anorexia, sweating, convulsions, and coma.

C. **Pharmacology and medicinal chemistry of adrenergic antagonists**

1. **Selective α-adrenergic antagonists.** Antagonists of the α-adrenergic receptors are primarily imidazoline or quinazoline derivatives.
   a. The imidazoline antagonists are represented by phentolamine (Regitine®) and tolazoline (not marketed), having a similar structure to imidazoline α-agonists but lacking the lipophilic substitutions on the aromatic ring (*Figure 9-2*). They are unable to activate α-receptors and behave as competitive antagonists of both α_1- and α_2-adrenergic receptors.
   b. Blockade of α_1- and α_2-adrenergic receptors on the arteriolar beds leads to reduced peripheral vascular tone and systemic blood pressure and can be used to treat hypertension. They are also used to manage the hypertensive crisis resulting from catecholamine released by pheochromocytomas.
   c. Due to their actions to block inhibitory **presynaptic α_2-receptors** (see I.A.1), they often produce marked tachycardias as a result of increased NE release from cardiac sympathetic nerves. This can progress to cardiac ischemia, myocardial infarction (MI), or arrhythmias in susceptible individuals.

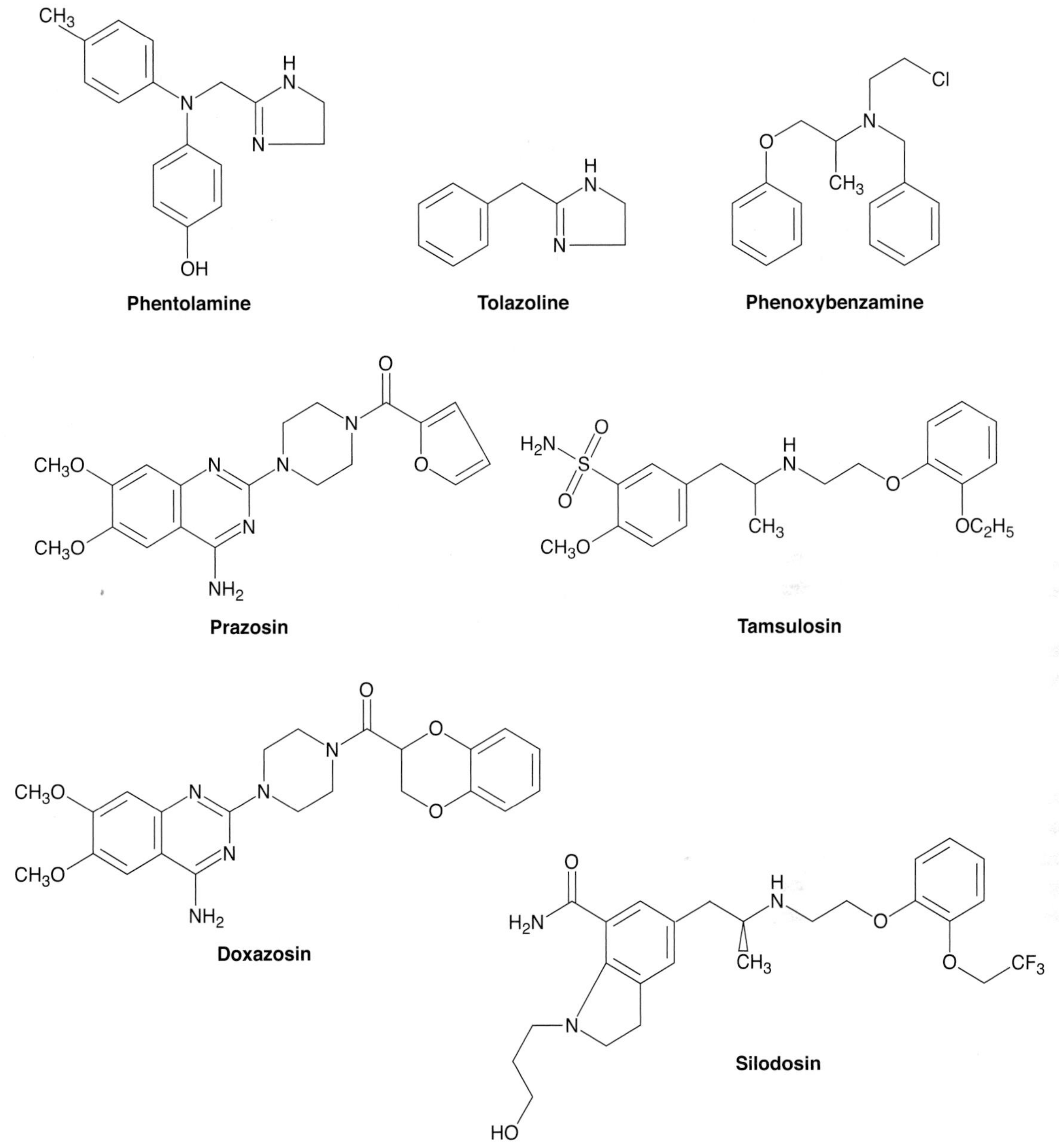

Figure 9-2. Structural formulas of the nonselective α-adrenergic antagonists phentolamine, tolazoline, and phenoxybenzamine. The α_1-selective antagonists are represented by prazosin and doxazosin, whereas tamsulosin and silodosin are α_{1A}-selective antagonists.

d. Blockade of α-receptors on veins increases venous pooling of blood and can result in **orthostatic or postural hypotension**. Additionally, blockade of gastrointestinal (GI) α-receptors can result in abdominal cramping, nausea, and exacerbation of peptic ulcers.

e. The β-haloalkylamine phenoxybenzamine (Dibenzyline®) is unique among α-antagonists in that the tertiary amine undergoes cyclization (with the loss of the chlorine atom, *Figure 9-2*) to form a reactive aziridinium intermediate. Cleavage of this ring results in the formation of a highly reactive carbonium ion that alkylates sulfhydryl, carboxyl, and amino groups on proteins. The covalent interaction of the drug with α-receptors results in irreversible inactivation of the receptor, which cannot be overcome even with very high catecholamine levels.

f. Phenoxybenzamine is used to manage metastatic pheochromocytoma, where high catecholamine levels would displace reversible antagonists such as phentolamine. Clinical doses of phenoxybenzamine probably antagonize both α_1- and α_2-receptors.

g. Prazosin (Minipress®), doxazosin (Cardura®; *Figure 9-2*), and terazosin (Hytrin®) belong to the quinazoline class and show increased selectivity for the α_1- versus α_2-receptors. Vasodilation of arteriolar beds results from antagonism of α-receptors that are tonically driven by innervating sympathetic nerves, with reduction in peripheral vascular resistance. A similar mechanism leads to venodilation, which reduces venous return to the heart and, in a sequential manner, decreases end-diastolic filling, myocardial contractility, and eventually cardiac output. Because both peripheral vascular resistance and cardiac output contribute to systemic blood pressure, a reduction of either parameter will decrease systemic blood pressure.

h. Quinazoline antagonists are important in the management of essential hypertension but are also used to manage **benign prostatic hyperplasia**, especially terazosin.

i. Adverse effects often seen with the use of prazosin and congeners are postural hypotension especially after the first dose, pupil constriction, nasal congestion, and impaired ejaculation.

j. Newer α-antagonists tamsulosin (Flomax®) and silodosin (Rapaflo®) have increased affinity for the α_{1A}-receptors of the prostate as compared to the α_{1B}-receptors of the vasculature, relaxing the prostate and the neck of the bladder without affecting systemic blood pressure.

k. Yohimbine (Yocon®) is the only clinically relevant α_2-selective antagonist currently on the market and is used to treat erectile dysfunction. It appears to improve this condition by blockade of α_2-receptors in the penile cavernosum, resulting in vasodilation and increased blood pooling.

2. **β-Adrenergic receptor antagonists.** Although all the drugs in this class are β-receptor antagonists, they are heterogeneous with regard to additional actions such as sodium/potassium channel blockade, having inverse or partial agonist activity and blockade of α-receptors.

a. Propranolol (Inderal®), the prototypical drug in this class, is an aryloxypropanolamine (*Figure 9-3*), derived from modifications of earlier antagonists such as dichloroisoproterenol and pronethalol. Generally, an arylethylamino or similar large hydrophobic group, without phenolic hydroxyls, is required for antagonistic activity at both β_1- and β_2-receptors, for example, timolol (Timoptic®), nadolol (Corgard®), and carteolol (Ocupress®) (*Figure 9-3*).

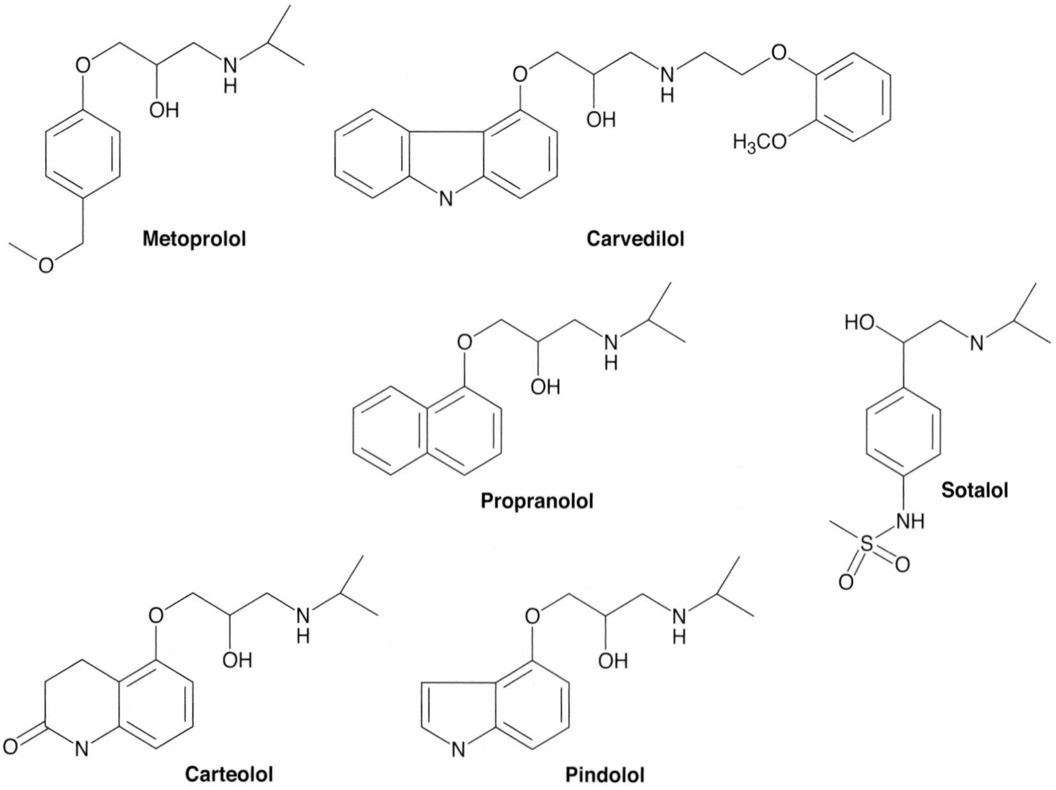

Figure 9-3. Propranolol and carteolol are β-nonselective antagonists, whereas metoprolol is β_1-selective. Pindolol is a β-nonselective partial agonist; carvedilol is also β-nonselective and blocks α_1-receptors as well. Sotalol is a β-nonselective antagonist with prominent K^+ channel blocking activity.

Table 9-2 SELECTIVE AND NONSELECTIVE β-RECEPTOR ANTAGONISTS

β–Antagonist	Partial Agonist Activity	Local Anesthetic Activity	Other Activity
Subtype nonselective			
Propranolol	No	Yes	
Nadolol	No	No	
Pindolol	Yes	Yes	
Sotalol	No	No	K^+ channel blocker
Timolol	No	No	
Carvedilol	No	No	α_1-Blocker
Carteolol	Yes	No	
Labetalol	Yes	Yes	α_1-Blocker
β_1-Selective			
Acebutolol	Yes	Yes	
Atenolol	No	No	
Betaxolol	No	Low	
Esmolol	No	No	
Metoprolol	No	Yes	

b. Substitutions *para* to the phenoxy position increase the relative β_1-selectivity of these agents, for example, metoprolol (Toprol-XL®; *Figure 9-3*), atenolol (Tenormin®), and acebutolol (Sectral®). Pindolol (Visken®) and carteolol possess significant agonistic activity at β-receptors and are more appropriately partial agonists than antagonists. The S-isomers of labetalol (Trandate®) and carvedilol (Coreg®; *Figure 9-3*) appear to have significant α_1-receptor antagonist activity in addition to β-blocking actions.

c. Propranolol and carvedilol have the ability to block voltage-dependent sodium channels, whereas sotalol (Betapace®) is primarily used for its potassium-channel blocking/antiarrhythmic actions rather than its β-blocking activity.

d. β-Receptor antagonists are used to manage several diverse conditions such as hypertension, post-MI cardiac arrhythmias, angina, congestive heart failure (CHF), stage fright, hand tremors, and glaucoma. Their use in hypertension has been largely supplanted by more effective agents; however, they have been shown to be effective in preventing a second MI, slow down the progression of CHF, and decrease the incidence of stable angina.

e. For the most part, there appears to be no clinical benefit of using β_1-selective agents over nonselective antagonists except in special populations: β_1-selective agents (e.g., metoprolol) may be less likely to cause bronchospasms in asthmatic patients; partial agonists (e.g., pindolol) may be better tolerated in bradycardic conditions. *Table 9-2* summarizes several important pharmacological actions of β-receptor antagonists.

3. The parasympathetic nervous system is able to produce discreet changes in specific organs to mediate processes such as lacrimation, salivation, or emptying of the bladder. These functions are initiated by preganglionic parasympathetic nerves originating from the tectal brainstem or sacral portions of the spinal cord and end in ganglia close to the innervated organ. Postganglionic nerves from these structures innervate relevant organs and modify their functions by activating **muscarinic-cholinergic (M)** receptors through the release of acetylcholine (ACh). The actions of released ACh are terminated by **acetylcholinesterase (AChE)** found in the synaptic space. *Table 9-3* summarizes the organs innervated by the parasympathetic nerves, the receptors activated, and the resulting biological effects.

D. Pharmacology and medicinal chemistry of cholinomimetic agents

1. Direct-acting cholinergic agonists. ACh is considered the prototypical cholinergic agonist having actions at all muscarinic and nicotinic receptor subtypes (*Figure 9-4*).

a. Agonist activity is tightly constrained and requires that there be no more than five atoms between the nitrogen and terminal hydrogen on the acyloxy group (*Figure 9-4*). Substitution of

Table 9-3 CHOLINERGIC RECEPTORS AND THEIR MAJOR PHYSIOLOGICAL EFFECTS

Organ/Tissue	Cholinergic Receptor	Major Effect
Eye		
Iris radial muscle	M_3	Pupillary constriction
Ciliary muscle	M_3	Contraction for near vision
Heart		
Sinoatrial, atrioventricular nodes	M_2	Decreased spontaneous depolarization
His-Purkinje system	M_2	Little effect
Atria, ventricles	M_2	Decreased contractility in atria
Blood vessels		
Arteries, arterioles	M_3	Increased NO release and vasodilation
Veins, venules	—	Little effect
Lungs		
Tracheal, bronchial muscle	M_3	Bronchoconstriction
Bronchial glands	M_2, M_3	Increased secretions
GI tract		
Salivary glands	M_2, M_3	Increased secretions
Stomach	M_2, M_3	Increased motility and secretions
Intestines	M_2, M_3	Increased motility
Kidneys	—	—
Urinary bladder		
Detrusor	M_3	Contraction, decreased capacity
Trigone, sphincter	M_2	Relaxation
Sex organs	M_3	Erection
Skeletal muscle	N_M	Muscle contraction
Liver	—	—
Pancreas	M_3, M_2	Increased digestive enzyme release
Fat cells	—	—

NO, nitric oxide.

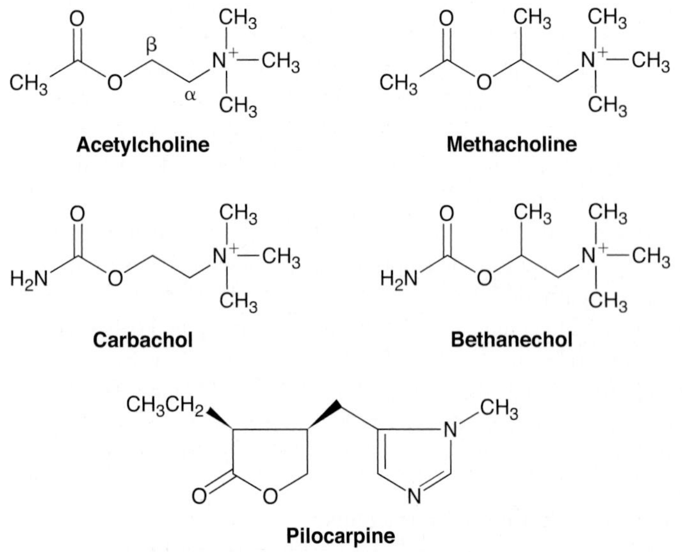

Figure 9-4. The structural formulas of the naturally occurring (acetylcholine, pilocarpine) and synthetic (methacholine, carbachol, bethanechol) muscarinic agonists.

the quaternary nitrogen with S or P usually reduces activity, but the positive charge is required for activity. If more than one of the methyl groups on the amine is altered by a larger alkyl substitution, marked reduction in activity is observed. Generally, the addition of a methyl group on the β-carbon results in increased selectivity for muscarinic versus nicotinic receptors (e.g., methacholine [Provocholine®; *Figure 9-4*]). This also reduces susceptibility to metabolism by cholinesterases, prolonging the duration of action.

b. The substitution of the methyl group on the acyloxy to an amino group (carbamate) provides additional resistance to cholinesterase metabolism for carbachol (Miostat®) and bethanechol (Urecholine®; *Figure 9-4*). Thus, the susceptibility to metabolism of the four agents follows the trend: ACh > methacholine > carbachol > bethanechol. Only bethanechol has significant oral activity, and the others have to be applied parenterally or topically for pharmacological action.

c. ACh and carbachol are applied as drops to produce brief miosis during eye surgery, and carbachol is also able to control increases in intraocular pressure after surgery. Inhaled methacholine has been used to assess bronchial hyperactivity in patients who do not exhibit clinical asthma. Bethanechol is indicated for urinary retention that occurs postoperative or postpartum and due to neurogenic atony of the bladder. By contracting the detrusor and relaxing the trigonal and sphincter muscle of the bladder, bethanechol is able to increase voiding action. As indicated in *Table 9-3*, the contractile effects are most likely mediated by M_3-receptors on the bladder wall, whereas the relaxant effects are due to the activation of M_2-receptors on the sphincters. Bethanechol has also been used to increase GI motility in postsurgical distention of the abdomen.

d. Pilocarpine (Ocusert Pilo-20®) applied topically is used to treat open-angle glaucoma and oral administration has been used to treat dry mouth resulting from head/neck radiation or due to Sjögren syndrome. Pilocarpine relieves glaucoma symptoms by activating muscarinic receptors on iris sphincter and longitudinal ciliary muscles, along with relaxing the suspensory ligaments on the lens, and allows for improved drainage of aqueous humor through the canal of Schlemm.

e. Because ACh and carbachol are applied topically, they are generally accompanied by relatively few systemic effects. Methacholine has caused profound bronchoconstriction in susceptible individuals when used as a diagnostic agent. The systemic use of bethanechol or pilocarpine may be associated with pupillary constriction, sweating, bradycardia, difficulty focusing the eyes, hypotension, and excessive salivation.

2. Indirect-acting cholinomimetics. Inhibition of AChE in the cholinergic synapse results in enhanced ACh levels in the synapse and increased muscarinic or nicotinic receptor activation. Thus, inhibition of ACh metabolism in the synapse mimics the stimulation of cholinergic nerves.

a. AChE inhibitors interact with the catalytic site of the enzyme in a reversible or irreversible manner and prevent the access of ACh to the same site. Agents such as tacrine (Cognex®), donepezil (Aricept®), and galantamine (Razadyne®) have high affinity for the AChE active site but interact via noncovalent bonds and can theoretically be displaced by excess ACh.

b. Carbamate derivatives of AChE inhibitors such as neostigmine (Prostigmin®), pyridostigmine (Mestinon®), and rivastigmine (Exelon®; *Figure 9-5*) form covalent, carbamoylated intermediates with a serine residue in the AChE active site. These inhibitors are often termed "suicide" inhibitors because they are destroyed in the process of covalently modifying AChE. These intermediates are only slowly hydrolyzed to regenerate the active site serine to metabolize ACh again.

c. The polar nature of quaternary amines (e.g., neostigmine, pyridostigmine) prevents them from crossing the blood–brain barrier and having CNS effects, whereas the tertiary amines (e.g., rivastigmine, donepezil, tacrine, and galantamine) have improved CNS penetration and activity.

d. The organophosphate inhibitors of AChE, such as echothiophate (Phospholine®; *Figure 9-5*), form much more stable phosphoester bonds with the serine residue and are extremely slowly hydrolyzed. Loss of one or both ethyloxy groups from echothiophate (a process known as aging) increases the stability of the phosphoester bond, and the enzyme is permanently inactivated.

e. The quaternary amine AChE inhibitors (e.g., neostigmine, pyridostigmine) are used to improve GI motility (e.g., after surgery) by increasing muscarinic stimulation on smooth muscle. They are also used to treat myasthenia gravis, where autoimmune reactions cause a marked loss

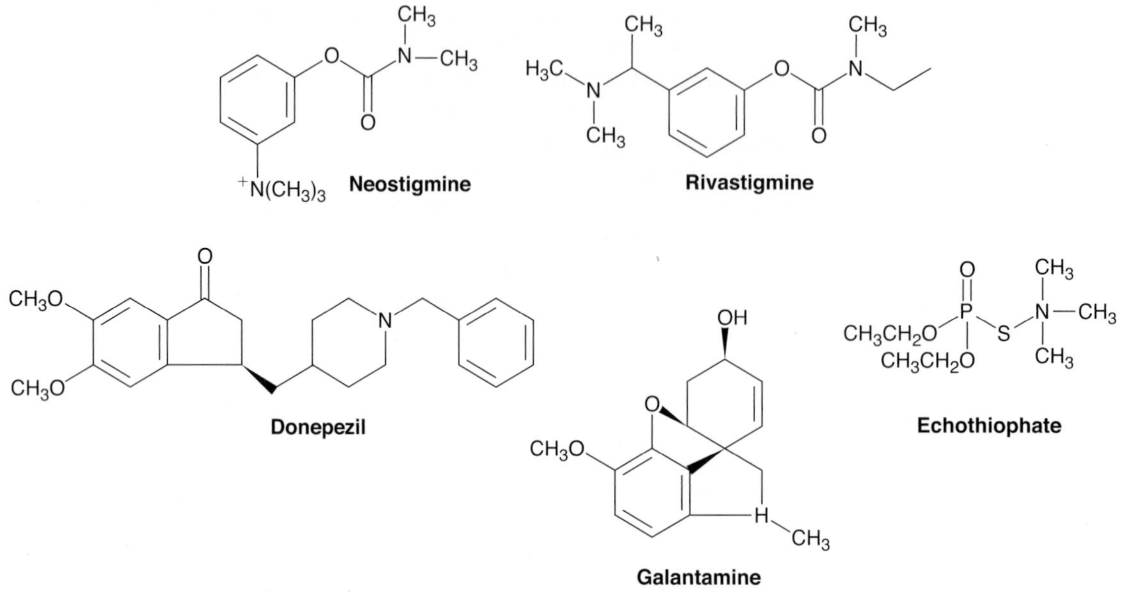

Figure 9-5. The structural formula of the carbamate (neostigmine, rivastigmine) and organophosphate (echothiophate) AChE inhibitors. Donepezil and galantamine do not covalently interact with AChE to inhibit its activity.

in nicotinic receptors at the motor end plate with resultant muscle weakness. Inhibition of AChE in the neuromuscular junction elevates ACh levels at the remaining nicotinic receptors to increase skeletal muscle contractions. Topical application of echothiophate and physostigmine can improve the drainage of aqueous humor in patients with open-angle glaucoma via indirect stimulation of muscarinic receptors. The carbamate AChE inhibitors have been used to reverse the poisoning by muscarinic antagonists such as atropine by indirectly elevating synaptic ACh. The tertiary amine inhibitors (e.g., rivastigmine, donepezil, galantamine) are primarily used to block AChE in the CNS to increase synaptic ACh and treat conditions such as Alzheimer dementia.

f. Systemic application of AChE inhibitors mimics generalized parasympathetic nervous system stimulation with patients experiencing pupillary miosis, loss of far vision, increased salivation and GI motility, and bradycardia.

E. Pharmacology and medicinal chemistry of cholinergic antagonists

1. Selective muscarinic antagonists. The prototypical muscarinic antagonist, atropine, was originally identified in extracts of the belladonna plant and is an ester of tropic acid and an organic base such as tropine (*Figure 9-6*).

a. The pharmacophoric structure indicated in *Figure 9-6* represents the wide variety of muscarinic antagonists (naturally occurring and synthetic) and can be grouped into amino alcohols, amino alcohol esters, amino ethers, and amino amides. Cyclic or heterocyclic rings at the R_1 and R_2 positions increase muscarinic receptor binding, whereas R_3 may be -H, -OH, or $-CH_2OH$. Position X may be an ester or ether (ester is more potent) group, whereas increased substitution of the terminal nitrogen improves receptor affinity such that the quaternary amine is most potent.

b. Most of the these agents are nonselective for the five muscarinic receptors found in the body; however, newer agents such as solifenacin (VESIcare®; *Figure 9-6*) and darifenacin (Enablex®) have some selectivity for M_3-receptors relative to M_1-and M_2-receptors.

c. Muscarinic antagonists are used to treat several conditions where receptor stimulation via the parasympathetic system needs to be decreased. Atropine and glycopyrrolate (Robinul®) are used to decrease the effects of vagal reflexes during surgery (bronchial secretions, bradycardia), whereas scopolamine is used to induce sedation and decrease motion sickness.

d. Atropine in preparations such as Lomotil® reduces GI motility associated with diarrhea.

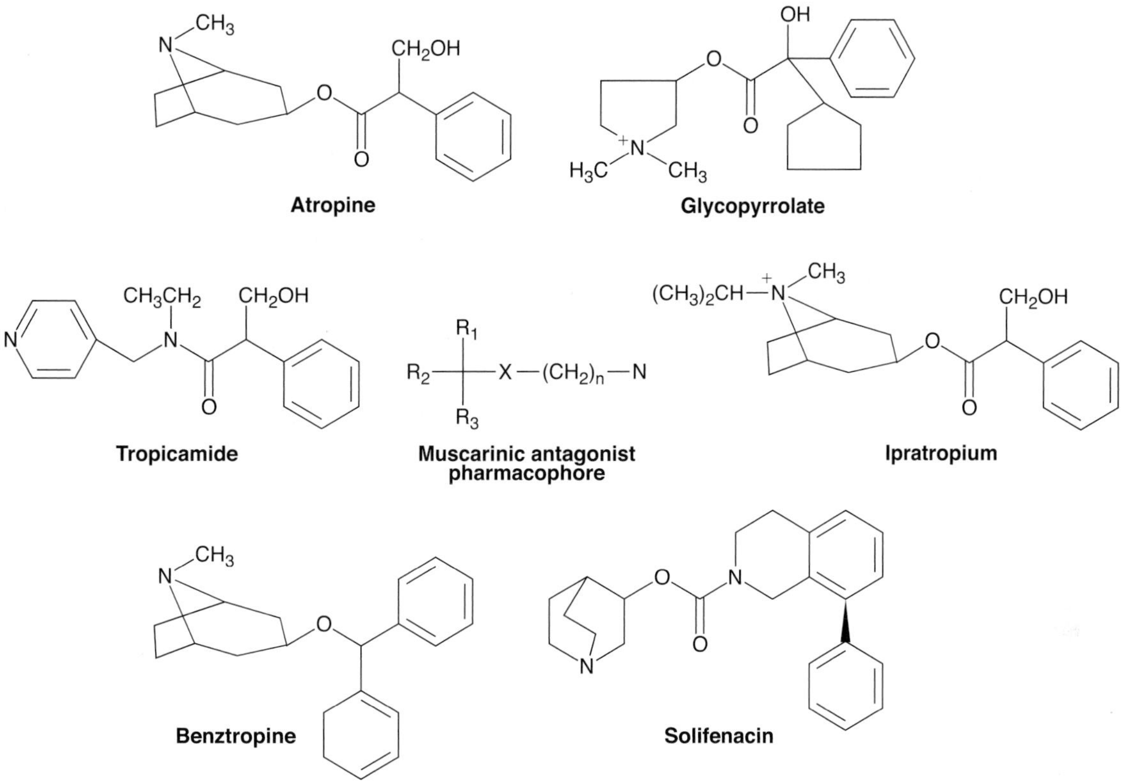

Figure 9-6. Structural formulas of muscarinic antagonist pharmacophore and the nonselective M-antagonists atropine, glycopyrrolate, tropicamide, benztropine, and ipratropium. Solifenacin has selectivity for the M_3-receptor.

e. Tropicamide (Mydriacyl®) applied topically is used most often to produce pupillary dilation during eye exams, whereas ipratropium (Atrovent®; *Figure 9-6*) and tiotropium (Spiriva®) are applied via metered-dose inhalers for the management of asthma and chronic obstructive pulmonary disease.

f. Blockade of M_3-receptors on the bladder decreases intravesicular pressure, increases bladder capacity, and reduces the frequency of spasms to effectively manage symptoms of overactive bladders. Oxybutynin (Ditropan®), trospium (Sanctura®), tolterodine (Detrol®), solifenacin, and darifenacin are the primary agents used to manage this condition.

g. Muscarinic antagonists are used to control movement disorders related to Parkinson disease or antipsychotic drug therapy (e.g., benztropine [Cogentin®] and trihexyphenidyl HCl [Artane®]).

h. The primary adverse effects related to the systemic use of muscarinic antagonists are dry mouth, tachycardia, constipation, mydriasis/photophobia, loss of accommodation, urinary retention, and CNS excitation. Ocular application of muscarinic antagonists can cause loss of accommodation and increased intraocular pressure.

III. DRUGS AFFECTING THE SOMATIC NERVOUS SYSTEM.

The somatic nerves that produce voluntary movement originate in the spinal cord and project their myelinated axons via the dorsal root to specific muscle bundles. These axons release ACh at the neuromuscular junction to activate **nicotinic–cholinergic (N)** receptors, causing the depolarization and contraction of muscle fibers. The actions of ACh at the nicotinic receptor are terminated by synaptic AChE and result in relaxation of the muscle fiber.

A. Drugs affecting the neuromuscular junction. The motor end plate of the neuromuscular junction contains cholinergic–nicotinic receptors (N_N subtype) that are voltage-gated sodium channels. Binding of ACh to these receptors opens the channel's gating mechanism, allowing a rapid influx of Na^+ ions that depolarize the end plate. This depolarization spreads longitudinal along the muscle fiber to open T-type calcium channels in the T tubule to allow a secondary calcium influx that triggers further calcium release from the sarcoplasmic reticulum to mediate muscle contraction. The N_N receptor is a pentamer of 2α, β, γ, and δ subunits arranged in the plasma membrane to form an ion channel. The binding of an ACh molecule to each α-subunit is thought to be necessary for optimal channel activation.

1. All the drugs in this class also appear to bind to the same sites on the α-subunits and can thus be classified as competitive ligands. Nicotinic antagonists are primarily divided into **non-depolarizing** and **depolarizing** agents, depending on whether they activate the ion channel to cause depolarization of the motor end plate or not. Nondepolarizing agents such as tubocurarine, atracurium (Tracrium®), pancuronium, and rocuronium (Zemuron®) (*Figure 9-7*) prevent the binding of ACh to the α-subunits of N_N receptor to prevent depolarization of the end plate, and a rapid paralysis ensues. Thus, these agents possess no inherent ability to activate ion conductance.

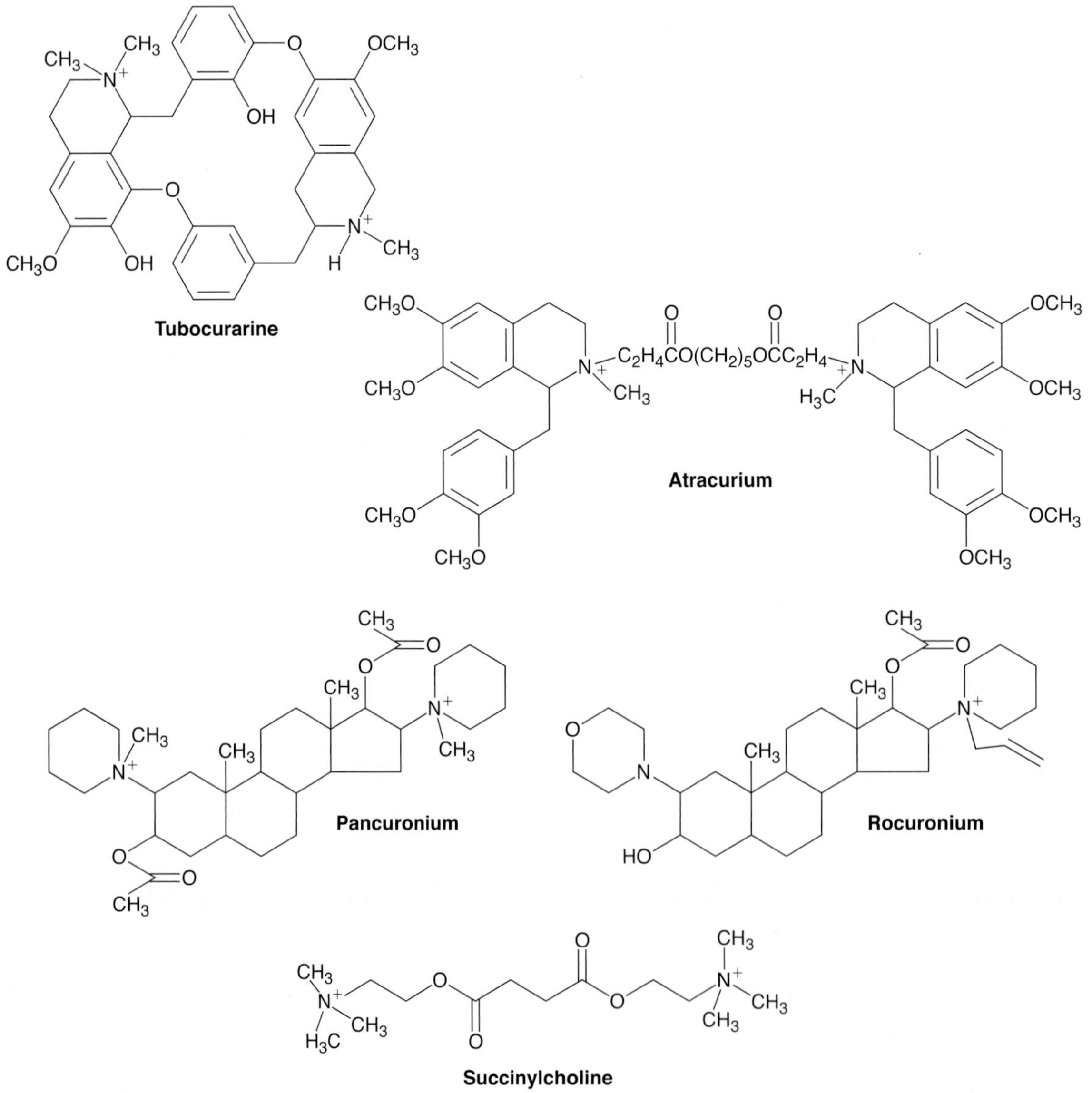

Figure 9-7. Structural formulas of the nondepolarizing (tubocurarine, atracurium, pancuronium, rocuronium) and depolarizing (succinylcholine) nicotinic antagonists.

2. Nondepolarizing antagonists can be subdivided into isoquinoline (e.g., tubocurarine, atracurium) or steroid (e.g., pancuronium, rocuronium) chemical classes; however, they all possess one or two quaternary amines, which mimic that on ACh and are required for binding to the receptor.
3. The depolarizing blocker succinylcholine (Anectine®; *Figure 9-7*) is essentially two ACh molecules attached at their acyloxy group. The drug binds to the same site as ACh to cause motor end plate depolarization and some muscle contraction initially. The inability of synaptic AChE to rapidly metabolize succinylcholine results in prolonged end plate depolarization and inactivation of the ion channel. Consequently, initial depolarization and muscle contraction is followed by a prolonged flaccid paralysis of muscle as the N-receptor is unable to reset and respond to subsequent agonist stimulation. Any ACh that binds to the receptors tends to further the depolarization/inactivation cycle to promote greater paralysis.
4. Application of an AChE inhibitor (neostigmine) can be used to reverse the paralysis induced by nondepolarizing agents, whereas the paralysis induced by succinylcholine will only be exacerbated by this strategy.
5. Nondepolarizing agents are used to produce prolonged skeletal muscle relaxation during surgery, whereas succinylcholine is used to induce short-term paralysis in procedures such as intubations, resetting of a fracture, and endoscopic investigations.
6. The major adverse effects observed with these agents are histamine release, hypotension, tachycardia, cardiopulmonary collapse, and malignant hyperthermia. Succinylcholine is also associated with hyperkalemia secondary to excessive K^+ release from skeletal muscle.

IV. DRUGS AFFECTING THE CENTRAL NERVOUS SYSTEM

A. Local anesthetic drugs affecting sensory nerves

1. The afferent sensory nerve fibers that transmit pain sensations to the CNS are located in the periphery, but secondary afferent neurons found in the spinal cord would also be involved in transmitting those signals to the brain.
2. Noxious stimuli initiate depolarizing currents at the sensory nerve ending that are transmitted up the axon by action potentials regulated by the sequential opening of voltage-gated sodium and potassium channels.
3. This action potential propagates up the axon carrying the sensory signal to the secondary afferent in the spinal cord. Local anesthetics can have actions on the primary or secondary sensory afferents, depending on where the drugs are applied.
4. The general chemical characteristics of local anesthetics are an aromatic ring connected to an ionizable tertiary amine via an ester or amide linkage (*Figure 9-8*). Examples of ester local anesthetics are procaine (Novocaine®) and benzocaine, whereas lidocaine (Xylocaine®) and ropivacaine (Naropin®) are examples of amides.
5. Due to the actions of tissue esterases, amide local anesthetics generally have longer durations of action when compared to esters. Although the uncharged form of these drugs penetrates through

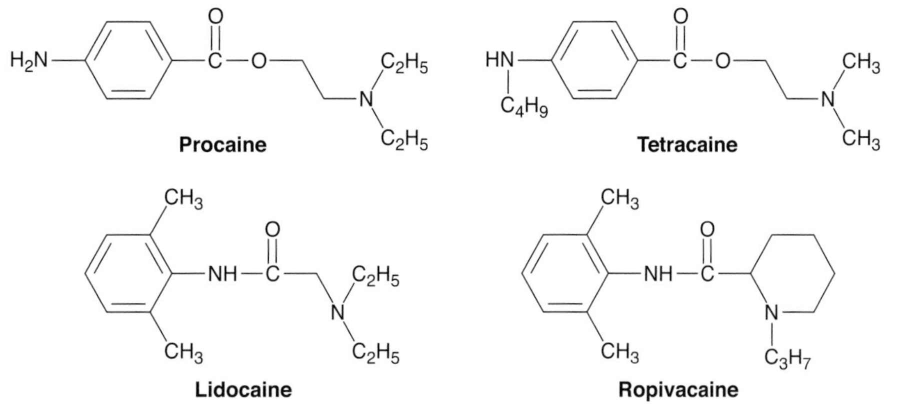

Figure 9-8. Formulas of the ester (procaine, tetracaine) and amide (lidocaine, ropivacaine) local anesthetics.

the plasma membrane, the inhibition of voltage-gated sodium channels on axons requires protonation of the tertiary amines.

6. During action potential propagation, sodium channels cycle between closed, open, and inactive states, and local anesthetics bind preferentially to the open and inactive states and stabilize the channel in the inactive state. Thus, local anesthetics display a use-dependent effect, whereby rapidly depolarizing axons are more readily blocked by the drug.
7. These agents are usually injected into the dermis surrounding sensory nerves to produce decreased nociception during procedures such as wound care, dental manipulation, and placement of sutures. However, they can also be administered at the site of nerve trunks or via intravenous route for regional anesthesia. Epinephrine is often coadministered with local anesthetic agents to produce a vasoconstriction that prolongs the duration of action and reduces systemic effects. Administration of local anesthetics into the epidural or subarachnoid space of the spinal cord is used for pain control during labor or C-section.
8. Systemic adverse effects may occur with high doses or repeated administrations of local anesthetic and include allergic reactions (especially to esters), cardiac arrhythmias, hypotension, methemoglobinemia, CNS depression, nystagmus, convulsions, and coma.

B. **General anesthetics.** Volatile and nonvolatile general anesthetics are used to induce analgesia, amnesia, loss of consciousness, and skeletal muscle relaxation during surgical procedures. Usually, anesthesia is accomplished by preoperative benzodiazepine (BDZ), induction of anesthesia by an intravenous agent, and maintenance of anesthesia by a combination of inhaled and intravenous agents.

1. **Intravenous general anesthetics** are a diverse group of agents used for induction and maintenance of anesthesia. This group includes barbiturates such as thiopental, BDZs such as midazolam (Versed®), phenols such as propofol (Diprivan®), opioids such as fentanyl (Sublimaze®), and carboxylated imidazoles such as etomidate (Amidate®). Thiopental, propofol, and etomidate (*Figure 9-9*) are able to produce a smoother and more rapid anesthesia as compared to inhaled agents and thus are often used for induction. In short-term procedures, these agents may also be used to maintain anesthesia without the addition of an inhaled agent. Opioids and BDZs are generally used as adjuvants for their antinociceptive and amnesic properties.
2. **Volatile or inhalation anesthetics** are drugs inhaled as gases or vapors. These diverse drugs are relatively simple lipophilic molecules.
   a. They include the inorganic agent nitrous oxide (N_2O) and the nonflammable halogenated hydrocarbons (e.g., halothane [Fluothane®]) and ethers (e.g., isoflurane [Forane®], desflurane [Suprane®], sevoflurane [Ultane®]; *Figure 9-9*). These agents produce a reversible loss in consciousness and skeletal muscle relaxation when administered via the inhalational route.
   b. The absorption of these agents from the lungs depends on their blood:gas partition coefficient such that the more water-soluble agents equilibrate much slower in the blood and thus

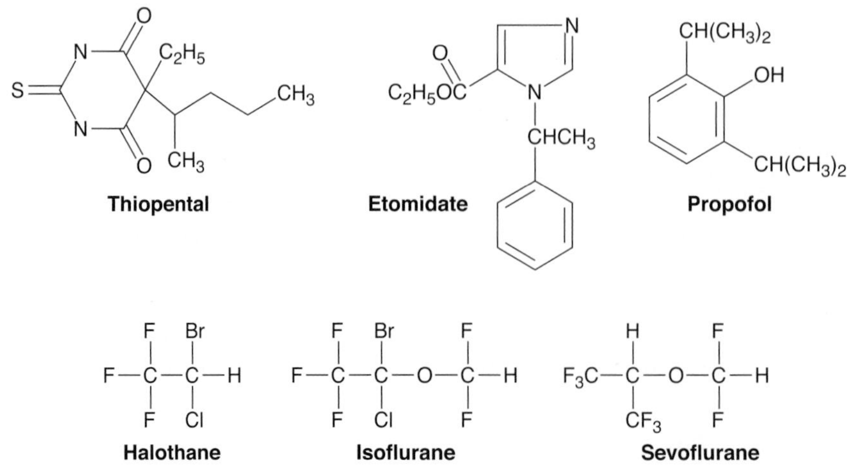

Figure 9-9. Structural formulas of the intravenous (thiopental, etomidate, propofol) and inhalational (halothane, isoflurane, sevoflurane) general anesthetics.

partition out of the blood into the CNS at slower rates. This chemical characteristic generally results in both induction and recovery from anesthesia to be slow.

c. It was previously thought that inhaled anesthetics altered membrane fluidity to produce anesthesia, but currently, it is understood that these agents modify $GABA_A$ channel function on neurons. Interaction of these agents with the transmembrane domains of the channel subunits leads to increased chloride conductance, membrane hyperpolarization, and decreased neuronal activity.

d. The adverse effects experienced during the use of volatile anesthetics have led to the greater reliance on the combination with intravenous agents. These effects include hepatotoxicity (especially with halothane), malignant hyperthermia, respiratory depression, cardiac arrhythmias, and hypotension.

C. Sedative hypnotics and anxiolytic agents. The ideal sedative would produce adequate CNS depression to reduce activity, decrease excitement, and generally have a calming effect. Hypnotic agents are used to produce drowsiness and initiate and maintain sleep. In many cases, a single agent can produce sedative effects at lower doses and hypnotic effects at successively higher doses. It is important to note that, for the most part, these agents do not produce CNS depression to the extent that leads to respiratory depression and death unless used in combination with other CNS depressants.

1. Benzodiazepines. The pharmacophore structure of the BDZ class of drugs is represented by 5-phenyl-1,4-benzodiazepine-2-one (*Figure 9-10*).

a. Pharmacological activity depends on ring A on the drug being aromatic, and this is further increased by having an electron-withdrawing group (Cl or nitro) at position 7 as in the case

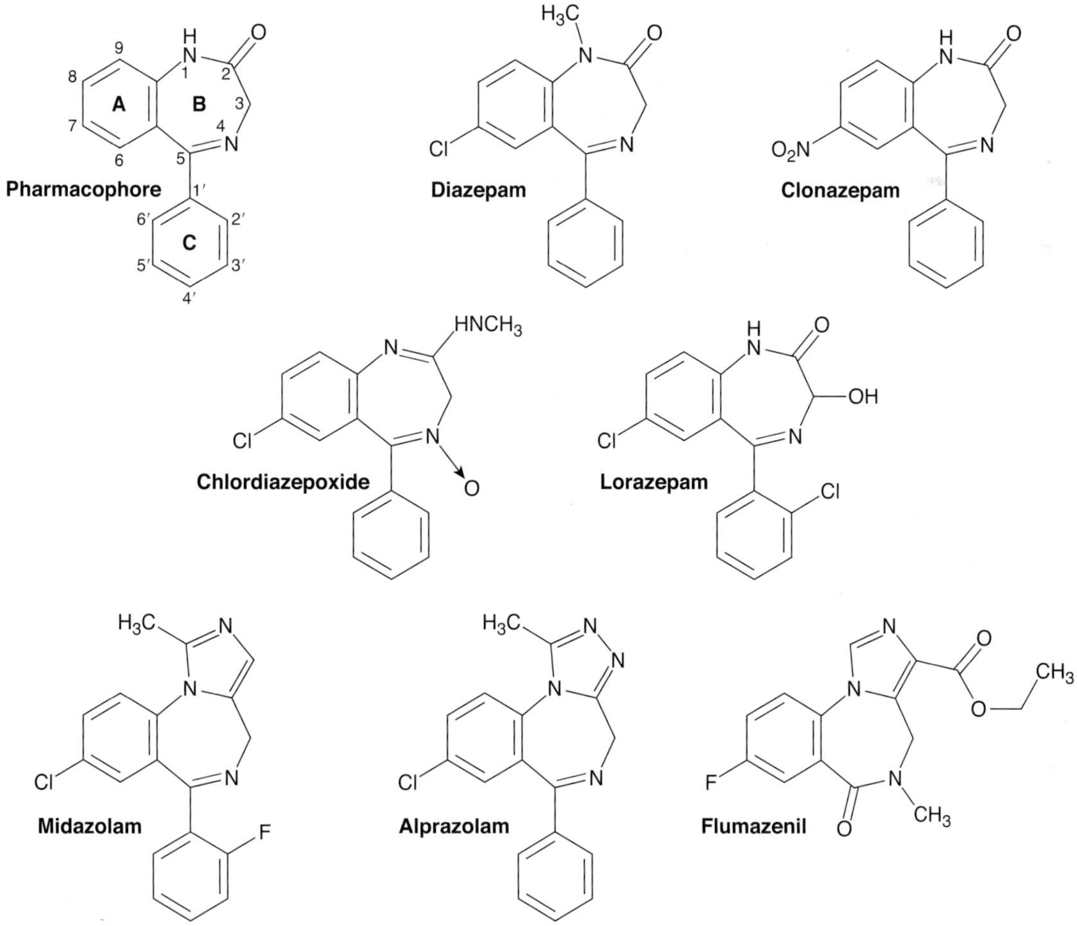

Figure 9-10. The benzodiazepine pharmacophore and representative agents in the class (diazepam, chlordiazepoxide, clonazepam, midazolam, lorazepam, alprazolam). Flumazenil is a selective benzodiazepine antagonist.

of diazepam (Valium®) and clonazepam (Klonopin®). Although the carbonyl group at position 2 is most often seen, this can be substituted with other proton-bond acceptors such as aminomethyl group as in the case of chlordiazepoxide (Librium®), a fused imidazole group at position 1 and 2 for midazolam (Versed®), or a fused triazole group at the position 1 and 2 as seen in alprazolam (Xanax®). Substitutions at position 1 or 3 may increase lipophilicity as in the case of diazepam or hydrophilicity as with lorazepam (Ativan®). Substitutions on ring C are only allowed at position 2 and are electron-withdrawing Cl or F (lorazepam, midazolam).

b. Removal of ring C results in loss of agonist activity, although high-affinity binding to the BDZ site on the $GABA_A$ receptor is maintained (flumazenil [Romazicon®]). The chemical structures of the BDZs discussed earlier are shown in *Figure 9-10.*

c. BDZs appear to produce their pharmacological effects by enhancing the binding of the neurotransmitter γ-aminobutyric acid (GABA) to the $GABA_A$ receptor, a multimeric, ligand-gated chloride channel. BDZs bind to a unique site on the receptor and require the presence of GABA to produce a biological effect; they can be regarded as modulators of GABA functions. The increased GABA-mediated chloride current into neurons of the spinal cord, hypothalamus, hippocampus, substantia nigra, and cortex causes generalized CNS depression leading to anxiolytic, sedative/hypnotic, and muscle relaxant effects. Other uses for BDZs include the emergency treatment of seizures (e.g., status epilepticus) and, as discussed earlier, midazolam is primarily used as a preanesthetic due to its rapid metabolism. They are also used to treat symptoms due to alcohol withdrawal.

d. With prolonged use, some dependence on the BDZs may result, and sudden withdrawal will result in a temporary increase in the symptoms such as insomnia or anxiety.

e. The antagonist flumazenil has no direct effect on GABA function and competes with BDZs for binding to the BDZ site on the channel. It is used in cases of BDZ overdose and to reverse the sedative effects of BDZs after a surgical or therapeutic procedure. Adverse effects with the use of BDZs include daytime sleepiness, mental confusion, amnesia, headache, blurred vision, nausea, vomiting, and diarrhea.

2. **Barbiturates.** Includes phenobarbital (Luminal®), secobarbital (Seconal®), and pentobarbital (Nembutal®). Historically, this class of drugs was used most often to treat anxiety and insomnia but has largely been replaced by the BDZs.

a. The pharmacophoric structure of barbiturates is shown in *Figure 9-11*, with barbituric acid having hydrogen at position 5. The electron-withdrawing nature of the carbonyl groups allows

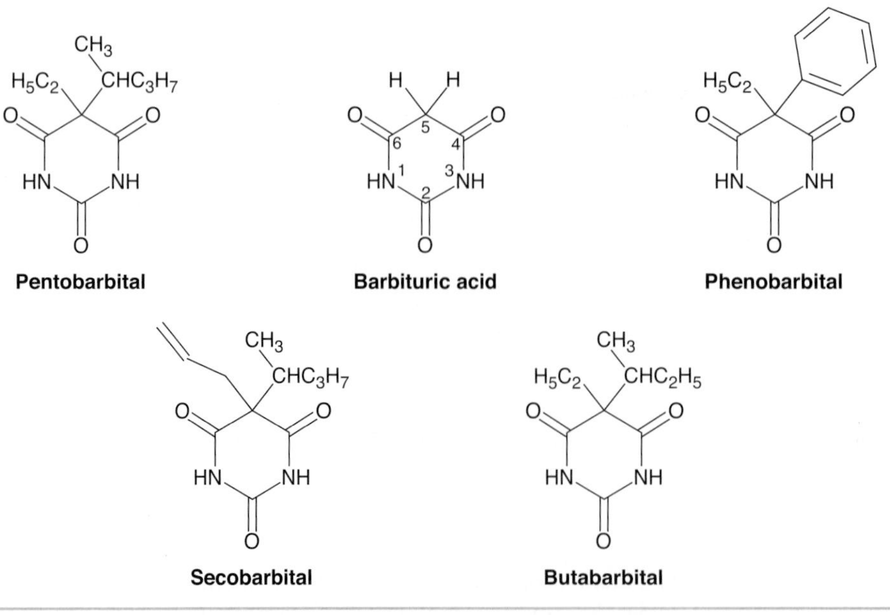

Figure 9-11. Chemical structure of barbituric acid and representative agents in the class.

the amines to behave as weak acids rather than bases, and alkyl or aryl substitutions at the C-5 position increases lipophilicity and duration of action (*Figure 9-11*).

b. At low doses, barbiturates appear to enhance GABA binding to its receptor and enhance chloride conductance into neurons. They also have inhibitory effects at AMPA-type glutamate receptors. These two effects combined are responsible for depression of nerve activity throughout the CNS to cause sedation and anxiolytic benefits. At higher doses, barbiturates appear to have direct actions to increase chloride conductance (even in the absence of GABA) and to block sodium and potassium channels. Thus, overdoses can have marked CNS depression leading to coma and death. Experimental data suggest that barbiturates interact with the $GABA_A$ receptor at a site distinct from that of BDZs.

c. With chronic use of barbiturates, tolerance to the sedative and anxiolytic effects can result. Pharmacokinetic tolerance develops quickly and is due to the induction of several cytochrome P450 enzymes responsible for barbiturate metabolism. Pharmacodynamic tolerance may continue to develop for several months and provides cross-tolerance to other CNS-depressant drugs.

d. Apart from anxiety and insomnia, barbiturates are also used to treat convulsions in emergencies such as those due to tetanus, eclampsia, convulsant drug overdose, and status epilepticus.

e. Adverse effects associated with barbiturate use include drowsiness, excitement or restlessness in elderly patients, allergic reactions, apnea, and hypotension.

3. Miscellaneous anxiolytic/sedative hypnotics. Drugs in this category are structurally diverse and may have distinct mechanisms of action.

a. Zolpidem (Ambien CR®), zaleplon (Sonata®), and eszopiclone (Lunesta®) have a similar mechanism of action as the BDZs and their actions can be blocked by flumazenil. These newer BDZ receptor agonists are used primarily to treat sleep disorders and appear less likely to cause dependency or rebound withdrawal symptoms.

b. Buspirone (BuSpar®) may exert its effects by behaving as a partial agonist at serotonin $5\text{-}HT_{1A}$-receptors but may also interact with central dopamine D_2-receptors. It is not associated with rebound anxiety and insomnia upon abrupt withdrawal, but its therapeutic effects may be delayed for 1 to 2 weeks.

c. Ramelteon (Rozerem®) is an agonist at the melatonin MT_1- and MT_2-receptors in the suprachiasmatic nucleus of the brain. It does not have the same abuse potential as BDZs and is used to treat generalized anxiety states and sleep disorders. The chemical structures of these agents are found on *Figure 9-12*.

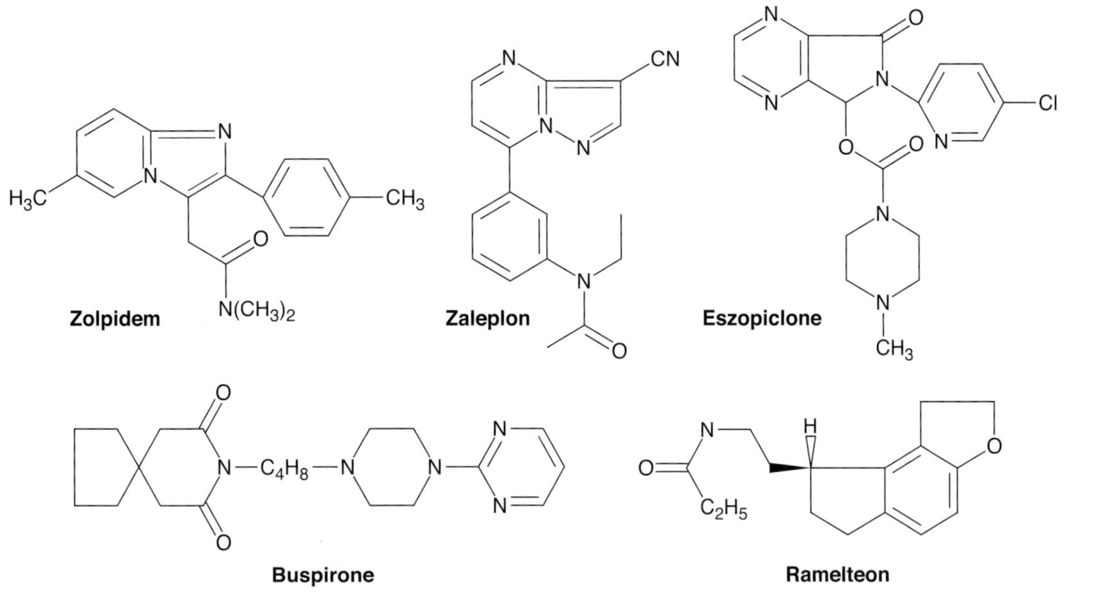

Figure 9-12. Structural formulas of miscellaneous anxiolytic/sedative-hypnotic agents.

D. Drugs to manage psychosis and mania. Drugs may be used to manage patients exhibiting several conditions such as schizophrenia, bipolar disorder (manic phase), psychotic depression, senile psychosis, and drug-induced psychosis. Psychotic conditions are usually characterized by delusions and auditory or visual hallucinations with some types (e.g., schizophrenia) having a genetic link. Currently, it is thought that altered serotonin, dopamine, and glutamate signaling in the brain are responsible for most symptoms displayed in psychotic behavior. The major antipsychotic drug classes that will be discussed are the phenothiazines, thioxanthenes, butyrophenones, dibenzapines, and benzamides.

1. **Phenothiazines.** This class of drugs is subdivided into aliphatic (e.g., chlorpromazine [Thorazine®]), piperidine (e.g., thioridazine [Mellaril®]), and piperazine (e.g., trifluoperazine [Stelazine®], fluphenazine [Prolixin®]) derivatives, depending on the type of substitution found at the R position on the phenothiazine nucleus (*Figure 9-13*).
   a. The tertiary amine of these substitutions is required for activity, and electron-withdrawing substitutions at the X position further enhance potency.
   b. All these agents have their therapeutic effect through the blockade of dopamine D_2-receptors of the mesolimbic and mesocortical pathways in the brain. However, their interaction with α-adrenergic, muscarinic, histamine, and 5-HT_2-receptors may be responsible for some of the beneficial effects and many adverse effects seen during treatment.
2. **Thioxanthenes.** This class of drugs has a similar tricyclic structure to the phenothiazines; however, only thiothixene (Navane®; *Figure 9-14*) is marketed in the United States. This agent displays high extrapyramidal effects but low sedative and autonomic effects.
3. **Butyrophenones.** This class of antipsychotics is represented by haloperidol (Haldol®; *Figure 9-14*) and pimozide (Orap®), which are thought to act via D_2-receptors to modify psychotic behavior. The tertiary amino group of the piperidine is required for binding to D_2-receptors, as is an aromatic ring para to the piperidine ring. The butyrophenone group (haloperidol) can be substituted with a diphenylbutyl (pimozide) and still have high selectivity for the receptor. These agents have low sedative and autonomic effects but high extrapyramidal effects.
4. **Dibenzapines.** This class contains clozapine (Clozaril®), loxapine (Loxitane®; *Figure 9-14*), olanzapine (Zyprexa®), and quetiapine (Seroquel®). These agents display relatively low extrapyramidal effects but can be sedating and have autonomic effects. They are considered atypical

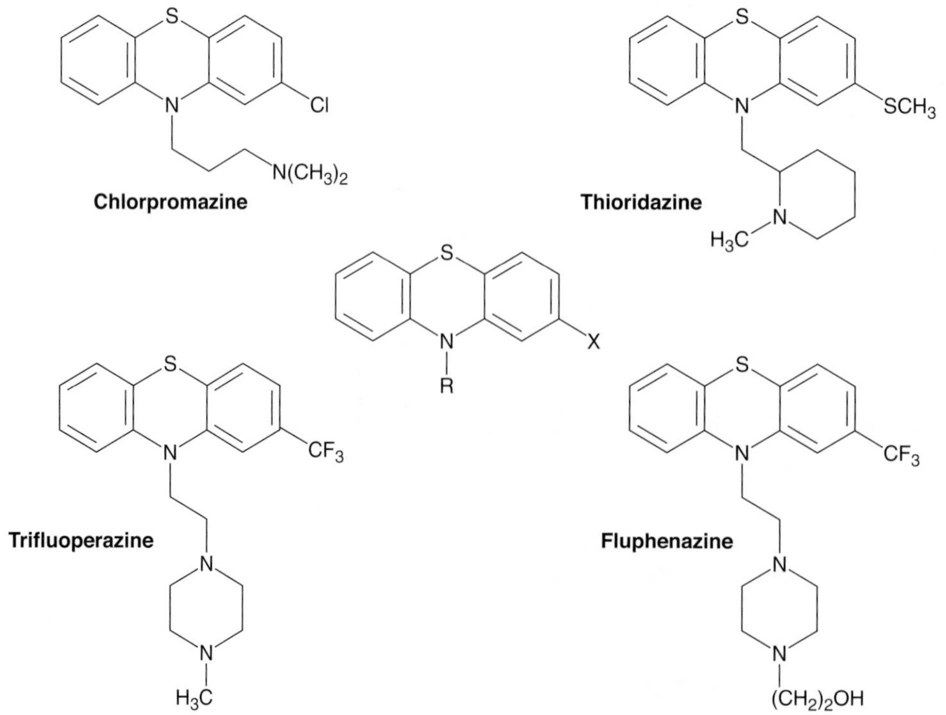

Figure 9-13. Structural formulas of the phenothiazine antipsychotic agents.

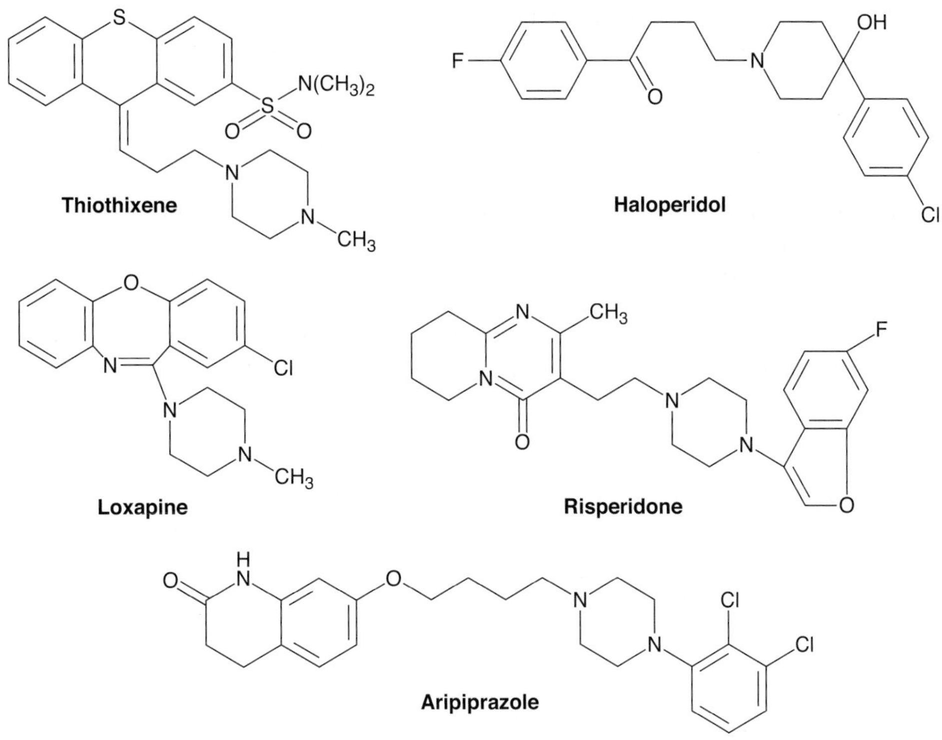

Figure 9-14. Structural formulas of thioxanthene (thiothixene), butyrophenone (haloperidol), and benzamide (risperidone, aripiprazole) antipsychotic agents.

to phenothiazines in their antipsychotic mechanism of action. They have CYP1A2 induction action, which can be a source of drug interactions; quetiapine dosing has to be increased in smokers because cigarettes also induce CYP1A2 expression. Clozapine is likely to cause leucopenia and eosinophilia, which may progress to agranulocytosis, requiring frequent monitoring with blood tests.

5. **Benzamides.** These are also considered atypical in the pharmacological action and are represented by remoxipride (Roxiam®), risperidone (Risperdal®; *Figure 9-14*), paliperidone (Invega®), ziprasidone (Geodon®), and aripiprazole (Abilify®; *Figure 9-14*).
   a. Although phenothiazines, thioxanthenes, and butyrophenones appear to produce their effects primarily by blocking D_2-receptors, the atypical agents appear to have more prominent effects as partial agonists at the 5-HT_{1A}-receptors. Thus, they tend to exhibit lower extrapyramidal effects but still have sedative (blockade of central M receptors) and autonomic (blockade of central α-adrenergic receptors) effects.
   b. Apart from schizophrenia, these agents are used to treat manic phases of bipolar disorder, Tourette syndrome, and psychotic depression.
   c. The major adverse effects seen with the use of these agents (especially the typical agents) are tardive dyskinesia, sedation, autonomic dysfunction (hypotension, orthostatic hypotension, decreased blood pressure), failure to ejaculate, hepatotoxicity, photosensitivity, and blurred vision.
   d. The atypical agents show less extrapyramidal effects but can cause weight gain and prolong the QT interval of the heart.
6. **Lithium in bipolar disorder.** Bipolar disorder is characterized by a manic phase where the patient is highly excitable, hyperactive, impulsive, requires little sleep, and has cognitive impairment. This manic phase is usually followed by a depressive phase similar to major depression.
   a. Lithium carbonate (Eskalith®) is used to manage the disorder (especially manic phase), but its popularity has decreased due to the introduction of valproate, aripiprazole, and benzamide antipsychotics. Usually, an antidepressant is used to treat the depressive phase of the disorder but has been associated with inducing the manic phase.

b. Lithium may have its mood-stabilizing effects by blocking inositol phosphate phosphatases to elevate inositol phosphates or reducing glycogen synthase kinase-3 activity in neuronal cells, but the precise mechanisms are unknown.

c. The primary adverse effects seen with the use of lithium are tremors, decreased thyroid function, nephrogenic diabetes insipidus (polyuria, polydipsia due to loss of sensitivity to antidiuretic hormone), edema, and bradycardia.

E. **Drugs used to treat depression.** Major depressive disorder is characterized by loss of interest or pleasure in daily activities most of the time for up to 2 weeks and usually exhibits as sleep and appetite disturbance, low energy levels, and decreased cognition. The causes of depression are not entirely clear but may include a decrease in monoamines (serotonin, norepinephrine) as well as neurotrophic and endocrine factors, such as brain-derived neurotrophic factor, in the brain. The primary classes of agents used to treat depression are selective serotonin reuptake inhibitors (SSRIs), serotonin–norepinephrine reuptake inhibitors (selective and tricyclic antidepressants), 5-HT_2-antagonists, MAO inhibitors, and several miscellaneous agents.

1. **Selective serotonin reuptake inhibitors.** The serotonin transporter (SERT) is glycoprotein inserted into the membrane of axon terminals of neurons that release serotonin (5-HT). Binding of 5-HT to SERT results in transport of the amine Na^+ and Cl^- into the nerve terminal with the 5-HT being released in the cytoplasmic side.

   a. SSRIs allosterically interact with SERT at a distinct extracellular site to 5-HT to inhibit the reuptake of the amine into nerve terminals. Presumably, this leads to a buildup of 5-HT in the synaptic space and greater activation of the complementary receptor on the postsynaptic nerve. The overall outcome of this action is a progressive inhibition of the central dopamine system. There is no evidence for the interaction of SSRIs with the NET or other transporters and receptors.

   b. The SSRIs are represented by a diverse group agents such as fluoxetine (Prozac®), paroxetine (Paxil®), sertraline (Zoloft®), atomoxetine (Strattera®), and escitalopram (Lexapro®), with chemical structures shown in *Figure 9-15*.

   c. SSRIs are used to manage major depression; anxiety disorders such as posttraumatic stress disorder (PTSD), panic disorder, and obsessive–compulsive disorder (OCD); premenstrual dysphoric disorder; and bulimia.

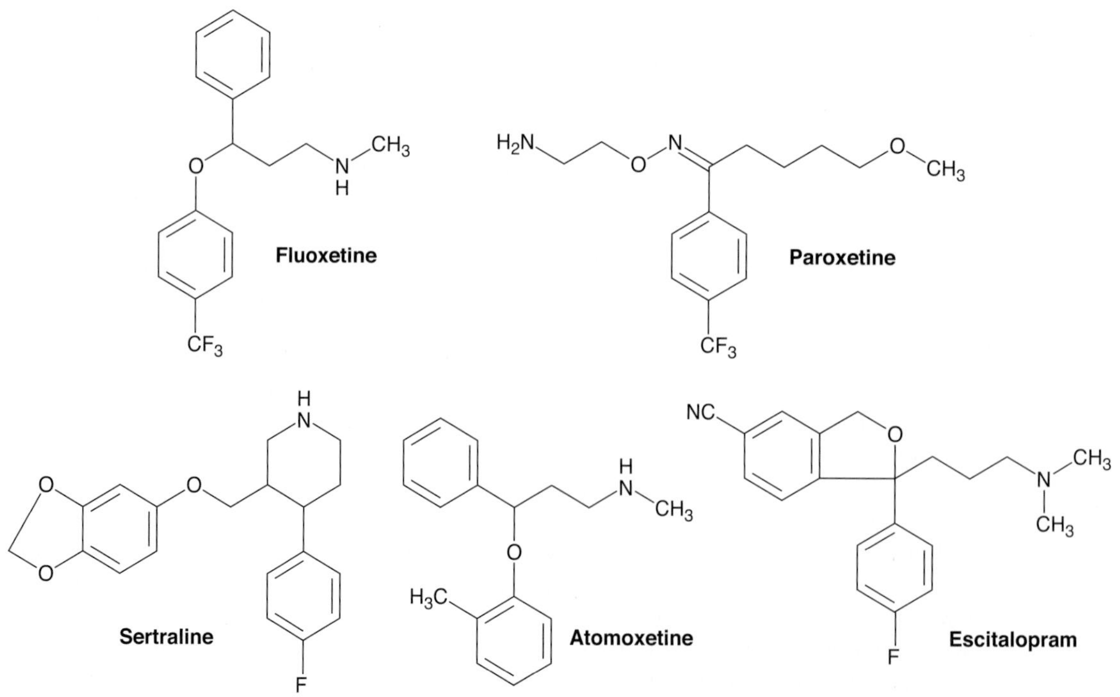

Figure 9-15. Structural formulas of the selective serotonin reuptake inhibitors (SSRIs).

d. The most frequent adverse events experienced by patients on SSRIs include nausea, GI upset, diarrhea, decreased sexual function, headaches, insomnia, and weight gain. Sudden discontinuation of SSRIs may result in a syndrome of effects such as dizziness and paresthesias.

2. **Serotonin–norepinephrine reuptake inhibitors (SNRIs).** These agents comprise the tricyclic antidepressants and selective SNRIs.

a. The tricyclic antidepressants were the mainstay of depression therapy for the decades preceding the introduction of SSRIs and include imipramine (Tofranil®), amitriptyline (Elavil®), amoxapine, doxepin (Sinequan®), and trimipramine (Surmontil®).

b. These agents have multiple pharmacological effects via the interaction with SERT, NET, α1- and α2-adrenergic, muscarinic, and histamine receptors; however, the mood-elevating effects may be attributed to increased α1- and 5-HT-receptor stimulation, secondary to buildup of NE and 5-HT in the synaptic space.

c. Imipramine serves as the prototypical tertiary amine tricyclic (*Figure 9-16*), which can be modified in several ways to retain antidepressant activity. Modifications of the propylamine at position 5 to a secondary amine (desipramine) or isobutylamine (trimipramine) produce drugs that have increased selectivity for the NET versus the SERT and reduced anticholinergic effects. Loss of the propylamino modification also retains more NET activity as in the case of amoxapine.

d. There is considerable flexibility for the composition of the seven-member ring where the N at position 5 can be replaced by a carbon (amitriptyline) or oxygen (amoxapine), and the carbon at position 10 or 11 can be replaced by nitrogen (amoxapine) or oxygen (doxepine). The fusion of a piperidine ring to position 10 and 11 also improves NET interaction (maprotiline [Ludiomil®]). Mirtazapine (Remeron®) lacks the propylamino modification and contains a fused tetracyclic ring (*Figure 9-16*) that retains bioamine reuptake blocking activity but increases α_2 and 5-HT-receptor blocking activity as well.

e. The nontricyclic agents with somewhat greater selectivity for the SERT versus NET are represented by venlafaxine (Effexor®), desvenlafaxine (Pristiq®), and duloxetine (Cymbalta®).

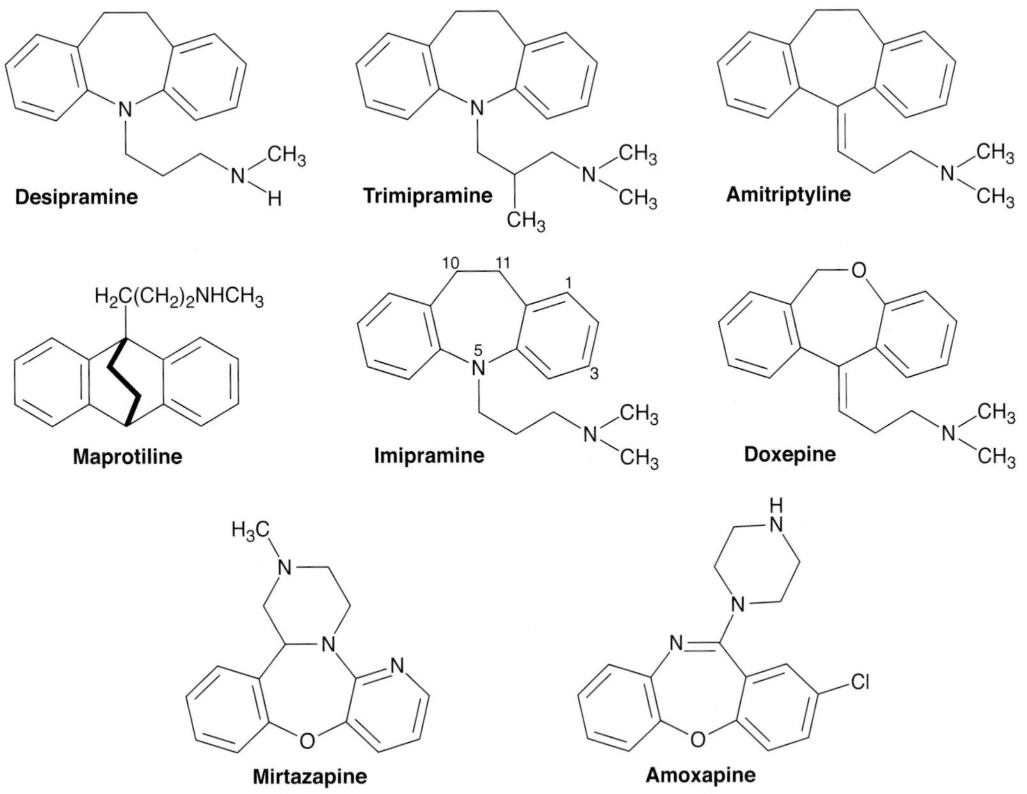

Figure 9-16. Structural formulas of the serotonin–norepinephrine reuptake inhibitors (SNRIs).

These drugs are chemically unrelated and have the advantage of having relatively few interactions with adrenergic, muscarinic, histaminic, and serotonergic receptors.

f. Adverse effects related to therapy with SNRIs include those with SSRIs (previously discussed) as well as increased blood pressure, heart rate, insomnia, anxiety, and agitation. Tricyclic agents have additional antimuscarinic effects (dry mouth, constipation, urinary retention), as well as orthostatic hypotension due to peripheral α_1-blockade. Most of the SNRIs are also associated with a serotonin-withdrawal syndrome as seen with SSRIs.

3. **Monoamine oxidase inhibitors (MAOIs).** MAOIs were some of the first pharmacological agents developed to treat major depression, but their use has decreased significantly due to the advent of newer agents (previously discussed) with better therapeutic and safety profiles.
   a. MAOIs are reserved for depression that is refractory to other agents, and currently, hydrazine (isocarboxazid [Marplan®], phenelzine [Nardil®]) and phenylcyclopropylamine (selegiline [Emsam®], tranylcypromine [Parnate®]) are marketed in the United States.
   b. These agents bind irreversibly to MAO-A and MAO-B isoforms in aminergic nerve terminals to prevent the metabolism of biogenic amines dopamine, norepinephrine, and serotonin. It is believed that this action leads to elevation of central biogenic amine neurotransmission to improve depressive mood disorders; however, this outcome usually takes several weeks to develop.
   c. Orthostatic hypotension, weight gain, sexual dysfunction, insomnia or sedation, restlessness, and confusion are some of the most common adverse effects experienced while on MAOIs.
   d. The consumption of tyramine-containing foods (cheese, beer, sausage, etc.) while on MAOIs can result in drastic increases in blood pressure, leading to stroke or myocardial infarction. Sudden withdrawal of MAOIs results in delirium, psychosis, and mental confusion.
4. **Miscellaneous antidepressants.** Serotonin 5-HT_2-receptor antagonists nefazodone and trazodone (Desyrel®) are rarely used to treat depression and have found use as sedatives. Bupropion (Wellbutrin®) may have NET-inhibiting activity but also appears to enhance catecholamine release from adrenergic nerves. It has little effect on the SERT or 5-HT-receptor systems.

F. **Drugs used to treat seizures.** Epilepsy is a complex of symptoms characterized by recurrent seizures due to abnormal discharge of electrical activity in the brain. The causes of seizures are myriad, from infection, head injury, or neoplastic disease; however, chronic seizures unrelated to these events may be due to genetic defects in neuronal voltage-dependent ion channels. Generally, the type of drug used to treat seizures is based on the type of disease displayed and may be localized to the cerebral cortex (partial seizures) or more generalized with sequential firing of neurons between the cortex and thalamus. Seizures can be of the convulsive and absence (nonconvulsive) types, with the convulsive form usually involving both hemispheres of the brain and resulting in loss of consciousness and often muscle spasms (myoclonic, tonic, tonic-clonic, etc.). Absence seizures are usually brief (< 20 secs), with loss of consciousness and rapid onset and cessation but with no muscle spasms.

1. **Agents for partial and generalized tonic-clonic seizures.** There are no common structural characteristics of these agents that account for their activity as antiseizure drugs and are composed primarily of sodium channel blockers and drugs modulating GABA and glutamate function.
   a. Phenytoin (Dilantin®) binds to sodium channels, stabilizes its inactive conformation, and reduces the excitability of neurons. The action is both voltage and use dependent because a greater proportion of the channels are in the inactive state. The resulting therapeutic benefit is the reduction in the tonic phase of seizures while the clonic phase may be enhanced.
   b. Adverse effects seen with phenytoin are cardiac arrhythmias, CNS depression, gingival hyperplasia, hirsutism, and hypersensitivity reactions.
   c. Carbamazepine (Tegretol®), lamotrigine (Lamictal®), lacosamide (Vimpat®), and topiramate (Topamax®) are all sodium channel blockers with a similar mechanism to phenytoin (*Figure 9-17*).
   d. Carbamazepine has additional actions to reduce synaptic transmission that may be responsible for the anticonvulsant effect of the drug. Its use has been associated with drowsiness, ataxia, blurred vision, aplastic anemia, and hypersensitivity reactions.
   e. Lamotrigine may also block N/P types of calcium channels and decrease glutamate release from excitatory nerves. Chronic use of lamotrigine can be accompanied by dizziness, ataxia, blurred vision, and rash.
   f. Lacosamide may also interfere with the function of neurotrophic factors such as brain-derived neurotrophic factor (BDNF) and NT3 on axonal/dendritic growth. Suicidal ideation is probably the adverse effect of most concern with the use of this drug.

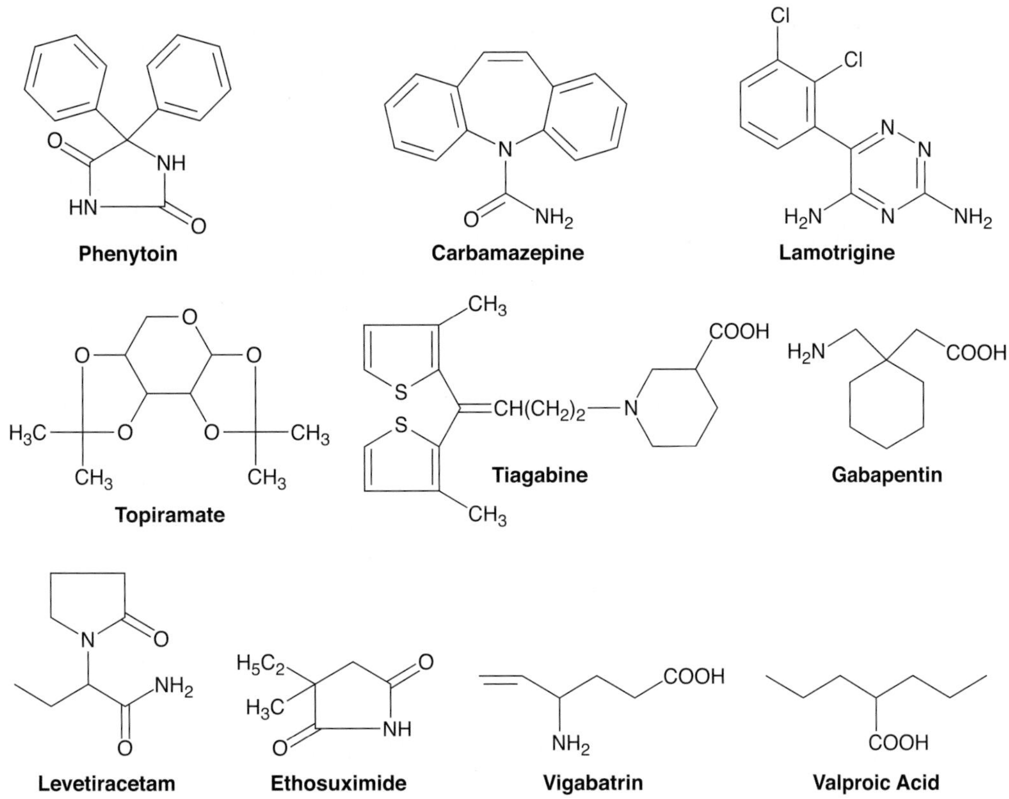

Figure 9-17. Structural formulas of several drugs used to treat seizure activity.

g. Apart from sodium channel blockade, topiramate may also potentiate GABA-induced chloride conductance and block kainate action on glutamate receptors. Drowsiness, fatigue, weight loss, and nervousness are the most common adverse effects reported with topiramate use. The chemical structures of these agents are shown in *Figure 9-16.*

h. Tiagabine (Gabitril®), gabapentin (Neurontin®), and vigabatrin (Sabril®) interfere with GABA neurotransmission to modify seizure activity (*Figure 9-17*).

i. Tiagabine was rationally designed to block GABA uptake into neurons to enhance its postsynaptic effect on $GABA_A$ receptors and consequent increase in chloride current. The most frequent adverse effects seen with tiagabine are somnolence, dizziness, and tremors.

j. Gabapentin is structurally similar to GABA and appears to increase GABA release into nerve synapses as well as block N-type calcium channels to decrease glutamate release. Gabapentin is also used to treat chronic pain, migraines, and bipolar disorder. Fatigue, dizziness, drowsiness, and ataxia are the most common adverse effects seen with gabapentin use.

k. Vigabatrin has the unique mechanism of action of irreversibly inhibiting the aminotransferase that degrades GABA. This results in maintained synaptic GABA levels to enhance receptor activation and tonic inhibition of neuronal activity. The primary adverse effects observed with vigabatrin use are drowsiness, dizziness, weight gain, mental confusion, and psychosis.

l. Levetiracetam (Keppra®; *Figure 9-17*) has an unknown mechanism of action but has been effective against generalized tonic-clonic seizures and juvenile myoclonic seizures. As with many other drugs in this category, ataxia, somnolence, dizziness, and agitation are its most common adverse effects.

2. **Drugs used to manage other generalized seizures**

a. Ethosuximide (Zarontin®) is a cyclic ureide that blocks low-threshold T-type calcium channels. Thalamic pacemaker currents that give rise to absence seizures can be depressed by T-channel blockers. Adverse effects with the use of ethosuximide are nausea, gastric pain, vomiting, lethargy, headache, and euphoria.

b. Valproic acid (Depakene®) may have actions on sodium channels (similar to phenytoin), as well as block *N*-methyl-D-aspartate (NMDA)-type glutamate ion channels. Additionally, it appears to increase GABA levels in the brain by a poorly defined mechanism and alters neuronal gene expression by inhibiting histone deacetylase. Valproate can be used to effectively manage absence seizures especially when the patient also exhibits generalized tonic-clonic seizures. The most common adverse effects seen with the use of valproate are nausea, vomiting, abdominal pain, weight gain, and hair loss. The agent also increases the risk of spina bifida in infants born to women who took valproate during pregnancy. The chemical structures of several antiseizure drugs discussed in this section are shown on *Figure 9-17*.

G. **Drugs to treat Parkinson disease and other movement disorders.** Parkinson disease is characterized by the loss of dopaminergic neurons that project from the substantia nigra into the corpus striatum due to poorly defined mechanisms. The consequence of this type of neuronal death is decreased inhibition of GABA-ergic neurons in the corpus striatum, leaving positive cholinergic input on GABA neurons unopposed. This imbalance leads to tremors of the extremities and with progression of the disease, rigidity, postural instability, slowed movement, and cognitive decline. Other movement disorders may be due to drug-induced toxicities (antipsychotics), other toxins (1-methyl-4-phenyl-1,2,3,6-tetrahydropyridine [MPTP]), or neuronal injuries. The general strategy of treating Parkinson-type disorder is to attempt the restoration of the balance of dopaminergic and cholinergic inputs on GABA-ergic neurons in the corpus striatum.

1. **Agents modifying the dopaminergic system**

a. Levodopa (Dopar®) is a dopamine precursor that is actively taken into the CNS via the amino acid transporter and converted by dopa decarboxylase to dopamine in neurons expressing the enzyme. Levodopa is often coadministered with carbidopa (Sinemet®), an inhibitor of peripheral dopa decarboxylase that ensures high blood levels of levodopa for CNS uptake.

b. Catechol-*O*-methyltransferase (COMT) is another enzyme that metabolizes levodopa, and its inhibition with agents such as tolcapone (Tasmar®) and entacapone (Comtan®) also potentiates levodopa activity. Levodopa ameliorates many of the symptoms of Parkinson disease, particularly the diminished or slowed movements.

c. The major adverse effects experienced by patients on levodopa are nausea and vomiting (especially when taken without carbidopa), cardiac arrhythmias, dyskinesias, depression, hallucinations, confusion, mydriasis, and glaucoma.

d. Dopamine receptor agonists used to directly modulate striatal GABA neuronal activity have also proven useful in managing Parkinson disease symptoms and are often better tolerated than levodopa. Bromocriptine (Parlodel®) and ropinirole (Requip®) are relatively selective dopamine D_2-receptor agonists that ameliorate Parkinson disease symptoms. Pergolide (Permax®) is both a D_1- and D_2–agonist, whereas pramipexole (Mirapex®) appears to have greater activity at the D_3-receptor. Ropinirole and pramipexole have also found use in the treatment of restless leg syndrome.

e. The potent dopamine agonist apomorphine (Apokyn®) is only used temporarily for the "off-periods" of patients on dopamine agonist therapy. The primary adverse effects of dopamine agonists are anorexia, nausea, vomiting, constipation, dyspepsia, acid reflux, postural hypotension, cardiac arrhythmias, dyskinesias, hallucinations, delusions, poor impulse control, and narcolepsy.

2. **Anticholinergic agents for Parkinson disease.** The mechanism of action of these agents has been discussed previously in the muscarinic antagonist section. They essentially reduce cholinergic input onto GABA-ergic neurons in the basal ganglia.

H. **Opioid agonists and antagonists.** Opioid alkaloids from *Papaver somniferum* have been known for their analgesic properties for thousands of years, and the principle agent in the extract, morphine, is considered the prototypical analgesic opiate. The pharmacology of opiates led to the discovery of the endogenous opioid peptides that specifically interacted with opioid receptors in the periphery as well as the CNS. These peptides, endorphins, enkephalins, and dynorphins, interact selectively with μ-, δ-, and κ-opioid receptors, respectively. These receptors are located on primary sensory afferent fibers as well as dendrites of the secondary afferent neurons in the spinal cord and on multiple afferent neurons along the pain sensory pathway that ends in the cerebral cortex. The opioid peptides are thought to be released during stressful periods to activate μ, δ, or κ receptors to increase the threshold for pain sensory transmission and thereby decrease pain sensation by the cortex.

1. **Chemistry.** Morphine's phenolic hydroxyl group is extremely important for activity; however, analgesic activity appears to depend on a *p*-phenyl-*N*-alkylpiperidine moiety (in bold, *Figure 9-18*), in which the piperidine ring is in the chair form and is perpendicular to the aromatic ring. The alkyl group at position 17 is usually methyl. The **morphine molecule** can be altered in various ways to retain analgesic activity, and related compounds also can be synthesized from other starting materials.

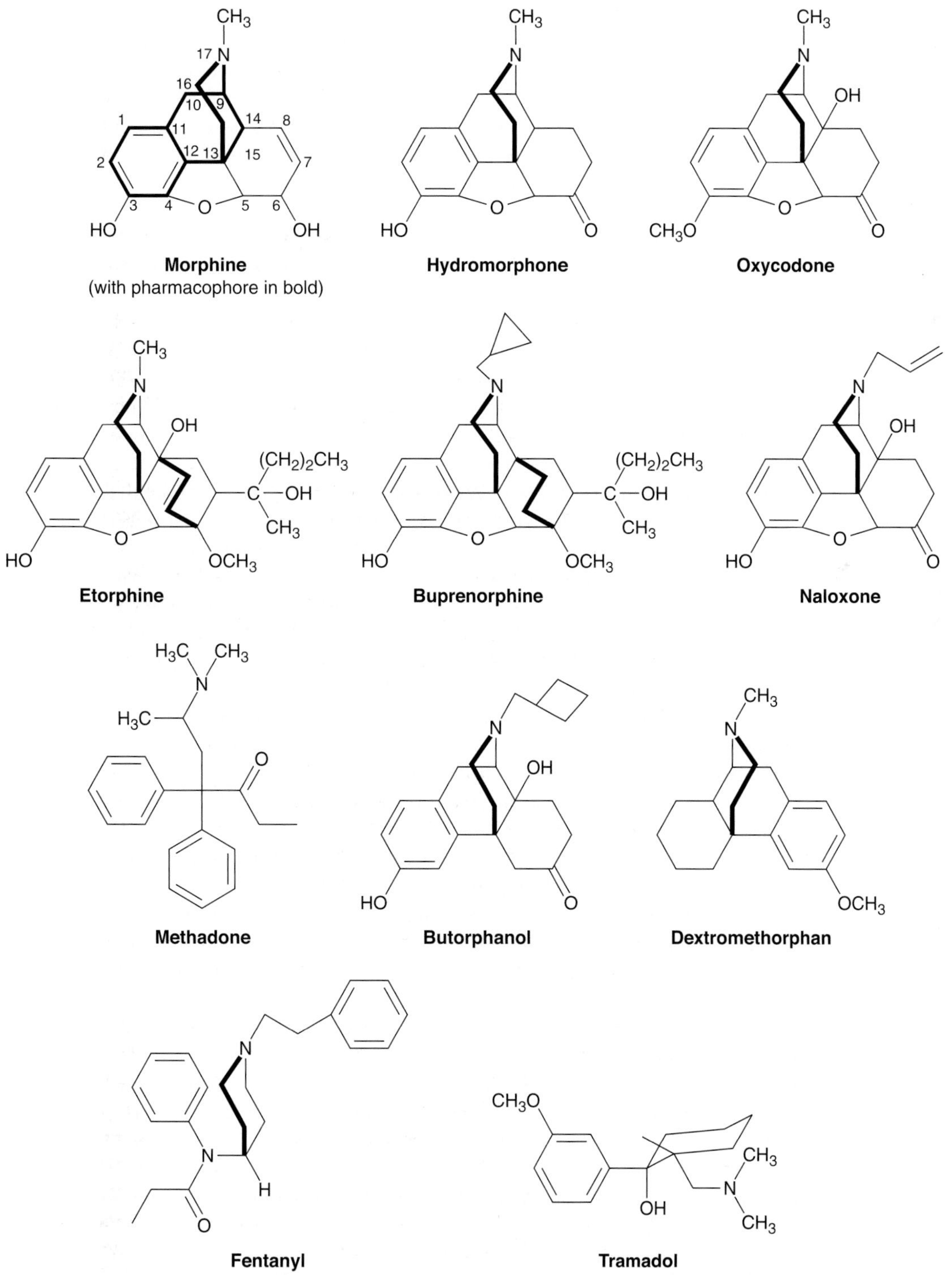

Figure 9-18. Structural formulas of the morphine (with pharmacophore in bold) and other opioid ligands. Naloxone has only antagonist activity at the opioid receptors.

a. **Natural or synthetic opioids** may be classified into four chemical groups (*Figure 9-18*):

(1) *Phenanthrenes* such as morphine (MS-Contin®), hydromorphone (Dilaudid®), codeine, and hydrocodone (Vicodin®) are considered full agonists at the μ-receptor although their analgesic potencies vary. Methylation of the phenolic 3-hydroxyl group with or without modification of the 6-hydroxyl group of morphine yields agents with reduced agonist potency but enhanced oral bioavailability (e.g., codeine, hydrocodone, oxycodone [OxyContin®]). Cyclopropylmethyl or cyclobutylmethyl substitutions at the amine as well as large substitutions at position 7 produce opioids that are partial agonists at the μ-receptor (e.g., nalbuphine [Nubain®], buprenorphine [Buprenex®]).

(2) *Phenylheptylamines,* represented by methadone (Dolophine®), is a bisphenyl derivative of heptylamine that has strong high agonist potency and excellent oral bioavailability.

(3) *Phenylpiperidines,* which include meperidine (Demerol®), fentanyl (Sublimaze®), and sufentanil (Sufenta®), are potent parenteral μ-agonists. This class also includes diphenoxylate (in Lomotil®) and loperamide (Imodium®) that have lower affinity for opioid receptors, have poor CNS penetration, and thus have lower abuse potential.

(4) *Morphinans* such as levorphanol (Levo Dromoran®) and butorphanol (Stadol®) lack the oxygen bridge between C4 and C5. This results in agonists with increased potency versus morphine, high oral bioavailability, and increased activity at κ-receptors.

b. ***Opioid antagonists*** are derived by replacing the methyl group on the nitrogen atom with more bulky substitutions. Therefore, cyclopropylmethyl or allyl substitutions at the amine, along with alterations of the 6-OH to carbonyl or methylene groups, result in pure μ-antagonists such as naltrexone (Revia®), naloxone (Narcan®), and nalmefene hydrochloride (Revex®).

c. Agents having both a free phenolic hydroxyl group and a tertiary amine function (e.g., morphine and nalbuphine) are chemically amphoteric. Amphotericity probably accounts for the erratic absorption of morphine when administered orally.

d. The newer opioid analgesic agent, **tramadol** (Ultram®), may be considered an open-ring codeine analog with weak μ-opioid agonist activity but increased activity as a SERT blocker.

2. **Pharmacology of opioid drugs.** Most of the opioid drugs on the market appear to produce their pharmacological effects through the activation of μ-opioid receptors in the pain sensory pathway. Exceptions to this paradigm are partial agonists (at μ-receptors) with higher affinity for κ-receptors (e.g., pentazocine [Talwin®]). Additionally, butorphanol and nalbuphine have antagonist activity at μ-receptors but maintain agonist activity at κ-receptors. Tramadol and tapentadol (Nucynta®) have low to modest μ-receptor agonist activity but enhanced blockade of SERT and NET, respectively. These agents appear to have low abuse potential and, in fact, the latter is not a controlled substance.

a. Opioid drugs are primarily used for the following:

(1) Constant chronic pain after surgical procedures or due to acute biliary or renal colic and cancer-related disease.

(2) Obstetric pain, although respiratory depression in the neonate may be of concern because these agents can cross the placenta.

(3) Acute pulmonary edema accompanying MI when respiratory depression is not of concern.

(4) Suppression of cough is achieved at codeine doses lower than that required for analgesia. Over-the-counter preparations of the opioid derivative dextromethorphan are effective antitussives with no analgesic activity and little abuse potential.

(5) Most cases of diarrhea can be managed with various preparations containing diphenoxylate and loperamide.

(6) Analgesia, anti-anxiety and sedative effects can be produced by fentanyl and its derivatives when used as adjuncts to anesthesia. They have also been used as regional analgesics when applied to the epidural space of the spinal cord (e.g., management of the obstetric or postsurgical patient).

b. The primary concern with opioid use during surgical procedures and overdose is the potential for significant respiratory and CNS depression leading to coma; this can be managed by the administration of opioid antagonists such as naloxone.

c. A psychological dependence characterized by euphoria, sedation, and high tolerance to stimuli can develop in susceptible individuals, and this may be reinforced by a physical dependence on the drug.

d. Chronic opioid use may lead to tolerance (requiring higher doses to produce adequate analgesia) and physical dependence that is characterized by tearing, piloerection, hyperventilation, vomiting, diarrhea, anxiety, and hostility upon withdrawal of the drug. Administration of antagonists (e.g., naloxone) or partial agonists (e.g., pentazocine) in a physically dependent patient can suddenly precipitate these symptoms.

e. Opioid analgesics are associated with the following adverse effects:

(1) CNS effects, including CNS depression, miosis, dizziness, sedation, confusion, disorientation, and coma

(2) GI effects, including nausea, vomiting, constipation, biliary spasm, and increased biliary tract pressure

(3) Cardiovascular effects, such as orthostatic hypotension, peripheral circulatory collapse, dysrhythmias, and cardiac arrest

(4) Bronchoconstriction

(5) Psychiatric effects, such as euphoria, dysphoria, and hallucinations

(6) Abuse potential and dependence

(7) Classic opioid analgesics can also prompt the release of histamine, causing intense pruritus, vasodilation, and bronchoconstriction, which can be confused with a true allergic reaction.

(8) Tramadol appears to have significantly fewer respiratory depressant effects than the classic opioids. It also does not appear to cause the release of histamine. It has fewer cardiovascular effects with the exception of orthostatic hypotension, which is produced. Tramadol does possess the typical μ-receptor–mediated side effects of constipation, nausea, vomiting, and sedation.

Study Questions

Directions for questions 1–14: Each of the questions, statements, or incomplete statements in this section can be correctly answered or completed by **one** of the suggested answers or phrases. Choose the **best** answer.

1. Which of the following drugs would most likely be used in the treatment of bronchospasm that is associated with chronic obstructive pulmonary disease?

(A) edrophonium (Tensilon)
(B) ipratropium (Atrovent)
(C) rocuronium (Zemuron)
(D) propantheline (Pro-Banthine)
(E) homatropine

2. All of the following adverse effects are manifestations of cholinergic agonists *except*

(A) bradycardia.
(B) bronchoconstriction.
(C) xerostomia.
(D) lacrimation.
(E) myopic accommodation.

3. Which of the following drugs is considered to be the agent of choice for anaphylactic reactions?

(A) clonidine (Catapres)
(B) isoproterenol (Inderal)
(C) epinephrine
(D) phenylephrine
(E) terbutaline (Brethine)

4. Which of the following neuromuscular blocking agents can cause muscarinic responses such as bradycardia and increased glandular secretions?

(A) tubocurarine
(B) succinylcholine (Anectine)
(C) pancuronium
(D) decamethonium
(E) gallamine

5. Which of the following agents would *not* be appropriate in the treatment of glaucoma?

(A) atropine
(B) pilocarpine
(C) physostigmine
(D) timolol (Timoptic)
(E) epinephrine

6. Adverse reactions to atropine include all of the following *except*

(A) photophobia.
(B) dry mouth.
(C) sedation.
(D) diarrhea.
(E) tachycardia.

7. Which of the following drugs is a volatile substance that is administered by inhalation?

(A) thiopental (Pentothal)
(B) halothane
(C) alprazolam (Xanax)
(D) buspirone (Buspar)
(E) phenytoin (Dilantin)

8. Which of the following agents is used to treat anxiety?

(A) chlordiazepoxide (Librium)
(B) thioridazine
(C) alprazolam (Xanax)
(D) buspirone (Buspar)
(E) pentobarbital

9. Which of the following best describes the mechanism of diazepam to cause a sedative effect?

(A) The drug blocks glutamate receptor to decrease neuronal excitability.
(B) The drug blocks the uptake of GABA into the nerve to increase its action at the receptor.
(C) It increases the ability of GABA to produce chloride conductance into neurons.
(D) It prevents the metabolism of catecholamines by blocking monoamine oxidases.
(E) It blocks inositol phosphate metabolism in neurons.

10. Which of the following mechanisms of action is true and most likely contributes to the treatment of parkinsonism?

(A) The direct-acting dopaminergic agonist bromocriptine (Parlodel) mimics the activity of striatal dopamine.
(B) The antimuscarinic activity of entacapone (Comtan) contributes to the restoration of striatal dopaminergic–cholinergic neurotransmitter balance.
(C) Striatal H_1-receptors are blocked by levodopa.
(D) The ergoline bromocriptine stimulates the release of striatal dopamine from intact terminals.
(E) The ability of dopamine to cross the blood–brain barrier allows it to restore striatal dopaminergic–cholinergic neurotransmitter balance.

11. All of the following adverse effects are associated with the use of levodopa *except*

(A) increased intraocular pressure.
(B) orthostatic hypotension.
(C) delusions and confusion.
(D) dyskinesia.
(E) agranulocytosis.

12. The activity of which of the following drugs depends on a *p*-phenyl-*N*-alkylpiperidine moiety?

(A) phenobarbital
(B) chlorpromazine
(C) diazepam (Valium)
(D) imipramine (Tofranil)
(E) meperidine (Demerol)

13. Opioids are used for all the following conditions *except*

(A) cough.
(B) severe chronic pain.
(C) arthritis.
(D) severe diarrhea.
(E) preanesthetic.

14. Which of the following agents would *not* be an alternative to phenytoin in the treatment of tonic-clonic seizure?

(A) levetiracetam (Keppra)
(B) gabapentin (Neurontin)
(C) ethosuximide (Zarontin)
(D) lamotrigine (Lamictal)
(E) carbamazepine (Tegretol)

Directions for questions 15–19: The questions and incomplete statements in this section can be correctly answered or completed by **one or more** of the suggested answers. Choose the answer, **A–E**.

A if **I only** is correct
B if **III only** is correct
C if **I and II** are correct
D if **II and III** are correct
E if **I, II, and III** are correct

15. Cholinesterase inhibitors can be used therapeutically

I. as miotic agents in the treatment of glaucoma.
II. to increase skeletal muscle tone in the treatment of myasthenia gravis.
III. to decrease gastrointestinal (GI) and urinary bladder smooth muscle tone.

16. Antimuscarinic agents are used in the treatment of Parkinson disease and in the control of some neuroleptic-induced extrapyramidal disorders. These agents include

I. ipratropium (Atrovent).
II. benztropine.
III. trihexyphenidyl.

17. Certain drugs are sometimes incorporated into local anesthetic solutions to prolong their activity and reduce their systemic toxicity. These drugs include

I. dobutamine.
II. phenoxybenzamine.
III. epinephrine.

18. Improper administration of local anesthetics can cause toxic plasma concentrations that may result in

I. seizures and central nervous system (CNS) depression.
II. respiratory and myocardial depression.
III. circulatory collapse.

19. In addition to their anxiolytic properties, benzodiazepines are indicated for use

I. as preanesthetic medications.
II. as anticonvulsants.
III. during acute withdrawal from alcohol.

For questions 20–23: A 58-year-old white male who has a history of essential hypertension and bronchial asthma has recently been diagnosed with prostatic hypertrophy. His medication history includes the following drugs:

(A) propranolol (Inderal), for hypertension
(B) ipratropium (Atrovent), for asthma
(C) metaproterenol, for asthma
(D) finasteride (Proscar), for prostatic hypertrophy
(E) prazosin (Minipress), for hypertension

Directions: The following questions can be answered by **one** of the listed drugs. Choose the **best** answer, **A–E.**

20. Tamsulosin (Flomax) may replace this agent on the list.

21. Which agent would be most likely to cause postural hypotension?

22. Which agent acts selectively at β_2-receptors?

23. Which of the agents on the list would be counterproductive or inappropriate in a patient taking metaproterenol?

For questions 24–27: A 55-year-old black female has a history of moderate hypertension, glaucoma, and mild osteoarthritis. Her medication history includes the following drugs:

(A) metoprolol (Lopressor), for hypertension
(B) pilocarpine gel, for glaucoma
(C) dipivefrin (Propine) drops, for glaucoma
(D) echothiophate, for glaucoma
(E) timolol (Timoptic), for glaucoma

Directions: The following questions can be answered by **one or more** of the listed drugs. Choose the **best** answers, **A–E.**

24. Which of her glaucoma medicines acts via an indirect mechanism?

25. Which two agents could have an additive effect to produce excessive bradycardia?

26. Which two glaucoma agents could lessen the effects of the other?

27. Which of the aforementioned agents is a prodrug that is metabolized to its active form?

Directions for questions 28–31: Each statement in this section describes **one** of the following drugs. Choose the **best** answer, **A–E.**

(A) tranylcypromine (Parnate)
(B) imipramine (Tofranil)
(C) buspirone (Buspar)
(D) fluoxetine (Prozac)
(E) phenelzine (Nardil)

28. An anxiolytic drug that does not possess either hypnotic or anticonvulsant properties.

29. A prototype tricyclic antidepressant with significant antimuscarinic properties.

30. An antidepressant that inhibits serotonin reuptake and may cause adverse effects such as insomnia, sexual dysfunction, and GI distress.

31. Tyramine-containing foods may cause dangerous hypertension in patients on this agent.

Directions for questions 32–34: Each structure in this section can be described by **one** of the following pharmacological categories. Choose the **best** answer.

(A) general anesthetic
(B) local anesthetic
(C) antidepressant
(D) anxiolytic
(E) opioid antagonist

32.

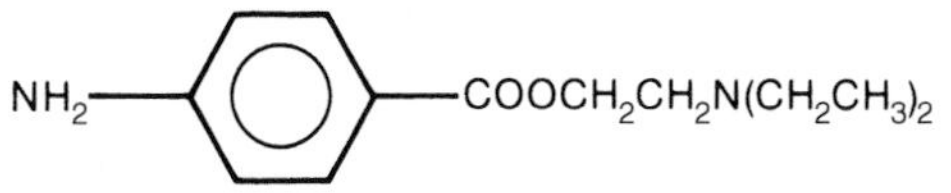

33.

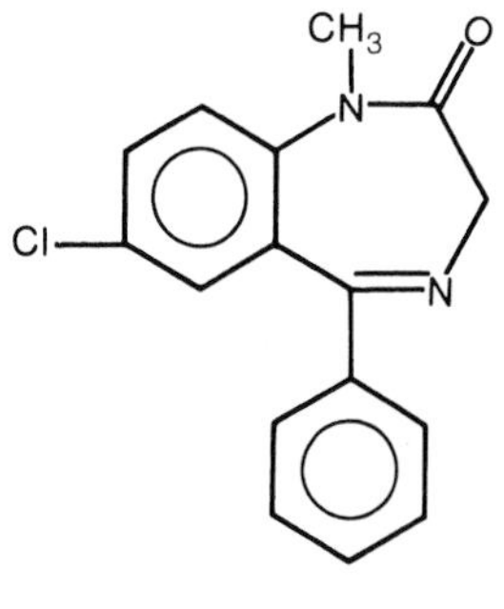

34.

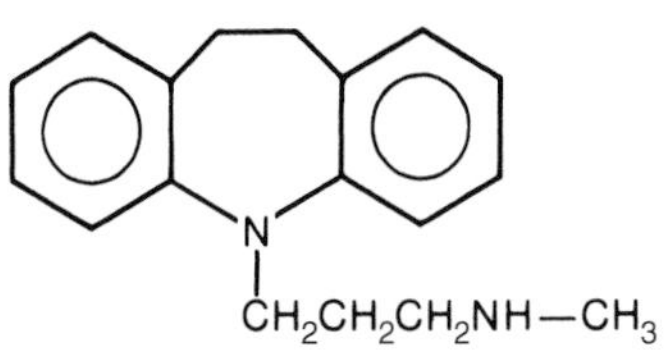

For questions 35–37: A 38-year-old man has a history of affective disorders, including schizophrenia, depression, obsessive–compulsive disorder, and situational anxiety. His past medications include thiothixene, chlorpromazine, amitriptyline, and diazepam. His current medication profile includes the following drugs:

(A) clozapine (Clozaril)
(B) fluoxetine (Prozac)
(C) buspirone (Buspar)
(D) amoxapine

Directions: The following questions can be answered by **one** of the listed drugs. Choose the **best** answer, **A–D.**

35. Which agent is most likely being used to treat his schizophrenic psychosis?

36. Which agent is most likely being used to treat depression and obsessive–compulsive disorder?

37. Which of these agents is able to selectively block the actions of the serotonin transporter?

Directions for questions 38–44: Each of the questions, statements, or incomplete statements in this section can be correctly answered or completed by **one** of the suggested answers or phrases. Choose the **best** answer.

38. Amphetamine exemplifies the pharmacologic mechanism of

(A) ganglionic blockade.
(B) inhibition of transmitter release.
(C) facilitation of transmitter release.
(D) interference with vesicular storage.
(E) blockade of transmitter reuptake.

39. Considering the general chemical structures of sympathomimetic amines, modification of the meta-hydroxyl group on the phenyl ring of norepinephrine would likely produce

(A) increased α-receptor potency.
(B) increased β-receptor potency.
(C) indirect sympathomimetic activity.
(D) decreased transport through the blood–brain barrier.
(E) loss of any biological activity in the nervous system.

40. Sometimes, combination treatment of Parkinson disease is warranted. Which of the following drug combinations could work cooperatively to enhance a clinical anti-parkinsonian response?

(A) amphetamine (Adderall) and reserpine
(B) levodopa and carbidopa
(C) carbidopa and tolcapone (Tasmar)
(D) amantadine (Symmetrel) and haloperidol (Haldol)
(E) dopamine and tyramine

41. Terazosin is able to facilitate micturition when used in the treatment of benign prostatic hypertrophy (BPH) because the drug

(A) relaxes the prostate gland.
(B) constricts the neck of the bladder.
(C) prevents penile erections associated with BPH.
(D) blocks seminal fluid production.
(E) blocks prostate cell growth.

42. BRL37344 is a β_3-agonist. It might be of interest to develop this agent into a clinically usable drug because of the expectation that β_3-agonists would

(A) constrict blood vessels and increase blood pressure in shock patients.
(B) induce lipolysis and decrease adipose cell mass in obese patients.
(C) increase glycogenolysis and prevent glycogen storage in liver cirrhosis.
(D) enhance renal vasodilation and increase urinary elimination of ethanol in alcoholics.
(E) cause bronchodilation and counteract the negative effects of asthma treatment agents.

43. The pharmacologic profile of carvedilol is most similar to that of

(A) esmolol.
(B) labetalol (Trandate).
(C) metoprolol (Lopressor).
(D) nadolol (Corgard).
(E) timolol (Timoptic).

44. The CNS and respiratory depression due to morphine overdose can be reversed by

(A) methadone (Dolophine).
(B) meperidine (Demerol).
(C) propranolol (Inderal).
(D) flumazenil (Romazicon).
(E) naloxone (Narcan).

Answers and Explanations

1. **The answer is B** *[see II.B.2.b].*
Ipratropium is an approved antimuscarinic agent used to treat bronchospasm. Propantheline and homatropine are antimuscarinic agents used as a gastrointestinal (GI) antispasmodic and as a mydriatic, respectively. Edrophonium and ambenonium are indirect-acting cholinergic agonists and, as such, would be expected to induce bronchospasm.

2. **The answer is C** *[see II.B.1].*
Xerostomia, or dry mouth, results from reduced salivary secretions and, therefore, is not a manifestation of cholinergic agonist activity. All of the other effects listed in the question are extensions of therapeutic effects of cholinergic agonists to the point of being adverse effects.

3. **The answer is C** *[see II.A.8.a].*
Of the adrenergic agonists listed in the question, only epinephrine, because of its broad, nonselective α- and β-activity, is an agent of choice for anaphylactic reactions. Epinephrine improves circulatory and respiratory function and counteracts the vascular effects of histamine-related anaphylaxis.

4. **The answer is B** *[see II.C.1.f].*
Neuromuscular blocking agents interact with nicotinic receptors at the skeletal neuromuscular junction. Succinylcholine is also capable of eliciting K^+ release from skeletal muscle due to muscle contractions.

5. **The answer is A** *[see II.B.1.a,b].*
Both direct-acting (e.g., pilocarpine) and indirect-acting (e.g., physostigmine) cholinergics may be used in glaucoma to increase cholinergic activity and facilitate outflow of aqueous humor. Similarly, both β-agonists (e.g., epinephrine) and antagonists (e.g., timolol) may be used, respectively, to increase outflow and decrease production of aqueous humor. Atropine is contraindicated in glaucoma because its anticholinergic effects can block the outflow of aqueous humor and, consequently, increase intraocular pressure.

6. **The answer is D** *[see II.B.2.a].*
Classic signs and symptoms of muscarinic blockade, as with atropine, include mydriasis, which may cause light sensitivity (photophobia); dry mouth and constipation by decreasing secretory activity and motility in the GI tract; and tachycardia by inhibiting the normal inhibitory cholinergic control of the cardiac system. Diarrhea is one of the common signs of cholinergic agonists (others signs include salivation, lacrimation and urination).

7. **The answer is B** *[see III.B.2.a].*
The general anesthetics are divided into two major classes of drugs: those that are gases or volatile liquids, which are administered by inhalation, and those that are nonvolatile salts, which are administered as intravenous solutions. Halothane is a halogenated hydrocarbon, which belongs to the former class. It has the advantage over older volatile anesthetics (e.g., ethyl ether, cyclopropane) of being nonflammable. Thiopental sodium, alprazolam, buspirone, and phenytoin are all nonvolatile substances that are administered orally or parenterally. Thiopental is a general anesthetic and is sometimes referred to as a basal anesthetic because it does not produce significant third-stage surgical anesthesia. Alprazolam and buspirone are anxiolytics, whereas phenytoin is an anticonvulsant.

8. **The answer is B** *[see III.C].*
Chlordiazepoxide, alprazolam, buspirone, and phenobarbital are all used as anxiolytic agents, whereas thioridazine is a phenothiazine antipsychotic.

9. **The answer is C** *[see III.C.1.c].*
Benzodiazepines like diazepam enhance the actions of GABA on the $GABA_A$ receptor to enhance chloride influx into neurons. Topiramate and valproate are able to decrease epileptic activity by blocking glutamate receptors, whereas tiagabine prevents GABA uptake into the nerve terminal. Diazepam is not a MAOI and does not block the metabolism of inositol phosphates like lithium.

10. **The answer is A** *[see III.G.1.d].*
Entacapone blocks peripheral COMT to enhance CNS penetration of levodopa, which is metabolized to dopamine but has no H_1-receptor activity. Bromocriptine directly stimulates dopamine receptors in the striatum to restore the balance between GABA-ergic and cholinergic neurons in Parkinson disease.

11. **The answer is E** *[see III.G.1.c].*
Levodopa is not associated with agranulocytosis.

12. **The answer is E** *[see III.H.1; Figure 9-17].*
The *p*-phenyl-*N*-alkylpiperidine moiety is common to the structurally specific opioid analgesics. Meperidine is an opioid analgesic and is an *N*-methyl-*p*-phenylpiperidine derivative. Its chemical name is ethyl 1-methyl-4-phenylpiperidine-4-carboxylate. Phenobarbital is a barbiturate sedative. Chlorpromazine is a phenothiazine antipsychotic. Diazepam is a benzodiazepine anxiolytic. Imipramine is a tricyclic dibenzazepine antidepressant.

13. **The answer is C** *[see III.H.2].*
Opioids are used to treat all the following conditions except arthritis, which is often treated with nonsteroidal anti-inflammatory drugs (NSAIDs) and immunosuppressants, depending on the type of disease and severity.

14. **The answer is C** *[see III.F.1].*
All these agents are used to treat partial or generalized tonic-clonic seizures except ethosuximide, which is more effective against absence seizures.

15. **The answer is C** *[see II.B.2.b].*
Cholinesterase inhibitors are indirect-acting cholinergic agonists useful in treating myasthenia gravis and glaucoma. Their effects on GI and urinary bladder smooth muscle would be to increase smooth-muscle tone, not decrease it.

16. **The answer is D** *[see II.B.2].*
All three compounds listed in the question are antimuscarinic agents; however, only benztropine and trihexyphenidyl are used to control parkinsonism and some neuroleptic-induced extrapyramidal disorders. Ipratropium is an approved agent for the treatment of bronchospasm.

17. **The answer is B** *[see II.A.8.c].*
Dobutamine is a β_1-selective adrenergic agonist. It would be inappropriate to use dobutamine to decrease blood flow at the site of local anesthetic administration. Epinephrine is a nonselective α- and β-agonist that can be used to limit the systemic absorption of local anesthetics and prolong their activity. Phenoxybenzamine is an α-selective antagonist that will only enhance the loss of the local anesthetic away from the site of application.

18. **The answer is E** *[see III.A.4].*
Careful administration of a local anesthetic by a knowledgeable practitioner is essential to prevent systemic absorption and consequent toxicity. This is especially important when the patient has cardiovascular disease, poorly controlled diabetes, thyrotoxicosis, or peripheral vascular disease.

19. **The answer is E** *[see III.C.1.c].*
Benzodiazepines can serve as induction agents for general anesthesia; they also have anxiolytic properties. In addition, intravenous diazepam is used to treat status epilepticus, whereas clonazepam is used orally for myoclonic and absence (petit mal) seizures. Benzodiazepines also diminish alcohol withdrawal symptoms.

20. **The answer is D** *[see II.A.9.a].*
Tamsulosin is an α_{1A}-selective antagonist that may be used in place of finasteride to treat benign prostatic hypertrophy (BPH).

21. **The answer is E** *[see II.A.9.a].*
Due to venodilatory actions, prazosin is associated with postural or orthostatic hypotension.

22. **The answer is C** *[see II.A.8.c].*
Of all of the agents, only metaproterenol is an agonist at the β_2-receptors.

23. **The answer is A** *[see II.A.9.b].*
The administration of propranolol, a nonselective antagonist of β-receptors, will antagonize β_2-receptors in the bronchioles of the patient to prevent the ability of metaproterenol to dilate the airways.

24. **The answer is D** *[see II.B.2.a].*
Pilocarpine acts directly at the muscarinic receptor, whereas dipivefrin eventually activates α_2-receptors. Timolol blocks β-receptors. Echothiophate inhibits the metabolism of ACh, indirectly increasing levels of the endogenous neurotransmitter.

25. **The answers are A and E** *[see II.A.9.b].*
Metoprolol, a β_1-selective agent, can cause bradycardia alone. The addition of topical timolol, while limiting systemic absorption, could have an additive β-blocking effect to decrease heart rate (negative chronotropy) and hypotension.

26. **The answers are C and E** *[see II.A.9.b; II.B.1.a,b].*
Pilocarpine and echothiophate cause the stimulation of muscarinic receptors (pilocarpine directly and echothiophate indirectly), so applying them together would not produce any additional benefit. However, dipivefrin (once activated, below) can compete with timolol for β-receptors on the ciliary body, reducing the effectiveness of timolol.

27. **The answer is C** *[see II.A.8.a].*
Dipivefrin is diacetylated epinephrine, which is readily metabolized to epinephrine to activate α_2-receptors on the ciliary body to reduce the production of aqueous humor.

28–31. **The answers are: 28-C** *[see III.C.3]*, **29-B** *[see III.E.2.e]*, **30-D** *[see III.E.1.d]*, **31-E** *[see III.E.3.d].*
Buspirone's mechanism of anxiolytic action is unknown. Unlike the benzodiazepines, buspirone lacks hypnotic and anticonvulsant properties. The tricyclic antidepressant imipramine is useful in the treatment of enuresis because the compound blocks muscarinic receptors mediating micturition. Fluoxetine is the serotonin uptake blocker and has the adverse effects listed. Phenelzine is a MAOI that enhances catecholamine content in the nerve terminal, and foods containing tyramine (e.g., cheese) would elicit greater catecholamine release to potentially cause hypertension.

32–34. The answers are: 32-B *[see Figure 9-8]*, **33-D** *[see Figure 9-10]*, **34-C** *[see Figure 9-15]*.

The structure shown in question 29 is that of procaine, which is a diethylaminoethyl *p*-aminobenzoate ester. It contains a hydrophilic amino group in the alcohol portion of the molecule and a lipophilic aromatic acid connected by the ester linkage. The procaine molecule is typical of ester-type local anesthetics.

The structure in question 30 is that of diazepam, which has a benzo-1,4-diazepine as its base nucleus. The widely used benzo-1,4-diazepine derivatives have significant anxiolytic, hypnotic, and anticonvulsant activities.

The structure in question 31 is that of desipramine, which has a dibenzazepine as its base nucleus. Dibenzazepine derivatives that have a methyl- or dimethylaminopropyl group attached to the ring nitrogen have significant antidepressant activity. Similarly, substituted dibenzocycloheptadienes also have antidepressant activity. Together, these two chemical classes make up most of the tricyclic antidepressants.

35. The answer is A *[see III.D.4]*.

Clozapine, although therapeutically defined as a general antipsychotic, is used almost exclusively in the treatment of schizophrenia.

36. The answer is B *[see III.E.1]*.

Fluoxetine is most likely being used in this patient in an attempt to treat depression and obsessive–compulsive disorder with the same drug. Clinical trials have shown fluoxetine to improve both conditions. The use of a single agent for both conditions will minimize the risk of drug–drug interactions, as well as reduce the chances of adverse effects.

37. The answer is B *[see III.E.1]*.

Fluoxetine produces its antidepressant actions by selectively blocking the SERT to enhance serotonin levels in the synapse.

38. The answer is C *[see II.A.8.d]*.

Amphetamine is an indirectly acting sympathomimetic that enters the nerve terminal and displaces norepinephrine from the storage vesicles, thus increasing the quanta of the transmitter released.

39. The answer is A *[see II.A.8.b]*.

Both aromatic hydroxyl functions are important for both α- and β-receptor binding; however, modification of the meta-hydroxyl to a methoxy derivative increases α- versus β-receptor selectivity.

40. The answer is B *[see III.G.1.a]*.

Although levodopa can cross the blood–brain barrier to gain access into the brain, a significant portion of an orally administered dose is converted into dopamine and norepinephrine at peripheral sites, leading to peripheral side effects and decreased brain bioavailability. Carbidopa, a dopa decarboxylase inhibitor that does not cross the blood–brain barrier, is coadministered with levodopa to decrease its peripheral conversion and increase central delivery of the drug and, hence, the therapeutic response.

41. The answer is A *[see II.A.9.a]*.

Terazosin blocks α-receptors on the prostate gland to cause a relaxant effect, which reduces the pressure exerted by the prostate on the urethra, thus easing urinary voidance.

42. The answer is B *[see Table 9-1]*.

Stimulation of β_3-receptors induces the metabolic breakdown of fat stores into free fatty acids that can be further catabolized by the body. The hope is that this category of pharmacologic agents could, with repeated use, lead to a decrease in the content and number of fat cells, and, hence, an antiobesity effect.

43. The answer is B *[see II.A.9.b; Table 9-2]*.

Like labetalol, carvedilol is a nonselective α- and β-receptor antagonist used in the treatment of hypertension. Blockade of vascular α (alpha-1)-receptors would cause vasodilatation and decreased peripheral vascular resistance, whereas blockade of myocardial β (beta-1)-receptors would decrease cardiac contractility. The resultant decrease in cardiac output would produce a fall in blood pressure (blood pressure = cardiac output × peripheral resistance).

44. The answer is E *[see III.H.1.b]*.

Only naloxone is able to effectively compete with morphine binding to central μ-opioid receptors to reverse the depressant effects of the opiate. Meperidine may have additive suppressive effects in this condition.

10 Pharmacology and Medicinal Chemistry of Cardiovascular and Diuretic Drugs

S. THOMAS ABRAHAM, MICHAEL L. ADAMS

I. INTRODUCTION. Cardiovascular diseases such as coronary heart disease (CHD), heart failure, and hypertension are some of the most widespread causes of mortality and morbidity in the world. CHD is more appropriately a disease of the coronary vasculature that can be exacerbated by thrombotic events to precipitate an acute myocardial infarction. Survivors of myocardial infarctions are often susceptible to heart failure and sudden cardiac death due to ventricular arrhythmias. Uncontrolled hypertension can also lead to CHD, heart failure, and stroke. Thus, several significant cardiovascular diseases have multiple causes, and patients are often treated for multiple, interconnected diseases using an array of agents.

II. ANTIHYPERTENSIVE AGENTS. Some of the drugs used to treat hypertension have been discussed in Chapter 9 and will not be addressed here in any detail. Antagonists of α_1- and β-adrenergic receptors (e.g., prazosin, propranolol, respectively) and α_2-agonists (clonidine) are examples of some these agents. The other classes of drugs used to treat systemic hypertension include angiotensin-converting enzyme (ACE) inhibitors, renin inhibitors, angiotensin receptor antagonists, diuretics, calcium-channel blockers, and direct vasodilators. Pulmonary hypertension is managed by endothelin antagonists and PDE5 inhibitors.

A. Drugs that modify the renin-angiotensin-aldosterone system

1. The renin-angiotensin system is an important regulator of systemic blood pressure and may be a contributing factor in about one-third of the cases of essential hypertension. In response to low renal tubular sodium or sympathetic nervous system stimulation, the renal juxtaglomerular cells release renin into the afferent arterioles.
2. Renin converts circulating angiotensinogen to angiotensin I, which is rapidly converted to angiotensin II by endothelial ACE, primarily in the pulmonary circulation (*Figure 10-1*). ACE is also responsible for the inactivation of the vasoactive peptide bradykinin.

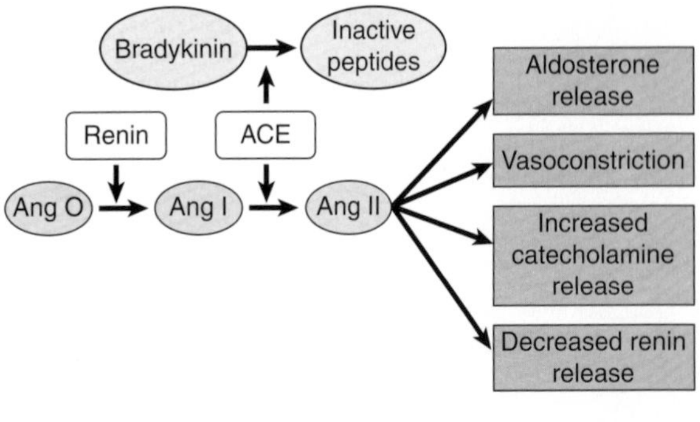

Figure 10-1. The renin-angiotensin-aldosterone system with sites for pharmacological intervention. *Ang 0*, angiotensinogen; *Ang I*, angiotensin I; *Ang II*, angiotensin II; *ACE*, angiotensin-converting enzyme.

3. Angiotensin II is a potent vasoconstrictor; it releases aldosterone from the adrenal cortex and increases catecholamine release from sympathetic nerves. Aldosterone increases sodium and water reabsorption from the renal tubules and has vasoconstrictor effects as well. These direct and indirect effects of angiotensin II increase peripheral vascular resistance and blood volume that eventually increases systemic blood pressure.
4. **Renin inhibitors** are represented by aliskiren (Tekturna®). Renin is an aspartate protease that catalyzes the rate-limiting conversion of angiotensinogen to angiotensin I (*Figure 10-1*). Aliskiren (*Figure 10-2*) is considered a peptidomimetic amide hydrolysis transition state analog that results in a high affinity interaction with renin. Its actions on preventing the production of angiotensin I cause a decrease in circulating angiotensin II and subsequent lowering in aldosterone. The loss of both aldosterone and angiotensin II leads to significant decreases in peripheral vascular resistance and systemic blood pressure. Currently, aliskiren is used as a second-line therapy for the management of hypertension.
5. **Angiotensin-converting enzyme inhibitors (ACEIs)**
   a. These agents are also transition-state analogs with the general structure shown in *Figure 10-2*. Binding to ACE requires a nitrogen-containing heterocyclic ring that also has a carboxylate group, as well as zinc-binding domain that may be a sulfhydryl, carboxylate, or a phosphinic acid.
   b. Generally, the esterification of this carboxylate or phospho group improves oral activity but requires hydrolysis to the acid form for inhibitory action. Captopril (Capoten®; *Figure 10-2*) is an

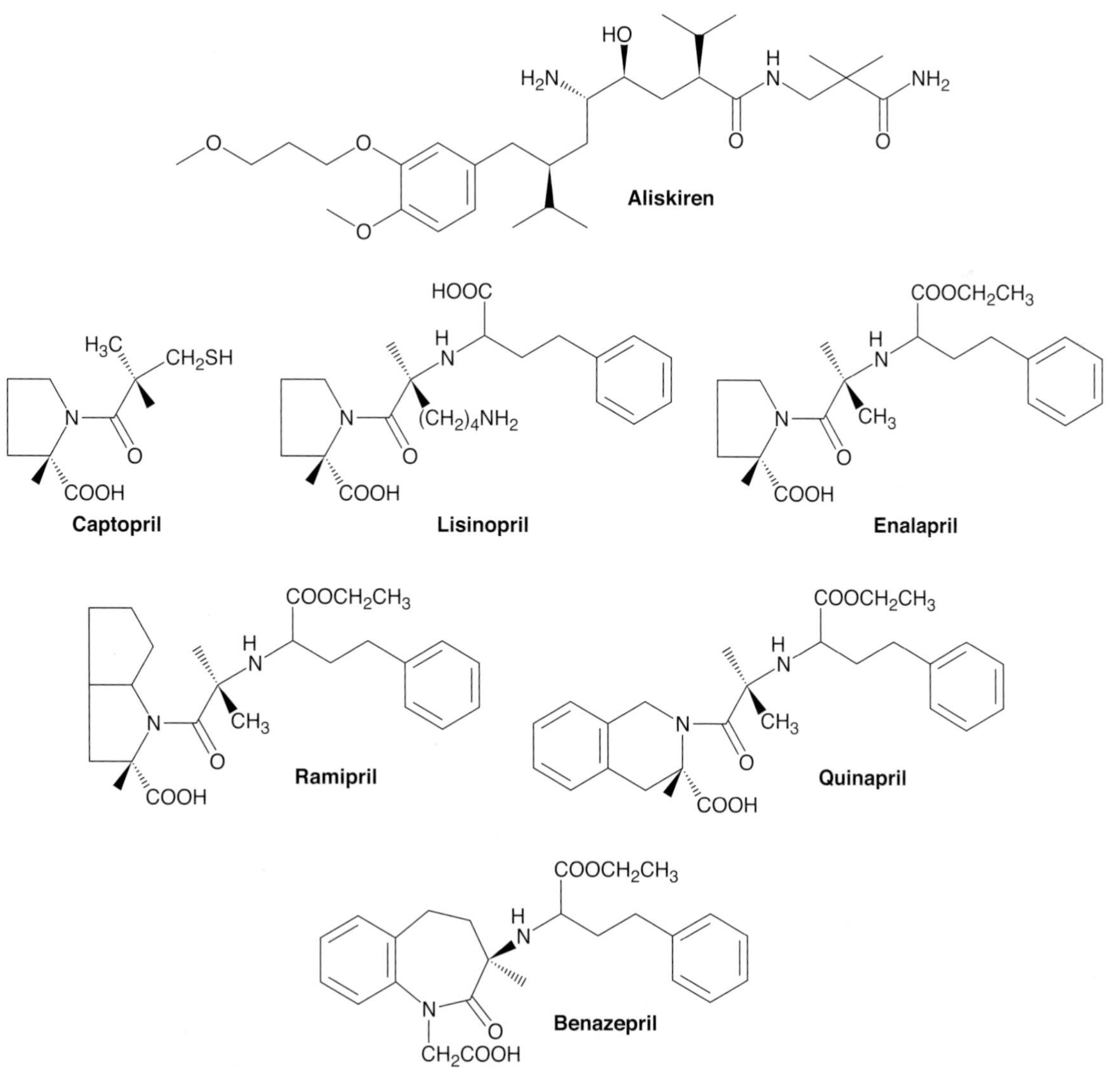

Figure 10-2. Structural formulas of aliskiren (a renin inhibitor) and the ACE inhibitors captopril, enalapril, lisinopril, benazepril, ramipril, and quinapril.

example of sulfhydryl-containing drug with not only high affinity for ACE but also increased incidence of skin rash and dysgeusia due to this moiety. Lisinopril (Zestril®) and enalapril (Vasotec®) are carboxylate variant of ACEIs with enalapril being hydrolyzed by esterases to the active form enalaprilat. Other carboxylate derivatives of ACEIs are trandolapril (Mavik®), benazepril (Lotensin®), moexipril (Univasc®), perindopril (Aceon®), quinapril (Accupril®), and ramipril (Altace®).The phosphoester fosinopril (Monopril®; *Figure 10-2*) is converted by ester hydrolysis to fosinoprilat.

c. Inhibition of ACE activity systemically leads to reduced circulating angiotensin II with the consequent reductions in blood pressure. Inhibition of ACE and reduction in circulating angiotensin II and aldosterone also ameliorate cardiac and vascular remodeling and hypertrophy seen in hypertension and cardiomyopathies. ACEIs are used to treat hypertension, especially those prone to diabetic nephropathy, congestive heart failure, dilated cardiomyopathy, and the postmyocardial infarction patient.

d. Adverse effects of the ACEIs include cough and angioedema that are associated with an accumulation of bradykinin, which is also metabolized by ACE. Other adverse effects include hypotension, hyperkalemia, and acute renal failure.

6. Angiotensin receptor blockers

a. The angiotensin AT1 receptor is the predominant mediator angiotensin II's effects with regard to aldosterone release, vasoconstriction, catecholamine release, etc. Thus, blocking this receptor effectively reduces the untoward effects of this vasoactive peptide.

b. These drugs (losartan [Cozaar®], valsartan [Diovan®], telmisartan [Micardis®], azilsartan [Edarbi®], irbesartan [Avapro®], olmesartan [Benicar®], and candesartan [Atacand®]) are all biphenylmethyl derivatives except for eprosartan (Teveten®), which is a thienylmethylacrylate (*Figure 10-3*). The angiotensin receptor blockers (ARBs) are nonpeptide molecules that mimic the pharmacophore of angiotensin II to allow for AT1 receptor binding with no agonist activity. The ARBs have an acidic group that mimics either the carboxy terminal or the acidic tyrosine of angiotensin II. In the biphenyl compounds, the acidic functional group is either a carboxylic acid or a tetrazole in the ortho position on the second phenyl ring. The acidic group of the nonbiphenyl ARB eprosartan is attached in the para position of the only phenyl ring. The imidazole ring, or the amide bond in valsartan, mimics the histadine ring of angiotensin II, and the lipophilic substituents provide additional AT1 affinity.

c. Generally, these receptor antagonists interact with the receptor with a very slow off rate such that they behave as pseudo-irreversible antagonists. This has advantages in situations where a dose or two may be missed with no immediate reversal in hypotensive effect. Additionally, the buildup of angiotensin II due to the lack of negative feedback on the juxtaglomerular cells will be unable to effectively displace the antagonist.

d. The major pharmacological effect of these receptor antagonists is a lowering in systemic blood pressure without affecting cardiac output or initiating a baroreceptor reflex. Receptor antagonists also reduce smooth and cardiac muscle hypertrophy and decrease the progression of renal disease in diabetics. They have similar therapeutic use profile to the ACEIs and may be used in cases where the latter are poorly tolerated.

e. The major adverse effect of renin inhibitors, ACEIs, and angiotensin antagonists is first-dose hypotension, especially in patients with high plasma renin activity or are hypovolemic. Other prominent effects include acute renal failure in patients with renal artery stenosis, birth defects if taken during second/third trimesters, hyperkalemia, and liver toxicity. Additionally, angiotensin receptor antagonists are less likely to cause life-threatening angioedema and unproductive cough than ACEIs due to the inhibition of bradykinin metabolism observed with ACEIs (*Figure 10-1*).

7. Aldosterone antagonists

a. Although aldosterone antagonists have been historically grouped with the diuretics, their nondiuretic effects are more often relied upon to produce therapeutic benefit. Aldosterone is the primary mineralocorticoid released by the adrenal cortex in response to angiotensin II and high potassium levels. It functions in the renal collecting tubules to increase sodium and water reabsorption via the mineralocorticoid receptor (MR).

b. The antagonists spironolactone (Aldactone®) and eplerenone (Inspra®) are structurally analogous to aldosterone (*Figure 10-4*) and compete with it for the MR to prevent salt and water reabsorption. The result is a modest diuresis without concomitant wasting of potassium. This

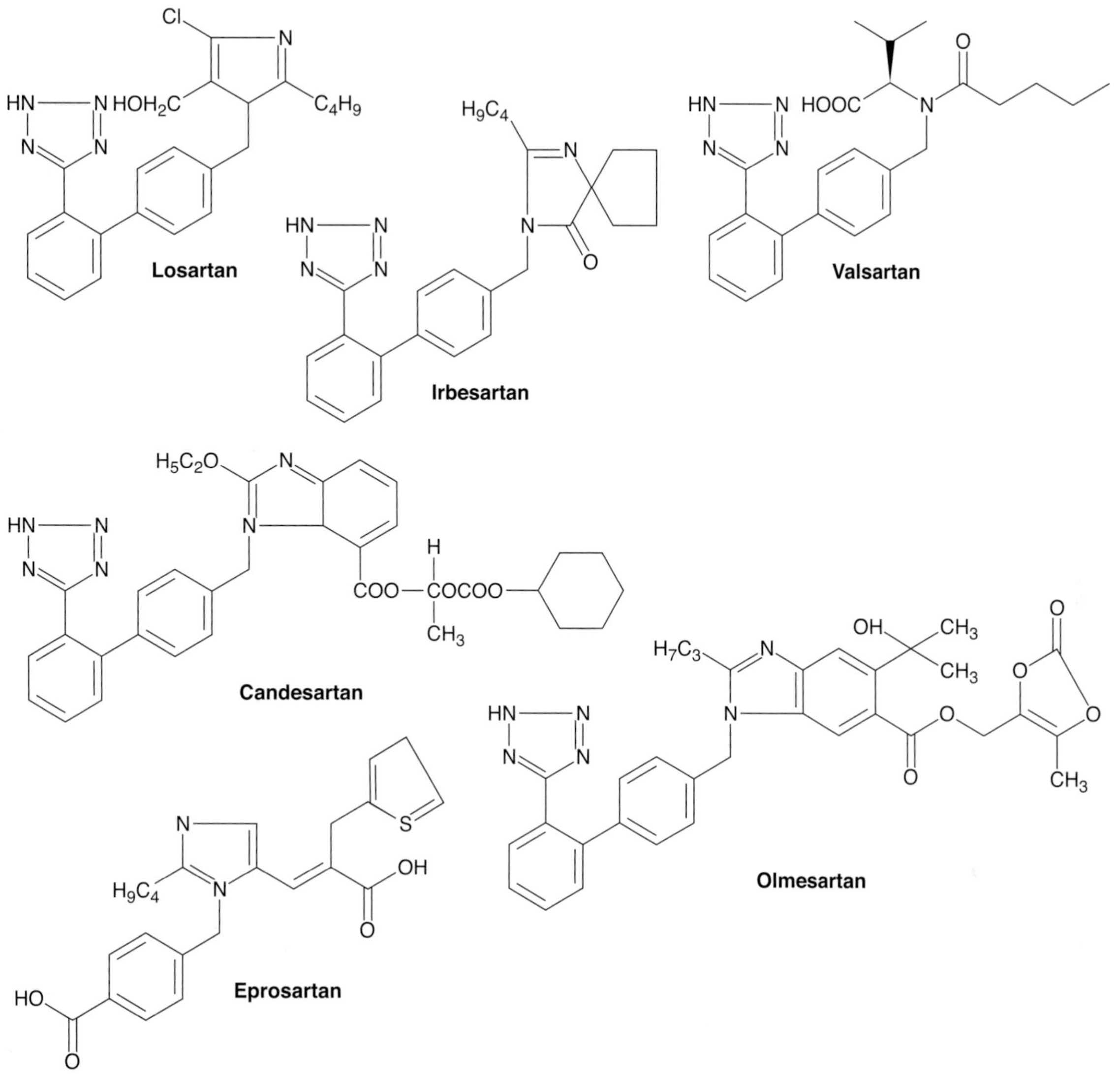

Figure 10-3. Structural formulas of the angiotensin receptor antagonists losartan, valsartan, candesartan, irbesartan, olmesartan, and eprosartan.

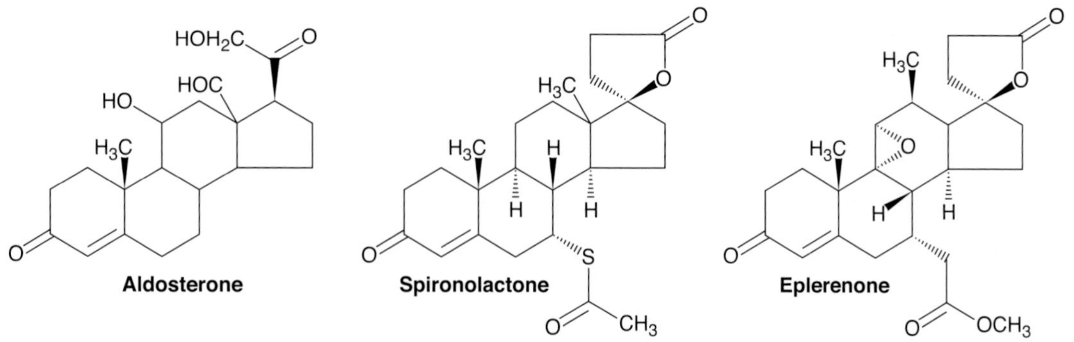

Figure 10-4. Structural formulas of the mineralocorticoid aldosterone and antagonists for its receptor spironolactone and eplerenone.

effect, coupled with a significant vasodilator effect on the arteriolar vascular beds, produces significant lowering in systemic blood pressure. Additionally, spironolactone and eplerenone have been found to reduce the cardiac and renal remodeling in congestive heart failure and diabetes. These agents are primarily used to treat heart failure patients, hyperaldosteronism, and diabetic nephropathy.

c. The adverse effects related to aldosterone antagonists are hyperkalemia, which may be proarrhythmic, and metabolic acidosis. Spironolactone is also likely to cause gynecomastia, menstrual irregularities, impotence, and benign prostatic hyperplasia due to its interactions with androgen and progesterone receptors.

B. Diuretic agents. The kidneys regulate salt and water balance to maintain systemic blood pressure and acid–base balance. Diuretic agents alter salt reabsorption in the renal tubules to modify the concomitant water reabsorption. The majority (> 60%) of sodium and chloride, the primary osmotic ions in the glomerular filtrate, are reabsorbed in the proximal convoluted tubules, whereas the remainder is taken up in the thick ascending loop of Henle (TAL, ~25%), the distal convoluted tubule (~10%), and collecting tubules (~5%). The most efficacious and therapeutically relevant diuretics function at sites distal to the proximal tubules.

1. Loop diuretics

a. Loop diuretics are anthranilic acid derivatives with a sulfonamide substituent (furosemide [Lasix®]; bumetanide [Bumex®]; torsemide [Demadex®]) or an aryloxyacetic acid without a sulfonamide substituent (ethacrynic acid [Edecrin®]; *Figure 10-5*).

b. These agents are secreted via the organic acid transporter into the proximal tubule and block the functions of the Na/K/2Cl-transport system in the TAL from the luminal side. This prevents the reabsorption of a large quantity of Na^+ and Cl^- in the TAL and most of this is lost along with water in the urine. The loop diuretics also induce cyclooxygenase expression that leads to PGE2-mediated inhibition of salt transport in the TAL. Prostaglandin production may also be responsible for the vasodilator effects of loop diuretic and decreases in peripheral resistance.

c. Loop diuretics are used when a large, rapid diuresis is required, as in the case of pulmonary congestion due to heart failure, other edematous diseases, hyperkalemia, hypercalcemia, acute renal failure, and fluoride/iodide overdose.

d. Loop diuretics tend to cause large losses in K^+ as the collecting tubules attempt to recover some of the sodium load through the actions of aldosterone. This potassium-wasting effect can lead to hypokalemia and potential arrhythmogenic activity. Loss of magnesium absorption in the TAL due to diuretic action can result in hypomagnesemia. Ethacrynic acid is associated

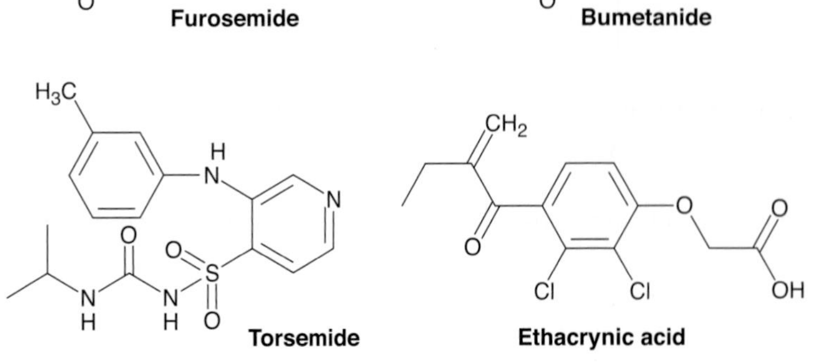

Figure 10-5. Structural formulas of the loop or high ceiling diuretics.

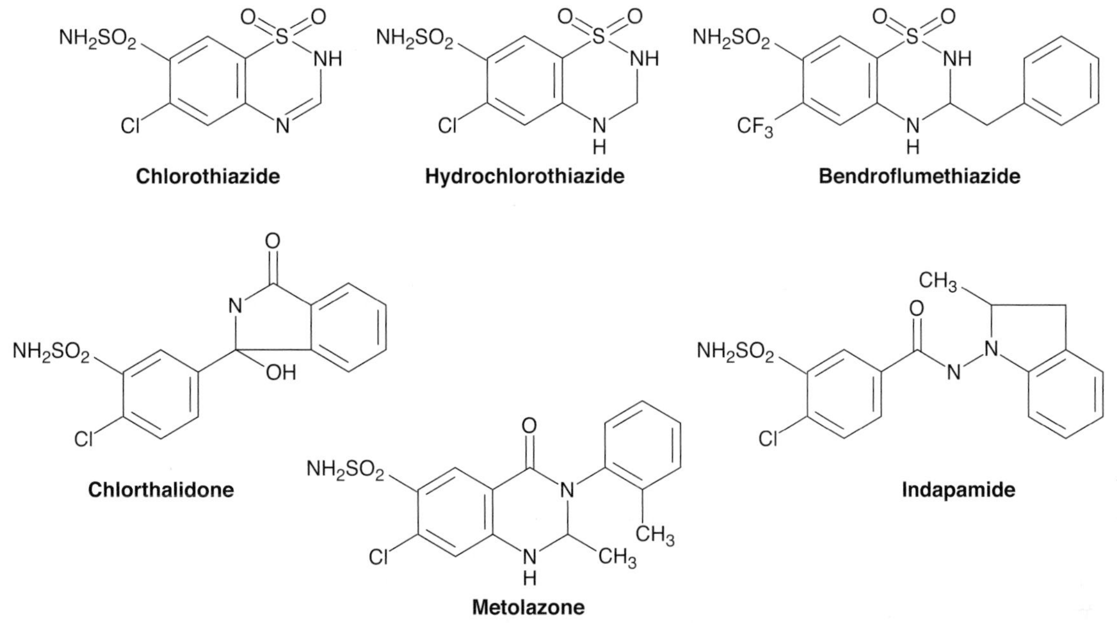

Figure 10-6. Structural formulas of the thiazide (chlorothiazide, hydrochlorothiazide, and bendroflumethiazide) and thiazide-like (chlorthalidone, metolazone, and indapamide) diuretics.

with ototoxicity, especially when combined with aminoglycoside antibiotics. The sulfonamide moiety of loop diuretics (except ethacrynic acid) may result in allergic reactions in susceptible patients.

2. **Thiazide and thiazide-like agents**
   a. These agents are substituted benzothiadiazines with the general structure shown in *Figure 10-5* and represented by chlorothiazide (Diuril®), hydrochlorothiazide (HydroDIURIL®), bendroflumethiazide (Naturetin®; *Figure 10-6*), and methylchlorothiazide (Enduron®). These agents require an unsubstituted sulfonamide at position 7 as well as an electron-withdrawing group at position 6 for activity. Additionally, the saturation of the C3–C4 bond, lipophilic substitutions on C3, and alkylation of the nitrogen at position 2 improve the potency and duration of action.
   b. The thiazide-like agents are structurally similar except that the cyclic sulfonamide is replaced by an amide (e.g., chlorthalidone [Thalitone®], metolazone [Mykrox®], indapamide [Lozol®]; *Figure 10-6*).
   c. The agents in this class are organic acids that are secreted into the proximal tubular lumen to eventually inhibit the actions of the Na^+/Cl^- symporter in the early distal convoluted tubule (DCT). Inhibition of the symporter reduces salt reabsorption at this location and osmotically draws water with it as it is eliminated in the urine. Loss of water in the renal filtrate lowers blood volume, which ultimately decreases systemic blood pressure. Thiazide diuretics are a mainstay in the treatment of hypertension and congestive heart failure, calcium renal stones, and nephrogenic diabetes insipidus.
   d. The decrease in intracellular Na^+ increases Ca^{2+} reabsorption at the DCT to potentially cause hypercalcemia. As with the loop diuretics, the delivery of high Na^+ to the collecting tubules can cause excessive K^+ loss as aldosterone-stimulated Na^+ reabsorption takes place. Note that the Na^+ reabsorption capacity of the collecting tubules is limited and will not significantly counter the natriuresis seen with loop or thiazide diuretics.
   e. Apart from the hypokalemia, thiazides can cause hyponatremia, hypercalcemia, and sulfonamide-related sensitivity reactions. Hyperglycemia may be seen in diabetic patients and some increases in low density lipoprotein (LDL) levels may be observed.
3. **Potassium-sparing diuretics**
   a. These include the structurally dissimilar amiloride (Midamor®), triamterene (Dyrenium®; *Figure 10-7*), and spironolactone and eplerenone (see II.A.4 for discussion).

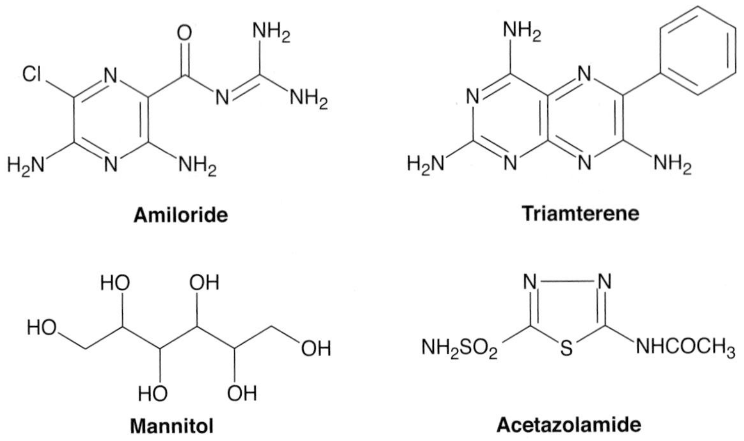

Figure 10-7. Structural formulas of the potassium-sparing diuretics (amiloride and triamterene), osmotic diuretic (mannitol), and the carbonic anhydrase inhibitor (acetazolamide).

- **b.** Amiloride and triamterene block the Na^+ channel through which the ion is absorbed into the principal cells of the collecting tubule leading to a small natriuresis and diuresis. Normally, Na^+ reabsorption here is electrically coupled to K^+ elimination, but these agents are able to produce a natriuresis without K^+ wasting, hence their designation as "K^+-sparing". Amiloride and triamterene are used to minimize K^+-wasting induced by loop and thiazide diuretics, reduce symptoms of cystic fibrosis, and treat Liddle syndrome and lithium-induced diabetes insipidus.
- **c.** These agents can cause hyperkalemia (and consequent arrhythmias), metabolic acidosis, and precipitate acute renal failure.

4. Miscellaneous diuretics

- **a.** The osmotic diuretic mannitol (Osmitrol®; *Figure 10-7*) is freely filtered into the renal tubules to produce an osmotic pressure resulting in a rapid diuresis. This agent is use to rapidly reduce intracranial or intraocular pressure in emergency situations.
- **b.** The carbonic anhydrase inhibitor acetazolamide (Diamox®; *Figure 10-7*) reduces Na^+ reabsorption in the proximal convoluted tubules but has low efficacy because the amount of natriuresis produced is marginal and short-lived. The primary use of acetazolamide is to reduce aqueous humor production to treat glaucoma, metabolic alkalosis, and acute altitude sickness.

C. Calcium-channel blockers and other vasodilators

1. Calcium is a fundamental signaling molecule in biological processes and is necessary for the orderly contraction of smooth, cardiac, and skeletal muscle. The activation of α-adrenergic receptors on vascular smooth muscle cells (*Table 9-1*) initiates an influx of calcium, through voltage-dependent calcium channels, that promotes contractile response. Cardiac conduction cells and muscle also contain similar calcium channels and are most often designated as L-type channels. These channels participate in spontaneous depolarization of the sinoatrial (SA) and atrioventricular (AV) nodes and provide the trigger calcium for sarcoplasmic calcium release and contraction of myocardial cells.
2. The major use of all the aforementioned calcium-channel blockers (CCBs) is in the therapy of hypertension, angina, and Raynaud syndrome. Verapamil and diltiazem are also used to treat supraventricular arrhythmias.
3. CCBs belong to the dihydropyridine, phenylalkylamine, and benzothiazepine classes.
   - **a. Dihydropyridines** contain a 1,4-dihydropyridine (DHP) ring that is required for channel blocking activity, and generally ester groups at the C3 and C5 positions improve activity (e.g., nifedipine [Procardia®], amlodipine [Norvasc®], nicardipine [Cardene®]; *Figure 10-8*). Additionally, electron-withdrawing ortho or meta substitutions on the phenyl ring improve channel blocking activity. DHPs interact preferentially with the inactive form of the calcium channel and maintain that conformation to prevent its opening during membrane depolarization. At therapeutic doses, DHPs preferentially inactivate vascular versus cardiac calcium channels to produce greater vasodilation than negative ionotropic and chronotropic effects. The drop in blood pressure can elicit a baroreceptor reflex increase in heart rate and contractility that can lead to angina attacks.
   - **b. Phenylalkylamines** are represented by verapamil (Calan®; *Figure 10-8*). Verapamil diffuses through the plasma membrane and interacts on the cytoplasmic domain of the calcium

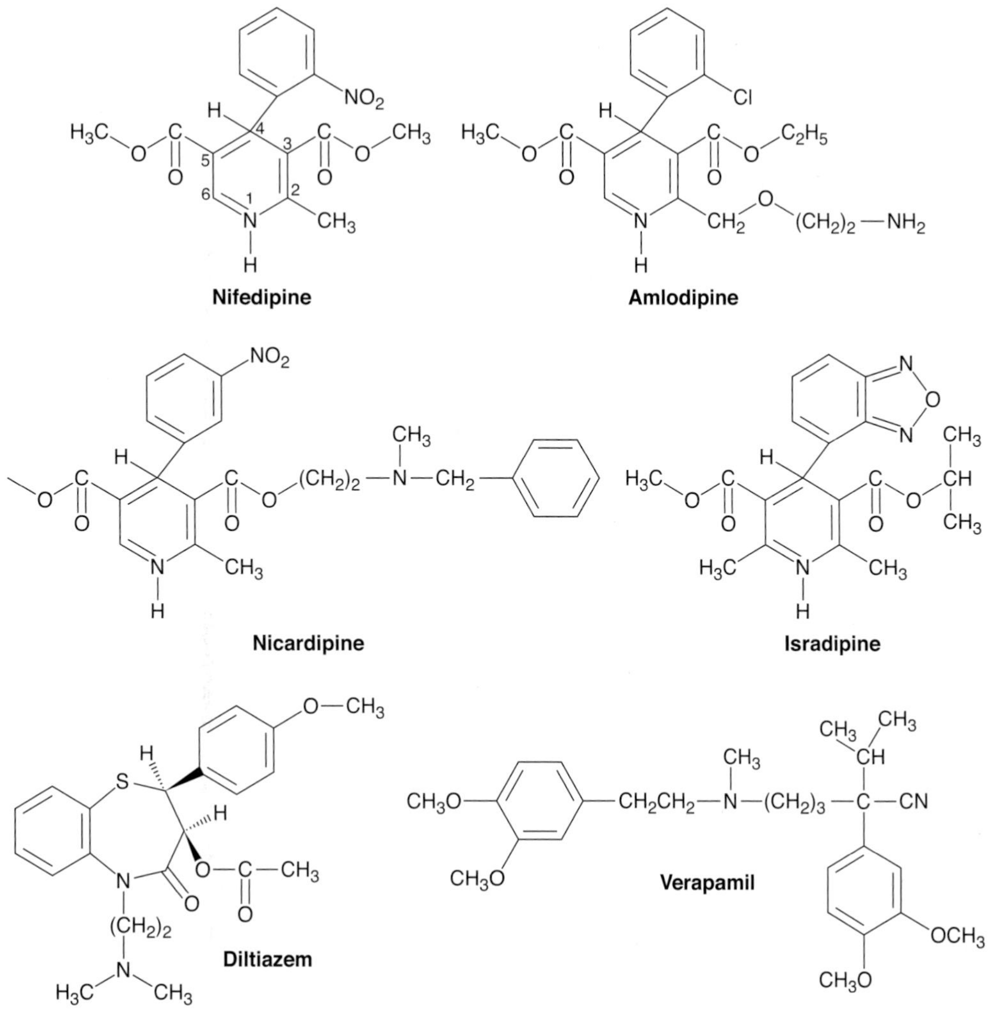

Figure 10-8. Structural formulas of the dihydropyridine (nifedipine, nicardipine, amlodipine, and isradipine), phenylalkylamine (verapamil), and benzothiazepine (diltiazem) calcium-channel blockers.

channel. Verapamil has equivalent actions on vascular and cardiac calcium channels to produce vasodilation and decreased cardiac output to decrease blood pressure.

c. **Benzothiazepines** are represented by diltiazem (Cardizem CD®; *Figure 10-8*). Diltiazem has a similar mechanism of action as verapamil to reduce blood pressure.

4. Adverse effects related to the use of CCBs are hypotension, headache, peripheral edema, constipation, cough, and wheezing. Verapamil and diltiazem are also prone to cause bradycardia, AV block, and transient sinus arrest.
5. **Miscellaneous vasodilators** are a diverse group of agents with distinct vasodilator or hypotensive actions.
   a. Nitroprusside (Nitropress®) is an intravenous agent for the rapid reduction in blood pressure. Nitroprusside is a potent nitric oxide (NO) donor that relaxes vascular smooth muscle cells to decrease systemic blood pressure.
   b. Hydralazine (Apresoline®) is a direct vasodilator that may be administered parenterally or orally to manage hypertension that is not responsive to other agents.
   c. Minoxidil (Loniten®) is metabolized to a glucuronide conjugate that is a potent K^+ATP channel activator. This action results in hyperpolarization of smooth muscle membranes, reduced calcium influx, and vasodilation. Minoxidil is used to treat hypertension resistant to standard therapy and also increases hair growth when applied topically (Rogaine®).
   d. These agents can also be used to manage the congestive heart failure patient.

e. All three agents may cause edema, tachycardia, angina, and hypotension. Hydralazine is also associated with lupus-like sensitivity reactions, whereas minoxidil may also increase pulmonary artery pressure and hirsutism. Nitroprusside may also cause lactic acidosis secondary to cyanosis with sustained use.

D. Agents used to treat pulmonary arterial hypertension (PAH)

Pulmonary hypertension is characterized by elevated pulmonary artery pressure leading to dyspnea, dizziness, fatigue, right ventricular failure, and edema.

1. The potent vasoactive protein endothelin appears to be elevated in the pulmonary circulation of patients with PAH. Endothelin activates its receptors (ET_A and ET_B) on pulmonary vascular cells to cause vasoconstriction and subsequent hypertension. The endothelin receptor antagonists bosentan (Tracleer®) and ambrisentan (Letairis®) are able to prevent endothelin's actions and the result is arterial vasodilation. These agents have little effect on systemic blood pressure but have been associated with hepatotoxicity and fetal death if taken by pregnant women. Less serious adverse effects include nasal congestion, flushing, edema, headaches, and gastric cramps.
2. The **type 5A phosphodiesterase (PDE5A)** is the target for sildenafil (Revatio®) and tadalafil (Adcirca®), which are also used to treat PAH. Guanylyl cyclase in vascular smooth muscle cells of the pulmonary circulation convert guanosine triphosphate to cyclic guanosine monophosphate that reduces intracellular calcium and leads to vasodilation (details discussed later in this chapter). The PDE5A inhibitors prevent the metabolism of cGMP; maintain its intracellular concentrations; and, thus, preserve its vasodilatory actions on smooth muscle. Sildenafil and tadalafil are also used to treat erectile dysfunction, so priapism is a potential adverse effect and other effects may include headache, nausea, mild hypotension, visual disturbances, and flushing of the skin.
3. Prostanoids such as epoprostenol (Flolan®), iloprost (Ventavis®), and treprostinil (Remodulin®) are also used to treat PAH and are discussed in more detail in Chapter 11.

III. AGENTS USED TO MANAGE ANGINA.

Angina is characterized by chest pain either upon exertion (stable angina) or even at rest (unstable or vasospastic form). The symptoms are due to the lack of myocardial oxygenation secondary to atherosclerotic disease of the coronary vasculature (stable), spontaneous vasoconstriction of the coronary vessels (vasospastic), and episodic thrombotic events in the cardiac vessels (unstable). The general strategy for the treatment of acute or chronic angina is to increase oxygen supply or reduce myocardial oxygen demand.

A. Nitrate vasodilators are polyol esters of nitric acid nitrite (amyl nitrite) or nitrate (isosorbide dinitrate [Isordil®], nitroglycerin [Nitro-Dur®], isosorbide mononitrate [Ismo®]; *Figure 10-9*).

1. The fully nitrated polyols are nonpolar and lipid soluble, allowing rapid absorption from inhalational, dermal, sublingual, and oral routes. These routes (except for the oral) avoid first-pass metabolism to produce rapid antianginal effects, especially nasal and sublingual administration.
2. The systemic actions of these agents occur after a reductase-catalyzed (glutathione functioning as cofactor) production of nitric oxide (NO) in the vasculature. The potency and duration of action of these agents increase with the number of reducible nitrate groups found on the molecule. Higher reductase activity in veins than arteries is thought to produce greater venous rather than arterial effects of usual doses of nitrate derivatives.

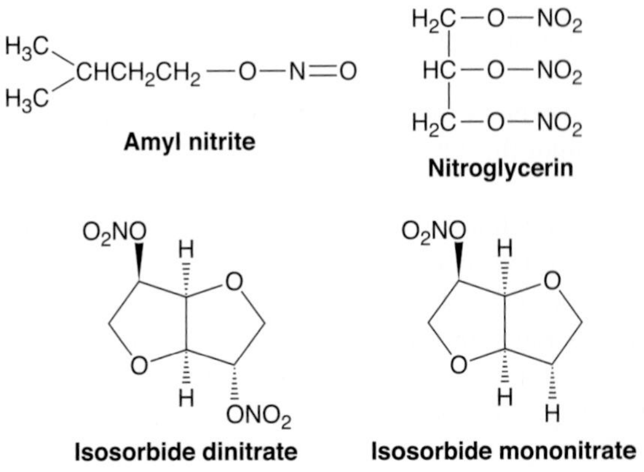

Figure 10-9. Structural formulas of the nitrite (amyl nitrite) and nitrate (nitroglycerin, isosorbide dinitrate, and isosorbide mononitrate) vasodilators.

3. NO produced in vascular smooth muscle cells activates soluble guanylyl cyclase that converts GTP to cGMP, which in turn activates protein kinase G (PKG). PKG is thought to reduce smooth muscle contraction by reducing cytoplasmic calcium levels and decreasing actin-myosin interactions.
4. Venodilation results in reduced venous return and decreased myocardial filling, which ultimately decreases myocardial work and oxygen demand. Reduced end-diastolic pressure also has the ability to improve subendocardial blood flow to increase oxygen supply to ischemic regions. Modest arterial dilation produced at these doses may also contribute to these two mechanisms.
5. Tolerance to nitrates occurs with chronic use and may be due to depletion of vascular glutathione; a withdrawal period is often required to restore sensitivity.
6. The most frequent adverse effects associated with nitrate use are flushing, headache, orthostatic hypotension, tachycardia, and dizziness.

B. **Ranolazine (Ranexa®)** is a relatively new agent used in the treatment of angina due to ischemic disease. Its mechanism of action is not entirely clear but may reduce myocardial contractility (and consequently oxygen demand) by blocking the late sodium current. The most common adverse events related to its use are dizziness, nausea, constipation, headache, and bradycardia.

C. **CCBs** prevent vasospastic angina by dilating coronary vessels to improve blood supply to the ischemic myocardium. The CCBs have been discussed in the previous section (see II.C).

D. **β-Adrenergic antagonists** reduce myocardial work by decreasing catecholamine-induced changes in heart rate and contractility. These agents primarily reduce myocardial oxygen demand and have been discussed in Chapter 9 (see II.B.3).

E. **Antiplatelet agents** reduce thrombotic events in the coronary circulation to prevent episodic reductions in myocardial blood flow and thus improve oxygen supply. These agents are discussed in the succeeding antiplatelet section.

IV. AGENTS FOR THE TREATMENT OF CONGESTIVE HEART FAILURE.

Congestive heart failure (CHF) is the reduction in cardiac output at normal filling pressures and may be secondary to a myocardial infarction or uncontrolled hypertension but may be the result of underlying myopathies of cardiac tissue. Generally, the treatment strategy is to alleviate the pulmonary and peripheral congestion due to edema and enhance cardiac pump function. Thus, diuretics and positive ionotropic agents are critical to CHF management; however, other agents that reduce cardiac remodeling and lower the work of the myocardium have also been found to be useful.

A. **Positive ionotropic agents** include several diverse agents used to manage acute and chronic pump failure.

1. Digoxin (Lanoxin®)
   a. Digoxin belongs to the cardiac glycoside family of positive ionotropic agents and is composed of a steroidal nucleus, an unsaturated lactone ring, and three sugars attached via glycosidic linkage (*Figure 10-10*). The glycoside portion is required for function, and bacterial cleavage of the glycosidic bond in the gastrointestinal (GI) tract reduces efficacy in about 10% of the population.
   b. Digoxin inhibits the actions of the electrogenic Na^+/K^+-ATPase resulting in increased intracellular Na^+ and consequent increase in intracellular calcium via actions of the coupled Na^+-Ca^{2+} exchanger. This intracellular calcium is stored in the sarcoplasmic reticulum until myocardial depolarization produces greater calcium-induced calcium release, which produces enhanced cardiac contractility.
   c. Improved cardiac contractility leads to increased cardiac output, better tissue perfusion, and enhanced renal function and urine output. This promotes greater water loss and reduces pulmonary congestion and edema of the extremities.
2. Infusions of dopamine or dobutamine (*Figure 10-10*) are used to manage acute heart failure via the activation of β_1-adrenergic receptors on the myocardium (discussed in Chapter 9). Activation of β_1-adrenergic receptors initiates the cAMP-protein kinase A (PKA) pathway (*Figure 58-1*) to increase myocardial calcium levels and subsequent increases in contractility and cardiac output. Dopamine also improves renal blood flow to enhance urine output and reduce edema.
3. The bipyridine phosphodiesterase type 3 (PDE3) inhibitors, milrinone (Primacor®; *Figure 10-10*) and inamrinone (Inocor®; not currently marketed), are also used intermittently in acute heart failure (*Figure 10-10*). Inhibition of PDE3 prevents the metabolism of cAMP to AMP that results

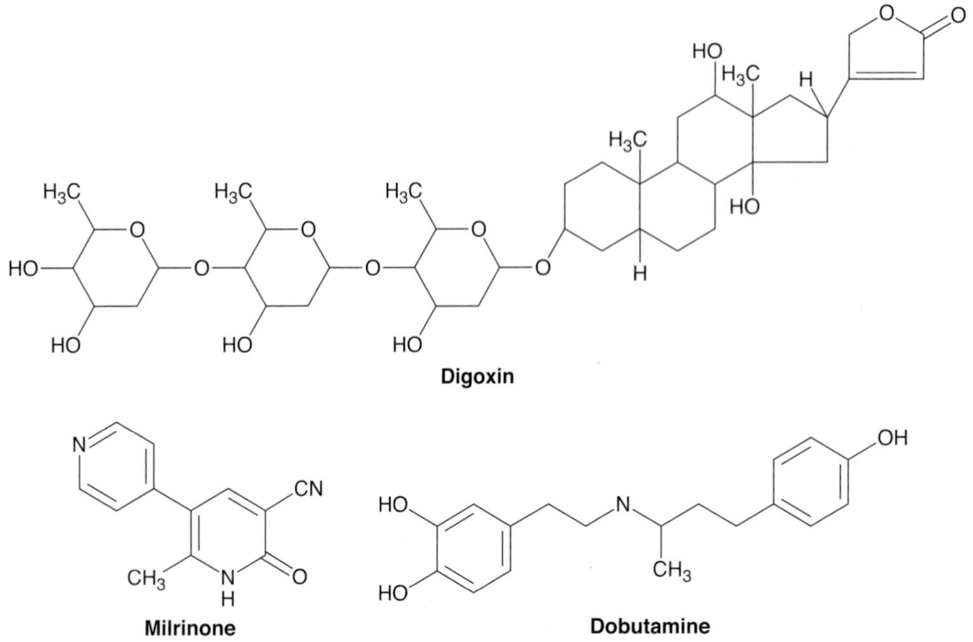

Figure 10-10. Structural formulas of the positive ionotropic agents digoxin, milrinone, and dobutamine.

in greater PKA activation and an ionotropic effect. Elevated cAMP-PKA in vascular smooth muscle also results in vasodilation and reduced systemic pressure to improve cardiac output.

4. A common adverse effect of all these positive ionotropic agents is the possibility of inducing ventricular arrhythmias during treatment. Nausea, vomiting, and visual disturbances are seen with digoxin, whereas PDE3 inhibitors are associated with thrombocytopenia and liver toxicity.

B. **β-Receptor antagonists.** In an apparently paradoxical manner, these drugs can be used to effectively manage chronic heart failure if they are carefully titrated. Blocking the β_1-receptors on the myocardium agents such as metoprolol, atenolol, and carvedilol can reduce the sympathetically driven heart rate and myocardial remodeling seen in CHF patients. Reduction in heart rate coupled with the lowering in peripheral resistance allows for better ventricular filling and improved ejection fraction to diminish the congestive symptoms.

C. **Inhibitors of renin-angiotensin-aldosterone system.** The high blood pressures seen in compensated heart failure and chronic cardiac remodeling can be reduced by ACEIs, ARBs, and aldosterone antagonists (e.g., eplerenone). The mechanisms for these effects are discussed in the previous section.

D. **Vasodilators.** Agents such as hydralazine and isosorbide dinitrate can reduce systemic blood pressure in the CHF patient to improve ventricular ejection and reduce pulmonary congestion. The combination of these two drugs (BiDil®) has been found to be beneficial in patients of African origin.

E. **Diuretics.** The extensive pulmonary congestion and peripheral edema experienced by CHF patients can be managed by the use of thiazide (e.g., hydrochlorothiazide) and loop (e.g., furosemide) diuretics.

F. **Nesiritide (Natrecor®)** is a recombinant form of brain natriuretic peptide that activates guanylyl cyclase A receptors on vascular smooth muscle cells to produce vasodilation and improve natriuresis and diuresis in the kidneys. Infusions of nesiritide are used to manage congestive symptoms in advanced heart failure.

V. ANTIARRHYTHMIC AGENTS.

Cardiac arrhythmias are often the result of underlying organic disease secondary to myocardial infarction or genetic mutations in the specific ion channels responsible for cardiac electrical activity.

A. The orderly movement of electrical activity from the SA node, through the atrial body to the AV node, and through the His-Purkinje system to the myocardium, is responsible for the organized contraction of the heart.

1. Arrhythmias result in uncoordinated atrial and ventricular contractions that reduce cardiac output and systemic blood pressure.
2. SA nodal pacemaker cells are able to spontaneously depolarize due to the leakiness of these cells to Na^+ (via the I_f channel) and Ca^{2+} (via L-type channels), producing a characteristic action potential (*Figure 10-11*). AV nodal cells are also leaky to Na^+/Ca^{2+} ions to spontaneously depolarize, but more often, they conduct atrial impulses through the His-Purkinje system.
3. Atrial, His-Purkinje, and ventricular myocardial cells are much less permeable to cations and are triggered to depolarize by electrical impulses from the SA nodes or AV nodes, respectively. Once triggered, voltage-dependent Na^+ channels open to depolarize the cells (phase 0), which is followed by rapid opening of outward K^+ channels (phase 1) and slower inward L-type (Ca^{2+}) currents to produce the phase 2 portion of the action potential (*Figure 10-11*). These cells are repolarized by the opening of delayed rectifier K^+ channels in phase 3 to reset the voltage-dependent Na^+ channels from inactive to the closed state in preparation for depolarization.
4. Generally, L-type channel blockers will preferentially affect SA and AV nodal cells due to their dependence on calcium currents for depolarization, whereas sodium channel blockers will decrease the activity of atrial and ventricular myocardial cells as well as those of the His-Purkinje conduction system. Potassium channel blockers decrease the rate of repolarization of all cells in the heart and can affect myocardial and conduction system cells.
5. Cardiac electrical activity is assessed by the use of surface chest electrodes connected to an amplification system that generates the recognizable electrocardiogram (ECG). The components of the ECG that are important for diagnosis of disease, as well as efficacy of antiarrhythmic drugs, are the P wave, PR interval, R wave, QRS interval, T wave, and QT intervals (*Figure 10-11*).

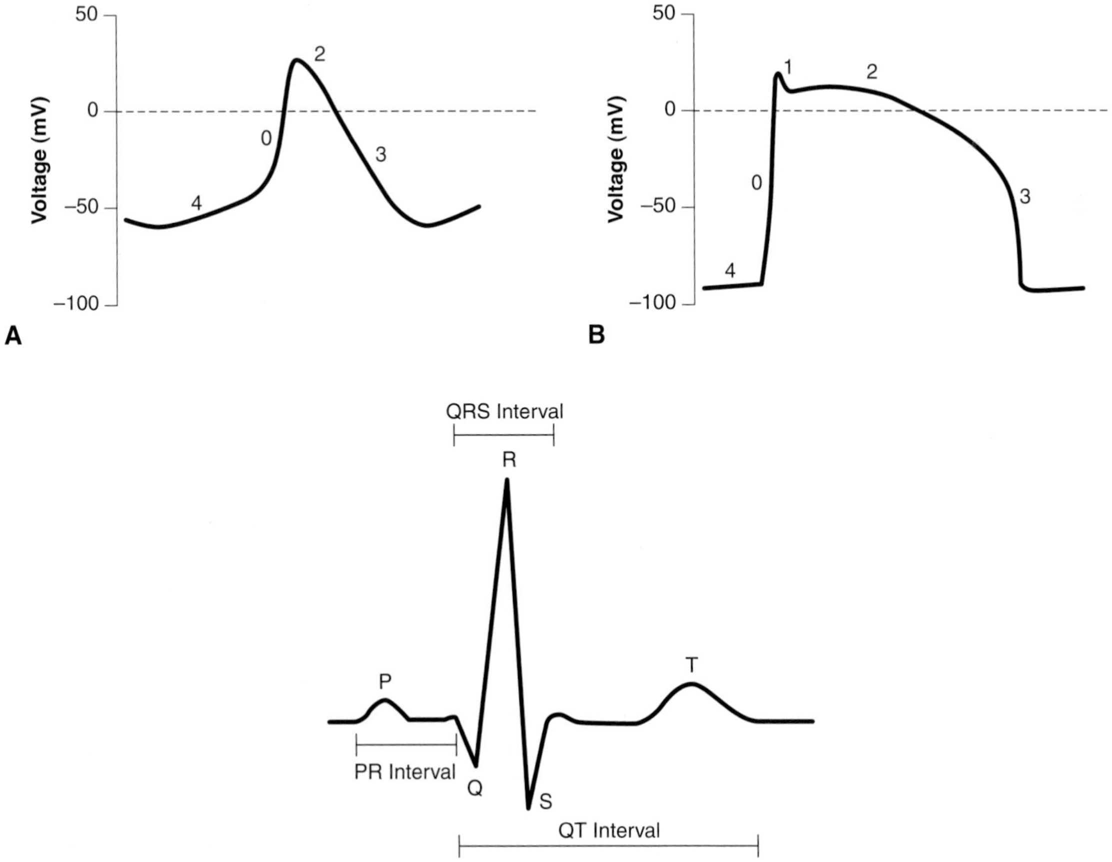

Figure 10-11. **A.** Action potential of an SA nodal cell with slow depolarization (phase 4), rapid depolarization (phase 0), plateau (phase 2), and rapid depolarization (phase 3). **B.** Action potential of a myocardial Purkinje cell with slow depolarization (phase 4), rapid depolarization (phase 0), rapid repolarization (phase 1), plateau (phase 2), and slow repolarization (phase 3). **C.** A typical electrocardiogram indicating atrial depolarization (P wave), ventricular depolarization (QRS wave), and ventricular repolarization (T wave).

a. The P wave is indicative of the depolarization of the atria, whereas the PR interval is the time taken for the impulses to travel through the atria to the ventricles.
b. The electrical activity of the AV node is the largest contributor to the PR interval, and drugs that affect the excitability of the AV node would tend to widen the PR interval (e.g., CCBs).
c. The QRS interval indicates the time taken for electrical impulses to travel through the His-Purkinje and ventricular cells, whereas the QT interval represents the cardiac repolarization time. Drugs that affect Na^+ channels would slow electrical conduction through the His-Purkinje–ventricular pathway to prolong the QRS interval.
d. Agents that slow down repolarization by interacting with K^+ channels have the effect of prolonging the PR, QRS, and QT intervals by increasing the refractory period of Ca^{2+} or Na^+ channels.
e. Most antiarrhythmic agents are Na^+, Ca^{2+}, or K^+ channel blockers that reduce the excitability of various cells of the cardiac conduction system. β-Adrenoreceptor antagonists are the fourth class of antiarrhythmic agents used to reduce the impact of the sympathetic nervous system on aberrant electrical activity.

6. Arrhythmias are due to defects in action potential initiation such as sinus bradycardia or premature ventricular beat, or defects in the conduction of electrical activity through the heart (e.g., reentrant supraventricular arrhythmias or torsades de pointes).

B. Sodium channel blocking antiarrhythmics

1. Quinidine, procainamide (Pronestyl®), and disopyramide (Norpace®; *Figure 10-12*) have dissimilar structures but similar Na^+ channel blocking activity to reduce excitability in atrial fibrillation and flutter, and also to decrease the recurrence of ventricular arrhythmias. Quinidine also has significant K^+ channel blocking activity as well as α-adrenergic blocking activity. Procainamide is metabolized to *N*-acetyl procainamide that has more prominent K^+-channel blocking activity, whereas disopyramide has the ability to block K^+-channels and depress cardiac contractility. The K^+-channel blocking activity of these three agents can predispose to torsades de pointes type of arrhythmias, whereas quinidine is associated with hypotension and syncope and disopyramide may precipitate heart failure. Procainamide is associated with lupus-like reactions, especially in patients who are unable to acetylate the drug effectively.
2. Lidocaine (Xylocaine®) and mexiletine (Mexitil®; *Figure 10-12*) have much more selective Na^+ channel blocking activity than the agents discussed in (V.B.1) above. The chemistry of lidocaine with respect to Na^+ channel interaction has been addressed in Chapter 9. Intravenous lidocaine can be used for the treatment of ventricular fibrillation, especially rapidly paced arrhythmias. Due to its high affinity for Na^+ channels in the inactive state, it binds preferentially to the channels on arrhythmic tissues but dissociates readily as the channels transition to the closed state. Thus, lidocaine has less effect on normal myocardial cells and, thus, only small changes in the overall ECG are seen with its use. Mexiletine is an oral derivative of lidocaine that can be used to prevent the occurrence of ventricular arrhythmias. Adverse effects related to the use of these agents are seizures, tremors, nystagmus, and heart block.
3. Flecainide (Tambocor®) and propafenone (Rhythmol®; *Figure 10-12*) are less selective Na^+ channel blockers than lidocaine that are used to manage supraventricular tachycardias such as atrial fibrillation and have some activity against ventricular arrhythmias. Both agents may have activity at K^+ channels, and propafenone has some β-adrenoreceptor antagonist activity as well. Adverse effects related to their use are worsening of heart failure symptoms, and flecainide may initiate lethal ventricular arrhythmias in patients with ischemic disease.

C. Potassium channel blockers. Sotalol (Betapace®), amiodarone (Cordarone®), dronedarone (Multaq®), ibutilide (Corvert®), and dofetilide (Tikosyn®; *Figure 10-13*) are generally recognized as K^+ channel blockers; however, they have other significant pharmacological action.

1. The levorotary isomer of sotalol has prominent β-adrenoreceptor antagonist activity, whereas amiodarone is known to also interact with Na^+ and Ca^{2+} channels and may interfere with thyroid hormone function in the myocardium. Ibutilide may activate Na^+ channels.
2. All these agents are used to maintain normal sinus rhythm in patients with atrial fibrillation or flutter, whereas amiodarone may also be useful in treating ventricular arrhythmias.
3. The most significant adverse effect of these agents is the potential to cause torsades de pointes arrhythmias by virtue of their K^+ channel blocking activity. Amiodarone has also caused lethal pulmonary fibrosis, microcrystalline corneal deposits, and photosensitivity. Dronedarone may be associated with hepatotoxicity, whereas amiodarone, dronedarone, and sotalol may also cause heart block and bradycardia and exacerbate heart failure.

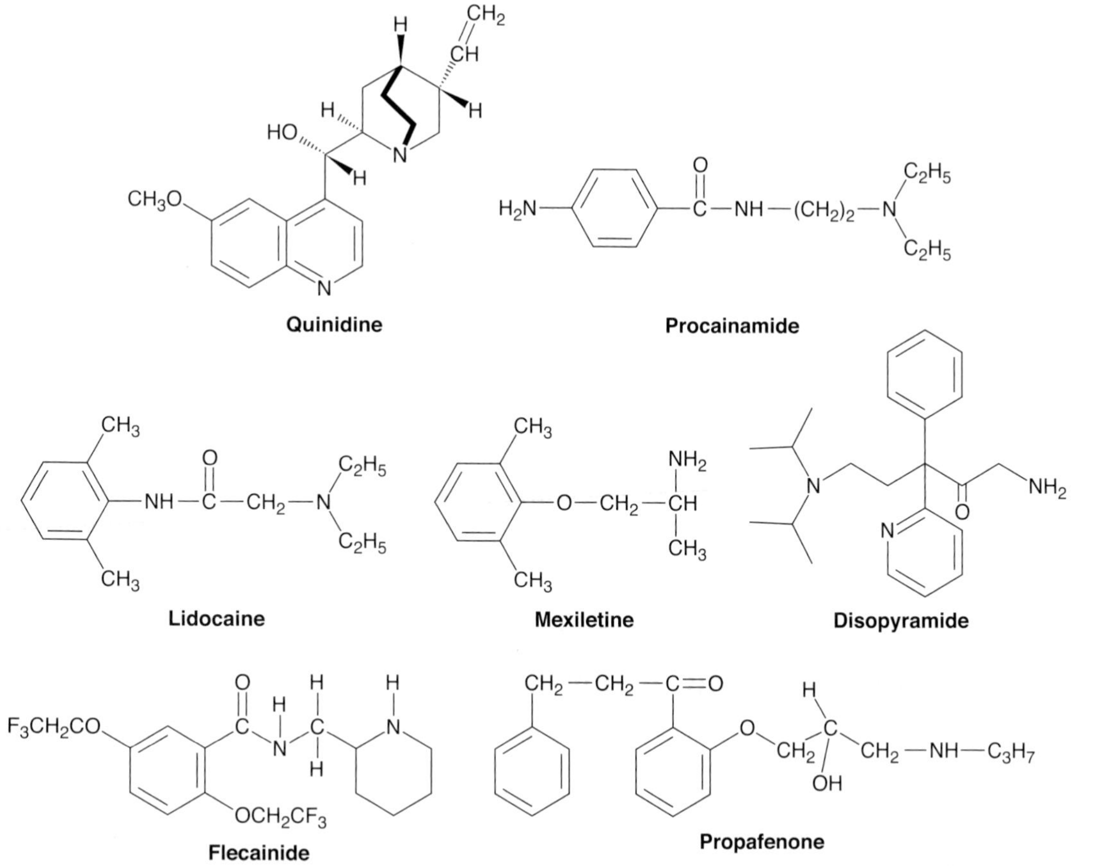

Figure 10-12. Structural formulas of antiarrhythmic agents with predominant Na^+ channel blocking activity.

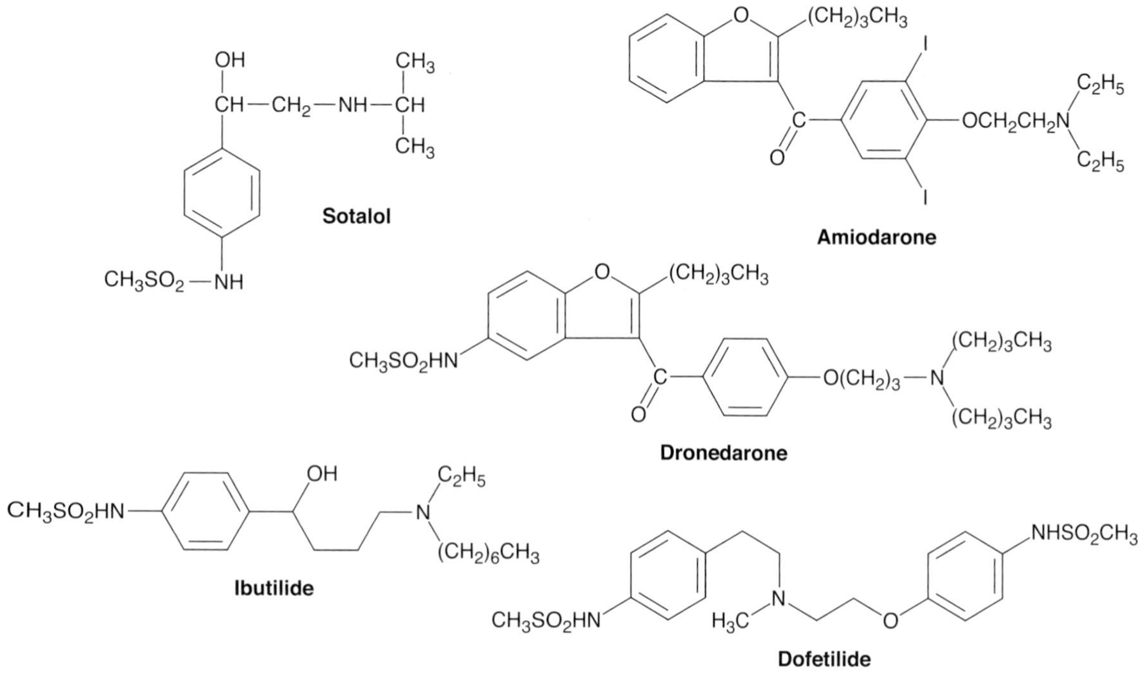

Figure 10-13. Structural formulas of antiarrhythmic agents with predominant K^+ channel blocking activity.

11 Pharmacology and Medicinal Chemistry of Autacoids, Nonsteroidal Anti-inflammatory Drugs, and Antihistamines

MICHAEL L. ADAMS, S. THOMAS ABRAHAM

I. AUTACOIDS are classified as substances that are released at or near their site of action and have a short duration of activity. Autacoids, such as **prostaglandins**, **leukotrienes**, kallidin, bradykinin, **serotonin**, and **histamine**, have varied structures and physiological activities that are modulated by several different drugs. Although some autacoids (histamine and serotonin) function as neurotransmitters, their autacoid functions will be covered here. Currently, there are no agents that specifically modulate the function of bradykinin or kallidin; however, drugs or analogs that mimic, block, or modulate other autacoid functions and/or synthesis have important therapeutic roles.

II. PROSTAGLANDINS (PGs) are autacoids with diverse pharmacological activities, including the initiation of inflammation.

A. **PGs** are derivatives of prostanoic acid, a 20-carbon fatty acid containing a 5-carbon ring (*Figure 11-1*). In the body, PGs are principally synthesized from arachidonic acid, which is formed from membrane phospholipids by the action of phospholipase A2. Specifically, PGs are synthesized from arachidonic acid by the enzyme cyclooxygenase (COX). Note that the products of COX are then converted into

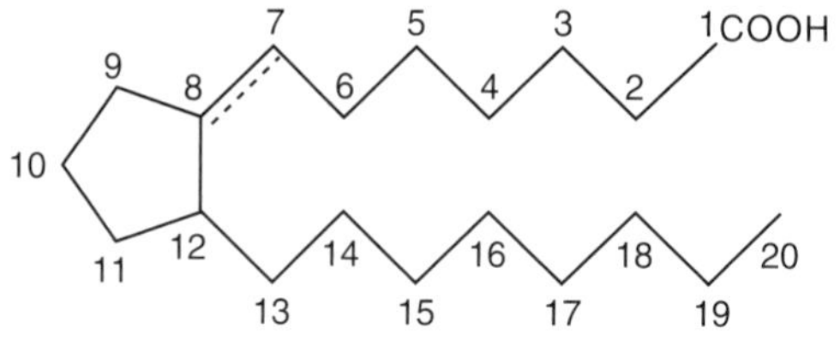

Figure 11-1. Structural formula of prostanoic acid, from which the prostaglandins are derived.

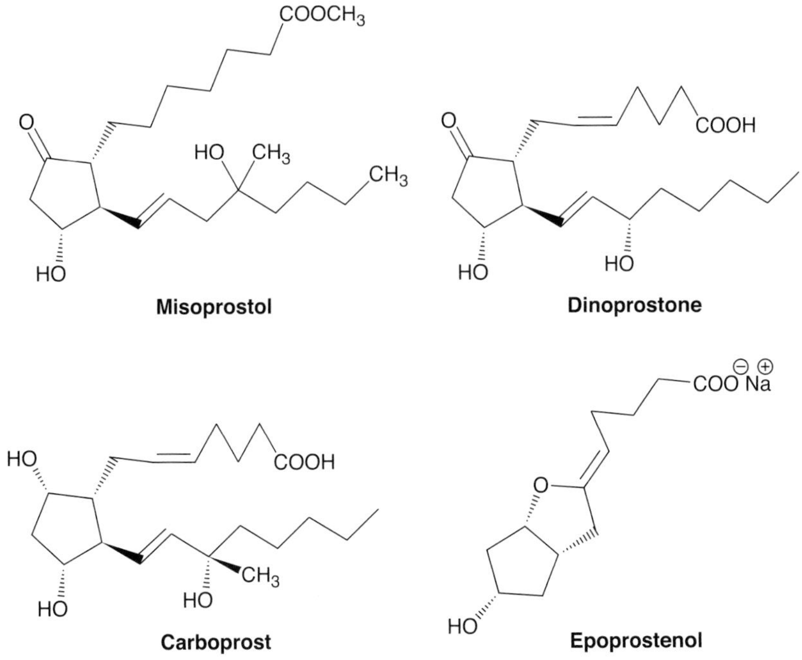

Figure 11-2. Prostaglandin analogs including misoprostol (PGE_1), dinoprostone (PGE_2), carboprost ($PGF_{2\alpha}$), and epoprostenol (PGI_2).

either PGs by PG synthase or thromboxanes by thromboxane synthase. The thromboxanes differ from the PGs mainly by the substitution of a tetrahydropyran ring structure for the pentane ring found in PGs. The only clinically relevant thromboxane currently identified is thromboxane A2 (TxA2), which causes platelet aggregation.

B. Classification of PGs as prostaglandin A (PGA), prostaglandin B (PGB), prostaglandin E (PGE), and so forth relates to the presence or absence of keto or hydroxyl groups at positions 9 and 11 (*Figure 11-1*). Subscripts relate to the number and position of double bonds in the aliphatic chains (*Figure 11-2*).

C. PGs produce **diverse physiological and pathological effects** by activating specific PG receptors on relevant tissues. The physiological responses to PGs include **vasodilation** in most vascular beds, although vasoconstriction can occur in some others. In general, PGs increase renal blood flow, promote diuresis, natriuresis, and kaliuresis. The PGs are also important regulators of renin release from juxtaglomerular cells. Specific activities for the individual PGs and their respective receptors are summarized in the following.

1. **PGEs inhibit platelet aggregation, relax bronchial and gastrointestinal (GI) smooth muscle, contract uterine smooth muscle, and inhibit gastric acid secretion.** Most of these effects are mediated by PGE (EP)-type receptors on smooth muscle and secretory cells.
2. **PGDs and PGFs contract bronchial, iris sphincter, and GI smooth muscle by activating PGD (DP)- or PGF (FP)-type receptors, respectively.**
3. **PGI_2**, also called prostacyclin, **inhibits platelet aggregation**, **is a potent vasodilator**, and **stimulates gastric release of bicarbonate** and **mucus**. These effects are dependent on the PGI2 (IP)-type PG receptors on vascular smooth muscle, platelets, and gastric mucosal cells.

D. By selectively activating various PG receptors, several PG derivatives are used to manage diverse conditions or disease states.

1. PGE_1 analogs
   - **a.** Alprostadil (PGE_1) is the endogenous PG marketed in various forms for different indications (*Figure 11-2*).
     - **(1)** Alprostadil (Prostin VR Pediatric) is used for the **temporary maintenance of a patent ductus arteriosus** until corrective surgery for the congenital heart defect can be performed.
     - **(2)** Alprostadil (Caverject, Edex) and alprostadil (Muse) are marketed as an intracavernosal injection and urethral suppository, respectively, for the **treatment of erectile dysfunction** (*Figure 11-2*).

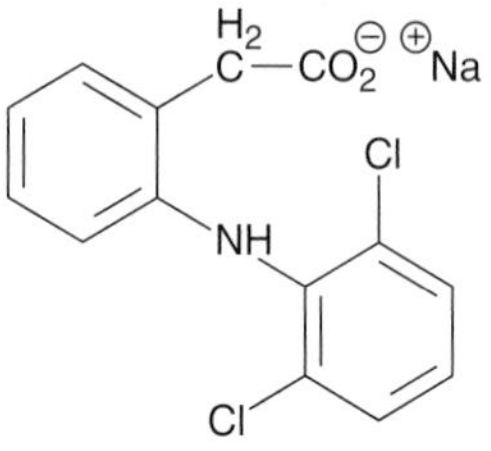

Diclofenac sodium

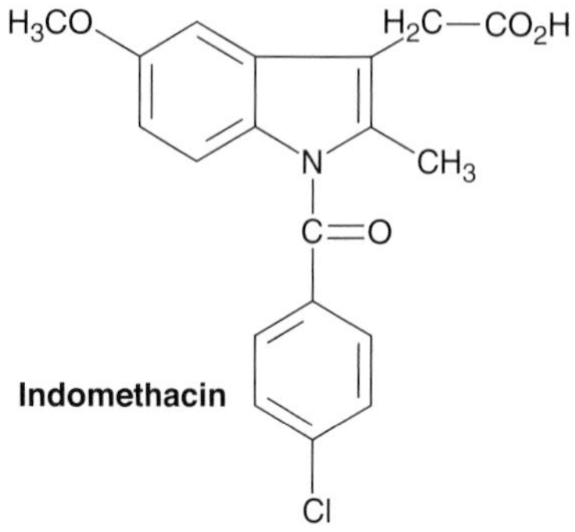

Indomethacin

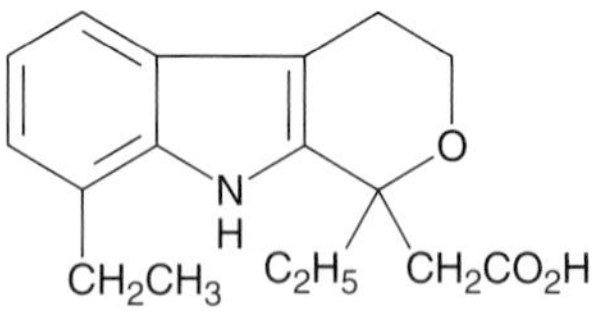

Etodolac

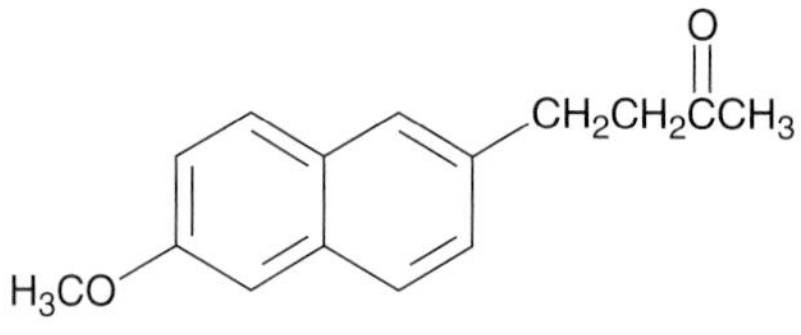

Nabumetone

Figure 11-4. The acetic acid derivative NSAIDs including diclofenac, indomethacin, etodolac, and the prodrug nabumetone.

C. NSAIDs are the agents of choice for the treatment of **rheumatoid arthritis**, **osteoarthritis**, and **ankylosing spondylitis**.
   1. NSAIDs may also be used to relieve musculoskeletal pain, headache, and gouty arthritis.
   2. NSAIDs have **antipyretic effects** for the relief of fever. The salicylates should not be used in children with varicella or influenza-type viral infections because of the observed association between salicylate use in these situations and Reye syndrome.
   3. Aspirin is also indicated for prophylaxis and initial treatment of myocardial infarction based on its ability to inhibit platelet aggregation (see Chapter 10).

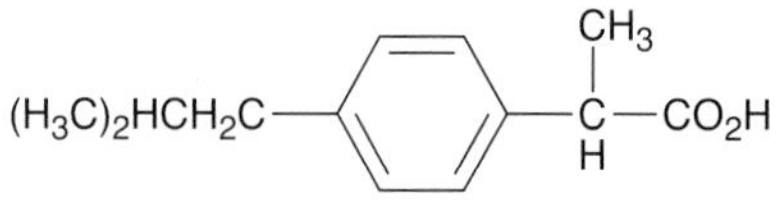

Ibuprofen

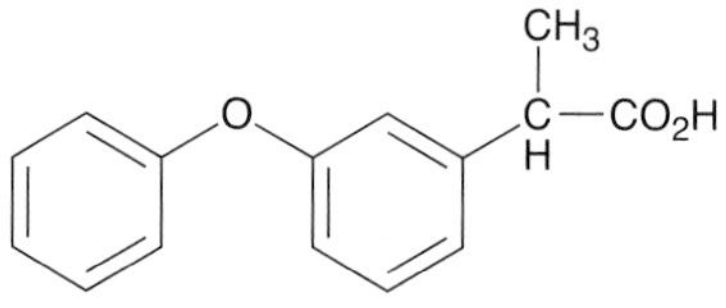

Fenoprofen calcium

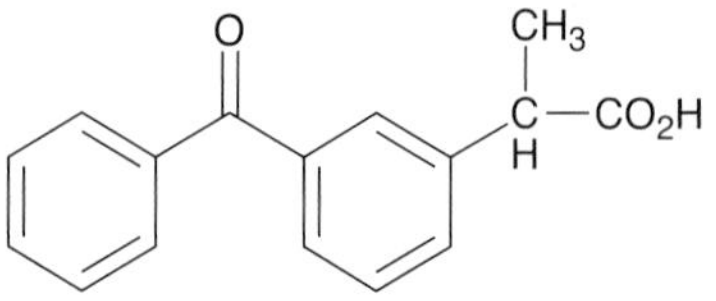

Ketoprofen

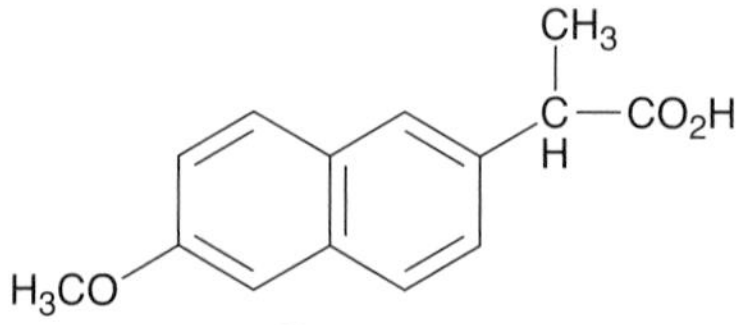

Naproxen

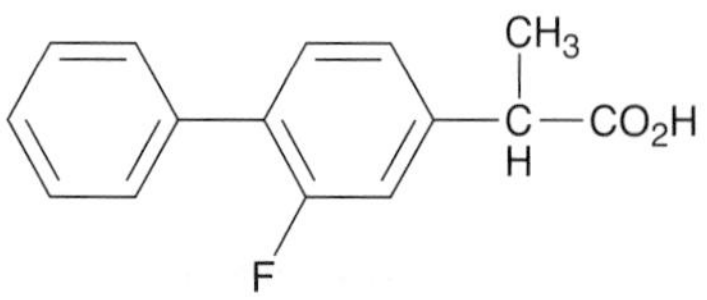

Flurbiprofen

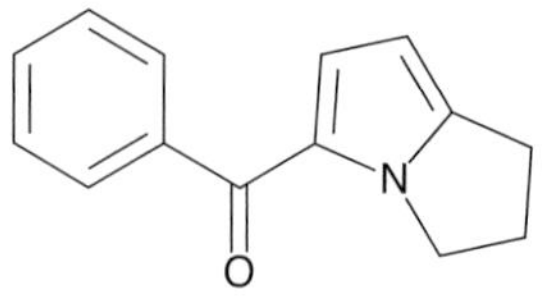

Ketorolac

Figure 11-5. The propionic acid derivative NSAIDs including ibuprofen, fenoprofen, ketoprofen, naproxen, flurbiprofen, and ketorolac.

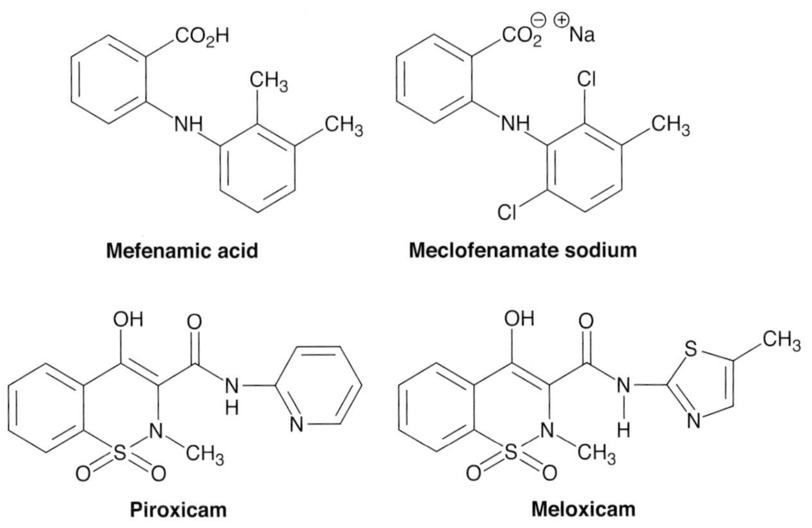

Figure 11-6. The *N*-arylanthranilic acid derivative NSAIDs including mefenamic acid and meclofenamate. The oxicams or enolic acid derivatives of NSAIDs including piroxicam and meloxicam.

D. NSAIDs are associated to varying degrees, depending on the agent, with the following adverse effects.

1. **GI effects**, such as GI distress, irritation, erosion of the gastric mucosa, nausea, vomiting, and dyspepsia are the most commonly observed effects and are attributed to the **acidic nature of the molecules** and the **decreased synthesis of gastric mucosa** secondary to inhibition of COX-1. Serious GI toxicity including bleeding and gut perforation is also possible.
2. **CNS (central nervous system) effects**, such as CNS depression, drowsiness, headache, dizziness, visual disturbances, ototoxicity, and confusion are observed.
3. **Cardiovascular events** associated with NSAIDs include an increased risk of myocardial infarction and stroke that increases with longer duration of therapy. These risks are addressed in a black box warning on all NSAIDs.
4. **Hematologic effects** observed include thrombocytopenia, altered platelet function, and prolonged bleeding time, which are commonly called antiplatelet effects.
5. **Nephrotoxicity** in the form of renal failure, hyperkalemia, and proteinuria are also possible adverse effects.
6. Other adverse effects include skin rashes, rare liver failure, asthma, and fluid retention.
7. In addition, the salicylates are associated with increased depth of respirations, excessive bleeding due to inhibition of thromboxane synthesis, and Reye syndrome in children with viral infections. Salicylate overdose is called salicylism and is characterized by tinnitus, nausea, and vomiting.

E. The family of NSAIDs also includes the **COX-2 selective inhibitors**.

1. The COX-2 inhibitors selectively inhibit the inducible form of COX to reduce PG synthesis associated with the inflammatory response. Their ability to decrease pain and inflammation associated with arthritic diseases is approximately equal to that produced by the nonselective or traditional NSAIDs. The theoretical advantage of this selectivity is to **reduce the GI adverse effects** caused by the inhibition of the constitutive COX-1.
2. The only compound marketed in the United States as a COX-2 selective inhibitor is celecoxib (Celebrex), a diarylheterocycle containing a sulfonamide (*Figure 11-7*). Rofecoxib (Vioxx) and valdecoxib (Bextra) were removed from the U.S. market after concerns over adverse effects (see III.E.4.).
3. Celecoxib (Celebrex) is approved for the treatment of acute pain, ankylosing spondylitis, osteoarthritis, rheumatoid arthritis, primary dysmenorrhea, and familial adenomatous polyposis.
4. Celecoxib does not appear to cause as great an incidence of GI ulceration or antiplatelet effects as the traditional NSAIDs, but **GI upset** and bleeding is still a significant side effect. The risk of adverse GI events increases with increasing dose and duration of therapy. Additionally, **adverse cardiovascular events** observed with the potent COX-2 inhibitors rofecoxib (Vioxx) and valdecoxib (Bextra) resulted in their market withdrawal. These risks included an increased risk of heart attack and stroke in patients taking rofecoxib (Vioxx) and valdecoxib (Bextra) compared to patients taking the traditional NSAIDs.

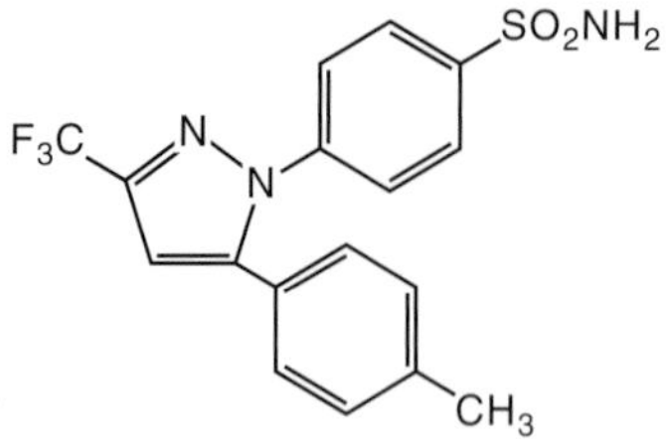

Celecoxib

Figure 11-7. Structural formula of celecoxib, a COX-2–specific inhibitor.

IV. NONNARCOTIC ANALGESICS AND ANTIPYRETICS lack the anti-inflammatory properties of the NSAIDs but remain useful as analgesics and antipyretics.

A. **Acetaminophen** (paracetamol, Tylenol, and various combination drugs) is a *p*-aminophenol derivative, which is the active metabolite of the older, no longer used agents phenacetin and acetanilide (*Figure 11-8*).

B. Acetaminophen does not significantly inhibit peripheral COX-1 or COX-2; therefore, it is not useful as an anti-inflammatory agent but has a similar antipyretic and analgesic potency when compared to aspirin. These activities of acetaminophen are proposed to be related to inhibition of COX in the CNS and potentially the controversial COX-3 enzyme.

C. Acetaminophen is indicated for use as an **antipyretic** and **mild analgesic** for minor aches and pains. Acetaminophen is the antipyretic of choice in children because there is no association between acetaminophen use in children with viral infections and Reye syndrome.

D. Acetaminophen is usually well tolerated, but the following adverse effects have been reported:

1. Hypersensitivity, including a rash
2. Rare methemoglobinemia
3. Renal dysfunction
4. **Hepatotoxicity**
   a. **Mild increases in liver function enzymes** may be observed with therapeutic doses, but these elevations are reversible upon drug withdrawal.
   b. **Acute overdose** and **chronic excessive doses** of acetaminophen results in significant **hepatotoxicity** characterized by **centrilobular necrosis** with potential for fulminant hepatic failure requiring a liver transplant.
   c. **Acetaminophen hepatotoxicity** is dependent on the **CYP metabolism** to the reactive metabolite *N*-acetyl-*p*-benzoquinone imine (NAPQI). NAPQI is inactivated by glutathione but covalently binds to cellular proteins as glutathione is depleted.
   d. Acetaminophen hepatotoxicity is treated orally or IV with ***N*-acetylcysteine** (Mucomyst, Acetadote), which restores the glutathione levels in the hepatocytes (see *Figure 8-5*).

V. GOUT is the result of an inflammatory response to deposition of sodium urate crystals in the joint formed by the breakdown of purine nucleotides from DNA. Treatments for gout reduce plasma uric acid concentration or inhibit the inflammatory response.

A. NSAIDs, except aspirin, salicylates, and tolmetin, are useful in the treatment of gout. Additionally, oxaprozin is a good choice due to its uricosuric properties (i.e., the ability to lower serum uric acid levels).

B. **Colchicine** (Colcrys) is an alkaloid isolated from the **autumn crocus plant** and is useful in the treatment of the symptoms of **gouty arthritis** (*Figure 11-9*).

1. Multiple pharmacological activities for colchicine have been identified, but the presumed mechanism useful in the treatment of gout is related to **inhibition of tubulin polymerization into**

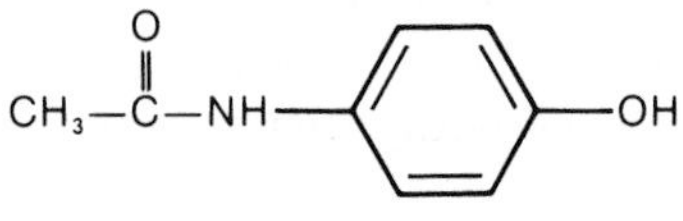

Figure 11-8. Structural formula of acetaminophen, the prototypical *p*-aminophenol derivative.

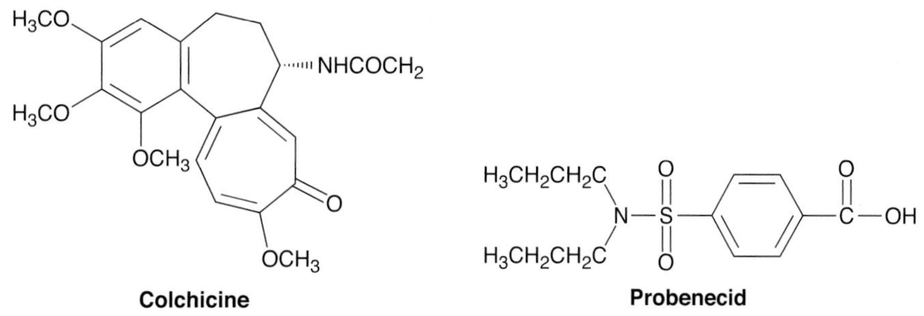

Figure 11-9. Colchicine and probenecid are both used to treat gout.

microtubules. This process is required for the movement and phagocytosis of uric acid by leukocytes that play a role in the initiation of the inflammatory process. Colchicine also reduces the production of lactic acid by the leukocytes. Lactic acid production lowers the pH and causes more uric acid crystals to precipitate.

2. Colchicine is used for the treatment of **acute gout attacks** and usually provides relief to the pain and inflammation within 24 hrs. Colchicine is also marketed in combination products with probenecid (see section V.C) for the treatment of gout.
3. The majority of the **side effects** of colchicine are **related to the inhibition of tubulin microtubules** required for cell division in rapidly dividing cells.
   a. GI effects including nausea, vomiting, abdominal pain, and diarrhea are the most common side effects and may be the early signs of colchicine toxicity characterized by hemorrhagic gastropathy.
   b. Other serious side effects include agranulocytosis, aplastic anemia, myopathy, hair loss, and peripheral neuritis.

C. The benzoic acid derivative **probenecid** (Benemid, Probalan) is useful in the treatment of chronic gout (*Figure 11-7*).
   1. Probenecid, a uricosuric agent, **inhibits the proximal tubular reabsorption of uric acid**, increasing uric acid excretion, thus reducing plasma uric acid levels.
   2. Probenecid is used to treat **chronic tophaceous gout**. It is also used in smaller doses to prolong the effectiveness of penicillin-type antibiotics by inhibiting their tubular secretion. Probenecid is also marketed in combination products containing colchicine for the treatment of gout.
   3. Side effects for probenecid include GI irritation and less frequently, hemolytic anemia, rash, and renal stones caused by increased excretion of uric acid.

D. **Decreasing the synthesis of uric acid** is another approach to the treatment of gout.
   1. **Allopurinol** (Zyloprim) is an isopurine and **febuxostat** (Uloric) is a nonpurine analog (*Figure 11-10*). Both **inhibit xanthine oxidase** to slow the conversion of the purine metabolites xanthine and hypoxanthine to uric acid.
      a. Allopurinol is a **competitive inhibitor of xanthine oxidase** at low concentration and noncompetitive at high concentration. The active metabolite of allopurinol, oxypurinol, is produced by xanthine oxidase and is a noncompetitive inhibitor of xanthine oxidase.
      b. Febuxostat (Uloric) inhibits xanthine oxidase through the formation of a stable complex with xanthine oxidase.

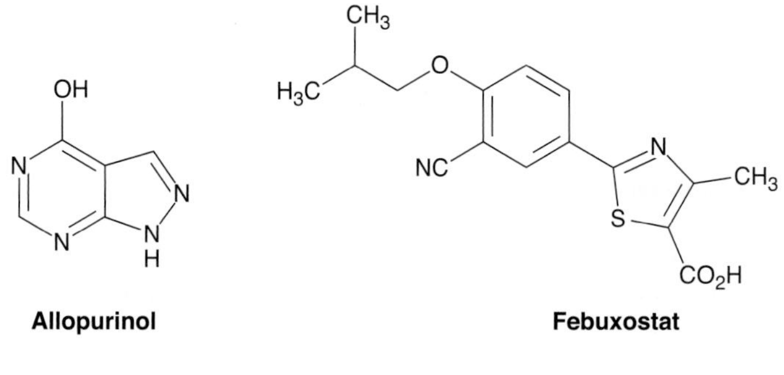

Figure 11-10. Xanthine oxidase (XO) inhibitors allopurinol and febuxostat.

2. Allopurinol is indicated for **gouty arthritis**, the treatment of tophaceous gout, whereas febuxostat is indicated for patients experiencing **gouty arthritis with hyperuricemia**. Neither agent is indicated for asymptomatic hyperuricemia.
3. Allopurinol and febuxostat are associated with the following adverse effects, although febuxostat generally has a better adverse effect profile.
   a. Precipitation of an acute gout attack with initiation of therapy due to mobilization of stored urate
   b. GI intolerance, including GI distress, nausea, vomiting, and diarrhea
   c. Rarely, aplastic anemia and hepatotoxicity have been reported.
   d. Peripheral neuritis and necrotizing vasculitis, bone marrow depression, skin rash, and Stevens-Johnson syndrome are also seen in rare instances of allopurinol use.

E. **Pegloticase** (Krystexxa) and **rasburicase** (Elitek) are recombinant uricase or urate-oxidase, enzymes responsible for the final step in the breakdown of purines. Uric acid is converted to allantoin, a more water-soluble metabolite by urate-oxidase. Whereas pegloticase (Krystexxa) is indicated for **gout refractory to conventional therapy**, rasburicase (Elitek) is indicated for the **treatment of hyperuricemia secondary to anticancer therapy** in patients with leukemia, lymphoma, and solid tumor malignancies but is used off-label for refractory, non–malignancy-related gout. Major side effects including anaphylaxis, hemolysis, and methemoglobinemia and excessive cost for these parenterally administered products will most likely limit their use to the treatment of last resort for gout.

VI. LEUKOTRIENES (LTs) are autacoids with diverse pharmacological activities, including **inflammation** and **bronchoconstriction**.

A. The LTs are **20-carbon derivatives of the fatty acids** that are formed via the enzymatic catalysis of arachidonic acid by **lipoxygenase**. Unlike the PGs, they contain no ring structure and are covalently linked to two or three amino acids. The two most important LTs identified to date (LTC_4 and LTD_4) differ only by the presence of a glutamine residue. The nomenclature of the LTs is similar to that used for the PGs (*Figure 11-11*).

B. LTs play a role in the immune response to antigen challenge and were initially called the slow-reacting substances of anaphylaxis. Specific actions of the LTs that are targets for pharmacological modulation include their **potent chemotactic** action on neutrophils and eosinophils and significant **bronchoconstriction** and **mucus secretion**. These activities are readily seen in asthmatic patients and are specifically targeted by inhibitors of LT synthesis or antagonists of LT receptors.

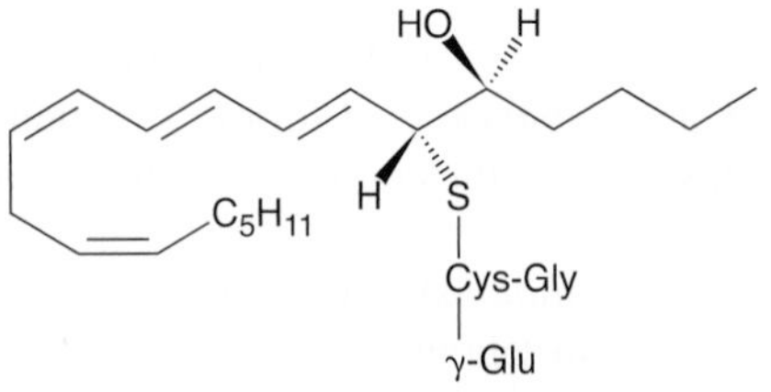

Leukotriene C_4(LTC_4)

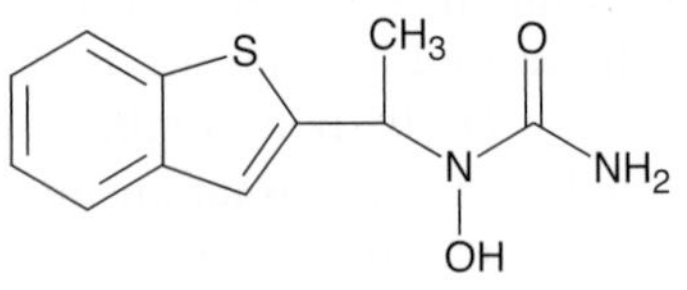

Zileuton

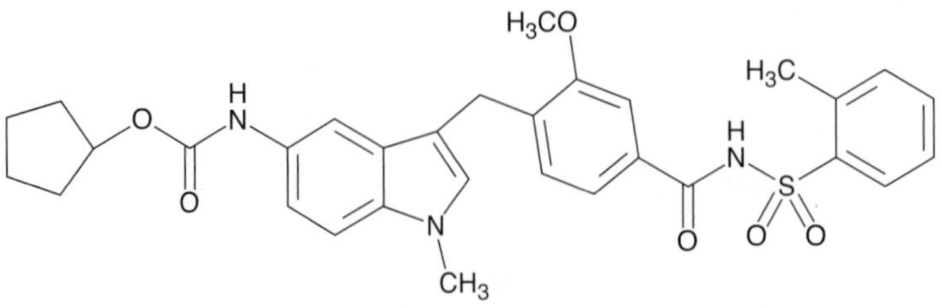

Zafirlukast

Figure 11-11. Endogenous leukotriene C_4 and two modulators of leukotriene activity. Zileuton inhibits the synthesis of leukotrienes by inhibiting 5-lipoxygenase, and zafirlukast is an antagonist of the $cysLT_1$-receptor that blocks the effects of leukotrienes.

C. Specific **inhibition of LT synthesis** can be achieved to reduce the tissue content of these inflammatory mediators. Zileuton (Zyflo) is an orally administered benzothiophene derivative **inhibitor of lipoxygenase** (*Figure 11-11*).

1. The inhibition of lipoxygenase prevents the synthesis of LTs, thereby preventing their contribution to various inflammatory processes. Because the lungs are sensitive to LT-induced bronchoconstriction, zileuton (Zyflo) is indicated for **prophylactic treatment of asthma**. It is not, however, effective in the management of acute asthma attacks.
2. Adverse effects of zileuton include GI effects, including dyspepsia and nausea, and headache. Reports of elevated liver enzymes in the plasma and neuropsychiatric events, including sleep disorders and behavior changes, require continued monitoring with zileuton treatment.

D. Antagonism of LT receptors prevents the consequence of immune-related production of LTs. Zafirlukast (Accolate) and montelukast (Singulair) are nonstructurally related molecules with hydrophobic regions and an acidic functional group (i.e., sulfonamide and carboxylic acid, respectively) required for their **antagonist activity at the leukotriene CysLT$_1$-receptor** (*Figure 11-11*).

1. By acting as **competitive antagonists**, zafirlukast and montelukast **inhibit bronchoconstriction** and **pulmonary edema** induced by endogenously produced LTs.
2. Zafirlukast may produce GI upset and liver dysfunction but to a lesser extent than zileuton. Zafirlukast is a substrate and an **inhibitor of CYP2C9** and may result in drug–drug interactions. Interactions have been reported with warfarin, erythromycin, and theophylline. Rare cases of **Churg-Strauss syndrome** or eosinophilic vasculitis have been reported in association with reduction of oral steroid therapies.
3. Montelukast has adverse effects similar to zafirlukast without significant reports of hepatotoxicity. CYP450 induction increases the clearance of montelukast leading to the potential for therapeutic failure.

VII. SEROTONIN, in addition to being a neurotransmitter, is also an autacoid with various effects, including **vasoconstriction** and **platelet aggregation**.

A. **Serotonin** (5-hydroxytryptamine, 5-HT) is a bioamine that is synthesized from the amino acid **tryptophan** by a two-step enzymatic process catalyzed by tryptophan hydroxylase and L-amino acid decarboxylase (*Figure 11-12*).

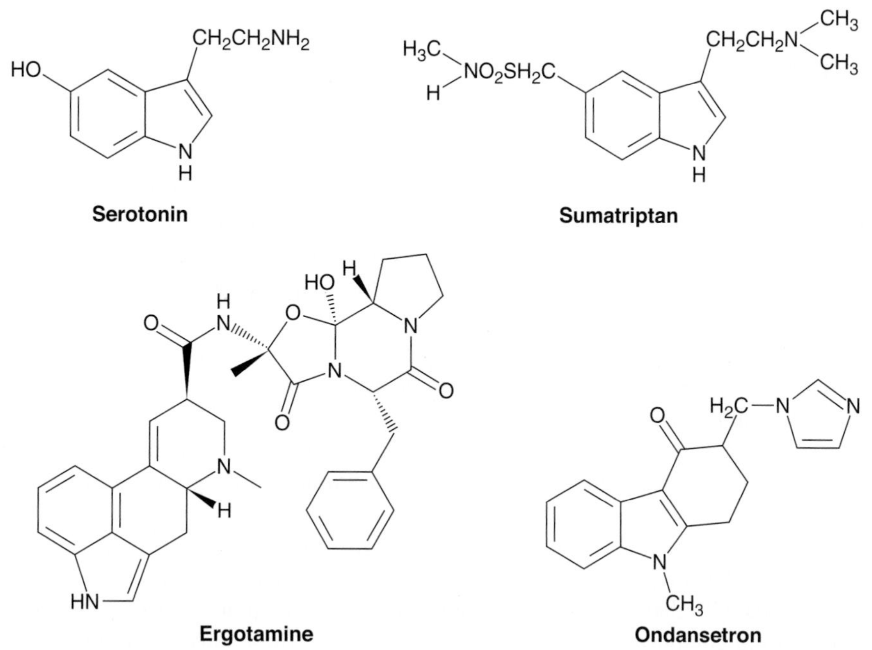

Figure 11-12. Structures of serotonin and representative serotonin agonists sumatriptan, ergotamine, and the serotonin antagonist ondansetron.

B. Serotonin exerts a wide range of effects via a family of seven receptors with several subtypes. Major physiological effects of serotonin include **vasoconstriction** (5-HT_2); **platelet aggregations** (5-HT_2); **increased release of acetylcholine** in the enteric nervous system (5-HT_3, 5-HT_4); **nausea/emesis** (5-HT_3); and CNS actions that influence anxiety, depression, aggression, impulsivity, and appetite (5-HT_1, 5-HT_2, 5-HT_3). In addition, the 5-HT_1-receptor acts presynaptically at both serotonergic and adrenergic neurons to reduce neurotransmitter release. Based on these numerous effects, the serotonergic system is a rich pharmacologic target to modulate. Many **CNS drugs** modulate the **serotonergic system** to treat conditions such as **anxiety** (buspirone [Buspar]) and **depression** (fluoxetine [Prozac]), which are discussed in more detail in Chapter 9.

C. **5-HT_1-receptor agonists** are **indole derivatives** with structural similarity to serotonin (*Figure 11-12*) and include sumatriptan (Imitrex), rizatriptan (Maxalt), naratriptan (Amerge), zolmitriptan (Zomig), almotriptan (Axert), eletriptan (Relpax), and frovatriptan (Frova).

1. **5-HT_1-receptor agonists** mimic the actions of serotonin at this receptor to produce **direct vasoconstriction** of cerebral vessels, **decrease the release of inflammatory** and **vasodilating substances** (neurokinin A, substance P), and have **antinociceptive activities.** These actions are thought to contribute to the efficacy of these drugs in the treatment of pain and nausea associated with migraine headaches.
2. Adverse effects of the 5-HT_1-receptor agonists include feeling warm, paresthesias, dizziness, and tightness or heaviness in the chest. Rarely, patients may experience chest pain. Because these agents may cause **coronary vasoconstriction**, they are contraindicated in angina patients and should be used cautiously in patients with hypertension or other risk factors for ischemic heart disease.

D. **Ergot alkaloids** are derived from the *Claviceps purpurea* fungus that infects grains and contains a tetracyclic ergoline nucleus (*Figure 11-12*). The activity of the ergot alkaloids is complex and includes serotonin receptor agonist activity for some alkaloids and serotonin receptor antagonist activity for other alkaloids in addition to mixed activities at the α-adrenergic receptors and the dopamine receptors. The specific pharmacological response depends on the specific alkaloid drug and the animal model.

1. Ergotamine (Ergomar) and dihydroergotamine (injection [D.H.E. 45], intranasal [Migranal]) are used for the treatment of **migraine headaches** via 5-HT_1-receptor and α-adrenoreceptor agonist activity.
2. Other ergotamine alkaloids including ergonovine (Ergotrate) and methylergonovine (Methergine) are used to **prevent postpartum hemorrhage** through both **vasoconstrictive** and **uterine contractile actions** of 5-HT_2 and α-adrenoreceptor activities. Bromocriptine (Parlodel), through its dopaminergic activity, is also used to prevent postpartum breast engorgement.
3. Adverse effects of the ergot alkaloids include GI upset and cold extremities. With increasing doses, the patient may experience emesis, diarrhea, peripheral pain secondary to local ischemia, and hallucinations or delusions.

E. **5-HT_3-antagonists** are indole or indole-like derivatives that block the ligand-gated ion channel, which is the 5-HT_3-receptor. This prevents serotonin from causing **nausea** and/or **emesis** both locally at the GI track and centrally in the area postrema. In addition, activation of peripheral 5-HT_3-receptors will increase pain, abdominal distention, and motor responses of the intestinal tract.

1. 5-HT_3-antagonists indicated for **nausea and vomiting,** including that due to radiation or **cancer chemotherapy,** are ondansetron (Zofran), dolasteron (Anzemet), granisetron (IV or PO [Kytril], transdermal [Sancuso]), and palonosetron (Aloxi) (*Figure 11-12*).
2. Alosetron (Lotronex) is also a 5-HT_3-antagonist at the peripheral receptors that **slows GI motility**, making it useful in certain cases of **irritable bowel syndrome** (IBS) when diarrhea is predominant.
3. 5-HT_3-antagonists will produce headache, constipation, and dizziness. In addition, granisetron (Kytril) has been reported to produce somnolence and diarrhea. The use of alosetron (Lotronex) in patients with diarrhea-associated IBS has resulted in some cases of ischemic colitis and life-threatening complications from severe constipation. These adverse events have resulted in the development of a risk evaluation and mitigation strategy (REMS) that requires prescribers be specially certified to prescribe alosetron (Lotronex).

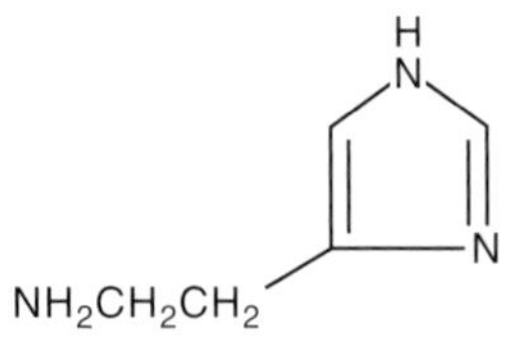

Figure 11-13. Structural formula of histamine, an autacoid.

VIII. ANTIHISTAMINES

A. **Histamine** is a bioamine derived principally from dietary histidine, which is decarboxylated by L-histidine decarboxylase (*Figure 11-13*). Histamine is synthesized throughout the body but is highly concentrated in the granules of basophils and mast cells. The physiological functions of histamine are numerous and include **allergic responses**, **cell proliferation**, **cell differentiation**, **hematopoiesis**, and neurotransmission related to **wakefulness** and **memory**. This wide array of responses to histamine is mediated by different histamine receptor types and their tissue localization.

B. One approach to manage the effects of histamine is to **inhibit the release of histamine from mast cells**. Cromolyn, the prototype for mast cell stabilizers, is marketed as an intranasal (Nasalcrom), ophthalmic (Crolom), and inhalation (Intal) product for the treatment of **allergic rhinitis**, **allergic conjunctivitis**, and **asthma**, respectively (*Figure 11-14*). Cromolyn is also available in an oral formulation (Gastrocrom) for mastocytosis. Other ophthalmic mast cell stabilizing agents for the treatment of allergic conjunctivitis include lodoxamide (Alomide), nedocromil (Alocril), and pemirolast (Alamast). The adverse effects of the mast cell stabilizers are generally related to the route of administration and include burning or irritation of the tissue.

C. **Four different histamine receptors** (i.e., H_1, H_2, H_3, and H_4) have been characterized thus far as **G protein couples receptors**. H_1 and H_2 receptors are therapeutically modulated and will be discussed further in the following. The H_3 receptor is found presynaptically in the brain and is thought to act as an autoreceptor to modulated histamine release in the CNS. The H_4 receptor is found on eosinophils, neutrophils, and CD4 T cells and has effects on the chemotactic function of eosinophils and mast cells.

1. The **H_1-receptors** mediate typical **allergic** and **anaphylactic responses** to histamine release, such as **bronchoconstriction**, **vasodilation**, **increased capillary permeability**, and **spasmodic contractions of GI smooth muscle**.

   a. **H_1-receptor antagonists** have been historically believed to competitively antagonize the receptor, but the observation that H_1-receptors have constitutive activity allows for the possibility that some of these agents act as inverse agonists rather than pure antagonists (see Chapter 58). Regardless of this pharmacological distinction, the H_1-receptor antagonists block the physiological response to histamine release, thereby limiting its effects on bronchial smooth muscle, capillaries, and GI smooth muscle. Additionally, the antagonists prevent histamine-induced pain and itching of the skin and mucous membranes; therefore, they are useful in providing **symptomatic relief of allergic symptoms** (i.e., seasonal rhinitis and conjunctivitis) or the common cold caused by **rhinoviral infections**. Their antihistaminic effects also make them useful for symptomatic **relief of urticaria**. Because of the **anticholinergic activities** of several of the H_1-receptor antagonists, some agents have utility as **antiemetics** and **anxiolytics**.

   b. The H_1-receptor antagonists, or antihistamines, are divided into **first-** and **second-generation** agents based on the sedating activities of the agents secondary to CNS access and distribution (*Figure 11-14*).

      (1) The classic, first-generation antihistamines include the chemical classes of

         (a) the **ethanolamines**: carbinoxamine (Arbinoxa, Palgic), clemastine (Tavist), diphenhydramine (Benadryl), and doxylamine (Unisom);

         (b) the **alkylamines**: brompheniramine (Dimetane, Brovex, Lodrane), chlorpheniramine (Chlor-Trimeton), dexbrompheniramine (Drixoral, Ala-Hist IR), dexchlorpheniramine (Polaramine), and triprolidine (Zymine, Actidil, Tripohist);

         (c) the **piperazine**: hydroxyzine (Atarax, Vistaril);

         (d) the **piperidine**: cyproheptadine (Periactin);

         (e) the **phenothiazine:** promethazine (Phenergan).

Study Questions

Directions: Each of the questions, statements, or incomplete statements in this section can be correctly answered or completed by **one** of the suggested answers or phrases. Choose the **best** answer.

1. A 45-year-old long-haul trucker suffers from seasonal allergies. He asks advice on which over-the counter product is best to relieve his symptoms. Which of the following choices is the best recommendation for this patient?

(A) diphenhydramine
(B) promethazine
(C) clemastine
(D) chlorpheniramine
(E) loratadine

2. Which of the following choices would be most appropriate in treating nausea and vomiting associated with motion sickness?

(A) diphenhydramine
(B) brompheniramine
(C) ondansetron
(D) omeprazole
(E) ranitidine

3. Omeprazole would *not* be effective in the treatment of

(A) gastroesophageal reflux disease.
(B) peptic ulcer disease.
(C) Zollinger-Ellison syndrome.
(D) heartburn.
(E) urticaria.

4. Which of the following antiulcer medications is most likely to cause drug interactions and endocrine side effects?

(A) ranitidine
(B) omeprazole
(C) lansoprazole
(D) cimetidine
(E) famotidine

5. A patient has just been diagnosed with recurrent migraine headaches. Which of the following preexisting conditions would preclude the use of sumatriptan for this patient?

(A) liver disease
(B) renal failure
(C) ischemic heart disease
(D) irritable bowel syndrome (IBS)
(E) gouty arthritis

6. Aspirin is best described as a(n)

(A) acetyl ester of salicylic acid.
(B) acetic acid derivative.
(C) propionic acid derivative.
(D) *N*-arylanthranilic acid derivative.
(E) enolic acid derivative.

7. Which of the following prostaglandin analogs is used specifically for the treatment of glaucoma?

(A) alprostadil
(B) latanoprost
(C) carboprost
(D) dinoprostone
(E) epoprostenol

8. The use of misoprostol to prevent nonsteroidal anti-inflammatory drug–induced ulcers could cause all of the following side effects *except*

(A) fever.
(B) gastrointestinal cramping.
(C) hypertension.
(D) headache/pain.
(E) diarrhea.

9. Which of the following asthma therapies has been associated with an acute vascular syndrome that is associated with sudden withdrawal of corticosteroid anti-inflammatory drugs?

(A) zafirlukast
(B) zileuton
(C) montelukast
(D) cetirizine
(E) ranitidine

10. Which of the following asthma therapies is effective by decreasing the amounts of released leukotrienes?

(A) zafirlukast
(B) zileuton
(C) montelukast
(D) alprostadil
(E) bimatoprost

11. Rizatriptan is effective in treating migraine headache by all of the following *except*

(A) directly vasoconstricting involved blood vessels.
(B) inhibiting the roles of inflammatory neurotransmitters.
(C) directly blocking pain transmission.
(D) inhibiting platelet aggregation.
(E) inhibiting the release of vasodilating substances.

12. Which of the following drugs, based on its mechanism of action, is effective in treating diarrhea-predominant irritable bowel syndrome (IBS)?
    (A) misoprostol
    (B) naratriptan
    (C) alosetron
    (D) cetirizine
    (E) rabeprazole

13. The second-generation antihistamines (H_1-receptor antagonists) are generally considered nonsedating because they
    (A) are more selective for H_1 receptors than the first-generation agents.
    (B) are metabolized faster than the first-generation agents.
    (C) actually function as H_1 receptor inverse agonists.
    (D) do not cross the blood–brain barrier as easily as the first-generation agents.
    (E) are only applied topically and therefore do not enter the systemic circulation.

14. Aspirin exerts its antiplatelet effect by inhibiting
    (A) cyclooxygenase (COX) 1.
    (B) COX-2.
    (C) COX-3.
    (D) prostaglandin synthesis.
    (E) leukotriene synthesis.

15. Acetaminophen has advantages over aspirin or other nonsteroidal anti-inflammatory drugs by virtue of all of the following *except*
    (A) relative lack of antiplatelet effects.
    (B) relative lack of gastrointestinal ulcerative effects.
    (C) being a safe alternative for children with viral infections.
    (D) no hepatotoxicity.
    (E) absence of adverse cardiovascular effects.

16. Acetaminophen toxicity is characterized by
    (A) profound vasoconstriction and pain.
    (B) severe abdominal cramping and diarrhea.
    (C) central nervous system stimulation and seizures.
    (D) profound liver damage and failure.
    (E) tinnitus.

17. Which of the following antigout medications is specifically used in acute attacks?
    (A) colchicine
    (B) allopurinol
    (C) probenecid
    (D) pegloticase
    (E) febuxostat

18. Which of the following antigout medications acts by decreasing serum levels but increasing urine levels of uric acid, thus increasing the risk of kidney stone development?
    (A) colchicine
    (B) allopurinol
    (C) probenecid
    (D) rasburicase
    (E) pegloticase

19. The nonsteroidal anti-inflammatory drugs, as a class, are anti-inflammatory primarily through their ability to inhibit
    (A) cyclooxygenase (COX) 1.
    (B) COX-2.
    (C) COX-3.
    (D) leukotriene synthesis.
    (E) thromboxane synthesis.

20. The selective cyclooxygenase (COX) 2 inhibitors have been associated with which of the following adverse drug reactions?
    (A) severe ischemic colitis
    (B) torsades de pointes
    (C) cardiovascular thrombotic events
    (D) acute liver failure
    (E) Churg-Strauss syndrome

21. Which of the following antihistamines is used for the treatment of emesis?
    (A) fexofenadine
    (B) doxylamine
    (C) chlorpheniramine
    (D) promethazine
    (E) desloratadine

22. Which of the following agents would produce a long-term inhibition of reduced gastric acid secretion through an irreversible mechanism?
    (A) rabeprazole
    (B) cimetidine
    (C) famotidine
    (D) nizatidine
    (E) nedocromil

23. Which of the following is an indole derivative that antagonizes the 5-HT_1-receptor?
    (A) ergotamine
    (B) sumatriptan
    (C) granisetron
    (D) buspirone
    (E) methylergonovine

24. Each of the following is classified as an NSAID *except*
    (A) piroxicam
    (B) ketorolac
    (C) oxaprozin
    (D) acetaminophen
    (E) indomethacin

25. Which one of the following side effects is the topic of a black box warning on all NSAIDs?
    (A) liver failure
    (B) asthma
    (C) cardiovascular events
    (D) nephrotoxicity
    (E) CNS depression

Answers and Explanations

1. **The answer is E** *[see VIII.C.1.b]*.
   Diphenhydramine, promethazine, and clemastine all possess moderate to strong anticholinergic activity. This will increase the risk of sedation, which could prove dangerous in this patient. Chlorpheniramine, although the least sedating of the first-generation drugs, still may cross the blood–brain barrier and cause some sedation. Loratadine, as a second-generation drug that has minimal anticholinergic activity and does not cross the blood–brain barrier (thus producing no central effects), is least likely to cause sedation and thus affect his job.

2. **The answer is A** *[see VIII.C.1.b.(2)]*.
   Although ondansetron is used for nausea associated with chemotherapy and anesthetics, it is not typically used for nausea associated with motion or vertigo. Diphenhydramine, which possesses a high degree of anticholinergic activity, is effective in reducing nausea and vomiting associated with vestibulocochlear activity, vertigo, and motion sickness. None of the other choices directly reduces nausea or vomiting; therefore, diphenhydramine is the best choice.

3. **The answer is E** *[see IX.A]*.
   Because choices A–D are all disease states that represent some action of excessive acid secretion, omeprazole, which also blocks the proton or acid pump, would be effective in reducing the acid-induced pain and damage associated with gastroesophageal reflux disease (GERD), peptic ulcer disease (PUD), Zollinger-Ellison syndrome, and heartburn. Urticaria is best treated with a H_1-receptor antagonist.

4. **The answer is D** *[see VIII.C.2.c]*.
   Of the drugs listed, and specifically, of the H_2 antagonists, cimetidine is the only drug that inhibits the hepatic microsomal metabolizing system (specifically, the 3A4 isozyme) and the only drug that exhibits weak androgenic activity. The former is responsible for numerous drug interactions and some side effects, whereas the latter is responsible for endocrine (specifically, androgen-like) side effects.

5. **The answer is C** *[see VII.C.2]*.
   Sumatriptan (and other drugs in the class) specifically causes vasoconstriction. This effect, when present in coronary vessels, can cause chest tightness or pain as a normal side effect of the drug. However, in patients with ischemic heart disease, angina, or a risk for coronary artery disease, this action could precipitate attacks of angina or potentially cause myocardial infarction and should not be used in those patients.

6. **The answer is A** *[see III.B.1–5]*.
   Aspirin is the acetyl ester of salicylic acid or a salicylate member of the NSAIDs. Diclofenac is an example of an acetic acid derivative, whereas ibuprofen is an example of a propionic acid. Meclofenamate sodium is an example of an *N*-arylanthranilic acid or fenamic acid. Meloxicam is an example of an enolic acid derivative or an oxicam.

7. **The answer is B** *[see II.D.3.b]*.
   Although most prostaglandin analogs are nonspecific in their sites of action and may produce similar physiological effects, latanoprost is specifically formulated and marketed for use in the treatment of glaucoma. The relative selectivity of latanoprost for the $PGF_2\alpha$ receptor is responsible for its ability to lower intraocular pressure and therefore its benefit in treating glaucoma.

8. **The answer is C** *[see II.D.1.c]*.
   As noted in the answer to question 7, most prostaglandin analogs have activity at receptors throughout the body, causing a prostaglandin-like effect on numerous organ systems. Misoprostol, as a relatively nonselective agonist, would cause contraction of gastrointestinal smooth muscle, stimulate pain fibers, and reset the thermoregulatory center of the CNS, thus causing all the potential side effects listed except hypertension. Hypotension is more commonly observed.

9. The answer is A *[see VI.D.2].*
Zafirlukast is the only drug that has been associated with Churg-Strauss syndrome, a condition of eosinophilic vasculitis that occurs when a patient who is on both zafirlukast and corticosteroid therapy suddenly discontinues the corticosteroid. This effect has not been observed with the pharmacologically similar drug montelukast. Note that slow withdrawal of the corticosteroid (which should be done anyway, to minimize acute adrenal insufficiency) will prevent this adverse drug reaction. Neither ranitidine nor cetirizine are indicated for the treatment of asthma.

10. The correct answer is B *[see VI.C.1].*
Zafirlukast and montelukast exert their effect by blocking leukotrienes at their receptor. Zileuton, which acts by inhibiting lipo-oxygenase, will decrease the synthesis of these inflammatory mediators. Therefore, it is the only drug listed that will decrease the synthesis and, consequently, the release of leukotrienes. Alprostadil and bimatoprost are both prostaglandin analogs.

11. The answer is D *[see VII.C.1; II.C.3].*
Rizatriptan (and other drugs in the class) are 5-HT_1-agonists. This mechanism results in three distinct and beneficial pharmacodynamic effects. First, it causes direct vasoconstriction, which returns the blood vessel to its preheadache diameter. Second, by acting on neuronal receptors, it inhibits the release of additional vasodilating and pain-transmitting substances, such as neurokinin A and substance P. Third, this action has been shown to have a direct antinociceptive action, preventing the firing of pain neurons directly. Therefore A, B, C, and E are correct answers that describe the benefit of rizatriptan. Platelet aggregation is inhibited by PGI and its analogs along with some of the NSAIDs but not by the 5-HT_1-agonists.

12. The correct answer is C *[see VII.E.2; II.D.1.b; VIII.C.1.a and b.(2)].*
Alosetron is the agent useful in treating diarrhea-predominant IBS. By blocking the 5-HT_3-receptor, it inhibits the serotonin-induced increase in intestinal motility, thus slowing peristalsis and gut movement. Naratriptan, acting as a 5-HT_1-agonist, has little effect on GI motility. Misoprostol is a PGE_1 analog that causes diarrhea. Cetirizine is a second-generation antihistamine with minimal anticholinergic activity or effects on GI motility. Rabeprazole is a proton pump inhibitor used to decrease gastric acid secretion that has little effect on GI motility.

13. The correct answer is D *[see VIII.C.1.b; VIII.C.1.b.(4)].*
The division between first- and second-generation antihistamines is the sedating properties of the first-generation agents that are a result of the antagonism of histamine receptors in the CNS. The second-generation agents do not access the CNS as easily as the first-generation agents. The second-generation agents are more selective for the H_1 receptor that reduces the anticholinergic side effects but does not affect sedation.

14. The correct answer is A *[see III.A].*
Recall that in prostaglandin and thromboxane synthesis, COX-1 is responsible for much of the daily production of maintenance eicosanoids. COX-2, while also contributing to daily production of prostaglandins and thromboxanes, is more important in inflammation. COX-3 is the debated splice variant that may be the central source of prostaglandins that contributes to CNS function of the eicosanoids. Also recall that it is thromboxane that specifically has platelet-aggregating ability. Therefore, it is through inhibition of COX-1 and the subsequent decrease in thromboxane (not prostaglandin or leukotriene) synthesis that the antiplatelet effect of aspirin is effected.

15. The correct answer is D *[see III.D; IV.D.4].*
Acetaminophen does not possess any antiplatelet activity or reduce the synthesis of gastric cytoprotective prostaglandins, so it does not interfere with platelet function or other antiplatelet therapies, and it would not be prone to cause gastric ulceration. In addition, the relationship between aspirin and Reye syndrome in children with viral infections does not apparently exist with acetaminophen, making it a safe antipyretic to use in those patients. Acetaminophen does have a significant risk of hepatotoxicity with overdose or chronic use, but, to date, no correlation to increased risk of cardiovascular disease has been identified.

16. The correct answer is D *[see IV.D.4].*
Acetaminophen toxicity is characterized by a profound hepatotoxicity, which is mediated by a reactive intermediary formed on saturation and depletion of the normal metabolic pathways. This does not affect the vasculature (as with the ergot derivatives), thus no vasoconstriction is observed. Neither is severe GI upset evident (although mild GI upset may occur early in toxicity), nor does profound CNS stimulation occur, as it does with aspirin toxicity. Tinnitus is a sign of salicylate overdose. Therefore, answer D is correct.

17. The correct answer is A *[see V.B.2].*
Allopurinol, probenecid, pegloticase, and febuxostat, although effective in preventing attacks of gouty arthritis by lowering circulating levels of uric acid, are not effective in treating the acute inflammatory situation that characterizes an acute attack. Colchicine, by inhibiting the migration of proinflammatory cells into the affected joint, will reduce the inflammatory process, thus alleviating the pain and edema associated with acute attacks of gouty arthritis.

18. **The correct answer is C** *[see V.C.3, D, and E]*.
Probenecid, as a uricosuric and promoting the excretion of uric acid, will effectively lower plasma concentration of urate. However, it also increases the urinary levels of uric acid. If this concentration exceeds the solubility constant of uric acid in the urine, then it may crystallize and precipitate out, causing stone formation or urinary lithiasis. For this reason, patients taking probenecid should always be counseled to drink copious amounts of water. Pegloticase and rasburicase are recombinant uricase enzymes that metabolize uric acid to allantoin, which is more water soluble.

19. **The correct answer is B** *[see III.A.2]*.
The roles of COX-1, -2, and -3 are reviewed in the answer to question 14. It is through their inhibition of inflammatory prostaglandin synthesis by inhibiting COX-2 that the NSAIDs exert their anti-inflammatory actions.

20. **The correct answer is C** *[see III.E.4]*.
The primary side effects that have been associated with the COX-2–specific inhibitors are gastrointestinal bleeding and, more recently, potentially fatal thrombotic events. The latter is thought to reflect a toxicodynamic effect that results from inhibition of vascular COX-2, which contributes to the daily control of platelet and/or vascular function. Severe ischemic colitis has been reported with alosetron; torsades de pointes, with older second-generation antihistaminics and cisapride, which is no longer available for use; acute liver failure, with acetaminophen overdose; and Churg-Strauss syndrome, with zafirlukast and corticosteroid withdrawal. None of these adverse drug reactions has been associated with the COX-2–specific inhibitors.

21. **The correct answer is D** *[see VIII.C.1.b.(2)]*.
Promethazine (Phenergan) is an H_1-receptor antagonist, which is useful as an antiemetic. Diphenhydramine, marketed as Dramamine, is also used as an antiemetic. Other antihistamines do not have significant antiemetic effects.

22. **The correct answer is A** *[see IX.A; VIII.C.2.a]*.
Rabeprazole is a proton pump inhibitor that works by covalently binding to the proton pump for an irreversible inhibition of acid secretion. This irreversible inhibition of the proton pump produces a longer term inhibition of gastric acid secretion compared to the H_2-receptor antagonists (i.e., cimetidine, ranitidine, famotidine, and nizatidine). Nedocromil is a mast cell stabilizer used ophthalmically for the treatment of allergic conjunctivitis, not acid reduction.

23. **The correct answer is B** *[see VII.C.1]*.
Sumatriptan (Imitrex) is a 5-HT_1-receptor agonist and indole derivative that causes direct vasoconstriction and decrease in the release of inflammatory and vasodilating substances that contributes to the efficacy of sumatriptan as a migraine headache medication. Both ergotamine and methylergonovine are ergot alkaloids that have 5-HT_1-receptor agonist activity as a contributor to its mechanism of action, but the ergotamine derivatives are not indoles. Granisetron (Kytril) is a 5-HT_3-receptor antagonist used to manage nausea and vomiting. Buspar is an anxiolytic agent that modulates the CNS serotonergic system but lacks efficacy in the treatment of migraine headaches.

24. **The answer is D** *[see IV; III.B]*.
Acetaminophen is not an NSAID because it has no anti-inflammatory properties. Acetaminophen does have antipyretic and analgesic activities similar to aspirin, the prototypical NSAID. Each of the other drugs listed are anti-inflammatory agents.

25. **The answer is C** *[see III.D.1–6; III.E.4]*.
There is an increased risk of cardiovascular events, which may include thrombotic events, myocardial infarction, or stroke, with the use of NSAIDs. This was also observed with the COX-2–specific NSAIDs. Adverse GI effects are also included in a black box warning in the NSAIDs. Each of the other side effects listed are associated with NSAID use but are not specifically addressed in a black box warning.

12

Pharmacology and Medicinal Chemistry of Endocrine and Related Drugs

MICHAEL L. ADAMS, S. THOMAS ABRAHAM

I. INTRODUCTION.

Hormones are substances secreted by specific tissues and transported via the blood to distant tissues where they exert their effects. Hormones can be obtained from natural substances (animal preparations) or they may be synthetic or semisynthetic compounds resembling the natural products. They are often used for replacement therapy (e.g., exogenous insulin for treatment of diabetes mellitus). However, they can also be used for a variety of other therapeutic and diagnostic purposes. Certain drugs (e.g., thyroid hormone inhibitors, oral antidiabetic agents) are not hormones themselves but rather influence the synthesis, secretion, or activity of hormones. Therapeutically important hormones include the pituitary hormones, the gonadal hormones, the adrenocorticosteroids, the thyroid hormones, the parathyroid hormones, and insulin. Some of these hormone systems are modified by antagonists, inhibitors, and release modifiers.

II. PITUITARY HORMONES

are synthesized in the pituitary gland. The pituitary gland is divided into two anatomical lobes called the **anterior lobe** (adenohypophysis) and the **posterior lobe** (neurohypophysis).

A. The two **posterior pituitary hormones**, oxytocin (Pitocin) and vasopressin (Pitressin), are closely related nonapeptides that differ only in two of their nine amino acids. Both oxytocin and vasopressin exert their physiological effects through distinct G protein coupled receptors.

1. **Oxytocin** (Pitocin) **stimulates uterine contraction** and plays an important role in the **induction of labor**. It is used to initiate and maintain uterine contractions in near-term pregnancies and to control postpartum bleeding or hemorrhage. Adverse effects of prolonged and excessive oxytocin administration include uterine hypertonicity with spasms, uterine or placental rupture, fluid retention, hyponatremia, heart failure, and seizures. Fetal effects such as bradycardia, neonatal jaundice, and cardiac arrhythmias have been observed.
2. **Vasopressin** (Pitressin, arginine vasopressin [AVP]) also called **antidiuretic hormone (ADH)** produces most of its effects through V1 and V2 receptors.
   a. Through V1 receptors located on the vasculature, AVP produces a potent vasoconstriction to increase blood pressure. Intravenous infusion of AVP can be useful in hypotensive conditions requiring emergency support (e.g., ventricular arrhythmias or asystole).
   b. AVP and **desmopressin** (DDAVP, Minirin, Stimate) can also activate V2 receptors in the renal collecting tubules to reduce the amount of water lost in the urine (antidiuretic function). DDAVP is a **vasopressin analog** that has been modified at the N-terminal and by the replacement of L-arginine with D-arginine at position 8. These modifications increase the oral and nasal bioavailability, duration of action, and provide selectivity for V2 receptors over

V1 receptors. Both AVP and DDAVP can be used to treat central **diabetes insipidus**, **nocturnal enuresis** (bed wetting), and manage bleeding in hemophilia A patients.

c. The most likely adverse effects of AVP and DDAVP use are headaches, nausea, gastrointestinal (GI) cramps, central nervous system (CNS) agitation, and allergic reactions. AVP may also increase blood pressure and increase the likelihood of cardiovascular events and strokes.

d. The **vasopressin antagonists** conivaptan (Vaprisol) and tolvaptan (Samsca) are used to **manage conditions where excessive AVP** is involved in pathological conditions. Conivaptan is a V1/V2 antagonist that is administered intravenously, whereas tolvaptan is an orally active, selective V2 antagonist. These agents are used primarily to control hyponatremia secondary to hypovolemic states such as congestive heart failure and hepatic cirrhosis. A specific use of these agents is in the management of syndrome of inappropriate ADH where excessive AVP is released by the posterior pituitary.

e. Adverse effects associated with conivaptan and tolvaptan are headache, constipation, diarrhea, thirst, fever, and polyuria. Additionally, conivaptan can cause severe injection site reactions and phlebitis.

B. The **anterior pituitary hormones** are required for the maintenance of **thyroid function**, **adrenal function**, and **ovulation** (gonadotropins).

1. **Adrenocorticotropic hormone** (ACTH) is a 39-amino acid polypeptide that stimulates the adrenal cortex to produce and secrete adrenocorticosteroids (see section IV). The activity of ACTH is mimicked by corticotropin (Acthar HP), which can be used as a diagnostic agent to test adrenocortical function and differentiate between primary and secondary adrenal insufficiency. Adverse effects of corticotropin are rare but include hypersensitivity and corticosteroid excess.

2. **Thyroid-stimulating hormone** (TSH) is a protein with a molecular weight of 28,000 Da that stimulates the thyroid to produce T_4 and T_3 (see section V). Thyrotropin-α (Thyrogen) is human recombinant TSH that is used diagnostically with thyroglobulin and radioiodine imaging to monitor thyroid cancer. Adverse effects are similar to hyperthyroid symptoms.

3. **Growth hormone**, also called **somatropin**, is a protein of 191 amino acids that stimulates protein, carbohydrate, and lipid metabolism to promote increased cell, organ, connective tissue, and skeletal growth, causing a rapid increase in the overall rate of linear growth. Somatropin (Genotropin, Humatrope, Norditropin, Nutropin, Omnitrope, Saizen, Serostim, Tev-tropin, Valtropin, Zorbtive) is indicated for long-term treatment of children whose **growth failure** is the result of **lack of endogenous growth hormone secretion**. Adverse effects are limited to the formation of nonbinding antibodies to growth hormone but antibody development does not interfere with continued use.

4. **Anterior pituitary gonadotropins** include **follicle-stimulating hormone** (FSH), **luteinizing hormone** (LH), and **prolactin** or **luteotropic hormone** (LTH). Only recombinant FSH is used therapeutically; however, several related nonpituitary gonadotropins have FSH-like or LH-like actions. These include the following agents that can be used to induce ovulation.

a. **Menotropins** (Menopur, Repronex), also known as human menopausal gonadotropin (hMG), are **high in FSH-like** and **LH-like activity** and are obtained from the urine of postmenopausal women. In men, menotropins are used to induce spermatogenesis.

b. **Urofollitropin** (Bravelle) is obtained from the urine of postmenopausal women and has **significant FSH-like activity**. Two recombinant DNA forms, follitropin alfa (Gonal-f) and follitropin beta (Follistim AQ), are also available. These agents can also **induce spermatogenesis** in men.

c. **Human chorionic gonadotropin** (Novarel, Pregnyl), produced by the placenta, is isolated from the urine of pregnant females, and choriogonadotropin alfa (Ovidrel) is recombinant human chorionic gonadotropin. Human chorionic gonadotropin is indicated for the treatment of some cases of **hypogonadism** in males in addition to **inducing ovulation**. The presence of human chorionic gonadotropin in the urine is the basis for home pregnancy tests.

III. GONADAL HORMONES

are hormones produced in the gonads (i.e., ovary or testis). Most natural and synthetic gonadal hormones are derivatives of **cyclopentanoperhydrophenanthrene** with various changes in strategic positions (*Figure 12.1*). The steroid hormones contain this 17-carbon fused-ring system that uses a common numbering system.

A. **Estrogens** are the female sex hormones responsible for the development of female sex organs and secondary sexual characteristics.

1. Both **natural** and **semisynthetic estrogens** are marketed for clinical use. The basic nucleus of the natural estrogens has a methyl group designated as C-18 on position C-13 of the

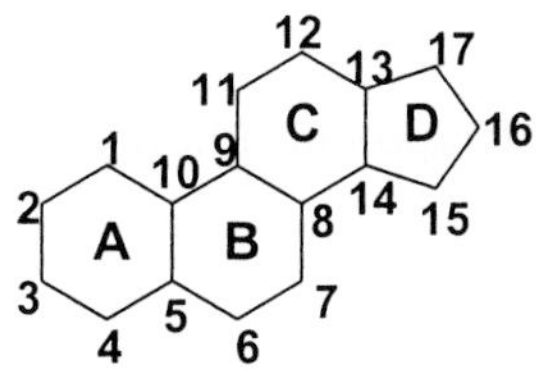

Figure 12-1. Structural formula of cyclopentanoperhydrophenanthrene, from which the gonadal hormones are derived. *A–D* rings, which may be modified during subsequent conversions; *1–17*, carbon atom positions on the rings.

cyclopentanoperhydrophenanthrene and is known as estrane. Unlike other steroid hormones, **all estrogens have an aromatic A-ring** (*Figure 12-2*).

a. **Estradiol**, the principal estrogenic hormone, exists in the body in equilibrium with estrone, which is converted to estriol before excretion (*Figure 12-2*).
b. The various routes of administration for estradiol include oral (Estrace), vaginal cream (Estrace), vaginal ring (Estring, Femring), vaginal tablet (Vagifem), transdermal patch (Climara, Estraderm, Alora), and topical emulsion (Estrasorb) or gel (Estrogel, Divigel). Estradiol is **only weakly active when administered orally due to extensive first-pass metabolism**.
c. Several synthetic estradiol esters, such as estradiol cypionate (Depo-Estradiol) and estradiol valerate (Delestrogen) (*Figure 12-3*), are prepared as intramuscular injections in oil to prolong their action. These estradiol esters are slowly absorbed into the circulation, hydrolyzed to estradiol to act on the target tissue. Before hydrolysis, these compounds do not have estrogenic activity and thus are considered to be prodrugs. Another prodrug, estradiol acetate, is available for oral (Femtrace) and vaginal ring (Femtrace) administration.
d. The addition of a 17 α-ethinyl to estradiol increases resistance to first-pass metabolism and enhances oral effectiveness. The estradiol derivatives, ethinyl estradiol and its 3-methyl ether mestranol, are used principally as the estrogenic components of serial-type oral contraceptives (*Figure 12-4*). Mestranol is a prodrug and is metabolized to ethinyl estradiol after its oral administration.
e. Conjugated estrogens or esterified estrogens are a mixture of estrogen metabolites, most often estrogen sulfates from plant or animal sources, that can be administered orally. Brand names included in this class are Premarin, Cenestin, Menest, and Enjuvia. Estropipate (Ogen) is a single-component conjugated estrogen sulfate.

2. Estrogens exert their actions through ERα- and ERβ-type **estrogen receptors** in estrogen-responsive tissues (e.g., vagina, uterus, mammary glands, anterior pituitary, hypothalamus). The estrogen receptors are localized in the nucleus bound to stabilizing proteins. When estrogen or an estrogen analog binds to the estrogen receptor, the receptor forms a dimer that increases its affinity for DNA, and increases the expression of specific genes. This ultimately leads to an increase in protein synthesis and a biological response.
3. The **therapeutic indications** for the estrogens vary and include the following:
   a. **Oral contraceptives** (in combination with progestins)
   b. **Treatment of menopausal symptoms** including vasomotor disorder, vaginal dryness, urogenital atrophy, and psychological disorder. It is not recommended to use estrogens, with or without progestins, for the prevention of cardiovascular disease or dementia.
   c. **Acne**
   d. **Osteoporosis**, both senile and postmenopausal osteoporosis

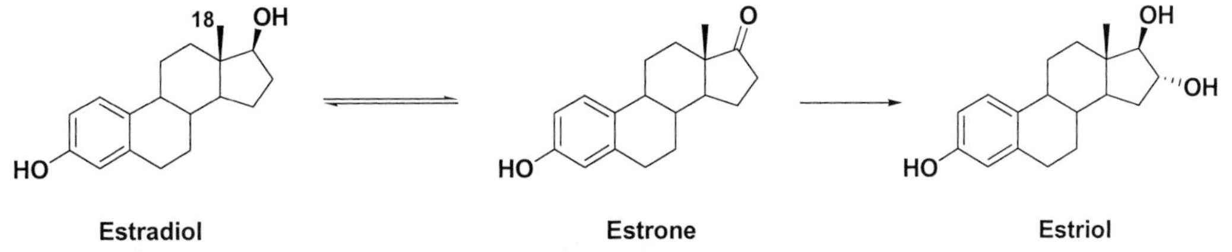

Figure 12-2. Structural formula of estradiol, which exists in the body in equilibrium with estrone, which in turn is converted to estriol before excretion.

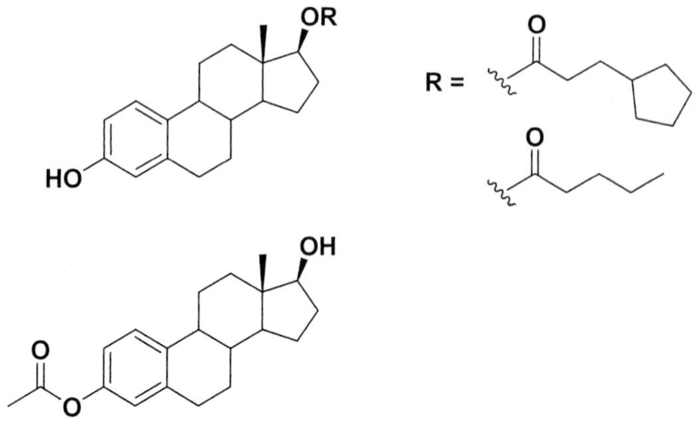

Cypionate (Depo-estradiol)

Valerate (Delestrogen)

Estradiol acetate

Figure 12-3. Structural formulas of estradiol cypionate (Depo-Estradiol), estradiol valerate (Delestrogen), and estradiol acetate.

4. The adverse effects from the pharmacological use of estrogens include the following:
   a. **GI effects**, including GI distress, nausea, vomiting, anorexia, and diarrhea.
   b. **Cardiovascular effects**, including hypertension and an increased incidence of thromboembolic diseases, stroke, and myocardial infarction.
   c. **Fluid and electrolyte disturbances**, including increased fluid retention and increased triglyceride levels.
   d. An increased incidence of endometrial cancer and hepatic adenomas (associated with long-term use).

B. **Antiestrogens** antagonize the effects of estrogens at various tissues.
   1. The **nonsteroidal antiestrogens** (i.e., **estrogen antagonists**) clomiphene (Clomid), tamoxifen (Nolvadex), and toremifene (Fareston) are triphenylethylene derivatives with an important basic amine side chain (*Figure 12-5*). These agents are structurally related to nonsteroidal synthetic estrogens with a stilbene-like structure. Raloxifene (Evista) is a benzothiophene with structural similarity to the triphenylethylethylene derivatives and fulvestrant (Faslodex) is a potent steroidal antiestrogen (*Figure 12-5*). Except for fulvestrant, these behave as agonists or antagonists of estrogen response, depending on the site of action and are often called selective estrogen response modifiers. Fulvestrant appears to behave as a pure estrogen receptor antagonist regardless of the tissue or organ.
   2. Pharmacology
      a. **Tamoxifen** and **toremifene** are predominantly **estrogen antagonists** and inhibit the action of estrogens by competitively binding to estrogen receptors in **breast tissue**. These agents have a **weak estrogen agonist effect on the endometrium, bone, and lipid levels.**
      b. **Clomiphene** has **estrogenic and antiestrogenic activity** and **induces ovulation** by causing an increase in the secretion of the pituitary gonadotropins FSH and LH.
      c. **Raloxifene** has estrogenic activities and antiestrogenic activities at certain tissues. Raloxifene is an **agonist in bone** and **antagonist in uterine and breast tissue**.
      d. Fulvestrant inhibits the action of estrogen by competitively binding to estrogen receptors and preventing estrogen-like responses to receptor binding (i.e., changes in gene expression).

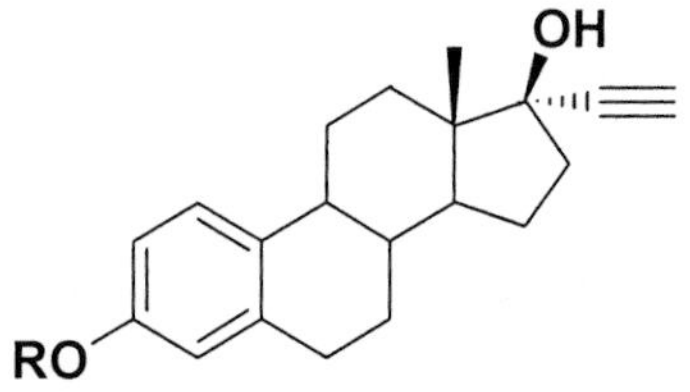

R = H, Ethinyl estradiol
R = CH_3, Mestranol

Figure 12-4. Structural formulas of ethinyl estradiol and mestranol.

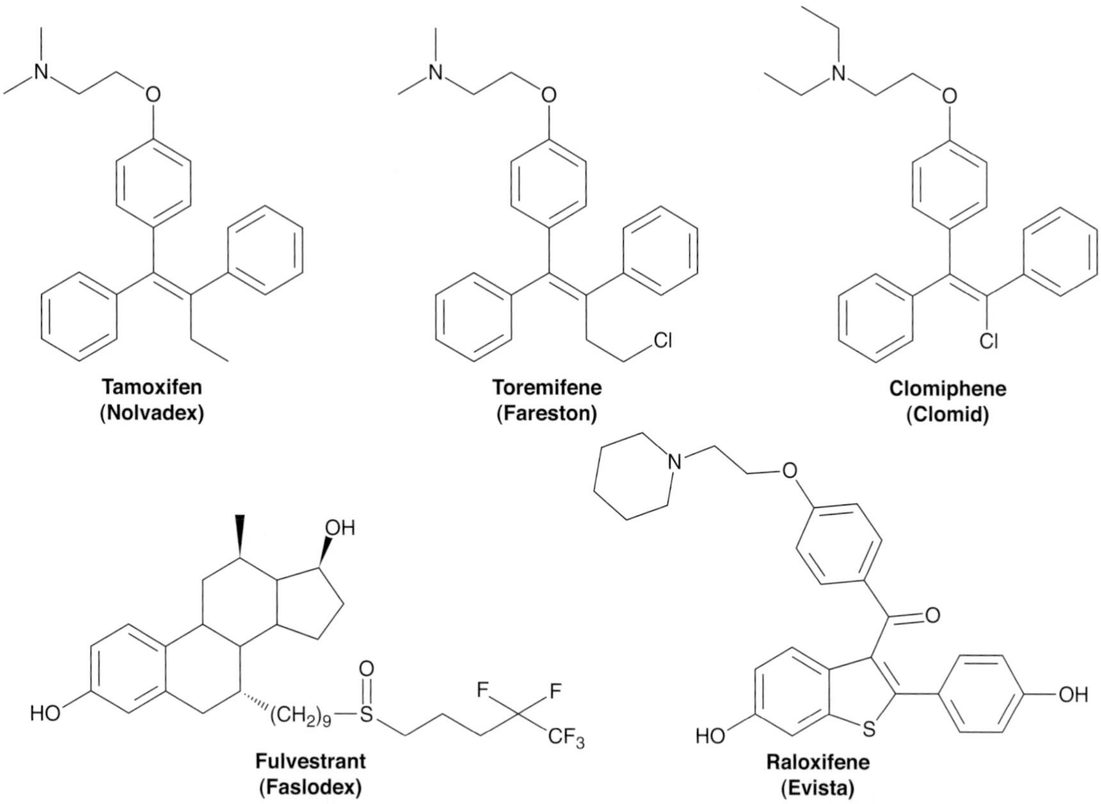

Figure 12-5. Structural formulas of the antiestrogens tamoxifen, toremifene, clomiphene, raloxifene, and fulvestrant. Clomiphene, tamoxifen, toremifene, and raloxifene are structurally similar, whereas fulvestrant is a larger and more lipid-soluble analog of estradiol. Raloxifene is a SERM used to treat osteoporosis.

3. Therapeutic indications
   a. Tamoxifen, toremifene, and fulvestrant are used to treat **estrogen-dependent breast cancer**.
   b. Clomiphene is used to **induce ovulation** in women who have ovulation failure.
   c. Raloxifen is used to **treat and prevent osteoporosis** in postmenopausal women.
4. Adverse effects of the antiestrogens include hot flashes, nausea, and vomiting.

C. **Aromatase inhibitors** decrease endogenous estrogen synthesis. Aromatase, a cytochrome P450 enzyme, is responsible for generating the **aromatic A-ring** that distinguishes estrogen from the progesterones and androgens (e.g., androstenedione and testosterone). Inhibition of aromatase dramatically **decreases the amounts of estrogen in circulation.**
1. Anastrozole (Arimidex) and letrozole (Femara) are potent and selective triazole containing **nonsteroidal inhibitors of aromatase** (*Figure 12-6*). Exemestane (Aromasin) is the **only steroidal irreversible inhibitor of aromatase.**
2. Aromatase inhibitors are indicated for the treatment of **advanced estrogen-dependent breast cancer.**
3. Adverse effects are similar to the antiestrogens, including hot flashes.

D. **Progestins.** Endogenous progestins are produced by the corpus luteum after normal ovulation to prevent further ovulation and maintain pregnancy if fertilization occurs.
1. The naturally occurring progestin progesterone is a C-21 steroid. Its basic nucleus is known as pregnane (*Figure 12-7*). The routes of administration for progesterone include oral, vaginal gel, and intramuscular injection. Progesterone has a half-life of 5 to 10 mins because of rapid liver metabolism at C-5 and C-20.
2. Synthetic steroidal progestins have structural features that hinder metabolism at C-5 and C-20. They consist of three types:
   a. The 17α-hydroxyprogesterone derivatives (e.g., medroxyprogesterone acetate [Provera, Depo-Provera], megestrol acetate [Megace]) typically introduce a methyl group at position

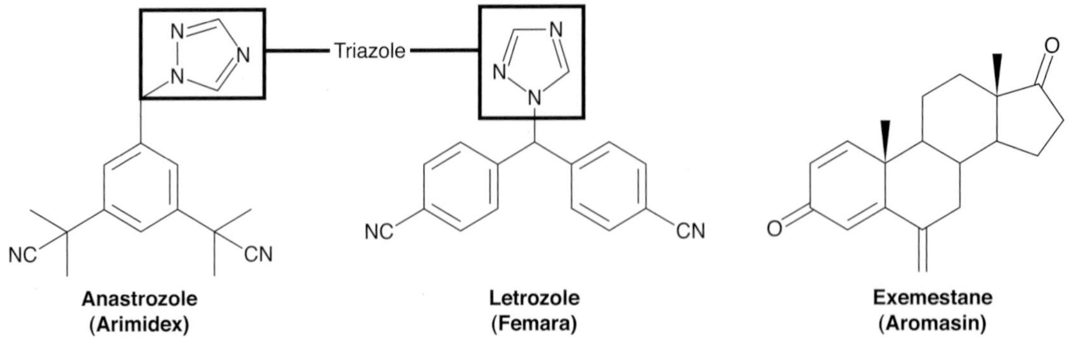

Figure 12-6. Structures of the triazole containing aromatase inhibitors anastrozole and letrozole and the only steroid-based aromatase inhibitor, exemestane.

C-6 of progesterone and an acetoxyl group at position C-17. These substitutions **increase lipid solubility** and **decrease first-pass metabolism**, enhancing oral activity and the progestin effect (*Figure 12-8*).

b. The second group of progestins is 19-nortestosterone derivatives (17α-ethinylandrogens). They are structurally classified as androgens because they lack the 19-methyl group. Although these compounds have progestational and androgenic activity, their primary activity is progestational.

(1) The absence of the 19-methyl group increases progestational activity.

(2) The 17α-ethinylandrogens are **more lipid soluble** than progesterone and undergo **less first-pass metabolism**. The 17α-ethinyl substituent increases progestational activity relative to androgenic activity in addition to **blocking metabolism at C-17** as with ethinyl estradiol.

(3) These agents, with a **17α-ethinyl group**, have **potent oral activity** and are extensively used as **oral contraceptives** in combination with ethinyl estradiol (*Figure 12-9*). Other orally active 17α-ethinylandrogens include the positional isomer of norethindrone, norethindrone acetate, norethynodrel, its 18-methyl homolog norgestrel, and its 3,17-diacetate analog ethynodiol diacetate. Norgestimate is an orally active 3-oxime prodrug that is metabolically deacetylated and oxidized to norgestrel. Desogestrel is a prodrug that is metabolically oxidized to the 3-ketone.

(4) Norelgestromin (Ortho-Evra) and etonogestrel (NuvaRing) are also used as contraceptive agents given in combination with ethinyl estradiol (*Figure 12-9*). Norelgestromin is administered as a **transdermal patch** to **avoid first-pass metabolism**, and etonogestrel is formulated in a vaginal ring.

c. Drospirenone is a progestin that is structurally different from the other progestins in that it is a structural analog of the aldosterone antagonist spironolactone with minimal androgenic activity. Drospirenone is used in the oral contraceptive agents Yasmin and Yaz in combination with ethinyl estradiol or estradiol, respectively (*Figure 12-9*).

3. The mechanism of action of progestins is similar to estrogen. Progestins bind to nuclear progesterone receptors that dimerize to bind to the DNA in progestin-responsive tissues. The formation of the progestin-receptor complex results in an increase in the synthesis of mRNA and specific enzyme or protein synthesis.

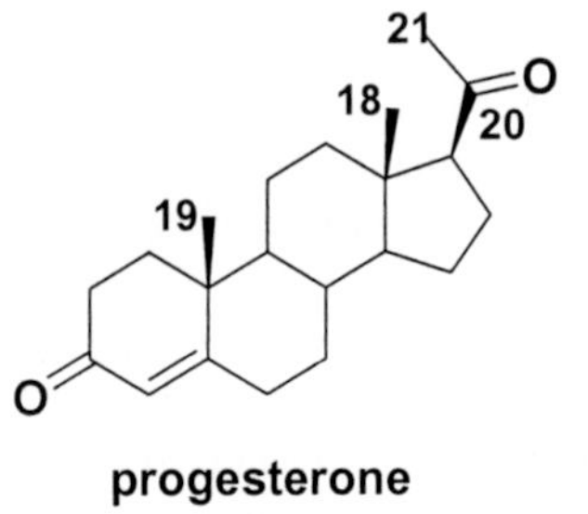

Figure 12-7. Structural formula of progesterone, which is a derivative of pregnane.

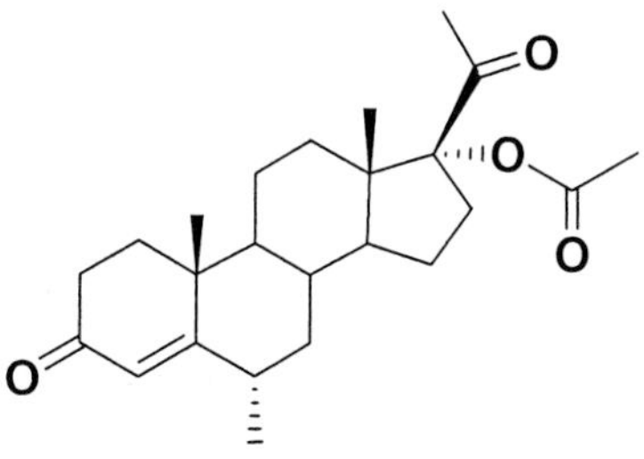

Medroxyprogesterone acetate

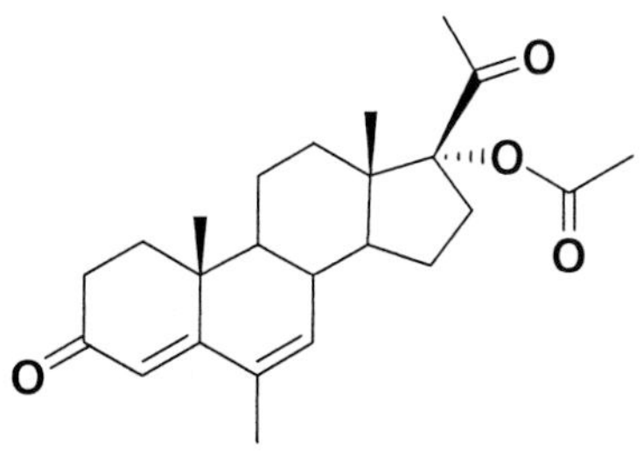

Megestrol acetate

Figure 12-8. Structural formulas of medroxyprogesterone acetate (Provera) and megestrol acetate (Megace), synthetic progestins.

4. Progestins have various therapeutic uses.
   a. The progestins are predominantly used as **oral contraceptive agents**. Progestins can be given alone (progestin only such as norethindrone acetate) or in combination with estrogens as monophasic, biphasic, and triphasic combinations. Extended oral contraception (Seasonale, Seasonique) is also available for a 91-day cycle.
   b. Progestins are also used for **emergency contraception** in the form of levonorgestrel (Plan B) and levonorgestrel with ethinyl estradiol (Preven).
   c. **Endometriosis** and **menstrual disorders** including dysfunctional uterine bleeding and dysmenorrhea can also be treated with progestins.
5. Adverse effects of the progestins include irregular menses, breakthrough bleeding, amenorrhea, weight gain, edema, and exacerbation of breast carcinoma.

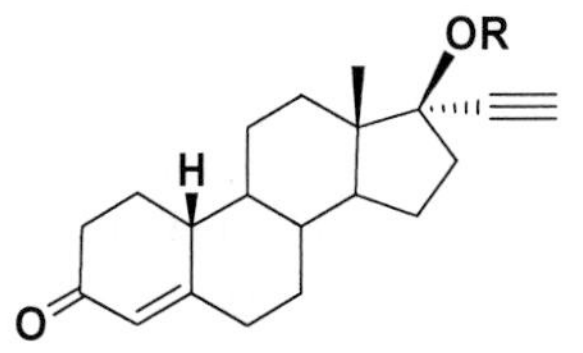

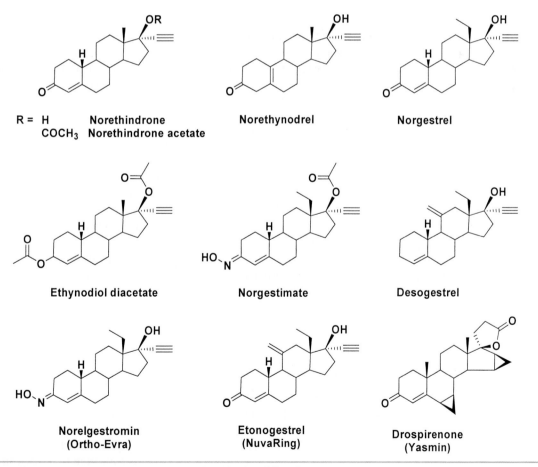

R = H Norethindrone
$COCH_3$ Norethindrone acetate

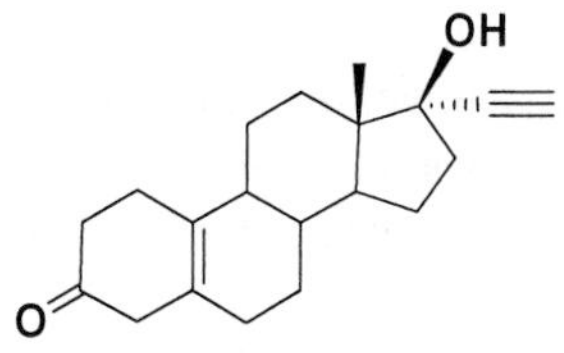

Norethynodrel

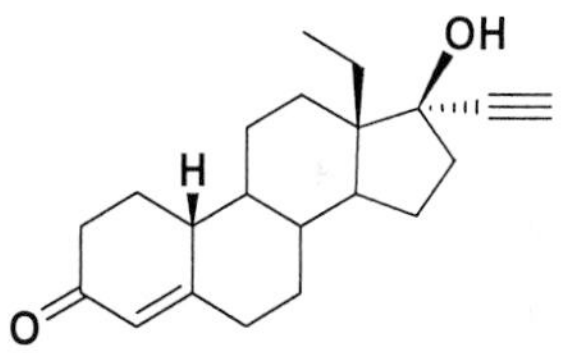

Norgestrel

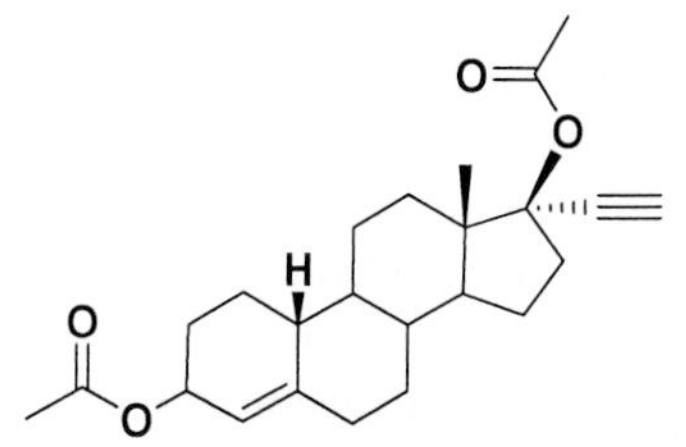

Ethynodiol diacetate

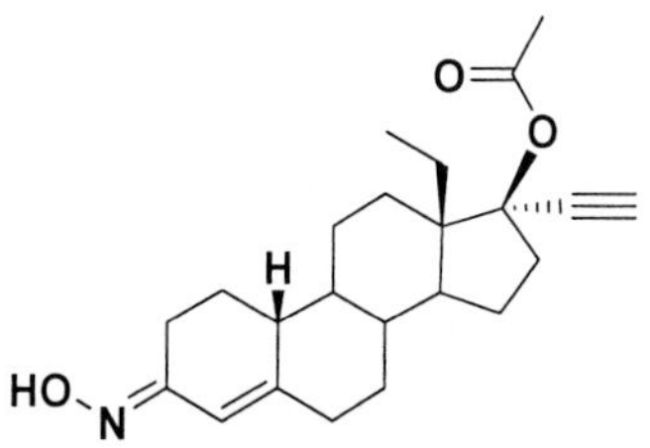

Norgestimate

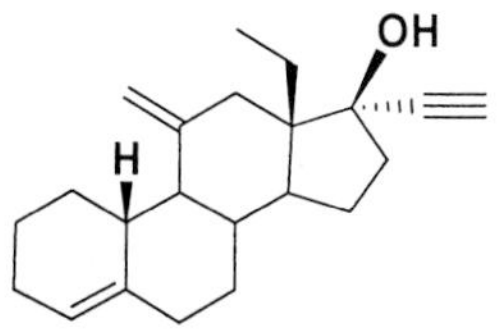

Desogestrel

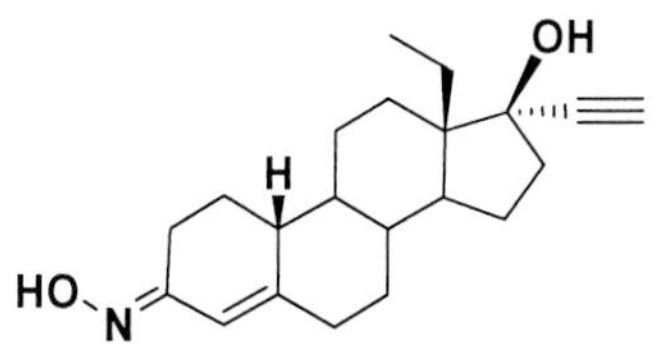

Norelgestromin (Ortho-Evra)

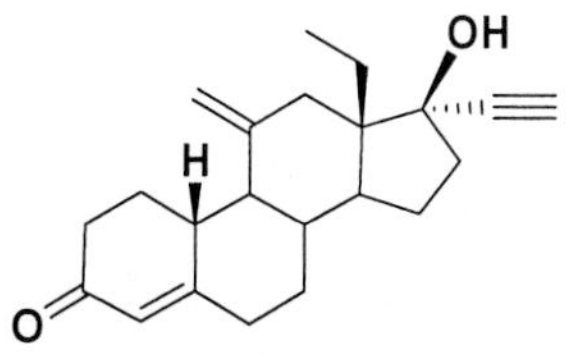

Etonogestrel (NuvaRing)

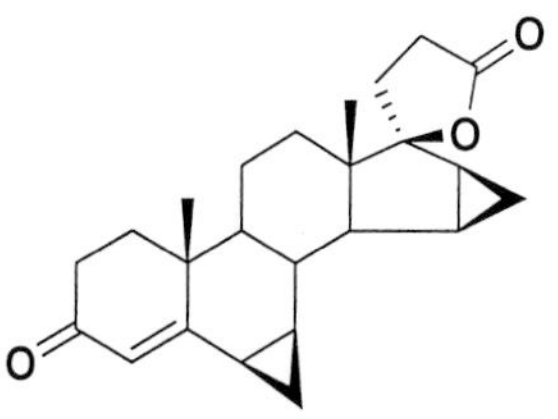

Drospirenone (Yasmin)

Figure 12-9. Structural formulas of norethindrone, norethindrone acetate, norethynodrel, norgestrel, ethynodiol diacetate, norgestimate, desogestrel, norelgestromin, etonogestrel, and drospirenone.

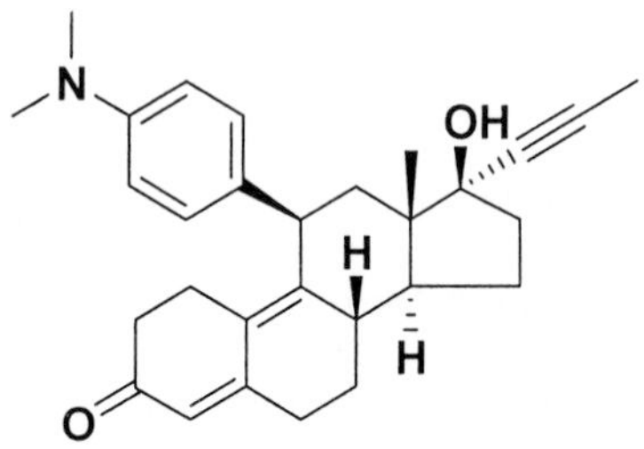

Figure 12-10. Structural formula of the antiprogestin mifepristone (Mifeprex).

E. **Antiprogestins** antagonize the effects of endogenous progestins.

1. Mifepristone (Mifeprex) is a **steroidal progestin receptor antagonist** that can be used to medically terminate pregnancy through 49 days (*Figure 12-10*). At 2 days after administration of mifepristone, a health care provider will administer the prostaglandin E_1 (PGE_1) analog misoprostol.
2. Mifepristone inhibits the action of progestins by competitively binding to progestin receptors. Misoprostol induces uterine contractions. This activity is used to terminate intrauterine pregnancy.
3. Adverse effects include the expected vaginal bleeding and uterine cramping but vaginal bleeding is generally heavier than a menstrual period. Additional adverse effects include nausea, vomiting, and diarrhea.

F. **Androgens and anabolic steroids.** Androgens are responsible for the development and maintenance of the male sex organs and secondary male characteristics including deep voice, and growth of hair on face, arms, legs, and pubic areas. Androgens also have anabolic activities that result in increased tissue growth including bone and muscle. The anabolic steroids have a much greater capacity to increase tissue growth (i.e., muscle) than the natural androgens.

1. The primary natural androgen is **testosterone**, a C-19 steroid with various routes of administration (buccal [Striant], transdermal gel [AndroGel, Fortesta, Testim], transdermal patch [Androderm], subcutaneous pellets [Testopel], intramuscular [Depo-Testosterone]) (*Figure 12-11*). **Testosterone has two physiological effects: androgenic and anabolic effects.**
   a. Compounds used for **androgenic** effects
      (1) Esters of testosterone, such as testosterone 17-enanthate (Delatestryl) and testosterone cypionate (Depo-Testosterone), are prodrugs and provide increased duration of action when administered intramuscularly owing to slow absorption and ester hydrolysis to the active testosterone (*Figure 12-12*).
      (2) Introduction of a 17α-methyl group results in potent, orally active androgens, such as methyltestosterone (Android, Testred) and fluoxymesterone (Androxy) (*Figure 12-12*). The **17α-methyl group decreases first-pass oxidative metabolism** to the 17-ketone.
   b. Compounds used for anabolic effects include drugs resulting from structural modifications of testosterone. These drugs have a **much enhanced anabolic-androgenic activity ratio** and a 17α-methyl group providing **oral activity** (e.g., oxymetholone [Anadrol-50], oxandrolone [oral-Oxandrin]; *Figure 12-13*).

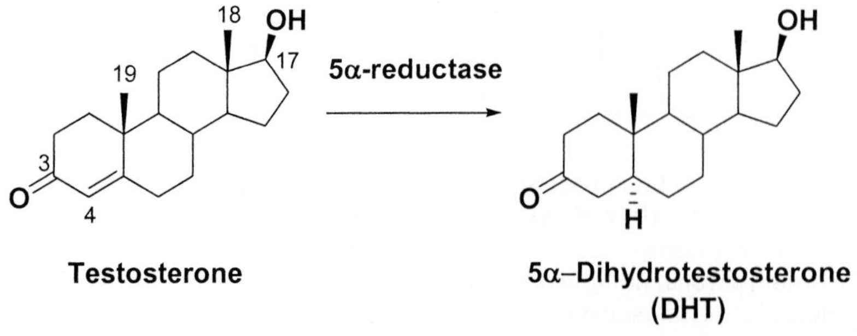

Figure 12-11. Testosterone is converted to 5α-dihydroxy-testosterone (DHT) by the enzyme 5α-reductase.

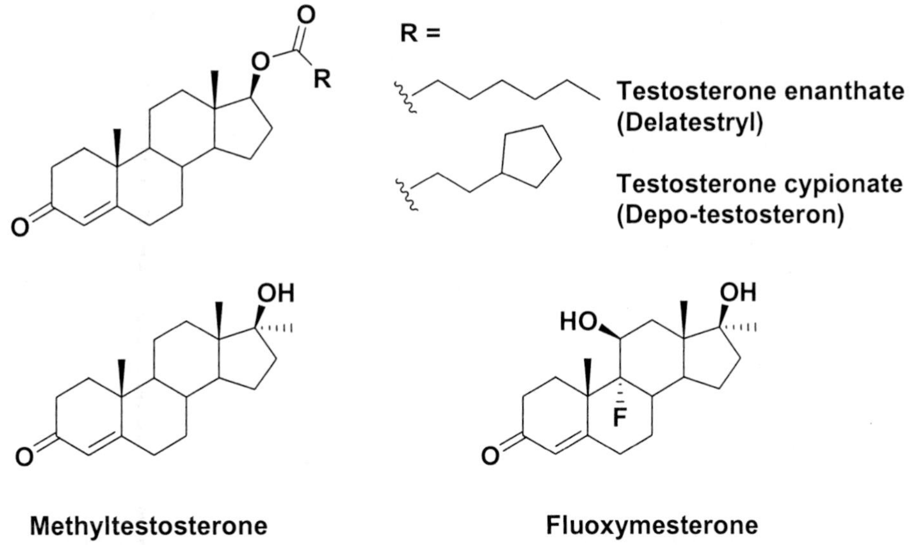

Figure 12-12. Structural formulas of testosterone enanthate, testosterone cypionate, methyltestosterone, and fluoxymesterone.

c. Danazol (Danocrine), a weak androgen, suppresses the pituitary–ovarian axis (i.e., LH and FSH release) and is used for treatment of **endometriosis** and **fibrocystic breast disease** (*Figure 12-13*). The 17α-ethinyl group provides for **oral bioavailability**.

2. The mechanism of action of androgens is similar to that of estrogen. Testosterone is converted to **5α-dihydroxytestosterone** (DHT) in the cytoplasm of androgen-responsive tissue by the enzyme **5α-reductase** (*Figure 12-11*). **DHT binds** to the cytoplasmic androgen receptor **with higher affinity** than testosterone and also acts as an agonist. The formation of androgen-receptor complex results in translocation to the nucleus and an increase in the synthesis of mRNA and eventually protein synthesis.
3. The androgens are used for **androgen-replacement therapy**, **breast cancer**, **endometriosis**, **female hypopituitarism** (with estrogen therapy), **anabolic therapy**, and **anemia**.
4. The adverse effects of the androgens include fluid retention, increased low density lipoprotein (LDL), decreased high density lipoprotein (HDL), psychological changes, liver disorders, decreased male fertility (i.e., **azoospermia**), and development of masculine features in the female.

G. **Antiandrogens** antagonize the effects of endogenous testosterone or DHT.

1. Most of the antiandrogens are **nonsteroidal** in nature. They include flutamide (Eulexin), bicalutamide (Casodex), and nilutamide (Nilandron) (*Figure 12-14*).
2. Flutamide, bicalutamide, and nilutamide inhibit the action of androgens by **competitively binding to the androgen receptors** and acting as **antagonists** in the target tissue.

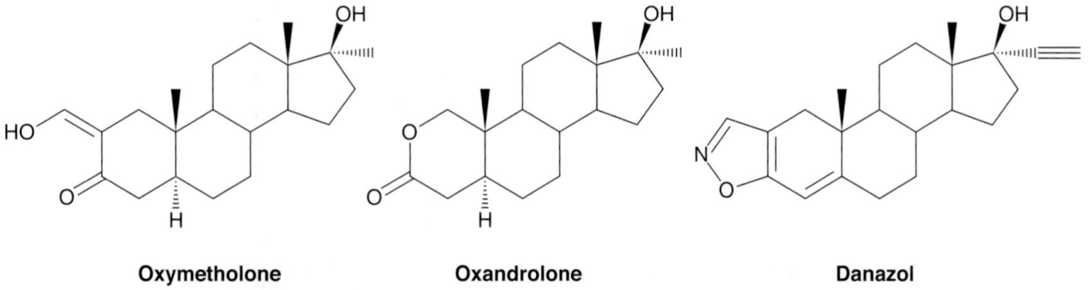

Figure 12-13. Structural formulas of the anabolic steroids oxymetholone, and oxandrolone, and the weak androgen danazol.

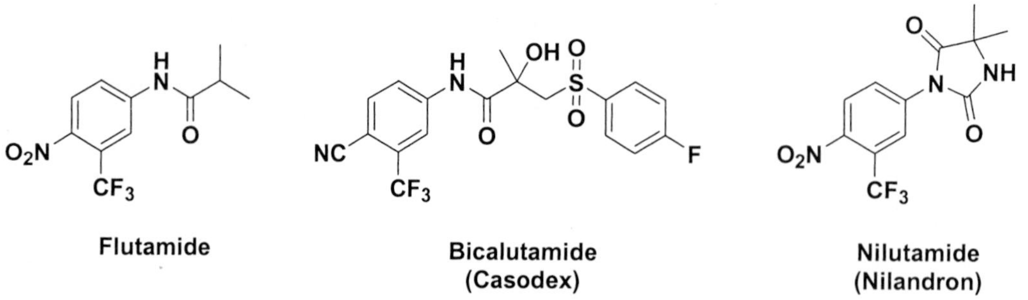

Figure 12-14. Structures of the antiandrogens flutamide, bicalutamide, and nilutamide.

3. The antiandrogens are used to treat **prostate cancer**. Flutamide and bicalutamide are given in combination with luteinizing hormone-releasing hormone (LHRH) agonists.

H. **5α-Reductase inhibitors** decrease the synthesis of the potent tissue androgen DHT.

1. Finasteride (Proscar, Propecia) and dutasteride (Avodart; *Figure 12-15*) are **competitive inhibitors of the 5α-reductase**, the enzyme in target tissues that converts testosterone to the potent androgen DHT.
2. The 5α-reductase inhibitors are used to treat **benign prostatic hyperplasia** (BPH). Finasteride, marketed as Propecia, is used for **androgenic alopecia** at one-fifth the dose used in BPH.

IV. ADRENOCORTICOSTEROIDS

ADRENOCORTICOSTEROIDS are synthesized in the adrenal cortex. Adrenocorticosteroids are divided into two classes, **mineralocorticoids** and **glucocorticoids**, based on their physiological activities. Most naturally occurring adrenocorticosteroids have some degree of both mineralocorticoid and glucocorticoid activity. All adrenocorticosteroids are derived from the C-21 pregnane nucleus.

A. **Mineralocorticoids** cause the **retention of sodium** and the **excretion of potassium** in the kidney. **Aldosterone** is the endogenous, prototypical mineralocorticoid, which is formed in the outer (glomerular) layer of the adrenal cortex.

1. Mineralocorticoids act by binding to **cytoplasmic receptors** that are then translocated to the nucleus to stimulate the production of mineralocorticoid-responsive mRNA to change the expression of target proteins. The mineralocorticoids also act in the feedback regulation of pituitary corticotropin.
2. **Fludrocortisone** acetate (Florinef) has significant **mineralocorticoid activity** and it is therefore used to treat **Addison's disease** (*Figure 12-16*).
3. Mineralocorticoid receptor antagonists, **spironolactone** (Aldactone) and **eplerenone** (Inspra), are **steroidal aldosterone-receptor (mineralocorticoid) antagonists** used to treat cardiovascular disorders (see Chapter 10).

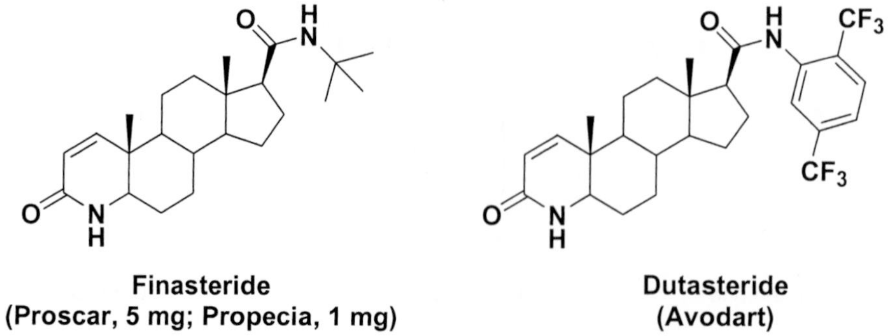

Figure 12-15. Structures of 5α-reductase inhibitors finasteride and dutasteride.

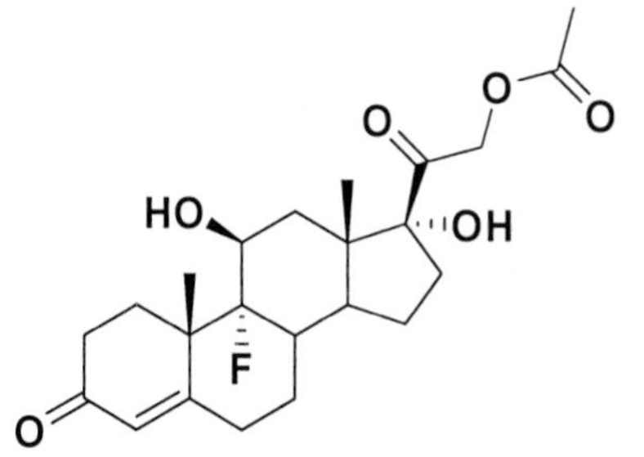

Fludrocortisone Acetate

Figure 12-16. Structural formula of fludrocortisone acetate, the clinically useful mineralocorticoid.

B. Glucocorticoids have anti-inflammatory, protein-catabolic, and immunosuppressant effects.

1. **Cortisone** and **hydrocortisone** (Cortisol), the **prototypical glucocorticoids**, are formed in the middle (fascicular) layer of the adrenal cortex (*Figure 12-17*).
   a. The 17β-ketol side chain (-COCH2OH), the 4-ene, and the 3-ketone structures are found in all clinically useful adrenocorticosteroids (*Figure 12-17*).
   b. Many natural, semisynthetic, and synthetic glucocorticoids are available. Modifications of the prototypes cortisone and hydrocortisone represent attempts to **increase glucocorticoid activity** while **decreasing mineralocorticoid activity**.

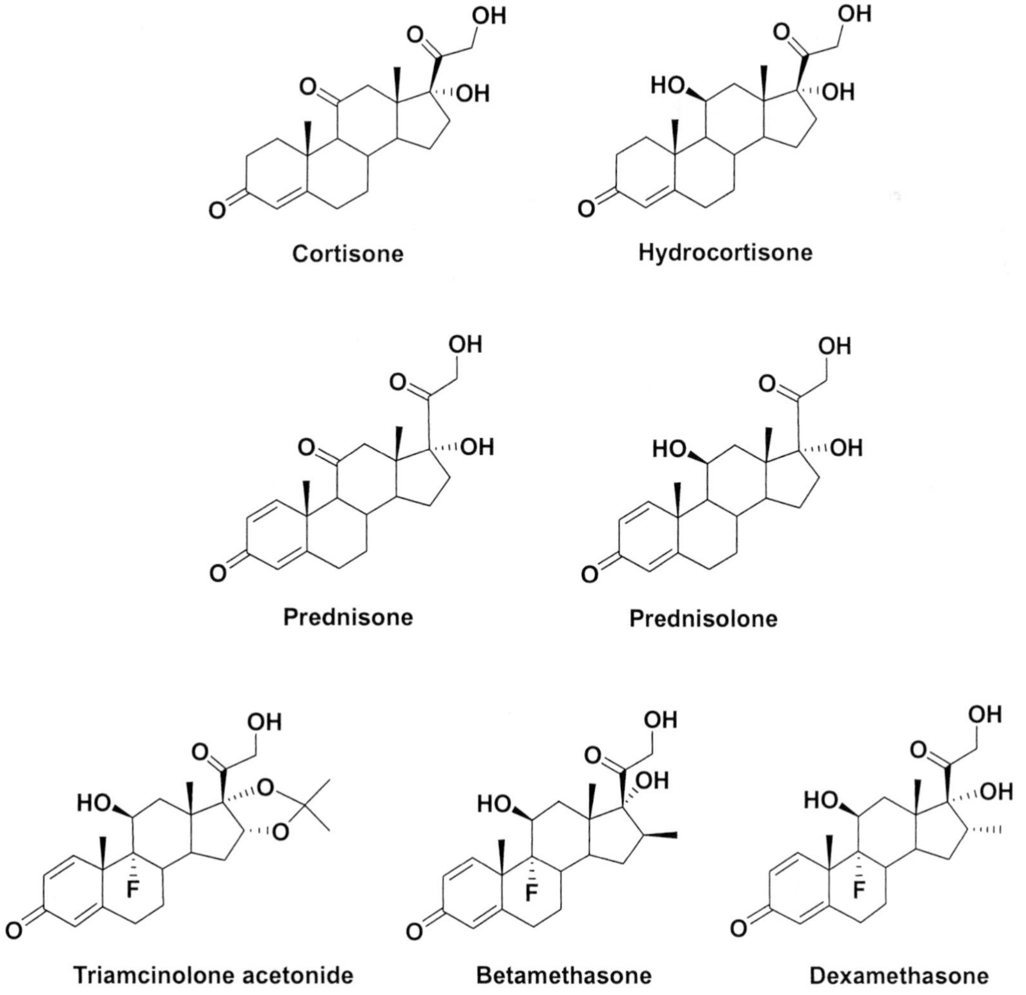

Figure 12-17. Structural formulas of cortisone, hydrocortisone, prednisone, prednisolone, triamcinolone acetonide, betamethasone, and dexamethasone.

(1) The **oxygen atom at position C-11** is essential for glucocorticoid activity.

(2) A **double bond between positions C-1 and C-2** increases glucocorticoid activity without increasing mineralocorticoid activity as with prednisone (Deltasone) and prednisolone (Delta-Cortef; *Figure 12-17*).

(3) Fluorination at position **C-9 greatly increases both mineralocorticoid** and **glucocorticoid activity**, as with fludrocortisone (*Figure 12-16*); whereas fluorination at position **C-6 increases glucocorticoid activity** with less effect on mineralocorticoid activity (*Figure 12-17*).

(4) A **17α-hydroxyl group** in combination with either a **16α-hydroxyl group** forming an acetonide, as with triamcinolone, or a 16-methyl group, as with betamethasone or dexamethasone, enhances glucocorticoid activity and abolishes mineralocorticoid activity (*Figure 12-17*).

2. The cellular activity of the glucocorticoids is exactly as the mineralocorticoids (see previous section) except they bind to the glucocorticoid receptors. The therapeutic uses of the glucocorticoids include **metabolic**, **anti-inflammatory**, and **immunosuppressive** activities. More specifically, glucocorticoids are useful for the last resort management of severe, disabling arthritis; severe allergic reactions; seasonal allergic rhinitis; bronchial asthma; chronic ulcerative colitis; rheumatic carditis; nephrotic syndrome; collagen vascular disease; cerebral edema; and topically for inflammatory disorders.

3. The adverse effects of the glucocorticoids include **suppression of the pituitary–adrenal axis** that requires dose tapering while withdrawing the drug. **GI effects** are also common adverse effects and may include **peptic ulcer**, **GI hemorrhage**, ulcerative esophagitis, and acute pancreatitis. Characteristic effects of glucocorticoids include **weight gain**, **osteoporosis**, **hyperglycemia**, acne, increased susceptibility to infection, and **cushingoid "moon face"** and **"buffalo hump."** Other adverse effects include headache, vertigo, increased intraocular and intracranial pressures, muscle weakness, psychological disturbances, edema, and hypertension.

V. THYROID HORMONES are responsible for the development and regulation of metabolic homeostasis.

A. **Synthesis** of thyroid hormones is a four-step process beginning with the concentration of iodide in the thyroid gland. The enzyme **iodoperoxidase** then catalyzes steps two and three: iodination of tyrosine residues located on thyroglobulin, a 650,000 Da molecular weight glycoprotein located within the thyroid gland, and coupling of the iodinated tyrosine precursors. Finally, proteolysis of thyroglobulin produces the two naturally occurring thyroid hormones: **thyroxine (levothyroxine; T_4)** and **triiodothyronine (liothyronine; T_3)** in a ratio of 4:1 (*Figure 12-18*).

1. Levothyroxine is **less potent** than liothyronine but possesses a **longer duration of action** (6 to 7 days vs. 1 to 2 days).
2. **Peripheral deiodination** by 5′-deiodinase converts T_4 to T_3.
3. Regulation of thyroid hormone production involves a **hypothalamic-pituitary-thyroid feedback system**. Thyrotropin-releasing hormone (TRH) is secreted by the hypothalamus and stimulates the release of TSH (thyrotropin) from the anterior pituitary. Thyrotropin stimulates the thyroid gland to produce T_4 and T_3. T_3 and T_4 hormones then regulate their own synthesis by binding to specific sites in the anterior pituitary and inhibiting the release of TSH.

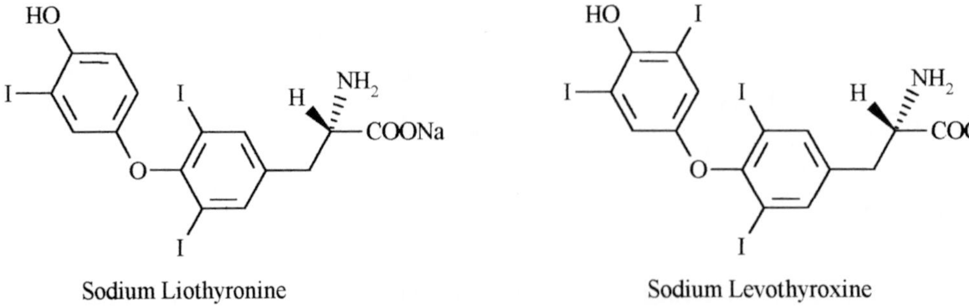

Figure 12-18. Sodium salt forms of the naturally occurring thyroid hormones, liothyronine (T_3) and levothyroxine (T_4).

B. Various forms of thyroid hormones are used therapeutically including the sodium salts of liothyronine (T_3) and levothyroxine (T_4) either alone or together.

1. **Thyroid *USP*** or porcine-derived thyroid desiccated (Armour Thyroid) is made from dried, defatted thyroid glands from pigs and is standardized based on iodine content.
2. **Liotrix** (Thyrolar) is a **4:1 mixture of levothyroxine sodium to liothyronine sodium**, which is equivalent to but offers no advantages over levothyroxine alone.
3. Administration of **levothyroxine** or T_4 (Synthroid, Levoxyl) alone will produce the natural 4:1 ratio of T_4 to T_3.
4. **Liothyronine** (T_3, Cytomel, Triostat) has a **rapid onset** and **short duration of action** compared to levothyroxine sodium and may have utility in patients who may be sensitive to the adverse effects of thyroid medication, but the rapid changes in T3 levels may be more of a disadvantage.

C. Thyroid hormone preparations mimic the activity of endogenous thyroid hormones. These hormones regulate growth and development, have calorigenic and metabolic activity, and (through sensitization of the β-adrenergic receptors) have positive inotropic and chronotropic effects on the myocardium. The major indication for the thyroid hormone preparations are **hypothyroidism** (i.e., **myxedema**), myxedema coma, cretinism, and simple goiter. Other indications include endemic goiter and thyrotropin-dependent carcinoma.

D. The adverse effects of the thyroid preparations are rarely observed. An overdose can cause palpitations, nervousness, insomnia, and weight loss.

E. Drug interactions with thyroid hormones

1. Bile acid sequestrants (BAS), calcium, ferrous sulfate, sucralfate, iron, and aluminum hydroxide antacids **can decrease the absorption of thyroid hormones**. An appropriate solution to this problem is to adequately space the administration of these agents (e.g., take the thyroid hormone 1 hr before or 4 hrs after taking the BAS).
2. Several drugs, including phenytoin, carbamazepine, and rifampin, accelerate thyroid metabolism. An appropriate solution to this problem is to increase the dose of thyroid hormone.

F. Thyrotropin (TSH; Thyrogen) is marketed as a highly purified and lyophilized thyrotropic hormone isolated from bovine anterior pituitary glands and used as an **adjunct in the detection and treatment of thyroid cancer**. Adverse effects associated with thyrotropin include nausea, vomiting, headache, urticaria, anaphylaxis, thyroid gland swelling, transient hypotension, tachycardia, and arrhythmias.

G. Inhibitors of thyroid function directly or indirectly interfere with the synthesis of thyroid hormones and have use in the **treatment of hyperthyroid**. These agents include potassium or sodium iodide, radioactive iodine (e.g., $Na^{131}I$ [Hicon]), and the thioamides (e.g., propylthiouracil [PTU; generic], methimazole [Tapazole]; *Figure 12-19*).

1. **Iodides in high concentrations** (e.g., Lugol's solution) **have profound effects in all aspects of thyroid hormone synthesis, release, and metabolism**. Iodides limit their own transport, inhibit the synthesis of both iodotyrosine and iodothyronine, and most importantly, inhibit the release of thyroid hormones.
   a. **Lugol's solution** is used **before thyroid surgery** to make the thyroid gland firmer and reduce its size.
   b. Adverse effects include **iodism** characterized by increased salivation, brassy taste, sore teeth and gums, swollen eyelids, inflamed larynx and pharynx, frontal headache, skin lesions, and skin eruptions. Hypersensitivity reactions including fever, arthralgia, eosinophilia, and angioedema are also observed. Large doses of iodides given over long periods can cause goiter and hypothyroidism, which can be corrected by the administration of thyroid hormone.

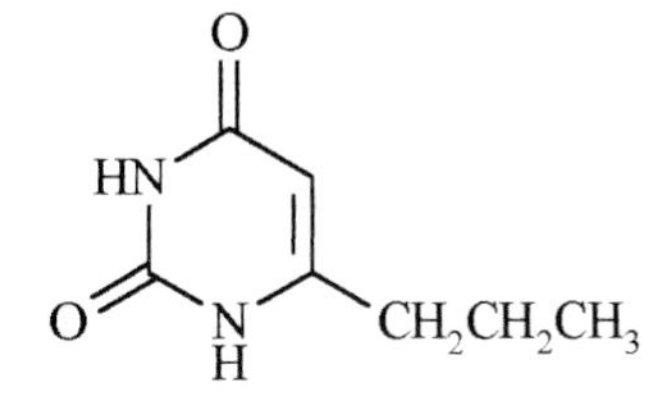

Propylthiouracil (PTU)

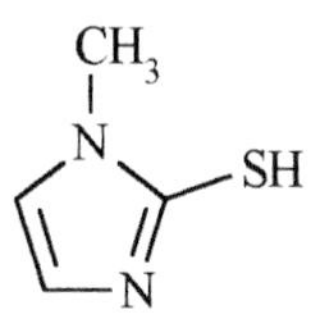

Methimazole

Figure 12-19. Structures of the thiourylene class of antithyroid hormones.

longer half-life and therefore is clinically useful in the treatment of **Paget's disease**, **hypercalcemia**, and **osteoporosis**.

E. **Bisphosphonates** are pyrophosphate analogs with a bioisosteric substitution of a carbon in place of an oxygen between the two phosphonate groups (*Figure 12-22*). The net result of this substitution is that bisphosphonates slow the formation and dissolution of hydroxyapatite crystals in the bone and elsewhere in the body by inhibiting the activity of osteoclasts.

1. Alendronate (Fosamax), etidronate (Didronel), ibandronate (Boniva), pamidronate (Aredia), risedronate (Actonel, Atelvia), tiludronate (Skelid), and zoledronic acid (Reclast, Zometa) are marketed bisphosphonates used for the **treatment of hypercalcemia** associated with malignancy, **Paget's disease**, and **osteoporosis**.
2. Bisphosphonates are generally well tolerated but side effects related to their structure and acidic nature include **gastric irritation**, **heartburn**, and **esophageal irritation**. Osteonecrosis of the jaw is rare but has been reported, mostly with the parenteral administration, with bisphosphonates.

F. Other agents that influence bone mineral homeostasis.

1. **Cinacalcet** (Sensipar) is a **calcimimetic drug** that acts as an agonist at the calcium-sensing receptor on the parathyroid gland that regulates PTH secretion. PTH release is inhibited when the calcium-sensing receptor is activated. Cinacalcet is used to treat **hyperparathyroidism secondary to renal failure** and **hypercalcemia caused by parathyroid carcinoma**. Hypocalcemia is the primary adverse effect observed.

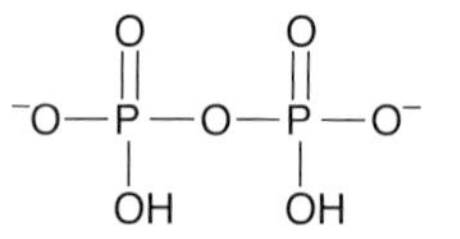

Pyrophosphate

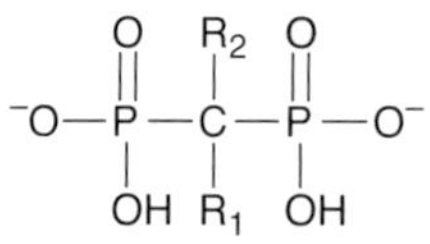

Bisphosphonate

Agent name	R_1	R_2
Etidronate	—OH	$—CH_3$
Tiludronate	—OH	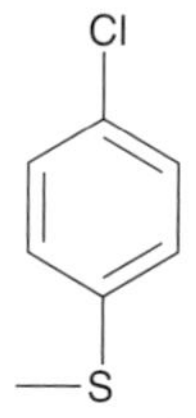
Pamidronate	$—CH_2CH_2NH_2$	—OH
Alendronate	$—CH_2CH_2CH_2NH_2$	—OH
Ibandronate	$—CH_2CH_2—N(CH_3)—(CH_2)_4—CH_3$	—OH
Risedronate	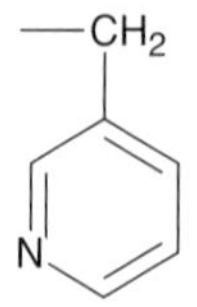	—OH
Zoledronic acid	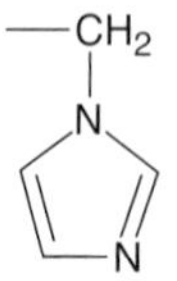	—OH

Figure 12-22. Structures of pyrophosphate and the pyrophosphate analog bisphosphonates.

2. **Denosumab** (Prolia) is a monoclonal antibody that binds the receptor activator of nuclear factor kappa B ligand (RANKL). RANKL binds to osteoclasts to allow proper osteoclast development and activity. With denosumab bound, RANKL cannot stimulate the osteoclasts appropriately, therefore **inhibiting osteoclast activity**.
3. **Glucocorticoids** stimulate the excretion of calcium from the kidney and calcium resorption from bone and decrease calcium absorption from the GI track, and therefore can **precipitate osteoporosis with chronic use**. These effects can be useful in the management of **hypercalcemia** secondary to lymphoma but are more commonly a limitation to long-term use as anti-inflammatory agents.
4. **Estrogens** have use in **slowing postmenopausal bone loss** through a mechanism that is not completely understood. The negative effects of long-term estrogen administration (i.e., breast cancer and cardiovascular events) limit the use of estrogens for the treatment of osteoporosis, but **selective estrogen receptor modulators** (SERMs) such as raloxifene (Evista) have been approved for the treatment of osteoporosis because they are estrogen agonists at the bone but not in breast and uterine tissue. A major side effect of raloxifene is hot flashes that are related to its antiestrogenic activities (see III.B.2.c).
5. **Thiazide diuretics** work at the kidney to **prevent the excretion of calcium** and, as a result, slow bone resorption in the hypercalcemic patient. The thiazides may be more useful in the prevention of the formation of calcium stones in the urine.

VII. ANTIDIABETIC AGENTS.

There are many different treatment options for the management of diabetes, including **insulin replacement** and various other agents that **lower blood glucose** or **increase glucose utilization**.

A. Parenteral antidiabetic agents

1. **Insulin** is an endocrine hormone secreted by the β-cells of the pancreas. It is a 51-amino acid protein composed of two polypeptide chains: an A-chain of 21 amino acids and a B-chain of 30 amino acids. Two interchain disulfide bonds connect the A- and B-chains, and a third intrachain disulfide bond is found between Cys6 and Cys11 of the A-chain. Insulin is derived from an 86-amino acid precursor known as proinsulin. At one time, insulin was available as bovine insulin (which differs from human insulin by three amino acids), and porcine insulin (which differs from human insulin only in one terminal amino acid); however, currently, only recombinant human insulin and its analogs are marketed. Exogenous insulin mimics the activity of endogenous insulin, which is required for the **proper use of glucose** in normal metabolism in insulin-sensitive tissues. Insulin monomers interact with a specific cell surface insulin receptor on multiple tissues (i.e., liver, muscle, and adipose tissue) to increase the expression of the GLUT-4 transporter responsible for the transport of glucose into the cells.
   a. **Human insulin** (Novolin, Humulin) is prepared by means of **recombinant DNA technology** using yeast (Novolin) or bacteria (Humulin).
      (1) Various preparations with **differences in their onset, duration, and intensity of action after subcutaneous administration** are manufactured for clinical use. These differences depend on the physical state of the insulin, the zinc content, the nature of the buffer, and the protein content.
      (2) **Regular insulin** (Novolin R, Humulin R) is a soluble insulin prepared at neutral pH. It can be mixed with most other insulins (with the exception of glargine and detemir) and is traditionally the only type of insulin that could be given **intravenously**. Novolog (see VII.A.1.b.[1–2]) is a short-acting, fast onset agent that is also approved for IV administration.
      (3) **Insulin isophane** (Novolin N, Humulin N) is an **intermediate-acting insulin**, which is a combination of recombinant human insulin with protamine (neutral protamine Hagedorn [NPH]) and zinc in stoichiometric amounts. The presence of the protamine enhances the aggregation of the insulin into inactive dimers and hexamers after subcutaneous injection and prolongs its duration of action. In vivo, the dimers and hexamers dissociate to form the active insulin monomers.
   b. Three **analogs of insulin** provide a **shorter onset of activity** (15 to 30 mins) and duration (3 to 4 hrs) than regular insulin due to alteration in the C-terminal of the B-chain responsible for the tendency of insulin to self-associate into hexamers. By hindering the formation

of hexamers, the pharmacologically functional monomer is released more quickly into the circulation. These analogs are used on insulin pumps and can be administered 15 mins before a meal. When compared with regular insulin, these analogs have a lower propensity to cause hypoglycemia, thus reducing the need for snacks between meals.

(1) **Insulin lispro** (Humalog) differs from normal insulin in that the Lys29 and Pro28 residues of the B-chain are reversed. Insulin lispro is also formulated with protamine (see VII.A.1.a.[3]) and marketed as Humalog Mix 75/25 and Humalog Mix 50/50, which is 75% and 50% insulin lispro protamine, respectively, with the balance being insulin lispro to provide a fast onset and a longer duration of action.

(2) **Insulin aspart** (NovoLog) differs from normal insulin in that the Pro28 residue of the B-chain is replaced with Asp. Insulin aspart is approved for intravenous administration. Insulin aspart is also formulated with protamine (see VII.A.1.a.[3]) and marketed as Novolog Mix 70/30, which is 70% insulin aspart protamine and 30% insulin aspart to provide a longer duration of action and fast onset, respectively.

(3) **Insulin glulisine** (Apidra) differs from normal insulin in two ways. First, Asn3 of the B-chain is replaced with Lys, and second, Lys29 of the B-chain is replaced by Glu.

c. **Long-acting insulin analogs** allow for a once daily administration that produces a constant concentration/time profile that more closely mimics endogenous basal insulin secretion.

(1) **Insulin glargine** (Lantus) differs from normal insulin in that Gly replaces the Asn21 residue of the A-chain and a basic Arg-Arg dipeptide replaces Thr30 of the B-chain. These structural alterations cause a **decrease in the solubility at physiological pH, precipitation,** and **delayed absorption after subcutaneous injections**, resulting in an increased duration of action for once daily dosing.

(2) **Insulin detemir** (Levemir) differs from normal insulin in two ways. **A 14-carbon fatty acid (myristic acid)** is covalently bound to Lys29 of the B-chain and Thr30 of the B-chain is removed. In circulation, the myristic acid addition **binds to albumin**, resulting in a longer half-life that mimics endogenous basal insulin secretion.

d. The various insulin preparations are used to **treat type 1,** or **insulin dependent, diabetes** by replacing insulin not produced by the nonfunctional β-cells of the pancreas. Insulin can also be used to treat type 2, or noninsulin dependent, diabetes that is not adequately controlled by either diet or oral antidiabetic agents. Insulin therapy aims to mimic the natural release of insulin in response to meals. This can be accomplished by administration through continuous infusion pumps with a bolus at meals or multiple daily injections of the different insulin formulations.

e. The most common adverse effect of insulin is **hypoglycemia**, which is characterized by sweating, tachycardia, and hunger. Severe hypoglycemia can progress to shock with hypoglycemic convulsions or coma. Hypersensitivity reactions and injection site irritation are also reported.

2. **Peptide mimetics** are used as adjunct therapy in combination with either insulin or oral antidiabetic agents to control hyperglycemia.

a. **Exenatide** (Byetta) is an **incretin mimetic peptide**. **Incretins** are endogenous compounds, such as glucagon-like peptide 1 (GLP-1), that are **released from the stomach** and **improve glycemic control**. Exenatide is isolated from the salivary gland of the lizard *Heloderma suspectum* (Gila monster) and has a **longer duration of action** than endogenous incretins.

(1) Exenatide binds and **activates the human GLP-1 receptor**. This stimulates glucose-dependent insulin synthesis, **enhances insulin secretion** by the pancreatic β-cells, **suppresses inappropriately elevated glucagon secretion**, and **slows gastric emptying**. These actions improve glycemic control in **type 2 diabetic patients** that are not adequately controlled by other therapies.

(2) Exenatide is associated with **significant GI side effects** including nausea, vomiting, diarrhea, dyspepsia, and anorexia that are thought to contribute to some of the **weight loss** observed with exenatide treatment. Other adverse effects include hypoglycemia, excessive sweating, asthenia, dizziness, restlessness, and tremors. Additionally, the slowing of gastric emptying by exenatide can decrease the rate and/or extent of oral absorption of other drugs. The coadministration with agents that slow gastric motility (i.e., antimuscarinics) should be avoided.

(3) **Liraglutide** (Victoza) is also a **GLP-1 analog** that has been modified by the **addition of a 16-carbon fatty acid**. The fatty acid addition binds liraglutide to albumin in circulation and slows the metabolism of liraglutide by dipeptidyl peptidase-IV (see VII.B.6). Because the mechanism of action for liraglutide is similar to that of exenatide, the use and side effects are also similar.

b. Pramlintide (Symlin) is a synthetic analog of **human amylin**. Amylin is a 37-amino acid neuroendocrine peptide that is secreted by the pancreatic β-cells in response to food intake. Pramlintide contains proline in place of Ala25, Ser28, and Ser29 normally present in amylin. This decreases the viscosity, instability, and aggregation that occur if amylin is placed in solution.

(1) **Amylin** and the amylin analog, pramlintide, **slow gastric emptying** without altering the overall absorption of nutrients. Amylin also **suppresses the postprandial glucagon secretion** and results in a **decreased appetite** and **caloric intake**. Pramlintide is used as an adjunct to mealtime insulin in patients with either type 1 or type 2 diabetes mellitus.

(2) Adverse effects associated with pramlintide include allergic reactions, dizziness, fatigue, headache, abdominal pain, anorexia, nausea, vomiting, arthralgia, cough, and pharyngitis. Because of the slowing of gastric emptying, pramlintide has similar motility concerns as discussed with exenatide.

B. Oral antidiabetic agents

1. The **sulfonylureas** are acidic compounds that are divided into first- and second-generation agents based on potency and substitutions on the aromatic ring (*Table 12-1*).

a. Sulfonylureas **block adenosine triphosphate (ATP)-sensitive potassium channels**, which **stimulate the release of insulin from the pancreatic β-cells**. Sulfonylureas are also called **secretagogues** because of their ability to induce insulin secretion. The sulfonylureas may also have a peripheral or extrahepatic activity that results in increased tissue sensitivity to insulin although this is not well established. Because of their activity on the β-cells, the sulfonylureas are used, either alone or in combination with other oral antidiabetic agents, to **treat type 2 diabetes mellitus** that cannot be adequately controlled by diet alone.

b. The sulfonylureas are divided into first- and second-generation agents (see *Table 12-1*).

(1) The first-generation agents are tolbutamide (Orinase), chlorpropamide (Diabinese), tolazamide (Tolinase), and acetohexamide (Dymelor).

(2) The second-generation agents are glyburide (DiaBeta, Micronase), glipizide (Glucotrol), and glimepiride (Amaryl).

c. The sulfonylureas increase the release of insulin regardless of the presence of glucose. As a result of this action, **hypoglycemia**, particularly with longer acting agents (i.e., chlorpropamide) or in patients with renal or hepatic insufficiency, is a significant concern. **Cross-sensitivity (i.e., hypersensitivity) among the sulfonylureas with the benzene sulfonamide functional group found in the sulfonamide antibiotics, thiazide, and loop diuretics is a possibility**. Chlorpropamide can cause hyponatremia due to the potentiation of the effects of antidiuretic hormone. Other potential side effects include blood dyscrasias (i.e., leukopenia, thrombocytopenia, agranulocytosis, and hemolytic anemia), cholestatic jaundice, and GI effects such as nausea, vomiting, diarrhea, and constipation.

d. The sulfonylureas are **highly plasma protein bound** with potential for the drug–drug interactions through plasma protein displacement (e.g., fibrates, sulfonamides). Additionally, drugs that influence cytochrome P450, as either an inhibitor or inducer, can affect the clearance of the sulfonylurea.

2. The **meglitinides** are acidic compounds that act as **secretagogues**.

a. Meglitinides are similar to the sulfonylureas in that they lower blood glucose levels by stimulating the release of insulin by **blocking the ATP-sensitive potassium channels in pancreatic β-cells**. They differ from the sulfonylureas in that they have a **more rapid onset of action and a shorter duration of action**. The meglitinides are indicated for the treatment of **type 2 diabetes** not controlled by diet alone.

b. The meglitinides include repaglinide (Prandin) and nateglinide (Starlix; *Figure 12-23*).

Table 12-1 ORAL HYPOGLYCEMIC AGENTS: THE SULFONYLUREAS

General Sulfonylurea Structure

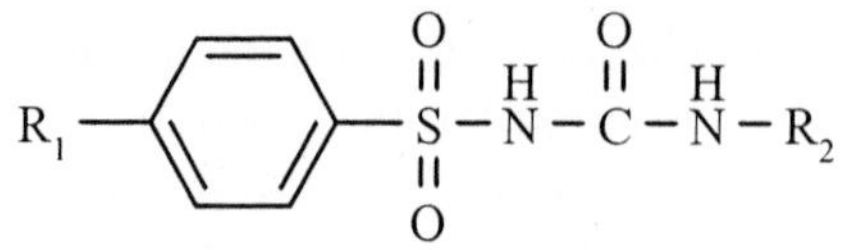

Drug	R_1 Substituent	R_2 Substituent
First-generation agents		
Tolbutamide (Orinase)	CH_3	$CH_2CH_2CH_2CH_3$
Chlorpropamide (Diabinese)	Cl	$CH_2CH_2CH_3$
Tolazamide (Tolinase)	CH_3	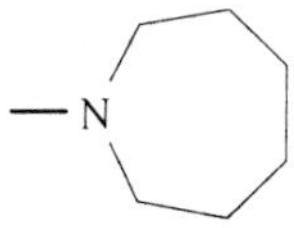
Acetohexamide (Dymelor)	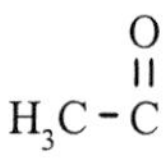	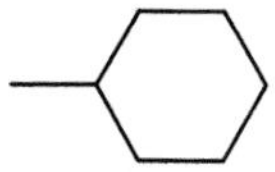
Second-generation agents		
Glyburide (DiaBeta, Micronase)	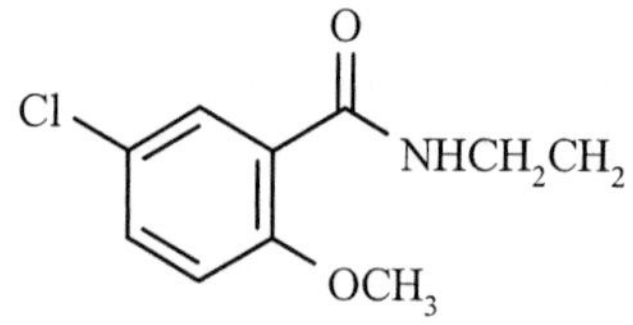	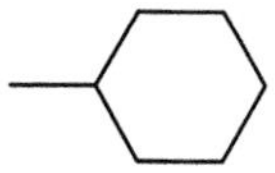
Glipizide (Glucotrol)	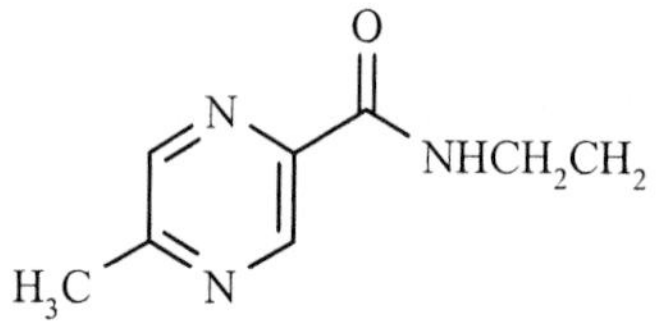	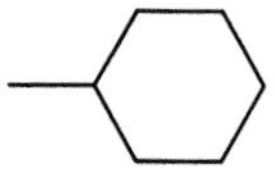
Glimepiride (Amaryl)	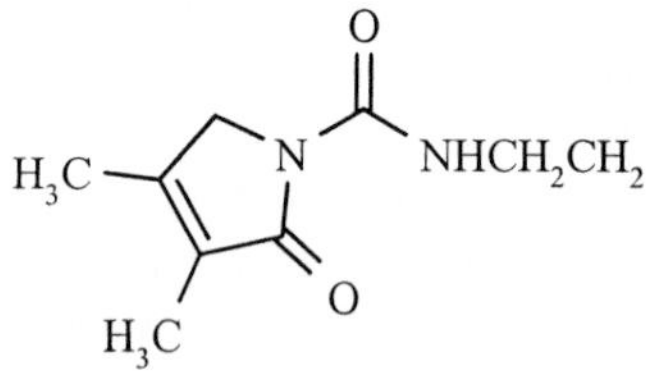	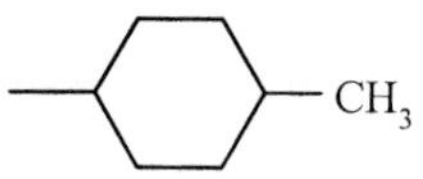

c. Like the sulfonylureas, the meglitinides are associated with **hypoglycemia**, but because of their short duration of action, the incidence is much lower. Repaglinide is also associated with upper respiratory infection, rhinitis, bronchitis, headache, and back pain.

d. Like the sulfonylureas, the meglitinides are highly protein bound so the potential for drug displacement exists. Additionally, nateglinide is metabolized by CYP2C9 and CYP3A4, whereas repaglinide is only metabolized by CYP3A4. The potential for drug–drug interactions is possible with agents that affect the activity of CYP2C9 and/or CYP3A4.

3. **Biguanides** are insulin-sensitizing agents that contain the basic biguanide functional group.

a. The exact mechanism of action for the biguanides is not known, but they do not stimulate the release of insulin or cause hypoglycemia, and thus are best described as **antihyperglycemic** or **euglycemic agents**. The regulation of blood glucose levels seen with these agents may be due to inhibition of hepatic glucose production by the inhibition of AMP-activated protein kinase.

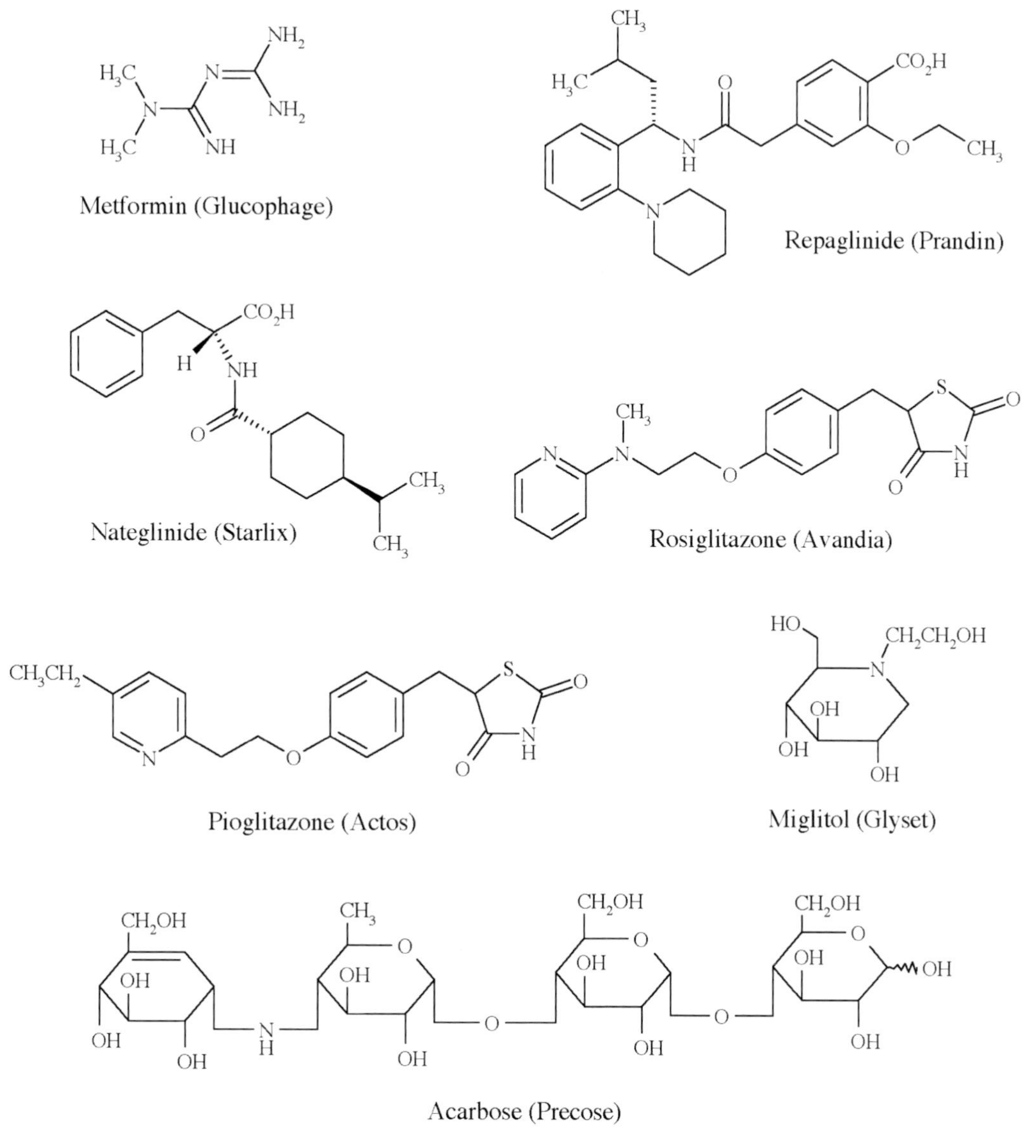

Figure 12-23. Structures of oral hypoglycemic agents: biguanides (metformin), meglitinides (repaglinide and nateglinide), thiazolidinediones (pioglitazone and rosiglitazone), and α-glucosidase inhibitors (miglitol and acarbose).

The biguanides may also increase tissue insulin sensitivity. Because of these actions, the biguanides are the **first-line therapy for type 2 diabetes**, either alone or in combination with other antidiabetic agents.

b. Phenformin was the originally marketed biguanide, but it was withdrawn from market in 1977 because of a high incidence of **fatal lactic acidosis**. Metformin (Glucophage) is the only biguanide currently marketed (*Figure 12-23*). It is also available in many combination products with sulfonylurea, thiazolidinediones, and DPP4 inhibitors.

c. Adverse effects associated with metformin include epigastric distress, nausea, vomiting, diarrhea, anorexia, and a metallic taste. **Lactic acidosis**, as observed with phenformin, has also been reported with metformin, but occurs with a much lower incidence. Most cases of **metformin-associated lactic acidosis are related to use in patients with contraindications** (i.e., congestive heart failure, hepatic or renal dysfunction) for the use of metformin.

7. In comparing levothyroxine to liothyronine, which of the following statements is *not* correct?
   (A) Both levothyroxine and liothyronine are naturally occurring thyroid hormones.
   (B) Liothyronine can be converted in the peripheral circulation to levothyroxine.
   (C) Liothyronine is more potent than levothyroxine.
   (D) The plasma concentration of liothyronine is less than that of levothyroxine.
   (E) Liothyronine has a shorter duration of action than levothyroxine.

8. Which of the following classes of compounds directly stimulates the release of insulin from pancreatic β-cells?
   (A) progestins
   (B) biguanides
   (C) α-glucosidase inhibitors
   (D) DPP-4 inhibitors
   (E) sulfonylureas

9. Which of the following compounds is incorrectly matched with its mechanism of action?
   (A) flutamide: competitively blocks the binding of androgens to their receptor
   (B) finasteride: inhibits 5α-reductase
   (C) miglitol: inhibits α-glucosidase
   (D) pioglitazone: competitively blocks the binding of estrogens to their receptor
   (E) anastrozole: inhibits aromatase

10. Which of the following compounds is incorrectly matched with one of its therapeutic uses?
   (A) raloxifene: ovulation induction
   (B) metformin: type 2 diabetes mellitus
   (C) finasteride: benign prostatic hyperplasia
   (D) propylthiouracil: hyperthyroidism
   (E) tamoxifen: estrogen-dependent breast cancer

11. Which of the following compounds would be most likely to cause hypoglycemia?
   (A) miglitol (Glyset)
   (B) metformin (Glucophage)
   (C) pioglitazone (Actos)
   (D) sitagliptin (Januvia)
   (E) glipizide (Glucotrol)

12. Which of the following compounds has a mechanism of action most similar to exenatide (Byetta)?
   (A) insulin (Humulin R)
   (B) saxagliptin (Onglyza)
   (C) pramlintide (Symlin)
   (D) repaglinide (Prandin)
   (E) metformin (Glucophage)

13. Anastrozole (Arimidex) as to aromatase as ______________ is to 5α-reductase.
   (A) flutamide (Eulexin)
   (B) tamoxifen (Nolvadex)
   (C) mifepristone (Mifeprex)
   (D) finasteride (Proscar)
   (E) testosterone

14. All of the following can be used to treat hypothyroid *except*
   (A) thyroid USP (Armour Thyroid).
   (B) liotrix (Thyrolar).
   (C) methimazole (Tapazole).
   (D) levothyroxine (Synthroid).
   (E) liothyronine (Cytomel).

Directions for questions 15–17: The questions and incomplete statements in this section can be correctly answered or completed by **one or more** of the suggested answers. Choose the answer, **A–E.**

A if **I only** is correct
B if **III only** is correct
C if **I and II** are correct
D if **II and III** are correct
E if **I, II, and III** are correct

15. Hormones that form lipophilic esters without prior structural modifications include
   I. hydrocortisone.
   II. testosterone.
   III. progesterone.

16. Insulin preparations that contain a modifying protein include
   I. insulin glargine.
   II. regular insulin.
   III. isophane insulin (neutral protamine Hagedorn [NPH]).

17. Agents used to treat hypercalcemia include
   I vitamin D.
   II calcitonin.
   III aledronate.

Directions for questions 18–20: Each statement in this section is most closely related to **one** of the following hormones. The hormones may be used more than once or not at all. Choose the **best** answer, **A–E.**

A Testosterone
B Insulin
C Corticotropin
D Estradiol
E Vasopressin

18. Secreted by pancreatic β-cells to facilitate glucose and amino acid transport for normal cellular metabolic processes.

19. Initiates and controls male sexual development and maintains the integrity of the male reproductive system.

20. Promotes the reabsorption of water at the renal collecting tubule.

Directions for questions 21–23: Each statement in this section is most closely related to **one** of the following drug classes. The drug classes may be used more than once or not at all. Choose the **best** answer, **A–E.**

A Antithyroid agents
B Sulfonylureas
C Adrenocorticosteroids
D Progestins
E Androgens

21. Peptic ulceration and gastrointestinal hemorrhage; hyperglycemia, hypertension, and edema; "buffalo hump" and "moon face"; psychological disturbances; and increased susceptibility to infection

22. Agranulocytosis and other blood dyscrasias, cholestatic jaundice, nausea and vomiting, hypoglycemia, and hypersensitivity reactions

23. Rare adverse effects include drug fever, hepatitis, nephritis, and systemic lupus erythematosus–like syndrome.

Answers and Explanations

1. The answer is A *[see III.A.1; Figure 12-2].*
Ring A is aromatic. Because the only type of steroidal hormone that has an aromatic A-ring is an estrogen, this structure represents an estrogen. Other structural characteristics of estrogens include the fact that the structure contains 18 carbon atoms; thus it is an estrane and contains a β-alcohol group in position 17.

2. The answer is B *[see II.B.1–4].*
hCG is produced by placental tissue and serves to stimulate the secretion of progesterone during pregnancy. Growth hormone (somatotropin), FSH, TSH, and ACTH are all secreted by the anterior pituitary gland.

3. The answer is C *[see II.B.4.c].*
hCG is a proteinaceous tropic hormone that is secreted by chorionic (e.g., placental) tissue. Thus, hCG is present in the urine only after conception has occurred.

4. The answer is C *[see III.A.1; III.D.1; III.F.2; IV.B.1.b.(2); Figures 12-12, 12-17, and 12-18].*
Liothyronine is a thyroid hormone. Thyroid hormones consist of iodinated aromatic amino acids and are not steroidal in nature. Ethinyl estradiol is a steroidal estrogen, norethindrone is a steroidal 19-norprogestin, prednisolone is an adrenocorticosteroid, and fluoxymesterone is a steroidal androgen.

5. The answer is D *[see IV.B.1.b.(4); Figure 12-17].*
Glucocorticoids have varying degrees of mineralocorticoid activity. This mineralocorticoid activity, which can result in sodium and fluid retention, can be blocked by the introduction of a methyl or hydroxyl group in position 16 of the steroidal nucleus. Dexamethasone has a 16α-methyl substituent.

6. The answer is A *[see VII.A.1.a.(2)].*
Most insulin preparations are suspensions; thus, they contain particulate matter. Only clear solutions may be administered intravenously. Regular insulin, which consists of water-soluble crystalline zinc insulin, is therefore suitable for intravenous administration. Insulin aspart (Novolog) is also approved for intravenous administration. All other insulin preparations are normally injected subcutaneously.

7. The answer is B *[see V.A.1].*
The thyroid gland produces both levothyroxine (T_4) and liothyronine (T_3). The natural ratio of these compounds is 4:1 in favor of levothyroxine; therefore, liothyronine is normally present at a lower concentration than levothyroxine. Liothyronine is more potent than levothyroxine, but has a shorter duration of action. Peripheral conversion involves deiodination; thus, levothyroxine is converted to liothyronine. The reverse process is not possible.

8. The answer is E *[see VII.B.1.a; VII.B.3.a; VII.B.5.a; VII.B.6.a].*
Of the five classes of compounds listed, only biguanides, α-glucosidase inhibitors, and sulfonylureas are used in the treatment of type 2 diabetes mellitus. These classes provide their beneficial effects through different mechanisms of action. Biguanides enhance the peripheral use of insulin, suppress gluconeogenesis, and are often referred to as antihyperglycemic agents. α-Glucosidase inhibitors decrease the absorption of glucose. Sulfonylureas and the structurally unrelated compounds, repaglinide and nateglinide, stimulate the secretion of insulin from pancreatic β-cells.

2. **Pharmacodynamic** interactions occur when the pharmacodynamic effect of the drug is altered by another drug, chemical, or food element, producing an antagonistic, synergistic, or additive effect.
3. **Pharmaceutical** interactions are caused by a chemical or physical incompatibility when two or more drugs are mixed together. Pharmaceutical interactions can occur during extemporaneous compounding of drugs, including the preparation of intravenous (IV) solutions. For example, an IV solution of sodium bicarbonate has an alkaline pH and should not be mixed with such drugs as dobutamine, ciprofloxacin, or magnesium sulfate, which decompose or precipitate in alkaline pH. Phenytoin sodium will precipitate from a solution that has an acid pH, such as dextrose 5%. Pharmaceutical interactions are usually considered during the development, manufacturing, and marketing of the drug product. Only drug interactions involving pharmacokinetic, pharmacodynamic, or pharmacogenetic processes will be considered in this chapter.

II. PHARMACOKINETIC INTERACTIONS

A. **Gastrointestinal absorption.** Drug interactions can affect the **rate** and the **extent** of systemic drug absorption (bioavailability) from the absorption site, resulting in increased or decreased drug bioavailability. Most drugs are given orally with drug absorption from the gastrointestinal (GI) tract. Additional sites of absorption drug interactions include skin, lung, nasal, and sublingual areas.

1. **Changes in gastric pH** can increase or decrease GI drug absorption in several different ways depending on the formulation of the drug and whether the drug is a weak electrolyte (e.g., weak base or weak acid).
   a. Agents, which decrease in gastric pH, include certain acidic foods, such as fruit juices, and drugs, such as aspirin and ascorbic acid. Weak acid drugs are less ionized in an acidic environment, becoming more lipid soluble, resulting in an increased absorption from the stomach. Examples include aspirin, the combination of aspirin/dipyridamole, diazepam, and furosemide.
      (1) Drugs, which are weak bases, have enhanced absorption in an alkaline or more neutral stomach environment, such as indomethacin and tetracycline.
      (2) An acid environment, which can develop when eating or when acidic drugs such as ascorbic acid are taken, can cause increased absorption of weak acid drugs such as aspirin or dipyridamole.
   b. Increasing gastric pH produces a more basic stomach environment, which enhances absorption of weak bases and impairs absorption of acidic drugs. Drugs such as antacids and bicarbonate salts increase the gastric pH. In addition, proton pump inhibitors such as omeprazole (Prilosec) will also increase gastric pH. Enteric drug products are formulated with coatings that maintain integrity in an acid environment of the stomach, and then dissolve in the more alkaline environment of the duodenum, releasing the drug. If the gastric pH is increased, the coating dissolves in the stomach rather than the duodenum and the drug is released in the stomach. Some enteric-coated drugs such as aspirin and diclofenac are highly irritating to the stomach linings if the coat is removed in the stomach.
2. **Complexation and chelation** of drugs can cause precipitation of a drug and prevent absorption. Complexation, or binding of a drug, can cause the drug, though not chelated, to be poorly absorbed as it moves through the GI tract.
   a. Chelation of a drug is a form of complexation in which a molecule or atom is trapped in a second molecule. Insoluble chelates such as a calcium-tetracycline complex are not well absorbed. Examples of chelation include calcium, magnesium, aluminum, or iron preparations given with fluoroquinolones or tetracycline. Milk is a source of calcium. Other common divalent anions are in antacids and vitamins/mineral combinations and iron supplementation.
   b. Resins, binders, and certain fiber products can bind various drugs and reduce their absorption. Resins such as cholestyramine, which binds bile, can also bind digoxin and warfarin, reducing the bioavailability of these drugs. Sodium polystyrene sulfonate also binds cations in antacids causing reduced renal clearance of bicarbonate, resulting in systemic acidosis. Fiber products such as Metamucil, which are used to treat constipation, can cause binding of warfarin, digoxin, and salicylates.

   c. Activated charcoal is specifically formulated to adsorb various drugs to prevent absorption of the drug and reduce the risk of toxicity in overdose. Activated charcoal does not adsorb simple chemical compounds such as iron sulfate.
   d. Sevelamer, which binds dietary phosphates, is also known to bind ciprofloxacin and levothyroxine.
3. **Increased GI motility** reduces drug residence time or the amount of time spent in the optimal environment for absorption of particular drugs.
   a. Drugs that increase GI motility include laxatives and cathartics such as bisacodyl, cascara, senna laxatives, and sorbitol.
   b. Psyllium and fiber taken with sufficient fluid can also cause an increase in GI motility and decrease the time available for coadministered drugs to be absorbed.
   c. Drugs that are specifically developed to pharmacologically stimulate the GI tract can also reduce the time available for absorption of coadministered drugs. These include tegaserod (a 5HT-partial antagonist available for compassionate use through the U.S. Food and Drugs Administration [FDA]), methylnaltrexone (opioid antagonist in the GI tract only), alvimopan (peripheral mu-opioid antagonist), metoclopramide, erythromycin, and cisapride (a prokinetic available by a registration system by the FDA).
4. **Decreased GI motility** increases the time a drug spends in its absorptive environment, which can lead to excessive absorption and toxicity, including local irritation to the GI mucosal cells or possible disruption to flora in the large bowel.
   a. Drugs that show anticholinergic activity and slow GI transit include diphenhydramine, hyoscyamine, tricyclic antidepressants, propantheline, and opioid narcotics.
5. **Alteration of intestinal flora** can change the availability of drugs by metabolism that takes place in the GI tract itself. Flora metabolize various drugs that have metabolites that are absorbed and are pharmacologically active. Flora also metabolize drugs into inactive metabolites, reducing the amount of parent drug available, or by metabolizing enterohepatically circulated drugs into inactive compounds. Disruptions in flora change the amounts of drug available.
   a. Decrease in intestinal flora usually occurs as a result of antibiotic treatment. Bacterial flora are the prime metabolizers of several drugs. Colonic cleansing may also reduce intestinal flora, causing GI distress such as diarrhea.
   b. Drugs that are metabolized in the GI by intestinal flora include estrogen contraceptives, which are metabolized to active metabolites. The reduction of GI flora could result in contraceptive failure. Digoxin is metabolized by bacterium into inactive metabolites. Coadministration of antibiotics can cause an increase in digoxin levels.
   c. Antibiotics can also reduce the GI flora, which synthesize vitamin K. Reduction of GI flora by antibiotics can result in too little vitamin K off-setting warfarin therapy, resulting in excessive anticoagulation.
6. **Competition for P-glycoprotein efflux pumps (P-GP)** affects enterohepatic circulation. The pumps, or "transporter proteins," can be activated or inactivated (induced or inhibited) in much the same way CYP450 isoenzymes can be induced or inhibited. If the pumps are inhibited, the systemic circulation of the substrate drug can increase as therapy is continued and elimination is reduced, and toxicity could result. If the pumps are induced, the systemic circulation of the substrate drug is increased and systemic levels of the substrate are decreased, which could lead to subtherapeutic levels. These pumps are located in both the lumen of the GI system and in the renal system.
   a. Known substrates of the P-GP efflux pumps include digoxin and linezolid.
   b. Known inhibitors of the P-GP efflux pumps include erythromycin, itraconazole, cyclosporin, ritonavir, verapamil, ketoconazole, amiodarone, and clarithromycin.
   c. Known inducers of the P-GP efflux pumps include rifampin and St. John's wort.
7. **Ethanol-induced "dose dumping" syndrome** affects the bioavailability of drugs in delayed-distribution or extended-release formulation. Studies involving coadministered ethanol in strengths of 40% and 20% lead to an increase in C_{max} of fivefold and twofold, respectively. The primary mechanism leading to the increase in therapeutic drug relates to the drug dissolution characteristics in ethanol.
   a. An FDA study reported a 16-fold increase in average peak hydromorphone concentration from a modified-release preparation when ingested with 40% ethanol as compared to water. A similar effect has been described with the coadministration of ethanol and controlled-released diazepam.

b. The effect is similar to food-induced "dose dumping" caused by the effect of food on pH or on the drug itself. Enteric-coated products are sensitive to pH, and a high gastric pH due to food or due to a drug such as omeprazole can disrupt the enteric coating, causing rapid release of the drug. Similarly, the sustained-release mechanism may be compromised, causing the immediate release of the entire drug amount in the dosage form. This has been observed in sustained-release theophylline, and has resulted in guidance by the FDA on drug delivery design.

c. In the absence of consistent FDA guidance, concomitant ethanol ingestion should be discouraged because it may result in "dose dumping" syndrome and toxicity.

8. **Alteration of intestinal blood flow** caused by the precipitant drug. In congestive heart disease, the blood flow to the GI tract is poor and an orally administered drug can have a slower rate of absorption. After digoxin therapy, the perfusion of the GI tract is improved along with bioavailability of the object drug.

B. Transdermal absorption

1. Transdermal medications are formulated for absorption through the hydrophobic and hydrophilic layers of the skin. The vehicle chosen determines the best placement of the drug on the skin—considering the pharmacokinetic properties of the vehicle.
2. Alterations in blood flow to the area of application can change the amount and extent of drug absorption.
   a. Vasoconstrictors such as epinephrine can decrease blood flow to the area. In combination with lidocaine, this allows local anesthesia with minimal bleeding and without systemic absorption of the lidocaine while repairing a skin wound.
   b. Vasodilators such as irritants like menthol creams, or local application of heat can increase blood flow to the area and increase drug absorption. This can result in toxicity if the dosage form is a controlled-release fentanyl or morphine patch.

C. Pulmonary absorption

1. Drug delivery by inhalation or by nebulizer is becoming more common. Drugs that inhibit lung absorption can theoretically reduce the amount of drug absorbed. Drugs that are bronchodilators may enhance absorption. Drugs that affect viscosity of pulmonary fluids can inhibit or block pulmonary absorption of the therapeutic drug. Vehicles for the nebulized drugs can influence the depth of penetration of the therapeutic drug into the pulmonary tree. The order in which several nebulized drugs are given can affect the absorption extent of the therapeutic drugs. For example, a nebulized bronchodilator dose theoretically may enhance penetration and absorption of a nebulized dose of morphine.

D. Distribution. Distribution can be affected by various protein cells in the body that are used for transportation, efflux and influx, and storage. Some of these glycoproteins are also thought to be involved in limited drug metabolism. Drugs that are highly bound ($> 70\%$) to a carrier protein can be displaced if the second drug introduced has a higher binding affinity to the carrier protein.

1. The following conditions must apply if a drug is to be displaced from its carrier protein by another drug.
   a. The displaced drug must be highly protein bound, greater than 90%.
   b. The drug has very potent pharmacodynamic activity (e.g., warfarin).
   c. Both drugs must bind to a common binding site.
   d. The displacing drug must have a higher affinity for the binding site than the drug being displaced—or the free concentration of the displacing drug must be higher than that of the drug being displaced.
      (1) **Albumin** is quantitatively the primary protein in the serum. It is the major binder and transporter for many drugs. It is synthesized by the liver and the concentration in blood is affected by various diseases, including hepatic and renal disease. If the concentration of serum albumin is substantially decreased, the concentration of "free" drug may increase multiple-fold, resulting in an adverse response.
         (a) Albumin is basic and binds primarily acidic and neutral drugs. Drugs that are highly bound to albumin include warfarin, salicylates, digoxin, fluoxetine, ibuprofen, citalopram, ketoconazole, phenytoin, prednisolone, and nafcillin.
      (2) **Alpha-1 acid glycoprotein (AAG)** is a carrier protein that circulates in the plasma. AAG is a carrier of basic and neutrally charged lipophilic molecules such as carbamazepine, lidocaine, lopinavir, methadone, prazosin, quinine, cocaine, and erythromycin.

(3) **Organic anion transporting polypeptides (OATPs)** are a family of proteins that provide membrane influx transport for anionic drugs across various tissues. Some of these influx transporters provide uptake through hepatocyte membranes, providing access for liver metabolism of substrate drugs. The extent to which drugs interact with particular OATP transporters depends on the physiochemical properties of the substrate and the size, lipophilicity, and degree of ionization of the drugs. Pharmacogenetic polymorphisms (genetic variabilities) can affect the extent of activity of these transporters in much the same way they affect the activity of CYP450 isoenzymes.

(a) OATPs are a family of 11 membrane influx transporters that regulate uptake for substrates into cells.

(b) OATP transporters can be in limited distribution, such as OATP4C1 being limited to the kidney, or may be found in tissues throughout the body. These tissues include hepatic, brain, kidney, intestinal, and skin tissues, among other sites. The most significant of these in terms of drug interactions are
OATP1A2 distributes to brain, kidney, liver, intestines;
OATP1B1 distributes to the liver;
OATP1B3 distributes to the liver;
OATP2B1 distributes to the liver, placenta, intestines, heart, and skin.

(c) Drugs that are substrates for the OATP transport proteins can also be substrates for other metabolic processes, so determining the exact drug–drug interaction site among involved proteins and enzymes can be difficult (*Table 13-1*).

E. Drug elimination and clearance

1. Drug metabolism and hepatic clearance

a. Drug metabolism (hepatic clearance) can be affected by enzyme induction, enzyme inhibition, substrate competition for the same enzyme, and changes in hepatic blood flow (*Table 13-2*).

b. Many drugs that share the same drug-metabolizing enzymes have a potential for a drug interaction. For example, fluconazole inhibits the hepatic metabolism of warfarin, causing increased risk of bleeding. Carbamazepine is both a substrate and an inducer of the CYP3A4 isoenzyme, thereby inducing its own metabolism and taking 3 to 5 weeks to reach stable blood levels. (*Table 13-3*). Phenytoin is also a substrate of the CYP3A4 and induces its own metabolism.

c. Over-the-counter (OTC) drugs and herbal preparations can also be involved in CYP450 isoenzyme metabolism and can cause serious drug–herbal interactions. For example, St. John's wort may induce CYP3A4 isoenzymes and decrease cyclosporine to subtherapeutic levels. Tobacco use (smoking) can induce the CYP1A2 isoenzyme and decrease clozapine levels, increasing the risk of therapeutic failure in treating obsessive–compulsive disorder (OCD).

d. Foods may also interfere with hepatic drug metabolism. For example, grapefruit juice is a powerful inhibitor of the CYP3A4 isoenzyme and will increase blood levels of CYP3A4 substrates such as ritonavir, methadone, amlodipine, alprazolam, cyclosporine, and diltiazem if taken together. Apple juice and orange juice are also implicated in inhibiting function of OATP transporter proteins.

Table 13-1 OATP TRANSPORTER DRUG–DRUG INTERACTIONS

OATP	Inhibitors	Substrates
OATP1B1	Carbamazepine, caspofungin clarithromycin, digoxin erythromycin, ketoconazole statins, tacrolimus, methotrexate, rifampicin sildenafil, valsartan cyclosporine, gemfibrozil	Bile acids, conjugated steroids, statins, ACE inhibitors, angiotensin II receptor blockers, caspofungin, repaglinide
OATP1A2	Apple, grapefruit, and orange juices; rifampicin; verapamil	Erythromycin, levofloxacin, imatinib levofloxacin, rocuronium, saquinavir
OATP1B3	Clarithromycin, cyclosporine erythromycin, rifampicin	Digoxin, docetaxel, statins, thyroxine valsartan, erythromycin, enalapril
OATP2B1	Cyclosporine, gemfibrozil	Statins, benzylpenicillin, bosentan fexofenadine

ACE, angiotensin-converting enzyme.

Table 13-2 DRUG INTERACTIONS THAT AFFECT THE DRUG METABOLISM

Drug Interaction	Examples (Precipitant Drugs)	Effect (Objective Drugs)
Enzyme induction		
	Smoking (polycyclic aromatic hydrocarbons)	Smoking increases duloxetine metabolism and decreases duloxetine levels
	Phenytoin	Tacrolimus levels are decreased because of increased metabolism
Enzyme inhibition		
Mixed function oxidase	Cimetidine	Decreased atorvastatin clearance and increased drug levels
Induction of UDP-G metabolism	Phenytoin, cimetidine, midazolam, rifabutin	Decreased posaconazole levels due to induction of metabolism
Nonhepatic enzymes	Monoamine oxidase inhibitors (MAOIs) (e.g., pargyline, tranylcypromine)	Serious hypertensive crisis can occur following ingestion of foods with a high content of tyramine or other pressor substances (e.g., cheddar cheese, red wines, avocados) and catecholamines
Inhibition of drug metabolism by intestinal cells	MAOIs such as phenelzine and tranylcypromine	MAOIs inhibit metabolism of albuterol and levalbuterol, leading to hypertension
Alteration of intestinal flora	Antibiotics	Digoxin has better bioavailability when taken after erythromycin. Erythromycin administration reduces bacterial inactivation of digoxin.
		Estrogen/progestin birth control requires intestinal flora to facilitate enterohepatic circulation. Antibiotics reduce intestinal flora and reduce estrogen/progestin levels, resulting in failure of ovulation suppression and menstrual changes.

MAOIs, monoamine oxidase inhibitors; *UDP-G*, Uridine 5'-diphosphate glucose.

e. Nonhepatic enzymes can be involved in drug interactions. For example, *serotonin syndrome* has been reported in patients receiving antidepressants such as amitriptyline or citalopram (a selective serotonin reuptake inhibitor [SSRI]) in combination with a monoamine oxidase inhibitor (MAOI), such as linezolid. A considerable portion of the CYP3A4 enzymes are found not only in the liver but also in the GI tract, where some of these substrates are metabolized.

f. A decrease in the hepatic blood flow can decrease the hepatic clearance for high extraction drugs, such as propranolol and morphine.

2. **Renal drug clearance** can be affected by changes in glomerular filtration, tubular reabsorption, active drug secretion, and renal blood flow and nephrotoxicity (*Table 13-4*).

III. PHARMACODYNAMIC INTERACTIONS

A. Drugs that have similar pharmacodynamic actions may produce an excessive pharmacodynamic response or a **toxic response**.

1. For example, central nervous system depressants, such as the combination of opioids, alcohol, and antihistamines (e.g., diphenhydramine, chlorpheniramine), can produce increased drowsiness in the patient.
2. Drugs with anticholinergic effects, such as promethazine and OTC antihistamines, can cause excessive dryness of the mouth, blurred vision, and urinary retention.
3. Drugs that prolong the QTc interval, such as paliperidone, amiodarone, sotalol, moxifloxacin, and atypical antipsychotics such as ziprasidone, have a much greater risk of causing QTc interval arrhythmias when given together.

Table 13-3 DRUG/HERB/FOOD ACTIONS WITH CYTOCHROME P450 ENZYMES

Enzyme	Inhibitor	Inducer	Substrate
CYP1A2	Ciprofloxacin	Phenytoin	Naproxen
	Levofloxacin	Carbamazepine	Amitriptyline
	Cimetidine	Charbroiled foods	Verapamil
	Citalopram	Tobacco	Clopidogrel
	Ketoconazole	Ritonavir	Duloxetine
	Paroxetine	St. John's wort	Ramelteon
CYP2C9	Cimetidine	Rifampin	Tamoxifen
	Fluoxetine	Carbamazepine	Losartan
	Voriconazole	Phenytoin	S-Warfarin
	Fluconazole		Celecoxib
	Amiodarone		Phenytoin
	Efavirenz		Carvedilol
	Metronidazole		Voriconazole
			Glyburide
			Sildenafil
CYP2C8	Gemfibrozil	Phenobarbital	Paclitaxel
	Nicardipine	Rifampin	Carbamazepine
	Atazanavir	Carbamazepine	Amiodarone
	Trimethoprim		Pioglitazone
CYP2C19	Ketoconazole	Rifampin	Diazepam
	Omeprazole	Carbamazepine	Phenytoin
	Topiramate	Phenytoin	Citalopram
	Fluoxetine		Omeprazole
	Fluvoxamine		Diphenhydramine
			Duloxetine
			R-Warfarin
CYP2D6	Methadone	Carbamazepine	Amitriptyline
	Cimetidine	Phenytoin	Metoprolol
	Fluoxetine	Ethanol	Paroxetine
	Ritonavir	St. John's wort	Duloxetine
	Haloperidol	Ritonavir	Haloperidol
	Amiodarone		Venlafaxine
	Paroxetine		Tramadol
	Quinidine		Trazodone
	Sertraline		Narcotic analgesics
CYP2E1	Cimetidine	Ritonavir	Acetaminophen
	Disulfiram	Isoniazid	Caffeine
		Ethanol	Venlafaxine
CYP3A family	Erythromycin	Carbamazepine	Atorvastatin
	Ketoconazole	Phenobarbital	Warfarin
	Saquinavir	St. John's wort	Lidocaine
	Verapamil	Nevirapine	Ethyl estradiol
		Efavirenz	
	Metronidazole	Carbamazepine	Cyclosporine
	Amiodarone	Rifampin	Alprazolam
	Cimetidine	Garlic supplements	Ziprasidone
	Diltiazem	Grapefruit	Doxorubicin
	Posaconazole	Seville orange	Amitriptyline
	Metronidazole	Bitter orange	Methadone

(Continued on next page)

Table 13-6 ST. JOHN'S WORT DRUG INTERACTIONS

Pharmacokinetic Process	Site	Action	Results in	Drug
Metabolism	CYP3A4	Induces	Lower levels of	NNRTI Protease inhibitors Benzodiazepines Calcium-channel blockers Carbamazepine Cyclosporine Irinotecan Digoxin
	CYP2C9	Induces	Lower levels of	Warfarin
	CYP1A2	Induces	Lower levels of	Warfarin
Transporter proteins	Intestinal P-glycoprotein transporter proteins	Increased catalyzed efflux of substrate drug	Lower levels of	Digoxin calcium-channel blockers Simvastatin
Pharmacodynamic toxicity	Serotonin reuptake receptor sites	Inhibits serotonin reuptake	Additive SSRI activity	SSRIs
	Serotonin reuptake receptor sites	Serotonin agonist activity	Additive serotonin toxicity	Serotonin agonists (e.g., fenfluramine) and "triptans"
	MAO receptor sites	Increased MAOI and serotonin activity	Additive serotonin toxicity	MAOIs
Pharmacokinetic	Serotonin and norepinephrine reuptake sites	Inhibits reuptake of norepinephrine and serotonin	Norepinephrine and serotonin toxicity	Nefazodone
	DNA-binding sites in human leukemia cells	Distorts DNA-binding sites	Reverses etoposide-stabilized cleavage complexes	Antagonizes chemotherapy effect of etoposide (in vitro)

MAOI, monoamine oxidase inhibitor; *NNRTI*, nonnucleoside reverse transcriptase inhibitor; *SSRI*, selective serotonin reuptake inhibitor.

V. FOOD–DRUG INTERACTIONS

A. Food can increase, decrease, or not affect the absorption of drugs (*Table 13-8*).

B. Food can influence the bioavailability of a drug from both modified-release dosage and immediate-release dosage forms, depending on the physical and chemical characteristics of the drug.

1. Generally, oral systemic absorption of lipid-soluble drugs is increased in the presence of fatty foods, whereas water-soluble drugs are decreased and possibly delayed due to delayed gastric emptying time.
2. Oral modified-release dosage forms such as controlled-release, delayed-release (enteric coated), or extended-release dosage forms may be adversely affected by food because these products may stay within an area of the GI tract to release drug over a period (e.g., 12-hour release product).

C. Complexation and adsorption of the drug in the GI tract with another food element is a common drug interaction that reduces the extent of drug absorption; for example, quinolone antibiotics complex with calcium (found in milk products) and magnesium.

1. Quinolone antibiotics will complex with calcium from the diet and the result will be reduced quinolone antibiotic.

Table 13-7 TABLE OF COMMON HERBS AND POTENTIAL DRUG INTERACTIONS

Herb	Drug/Drug Class	Interaction	Effect
Black cohosh	Antihypertensives	Pharmacodynamic potentiation	Increased effect of antihypertensives (hypotension)
Coenzyme Q10	Warfarin	Pharmacodynamic antagonism	Vitamin K antagonism (increased INR and risk of bleed)
Dong quai	β-blockers	Inhibition of CYP450 enzymes	Increased level of β-blockers (increased hypotension)
	Benzodiazepines	Inhibition of CYP450 enzymes	Increased benzodiazepine levels (increased drowsiness and CNS depression)
Echinacea	Immunosuppressants Monoclonal antibodies	Pharmacodynamic antagonism	Decreased immunosuppression (flair of autoimmune disease, transplant graft rejection)
Ephedrine Ma Huang	β-blockers	Pharmacodynamic antagonism	Sympathomimetic effect (hypertension)
	MAOIs	Blocked metabolism	Increased and prolonged sympathomimetic effect (hypertensive crisis)
	Corticosteroids	Increased metabolism Induced hepatic metabolism	Decreased corticosteroid levels (decreased steroid effectiveness)
Evening primrose oil	Antiplatelets	Pharmacodynamic potentiation	Decreased platelet aggregation (increased risk of bleed)
	Phenothiazines	Additive toxicity	Reduced seizure threshold (seizures)
Ginkgo biloba	Warfarin, LMWH	Pharmacodynamic potentiation	Increased inhibition of platelet aggregation (increased risk of bleed)
Ginseng	MAOI	Pharmacodynamic effect	Increased GABA metabolism and increased dopamine levels (mania symptoms)
Kava kava	Acetaminophen Azole antifungals Statins	Additive toxicity	Increased potential for hepatic toxicity (elevated LFT, hepatic failure)
	Barbiturates Benzodiazepines	Synergy	Increased GABA receptor binding affinity (increased drowsiness, CNS depression)
	Levodopa	Antagonism	Dopamine blockade (decreased effectiveness of levodopa)
Soy	Levothyroxine	Impaired absorption	Decreased levels of levothyroxine (hypothyroid symptoms)
St. John's wort	Irinotecan	Induced CYP3A4 Metabolism	Reduced levels of active irinotecan metabolite for chemotherapy (decreased myelosuppression)
Valerian	Sedatives	Pharmacodynamic	Increased CNS depression (drowsiness and sedation)
	Benzodiazepines	Displacement from binding sites	Displaced benzodiazepine but additive CNS depression (possible increased drowsiness)

CNS, central nervous system; *GABA*, gamma-aminobutyric acid; *INR*, international normalized ratio; *LFT*, liver function test; *LMWH*, low-molecular-weight-heparin; *MAOI*, monoamine oxidase inhibitor.

Table 13-11 THE EFFECT OF INHIBITION OF EM/UM AND PM ON CYP2D6 SUBSTRATES[a]

Enzyme	Inhibitor	Substrate	Effect of EM/UM on the Substrate	Effect of PM on the Substrate
CYP2D6	Diphenhydramine	Metoprolol	Increased 61%	Little change
CYP2D6	Quinidine	S-venlafaxine	Increased 4x	Little change
CYP2D6		R-venlafaxine	Increased 12x	No change
CYP2D6	Diphenhydramine	Venlafaxine	Increased 2x	Little change
CYP2D6	Fluoxetine	Risperidone	Increased 4x	Increase 1.3x

[a]Adapted from Lee LS et al. Evaluation of inhibitory drug interactions during drug development: Genetic polymorphisms must be considered. *Clin Pharmacol Ther.* 2005;78:1–6.
EM, extensive metabolizer; *PM*, poor metabolizer; *UM*, ultra-rapid metabolizer.

significant elevations in the active (substrate) drug. The substrate levels rise dramatically because the effect of the inhibitor is much greater in an EM. The drug interaction may occur to a greater extent than it would in normal metabolizers (*Table 13-11*).

2. In a **PM**, the level of substrate drug remains high because the metabolism of the substrate is much less than normal. When an **inhibitor** is added to the regimen, the additional inhibition of metabolism is not much greater than is already occuring in a PM. Therefore, the effect of an inhibitor on a PM is less than it would be in normal metabolizers. The drug interaction may not occur.
3. In an **EM**, the level of substrate drug is again lower than expected in a normal metabolizer because of the rapid metabolism. The addition of an **inducer** does not cause a great difference in the level of substrate because the metabolism is already increased greatly. The drug interaction may not occur.
4. In a **PM**, the level of substrate drug is again higher than expected in a normal metabolizer because of the lower metabolism of the substrate. The addition of an **inducer** will cause a significant increase in the metabolism of the substrate and cause a much lower level of substrate than expected in a normal metabolizer. The drug interaction may occur to a greater extent than in normal metabolizers, or the drug interaction may result in substrate levels similar to those of normal metabolizers.
5. As a general rule, the effect of inhibitors is greater in EMs than in PMs. The effect of inducers is greater in PMs than in EMs.
6. The addition of an inhibitor to a UM is expected to show an even greater drug reaction than would be seen with an EM.
7. Complex drug interactions can be seen when a substrate is metabolized through more than one enzyme system where one or more enzymes are affected by polymorphism. In these cases, the substrate is metabolized through a polymorphic enzyme and becomes an active metabolite and an inhibitor or inducer in a second system. Polymorphism in the first enzyme can cause the level of the inhibitor or inducer to be greater or less than expected, thus causing the extent of the expected inhibition or induction of the second enzyme to be significantly changed.

C. Some examples of specific pharmacogenomic drug interactions include the following:

1. **Omeprazole.** Omeprazole affects the pharmacokinetics of moclobemide according to the genetic polymorphism of CYP2C19. The effect of omeprazole inhibition of moclobemide metabolism varied according to the degree of genetic polymorphism, for example, extensive metabolizers (EM) and poor metabolizers (PM). In EM patients, the AUC level of the substrate moclobemide almost doubled, reflecting the greater effect of omeprazole inhibition on moclobemide, which is normally extensively metabolized. In comparison, PM subjects have poor metabolism of the moclobemide. Thus, inhibition of the 2C19 enzyme by omeprazole in PM did not show an extensive change in the AUC levels of moclobemide, because normal metabolism in these patients was already impaired.
2. **Fluvoxamine.** Fluvoxamine inhibits the metabolism of diphenhydramine by inhibiting the CYP2C19 isoenzyme. When EM patients on diphenhydramine were given fluvoxamine, the AUC and C_{max} levels of diphenhydramine were increased significantly. When PM patients on diphenhydramine were given fluvoxamine, the AUC and C_{max} of diphenhydramine did not change significantly. The effect of inhibition of CYP2C19 in an EM patient was greater than the effect of inhibition of CYP2C19 in PM patients. This demonstrates that the degree of inhibition varies by genotype. Homozygous EMs showed greater reduction in enzyme activity than

heterozygous EMs. EMs show greater inhibition than PMs because PMs already have reduced enzyme activity and will not show a great change in C_{max} or AUC, even with concurrent administration of an inhibitor such as fluvoxamine.

3. **Diphenhydramine.** Diphenhydramine inhibits the metabolism of metoprolol. In EM in the CYP2D6, the C_{max} and AUC of diphenhydramine increased by 16% and 61%, respectively, as compared to nonpolymorphisms. The inhibitor diphenhydramine decreased conversion of metoprolol to its metabolite by a factor of 3. In the PM, the change in metoprolol conversion was insignificant. Again, the effect of inhibition on the substrate in the EM was greater than in PM. There is significant interaction between the nonprescription antihistamine diphenhydramine and the CYP2D6 substrate metoprolol in healthy men with high or low CYP2D6 activity.
4. **Diphenhydramine.** Diphenhydramine inhibits the metabolism of venlafaxine by the CYP2D6 isoenzyme. When diphenhydramine is given to an EM who is taking venlafaxine, the levels of venlafaxine rise twofold. Diphenhydramine given to a PM who is taking venlafaxine causes insignificant change in the levels of venlafaxine. As with the previous example with metoprolol, the extent of inhibition in EM is much greater than in PM.

D. The effect of polymorphism on drug development and drug safety

1. Pharmacogenomic testing during drug development can identify the dosing variables in certain polymorphic populations and could lead to a greater safety in the use of these drugs. Clinical trials in warfarin therapy with genetic testing for polymorphisms in CYP2C9, such as the CYP2C9*2 and CYP2C9*3.
2. In small studies, or in studies of genetically homogeneous subjects, the pharmacokinetics described for the drug may be skewed toward the polymorphisms prevalent in the subject population. This can occur when, for example, Asians are the primary subject population for pharmacokinetic studies for a drug metabolized by CYP2C19. CYP2C19 polymorphisms occur in 20% to 25% of the Asian population.
3. When polymorphisms and pharmacogenomics are not considered during drug development, the result can be the development of some drugs that have shown toxicity in certain populations after FDA approval. Drugs that had to be withdrawn after market approval due to polymorphism include troglitazone (Rezulin) and mibefradil.
4. The identification of polymorphic factors in a specific drug under development may limit the clinical use of that drug to certain pharmacogenomic populations. Therefore, the FDA may make recommendations or require labeling for genetic testing of patients to determine polymorphisms that affect drug metabolism or transport. Some tests include the following:
   a. The Invader UGT1A1 molecular assay for UGT1A1 detects polymorphisms that can reduce the metabolism of irinotecan, a chemotherapy for colorectal cancer.
   b. The FDA has cleared the AmplicChip cytochrome P450 genotyping test for polymorphisms in the CYP450 isoenzyme system, which is extensively involved in drug metabolism.
   c. The FDA has added labeling to various drugs to test for genetic polymorphisms that affect metabolism, such as antiepileptic drugs.
   d. The FDA has also mandated the testing of HIV strains for guidance in using maraviroc.

VIII. CLINICAL SIGNIFICANCE AND MANAGEMENT OF DRUG INTERACTIONS

A. Potential drug interactions

1. **Multiple-drug therapy**, including both **prescription** and **nonprescription** (OTC) medication, can potentially lead to drug interactions. The more drugs used by a patient, the greater the potential for a drug interaction.
2. **Multiple prescribers.** Patients can be seen by different prescribers who prescribe interacting medication.
3. **Patient compliance.** Patients need to follow proper instructions for taking medications. For example, a patient might take tetracycline with food rather than before meals.
4. **Patient risk factors**
   a. Older patients are at more risk for drug interactions than younger patients. Older patients might have changes in their physiological and pathophysiological condition that lead to altered body composition, altered GI transit time and drug absorption, decreased protein

Study Questions

Directions for questions 1–2: Each question contains three suggested answers, of which **one** or more is correct. Choose the answer, **A–E**.

A **I only** is correct
B **III only** is correct
C **I and II** are correct
D **II and III** are correct
E **I, II, and III** are correct

1. Drug interactions may be classed as

I. pharmacokinetic interactions
II. pharmacodynamic interactions
III. pharmaceutical interactions

2. Situations that can potentially lead to drug interactions include

I. multiple-drug therapy
II. multiple prescribers
III. patient compliance

Directions for questions 3–10: Each question is followed by four suggested answers. Select the **one** lettered answer that is the **best** response to the question.

3. Which of the following statements regarding drug interactions is true?

(A) All drug interactions can potentially cause an adverse response in the patient.
(B) The clinical significance for each potential drug interaction must be considered individually.
(C) A precipitant drug that inhibits the metabolism of the object drug causes a more serious drug interaction compared to a precipitant drug causing an increase in the bioavailability of the object drug.
(D) If the patient is prescribed drugs that can potentially interact, the prescriber should be called, and a different precipitant drug should be suggested.

4. A patient on indinavir antiretroviral therapy (ART) begins taking St. John's wort for depression and suffers unexpected reduction in CD4 count. This is most likely due to

(A) pharmacodynamic interaction producing additive toxicity.
(B) pharmacodynamic interaction producing antagonistic therapeutic effect.
(C) enzyme induction by St. John's wort causing increased metabolism of ART.
(D) enzyme inhibition by St. John's wort causing toxic levels of ART.

5. Which of the following is a valid therapeutic use of a drug interaction?

(A) The use of probenecid with penicillin G to prolong high penicillin levels to treat a sexually transmitted disease
(B) Giving aspirin with warfarin to enhance anticoagulation
(C) Instructing the patient to take levofloxacin with milk or antacid to decrease GI intolerance to oral therapy
(D) The treatment of depression with a combination of citalopram and a MAOI

6. Which of the following is not a harmful food–drug interaction?

(A) Raw green salads for patients on warfarin deep vein thrombosis (DVT) prophylaxis
(B) Grapefruit juice and cyclosporine to prevent graft-versus-host rejection of a transplanted kidney
(C) Omeprazole beads in applesauce for a patient with problems swallowing capsules secondary to gastroesophageal reflux disease (GERD)
(D) Milk with doxycycline to treat *Helicobacter pylori*

7. Which of the following statements regarding pharmacogenetic polymorphisms is not true?

(A) An EM taking metoprolol for hypertension begins to take OTC Tagamet® regularly for heartburn. He or she is at increased risk for bradycardia and cardiac arrhythmias.
(B) An EM taking methadone begins taking Tegretol® for neuropathic pain. He or she is at risk for treatment failure and pain crisis.
(C) A PM taking atorvastatin for hyperlipidemia is placed on ketoconazole for a fungal infection. He or she is at increased risk for myalgia and rhabdomyolysis.
(D) A PM taking metoprolol for tachycardia begins taking Benadryl® for sleep. He or she is not at risk for significant bradycardia and cardiac block.

8. Asians are at greatest risk of all racial groups for genetic polymorphism in which one of the following CYP450 isoenzymes?

(A) CYP2D6
(B) CYP3A4
(C) CYP2C19
(D) CYP1A2

9. Which of the following statements regarding pharmacogenetics is false?

(A) Polymorphisms occur only in the CYP450 hepatic enzymes.
(B) Polymorphisms result in many variations of an isoenzyme.
(C) The overall expression of the combined alleles is the phenotype of the enzyme.
(D) Single-nucleotide polymorphisms (SNPs) can occur as errors of transcription, defective splicing, start and stop codones, and amino acid changes.

10. Which of the following statements regarding allele polymorphisms is false?

(A) Wild-type alleles encode for "normal" metabolism.
(B) Ultra-rapid metabolizers (UMs) have two or more amplified alleles.
(C) Poor metabolizers (PMs) carry one defective allele and one amplified allele.
(D) Extensive metabolizers (EMs) with heterozygous alleles have slower metabolism than metabolizers with homozygous alleles.

Answers and Explanations

1. The answer is E *[see I.B]*.
Most drug interactions in vivo are caused by pharmacokinetic and pharmacodynamic interactions. Pharmaceutical interactions can occur during extemporaneous compounding, preparation of IV admixtures, and improper dosing, as in the case of giving aspirin with acidic juices (e.g., orange, cranberry).

2. The answer is E *[see IV.A.1–3]*.
Patient profiles might not contain all the drug history information of the patient. Patients who take nonprescription (OTC) medications and who go to several different physicians or purchase drugs at various pharmacies may neglect to inform the pharmacist of all the medications being taken.

3. The answer is B *[see IV.B]*.
Not all drug interactions are clinically significant. Some potential clinically significant drug interactions can be prevented by proper patient instruction and compliance. The potential for a clinically significant drug interaction should be documented before calling a physician concerning the prescribed medication.

4. The answer is C *[see II.E.1.c; Table 13-3]*.
St. John's wort induces CYP3A4 isoenzymes, increasing the metabolism of the indinavir and resulting in low indinavir levels and therapeutic failure of ART. St. John's wort itself has no direct effect on CD4.

5. The answer is A *[see II.E.2; Table 13-4]*.
Probenecid is given with penicillin and some cephalosporins in the treatment of some sexually transmitted diseases. Probenecid competes with penicillins for renal elimination, prolonging the half-life of the penicillin. Aspirin and warfarin cause additive anticoagulation, leading to bleeding. Levofloxacin taken with milk to decrease GI irritation causes complexation of the levofloxacin with the calcium in the milk and results in decreased levofloxacin to be available. Concomitant treatment of depression of citalopram and MAOI results in serotonin syndrome, an additive toxicity.

6. The answer is C *[see V.B]*.
Omeprazole beads are enteric coated. Giving an enteric-coated bead with an acidic food such as applesauce preserves the enteric coating and allows the drug to pass intact through the acidic stomach environment and into the basic duodenum environment where it is absorbed. The result is improved drug absorption and decreased drug destruction in the acidic stomach than if the beads were not in an acidic food.

7. The answer is C *[see VII.C.2]*.
The PM already has inhibited metabolism of atorvastatin. Additional inhibition will not significantly increase the blood levels of atorvastatin. Therefore, dose-related toxicity is unlikely. The EM taking metoprolol and Tagamet® (cimetidine) will show a greater increase in the metoprolol levels due to the exaggerated effect of the inhibitor in EM. The EM taking methadone and Tegretol® (carbamazepine) will have increased enzyme induction and metabolism of the methadone, lowering methadone levels and putting the patient at risk for treatment failure of his pain. The PM taking metoprolol and Benadryl® (diphenhydramine) will show inhibition of the metabolism of the metoprolol and increased levels of metoprolol, leading to a higher risk of bradycardia and cardiac block.

8. The answer is A *[see VII.A.3]*.
Polymorphism is highest in the CYP2D6 isoenzyme in Asians, reaching incidence of greater than 50%.

9. The answer is A *[see VII.A.2]*.
Polymorphisms can occur in any enzyme system including mixed oxidase and *N*-acetyl transferase systems as well as the CYP450 hepatic enzyme system.

10. The answer is C *[see VII.B.3.a]*.
PMs carry a normal allele combined with a defective or deleted allele.

14 Drug Information Resources

PAUL F. SOUNEY, CONNIE LEE BARNES, VALERIE B. CLINARD

I. DEFINITION. Drug information is current, critically examined, relevant data about drugs and drug use in a given patient or situation.

A. **Current information** uses the most recent, up-to-date sources possible.
B. **Critically examined information** should meet the following criteria:
   1. More than one source should be used when appropriate.
   2. The extent of agreement of sources should be determined; if sources do not agree, good judgment should be used.
   3. The plausibility of information, based on clinical circumstances, should be determined.
C. **Relevant information** must be presented in a manner that applies directly to the circumstances under consideration (e.g., patient parameters, therapeutic objectives, alternative approaches).

II. DRUG INFORMATION RESOURCES. There are three sources of drug information: journals/clinical trials (primary sources), indexing and abstracting services (secondary sources), and textbook and databases (tertiary sources).

A. **Primary sources**
   1. **Benefits.** Clinical trials provide the most current information about drugs and, ideally, should be the source for answering therapeutic questions. Journals enable pharmacists to:
      a. Keep abreast of professional news
      b. Learn how another clinician handled a particular problem
      c. Keep up with new developments in pathophysiology, diagnostic agents, and therapeutic regimens
      d. Distinguish useful from useless or even harmful therapy
      e. Enhance communication with other health care professionals and consumers
      f. Obtain continuing education credits
      g. Share opinions with other health care professionals through letters to the editor
      h. Prepare for the board certification examination in pharmacotherapy, nutrition support, oncology, and so forth.
   2. **Limitations.** Although publication of an article in a well-known, respected journal enhances the credibility of information contained in an article, this does not guarantee that the data are accurate. Many articles possess inadequacies that become apparent as the ability to evaluate drug information improves.
   3. **Review articles (narrative reviews and systematic reviews), articles of opinion, correspondence, and special reports.** All material included in a journal is not considered a primary resource. Original clinical trials are considered primary literature; however, review articles, articles of opinion, correspondence, and special reports are not.
B. **Secondary sources**
   1. **Benefits.** Indexing and abstracting services are valuable tools for quick and selective screening of the primary literature for specific information, data, citation, and articles (*Table 14-1*). In some cases, the sources provide sufficient information to serve as references for answering drug information requests.

Table 14-1 EXAMPLES OF ABSTRACTING AND INDEXING SERVICES

Secondary References	Journals Indexed
CINAHL*	2999
ClinAlert	150
Current Contents/Clinical Medicine	1120
Embase	7500
Medline/PubMed	5516
International Pharmaceutical Abstracts	800
Iowa Drug Information System	353
Pharmaceutical News Index	—
Reactions Weekly	—
Science Citation Index	3700

*Cumulative Index to Nursing and Allied Health Literature.

2. **Limitations.** Each indexing or abstracting service reviews a finite number of journals. Therefore, relying on only one service can greatly hinder the thoroughness of a literature search. Another important fact to remember is the substantial difference in lag time (i.e., the interval between the publication of an article and the citation of that article in an index) among the available services. For example, the approximate lag time for PubMed may be less than 1 week, whereas the approximate lag time for the Iowa Drug Information Service may be 30 to 60 days.
   a. Secondary sources usually **describe** only articles and clinical studies from journals. Frequently, readers respond to, criticize, and add new information to published articles and studies through letters. Services such as Medline/PubMed or the Iowa Drug Information Service generally do include pertinent letters to the editor within the scope of coverage.
   b. Indexing and abstracting services are primarily used to **locate** journal articles. In general, abstracts should not be used as primary sources of information because they are typically interpretations of a study and may be a misinterpretation of important information. Additionally, abstracts may not include enough information to critically evaluate the study. Thus, pharmacists should obtain and evaluate the original clinical trial instead of relying on the abstract alone.

C. **Tertiary sources**
1. **Benefits**
   a. **Textbooks.** General reference textbooks can provide easy and convenient access to a broad spectrum of related topics. Background information on drugs and diseases is often available. Although a textbook might answer many drug-related questions, the limitations of these sources should not be overlooked.
      (1) It could take several years to publish a text, so information available in textbooks might not include the most recent developments in the field. Other resources should be used to update or supplement information obtained from textbooks.
      (2) The author of a textbook might not have conducted a thorough search of the primary literature, so pertinent data could have been omitted. An author also might have misinterpreted the literature. Reference citations should be available to verify the validity and accuracy of the data.
   b. **Databases.** Computer databases are convenient, easy to use, and often referenced. These resources are similar to textbooks, but are typically updated more frequently. Computer databases are easy to search and are often useful resources for drug monographs, pill identifications, drug interactions, drug compatibility, and various therapeutic calculations. Additionally, computer databases may address clinical questions. In some instances, a mobile version of the database is available. Examples include Clinical Pharmacology Mobile, Clinical Xpert, Lexicomp On-Hand, and Epocrates Rx or Epocrates Essentials.

2. **General considerations** when examining and using textbooks and/or databases as sources of drug information consider the following:
   a. The author, publisher, or both: What are the author's and publisher's areas of expertise?
   b. The year of publication (copyright date) or last revision date?
   c. The edition of the text: Is it the most current edition?
   d. The presence of a bibliography: If a bibliography is included, are important statements accurately referenced? When were the references published?
   e. The scope of the textbook or database: How accessible is the information?
   f. Alternative resources that are available (e.g., primary and secondary sources, other relevant texts)

III. INTERNET

A. **Benefits.** The Internet expands the ability to search therapies that have been recently published or discussed in the media. An Internet search may be used for the following: company-specific information, issues currently in the news, alternative medicine, or U.S. government information. One of the many available search engines can be used to find available data.

B. **Limitations**
   1. Unlike information published in journals and textbooks, information obtained from the Internet may not be peer reviewed or edited before release.
   2. Information received from the Internet may be only as reliable as the person who posted it and the users who read and comment on its content. A Web site should be evaluated by its source (author) of information. The name, location, and sponsorship should be disclosed. Also, a reputable site will provide easy access to information and references to support the information provided. Pharmacists should use traditional literature evaluation skills to determine whether information on the Web site is clear, concise, unbiased, relevant, and referenced. A selection of several reliable Web sites is provided in *Table 14-2.*
   3. Web sites are always changing and may not exist after several years. It is important to document when and where information from the Internet was found.

IV. STRATEGIES FOR EVALUATING INFORMATION REQUESTS.

It is important to obtain as much information as possible about drug information requests before beginning a literature search. Both time and money can be lost doing a vast search. The following are important questions to ask the inquirer or to evaluate before a manual or computerized search.

A. **Converse with the inquirer.** Before spending time searching for information, talk to the person who is requesting the information and acquire any necessary additional information.
   1. **Determine the reason for the inquiry.** Find out where the inquirer heard or read about the drug. Is he or she taking the medication? If so, why? Because the search can be done by the drug or disease name, determine whether the inquirer has a medical condition. Ascertaining the reason for the inquiry helps determine what additional information should be provided. For example, if the inquiry concerns a foreign drug, the inquirer might ask for a domestic equivalent.
   2. **Clarify the drug's identification and availability.** Make sure that the drug in question is available and double-check information about the drug, such as the following:
      a. The **correct spelling** of the drug's name
      b. Whether it is a **generic** or **brand name drug**
      c. What **pharmaceutical company** manufactures the drug and in what **country** the drug is manufactured
      d. Whether the drug is **prescription** or **nonprescription**
      e. Whether the drug is still **under investigation** and, if it is on the market, **the length of time on the market**
      f. The **dosage form** of the drug
      g. The **purpose** of the drug (i.e., what medical condition or symptom the drug is intended to alleviate; this information helps narrow the search if products with similar names are found)

B. To **identify** or **assess product availability**, consider using the following resources (see also Appendix E). Some of these resources are available in an electronic format or in an Internet/intranet version.
   1. For drugs manufactured in the **United States**, the following resources are available:
      a. *The American Drug Index*
      b. *Drug Facts and Comparisons/Facts and Comparison E Answers*

Table 14-2 SELECTED WEB SITES

Site	URL (Web Address)
Agency for Healthcare Research and Quality	http://www.ahrq.gov
American Association of Colleges of Pharmacy	http://www.aacp.org
American Cancer Society	http://www.cancer.org
American Diabetes Association	http://www.diabetes.org
American Heart Association	http://www.heart.org
American Society of Health-System Pharmacists	http://www.ashp.org
Centers for Disease Control and Prevention	http://www.cdc.gov
Clinical Trial Results	http://www.clinicaltrialresults.org
Clinical Trials	http://www.clinicaltrials.gov
Drug Infonet	http://www.druginfonet.com
eMedicine	http://www.emedicine.com
Evidence Medicine	http://www.evidmed.com
Healthfinder	http://www.healthfinder.gov
Health on the Net Foundation	http://www.hon.ch
Mayo Clinic	http://www.mayo.edu
Medscape	http://www.medscape.com
MedWatch	http://www.fda.gov/medwatch
National Cancer Institute	http://www.cancer.gov
National Guideline Clearinghouse	http://www.guideline.gov
National Heart, Lung, and Blood Institute	http://www.nhlbi.nih.gov
National Institutes of Health	http://www.nih.gov
Pharmaceutical Research and Manufacturers of America	http://www.phrma.org
PharmacyOneSource	http://www.pharmacyonesource.com
RxList	http://www.rxlist.com
RxMed	http://www.rxmed.com
U.S. Department of Health and Human Services	http://www.hhs.gov
U.S. Food and Drug Administration	http://www.fda.gov
U.S. National Library of Medicine	http://www.nlm.nih.gov
WebMD	http://www.webmd.com

   c. *Red Book*
   d. *Physician's Desk Reference (PDR)*
   e. *American Hospital Formulary Service (AHFS) Drug Information*
   f. *Martindale: The Complete Drug Reference*
   g. *Lexicomp Online*
   h. *Clinical Pharmacology*
   i. *Micromedex*
2. For drugs manufactured in **foreign countries**, the following resources are available:
   a. *Martindale: The Complete Drug Reference*
   b. *Index Nominum*
   c. *USP Dictionary of United States Adopted Names (USAN) and International Drug Names*
   d. *Lexi-Drugs International Online (Lexicomp Online)*
3. For **investigational drugs**, the following resources are available:
   a. *Martindale: The Complete Drug Reference*
   b. *Drug Facts and Comparisons/Facts and Comparison E Answers*
   c. *The Pink Sheet* published by FDC Reports
   d. *The NDA Pipeline* published by FDC Reports
4. For **orphan drugs**—that is, drugs that are used to prevent or treat a rare disease (affects fewer than 200,000 people in the United States, or affects more than 200,000 people but the

products are not expected to recover the costs required for developing and marketing the drug) and for which the U.S. Food and Drug Administration (FDA) offers assistance and financial incentives to sponsors undertaking the development of the drugs—the following resources are available:

a. *Drug Facts and Comparisons/Facts and Comparison E Answers*
b. The FDA Office of Orphan Products Development (OOPD)
c. The National Institutes of Health (NIH) Office of Rare Diseases
d. National Organization for Rare Disorders

5. For an **unknown drug** (i.e., one that is in hand but not identified), chemical analysis can be performed or the drug can be identified by physical characteristics, such as color, special markings, and shape. Consult the following sources for help:
   a. *PDR, Drug Facts and Comparisons, Facts and Comparison E Answers, Red Book, Ident-A-Drug Reference*
   b. *Identidex (Micromedex)*
   c. The manufacturer
   d. A laboratory
   e. *Lexicomp Online (Lexi-Drug ID)*
   f. *Clinical Pharmacology Product Identification*
6. For a **natural product**, the following resources are available:
   a. *Facts and Comparison E Answers*
   b. *Natural Medicines Comprehensive Database*
   c. *Natural Standards*
   d. *Natural Products Database (Lexicomp Online)*
   e. *Clinical Pharmacology*

V. SEARCH STRATEGIES.

To develop an effective search strategy for locating drug information literature, the following tactics should be followed after determining whether primary or secondary sources are desired.

A. Determine whether the question at hand is **clinical** or **research related**. **Define the question** as specifically as possible. Also, identify appropriate index terms (also called keywords or descriptors) with which to search for the information.

B. Determine the **type of information** and **how much** is needed (i.e., only one fact, the most recent clinical trials, review articles, or a comprehensive database search).

C. **Ascertain as much information as possible** about the drug being questioned and the **inquirer's association** with it. Remember that data on adverse drug effects or drug interactions are often fragmented and inadequately documented. See IV.A.2 for the specific drug information that should be acquired. Determine the answers to the following questions:

1. What is the indication for the prescribed drug?
2. Is the drug's use approved or unapproved? This information can be found in the following resources (remember to check how often these resources are updated to ensure having the latest information).
   a. **Approved uses** of drugs can be checked in the following:
      (1) *AHFS Drug Information*
      (2) *Drug Facts and Comparisons/Facts and Comparison E Answers*
      (3) *PDR*
      (4) *USP Drug Information*
      (5) *Drugdex (Micromedex)*
      (6) *Clinical Pharmacology*
      (7) *Drug Information Handbook/Lexi-Drugs Online (Lexicomp Online)*
   b. **Unapproved uses** of drugs can be found in the following:
      (1) *AHFS Drug Information*
      (2) *Drug Facts and Comparisons/Facts and Comparison E Answers*
      (3) *Martindale: The Complete Drug Reference*
      (4) Medline
      (5) *Drugdex* (Micromedex)

(6) *USP Drug Information*
(7) *Clinical Pharmacology*
(8) *Drug Information Handbook/Lexi-Drugs Online (Lexicomp Online)*

3. What is the age, sex, and weight of the patient in question?
4. Does the patient have any other medical conditions or renal or hepatic disease?
5. Is the patient taking any other medications?
6. What drugs has the patient taken during the past 6 months, and what were the dosages?
7. Did the patient experience any signs or symptoms of a possible adverse drug reaction? If so,
   a. How severe was the reaction?
   b. When did the reaction appear?
   c. Has the patient (or any member of the patient's family) experienced any allergic or adverse reactions to medications in the past?
   d. Consult the following resources for more information:
      (1) *Meyler's Side Effects of Drugs*
      (2) A general drug reference (e.g., *PDR*, *Clinical Pharmacology*)
      (3) Medline
   e. The manufacturer of the drug may be a useful source for missing information. Most companies request further information regarding a suspected adverse drug reaction.
8. Did the patient experience any signs or symptoms of a drug interaction? If so,
   a. What were the specific drugs in question?
   b. What were the respective dosages of the drugs?
   c. What was the duration of therapy?
   d. What was the length of the course of administration?
   e. What are the details of the events secondary to the suspected reaction?
   f. Consult the following resources for more information:
      (1) A drug interactions reference—for example, *Drug Interaction Facts/Facts and Comparisons E Answers, Hansten's Drug Interaction Analysis and Management, Evaluations of Drug Interactions (EDI)*
      (2) A general drug reference (e.g., *PDR*)
      (3) *Reactions Weekly*
      (4) Medline
      (5) *Lexi-International (Lexicomp Online)*
      (6) *Clinical Pharmacology*
      (7) *Micromedex*
9. What is the patient's current medication status?
10. Does the patient have any underlying diseases?
11. How has the patient been managed so far?
12. What is the stability of the drug? How is compatibility of the drug with other drugs? What are the administration techniques? What are appropriate containers for the product? Resources available with this information include the following:
    a. *Trissel's Handbook on Injectable Drugs*
    b. *King's Guide to Parenteral Admixtures*
    c. *Trissel's Stability of Compounded Formulations*
    d. *Handbook of Drug Administration via Enteral Feeding Tubes*
    e. *Extended Stability for Parenteral Drugs*

D. **Explore other possible information resources if necessary.** For example, it may be useful to find background material in textbooks or databases (tertiary references) or via the Internet, and then search the journal literature (primary references) for more current information.

VI. EVALUATING A CLINICAL STUDY.

Resource identification is followed by a critical assessment of the available information. This step is critical in developing an appropriate response for the inquirer.

A. **Evaluate the objective of the study.** Determine the aim of the research that was performed.
   1. What did the researchers intend to examine?
   2. Is this goal stated clearly (i.e., is the objective specific)?
   3. Was the research limited to a single objective, or were there multiple drugs or effects being tested?

B. Evaluate the subjects of the study. Determine the profile of the study population by assessing the following information:

1. Were healthy subjects or affected patients used in the study?
2. Were the subjects volunteers?
3. What were the criteria for selecting the subjects?
4. How many subjects were included, and what are the demographics of the subjects (age, sex, and race)?
5. If a disease was being treated, did any of the subjects have diseases other than that initially being treated? Were any additional treatments given? Were there any contraindications to the therapy?
6. What was the patient selection method and who was excluded from the study?
7. A patient selection review should be done. You will find that most groups of subjects are homogeneous (i.e., they all have comparable characteristics). If a disease state is studied, patients should exhibit similar severity of symptoms. Researchers aim to eliminate interpatient variability. By selecting patients with similar characteristics, researchers can avoid results that are caused by individual differences among patients. Strong individual differences can obscure the results of the experiment. If studying a group of patients who exhibit significant interpatient variability is necessary, researchers may divide the patients into groups according to the variables likely to be associated with responsiveness to therapy. This is known as stratification.

C. Evaluate the administration of the drug treatment. For each drug being investigated, determine the following information:

1. **Details of treatment** with the agent being studied:
   a. Daily dose
   b. Frequency of administration
   c. Hours of day when administered
   d. Route of administration
   e. Source of drug (i.e., the supplier)
   f. Dosage form
   g. Timing of drug administration in relation to factors affecting drug absorption
   h. Methods of ensuring compliance
   i. Total duration of treatment
2. **Other therapeutic measures** in addition to the agent being studied

D. Evaluate the setting of the study. Try to determine the environment of the study and the dates on which the trial began and ended. Assess the following information:

1. People who made the observations; various professionals who offer different and unique perspectives based on their backgrounds and interests (Were the same people making observations throughout the study?)
2. Whether the study was done on an inpatient or outpatient basis
3. Description of physical setting (e.g., hospital, clinic, ward)
4. Length of the study (i.e., dates on which the trial began and ended)

E. Evaluate the methods and design of the study. The method section of the research paper explains how the research was conducted. The study design (i.e., retrospective, prospective, blind, crossover) and the methods used to complete the study are important in judging whether the study and the results are reliable and valid. From the study, try to determine answers to the following questions:

1. Are the methods of assessing the therapeutic effects clearly described?
2. Were the methods standardized?
   a. **Retrospective versus prospective**
      (1) **Retrospective** studies evaluate events that have already occurred to find some common link among them, require reliance on patient memories and accurate medical records, and are unable to show cause and effect. Retrospective studies are useful for studying rare diseases (or effects) and can help a health care professional decide whether enough information exists to warrant prospective examination of a problem.
      (2) **Prospective** studies follow identified patients forward in time to answer a specific question. They can be observational or experimental (i.e., clinical trials).
   b. **Treatment allocation**
      (1) **Parallel** study design is a protocol in which two or more patient groups are studied concurrently. The groups are treated identically except for one variable, such as a drug therapy (*Figure 14-1*).

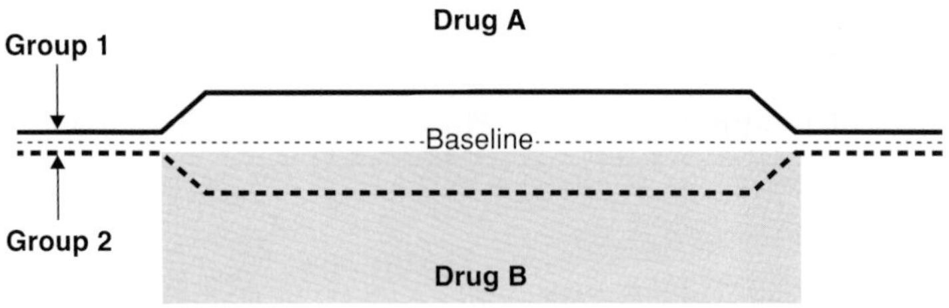

Figure 14-1. Parallel study design.

(2) **Crossover** design may be used as an additional control for interpatient and intrapatient variability (*Figure 14-2*). In this type of design, each patient group undergoes each type of treatment. However, the sequence in which the subjects undergo treatment is reversed for one group. Crossover design reduces the possibility that the results were strongly influenced by the order in which therapy was given. And because both groups of patients receive both types of treatment, any differences in responsiveness between the groups as a result of patient selection will be uncovered.

3. Were **control measures** used to reduce variation that might influence the results? Examples of such control methods include the following:
   a. Concurrent controls
   b. Stratification or matched subgroups
   c. A run-in phase
   d. The patient as his or her own control (i.e., crossover design)
   e. Identical ancillary treatment
4. Were controls used to reduce bias? Examples of such controls include the following:
   a. **Blind assessment**, which means that the people observing the patients do not know who is a subject and who is a control
   b. **Blind patients**, which means that the patients do not know whether they received the substance being studied or a placebo (**double-blind** combines this point with a point previously [VI.E.4.a]) (*Table 14-3*)
   c. **Random allocation**, which means that the patients involved in the study have an equal chance of being assigned to either the group of subjects receiving the active drug or the group receiving a placebo
   d. **Matching dummies**, which are placebos that are physically identical to the active agent being studied
   e. **Comparison** of a placebo or a therapy to a recognized standard practice (placebo-controlled)

F. **Evaluate the analysis of the study.** After assessing specific areas of the study separately, compile the information together to determine whether the trial is acceptable and the conclusions are justified by determining answers to the following questions (*Figure 14-3*):
   1. Were the subjects suitably selected in relation to the aim(s) of the study?
   2. Were the methods of measurement valid in relation to the aim(s) of the study?
   3. Were the methods adequately standardized?
   4. Were the methods sufficiently sensitive?
   5. Was the design appropriate?
   6. Were enough subjects enrolled?
   7. Was the dosage appropriate?

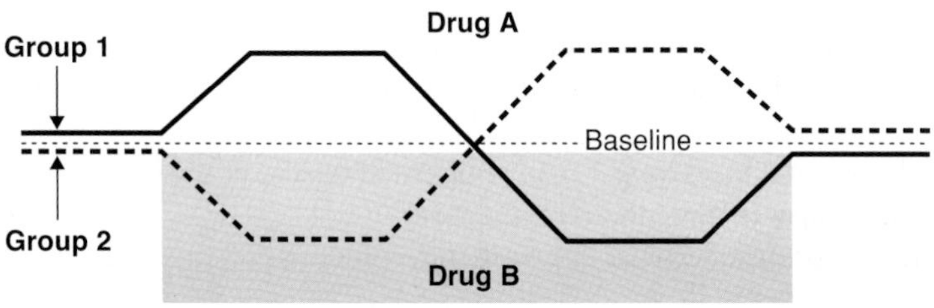

Figure 14-2. Crossover study design.

Table 14-3 TYPES OF BLIND STUDIES

Types of Blinds	Patient Aware of Treatment	Physician Aware of Treatment
Open label (nonblind)	✓	✓
Single-blind	—	✓
Double-blind	—	—

8. Was the duration of treatment adequate?
9. Were carryover effects avoided, or were compensations made for them? Did a wash-out period exist?
10. If no controls were used, were they unnecessary or overlooked?
11. If controls were used, were they adequate?
12. Was the comparability of treatment groups examined?
13. Are the data adequate for assessment?
14. If statistical tests were not done, were they unnecessary or overlooked?
15. If statistical tests are reported, assess the following:
    a. Is it clear how the statistical tests were done?
    b. Were the tests appropriately used?
    c. If results show no significant difference between test groups, were enough patients studied (i.e., statistical power)?

VII. GENERAL GUIDELINES FOR RESPONSES TO DRUG INFORMATION REQUESTS

A. **Do not guess!**

B. Responses to a member of the public must take several ethical issues into account.
1. Patient privacy must be protected.
2. Professional ethics must be maintained.
3. The patient–physician relationship cannot be breached.
4. A response is not necessary if the inquirer intends to misuse or abuse information that is provided. The inquirer often admits intent or offers clues to potential abuse, such as in the following examples:
    a. A patient asks how a certain drug is dosed (i.e., how much the drug can be increased, when it can be increased, what the maximum daily dose is). This kind of inquiry signals that the patient might be adjusting his or her own therapy.
    b. A patient asks a pharmacist to identify a tablet that is a prescription product known for a high rate of abuse.

C. Organize information before attempting to communicate the response to the inquirer. Responses should be concise and succinct. Anticipate additional questions.

D. Tailor the response to the inquirer's background. Also, consider the environment of the practice, institutional policy and procedure, and formulary.

E. Tell the inquirer where the information was found. Exercise caution when making statements such as, "There are no reports in the literature."

F. Use *extreme* caution when making statements such as, "I recommend . . ." Do not hesitate to refer consumers to their physicians.

G. Use more than abstracts to answer drug information questions. The information included in abstracts may be taken out of context and does not include all of the data available in the original article.

H. Alert the inquirer of a possible delay when it takes longer than anticipated to answer the question.

I. Ask if the information that is provided answers the inquirer's questions.

J. Ask if the inquirer would like to have reprints of articles or a written response.

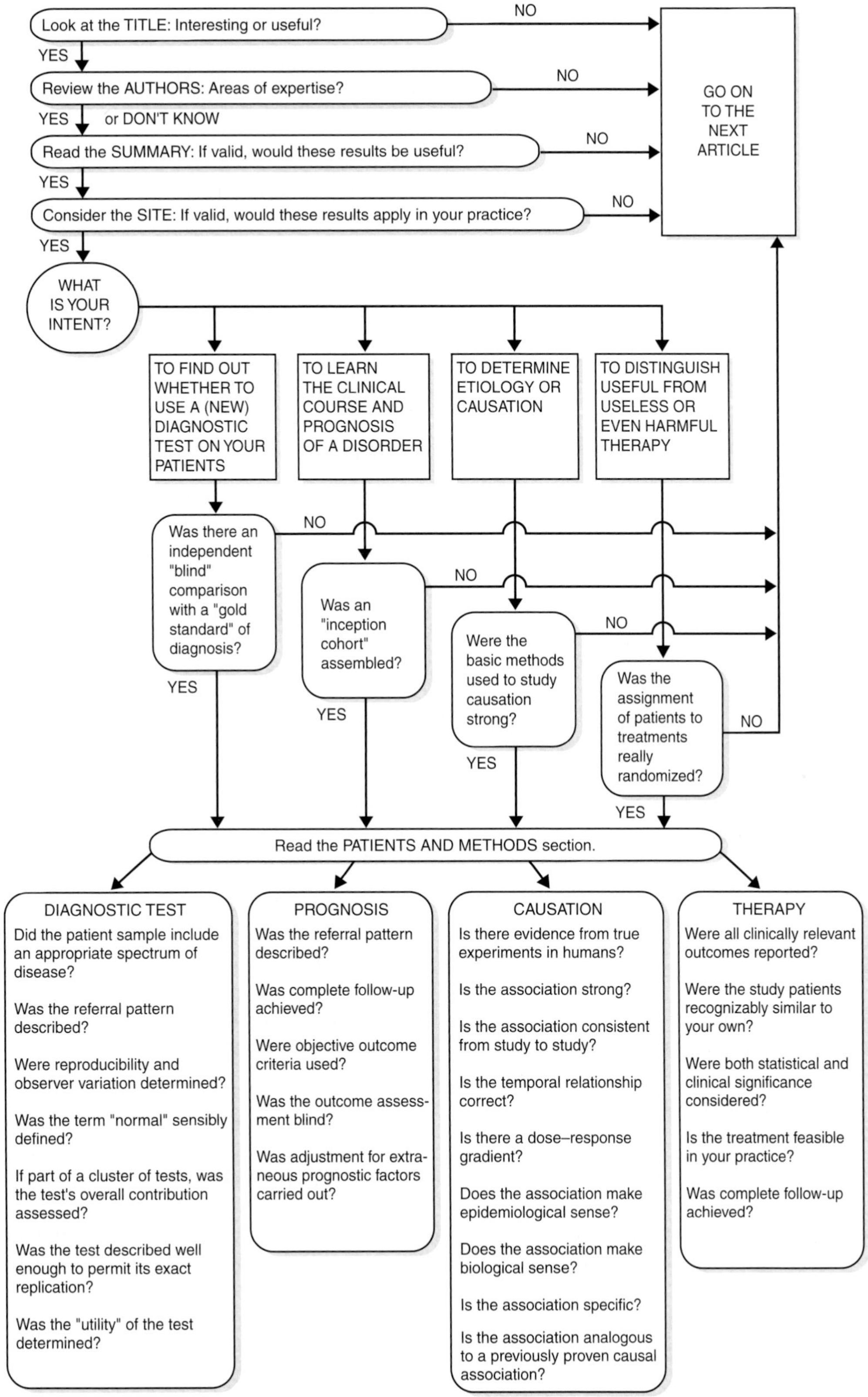

Figure 14-3. Evaluation of study analysis.

Study Questions

Directions: Each of the numbered items or incomplete statements in this section is followed by answers or completions of the statement. Select the **one** lettered answer or completion that is **best** in each case.

1. Primary literature includes which of the following?

(A) Original clinical trials
(B) Letters to the editor
(C) Systematic reviews
(D) Special reports

2. Which of the following statements is TRUE regarding tertiary resources?

(A) Tertiary resources include textbooks and computer databases.
(B) Textbooks typically include the most recent literature and/or information.
(C) Tertiary resources do not typically include a bibliography.
(D) The credentials of the editor of a tertiary resource are not considered important.

3. Which of the following should NOT be done when developing an effective search strategy?

(A) Determine if the question is clinical or research-related
(B) Identify appropriate search terms
(C) Disregard other medications the patient may be taking
(D) Ascertain if the inquirer is a health care professional

4. Which of the following resources would be appropriate for identifying a drug manufactured in a foreign country?

(A) *Martindale: The Complete Drug Reference*
(B) *Clinical Pharmacology*
(C) *Trissel's Stability of Compounded Formulations*
(D) *AHFS*

5. Which of the following resources would be appropriate for identifying the capsule with the imprint code of Watson 405?

I. *Facts and Comparison E Answers*
II. *Lexi-Drugs ID (Lexicomp Online)*
III. *Myler's Side Effects of Drugs*

(A) **I** and **II** only
(B) **I** and **III** only
(C) **II** and **III** only

6. Which of the following resources would be appropriate for determining the adverse effects of ginkgo biloba?

I. *Natural Medicines Comprehensive Database*
II. *Facts and Comparisons E Answers*
III. *Natural Standards*
IV. *Handbook on Injectable Drugs*

(A) **I** and **II** only
(B) **II** and **III** only
(C) **I**, **II**, and **III** only
(D) **II** and **IV** only

7. Which of the following resources would be appropriate for determining if Levaquin is compatible or stable in D_5W?

(A) *Evaluations of Drug Interactions (EDI)*
(B) *Trissel's Handbook on Injectable Drugs*
(C) *Red Book*
(D) *Nonprescription Products Therapeutics*

8. Which of the following resources can be used to determine unapproved uses of drugs?

(A) *Clinical Pharmacology*
(B) *PDR*
(C) *Index Nominum*
(D) *King's Guide to Parenteral Admixtures*

9. Which of the following is *not* important when evaluating a clinical study?

(A) Study objective
(B) Patient demographics
(C) Drug administration
(D) Number of authors

10. Which of the following statements is TRUE?

(A) Prospective studies evaluate events that have already occurred.
(B) Retrospective studies are useful for evaluating rare diseases.
(C) A run-in phase typically increases variation.
(D) Crossover design allows patients to undergo only one type of treatment.

11. Which of the following resources would be appropriate in evaluating the drug interaction between tramadol and citalopram?
    - **I.** *Evaluations of Drug Interactions (EDI)*
    - **II.** *Lexi-Interact (Lexicomp Online)*
    - **III.** *Trissel's Stability of Compounded Formulations*

    A. I and II only
    B. I and III only
    C. II and III only
    D. I, II, and III

12. Which of the following resources would be appropriate for determining whether ranitidine causes edema?
    - **I.** *Red Book*
    - **II.** *PDR*
    - **III.** *Myler's Side Effects of Drugs*

    A. I and II
    B. I and III only
    C. II and III only
    D. I, II, and III

13. What resource should be used when searching for the most current clinical trials on the use of atenolol for hypertension?

    A. *King's Guide to Parenteral Admixture*
    B. Medline
    C. *American Hospital Formulary Service (AHFS)*
    D. *The American Drug Index*

14. Which of the following resources would be appropriate for evaluating information on orphan drugs?
    - **I.** *Drug Facts and Comparisons/Facts and Comparison E Answers*
    - **II.** The FDA Office of Orphan Products Development (OOPD)
    - **III.** The National Institutes of Health (NIH) Office of Rare Diseases

    A. I and II only
    B. I and III only
    C. II and III only
    D. I, II, and III

15. Which of the following control methods are used in clinical trials to reduce bias?
    - **I.** Random allocation
    - **II.** Double-blind trial design
    - **III.** Matching dummies

    A. I and II only
    B. I and III only
    C. II and III only
    D. I, II, and III

Answers and Explanations

1. **The answer is A** *[see II.A.3]*.
   All material included in a journal is not considered a primary resource. Original clinical trials are considered primary literature; however, review articles, articles of opinion, correspondence, and special reports are not.

2. **The answer is A** *[see II, II.C]*.
   Tertiary resources include both textbooks and databases. Information available in textbooks may not include the most recent data because it could take several years to publish. A bibliography and reference citations should be present in both textbooks and databases so that the reader may refer to a specific reference if desired. Additionally, the areas of expertise for the author and/or publisher should be evaluated when using a tertiary resource.

3. **The answer is C** *[see V.A; V.C; VII.B; VII.D]*.
   One should determine whether the question is related to a clinical scenario or is research related to develop an effective search strategy. Appropriate index terms should be identified to assist in the literature search. Other medications, including herbal products, and disease states should be taken into consideration. The background of the inquirer should be determined so that the response can be tailored to the specific inquirer.

4. **The answer is A** *[see IV.B.2.a]*.
   Martindale: The Complete Drug Reference is one resource that may be used to identify a drug manufactured in a foreign country. Other resources for identifying drugs manufactured in a foreign country include *Index Nominum, Lexi-Drugs International Online (Lexicomp Online)*, and the *USP Dictionary of United States Adopted Names (USAN) and International Drug Names. Clinical Pharmacology, Trissel's Stability of Compounded Formulations,* and *AHFS* do not contain this type of information.

5. **The answer is A** *[see IV.B.5]*.
   For an unknown drug, the physical characteristics, including an imprint code, may be used to identify the drug. Several resources, including *Facts and Comparison E Answers* and *Lexi-Drugs Online (Lexicomp Online)* may be used.

6. **The answer is C** *[see IV.B.6]*.
For a natural product, the following resources are available: *Facts and Comparison E Answers*, *Natural Medicines Comprehensive Database*, *Natural Standards*, and *Natural Products Database (Lexicomp Online)*.

7. **The answer is B** *[see V.C.12]*.
The stability of a drug, the compatibility of a drug with other drugs and/or appropriate containers, and proper administration techniques are included in *Trissel's Handbook on Injectable Drugs*, *King's Guide to Parenteral Admixtures*, and *Trissel's Stability of Compounded Formulations*. Databases such as *Clinical Pharmacology*, *Micromedex*, *Lexicomp Online*, and *Facts and Comparison E Answers* may also be used for these types of questions.

8. **The answer is A** *[see V.C.2.b]*.
Unapproved uses of drugs can be found in *Clinical Pharmacology*. This information is not available in the *PDR*, *Index Nominum*, or *King's Guide to Parenteral Admixtures*.

9. **The answer is D** *[see VI.A; VI.B; VI.C]*.
A critical assessment of available information is important in developing an appropriate response. The study objective, the study subjects (via demographics and inclusion and exclusion criteria), and drug administration should be evaluated.

10. **The answer is B** *[see VI.E]*.
Retrospective studies evaluate events that have already occurred and are useful for studying rare diseases. Prospective studies follow identified patients forward in time to answer a specific question. Crossover design allows for each patient group to undergo each type of treatment. A run-in phase is a control measure used to reduce variation.

11. **The answer is A** *[see V.C.8.f]*.
The following resources may be helpful when evaluating drug–drug interactions: *Drug Interaction Facts*, *Hansten's Drug Interaction Analysis and Management*, *Evaluations of Drug Interactions (EDI)*, and a general drug reference such as the *PDR*. Medline may also be useful in identifying reports of drug interactions documented in the primary literature.

12. **The answer is C** *[see V.C.7.d]*.
Adverse drug reactions are documented in the *PDR*/package insert, *Myler's Side Effects of Drugs*, and in databases such as *Clinical Pharmacology*, *Micromedex*, *Facts and Comparison E Answers*, and *Lexicomp Online*. Additionally, Medline may be used to search the primary literature for case reports of adverse drug reactions.

13. **The answer is B** *[see II.B; Table 14-1]*.
Indexing and abstracting services, such as Medline, are helpful tools for searching the primary literature for specific information, data, citations, and articles. It is important to remember, however, that each indexing or abstracting service reviews a finite number of journals. Thus, multiple services must be used to conduct a thorough search of the available literature.

14. **The answer is D** *[see IV.B.4]*.
Orphan drugs are used to prevent or treat rare diseases. The following resources can be used for information on these drugs: *Drug Facts and Comparisons/Facts and Comparison E Answers*, The FDA Office of Orphan Products Development (OOPD), and The National Institutes of Health Office of Rare Disorders.

15. **The answer is D** *[see VI.E]*.
The methods used when completing a study are important when determining whether the results of the study are reliable and valid. Controls that are often used to reduce bias include blind assessment, patient blinding, random allocation, matching placebos, and controlled comparisons.

Biostatistics[1]

15

CHARLES HERRING

I. TYPES OF DATA[1]

A. Nonparametric (aka discrete) variables[1]
   1. Nominal: Numbers are purely arbitrary or without regard to any order of ranking of severity.[2–6] This includes dichotomous (binary) data (lived/died, yes/no, hospitalized/not hospitalized) and categorical data without order or inherent value (race, eye color, hair color, religion, blood type, acute renal failure [ARF]/congestive heart failure [CHF]/diabetes mellitus [DM]).[5,6]
   2. Ordinal: Categorical, but scored on a continuum, without a consistent level of magnitude of difference between ranks (pain scale, New York Heart Association [NYHA] class, trauma score, coma score).[2–8]

B. Parametric (aka continuous or measuring): Order and consistent level of magnitude of difference between data units (drug concentrations, glucose, forced expiratory volume in 1 second [FEV_1], heart rate, blood pressure [BP]).[2–6]

II. MEASURES OF CENTRAL TENDENCY[9]

A. Mean (aka average): "Sum of all values divided by the total number of values."[4] Mean is affected by outliers (extreme values) and is used for parametric data.[4,5,7,9] Mu (μ) is the population mean.[4,7] X-bar ($\overline{X}$) is the sample mean.[4,7,9]

B. Median (aka 50th percentile): The "mid-most" point. Median is not affected by outliers and may be used for ordinal or parametric data.[4,7,9]

C. Mode: The most common value.[4,7,9] Mode is not affected by outliers and may be used for nominal, ordinal, or parametric data.[4,7,9]

D. A weakness of measures of central tendency is that they do not describe variability or spread of data.[1]

III. MEASURES OF VARIABILITY: DESCRIBE DATA SPREAD AND CAN HELP INFER STATISTICAL SIGNIFICANCE[9]

A. Range: The interval between lowest and highest values. Range is simply descriptive and only considers extreme values, so it is affected by outliers.[3,4,7,9]

B. Interquartile range: The interval between the 25th and 75th percentiles, so it is not affected by outliers. Because it is directly related to median, it is typically used for ordinal data.[5,7,9]

C. Variance: Deviation from the mean, expressed as the square of the units used.[3,9]
   1. Variance = sum of (mean − data point) squared, divided by $n - 1$
   2. $\text{Variance} = \Sigma \dfrac{(\overline{X} - X_1)^2}{n - 1}$

D. Standard deviation (SD): Square root of variance. SD estimates data scatter around a sample mean. SD is only used for parametric data.[3–5,7,9] Sigma (σ) is the population SD.[3] S is the sample SD.[3]
   1. $SD = \sqrt{\text{variance}}$

E. Standard error of the mean (SEM) (aka standard error [SE]): SD divided by the square root of n. As a measure of variability, SEM is misleading. If one is provided SEM, SD and/or confidence intervals (CIs) should be calculated to see true sample variability.[3,4,7,9]
   1. $SEM = \dfrac{SD}{\sqrt{n}}$

F. CI: In medical literature, a 95% CI is most frequently used, and it is a range of values that "if the entire population could be studied, 95% of the time the true population value would fall within the CI estimated from the sample."[9] CIs are descriptive and inferential. All values contained in the CI are statistically possible.[4]
1. 95% CI = $\overline{X} \pm 1.96$ (SEM)
2. Interpretation of statistical significance for CI in superiority trials:
   a. For **differences** such as BP reduction, cholesterol reduction, fingerstick blood sugar (FSBS) or A1c reductions, relative risk reductions or increases, and absolute risk reductions or increases, if the 95% CI includes 0, then the results are not statistically significant (NSS).[4,7]
   b. For **ratios** such as relative risk (aka risk ratio), odds ratio, and hazards ratio, if the 95% CI includes 1, then the results are NSS.[5–7]

IV. HYPOTHESIS TESTING[10]

A. H_0 (null hypothesis) = For superiority trials, H_0 is that no difference exists between the populations studied.[4,5,10] H_1 (alternative hypothesis) = For superiority trials, H_1 is that a difference does exist between the populations studied.[5,10] Statistical significance is tested (hypothesis testing) to indicate whether H_0 should be accepted or rejected.[4,6,10]
1. For superiority trials, H_0 is "rejected" if a statistically significant difference between groups is detected (results unlikely due to chance). H_0 is "accepted" if no statistically significant difference is detected.[4,6,10]

B. A type 1 error occurs if one rejects H_0 when, in fact, H_0 is true.[5,10] For superiority trials, this occurs when one finds a difference between treatment groups when, in fact, no difference exists.[4–6,10] Alpha (α) is the probability of making a type 1 error.[5,6,10] H_0 is rejected when $P \leq \alpha$.[4,10] By convention, α is usually 0.05, which means that 1 time out of 20, a type 1 error will be committed. This is a consequence that investigators are generally willing to accept and is denoted in trials as a $P \leq 0.05$.[4–6,10]

C. A type 2 error occurs when one accepts H_0 when, in fact, H_0 is false.[4–6,10] For superiority trials, this is when one finds no difference between treatment groups when, in fact, a difference does exist.[5,6] Beta (β) is the probability of making a type 2 error.[5,6,10] By convention, β is $\leq$ 20% (0.2).[4,5,10]

D. Power is the ability of an experiment to detect a statistically significant difference between samples when a significant difference truly exists.[4–6,10] (Power = $1 - \beta$) Inadequate power may cause one to conclude that no difference exists when, in fact, a difference does exist (type 2 error).[10] Note that in most cases, power is an issue only if one accepts H_0. If one rejects H_0, there is no way that one could have made a type 2 error[1] (*Table 15-1*).

E. Clinical versus statistical significance
1. Just because one finds a statistically significant difference does not mean that the difference is clinically meaningful.[4,10] With enough patients, one can find all kinds of statistically significant differences that are *not* clinically meaningful. For example, with a large enough sample size, one could detect a statistically significant difference between one BP medication that decreases systolic BP by 10 mm Hg and another that decreases BP by 11 mm Hg. This would be statistically but not clinically significant. Also, lack of statistical significance does not mean the results are unimportant.[4,11] A nonstatistically significant difference is more likely to be accepted as being clinically significant in the instance of safety issues such as adverse effects.[1]
2. To help judge the clinical significance of a statistically significant data set, determine what others think is clinically significant by considering the effect used in the sample size calculation

Table 15-1 TYPE 1 AND 2 ERROR FOR SUPERIORITY TRIALS

	Reality	
Decision from statistical test	Difference exists (H_0 false)	No difference exists (H_0 true)
Difference found (Reject H_0)	Correct No error	Incorrect Type 1 error (aka false positive)
No difference found (Accept H_0)	Incorrect Type 2 error (false negative)	Correct No error

(if reported), the existing evidence-based or expert consensus statements, and any cost-effectiveness or decision analyses that have been performed.[8,12] Absent such guidance, require that the minimum worthwhile effect be large when the intervention is costly (e.g., in terms of time, money, or other resources), the intervention is high risk, a patient is risk averse, or the outcome is unimportant or has intermediate importance but with uncertain benefit to patients.[8,12] Accept the minimum worthwhile effect as small when the intervention is low cost, the intervention is low risk, the patient is risk taking, or the intervention is important and has an unambiguous outcome (e.g., death).[8,12]

V. STATISTICAL INFERENCE TECHNIQUES IN HYPOTHESIS TESTING FOR PARAMETRIC DATA[13]

A. *T* test
   1. Nonpaired *t* test. Observations between groups are independent as in a parallel trial.[4,13]
   2. Paired *t* test (aka matched or repeated measures data). Patients are their own control (i.e., observations between groups are dependent as in a pretest/posttest or crossover trial).[4,13]

B. The *t* test is the statistical test of choice when making a single comparison of parametric data between two groups. When making either multiple comparisons between two groups or a single comparison between multiple groups, type 1 error risk increases, and one should make an effort to keep the type 1 error risk ≤ 5% (i.e., ≤ 0.05). One of the best ways to help control for type 1 error risk when analyzing parametric data for multiple groups or comparisons is analysis of variance (ANOVA) testing.[1]

C. ANOVA tests for a statistically significant difference among a group's collective values.[13] ANOVA involves calculation of an F-ratio, which answers the question, "Is 'the variability between the groups large enough in comparison to the variability of data within each group to justify the conclusion that two or more of the groups differ?'"[5,13]

D. ANOVAs for independent (aka nonpaired) samples
   1. One-way ANOVA. Used if no confounders, the experimental groups differ in one factor (e.g., type of drug evaluated), and greater than or equal to three independent (i.e., nonpaired) groups are being evaluated.[3]

E. Multifactorial ANOVA for independent (aka nonpaired) samples. Any type of ANOVA controlling for one or more confounders (i.e., samples differ in greater than or equal to two factors). These include the following:
   1. Two-way ANOVA. Used if there is one confounder (i.e., samples differ in two factors at a time—drug and confounder) for two or more independent groups (nonpaired).[1]
      a. Example 1: Weight loss studies with at least two groups would use this because heavier patients lose weight faster than less heavy patients. This type of ANOVA will show if variability in results is attributable to either factor independently and/or the two factors are combined.[1]

F. Analysis of covariance (ANACOVA, ANCOVA) for independent (aka nonpaired) samples. Used if there are two or more confounders and two or more independent groups (nonpaired).[1]
   1. Three-way ANOVA. Used if there are two confounders (i.e., samples differ in three factors at a time—drug and two confounders) for two or more independent groups (nonpaired).[1]
   2. Four-way ANOVA. Used if there are three confounders (i.e., samples differ in four factors at a time—drug and three confounders) for two or more independent groups (nonpaired).
   3. . . . and so on . . .

G. ANOVAs for related (aka paired, matched, repeated) samples
   1. Repeated measures ANOVA. Used if there are no confounders and three or more related samples (paired). Subjects participate in more than one treatment group as in a crossover trial. [1]
   2. Two-way repeated measures ANOVA. Used if there is one confounder and two or more related samples (paired).[1]
   3. Repeated measures regression. Used if there are two or more confounders and two or more related samples (paired).[1]

H. ANOVA will indicate whether a difference exists between groups but will not indicate where this difference exists.[5] For this, one must use multiple comparison methods (MCMs). These are types of post hoc tests. MCMs are performed only after a statistically significant *F* test.[13]

VI. STATISTICAL INFERENCE TECHNIQUES IN HYPOTHESIS TESTING FOR NONPARAMETRIC DATA[14]

A. If data are not parametric, nonparametric statistical methods must be used.[14] We will start with nominal data. Chi-square and Fisher exact tests can be used for proportions and frequencies of nominal data matrices (e.g., prevalence).[14]

B. Chi-square tests are "used to answer questions about rates, proportions, or frequencies."[5,14] Used to determine whether a difference between populations or groups exists but will not indicate where the difference lies.[5,14]

1. Chi-square test of independence (aka test of association). Used to compare two or more groups ($\geq 2 \times 2$ table, i.e., 2×2, 2×3, 4, 5, 3×3, etc).[4,5,14] (Sample size must be > 20).[14] Chi-square test of independence "cannot be used for paired data."[14]
   - **a.** Example of a chi-square test: Might compare the Board of Pharmacy exam pass rates of candidates from three different pharmacy schools. This kind of table is a contingency table. It expresses the idea that one variable (such as passing or failing the examination) may be contingent on the other variable (such as which pharmacy school one attended).[1]

	Passing Scores	Failing Scores
School A	90	5
School B	120	9
School C	130	11

   - **b.** There are two possible results (passing vs. failing) for three schools of pharmacy. Therefore, this is called a 2×3 table or matrix.[1]

C. Once chi-square calculations (for greater than 2×2 contingency table) indicate a statistically significant difference, one must perform post hoc tests to determine which groups or treatments differ from one another.[5] These post hoc tests should only be performed if the chi-square test was significant.[1]

D. Fisher exact test may be used when the sample size for a nominal data set is between 20 and 40.[14] It may also be used for a 2×2 matrix when a nominal data set is 20 or less.[4,14] In addition, Fisher exact test may be used for matched or paired data (i.e., crossover or prepost test design).[1]

VII. STATISTICAL INFERENCE TECHNIQUES IN HYPOTHESIS TESTING FOR ORDINAL DATA[14]

A. Mann-Whitney U test and Wilcoxon rank sum test. These may be used when one comparison is being made with two nonpaired groups (which need not be of equal size).[5,14] These are not appropriate for grouping into a "cumulative frequency distribution."[14]

B. Kolmogorov-Smirnov test. This can also be used when one comparison is being made with two nonpaired groups.[14] However, this test is used when data are grouped into a "cumulative frequency distribution" (i.e., individual scores or data values are lumped together into groups for further analysis).[14] An example of a cumulative distribution grouping is the manner in which the Glasgow Coma Score is used to help determine trauma score.[14]

C. Wilcoxon signed rank test (not to be confused with Wilcoxon rank sum test). This may be used when one comparison is being made with two paired groups.[4,14]

D. Kruskal-Wallis test (for nonpaired data). This may be used when two or more comparisons are being made with three or more nonpaired groups.[4,14]

E. Friedman test (for paired data). This may be used when two or more comparisons are being made with three or more paired groups.[4,14]

1. As with chi-square and ANOVA tests for more than two groups, once Kruskal-Wallis or Friedman tests indicate a statistically significant difference, one must perform post hoc tests to determine which groups or treatments differ from one another.[5] These post hoc tests should only be performed if the Kruskal-Wallis or Friedman test was statistically significant.[1]

F. ANOVA rank tests are generally used to account for confounders in ordinal data with the exception of using repeated measures regression to account for two or more confounders in crossover design.[1]

VIII. CORRELATION[11] SIMPLY EXPLAINS THE STRENGTH OF A RELATIONSHIP BETWEEN TWO VARIABLES[4,11,15]

A. The sample correlation coefficient for parametric data is the Pearson correlation coefficient or Pearson product moment r.[5,11]
   1. r ranges from -1 to $+1$[5,11]
   2. -1 = perfect negative linear relationship[5,11]
   3. $+1$ = perfect positive linear relationship[5,11]
   4. zero = no relationship[5,11]
   5. H_0 is that $r = 0$ (i.e., no relationship between variables)[11]
   6. There is not a consistent level of magnitude of difference between r values.[15] Therefore, r of 0.25 is not half the relationship of an r of 0.5 and "an r of $\pm$ 0.5 does not imply that the strength of the relationship is 'half-way' between no correlation/relationship and a perfect correlation."[11,15]
   7. The strength of a relationship depends on the data being evaluated. In one field of study, an $r = 0.6$ may be a strong correlation, whereas in another field of study, an $r = 0.8$ may be required to indicate a strong correlation.[1]
   8. Some general guidelines are the following:
      a. $r < 0.25$: "doubtful" correlation[15,16]
      b. $r = 0.26–0.5$: "fair" correlation[15,16]
      c. $r = 0.51–0.75$: "good" correlation[15,16]
      d. $r > 0.75$: "superior" correlation[15,16]
   9. There is a P value associated with r and CIs can be calculated[5] [e.g., $r = 0.74$ (95% CI: $0.53 - 0.98$)].

B. The sample correlation coefficient for ordinal data is Spearman rho or Spearman rank order r.[5,11]

C. Most of the time, relationships are "confounded by extraneous variables."[11] This "adversely affects a 'perfect' correlation."[11]
   1. Example: There is an association with overuse of albuterol (ProAir HFA) and mortality. However, there are multiple confounders that prevent an absolute understanding of the relationship. Possible confounders include the type of controller medication being used, inhalation technique/medication compliance, concomitant disease states (chronic obstructive pulmonary disease [COPD], heart failure [HF]), concomitant medications (β-blockers), and one of many triggers.[1]

D. Correlation has many limitations. Although it does a good job of recognizing and measuring the strength of relationship(s) between variables, it does not establish causality.[11,15] Remember the ageless question of which came first, the chicken or the egg? A more relevant example is, does overuse of albuterol (ProAir HFA) lead to poorly responsive, severe asthma attacks? Or does poorly responsive, severe asthma lead to albuterol (ProAir HFA) overuse?[1]

E. Correlations do not have the ability to "predict" one variable based on another.[1]

IX. REGRESSION TAKES CORRELATION ONE STEP FURTHER

Regression not only recognizes and measures the strength of relationship(s) between variables, it also describes a relationship such that an equation for predicting one variable from another variable can be developed.[4,11]

A. With simple linear regression, where m = slope of the line, "y is the dependent variable, x is the independent variable," and "b is the y-intercept of the line."[11]

$$y = mx + b$$

B. r-squared (r^2) is known as the coefficient of determination. It "represents the percentage of variation in y that is accounted for by x."[8] For example, if a study produces a correlation/regression analysis between stroke and hypertension reporting an $r = 0.70$, then $r^2 = 0.49$, and one could say that 49% of stroke risk may be explained by BP.[1]

1. Conversely, $1 - r^2$ represents the proportion of the variation that is not related to the independent variables (i.e., the residual variation).[11] This is sometimes referred to as the *coefficient of nondetermination.*[15]
2. As with correlation, CIs can be calculated for regression analyses. Also, as with correlation, the existence of this kind of statistical association is not in itself evidence of causality. One must take into account what type of analysis is being performed (i.e., case control vs. cohort vs. randomized controlled trial [RCT]).[1]

C. Multiple regression. When more than one independent variable is used to predict a dependent variable, multiple (or multivariate) regression analysis (MRA) is used.[4,15] For example, the national cholesterol guidelines use multiple regression to help establish 10-year coronary heart disease (CHD) risk for patients based on population data. A patient's 10-year CHD risk is the dependent variable because its estimate "depends on" several independent variables. The independent variables include age, total cholesterol, high-density lipoprotein (HDL) cholesterol, smoking status, and systolic BP. All of these independent variables are used to help predict a patient's 10-year CHD risk.[1]

1. Multiple linear regression is "used with parametric (aka continuous) outcomes like BP" and lipid values.[17]
2. Logistic regression is used with nominal outcomes such as death and hospitalization.[8,17]
3. Cox proportional hazards regression is "used when an outcome is the length of time to an event."[17] For example, time until death or hospitalization or time until discharge.[5,17]

X. ERROR VERSUS BIAS.

Errors are "mistakes that do not systematically under- or overestimate effect size."[18] Biases are systematic errors/flaws in study design that lead to incorrect results.[5,6,18] More common types of biases include publication bias, investigator bias, compliance bias, selection bias, diagnostic or detection bias, recall bias, and channeling bias (aka confounding by indication).[5–7,18–20] The best way to minimize bias is through proper study design (e.g., randomization, inclusion/exclusion criteria, blinding, using controls and objective outcome measures).[5,6,8,18,19]

XI. CONFOUNDING.

Confounders are "causes, other than the one studied, which may be linked to the studied outcomes and/or the hypothesized cause."[5,7,19] Although these are sometimes difficult to detect, investigators should account for known confounders.[5,19] For example, atherosclerosis causes myocardial infarction (MI). There is an association between atherosclerosis and smoking, smoking and risk for an MI, and atherosclerosis and risk for an MI. The proposed cause is atherosclerosis. The potential confounder is smoking, so investigators need to account for any significant smoking differences among studied groups.[19]

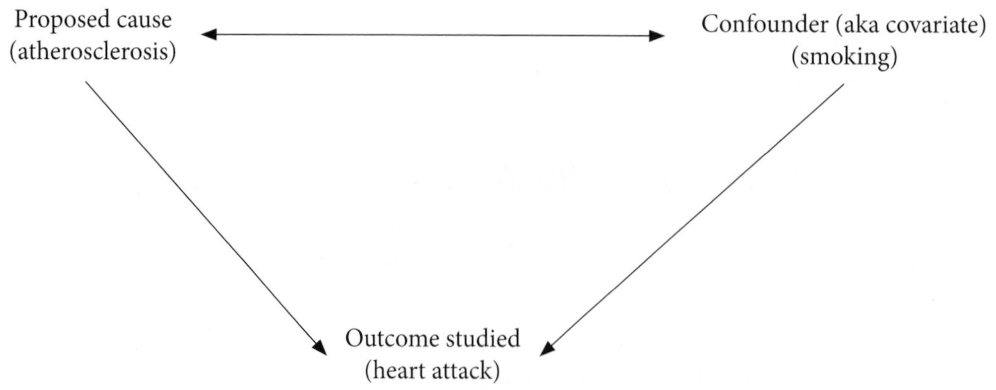

A. Ways of controlling for confounders include proper study design (e.g., randomization, inclusion/exclusion criteria, blinding, using controls and objective outcome measures) and proper statistical analysis (stratification, MRA, and use of ANOVA [for parametric data]).[5–8,18,19]

XII. CONTROLLED VERSUS NONCONTROLLED TRIALS

A. Controlled trials attempt to "keep the study groups as similar as possible and to minimize bias. Ideally the groups will differ only in the factor (treatment) being studied."[7]

B. Uncontrolled trials generally only evaluate one group[7] (i.e., no control group).[1]

C. Various types of controls

1. "Placebo control: One or more groups are given active treatment while the control group receives a placebo."[7]
2. "Historical Control: The data from a group of subjects receiving the intervention are compared to data from a group of subjects previously treated during a different time period, perhaps in a different place"[7] (experimental group vs. past group).
3. "Crossover control: Each subject serves as his/her own control. During a defined period of time, group A receives the experimental drug while group B receives the control. Then for the next defined period of time, group A receives the control and group B receives the experimental drug."[7]
4. "Standard Treatment (aka Active Treatment) Control: Control group subjects receive 'gold standard' treatment while the other group receives the experimental treatment."[7] These are mainly used when a placebo control would be unethical.[7]
5. "Within Patient Comparison Control: One part of the body is treated with the experimental treatment while another part of the body is treated with either the 'gold standard' or placebo." This is mainly used for dermatology trials.[7]

XIII. BLINDING DOES SEVERAL THINGS.

It helps minimize clinicians' treating/assessing one group differently from another, helps control for a placebo effect, and helps maximize equal patient compliance. Blinding is especially important if there is any degree of subjectivity associated with outcome assessment. Common types of blinding are listed in the following[1]:

A. Nonblinded trial: The investigator and subject know what treatment or intervention the subject is receiving. This is commonly referred to as an *open* or *open-label trial.*[7]

B. Single-blind trial: Someone (usually the patient) is unaware of what treatment or intervention the subject is receiving.[7]

C. "Double-blind trial: Neither the investigator nor the subject is aware of what treatment or intervention the subject is receiving."[7]

D. "Double-dummy trials are used if one is comparing two different dosage forms and doesn't want the patient or investigator to know in which arm the patient is participating. For example, if one is comparing intranasal sumatriptan (Imitrex) to injectable sumatriptan (Imitrex STATdose), one group would receive intranasal sumatriptan and a placebo injection, while the other group would receive intranasal placebo and a sumatriptan injection."[7]

XIV. VALIDITY

A. Internal validity. To what degree does a study appropriately test and answer the question(s) being asked and measure what is claimed to be measured? It "addresses issues of bias, confounding, and measurement of endpoints." [19] It directly affects external validity.[7,18,19]

B. External validity. Presuming internal validity, this assesses whether the results can be extrapolated to the general population, to other groups, patients, or systems.[7,18,19]

XV. ASSESSING RISK[1]

A. Absolute risk (AR) (aka incidence)

$$\text{AR} = \frac{\text{number who develop outcome during a specified period}}{\text{number available to develop outcome at the beginning of the study}}$$

1. Absolute risk reduction (ARR) = $\text{AR}_{\text{Control}} - \text{AR}_{\text{Experimental}}$
2. Numbers-needed-to-treat (NNT) = 1/ARR

B. Relative risk (RR) (aka risk ratio, rate ratio, or incidence rate ratio) = $\text{AR}_{\text{Experimental}}/\text{AR}_{\text{Control}}$

1. Relative risk reduction (RRR) = 1 − RR and RRR = $\text{ARR}/\text{AR}_{\text{Control}}$

XVII. REFERENCES

1. Herring C. *Quick Stats: Basics for Medical Literature Evaluation*. 3rd ed. Acton, MA: Copley; 2009.
2. Gaddis ML, Gaddis GM. Introduction to biostatistics: Part 1, basic concepts. *Ann Emerg Med.* 1990;19(1):86–89.
3. Glaser AN. *High Yield Biostatistics*. Media, PA: Williams & Wilkins; 1995.
4. DeYoung GR. *Biostatistics: A Refresher* (handout). 2000 Updates in Therapeutics: The Pharmacotherapy Preparatory Course.
5. Kaye KS. *Clinical Epidemiology and Biostatistics: Overview and Basic Concepts* (handout). Faculty Development Seminar, Campbell University School of Pharmacy, Department of Pharmacy Practice. 2001.
6. Kaye KS. *Clinical Epidemiology and Biostatistics, Part 2* (handout). Faculty Development Seminar, Campbell University School of Pharmacy, Department of Pharmacy Practice. 2001.
7. Berensen NM. *Statistics: A Review* (handout). 2001.
8. DeYoung GR. Understanding statistics: an approach for the clinician. In: *Pharmacotherapy Self-Assessment Program. Book 5: The Science and Practice of Pharmacotherapy 1*. 5th ed. Kansas, MO: American College of Clinical Pharmacy; 2005:1–17.
9. Gaddis GM, Gaddis ML. Introduction to biostatistics: Part 2, descriptive statistics. *Ann Emerg Med.* 1990;19(3):309–315.
10. Gaddis GM, Gaddis ML. Introduction to biostatistics: Part 3, sensitivity, specificity, predictive value, and hypothesis testing. *Ann Emerg Med.* 1990;19(5):591–597.
11. Gaddis ML, Gaddis GM. Introduction to biostatistics: Part 6, correlation and regression. *Ann Emerg Med.* 1990;19(12):1462–1468.
12. Froehlich GW. What is the chance that this study is clinically significant? A proposal for Q values. *Eff Clin Pract.* 1999;2:234–239.
13. Gaddis GM, Gaddis ML. Introduction to biostatistics: Part 4, statistical inference techniques in hypothesis testing. *Ann Emerg Med.* 1990;19(7):820–825.
14. Gaddis GM, Gaddis ML. Introduction to biostatistics: Part 5, statistical inference techniques for hypothesis testing with nonparametric data. *Ann Emerg Med.* 1990;19(9):1054–1059.
15. De Muth JE. *Basic Statistics and Pharmaceutical Statistical Applications*. 2nd ed. Boca Raton, FL: Chapman & Hall/CRC, Taylor & Francis Group; 2006.
16. Kelly WD, Ratliff TA, Nenadic CM. *Basic Statistics for Laboratories: A Prime for Laboratory Workers*. Hoboken, NJ: John Wiley and Sons; 1992:93.
17. Katz MH. Multivariable analysis: A primer for readers of medical research. *Ann Intern Med.* 2003;138:644–650.
18. Drew R. *Clinical Research Introduction* (handout). Drug Literature Evaluation/Applied Statistics Course. Campbell University School of Pharmacy. 2003.
19. DeYoung GR. *Clinical Trial Design* (handout). 2000 Updates in Therapeutics: The Pharmacotherapy Preparatory Course.
20. West PM. Literature evaluation. In: *Pharmacotherapy Self-Assessment Program. Book 5: The Science and Practice of Pharmacotherapy 2*. 5th ed. Kansas, MO: American College of Clinical Pharmacy; 2005.

Study Questions*

1. Which measure(s) of central tendency is/are sensitive to outliers?
   (A) Mean
   (B) Median
   (C) Mode
2. For what type of data can standard deviation (SD) be used?
   (A) Parametric data
   (B) Ordinal data
   (C) Nominal data
3. Which of the following is correct regarding measures of variability?
   (A) Range can be both descriptive and inferential.
   (B) Standard error of the mean (SEM) is always larger than SD.
   (C) All values contained in a confidence interval (CI) are statistically possible.
   (D) CI is a descriptive measure only.
4. A study was performed to determine the effect of a new antipsychotic agent (Drug A) on psychosis in patients with underlying schizophrenia as compared to placebo. A sample size of 300 patients was calculated to be needed based on an α of 0.05 and a β of 0.2. The double-blind, parallel, superiority trial was performed in 350 patients for 8 weeks. At the end of the 8-week period, the new antipsychotic agent was found to induce remission in 20% of patients as compared to 19% in the placebo group ($P = 0.04$). Which of the following statements is true based on the results of the study?
   (A) Drug A was found to have a statistically significant and clinically significant difference on remission of psychosis as compared to placebo.
   (B) Drug A was found to have a statistically significant difference but not a clinically significant difference on remission of psychosis as compared to placebo.
   (C) Drug A was found to have a clinically significant difference but not a statistically significant difference on remission of psychosis as compared to placebo.
   (D) Drug A was not found to have a clinically or statistically significant difference on remission of psychosis as compared to placebo.

(For the next two questions) A study of the effects of bupropion (Zyban) versus nicotine gum (Nicorette) on the primary end point of change in the number of cigarettes smoked per day in a parallel, randomized trial. The investigators plan to include 450 subjects (150 in each arm) to reach statistical significance based on a β of 0.2 and α of 0.05.

5. Which of the following statistical tests would be the most appropriate? (Hint: assume no confounders)
   (A) One-way ANOVA
   (B) Chi-square (χ^2)
   (C) Fisher exact test
   (D) Friedman test
   (E) *t* test
6. Which of the following statistical tests would be the most appropriate if the study had evaluated three groups instead of only two? (i.e., bupropion [Zyban] vs. nicotine patches [Nicoderm CQ] vs. nicotine gum [Nicorette])
   (A) One-way ANOVA
   (B) Chi-square (χ^2)
   (C) Fisher exact test
   (D) Friedman test
   (E) Student's *t* test
7. A study is designed to evaluate the change in blood pressure lowering between metoprolol tartrate (Lopressor®) and metoprolol succinate (Toprol XL®). The investigators decide to perform a parallel trial in 200 patients. There were significant baseline differences between the groups in diet and exercise. Which of the following statistical tests would be most appropriate?
   (A) One-way ANOVA
   (B) Chi-square (χ^2)
   (C) Fisher exact test
   (D) ANCOVA
   (E) Student's *t* test

* These study questions were composed by Melanie Pound, PharmD, BCPS and Rebekah Grube, PharmD, BCPS.

8. The makers of eplerenone (Inspra) want to design a study to compare their medication to the current standard of spironolactone (Aldactone) in the treatment of heart failure. They decide to perform a parallel trial of the two agents in 2000 patients with NYHA classes II to IV heart failure over 2 years. The primary end point is mortality. Which of the following statistical tests would be most appropriate to use?
   (A) ANOVA
   (B) Fisher exact test
   (C) Chi-square (χ^2)
   (D) Mann-Whitney U test
   (E) Student's *t* test

9. A retrospective study produces correlation/regression analysis between a high sodium intake (> 2.4 g/day) and hypertension (HTN) reporting an $r = 0.45$. Which of the following is correct?
   (A) 20% of HTN may be explained by high sodium intake.
   (B) 20% of HTN is not explained by high sodium intake.
   (C) 80% of HTN is explained by high sodium intake.
   (D) 55% of HTN is not explained by high sodium intake.
   (E) 45% of HTN may be explained by high sodium intake.

10. A study was performed to evaluate a possible correlation between the use of the herbal product Goldenseal and changes in pain relief (based on pain scale scores). Which type of correlation analysis should be used in this trial?
    (A) Pearson
    (B) Spearman
    (C) Linear
    (D) Cox

(For the next two questions) In the RE-LY trial, dabigatran (Pradaxa) was compared with warfarin (Coumadin) for the prevention of cerebrovascular accident (CVA) in atrial fibrillation (AF) patients. The primary outcome in this trial was CVA or systemic thromboembolism (TE). The results are presented as follows:

End point	Dabigatran (n = 6076)	Warfarin (n = 6022)	RR, 95% CI
CVA or TE	134 (2.2%)	159 (2.6%)	0.66 (0.53–0.82)
MI	89 (1.5%)	63 (1.0%)	1.38 (1.00–1.91)

11. What can be concluded about the outcome "CVA or TE"?
    (A) Dabigatran (Pradaxa) has a clinically significant lower risk than warfarin (Coumadin), although it is not statistically significant because the CI does not include 1.
    (B) Dabigatran (Pradaxa) has a clinically significant lower risk than warfarin (Coumadin), although it is not statistically significant because the CI does not include 0.
    (C) Dabigatran (Pradaxa) has a clinically significant higher risk than warfarin (Coumadin), and it is statistically significant because the CI does not include 0.
    (D) Dabigatran (Pradaxa) has a clinically significant lower risk than warfarin (Coumadin), and it is statistically significant because the CI does not include 1.

12. What can be concluded about the outcome "MI"?
    (A) Dabigatran (Pradaxa) has a higher MI risk than warfarin (Coumadin), although it is not statistically significant because the CI includes 1.
    (B) Dabigatran (Pradaxa) has a higher MI risk than warfarin (Coumadin), although it is not statistically significant because the CI does not include 0.
    (C) Dabigatran (Pradaxa) has a higher MI risk than warfarin (Coumadin), and it is statistically significant because the CI includes 1.
    (D) Dabigatran (Pradaxa) has a higher MI risk than warfarin (Coumadin), and it is statistically significant because the CI does not include 0.

13. A researcher was interested in examining the association between postmenopausal hormone replacement therapy (HRT) and development of heart disease. All women who were characterized as postmenopausal were approached regarding their interest in participating in the study by answering a questionnaire annually regarding their medication use and medical conditions. Of the 16,168 women who provided consent, the average length of follow-up was 12.5 years (range, 6 to 16 years). Which of the following best describes the study design?
    (A) Case-control study
    (B) Prospective cohort study
    (C) Randomized controlled trial
    (D) Meta-analysis

14. An investigator wishes to study a new drug for the treatment of hypertension in patients with diabetes. What is the best type of trial design the investigator should use for determining causality in this particular study?

(A) A case-control study
(B) A prospective cohort study
(C) A prospective, randomized, placebo-controlled trial
(D) A prospective, randomized, standard-of-care comparison trial
(E) A meta-analysis

15. Which of the following would be appropriate for a crossover design study?

(A) Effects of Drug A versus Drug B on hypertension in 100 patients
(B) Effects of varenicline (Chantix) compared to placebo on smoking cessation
(C) Effects of fluticasone/salmeterol (Advair) and budesonide/formoterol (Symbicort) on asthma exacerbations
(D) Effects of hydralazine and hydrochlorothiazide (Microzide) on all-cause mortality

Answers and Explanations

1. The answer is A *[see II.A]*.
Mean is the correct answer because it is affected by outliers. Median and mode are incorrect because they are not affected by outliers.

2. The answer is A *[see III.D]*.
Parametric (aka continuous) data is correct. Standard deviation is only meaningful for parametric data. It is not meaningful for nominal data. Measures of variability are not meaningful for nominal data. Standard deviation is usually not meaningful for ordinal data. Interquartile range is the preferred measure of variability for ordinal data.

3. The answer is C *[see III.F]*.
Answer C is correct because all values within a CI are statistically possible. Answer A is incorrect because range is descriptive only. Range is not inferential because one is unable to "infer" statistical significance for a data set based on range. Answer B is incorrect because SEM is always smaller than SD. Answer D is incorrect because CI is not only descriptive but also inferential since one is able to "infer" statistical significance for a data set based on CI.

4. The answer is B *[see IV.E]*.
Answer B is correct. The difference was statistically significant because the *P* value was .04. Based on this *P* value, there is a 4% chance that a type 1 error occurred, which is less than the prespecified acceptable risk of 5% (preset α was 0.05 or 5%). However, the difference was not clinically meaningful because there was only a 1% difference in the primary end point (induction of remission) between the treatment groups. For these reasons, answers A, C, and D are incorrect.

5. The answer is E *[see V.A–B]*.
Answer E is correct because a *t* test is the test of choice for evaluating statistical differences in parametric data (change in the number of cigarettes smoked daily) when only two groups are being evaluated and there are no detected confounders. Answer A is incorrect because one-way ANOVA is used for testing three or more groups. Answers B and C are incorrect because chi-square and Fisher exact test are used to test nominal data. Answer D is incorrect because Friedman test is used to test ordinal data.

6. The answer is A *[see V.C–D]*.
Answer A is correct because one-way ANOVA is used to test parametric data (change in the number of cigarettes smoked daily) when there are three independent groups and no detected confounders are present. Answers B and C are incorrect because chi-square and Fisher exact test are used to test nominal data. Answer D is incorrect because Friedman test is used to test ordinal data. Answer E is incorrect because *t* test is used for evaluating statistical differences in parametric data when only two groups are being evaluated.

7. The answer is D *[see V.F]*.
Answer D is correct because ANCOVA is used to test parametric data (change in BP) when two or more groups are being evaluated and two or more confounders (diet and exercise differences) are detected. Answer A is incorrect because one-way ANOVA is used when no detected confounders are present. Answers B and C are incorrect because chi-square and Fisher exact test are used to test nominal data. Answer E is incorrect because *t* test is used when no detected confounders are present.

8. **The answer is C** *[see VI.A–B]*.
Answer C is correct because chi-square is used to detect statistical differences for nominal data (mortality) when there are large numbers of patients in each treatment group. Answers A and E are incorrect because ANOVA and *t* test are used to test parametric data. Answer B is incorrect because Fisher exact test is used when there are small numbers of patients in each treatment group (< 40 patients). Answer D is incorrect because Mann-Whitney *U* test is used to test ordinal data.

9. **The answer is A** *[see IX.B]*.
Answer A is correct because $r = 0.45$, *r*-squared (r^2) $= 0.2$ or 20%. Therefore, 20% of one variable (hypertension) may be explained by the other variable (high-sodium diet). This would mean that $1 - 0.2 = 0.8$ or 80% of hypertension would not be explained by a high-sodium diet. Therefore, answers B, C, D, and E are incorrect.

10. **The answer is B** *[see VIII.B]*.
Answer B is correct because pain scale scores are ordinal data, and Spearman is the sample correlation coefficient for ordinal data. Answer A is incorrect because Pearson is the sample correlation coefficient for linear (parametric) data. Answer C is incorrect because pain scale is ordinal data, not linear (parametric). Answer D is incorrect because Cox is a type of regression analysis, not a form of correlation analysis.

11. **The answer is D** *[see III.F.1.b, IV.E, and XV.B]*.
Answer D is correct because the outcome measure is relative risk (RR). For ratios like relative risk, it is the difference from 1 that determines statistical significance. Answer A is incorrect because there is a statistically significant difference in CVA or TE because the 95% CI does not include 1. Answers B and C are incorrect because, for ratios like relative risk, it is the difference from 1 that determines statistical significance, not difference from 0.

12. **The answer is A** *[see III.F.1.b, IV.E, and XV.B]*.
Answer A is correct because for ratios like relative risk, it is the difference from 1 that determines statistical significance. The 95% CI included 1, so although this may be clinically meaningful, it is not statistically significant. Answers B and D are incorrect because for ratios like relative risk, it is the difference from 1 that determines statistical significance, not difference from 0. Answer C is incorrect because all values within the 95% CI are statistically possible and the 95% CI for MI contains 1. Therefore, it is statistically possible that there is no difference between dabigatran (Pradaxa) and warfarin (Coumadin) for the outcome of MI.

13. **The answer is B** *[see XVI.C.4]*.
Answer B is correct because postmenopausal women were identified based on exposure (medications they were taking, i.e., whether or not they were taking HRT) as is done in cohort studies. Answer A is incorrect because, for case-control studies, subjects are identified based on disease (heart disease in this case) rather than exposure (HRT), which was not the setup for this study. Answer C is incorrect because patients were not randomized to an intervention. Answer D is incorrect because meta-analyses include multiple studies, which is not the case in this example.

14. **The answer is D** *[see XII.C.4 and XVI.D.3]*.
Answer D is correct because the most robust and ethical way of determining differences between hypertension treatments and determining causality is through a randomized trial with a standard of care control. Answer A is incorrect because a case-control study is very weak at determining causality. Answers B and E are incorrect because cohort studies and meta-analyses are weaker than randomized trials for establishing causality. Answer C is incorrect because it would be unethical to treat hypertensive, diabetic patients with a placebo rather than an established therapy that has been shown to improve cardiovascular outcomes.

15. **The answer is A** *[see XVI.D.2.a]*.
Answer A is correct. Answer B is incorrect because it would be unethical to ask those who had stopped smoking in the first part of the trial to restart smoking in order to obtain data for the second part of the study. Answer C is incorrect because crossovers are not good for treatment evaluation in unstable diseases. Asthma severity may vary depending on seasons. Answer D is incorrect because those who died in the first part of the crossover trial could not be evaluated during the second part of the trial.

Clinical Toxicology

16

JOHN J. PONZILLO

I. OVERVIEW

A. This chapter is intended to provide the reader with an overview of the management of various toxic exposures. Emergency medical services (EMS) should be immediately contacted to provide advanced life support for patients with unstable vital signs resulting from a poisoning exposure. In addition, these patients should be referred to a hospital for follow-up. A nationwide toll-free poison center number became available. This number, 800-222-1222, is available 24 hr/day and should be used by health care professionals and the general public when dealing with exposures to potentially toxic substances.

B. Definitions

1. **Clinical toxicology.** Focuses on the effects of substances in patients caused by accidental poisonings or intentional overdoses of medications, drugs of abuse, household products, or various other chemicals
2. **Intoxication.** Toxicity associated with any chemical substance
3. **Poisoning.** A clinical toxicity secondary to accidental exposure
4. **Overdose.** An intentional exposure with the intent of causing self-injury or death
5. **Toxidromes.** A group of signs, symptoms, and laboratory findings that suggest a specific ingestion

C. Epidemiology. In 2007, a total of 27,658 unintentional drug overdose deaths occurred in the United States (more information can be found at the Centers for Disease Control and Prevention's [CDC] Web site, http://www.cdc.gov). Over the past several years, the number of poisoning exposures, emergency room visits, and subsequent costs has risen. Pharmacists are playing an increasing role in poison prevention and overdose management.

D. Information resources

1. **Computerized databases**
   - **a.** POISINDEX is a database that is updated quarterly and is a primary resource for poison control centers.
2. **Printed publications.** Textbooks and manuals provide useful information regarding the assessment and treatment of patients exposed to various substances, although their usefulness is limited by the lag time of information published in the primary literature reaching updated editions.
   - **a.** Ellenhorn MJ, ed. *Medical Toxicology: Diagnosis and Treatment of Human Poisonings.* 2nd ed. New York, NY: Elsevier Science; 1997.
   - **b.** Fraunfelder FT, Fraunfelder FW. *Drug-Induced Ocular Side Effects.* 5th ed. Little Rock, AR: Butterworth-Heinemann; 2001.
   - **c.** Fraunfelder FT, Fraunfelder FW, Wiley WA. *Clinical Ocular Toxicology.* 6th ed. Philadelphia, PA: Saunders; 2008.
   - **d.** Nelson L, Lewin N, Howland MA, et al. *Goldfrank's Toxicologic Emergencies.* 9th ed. New York, NY: McGraw Hill; 2010.
   - **e.** Grant WM. *Toxicology of the Eye.* 4th ed. Springfield, IL: Charles C Thomas; 1995.
   - **f.** Shannon MO, Borron SW, Burns M, et al. *Haddad and Winchester's Clinical Management of Poisoning and Drug Overdose.* 4th ed. Philadelphia, PA: Saunders; 2007.
   - **g.** Olson KR, Anderson IB, Benowitz NL, et al, eds. *Poisoning and Drug Overdose.* 5th ed. Stamford, CT: Appleton & Lange; 2006.

3. **Internet**[1]
   a. Centers for Disease Control and Prevention (CDC) at http://www.cdc.gov
   b. U.S. Food and Drug Administration (FDA) at http://www.fda.gov
   c. National Library of Medicine at http://www.nlm.nih.gov
   d. National Institute for Occupational Safety and Health (NIOSH) at http://www.cdc.gov/niosh
   e. American Society of Health–System Pharmacists at http://www.ashp.org
   f. Material Safety Data Sheets at http://www.msdssearch.com
   g. U.S. Environmental Protection Agency (EPA) at http://www.epa.gov
4. **Poison control centers** accredited by the American Association of Poison Control Centers (AAPCC) provide information to the general public and health care providers. These centers are the most reliable and up-to-date sources of information; thus, the AAPCC's phone number (800-222-1222) should be readily available. In Canada, call 1-800-268-0917.

II. GENERAL MANAGEMENT

A. **Supportive care and ABCs.** Evaluating and supporting the vital functions (airway, breathing, and circulation [ABCs]) are the mandatory first steps in the initial management of drug ingestions. After the patient is stabilized, the specific issue(s) of poison management should be addressed.[1]

B. **Treatment** for patients with depressed mental status includes the following:
   1. To rule out or treat hypoglycemia, 50 mL of 50% dextrose in adults and 1 mL/kg in children intravenously (IV)
   2. Thiamine 100 mg IV push (glucose can precipitate the Wernicke-Korsakoff syndrome in thiamine-deficient patients)
   3. Naloxone (Narcan) 0.4 to 2 mg IV push, if opiate ingestion is suspected. Naloxone may also be administered by the following routes: inhalation, intramuscular, and intranasal.

C. **Obtaining a history of exposure**
   1. **Identify** the substance(s) ingested, the route of exposure, the quantity ingested, the amount of time since ingestion, signs and symptoms of overdose, and any associated illness or injury. **Corroborate** history and other physical evidence (e.g., pill containers) from prehospital providers.
   2. **Neurological examination** evaluates any seizures, alterations in consciousness, confusion, ataxia, slurred speech, tremor, headache, or syncope.
   3. **Cardiopulmonary examination** evaluates any syncope, palpitations, cough, chest pain, shortness of breath, or burning or irritation of the upper airway.
   4. **Gastrointestinal (GI) examination** evaluates any abdominal pain, nausea, vomiting, diarrhea, or difficulty in swallowing.
   5. **Past medical history** should include
      a. Medications, including nonprescription (over-the-counter [OTC]) substances
      b. Use of herbal medications
      c. Alcohol or drug abuse
      d. Psychiatric history
      e. Allergies
      f. Occupational or hobby exposures
      g. Travel
      h. Prior ingestions
      i. Social history with potential for domestic violence or neglect
      j. Last normal menstrual period or pregnancy

D. **Routine laboratory assessment**
   1. Complete blood cell (CBC) count
   2. Serum electrolytes
   3. Blood urea nitrogen (BUN); serum creatinine (SCr)
   4. Blood glucose
   5. Urinalysis

[1]American Heart Association. Cardiac arrest in special situations: 2010 American Heart Association guidelines for cardiopulmonary resuscitation and emergency cardiac care. *Circulation* [Special issue] 2010;122:S829–S861.

6. Electrocardiogram (ECG)
7. Chest roentgenogram and/or kidneys, ureters, and bladder (**KUB**) x-ray

E. **Toxicology laboratory tests**
1. **Advantages**
   a. Confirm or **determine** the presence of a particular agent
   b. **Predict** the anticipated toxic effects or severity of exposure to some poisons
   c. Confirm or **distinguish** differential or contributing diagnosis
   d. Occasionally help **guide therapy**
2. **Disadvantages**
   a. These tests cannot provide a specific diagnosis for all patients.
   b. All possible intoxicating agents cannot be screened.
   c. In critically ill patients, supportive treatment is needed before laboratory results of the toxicology screen are available.
   d. Laboratory drug-detection abilities differ.
   e. In general, only a **qualitative determination** of a substance or substances is necessary; however, **quantitative levels** of the therapeutically monitored drugs may be necessary to guide therapy. Consult with your local laboratory for the availability of specific drug assays.

F. **Skin decontamination** should be performed when percutaneous absorption of a substance may result in systemic toxicity, or when the contaminating substance may produce local toxic effects (e.g., acid burns). The patient's clothing is removed, and the areas are irrigated with copious quantities of water. **Neutralization should not be attempted.** For example, neutralizing acid burns with sodium bicarbonate will produce an exothermic chemical reaction, thereby exacerbating the patient's condition.

G. **Gastric decontamination** may be attempted when supportive care is begun. GI decontamination involves removal of the ingestant with emesis or lavage, the use of activated charcoal potentially to bind any ingestants, and the use of cathartics to hasten excretion and thereby limit absorption.
1. **Emesis**
   a. **Contraindications**
      (1) Children younger than 6 months of age
      (2) Patients with central nervous system (CNS) depression or seizures
      (3) Patients who have ingested a strong acid, alkali, or a sharp object
      (4) Patients with compromised airway protective reflexes (including coma and convulsions)
      (5) Patients who have ingested some types of hydrocarbons or petroleum distillates
      (6) Patients who have ingested substances with an extremely rapid onset of action
      (7) Patients with emesis after the ingestion
   b. **Syrup of ipecac.** Owing to concerns of safety, efficacy, and the delay of antidote administration, syrup of ipecac is no longer recommended for general use. Ipecac may be administered within 30 mins of ingestion and **only on the advice of a poison control center.**[2]
2. **Gastric lavage**
   a. **Use.** Gastric lavage is infrequently used in patients who are not alert or have a diminished gag reflex. This procedure should also be considered in patients who are seen early after massive ingestions. This procedure is **contraindicated in patients who have ingested acids, alkalis, or hydrocarbons**. In addition, **patients should not receive gastric lavage if they are at risk for GI perforation or if they are combative.**
3. **Activated charcoal** adsorbs almost all commonly ingested drugs and chemicals and is usually administered to most overdose patients as quickly as possible (ideally, within 1 hr of ingestion). Commonly ingested substances not adsorbed include **ethanol**, **iron**, **lithium**, **cyanide**, **ethylene glycol**, **lead**, **mercury**, **methanol**, **organic solvents**, **potassium**, **strong acids**, and **strong alkalis**.
   a. **Dosage.** Activated charcoal (Actidose with sorbitol) is available as a colloidal dispersion with water or sorbitol. In **adults**, the dose of activated charcoal is 25 to 100 g; the dose in **children** 1 to 12 years of age is 25 to 50 g; the dose in children up to 1 year of age is 1 g/kg. Constipation has not been observed after the administration of a single dose of activated charcoal. **Multiple doses** of any cathartics should be avoided because they can cause electrolyte

[2]Manoguerra AS, Cobaugh DJ; Guidelines for the Management of Poisonings Consensus Panel. Guideline on the use of ipecac syrup in the out-of-hospital management of ingested poisons. *Clin Toxicol.* 2005;43:1–10.

imbalances and/or dehydration. Toxic ingestions with drugs having an enterohepatic circulation (e.g., carbamazepine, theophylline, phenobarbital, tricyclic antidepressants, phenothiazines, digitalis) generally require that the charcoal be readministered every 6 hrs to prevent reabsorption during recirculation.

b. **Adverse effects.** Charcoal aspiration and empyema have been reported in the literature. As such, charcoal should be withheld if patients are vomiting. Bowel obstruction may occur with multiple doses of activated charcoal and/or patients who are receiving concomitant therapy with neuromuscular-blocking drugs.[3]

H. **Whole bowel irrigation** has been shown to be effective under certain conditions, particularly when activated charcoal lacks efficacy. An isosmotic cathartic solution such as polyethylene glycol (GoLYTELY, Colyte) is used. The dosage is 1 to 2 L/hr given orally or by nasogastric tube until the rectal effluent is clear.

I. **Forced diuresis** and **urinary pH manipulation** may be used to enhance the elimination of substances, whose elimination is primarily renal, if the substance has a relatively small volume of distribution with little protein binding. However, the use of these methods is associated with fluid and electrolyte disturbances.

1. **Alkaline diuresis** promotes the ionization of weak acids, thereby preventing their reabsorption by the kidney, which facilitates the excretion of such weak acids. This procedure has been used in the management of patients who have ingested long-acting barbiturates such as phenobarbital or salicylic acid. Patients are given 50 to 100 mEq of sodium bicarbonate IV push, followed by a continuous infusion of 50 to 100 mEq of sodium bicarbonate in 1 L of 0.25% to 0.45% normal saline, maintaining a urine pH of 7.3 to 8.5. Urine output should be 5 to 7 mL/kg/hr. **Complications** include metabolic alkalosis, hypernatremia, hyperosmolarity, and fluid overload.

J. **Dialysis.** In patients who fail to respond to the measures of decontamination already outlined, hemodialysis, and to a lesser extent peritoneal dialysis, may enhance drug elimination. Substances that are removed by hemodialysis generally are water soluble, have a small volume of distribution (< 0.5 L/kg), have a low molecular weight (< 500 Da), and are not significantly bound to plasma proteins. Hemodialysis usually is indicated for life-threatening ingestions of ethylene glycol, methanol, or paraquat. This technique also has been used to enhance the elimination of ethanol, theophylline, lithium, salicylates, and long-acting barbiturates.

K. **Hemoperfusion** is a technique in which anticoagulated blood is passed through (perfused) a column containing activated charcoal or resin particles. This method of elimination clears substances from the blood more rapidly than hemodialysis, but it does not correct fluid and electrolyte abnormalities as does hemodialysis. Hemoperfusion, although more effective in removing phenobarbital, phenytoin, carbamazepine, methotrexate, and theophylline than hemodialysis, is less effective in removing ethanol or methanol. **Complications** of hemoperfusion include thrombocytopenia, leukopenia, hypocalcemia, hypoglycemia, and hypotension.

III. MANAGEMENT OF SPECIFIC INGESTIONS

A. **Acetaminophen (Tylenol)** is an antipyretic-analgesic that can produce fatal hepatotoxicity in untreated patients through the generation of a toxic metabolite.

1. **Available dosage forms.** Acetaminophen is available in a variety of OTC and prescription drug products.
2. **Toxicokinetics.** Acetaminophen is well absorbed from the GI tract and has a half-life between 2 and 3 hrs. Less than 5% is excreted unchanged in the urine; the remainder is metabolized in the liver by the cytochrome P450 system.
3. **Clinical presentation**
   a. **Phase I** (12 to 24 hrs postingestion). Nausea, vomiting, anorexia, and diaphoresis
   b. **Phase II** (1 to 4 days postingestion). Asymptomatic
   c. **Phase III** (2 to 3 days in untreated patients). Nausea, abdominal pain, progressive evidence of hepatic failure, coma, and death

[3]Chyka PA, Seger D. Position statement: Single-dose activated charcoal. American Academy of Clinical Toxicology; European Association of Poisons Centres and Clinical Toxicologists. *J Toxicol Clin Toxicol.* 1997;35:721–741.

4. **Laboratory data**
   a. **Serum acetaminophen levels.** Patients with levels greater than 150, 70, or 40 mg/mL at 4, 8, or 12 hrs after ingestion require antidotal therapy with *N*-acetylcysteine (NAC) according to the Rumack-Matthews nomogram.
   b. Baseline liver function tests should be done in all patients.
   c. Renal function tests, including a BUN and SCr, should be done.
   d. Coagulation studies include prothrombin time (PT), partial thromboplastin time (PTT), and bleeding time.
5. **Treatment**
   a. Adult patients who have ingested > 10 g or children who have ingested > 200 mg/kg require treatment. Elderly and alcoholic patients have an increased susceptibility to acetaminophen hepatotoxicity.
   b. The recommended treatment is GI decontamination with activated charcoal.
   c. Antidotal therapy with NAC is indicated for patients with toxic blood levels of acetaminophen.
      (1) **NAC dosage** is 140 mg/kg as a loading dose followed by 70 mg/kg every 4 hrs for a total of 17 doses. NAC is administered either orally or via a nasogastric tube. NAC (Mucomyst) 20% contains 200 mg/mL. Each dose must be diluted 1:3 in either cola or fruit juice to mask the unpleasant taste and smell. The dose of NAC should be repeated if the patient vomits within 30 mins of administration. Patients with severe nausea secondary to NAC may be pretreated with IV metoclopramide (Reglan) 10 mg every 6 hrs. Metoclopramide acts as an antiemetic while increasing the rate of NAC absorption.
      (2) **IV NAC** (Acetadote)
         (a) Loading dose: 150 mg/kg over 60 mins
         (b) Maintenance dose: 50 mg/kg over 4 hrs followed by 100 mg/kg over 16 hrs
         (c) Anaphylactoid reactions are observed in approximately 20% of patients. **Caution** should be exercised in patients with a history of **asthma**.

B. Alcohols[4]
1. **Ethylene glycol**
   a. **Available forms.** Ethylene glycol commonly is used in antifreeze and windshield de-icing solutions. This form is sometimes colorless and has a sweet taste.
   b. **Toxicokinetics.** Ethylene glycol is hepatically metabolized by alcohol dehydrogenase to glycolaldehyde, which is metabolized by aldehyde dehydrogenase to glycolic acid. Glycolic acid is converted to glyoxylic acid, whose most toxic metabolite is oxalic acid.
   c. **Clinical presentation**
      (1) **Stage I** (0.5 to 12 hrs postingestion). Ataxia, nystagmus, nausea and vomiting, decreased deep tendon reflexes, and severe acidosis (more severe overdoses: hypocalcemic tetany and seizures, cerebral edema, coma, and death)
      (2) **Stage II** (12 to 24 hrs postingestion). Tachypnea, cyanosis, tachycardia, pulmonary edema, and pneumonitis
      (3) **Stage III** (24 to 72 hrs postingestion). Flank pain and costovertebral angle tenderness; oliguric renal failure
   d. **Laboratory data** may reveal severe metabolic acidosis, hypocalcemia, and calcium oxalate crystals in the urinalysis.
   e. **Treatment**
      (1) **Gastric lavage** is performed within 30 mins of ingestion.
      (2) **IV ethanol (EtOH) is used in situations in which fomepizole is not available.**
         (a) **Indications** include an ethylene glycol level > 20 mg/dL, suspicion of ingestion pending level, or an anion gap metabolic acidosis with a history of ingestion, regardless of the level.
         (b) **EtOH dosage**
            (i) An EtOH level of at least 100 mg/dL should be maintained.
            (ii) Loading dose is 7.5 to 10 mL/kg of a 10% ethanol in dextrose 5% in water (D_5W) over 1 hr, followed by a maintenance infusion of 1.4 mL/kg/hr.
            (iii) Infusion rates may need to be increased in patients receiving hemodialysis.

---

[4]Megarbane B, Borron SW, Baud FJ. Current recommendations for the treatment of severe toxic alcohol poisonings. *Intensive Care Med.* 2005;31:189–195.

(3) **Fomepizole (Antizol)** is a potent inhibitor of alcohol dehydrogenase that can prevent the formation of the toxic metabolites of either methanol or ethylene glycol.
   (a) Administer a **loading dose** of 15 mg/kg (up to 1 g) in 100 mL of D_5W or 0.9% sodium chloride (NaCl) infused over 30 mins.
   (b) **Maintenance doses**: 10 mg/kg every 14 hrs for four doses, then increase to 15 mg/kg (to offset autoinduction phenomenon) until methanol or ethylene glycol levels are < 20 mg/dL.
(4) **Pyridoxine** (100 mg IV every day) and **thiamine** (100 mg IV every day) are cofactors that may convert glyoxylic acid to nonoxalate metabolites.
(5) **Sodium bicarbonate** is used as needed to correct the acidosis.
(6) **Hemodialysis.** Fomepizole must be continued, and the rate of administration may need to be increased. **Indications** include ethylene glycol level > 50 mg/dL, congestive heart failure, renal failure, and severe acidosis.

2. **Methanol**
   a. **Available forms** include gas-line antifreeze, windshield washer, and some sterno.
   b. **Toxicokinetics.** Alcohol dehydrogenase converts methanol to formaldehyde, which is then converted to formic acid.
   c. **Clinical presentation**
      (1) **Stage I.** Euphoria, gregariousness, and muscle weakness for 6 to 36 hrs, depending on the rate of formation of formic acid
      (2) **Stage II.** Vomiting, upper abdominal pain, diarrhea, dizziness, headache, restlessness, dyspnea, blurred vision, photophobia, blindness, coma, cerebral edema, cardiac and respiratory depression, seizures, and death
   d. **Laboratory data** include severe metabolic acidosis, hyperglycemia, and hyperamylasemia.
   e. **Treatment**
      (1) **Gastric lavage.** Charcoal has not been shown to absorb alcohols.
      (2) **IV EtOH (used in situations in which fomepizole is not available)**
         (a) **Indications** include any peak methanol level > 20 mg/dL, a suspicious ingestion with a positive history, or any symptomatic patient with an anion gap acidosis.
         (b) **Administration** is the same as per ethylene glycol (see III.B.1).
      (3) **Folic acid** administered at 1 mg/kg (maximum 50 mg) IV every 4 hrs for six doses increases the metabolism of formate.
      (4) **Fomepizole (Antizol)** (see III.B.1.e.[3])
      (5) **Sodium bicarbonate** is used for severe acidosis.
      (6) **Hemodialysis** is used for methanol levels > 50 mg/dL, severe and resistant acidosis, renal failure, or visual symptoms.

C. **Anticoagulants**[5]
   1. **Heparin/Low-Molecular-Weight Heparin (LMWH)**
      a. **Available dosage forms** include parenteral dosage forms for IV and subcutaneous administration.
      b. **Toxicokinetics.** Heparin has a half-life of 1 to 1.5 hrs and is primarily metabolized in the liver. The newer LMWHs—enoxaparin (Lovenox), dalteparin (Fragmin), tinzaparin (Innohep)—have a longer half-life, especially in patients with renal failure.
      c. **Clinical presentation**. Look for any signs or symptoms of bleeding or bruising.

---

[5]Full Text access to the American College of Chest Physician Guidelines Antithrombotic Therapy 8th Edition is available at: http://chestjournal.chestpubs.org/content/133/6_suppl

Ansell J, Hirsh J, Hylek E, et al; and American College of Chest Physicians. Pharmacology and management of the vitamin K antagonists: American College of Chest Physicians evidence-based clinical practice guidelines (8th edition). *Chest.* 2008;133(suppl 6):160s–198s.
Hirsh J, Bauer KA, Donati MB, et al; and American College of Chest Physicians. Parenteral anticoagulants: American College of Chest Physicians evidence-based clinical practice guidelines (8th edition). *Chest.* 2008;133(suppl 6):141s–159s.
Schulman S, Beyth RJ, Kearon C, et al; and American College of Chest Physicians. Hemorrhagic complications of anticoagulant and thrombolytic treatment: American College of Chest Physicians evidence-based clinical practice guidelines (8th edition). *Chest.* 2008; 133(suppl 6):257s–298s.
Van Ryn J, Stangier J, Haertter S, et al. Dabigatran etexilate—a novel, reversible, oral direct thrombin inhibitor: interpretation of coagulation assays and reversal of anticoagulant activity. *Thromb Haemost.* 2010;103:1–12.

d. **Laboratory data.** Obtain PTT, bleeding time, and platelet counts.

e. **Treatment**

(1) **Stopping heparin administration for 1 to 2 hrs and restarting therapy at a reduced dose can reverse mild over-anticoagulation.**

(2) **Severe overdoses** may require the administration of **protamine**.

(a) Protamine combines with heparin and neutralizes it: **1 mg protamine neutralizes 100 U heparin.**

(b) Protamine should be administered slowly, intravenously over 10 mins. The maximum dose of protamine is 50 mg in any 10-min period.

(c) Considerable controversy exists about the method of reversing the over-anticoagulation with LMWHs. Some sources recommend the administration of protamine to neutralize part of the effects of these anticoagulants, whereas case reports reported successes with recombinant factor VII (NovoSeven).

(d) These overdoses should be referred to a hematologist and/or the poison control center.

2. **Warfarin (Coumadin)**

a. **Available dosage forms** include oral tablets and a solution for parenteral administration.

b. **Toxicokinetics.** Warfarin is well absorbed after oral administration. Its mean half-life is 35 hrs; protein binding is 99%, with 5-day duration of activity. Vitamin K-dependent clotting factors begin to decline 6 hrs after administration, but therapeutic anticoagulation may require several days.

c. **Clinical presentation** includes minor bleeding, bruising, hematuria, epistaxis, and conjunctival hemorrhage. More serious bleeding includes GI, intracranial, retroperitoneal, and wound site.

d. **Laboratory data** include PT, international normalized ratio (INR), and bleeding time.

e. **Treatment**

(1) If **PT** or **INR** is **slightly elevated**, withhold warfarin for 24 to 48 hrs, then reinstitute therapy with a reduced dosage.

(2) If **PT** or **INR** is **elevated** and **bleeding**, administer 10 mg of phytonadione (vitamin K) over 30 mins. Patients who are bleeding may require the administration of blood products that contain clotting factors.

(3) For mild over-anticoagulation, follow American College of Chest Physicians (ACCP) guidelines.

(4) For patients with life-threatening bleeding or intracranial hemorrhage, the ACCP recommends the use of prothrombin complex concentrates or recombinant factor VIIa to immediately reverse the INR.

3. **Pradaxa (dabigatran)**

a. **Available dosage forms** include oral capsules.

b. **Toxicokinetics.** Dabigatran is poorly absorbed following oral administration, but it has a half-life of 12 to 17 hrs in healthy subjects with normal renal function.

c. **Clinical presentation** includes minor bleeding, bruising, hematuria, and epistaxis. More serious bleeding includes GI, intracranial, retroperitoneal, and wound site.

d. **Laboratory data** specialized hematologic monitoring may be required such as thrombin clotting time and ecarin clotting time.

e. **Treatment**

(1) **Mild bleeding.** Local treatment and withholding one dose

(2) **Moderate bleeding.** Consider blood product transfusion and/or hemodialysis

(3) **Severe bleeding.** As noted earlier with the additional consideration of charcoal filtration along with either recombinant factor VII or prothrombin complex concentrates. Dabigatran is the first FDA-approved oral direct-acting thrombin inhibitor. Many more compounds are in clinical trials and due to the paucity of overdose data with these drugs, consultation with a hematologist and/or a poison information specialist is highly recommended.

D. **Antidepressants**

1. Tricyclic antidepressants (TCAs)

a. **Available forms** include amitriptyline (Elavil), nortriptyline (Aventyl), imipramine (Tofranil), desipramine (Norpramin), doxepin (Sinequan), protriptyline (Vivactil), and clomipramine (Anafranil).

b. **Toxicokinetics.** The compounds are hepatically metabolized, undergo enterohepatic recirculation, are highly bound to plasma proteins, and have an elimination half-life of approximately 24 hrs.

c. **Clinical presentation.** Anticholinergic effects include mydriasis, ileus, urinary retention, and hyperpyrexia. **Cardiopulmonary toxicity** exhibits tachycardias, conduction blocks, hypotension, and pulmonary edema. **CNS manifestations** range from agitation and confusion to hallucinations, seizures, and coma.

d. **Laboratory data.** Blood level monitoring does not correlate well with clinical signs and symptoms of toxicity. Some authors suggest that electrocardiographic monitoring is a better guide to assessing the severity of ingestion.

e. **Treatment**

(1) **GI decontamination.** Syrup of ipecac is not recommended because patients may quickly become comatose, increasing the risk of aspiration. **Activated charcoal** is given every 6 hrs.

(2) **Alkalinization** with sodium bicarbonate 1 to 2 mEq/kg to maintain an arterial pH of 7.45 to 7.55 decreases the free fraction of the absorbed toxins, while reversing some of the cardiac abnormalities.

(3) **Phenytoin (Dilantin)** and/or **benzodiazepines** may be required to control seizures. Phenytoin must be administered at a rate not exceeding 25 mg/min because of hypotensive side effects. (**Fosphenytoin [Cerebyx]** may be used because it has a lower incidence of hypotension than phenytoin.)

(4) **Physostigmine** 2 mg IV over 1 min may be used to reverse **severe** anticholinergic toxicity owing to these drugs. **Because this antidote may cause asystole, the use of this antidote for TCA overdoses is declining.**

2. **Selective serotonin reuptake inhibitors (SSRIs)**

a. **Available forms** (nontricyclic agents) include fluoxetine (Prozac), sertraline (Zoloft), and paroxetine (Paxil).

b. **Toxicokinetics.** SSRIs are well absorbed after oral administration. Peak levels occur within 2 to 6 hrs. SSRIs are hepatically metabolized with a half-life between 8 and 30 hrs.

c. **Clinical presentation** includes mild symptomatology. Patients may become agitated, drowsy, or confused. Seizures and cardiovascular toxicity are rare.

d. **Laboratory data.** ECG monitoring is recommended. Blood level monitoring is not recommended.

e. **Treatment** includes gastric lavage and supportive treatment. Some toxicologists may recommend the use of cyproheptadine (Periactin) to manage the serotonin syndrome, which may manifest as a result of these ingestions.

E. **Benzodiazepines**

1. **Available forms** include chlordiazepoxide (Librium), diazepam (Valium), flurazepam (Dalmane), midazolam (Versed), lorazepam (Ativan), alprazolam (Xanax), and triazolam (Halcion).

2. **Toxicokinetics.** These drugs are hepatically metabolized.

3. **Clinical presentation** includes drowsiness, ataxia, and confusion. Fatalities are rare.

4. **Laboratory data.** Drug level monitoring is not indicated.

5. **Treatment**

a. **Supportive** treatment includes gastric emptying, activated charcoal, and a cathartic.

b. **Flumazenil** (Romazicon) is given 0.2 mg IV over 30 secs; repeat doses of 0.5 mg over 30 secs at 1-min intervals for a maximum cumulative dose of 5 mg.

(1) Flumazenil has a short elimination half-life.

(2) **Careful observation** for **resedation** is necessary, especially for ingestions of long-acting benzodiazepines.

(3) **Flumazenil is contraindicated in mixed overdose patients (particularly involving tricyclic antidepressants) in whom seizures are likely.**

F. **β-adrenergic antagonists**

1. **Available dosage forms.** Class examples include propranolol (Inderal), metoprolol (Lopressor), and atenolol (Tenormin). Oral and parenteral dosage forms are available.

2. **Toxicokinetics.** All of the members within this class differ in regard to renal versus hepatic elimination, lipid solubility, and protein binding. Patients may become toxic owing to changes in organ function.

3. **Clinical presentation** includes hypotension, bradycardia, and atrioventricular block. Bronchospasm may occur, particularly with noncardioselective agents.

4. **Laboratory data** include serum electrolytes and blood glucose (patients may become hypoglycemic).

5. **Treatment**
   a. **GI decontamination** includes gastric lavage and activated charcoal.
   b. **Glucagon** is given 50 to 150 mcg/kg as a loading dose over 1 min, followed by a continuous infusion of 1 to 5 mg/hr.
   c. **Epinephrine** should be used cautiously in β-blocker overdoses. Unopposed α-receptor stimulation in the face of complete β-receptor block may lead to profound hypertension.
   d. Calcium salts (see "Calcium Channel Antagonists")
   e. High-dose insulin dextrose (see "Calcium Channel Antagonists")

G. **Calcium channel antagonists**
1. **Available forms** include verapamil (Calan), diltiazem (Cardizem), and the dihydropyridine class (nifedipine derivatives [Procardia]).
2. **Toxicokinetics.** Onset of action is approximately 30 mins, whereas the duration is 6 to 8 hrs. Several compounds are available as sustained-release dosage forms, which may contribute to prolonged toxicity.
3. **Clinical presentation.** Hypotension is common to all classes. Bradycardia and atrioventricular block are more commonly seen with ingestions of verapamil or diltiazem. Pulmonary edema and seizures (verapamil) have been reported.
4. **Laboratory data** include ECG and serum electrolytes.
5. **Treatment**
   a. **GI decontamination** includes gastric lavage, activated charcoal, and whole-bowel irrigation (especially for ingestions with sustained-release products).
   b. **Calcium.** Calcium chloride 10% (10 to 20 mL) IV push is given for the management of hypotension, bradycardia, or heart block.
   c. **Glucagon** dosage is the same as for β-blocker overdose.
   d. **Combined insulin and dextrose administration** has been used in selected cases. The insulin dosages used are as follows: regular insulin 1 U/kg and a loading dose along with IV dextrose 0.5 g/kg. This should be followed with a continuous infusion of insulin at a rate of 0.5 to 2 U/kg/hr along with continuous dextrose infusions of 0.5 g/kg/hr to maintain serum glucose levels within a 100 to 250 mg/dL range. Insulin dosages are titrated to appropriate hemodynamic indices in an intensive care environment. This should be **used only in consultation with a poison control center**.
   e. Phosphodiesterase inhibitors. Inamrinone or milrinone.

H. **Cocaine**
1. **Available forms** include alkaloid obtained from *Erythroxylon coca*.
2. **Toxicokinetics.** Cocaine is well absorbed after oral, inhalational, intranasal, and IV administration. Cocaine is metabolized in the liver and excreted in the urine.
3. **Clinical presentation** includes CNS and sympathetic stimulation (e.g., hypertension, tachypnea, tachycardia, nausea, vomiting, seizures). Death may result from respiratory failure, myocardial infarction, or cardiac arrest.
4. **Laboratory data** include cocaine and cocaine metabolite urine screens.
5. **Treatment** is **supportive**: benzodiazepines for sedation seizure treatment, labetalol (Normodyne) for hypertension.

I. **Corrosives**
1. **Available forms** include strong acids or alkalis.
2. **Toxicokinetics.** Corrosives are well absorbed after oral and inhalational administration.
3. **Clinical presentation.** These compounds produce burns on contact.
4. **Laboratory data.** Arterial blood gases (ABGs), chest radiographs, and at least 6 hrs of observation are required for inhalation exposure.
5. **Treatment** is **decontamination.** Exposed skin must be irrigated with water. **Neutralization** should be **avoided** because these reactions are exothermic and will produce further tissue damage.

J. **Cyanide**
1. **Available forms** include industrial chemicals and some nail polish removers.
2. **Toxicokinetics.** The drug is rapidly absorbed after oral or inhalation exposure.
3. **Clinical presentation** includes headache, dyspnea, nausea, vomiting, ataxia, coma, seizures, and death.
4. **Laboratory data** include cyanide levels, ABGs, electrolytes, and an ECG.

5. **Treatment**
   a. Cyanide antidote kit
      (1) **Amyl nitrite.** Pearls are crushed and held under the patient's nostrils.
      (2) **Sodium nitrite** 10 mL IV push. Converts hemoglobin to methemoglobin, which binds the cyanide ion.
      (3) **Sodium thiosulfate** 50 mL of a 25% solution IV push. May be repeated if there is no response.
   b. **Oxygen**
   c. **Sodium bicarbonate.** As needed for severe acidosis
   d. Hydroxocobalamin (Cyanokit) adult dose is 5 g IV over 15 mins. Dose may be repeated for a total dose of 10 g. No data are available for pediatric dosing.[6]

K. **Digoxin (Lanoxin)**
1. **Available dosage forms** include oral and parenteral.
2. **Toxicokinetics.** Digoxin is well absorbed, is primarily renally eliminated, and has a half-life of 36 to 48 hrs. Its volume of distribution is 7 to 10 L/kg. Equilibration between serum level and myocardial binding requires 6 to 8 hrs.
3. **Clinical presentation** includes confusion, anorexia, nausea, and vomiting in mild cases. In more severe cases, cardiac dysrhythmias are seen.
4. **Laboratory data** include serum digoxin levels, electrolytes, particularly serum potassium levels, and an ECG.
5. **Treatment**
   a. **Decontamination** with activated charcoal is recommended.
   b. **Supportive therapy** includes managing hyperkalemia or hypokalemia and inotropic support as needed.
   c. **Digoxin-specific Fab antibodies (Digibind).** To determine the dosage, use the following formula:

$$\text{Dose (mg)} = [(\text{serum digoxin concentration [ng/mL]} \times \text{weight (kg)}/100]) \times (\text{mg/vial})$$

   Digibind 38 mg/vial or Digifab 40 mg/vial

L. **Electrolytes**
1. **Magnesium**
   a. **Available dosage forms** include oral, rectal, and parenteral. Magnesium-containing cathartics (e.g., magnesium citrate) have been reported to produce hypermagnesemia in patients receiving repetitive doses with activated charcoal.
   b. **Toxicokinetics.** Magnesium is found intracellularly and is renally eliminated.
   c. **Clinical presentation**
      (1) **Mild.** Deep tendon reflexes may be depressed; lethargy and weakness
      (2) **Severe.** Respiratory paralysis and heart block; prolonged PR, QRS, and QT intervals
   d. **Laboratory data**
      (1) **Mild:** > 4 mEq/L
      (2) **Severe:** > 10 mEq/L
   e. **Treatment** is **10% calcium chloride** 10 to 20 mL to temporarily antagonize the cardiac effects of magnesium. In severe cases, **hemodialysis** may be required.
2. **Potassium**
   a. **Available dosage forms** are oral and parenteral.
   b. **Toxicokinetics.** Potassium is primarily an intracellular cation. Changes in acid–base balance produce shifts in serum potassium values (e.g., a 0.1 U increase in serum pH produces a 0.1 to 0.7 mEq/L decrease in serum potassium values).
   c. **Clinical presentation** includes cardiac irritability and peripheral weakness with minor increases. Cardiac dysrhythmias, including bradycardia, may progress to asystole.
   d. **Laboratory data.** ECG data include **peaked T waves** and prolongation of the QRS complex.

[6] Hall AH, Dart R, Bogdan G. Sodium thiosulfate or hydroxocobalamin for the empiric treatment of cyanide poisoning? *Ann Emerg Med.* 2007;49:806–813.

e. **Treatment**
   (1) **Calcium.** Administer calcium chloride 10% 10 to 20 mL to antagonize the cardiac effects of hyperkalemia.
   (2) **Sodium bicarbonate.** 1 to 2 mEq/kg IV increases serum pH and causes an intracellular shift of potassium.
   (3) **Glucose and insulin.** 50 mL of 50% dextrose and 5 to 10 U of regular insulin are administered via IV push to shift potassium from the extracellular fluid into the cells.
   (4) **Cation exchange resins** bind potassium in exchange for another cation (sodium). **Sodium polystyrene sulfonate** (Kayexalate) is given 15 g/60 mL with 23.5% sorbitol in doses 15 to 30 g by mouth every 3 to 4 hrs as needed until the hyperkalemia resolves. Alternatively, 50 g of sodium polystyrene sulfonate can be given rectally in 200 mL of sodium chloride as a retention enema. There have been reports of colonic necrosis and other GI events. Some authors recommend other treatments before utilizing exchange resin therapy.[7]
   (5) **Hemodialysis** is reserved for life-threatening hyperkalemia that does not respond to the aforementioned measures.

M. **Iron (Fe)**
1. **Available dosage forms.** Numerous OTC products are available. Toxicity is based on the amount of elemental iron ingested: sulfate salt 20% elemental Fe; fumarate salt 33% elemental Fe; and gluconate salt 12% elemental Fe.
2. **Toxicokinetics.** Iron is absorbed in the duodenum and jejunum.
3. **Clinical presentation**
   a. **Phase I.** Nausea, vomiting, diarrhea, GI bleeding, hypotension
   b. **Phase II.** Clinical improvement seen 6 to 24 hrs postingestion
   c. **Phase III.** Metabolic acidosis, renal and hepatic failure, sepsis, pulmonary edema, and death
4. **Laboratory data** include serum Fe levels, total iron-binding capacity (TIBC; **is controversial**), ABGs, liver function tests (LFTs), hemoglobin, and hematocrit. Radiological evaluation of the abdomen notes the presence of radiopaque pills.
5. **Treatment**
   a. **Decontamination.** For ingestions $>$ 40 mg/kg. Gastric lavage using sodium bicarbonate is of questionable efficacy. Whole-bowel irrigation is used for large ingestions.
   b. **Supportive treatment**
   c. **Deferoxamine** (Desferal) is used to chelate iron. Administer at a rate of 15 mg/kg/hr up to a maximum dose of 6 to 8 g/day. Continue until patient is clinically stable.

N. **Isoniazid (INH)**
1. **Available dosage forms** include oral and parenteral.
2. **Toxicokinetics.** INH is well absorbed orally. Peak levels are within 1 to 2 hrs postingestion. Isoniazid is hepatically metabolized.
3. **Clinical presentation** includes nausea, vomiting, slurred speech, ataxia, generalized tonic–clonic seizures, and coma.
4. **Laboratory data** include severe lactic acidosis, hypoglycemia, mild hyperkalemia, and leukocytosis.
5. **Treatment**
   a. **Decontamination.** Avoid emesis because patients are at high risk for developing seizures; for severe ingestions, use activated charcoal gastric lavage.
   b. **Pyridoxine**, which reverses INH-induced seizures, is given in gram doses equivalent to the amount of isoniazid ingested. Pyridoxine is mixed as a 10% solution in D_5W and infused at 0.5 g/min until seizures stop, with the remainder infused over 4 to 6 hrs (maximum adult dose: 5 g).
   c. **Sodium bicarbonate** corrects the acidosis.

---

[7]Sterns RH, Rohas M, Bernstein P, Chennupati S. Ion-exhchange resins for the treatment of hyperkalemia: Are they safe and effective? *J Am Soc Nephrol.* 2010;21:733–735.

O. **Lead**

1. **Available forms** include lead-containing paint or gasoline fume inhalation.
2. **Toxicokinetics.** Lead has slow distribution, with a half-life of approximately 2 months.
3. **Clinical presentation** includes nausea, vomiting, abdominal pain, peripheral neuropathies, convulsions, and coma.
4. **Laboratory data** include anemia and an elevated blood-lead level.
5. **Treatment**
   a. **Edetate calcium disodium (Calcium Disodium Versenate)** is given 50 to 75 mg/kg/day intramuscularly (IM) or via slow IV in four divided doses.
   b. **Dimercaprol (BAL)** is given 4 mg/kg IM every 4 hrs for 3 to 5 days.
   Dimercaprol therapy is administered first. Following the second dose, concomitant edetate calcium disodium is initiated and both therapies are continued for up to 5 days. Oral chelation therapy is used for less severe cases.

P. **Lithium (Eskalith)**

1. **Available dosage forms** include liquid, capsules, and tablets (immediate and sustained release).
2. **Toxicokinetics.** Lithium is well absorbed after oral administration. It is not appreciably bound to plasma proteins and has a small volume of distribution (V_d) of 0.5 L/kg. Elimination is renal, with a half-life of 14 to 24 hrs.
3. **Clinical presentation**
   a. **Mild.** Polyuria, blurred vision, weakness, slurred speech, ataxia, tremor, and myoclonic jerks
   b. **Severe.** Delirium, coma, seizures, and hyperthermia
4. **Laboratory data**
   a. Therapeutic range: 0.6 to 1.2 mEq/L
   b. Mild toxicity: 1.5 to 2.5 mEq/L
   c. Moderate toxicity: 2.5 to 3.0 mEq/L
   d. Severe toxicity: $>$ 3.0 mEq/L
5. **Treatment**
   a. **Supportive** care, including basic life support and fluid and electrolyte replacement
   b. **Decontamination**
      (1) **Syrup of ipecac not recommended**
      (2) **Activated charcoal** ineffective
      (3) **Sodium polystyrene sulfonate** has been effective in experimental models. Need to monitor potassium levels.
      (4) **Whole-bowel irrigation** for large ingestions, especially those involving sustained-release products
      (5) **Hemodialysis** for severely symptomatic patients with acute exposure levels $>$ 2.5 mEq/L or chronic levels $>$ 1.5 mEq/L. **Note**: Lithium levels may rise after dialysis owing to a rebound effect.

Q. **Opiates**

1. **Available dosage forms** include oral immediate-release and sustained-release preparations as well as parenteral agents.
2. **Toxicokinetics.** Some agents have prolonged elimination half-lives (e.g., heroin, methadone).
3. **Clinical presentation** includes respiratory depression and a decreased level of consciousness. Rare effects include hypotension, bradycardia, and pulmonary edema. Seizures have been reported in patients with renal dysfunction in individuals who are receiving meperidine owing to the accumulation of the metabolite or meperidine.
4. **Laboratory data** include baseline ABGs and toxicology screens.
5. **Treatment**
   a. **Naloxone** is given 0.4 to 2.0 mg every 5 mins up to 10 mg and 0.03 to 0.1 mg/kg in pediatric patients. Naloxone has a very short half-life, and resedation is a concern in patients overdosing on long-acting opioids or sustained-release dosage forms.
   b. **Nalmefene (Revex)** has a half-life of 4 to 8 hrs. Initial dosages are 0.5 mg/70 kg. A follow-up dose 2 to 5 mins later is 1 mg/70 kg.

R. **Organophosphates**

1. **There are several available forms**; they are usually pesticides or chemical warfare agents.
2. **Toxicokinetics.** Organophosphates are absorbed through the lungs, skin, GI tract, and conjunctiva.

3. **Clinical presentation** includes excessive cholinergic stimulation.
4. **Laboratory data** include red blood cell acetylcholinesterase activity.
5. **Treatment**
   a. **Decontamination**
   b. **Atropine** is given 0.5 to 2.0 mg IV to reverse the peripheral muscarinic effects.
   c. **Pralidoxime (2-PAM; Protopam)** is given 1 g IV over 2 mins and repeated in 20 mins as needed.

S. **Salicylates**
1. **Available dosage forms** include several OTC products: oral, rectal, and topical.
2. **Toxicokinetics.** Salicylates are well absorbed after oral administration. The half-life is 6 to 12 hrs at lower doses. In overdose situations, the half-life may be prolonged to more than 20 hrs.
3. **Clinical presentation** includes nausea, vomiting, tinnitus, and malaise (mild toxicity). Lethargy, convulsions, coma, and metabolic acidosis appear in more severe overdoses. Potential **complications** from therapeutic and toxic doses include GI bleeding, increased PT, hepatic toxicity, pancreatitis, and proteinuria.
4. **Laboratory data** for the following 6-hr postingestion levels are:
   a. 40 to 60 mg/dL: tinnitus
   b. 60 to 95 mg/dL: moderate toxicity
   c. More than 95 mg/dL: severe toxicity
   d. With the presence of acidemia and aciduria, evaluate ABGs.
   e. In addition, laboratory evaluation may show leukocytosis, thrombocytopenia, increased or decreased serum glucose and sodium, hypokalemia, and increased serum BUN, creatinine, and ketones.
5. **Treatment**
   a. **Decontamination.** Repetitive doses of activated charcoal every 6 hrs, with one dose of cathartic for patients who ingested > 150 mg/kg. Whole-bowel irrigation for large ingestions.
   b. **Alkaline diuresis** is given as noted in decontamination section to enhance salicylate excretion. This is indicated for levels> 40 mg/dL.
   c. **Hemodialysis** is used for severe intoxications when serum levels are > 100 mg/dL. This method of decontamination is much better than repetitive doses of activated charcoal.
   d. **Fluid** and **electrolyte** replacement is administered as needed.
   e. **Vitamin K (Aquamephyton)** and **fresh frozen plasma** are used to correct any coagulopathy.

T. **Snake bites**
1. **Types.** There are numerous species of snakes found worldwide. The venomous snakes found in North America include the following: rattlesnake, cottonmouth, copperhead, and coral. Because patients may be exposed to more exotic snakes, a herpetologist should be consulted for a more definitive identification.
2. **Toxicokinetics.** Onset of symptomatology depends on the species of snake and the patient's underlying medical condition.
3. **Clinical presentation** includes nausea; vomiting; diarrhea; syncope; tachycardia; and cold, clammy skin. Local findings include pain, edema, and erythema. More severe envenomations can lead to severe tissue injury, compartment syndrome, and shock.
4. **Laboratory data**
   a. CBC and platelet count
   b. Coagulation profile
   c. Fibrin degradation products
   d. Electrolytes
   e. BUN, SCr, and urinalysis
5. **Treatment**
   a. **Supportive.** Move the patient away from striking distance of the snake. Ideally, the patient should be transported to a medical facility as soon as possible. Constrictive clothing, rings, watches, etc. should be removed. Tetanus immunization should be assessed, and surgical intervention may be necessary for severe cases.
   b. **Antivenoms**
      (1) Antivenin (Crotalidae) polyvalent is a horse-derived product that has been reported to produce allergic reactions. For mild bites, the recommended dose is 5 to 10 vials; moderate, 10–20; and severe envenomations may require 20 or more vials.

(2) Crotalidae polyvalent immune Fab is a polyvalent antivenin made from sheep sources. The initial dose is four to six vials diluted in 250 mL of 0.9% normal saline (NS) administered over 1 hr. Additional doses may be required for severe envenomations.

U. **Theophylline**

1. **Available dosage forms** include liquid, sustained-release tablets, and capsules as well as parenteral forms.
2. **Toxicokinetics.** Well absorbed orally with a V_d of approximately 0.5 L/kg. Theophylline is hepatically metabolized and has a half-life of 4 to 8 hrs. Theophylline clearance depends highly on age, concomitant disease states, and interacting drugs.
3. **Clinical presentation** includes nausea, vomiting, seizures, and cardiac dysrhythmias. Chronic toxicity carries a poorer prognosis than acute toxicity.
4. **Laboratory data.** Therapeutic theophylline levels are 5 to 20 μg/mL. Hyperglycemia and hypokalemia are seen with acute ingestions. Other useful laboratory tests include serum electrolytes, BUN, creatinine, hepatic function, and ECG monitoring.
5. **Treatment**
   a. **Supportive** therapy includes maintaining an airway and treating seizures and dysrhythmias as they occur.
   b. **Decontamination. Syrup of ipecac not recommended.**
   c. **Activated charcoal** (repetitive doses) to enhance elimination. **Whole-bowel irrigation** for massive ingestions (especially with sustained-release products). **Charcoal hemoperfusion** is used in unstable patients who are in status epilepticus. **Hemodialysis** is used when hemoperfusion is unavailable.
   d. **β-adrenergic antagonists** (e.g., esmolol, Brevibloc) are used to treat the hypotension, tachycardia, and dysrhythmias caused by elevated cyclic adenosine monophosphate levels.

Study Questions

Directions: Each of the questions, statements, or incomplete statements can be correctly answered or completed by **one** of the suggested answers or phrases. Choose the **best** answer.

1. A physician receives a call from the parent of a 2-year-old child who has ingested an unknown quantity of morphine controlled-release tablets and is now unconscious. The physician's initial recommendation is to
   (A) Call emergency medical services (EMS) and have the child taken to the hospital emergency department.
   (B) Administer 1 g/kg of activated charcoal with sorbitol.
   (C) Administer syrup of ipecac 15 mL by mouth to induce vomiting.
   (D) Suggest that the child receive emergency hemodialysis.
   (E) Suggest that the child receive acid diuresis with ammonium chloride.

2. A grandfather arrives at your pharmacy asking to purchase a bottle of syrup of ipecac to keep in his home in the event of a poisoning when grandchildren are visiting. What should you tell him?
   (A) Administer 15 mL of syrup of ipecac at the first sign of ingestion.
   (B) Syrup of ipecac is no longer recommended by the American Association of Poison Control Centers and the American Academy of Pediatrics.
   (C) Provide him with the toll-free number for the poison control center.
   (D) Both B and C.

3. An unconscious patient is brought into the emergency department. The patient is given 50 mL of 50% dextrose in water, thiamine 100 mg IV, followed by naloxone 1 mg, at which point he awakens. This patient most likely has overdosed on which of the following substances?
   (A) Methanol
   (B) Amitriptyline
   (C) Cocaine
   (D) Haloperidol
   (E) Heroin

4. Contraindications to the administration of syrup of ipecac include which of the following?
   (A) An unconscious patient
   (B) A patient who is experiencing a generalized tonic–clonic seizure
   (C) A patient who has ingested a caustic substance
   (D) All of the above
   (E) None of the above

5. An unconscious patient is brought to the emergency department with a history of an unknown drug overdose. Which of the following actions should the physician perform?
   (A) Administer 50 mL of 50% dextrose, thiamine 100 mg IV push, and naloxone 0.4 mg IV push.
   (B) Protect the patient's airway and ensure that vital signs are stable.
   (C) Order the following laboratory tests: complete blood count (CBC), electrolytes, and a toxicology screen.
   (D) All of the above.

6. A patient who overdoses on acetaminophen is admitted to the hospital for antidotal therapy with *N*-acetylcysteine (NAC). The patient has the following medication orders: NAC 140 mg/kg loading dose followed by 70 mg/kg for a total of 17 doses, ranitidine 50 mg IV every 8 hrs, prochlorperazine 10 mg IM every 6 hrs as needed for nausea, thiamine 100 mg IV every day for three doses, and Darvocet-N 100 one to two tablets every 4 hrs as needed for headache. What is the best course of action?
   (A) Call the physician to increase the dosage of ranitidine to 50 mg IV every 6 hrs.
   (B) Call the physician to have the Darvocet-N 100 discontinued.
   (C) Call the physician to initiate hemodialysis therapy.
   (D) Have the patient prophylactically intubated to protect the airway.
   (E) Administer ethanol 10% at a loading dose of 7.5 mL/kg over 1 hr, followed by a continuous infusion of 1.4 mL/kg/hr for 48 hrs.

7. Ethyl alcohol (EtOH) is administered to patients who have ingested either ethylene glycol or methanol because EtOH
   (A) helps sedate patients.
   (B) increases the metabolism of ethylene glycol and methanol.
   (C) blocks the formation of the toxic metabolites of ethylene glycol and methanol.
   (D) increases the renal clearance of ethylene glycol and methanol.
   (E) is not an antidote for ethylene glycol or methanol overdoses.

8. A patient with renal failure is inadvertently given three doses of potassium chloride 40 mEq IV in 100 mL of 0.9% sodium chloride over a 3-hr period. This error is immediately discovered, and a STAT serum potassium level is 8.0 mEq/L. The patient is bradycardic with a markedly prolonged QRS complex. The patient should receive which of the following?
   (A) Calcium chloride 10% 10 mL IV push
   (B) Sodium bicarbonate 50 mEq IV push
   (C) Insulin 10 U and 50% dextrose 50 mL IV push
   (D) Sodium polystyrene sulfonate 30 g by mouth every 3 hr for four doses
   (E) None of the above

9. Parenteral calcium is used as an antidote for which of the following situations?
   (A) Verapamil overdoses
   (B) Hyperkalemia
   (C) Cocaine intoxication
   (D) Verapamil overdoses and hyperkalemia

10. A 65-year-old woman with normal renal function is administered a 0.25 mg dose of digoxin IV push. A serum level obtained 1 hr after drug administration is 5 ng/mL. Your recommendation to the physician is which of the following?
   (A) Administer two vials of digoxin immune antibodies STAT.
   (B) Administer repetitive doses of activated charcoal.
   (C) Call a nephrologist, and put the patient on hemodialysis.
   (D) Repeat the serum digoxin level 6 to 8 hrs after the dose, and reassess the patient.

11. A 16-year-old woman is reported to have overdosed on 40 sustained-release theophylline tablets. She is transported to the emergency department, where gastric lavage was performed and she was given one dose of activated charcoal. An initial theophylline level is 42 μg/mL, but a follow-up level in the intensive care unit (ICU) is 95 μg/mL. What is the most appropriate course of therapy?
   (A) Charcoal hemoperfusion and multiple-dose activated charcoal
   (B) Syrup of ipecac administration
   (C) Forced alkaline diuresis
   (D) Nasogastric administration of sodium-polystyrene sulfonate

12. A 23-year-old man is admitted to the intensive care unit (ICU) after ingesting 20 acetaminophen tablets 500 mg with a six-pack of beer. He was initially awake and alert in the emergency department and was given one dose of activated charcoal. His initial acetaminophen level taken approximately 2 hrs after ingestion is 90 μg/mL. What would be the most appropriate course of action?
    (A) Administer repeated doses of activated charcoal and sorbitol.
    (B) Administer syrup of ipecac.
    (C) Administer a loading dose of *N*-acetyl-L-cysteine (NAC), and repeat the acetaminophen level in 4 hrs.
    (D) Discharge the patient to home.

13. An overdose victim presents to the emergency department with an elevated heart rate, decreased blood pressure, dilated pupils, and lethargy. Upon arrival to the intensive care unit (ICU), she has a generalized tonic–clonic seizure that is treated with IV diazepam and fosphenytoin. Which of the following is the most likely intoxicant?
    (A) Ethyl alcohol
    (B) Methanol
    (C) Acetaminophen
    (D) Oxycodone
    (E) Amitriptyline

14. A 37-year-old man is admitted to the ICU with an overdose of approximately 50 tablets of Depakote 500 mg sustained-release tablets. He never lost consciousness. He denies fevers, syncope, headache, vision changes, weakness, shortness of breath, chest pain, nausea, vomiting, or diarrhea. His initial valproic acid level was 41 mg/dL (therapeutic range 50 to 100 μg/mL). His ammonia level was elevated and therapy with intravenous levocarnitine was begun. At this point, you should recommend the following:
    (A) Discontinue levocarnitine.
    (B) Transfer the patient to in-patient psychiatry because the patient is asymptomatic.
    (C) Restart his home dose of valproic acid sustained-release tablets so that his level does not fall below the therapeutic range.
    (D) Recheck a follow-up valproic acid level and continue to observe in the ICU.

Answers and Explanations

1. **The correct answer is A** *[see I]*.
Patients with unstable vital signs should be taken to an emergency department for immediate treatment.

2. **The correct answer is D** *[see II.G.b]*.
Induced vomiting is no longer an acceptable option of managing poisonings at home because it is a relatively ineffective method of removing toxins and results in a delay in administering antidotal therapy. It is important to counsel patients on poison prevention and to give parents and other friends and relatives the toll-free number for the poison control center. Parents should also know basic first aid and cardiopulmonary resuscitation (CPR).

3. **The correct answer is E** *[see III.Q]*.
Naloxone reverses the effects of opioid receptor agonists, such as heroin, morphine, and propoxyphene.

4. **The correct answer is D** *[see II.G.a]*.
Contraindications to ipecac include the three Cs: caustics, conscious, and convulsions; see also the answer to question 2. The use of syrup of ipecac is reserved for rare circumstances and only under the direction of the poison control center and/or a physician. These are new recommendations, and many parents, relatives, and friends may have this product in their medicine cabinets.

5. **The correct answer is D** *[see II]*.
The management of unconscious overdose patients involves aggressive support of vital signs and the administration of empiric antidotal therapy, while obtaining various laboratory tests to determine the nature of the overdose.

6. **The correct answer is B** *[see III.a]*.
Darvocet-N 100 is an acetaminophen-containing product that should not be given to a patient with documented acetaminophen toxicity. Be aware particularly of OTC products containing acetaminophen.

7. **The correct answer is C** *[see III.b].*
Ethanol saturates alcohol dehydrogenase and prevents the formation of the toxic metabolites of either ethylene glycol or methanol; however, this antidote is falling out of favor owing to its adverse metabolic and central nervous system effects. Fomepizole (Antizol), a specific inhibitor of alcohol dehydrogenase, is becoming the preferred antidote for methanol or ethylene glycol overdoses. Ethanol may be used in situations in which fomepizole is not available.

8. **The correct answer is A** *[see III.L.2].*
All of the selections are used to manage hyperkalemia, although, in an unstable patient, the cardiac effects of hyperkalemia must first be reversed with intravenous calcium.

9. **The correct answer is D** *[see III.F & G].*
Parenteral calcium is used to reverse the cardiac effects of calcium-channel blocker overuse and hyperkalemia.

10. **The correct answer is D** *[see III.K].*
The plasma–tissue distribution phase for digoxin is 6 to 8 hrs postadministration. Sampling digoxin levels sooner may give a falsely elevated level. Only symptomatic patients should receive digoxin immune antibodies. Hemodialysis is of no value in managing digoxin overdoses.

11. **The correct answer is A** *[see III.U].*
Large ingestions of sustained-release products may act as drug reservoirs, necessitating aggressive measures to remove the toxin.

12. **The correct answer is C** *[see III.A].*
Large acetaminophen ingestions (> 140 mg/kg) may be fatal if unrecognized. The Rumack–Matthew nomogram requires a 4-hr level to accurately assess the potential for toxicity. If the 4-hr level is in the toxic range, the full course of NAC therapy should be administered.

13. **The correct answer is E** *[see III.D].*
Tricyclic antidepressant overdoses will produce seizures, hypotension, mydriasis, hypotension, and ventricular dysrhythmias. The cardiac and CNS effects of tricyclic antidepressant toxicity will respond to bicarbonate therapy. Opiates such as oxycodone will produce miosis.

14. **The correct answer is D** *[see II].*
The patient in this case ingested a sustained-release dosage form. Also from the history, it was estimated that the patient took 50 tablets that may produce a delayed release effect in and of itself. While the patient was asymptomatic, he may develop symptoms after a period as more drug are absorbed. In this case, a follow-up valproic acid level was 155 mg/dL, the patient was observed in the ICU, and carnitine therapy was continued. Carnitine has been shown to reverse the hyperaminemia induced by valproic acid and was continued while the patient was in the ICU. The next day, the valoproic acid level fell to 50 μg/dL, the patient remained asymptomatic, and he was transferred out of the ICU.

17 Sterile Products

CHRISTOPHER VITALE, CARYN DOMENICI BELISLE, JOHN FANIKOS

I. INTRODUCTION.

The *United States Pharmacopeia* (*USP*) and the National Formulary published practice standards for compounding sterile preparations after case reports of patient harm and fatality. The procedures and requirements outlined in *USP* Chapter 797 are intended to prevent patient harm resulting from ingredient errors and microbial contamination. This chapter includes compounding personnel responsibilities, training and evaluation requirements, medication preparation sterility and accuracy verification, classification of microbial contamination risk, and equipment and environmental quality and control. Although these standards apply to all facilities (hospitals, nursing homes, pharmacies) and all practitioners (physicians, nurses, technicians), they are especially important for pharmacists who are most often involved with sterile medication preparation. Because the standards require substantial investment in labor, equipment, and supplies, regulatory agencies (U.S. Food and Drug Administration, The Joint Commission on Accreditation of Health Care Organizations, U.S. state boards of pharmacy) are expecting implementation by January 2006, with evidence of long-term compliance and routine monitoring thereafter.

II. DEFINITIONS

A. **Sterility**, an absolute term, means the absence of living microorganisms.
   1. **Microbe** is a microscopic organism such as a bacterium, fungus, protozoon, or virus.
   2. **Pyrogens** are metabolic by-products of live or dead microorganisms that cause a pyretic response (i.e., a fever) upon injection.
   3. **Sterile products** are pharmaceutical dosage forms that are sterile. This includes products like parenteral preparations, irrigating solutions, and ophthalmic preparations (see Chapter 19). Sterile product compounding requires cleaner facilities, personnel training and testing, and a sound knowledge of sterilization and stability principals and practices.
   4. **Aseptic technique** refers to the sum total of methods and manipulations required to minimize the contamination of compounded sterile products and is of paramount importance when preparing such preparations.
   5. **Compounded sterile preparations** (CSPs) include
      a. Preparations that, when prepared according to manufacturer instructions, expose a sterile agent to potential microbial contamination.
      b. Preparations made from nonsterile ingredients that must be sterile before patient administration.
      c. Sterile or nonsterile biologicals (vaccines, immune globulins), diagnostics, medications, nutritionals, and radiopharmaceuticals that must be sterile prior to administration or use as an irrigation, bath, implant, inhalation, injection, or for use in the eye or ear.
   6. Beyond-use dating (BUD) is outlined by *USP* <797> subsection <71>, which defines the usability of CSPs postpreparation or after expiration of a punctured medication vial, based on product storage and microbial contamination risk levels (*Tables 17-1* and *17-2*).
      a. **Microbial contamination risk levels** are assigned according to the probability of contaminating a preparation with microbial organisms, endotoxins, or with foreign chemical or physical particulate matter.
         (1) **Low-risk level CSPs** are compounded by aseptically transferring a single sterile dosage form from a sterile ampoule, vial, bottle, or bag using sterile needles and syringes to a final sterile container or device for patient administration.

Table 17-1 MICROBIAL CONTAMINATION RISK LEVELS AND BEYOND USE DATING OF COMPOUNDED STERILE PREPARATIONS

	Beyond Use Date in the Absence of Sterility Testing (*USP* <71>)		
Type of CSP	**Room Temperature**	**Refrigeration**	**Frozen (≤ 10°C)**
Low risk	48 hrs	14 days	45 days
Medium risk	30 hrs	9 days	45 days
High risk	24 hrs	3 days	45 days
Immediate use	1 hr		

CSP, compounded sterile preparation; *USP*, United States Pharmacopeia.

(2) **Medium-risk level CSPs** are compounded by aseptically transferring multiple sterile dosage forms from sterile ampoules, vials, bottles, or bags using sterile needles and syringes to a single final sterile container or device for administration to multiple patients or to one patient on multiple occasions.

(3) **High-risk level CSPs** are compounded from nonsterile ingredients and are terminally sterilized prior to patient administration or sterile ingredients that are compounded under inferior air quality conditions.

(4) **Immediate-use CSPs** are compounded in emergency situations or where immediate patient administration is mandated to avoid harm that may result from delays in treatment.

7. **Compounded parenteral preparations** are pharmaceutical dosage forms that are injected through one or more layers of skin. Because the parenteral route bypasses the protective barriers of the body, parenteral preparations must be sterile. The pH of a solution may markedly influence the stability and compatibility of parenteral preparations.

III. DESIGN AND FUNCTION OF STERILE COMPOUNDING AREAS

A. **Clean rooms** are areas specially constructed and maintained to reduce the probability of environmental contamination of sterile products during the manufacturing process. Engineering controls to reduce the potential for airborne contamination include airflow through high-efficiency particulate-air (HEPA) filters, use of horizontal flow clean benches, vertical flow clean benches, biological safety cabinets, and barrier isolators. Clean rooms are traditionally designed in multicompartments or partitioned work areas for aseptic processing (*Figure 17-1*).

1. **Ante-area** provides a clean area for personal cleaning and for donning personal protective equipment such as hair covers, gloves, gowns, or full clean room attire. Supplies are removed from shipping cartons and decontaminated with a disinfecting agent. The area should provide at least an International Organization for Standardization (ISO) class 8 or better work environment.
2. **Buffer area** contains the work surfaces for the staging of supplies and equipment used in CSP preparation. It should provide at least an ISO class 7 work environment. The buffer area should

Table 17-2 BEYOND USE DATING OF PUNCTURED MEDICATION VIALS

Type of Vial	Beyond Use Date of Punctured Vials Under Refrigeration (*USP* <71>)
Single-dose vial	6 hrs after initial puncture within an ISO class 5 area or cleaner
Multi-dose vials containing an antimicrobial preservative	28 days
Ampoules	Requires immediate use

ISO, International Organization for Standardization; *USP*, United States Pharmacopeia.

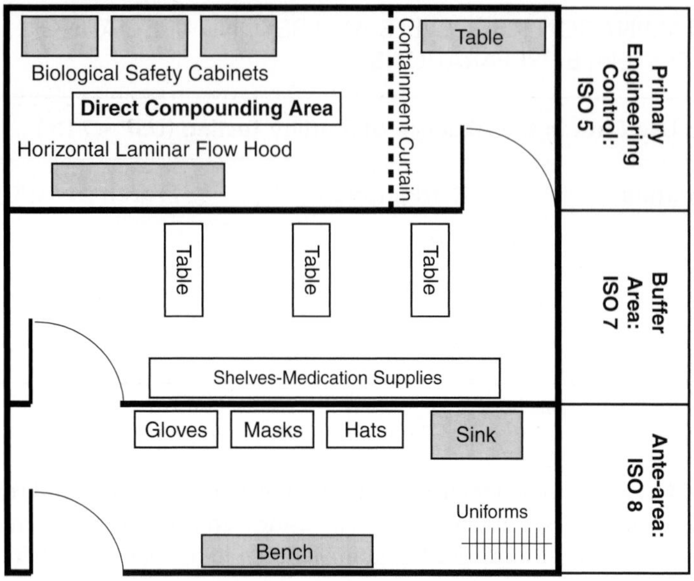

Figure 17-1. Clean room layout.

contain no sinks or drains and be free of objects that shed particles (cardboard, paper, cotton, etc.). Traffic flow in and out is minimized and restricted to qualified compounding personnel.

3. **Primary engineering control** is the room that provides the ISO class 5 environment for CSP preparation.
4. **Direct compounding area** is the critical area with the primary engineering control where compounding is performed and critical sites are exposed to HEPA-filtered air.
5. **HEPA filters** are used to cleanse the air entering the room. These filters remove all airborne particles 0.3 mm or larger, with an efficiency of 99.97%. The reference standards for HEPA-filtered rooms have changed to a metric-based system (*Table 17-3*). HEPA-filtered rooms are classified as ISO class 3 through 8. An ISO class 8 room contains no more than 3,520,000 particles of 0.5 μm or larger per cubic meter of air.
6. **Positive-pressure airflow** is used to prevent contaminated air from flowing into the clean room. In order to achieve this, the air pressure inside the clean room must be greater than the pressure outside the room, so that when a door or window to the clean room is opened, the airflow is outward.
7. **Counters** in the clean room are made of stainless steel or other nonporous, easily cleaned material.
8. **Walls, floors,** and **ceilings** do not have cracks or crevices and have rounded corners. All surfaces should also be nonporous and washable to enable regular disinfection. If walls or floors are painted, epoxy paint is used.

Table 17-3 INTERNATIONAL ORGANIZATION OF STANDARDIZATION (ISO) CLASSIFICATION OF PARTICULATE MATTER IN ROOM AIR

Class Name		Particle Size	
ISO Class	U.S. Federal Standard[a]	ISO (Particles per cubic meter)	U.S. Federal Standard[a] (Particles per cubic foot)
3	Class 1	35.2	1
4	Class 10	352	10
5	Class 100	3,520	100
6	Class 1000	35,200	1,000
7	Class 10,000	352,000	10,000
8	Class 100,000	3,520,000	100,000

[a]Federal Standard No. 209E, General Services Administration, Washington DC, 20407.

9. **Airflow.** As with the HEPA filters used in clean rooms, the airflow moves with a uniform velocity along parallel lines. The velocity of the airflow is 27 m/min (90 f).
10. **Critical site** is any opening providing a direct path between a sterile product and the environment or any surface coming in direct contact with the sterile product and the environment. Laminar flow work benches are used to provide an adequate critical site environment. *USP* Chapter 797 requires sterile preparation compounding be performed in at least an ISO class 5 quality air environment.

B. **Laminar flow work benches (LFWB)** are generally used in conjunction with clean rooms and are specially designed to create an aseptic environment for the preparation of sterile products. An ISO class 5 environment exists inside a certified horizontal or vertical LFWB.

1. **HEPA filter requirement**. Like clean rooms, laminar flow work benches use HEPA filters, but the benches use a higher efficiency air filter than do clean rooms.
2. **Types of laminar flow work benches**
   a. **Horizontal** laminar flow hoods (*Figure 17-2*) were the first hoods used in pharmacies for the preparation of sterile products. Airflow in horizontal hoods moves across the surface of the work area, flowing first through a prefilter and then through the HEPA filter. The major disadvantage of the horizontal hood is that it offers no protection to the operator, which is especially significant when antineoplastic agents are being prepared (see IX.D.2).
   b. **Vertical** laminar flow hoods (*Figure 17-3*) provide two major **advantages** over horizontal flow hoods.
      (1) The airflow is vertical, flowing down on the work space. This airflow pattern protects the operator against potential hazards from the products being prepared.
      (2) A portion of the HEPA-filtered air is recirculated a second time through the HEPA filter. The remainder of the filtered air is removed through an exhaust filter, which may be vented to the outside to protect the operator from chronic, concentrated exposure to hazardous materials.

C. **Biological safety cabinets (BSCs)** are vertical flow hoods with four major types available. They are differentiated by the amount of air recirculated in the cabinet, whether this air is vented to the room or outside, and whether contaminated ducts are under positive or negative pressure.

1. **Type A cabinets** recirculate 70% of cabinet air through HEPA filters back into the cabinet, the remainder is discharged through a HEPA into the clean room, and contaminated ducts are under positive pressure.
2. **Type B1 cabinets** recirculate 30% of cabinet air through HEPA filters back into the cabinet, the remainder is discharged through HEPA filters to the outside environment, and contaminated ducts are under negative pressure.

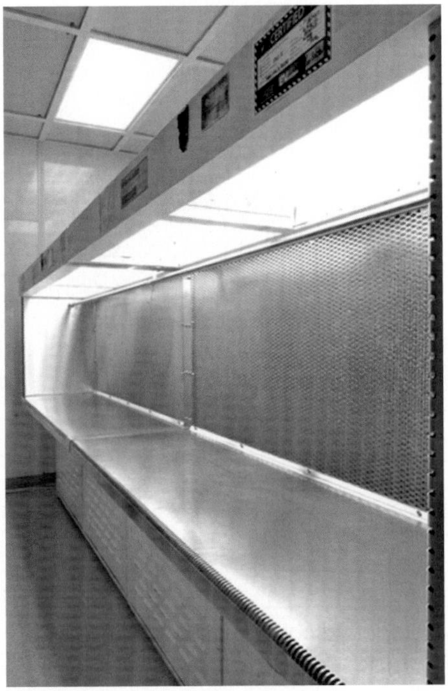

Figure 17-2. Horizontal laminar flow hood. (Courtesy of William Salkin.)

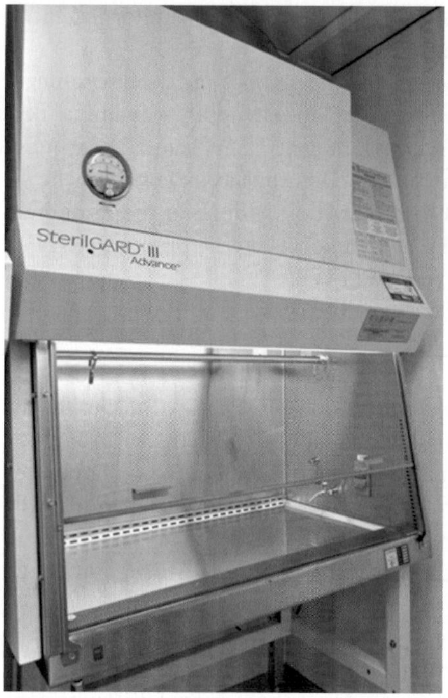

Figure 17-3. Vertical laminar flow hood. (Courtesy of William Salkin.)

3. **Type B2 cabinets** discharge all cabinet air through HEPA filters to the outside environment with contaminated ducts under negative pressure.
4. **Type B3 cabinets** recirculate 70% of cabinet air through HEPA filters back into the cabinet, 30% is discharged through HEPA filters to the outside, and contaminated ducts are under negative pressure.

D. **Compounding aseptic isolators (CAI)** provide an ISO class 5 environment for product preparation, with aseptic manipulations occurring inside a closed, pressurized environment accessible only via sealed gloves that reach into the work area (*Figure 17-4*).

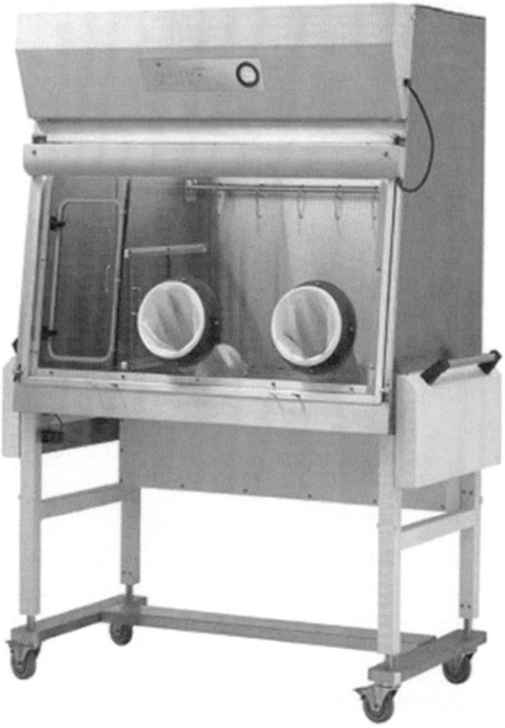

Figure 17-4. Compounding aseptic isolator. (Courtesy of William Salkin.)

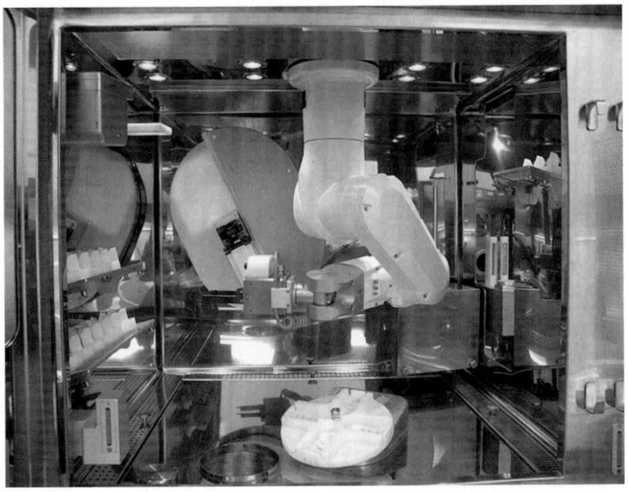

Figure 17-5. Advanced robotic automated compounding device. (Courtesy of William Salkin.)

E. **Compounding aseptic containment isolators** protect workers from exposure to undesirable or hazardous drugs during the compounding and material transfer processes. An isolator uses unidirectional or turbulent airflow to remove contaminants from the unit. It uses positive air pressure to keep external airborne particles out of the isolator. This technology represents an acceptable alternative to LFWBs in clean rooms for aseptic processing.

F. **Automated compounding devices (ACDs)** are important pieces of equipment used for the preparation of sterile products. ACDs provide accuracy, safety, and efficiency through technology. Portable ACDs are required to be in an ISO class 5 environment. **Advanced robotic ACDs** are available for compounding sterile syringes, chemotherapy and small-volume sterile products. Robotic devices are typically stand-alone machines housed within a fully enclosed ISO class 5 or better environment (*Figure 17-5*).

G. **Inspection and certification.** Clean rooms, LFWBs, BSCs, and barrier isolators are inspected and certified when they are first installed; at least every 6 months thereafter; and, in the case of LFWB, BSCs, and isolators, when moved to a new location.

1. **Inspections** should be conducted by National Sanitation Foundation (NSF)-accredited and certified technicians with expertise and training in contamination control technologies. Equipment used for testing has appropriate tolerance for the specified testing and is calibrated to National Institute of Standards and Technology (NIST) traceable standards.
2. **Testing** is performed per relevant industry standards and at minimum includes
   a. HEPA filter integrity testing
   b. Airflow testing: downflow and inflow where appropriate
   c. Particulate monitoring
   d. Pressurization monitoring (clean rooms and barrier isolators) ensures that no particle larger than 0.3 mm passes through the HEPA filter. In addition, an anemometer is used to determine airflow velocity, and a particle counter is used to determine the particle count.

IV. ASEPTIC MANIPULATIONS

A. **Aseptic technique** refers to the sum total of methods and manipulations required to minimize the contamination of compounded sterile products and is of paramount importance when preparing such preparations. Aseptic technique starts with proper gowning procedures, hand washing, and proper use of sterile gloves. A working knowledge and ability to perform appropriate manipulations of sterile compounding instrumentation such as syringes, needles, sterile vials, and infusion bags is also necessary to ensure sterility of the end product and thus patient safety.

B. **Full-body garb** has been shown to reduce the number of particles emitted from those working in a sterile environment. Proper gowning is required prior to entering the clean room and should take place in the ISO 8 Ante-Area. Gowning from "head-to-toe" should take place, including the use of hairnets or bonnets, surgical mask, shoe covers, sterile gloves, and sterile gown or full clean room attire (*Figure 17-6*).

C. **Hand antisepsis** has been shown to reduce the incidence of health care–associated infections by decreasing microbial transmission from patient to patient via the health care worker. This same

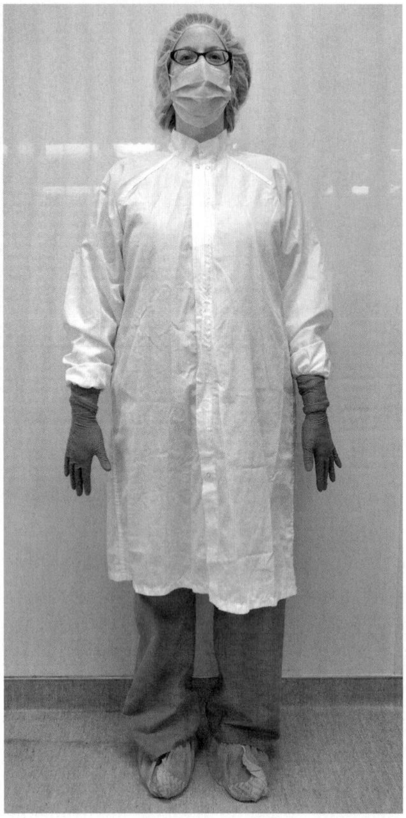

Figure 17-6. Full-body garb including hairnet, surgical mask, shoe covers, sterile gloves, and gown. (Courtesy of William Salkin.)

concept is applied to the preparation of CSPs, and thorough hand washing is required every time prior to entering the sterile environment. The following CDC guidelines for proper hand hygiene of the health care professional should be followed:

1. Removal of all artificial nails, nail polish, and jewelry.
2. Hands should be scrubbed with antimicrobial soap for 15 secs and rinsed with warm water. Dry thoroughly with a disposable towel. Alcohol-based hand sanitizers are alternatives to soap and water to disinfect **unsoiled** hands.
3. Washed hands that have been coughed or sneezed into, or that have come in contact with nonsterile surfaces, should be washed or sanitized again.

D. **Sterile gloves** should be donned after gowning and hand washing but prior to entering the ISO 5 direct compounding area and must be changed upon leaving the clean room. During CSP preparation, gloves should be rinsed frequently with an alcohol-based hand sanitizer and changed when their integrity is compromised by coming in contact with nonsterile surfaces or are coughed or sneezed into. The following steps should be taken when putting on a pair of sterile gloves:
   1. Open sterile glove packaging then paper wrapper around gloves, ensuring not to touch any outer portion of either glove.
   2. Place the first glove on one hand by only touching the folded, inner portion of the glove. Pull the glove up over the outer cuff of the sterile gown. Repeat.
   3. Pickup and discard the sterile glove packaging by touching only the sterile paper wrapper.

E. **Proper preparation of the laminar flow hood** (LAFW or BSC) and all supplies must be performed prior to the manufacturing of CSPs to ensure a biological and particulate-free work environment. When working in a laminar flow hood, all manipulations must take place at a minimum of 6 inches within the work surface (*Figure 17-7*). When preparing the work surface and supplies, the following steps should be followed:
   1. Remove all supplies from the work surface.
   2. Wash all surfaces of the laminar flow hood, excluding the HEPA filter grate, using 70% isopropyl alcohol. All surfaces should be wiped down with lint-free cleaning cloths by using side-to-side motions that extend entirely from one wall of the work surface to the other. Cleaning should always start in the back of the laminar flow hood and move toward the front in order to pull any debris out of the work area.

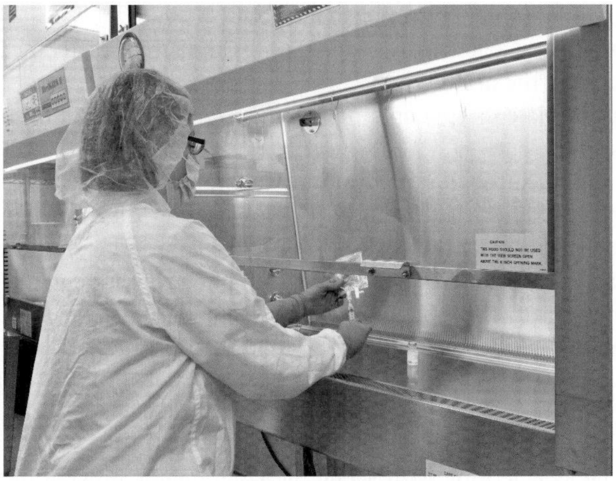

Figure 17-7. Working within a laminar flow hood. (Courtesy of Chistopher J. Belisle.)

3. All nonsterile supplies, such as vials and infusion bags, should be removed from their outer packaging and wiped down with 70% isopropyl alcohol and lint-free cleaning cloths prior to being placed within the laminar flow hood.
4. Instrumentation that is in sterile packaging such as needles and syringes should be opened within the laminar flow hood just prior to use. This packaging should always be "peeled" opened as intended as opposed to being torn open, to reduce the creation of particulate matter within the sterile environment. Place packaging to the side.
5. Place all sterilized supplies on the workbench in a manner that airflow is unobstructed from all vials and infusion bags.
6. Remove vial covers from all vials. Place to the side.
7. Use an alcohol swab to sterilize the rubber stoppers of the vials and the injection ports of the infusion bags by wiping thoroughly.

F. **Proper aseptic technique** must be used when preparing compounded sterile preparations, along with creating a slight negative pressure within the diluent and medication vials in order to prevent spray back from vial stoppers upon withdrawal of the needle. This can be accomplished by performing the following steps:
   1. Proper technique for **removing a needle cap** from a Luer-Lok needle that is attached to a syringe is necessary to reduce the risk of a finger stick, and includes the following steps (*Figure 17-8*):
      a. Hold the syringe with attached/capped needle in one hand like a pen.
      b. Place the heels of your hands together.

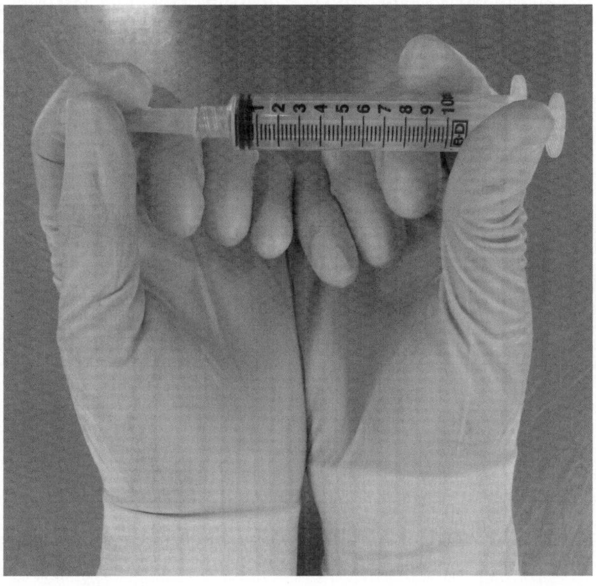

Figure 17-8. Proper technique for removing a needle cap from a Luer-Lok needle. (Courtesy of William Salkin.)

c. Grasp the needle cap with the finger and thumb of the opposite hand.
d. While keeping the heels of your hands firmly together, roll your thumbs away from each other until the needle cap is fully removed from the needle.
e. Place the needle and syringe in an appropriate sharps container after use. In order to minimize the risk of needle sticks, NEVER recap a needle.

G. **Anticoring technique:** While inserting a needle through a medication vial stopper, a small piece of the stopper can become sheared off or cored and left floating in the medication infusion bag. This core can easily go unnoticed due to its small size or if visualization is blocked by a medication label and can result in a foreign body being injected into the patient. Although coring is generally considered a low-frequency event, case reports have established it as a potential medical risk. In order to prevent coring when preparing compounded sterile preparations, the following technique should be used:
1. Position the needle on the vial stopper at about a 45 to 60 degree angle to the closure surface so that the bevel is facing upward (*Figure 17-9*).
2. Apply downward pressure on the needle as if writing with a pen, while gradually moving the needle to an upright position, reaching 90 degrees just before penetration is complete.

H. **Reconstituting powdered medication** (this step will be necessary only when working with lyophilized medication vials):
1. By pulling back on the syringe plunger, draw into the syringe a volume of air equal to about 1 mL less than the volume of diluent that will be used for reconstitution. This information can be found in the product package insert.
2. After penetrating the diluent vial, invert the vial by using the thumb and forefinger to hold the vial, and the little finger and the palm of the hand to hold the barrel of the syringe.
3. Using the other hand to manipulate the syringe plunger, use multiple small injections and withdrawals to transfer the air in the syringe and a slight excess of the diluent solution from the vial.
4. Prior to withdrawing the needle from the vial, remove all air bubbles by tapping the syringe and then adjust the syringe to the proper diluent volume.
5. Keeping the drug vial upright upon the work surface, insert the needle and use multiple small injections and withdrawals to transfer the diluent in the syringe and remove a volume of air from the vial equal to about 1 mL greater than the amount of diluent that was just added.
6. Swirl the vial according to the manufactures recommendations until the drug is fully dissolved.

I. **Reconstituted medications or medications that are already in solution:**
1. Using a new needle and syringe, draw into the syringe a volume of air equal to about 1 mL less than the volume of solution that will be used.
2. Withdraw the calculated amount of medication solution from the vial as previously described.
3. Transfer the drug solution in the syringe into a final container via the injection port. Cover the injection port with a protective cover.
4. Inspect the final container for integrity, evidence of particulates, and verification of product accuracy.

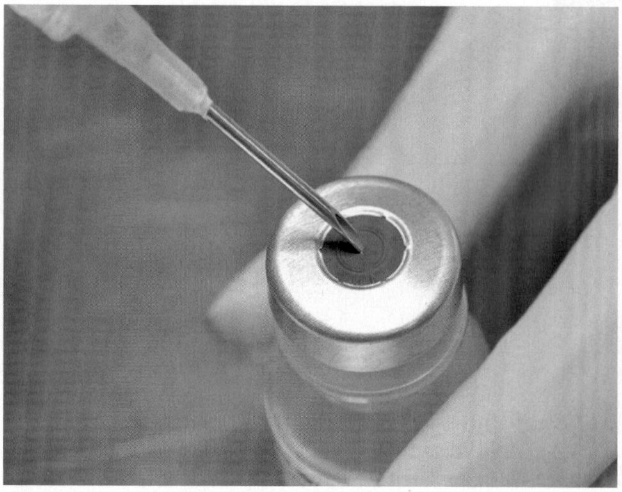

Figure 17-9. Anticoring technique. (Courtesy of William Salkin.)

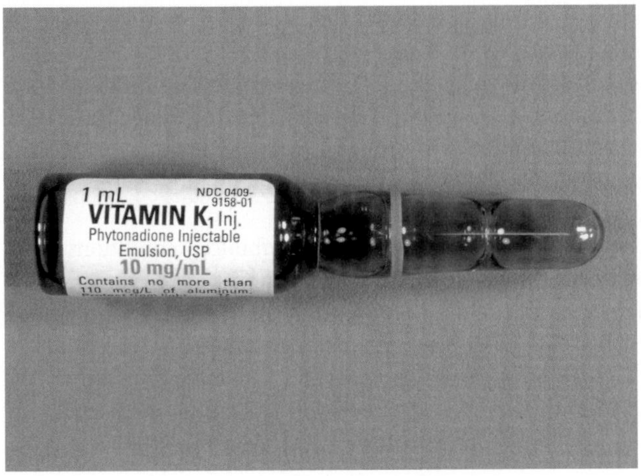

Figure 17-10. Glass medication ampoule. (Courtesy of Chistopher J. Belisle.)

J. **Ampoules** are small, sealed glass vials used to contain and preserve a medication (*Figure 17-10*). The following steps should be followed when using an ampoule:
   1. To open the ampoule:
      a. Hold upright and gently tap the top to remove any solution from the head space.
      b. Swab the neck of the ampoule with an alcohol swab.
      c. Grasp the top of the ampoule with the thumb and forefinger of one hand, while firmly holding the bottom of the ampoule with the other.
      d. By moving your hands away and out from you, quickly snap open the ampoule.
   2. To withdraw medication from the ampoule:
      a. Insert a 5 micron filter needle or straw into the ampoule while holding at a slight angle.
      b. Withdraw the appropriate amount of solution by positioning the needle or straw in the corner area of the ampoule, beveled edge down.
      c. Replace with new needle prior to transferring the solution to the final container.

V. QUALITY CONTROL AND QUALITY ASSURANCE

A. **Definitions**
   1. **Quality control** is the day-to-day assessment of all sterile compounding operations. This includes receipt of raw materials, preparation, storage, distribution, patient administration, and includes analytic testing of the finished product.
   2. **Quality assurance**, an oversight function, involves the auditing of quality control procedures and systems, with suggestions for changes as needed.

B. **Testing procedures.** Various types of tests are used to ensure that all sterile products are free of microbial contamination, pyrogens, and particulate matter.
   1. **Clarity testing** is used to check sterile products for particulate matter and leaks. Before dispensing a parenteral solution, pharmacy personnel should check it for particulates by swirling the solution and looking at it against both light and dark backgrounds, using a clarity testing lamp or other standard light source.
   2. **Compound accuracy checking** is a double check of the used drug products and supplies by a person other than the compounder. This includes an inspection of the label and syringes used to measure the additives.
   3. **Beyond use dating** represents the date and time beyond which a product should not be administered because of potency, sterility, or storage concerns. Beyond use dating should be assigned in accordance with the manufacturers' product labeling and should comply with *USP <797>* guidelines (*Table 17-1*, *Table 17-2*).
   4. **End product testing** is sterility and pyrogen testing that should be performed on all high-risk CSPs that are prepared in batches of 25 units or more, multidose vials, or preparations that are exposed longer than 6 to 12 hrs prior to sterilization.
      a. **Sterility testing** ensures that the process used to sterilize the product was successful. The **membrane sterilization method** is often used to conduct sterility testing. Test samples are

passed through membrane filters, and a nutrient medium is then added to promote microbial growth. After an incubation period, microbial growth is determined.

b. **Pyrogen testing** can be accomplished by means of qualitative fever response testing in rabbits or by in vitro limulus lysate testing. Commercial laboratories are available to perform these tests. People handling sterile products can attempt to avoid problems with pyrogens by purchasing pyrogen-free water and sodium chloride for injection from reputable manufacturers and by using proper handling and storage procedures.

C. **Environmental testing** includes air and surface sampling to measure microbiology conditions of the clean room and assesses the effectiveness of cleaning and sanitizing procedures.

1. **Viable air sampling** includes volumetric air collection in the controlled environment and evaluation of airborne microorganisms or collection of airborne organisms by exposing sterile nutrient plates containing tryptic soy broth (TSB) or tryptic soy agar (TSA) for a suitable time frame.
2. **Nonviable air sampling** is intended to evaluate the equipment that is used to create clean air. **Total particle counts** (*Table 17-3*) should be within established ISO classifications for a given compounding area.
3. **Surface sampling** uses TSA plates called replicate organism detection and counting (RODAC) plates to capture microorganism.
4. Both air and surface sampling plates are collected and incubated. The number of discrete colonies of organisms, colony forming units (CFUs), are counted and reported.

D. **Practical quality assurance programs** for noncommercial sterile products include training, monitoring the manufacturing process, personnel competency assessment, quality control check, and documentation.

1. **Training of pharmacists and technicians** in proper aseptic techniques and practices is the single most important aspect of an effective quality assurance program. Training should impart a thorough understanding of departmental policies and procedures.
2. By **monitoring the manufacturing process**, a supervisor can check adherence to established policies and procedures and take corrective action as necessary.
3. After training is completed, **competency assessment** through performance evaluation and reevaluation is required for routine tasks like hand washing, gowning, gloving, and aseptic manipulations. Evaluations should occur annually for personnel compounding and low- and medium-risk CSPs, and semi-annually for high-risk CSPs.

E. **Process validation** provides a mechanism for ensuring processes consistently result in sterile products of acceptable quality. This should include a written procedure to follow as well as evaluation of aseptic technique through process simulation.

F. **Process simulation testing or personnel evaluation** duplicates sterile compounding of low-, medium-, and high-risk level CSPs under most stressful conditions except that an appropriate growth media (Soybean-Casein Digest Medium) is used in place of the drug products. After preparation and incubation of the final product, no growth indicates proper aseptic techniques were followed.

G. **Quality control checking** includes monitoring the sterility of a sample of manufactured products. The membrane sterilization method is practically employed using a commercially available filter and trypticase soy broth media.

H. **Documentation** of training procedures, quality control results, laminar flow hood certification, and production records are required by various agencies and organizations.

VI. STERILIZATION METHODS AND EQUIPMENT.

Sterilization is performed to destroy or remove all microorganisms in or on a product. Sterilization can be achieved through thermal, chemical, radioactive, or mechanical methods.

A. **Thermal sterilization** involves the use of either moist or dry heat.

1. **Moist-heat sterilization** is the **most widely used** and reliable sterilization method.
   a. Microorganisms are destroyed by **cellular protein coagulation**.
   b. The objects to be sterilized are exposed to saturated steam under 1 atmosphere pressure at a minimum temperature of **121°C** for at least 20 to 60 mins.
   c. An **autoclave** is commonly used for moist-heat sterilization.
   d. Because it does not require as high a temperature, moist-heat sterilization causes **less product and equipment damage** compared to dry-heat sterilization.

2. **Dry-heat sterilization** is appropriate for materials that cannot withstand moist-heat sterilization. Objects are subjected to a temperature of at least **160°C** for **120 mins** (if higher temperatures can be used, less exposure time is required).

B. **Chemical (gas) sterilization** is used to sterilize surfaces and porous materials (e.g., surgical dressings) that other sterilization methods may damage.
   1. In this method, **ethylene oxide** is used generally in combination with heat and moisture.
   2. **Residual gas** must be allowed to dissipate after sterilization and before use of the sterile product.

C. **Radioactive sterilization** is suitable for the industrial sterilization of contents in sealed packages that cannot be exposed to heat (e.g., prepackaged surgical components, some ophthalmic ointments).
   1. This technique involves either **electromagnetic** or **particulate radiation**.
   2. Accelerated drug decomposition sometimes results.

D. **Mechanical sterilization (filtration)** removes but does not destroy microorganisms and clarifies solutions by eliminating particulate matter. For solutions rendered unstable by thermal, chemical, or radiation sterilization, filtration is the preferred method. A depth filter or screen filter may be used. Personnel should ensure the filter used either during compounding or administration is chemically and physically compatible with the CSP at the temperature and pressure conditions used.
   1. **Depth filters** usually consist of fritted glass or unglazed porcelain (i.e., substances that trap particles in channels).
   2. **Screen (membrane) filters** are films measuring 1 to 200 μm thick made of cellulose esters, microfilaments, polycarbonate, synthetic polymers, silver, or stainless steel.
      a. A **mesh** of millions of microcapillary pores of identical size filters the solution by a process of physical sieving.
      b. **Flow rate.** Because pores make up 70% to 85% of the surface, screen filters have a higher flow rate than depth filters.
      c. **Types of screen filters**
         (1) **Particulate filters** remove particles of glass, plastic, rubber, and other contaminants.
            (a) **Other uses.** These filters also are used to reduce the risk of phlebitis associated with administration of reconstituted powders. Filtration removes any undissolved powder particles that may cause venous inflammation.
            (b) The **pore size** of standard particulate filters ranges from 0.45 to 5 μm. Special particulate filters are required to filter blood, emulsions (e.g., fat emulsions), or colloidal dispersions or suspensions because these preparations have a larger particle size.
         (2) **Microbial filters** with a pore size of 0.22 μm or smaller ensure complete microbial removal and sterilization. This is referred to as cold sterilization.
         (3) **Final filters**, which may be either particulate or microbial, are often included as part of the tubing used in drug administration. They are referred to as in-line filters and are used to remove particulates or microorganisms from an intravenous (IV) solution during infusion.

VII. PACKAGING OF PARENTERAL PRODUCTS.

Parenteral preparations and other sterile products must be packaged in a way that maintains product sterility until the time of use and prevents contamination of contents during opening.

A. **Types of containers**
   1. **Ampoules**, the oldest type of parenteral product containers, are made entirely of **glass** (*Figure 17-10*).
      a. Intended for **single use only**, ampoules are opened by breaking the glass at a scored line on the neck.
      b. **Disadvantages.** Because glass particles may become dislodged during ampoule opening, the product must be filtered before it is administered. Their unsuitability for multiple-dose use, the need to filter solutions before use, and other safety considerations have markedly reduced the ampoule as a package form.

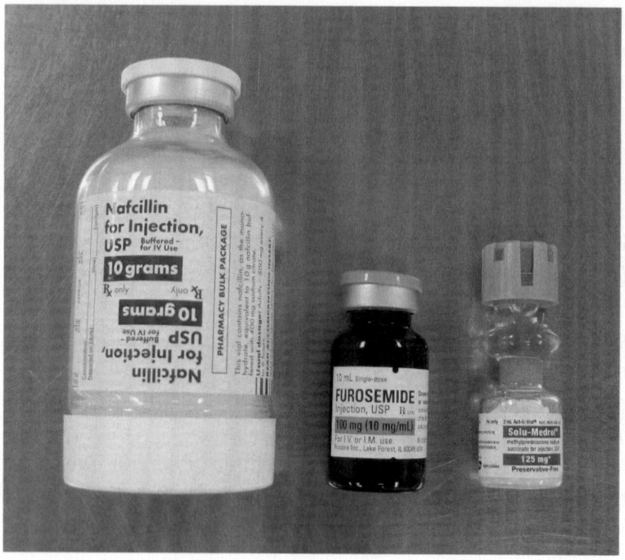

Figure 17-11. Medication vials. (Courtesy of Chistopher J. Belisle.)

2. **Vials** are glass or plastic containers closed with a rubber stopper and sealed with an aluminum crimp (*Figure 17-11*).
   a. Vials have several **advantages** over ampoules.
      (1) Vials can be designed to hold multiple doses (if prepared with a bacteriostatic agent).
      (2) The drug product is easier to remove from vials than from ampoules.
      (3) Vials eliminate the risk of glass particle contamination during opening.
   b. However, vials also have certain **disadvantages**.
      (1) The rubber stopper can become **cored**, causing a small bit of rubber to enter the solution (see IV.H).
      (2) Multiple withdrawals (as with multiple-dose vials) can result in microbial contamination.
   c. Some drugs that are unstable in solution are packaged in vials unreconstituted and must be **reconstituted** with a diluent before use. Sterile water or sterile sodium chloride for injection are the most commonly used drug diluents.
      (1) To accelerate the dissolution rate and permit rapid reconstitution, many powders are lyophilized (freeze dried).
      (2) Some of these drugs come in vials that contain a double chamber.
         (a) The top chamber, containing sterile water for injection, is separated from the unreconstituted drug by a rubber closure.
         (b) To dislodge the inner closure and mix the contents of the compartments, external pressure is applied to the outer rubber closure. This system eliminates the need to enter the vial twice, thereby reducing the risk of microbial contamination.
3. Some drugs come in vials that may be attached to a diluent-containing bag for reconstitution and administration, such as the **ADD-Vantage System** by Abbott or the **Mini-Bag Plus System** by Baxter (*Figure 17-12*). Premeasured drug and diluent may also be stored in separate compartments within a delivery system and then combined at the point of use, such as the **Duplex System** by B. Braun.
   a. The ADD-Vantage vial is screwed into the top of an ADD-Vantage diluent bag, and the rubber diaphragm is dislodged from the vial, allowing the diluent solution to dissolve the drug prior to administration.
   b. The Mini-Bag Plus System contains an adaptor that links standard 20 mm powdered drug vials with Baxter's Mini-Bag containers, allowing vial and bag to be attached without activation until time of administration.
   c. The Duplex systems has two compartments where a seal is broken and drug and diluent are mixed to form a solution prior to administration.
   d. The premixed piggyback contains drug solution that is prediluted and ready to be administered with no further preparation needed.

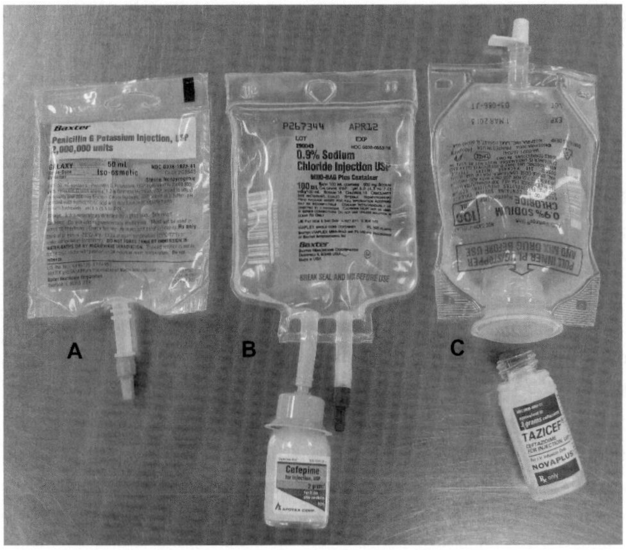

Figure 17-12. **A.** Prefilled intravenous medication piggyback dose. **B.** MiniBag Plus System by Baxter. **C.** ADD-Vantage System by Abbott. (Courtesy of Chistopher J. Belisle.)

4. **Prefilled syringes** and **cartridges** are designed for maximum convenience (*Figure 17-13*).
   a. **Prefilled syringes.** Drugs administered in an emergency (e.g., atropine, epinephrine) are available for immediate injection when packaged in prefilled syringes.
   b. **Prefilled cartridges** are ready-to-use parenteral packages that offer improved sterility and accuracy. They consist of a plastic cartridge holder and a prefilled medication cartridge with a needle attached. The medication is premixed and premeasured. Narcotics such as meperidine (Demerol) and hydromorphone (Dilaudid) are commonly available in prefilled cartridges.
5. **Infusion solutions** are divided into two categories: **small-volume parenterals** (SVPs), those having a volume less than 100 mL; and **large-volume parenterals** (LVPs), those having a volume of 100 mL or greater. Infusion solutions are used for the intermittent or continuous infusion of fluids or drugs.

B. **Packaging materials.** Materials used to package parenteral products include glass and plastic polymers.
   1. **Glass**, the original parenteral packaging material, has superior clarity, facilitating inspection for particulate matter. Compared to plastic, glass less frequently interacts with the preparation it contains.
   2. **Plastic polymers** used for parenteral packaging include polyvinylchloride (PVC) and polyolefin.
      a. **PVC** is flexible and nonrigid.
      b. **Polyolefin** is semirigid; unlike PVC, it can be stored upright.
      c. Both types of plastic offer several **advantages** over glass, including durability, easier storage and disposal, reduced weight, and improved safety.

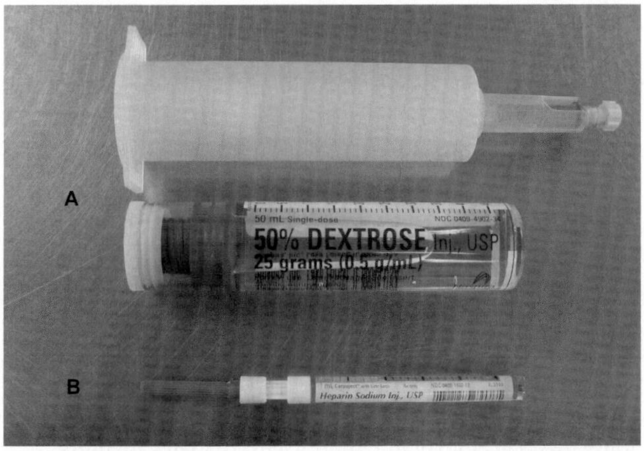

Figure 17-13. **A.** Prefilled syringe and medication cartridge. **B.** Prefilled medication Capuject by Hospira. (Courtesy of William Salkin.)

VIII. PARENTERAL ADMINISTRATION ROUTES.

Parenteral preparations may be given by a variety of administration routes.

A. **Subcutaneous (SC or SQ)** administration refers to injection into the subcutaneous tissue beneath the skin layers, usually of the abdomen, arm, or thigh. Insulin is an example of a subcutaneously administered drug.

B. **Intramuscular (IM)** administration means injection into a muscle mass. The mid-deltoid area and gluteus medius are common injection sites.

1. No more than 5 mL of a solution should be injected by this route.
2. Drugs intended for prolonged or delayed absorption such as medroxyprogesterone (Depo Provera) and methylprednisolone (Depo Medrol) commonly are administered intramuscularly.

C. **Intravenous (IV)** administration is the most important and most common parenteral administration route. It allows an immediate therapeutic effect by delivering the drug directly into the circulation. However, this route precludes recall of an inadvertent drug overdose. Antibiotics, cardiac medications, and many other drugs are given intravenously.

D. **Intradermal (ID)** administration involves injection into the most superficial skin layer. Because this route can deliver only a limited drug volume, its use generally is restricted to skin tests and certain vaccines.

E. **Intra-arterial (IA)** administration is injection directly into an artery. It delivers a high drug concentration to the target site with little dilution by the circulation. Generally, this route is used only for radiopaque materials, thrombolytic agents, and some antineoplastic agents.

F. **Intracardiac (IC)** administration is injection of a drug directly into the heart.

G. **Hypodermoclysis** refers to injection of large volumes of a solution into subcutaneous tissue to provide a continuous, abundant drug supply. This route occasionally is used for antibiotic administration in children.

H. **Intraspinal** administration refers to injection into the spinal column. Local anesthetics (e.g., lidocaine, bupivacaine) are frequently administered via this route during surgical procedures.

I. **Intra-articular** administration means injection into a joint space. Corticosteroids (e.g., methylprednisolone, hydrocortisone) use this route for the treatment of arthritis.

J. **Intrasynovial** administration refers to injection into the joint fluid.

K. **Intrathecal (IT)** administration is injection into the spinal fluid; it sometimes is used for antibiotics and cancer chemotherapy.

L. **Epidural (ED)** administration refers to the injection of medications, usually local anesthetics and/or narcotics near or outside the dura mater of the central nervous system. This route is frequently used during childbirth.

IX. PARENTERAL PREPARATIONS

A. **IV admixtures.** These preparations consist of one or more sterile drug products added to an IV fluid, generally dextrose or sodium chloride solution alone or in combination. IV admixtures are used for drugs intended for continuous infusion. Drugs that may cause irritation or toxicity when given as a rapid direct IV injection are also prepared as IV admixtures.

B. **IV fluids and electrolytes**

1. **Fluids** used in the preparation and administration of parenteral products include sterile water and sodium chloride, dextrose, and Ringer's solutions, all of which have multiple uses. These fluids serve as vehicles in IV admixtures, providing a means for reconstituting sterile powders. They serve as the basis for correcting body fluid and electrolyte disturbances and provide a caloric source in parenteral nutrition.

   a. **Dextrose (D-glucose) solutions** are the most frequently used glucose solutions in parenteral preparations.

   (1) **Uses.** Generally, a solution of dextrose 5% in water (D_5W) is used as a vehicle in IV admixtures. D_5W may also serve as a hydrating solution. In higher concentrations (e.g., a 10% solution in water), dextrose provides a source of carbohydrates in parenteral nutrition solutions.

   (2) **Considerations.** Because the pH of D_5W ranges from 3.5 to 6.5, instability may result if it is combined with an acid-sensitive drug.

   (a) Dextrose concentrations greater than 15% must be administered through a central vein.

   (b) Dextrose solutions should be used cautiously in patients with diabetes mellitus.

b. **Sodium chloride** usually is given as a 0.9% solution. Because it is isotonic with blood, this solution is called normal saline solution (NSS). A hypotonic solution of 0.45% sodium chloride is termed half-normal saline. A hypotonic solution of 0.225% sodium chloride is termed quarter-normal saline. Sodium chloride solutions greater than 0.9% concentration are hypertonic.
   (1) **Sodium chloride for injection**, which is a solution of 0.9% sodium chloride, is used as a vehicle in IV admixtures and for fluid and electrolyte replacement. In smaller volumes, it is suitable for the reconstitution of various medications.
   (2) **Bacteriostatic sodium chloride for injection**, which is also a 0.9% solution, is intended solely for multiple reconstitutions. It contains an agent that inhibits bacterial growth (e.g., benzyl alcohol, propylparaben, methylparaben), which allows for its use in multiple-dose preparations.

c. **Waters** are used for reconstitution and for dilution of such IV solutions as dextrose and sodium chloride. Waters suitable for parenteral preparations include sterile water for injection and bacteriostatic water for injection.

d. **Ringer's solutions**, which are appropriate for fluid and electrolyte replacement, commonly are administered to postsurgical patients.
   (1) **Lactated Ringer's injection** (i.e., Hartmann's solution, Ringer's lactate solution) contains sodium lactate, sodium chloride, potassium chloride, and calcium chloride. Frequently, it is combined with dextrose (e.g., as 5% dextrose in lactated Ringer's injection).
   (2) **Ringer's injection** differs from lactated Ringer's injection in that it does not contain sodium lactate and has slightly different concentrations of sodium chloride and calcium chloride. Like lactated Ringer's injection, it may be combined in solution with dextrose.

2. **Electrolyte preparations.** With ions present in both intracellular and extracellular fluid, electrolytes are crucial for various biological processes. Surgical and medical patients who cannot take food by mouth or who need nutritional supplementation require the addition of electrolytes in hydrating solutions or parenteral nutrition solutions.
   a. **Cations** are positively charged electrolytes.
      (1) **Sodium** is the chief extracellular cation.
         (a) **Importance.** Sodium plays a key role in interstitial osmotic pressure, tissue hydration, acid–base balance, nerve-impulse transmission, and muscle contraction.
         (b) **Parenteral sodium preparations** include sodium chloride, sodium acetate, and sodium phosphate.
      (2) **Potassium** is the chief intracellular cation.
         (a) **Importance.** Potassium participates in carbohydrate metabolism, protein synthesis, muscle contraction (especially of cardiac muscle), and neuromuscular excitability.
         (b) **Parenteral potassium preparations** include potassium acetate, potassium chloride, and potassium phosphate.
      (3) **Calcium**
         (a) **Importance.** Calcium is essential to nerve-impulse transmission, muscle contraction, cardiac function, bone formation, and capillary and cell membrane permeability.
         (b) **Parenteral calcium preparations** include calcium chloride, calcium gluconate, and calcium gluceptate.
      (4) **Magnesium**
         (a) **Importance.** Magnesium plays a vital part in enzyme activities, neuromuscular transmission, and muscle excitability.
         (b) **Parenteral preparation.** Magnesium is given parenterally as magnesium sulfate.
   b. **Anions** are negatively charged electrolytes.
      (1) **Chloride** is the major extracellular anion.
         (a) **Importance.** Along with sodium, it regulates interstitial osmotic pressure and helps to control blood pH.
         (b) **Parenteral chloride preparations** include calcium chloride, potassium chloride, and sodium chloride.
      (2) **Phosphate** is the major intracellular anion.
         (a) **Importance.** Phosphate is critical to various enzyme activities. It also influences calcium levels and acts as a buffer to prevent marked changes in acid–base balance.
         (b) **Parenteral phosphate preparations** include potassium phosphate and sodium phosphate.

(3) **Acetate**

(a) **Importance.** Acetate is a bicarbonate precursor that may be used to provide alkali to assist in the preservation of plasma pH.

(b) **Parenteral acetate preparations** include potassium acetate and sodium acetate.

C. **Parenteral antibiotic preparations** are available as sterile unreconstituted powders, which must be reconstituted with sterile water, normal saline, or D_5W, or as a sterile, ready-to-use liquid parenteral.

1. **Administration methods.** Parenteral antibiotics may be given intermittently by direct IV injection, short-term infusion, intramuscular injection, or intrathecal injection.
2. **Uses.** Parenteral antibiotics are used to treat infections that are serious and require high antibiotic blood levels or when the gastrointestinal tract is contraindicated, such as in ileus.
3. **Dosing frequencies** of parenteral antibiotics vary from once daily to as often as every 2 hrs, depending on the kinetics of the drug, seriousness of the infection, the site of infection, and the patient's disease or organ status (e.g., renal disease).

D. **Parenteral antineoplastic agents.** Studies suggest that these medications may be toxic to the personnel who prepare and administer them. The evidence is not conclusive, which necessitates special precautions to ensure safety and minimize risks. In response to concerns, the Occupational Safety and Health Administration (OSHA) has published a technical manual, "Controlling Occupational Exposure to Hazardous Drugs." Every facility must have a written plan that includes drug preparation precautions, storage, transport, personal protective equipment (gloves, gowns, masks), work equipment, waste disposal, spill management, and personnel medical surveillance.

1. **Administration methods.** Parenteral antineoplastics may be given by direct IV injection, short-term infusion, or long-term infusion. Some are administered by a non-IV route, such as the subcutaneous, intramuscular, intra-arterial, or intrathecal route.
2. **Safe antineoplastic handling guidelines.** All pharmacy and nursing personnel who prepare or administer antineoplastics should receive special training in the following guidelines to reduce the risk of exposure to these drugs.

a. A **vertical laminar flow hood** should be used during drug preparation, with exhaust directed to the outside (*Figure 17-3*).

b. All syringes and IV tubing should have **Luer-Lok fittings** (see XI.B).

c. **Clothing.** Personnel should wear personal protective equipment, including closed-front cuffed gowns resistant to liquid permeation and latex or nitrile gloves approved for use when handling chemotherapy (*Figure 17-6*). Double gloving is recommended.

d. **Final dosage adjustment** should be made into the vial, ampoule, or directly into an absorbent gauze pad.

e. **Priming equipment.** Special care should be taken when IV administration sets are primed. The IV tubing should be primed before adding the drug, or the tubing can be primed with drug-free fluid before connecting it to the chemotherapy drug container. If these are not available, prime the tubing into sterile gauze in a sealable plastic bag.

f. Proper procedures should be followed for **disposal** of materials used in the preparation and administration of antineoplastics.

(1) **Needles** should not be clipped or recapped.

(2) **Preparations** should be discarded in containers that are puncture-proof, leak-proof, and properly labeled.

(3) **Hazardous waste.** A color-coded system was created by the Environmental Protection Agency (EPA), of which use is required by facilities to ensure safe and proper disposal of hazardous waste (*Table 17-4*). Trace chemotherapy refers to any product that was exposed to a chemotherapy agent, such as a syringe, needle, or empty vial that once contained chemotherapy. All items with trace chemotherapy must be placed in a yellow container. All other hazardous waste that is not considered trace must be placed in a black container.

g. After removal of gloves, personnel should **wash hands** thoroughly.

h. Personnel and equipment involved in the preparation and administration of antineoplastic agents should be **monitored** routinely.

Table 17-4 ENVIRONMENTAL PROTECTION AGENCIES REQUIRED SYSTEM FOR PROPER DISPOSAL OF HAZARDOUS WASTE

Type of Waste	Container Color
Hazardous toxic Hazardous ignitable Hazardous infectious	Black
Trace chemotherapy	Yellow
Drain disposal	Sink/sewer
Nonregulated drugs	White with blue top or cream with purple top

3. **Patient problems.** Infusion phlebitis and extravasation are the most serious problems that may occur during the administration of parenteral antineoplastics.
   a. **Infusion phlebitis** (inflammation of a vein) is characterized by pain, swelling, heat sensation, and redness at the infusion site. Drug dilution and filtration can eliminate or minimize the risk of phlebitis.
   b. **Extravasation** (infiltration of a drug into subcutaneous tissues surrounding the vein) is especially harmful when antineoplastics with vesicant properties are administered. Proper measures must be taken immediately if extravasation occurs.

E. **Total parenteral nutrition (TPN)** are large-volume admixtures that are used when enteral nutrition cannot be tolerated.
   1. **Two in one admixture** contains both amino acids and dextrose.
   2. **Three in one admixture** contains amino acids, dextrose, and intralipid or "fat."
   3. **Formulas.** Most TPN admixtures contain various amounts of electrolytes and other additives such as insulin, H2 antagonists, and vitamins.
   4. **Calcium and phosphorus**-containing solutions form a precipitate when mixed together and are therefore deemed incompatible. This reaction is avoided when these ingredients are added non-consecutively to a TPN solution containing amino acid.
   5. **Administration.** TPN is most commonly administered through a central line. TPN can also be administered through a peripheral or femoral line. Osmolality must be taken into consideration when choosing the route of administration of TPN.

F. **Parenteral biotechnology products** are created by the application of recombinant technology to the generation of therapeutic agents, such as monoclonal antibodies, various vaccines, and colony-stimulating factors.
   1. **Uses** of these agents include cancer therapy, infections, transplant rejection, rheumatoid arthritis, inflammatory bowel disease, respiratory diseases, and malaria as well as vaccines against cancer, HIV infection, and hepatitis B.
   2. **Characteristics.** Protein and peptide biotechnology drugs that have a shorter half-life often require special storage such as refrigeration or freezing and must not be shaken vigorously to avoid destroying the protein molecules.
   3. **Administration.** Many biotechnology products require reconstitution with sterile water or normal saline and may be parenterally administered by direct IV injection or infusion, or by intramuscular or subcutaneous injection.

X. IRRIGATING SOLUTIONS.

Although these sterile products are manufactured by the same standards used to process IV preparations, they are **not intended for infusion into the venous system**. Labeling differences between irrigation solutions and injections are specified in the *United States Pharmacopeia* (*USP*) and reflect differences in acceptable particulate matter levels, volume of solution available for use, and the container design.

A. **Topical administration.** Irrigating solutions for topical use are packaged in pour bottles so that they can be poured directly onto the desired area. These solutions are intended for such purposes as irrigating wounds, moistening dressings, and cleaning surgical instruments.

B. **Infusion of irrigating solutions.** This procedure, using an administration set attached to a Foley catheter, is commonly used for many surgical patients. Surgeons performing urological procedures often use irrigating solutions to perfuse tissues in order to maintain the integrity of the surgical field, remove blood, and provide a clear field of view. To decrease the risk of infection, 1 mL of Neosporin G.U. Irrigant, an antibiotic preparation, often is added to these solutions.

C. **Dialysis.** Dialysates are irrigating solutions used in the dialysis of patients with such disorders as renal failure, poisoning, and electrolyte disturbances. These products remove waste materials, serum electrolytes, and toxic products from the body.

1. In **peritoneal dialysis**, a hypertonic dialysate is infused directly into the peritoneal cavity via a surgically implanted catheter. The dialysate, which contains dextrose and electrolytes, removes harmful substances by osmosis and diffusion. After a specified period, the solution is drained. Antibiotics and heparin may be added to the dialysate.
2. In **hemodialysis**, the patient's blood is transfused through a dialyzing membrane unit that removes the harmful substances from the patient's vascular system. After passing through the dialyzer, the blood reenters the body through a vein.

XI. NEEDLES AND SYRINGES

A. **Hypodermic needles** are stainless steel or aluminum devices that penetrate the skin for the purpose of administering or transferring a parenteral product (*Figure 17-14*).

1. **Needle gauge** is the outside diameter of the needle shaft; the larger the number, the smaller the diameter. Gauges in common use range from 13 (largest diameter) to 27. Subcutaneous injections usually require a 24-gauge or 25-gauge needle. Intramuscular injections require a needle with a gauge between 19 and 22. Needles between 18 gauge and 20 gauge are commonly used for compounding parenterals.
2. **Bevels** are slanting edges cut into needle tips to facilitate injection through tissue or rubber vial closures.
   a. **Regular-bevel needles** are the most commonly used type, and they are suitable for subcutaneous and intramuscular injections and hypodermoclysis.
   b. **Short-bevel needles** are used when only shallow penetration is required (as in IV injections).
   c. **Intradermal-bevel needles** are designed for intradermal injections and have the most beveled edges.
3. **Needle lengths** range from ¼ inch to 6 inches. Choice of needle length depends on the desired penetration.
   a. For **compounding parenteral preparations**, 1 ½-inch-long needles are commonly used.
   b. **Intradermal and subcutaneous injections** necessitate a short needle length, usually ¼ inch to ⅝ inch.
   c. **Intraspinal injection** requires a needle length of 3 ½ inches.
   d. **IV infusion** requires needles that range in length from 1 ¼ inches to 2 ½ inches.

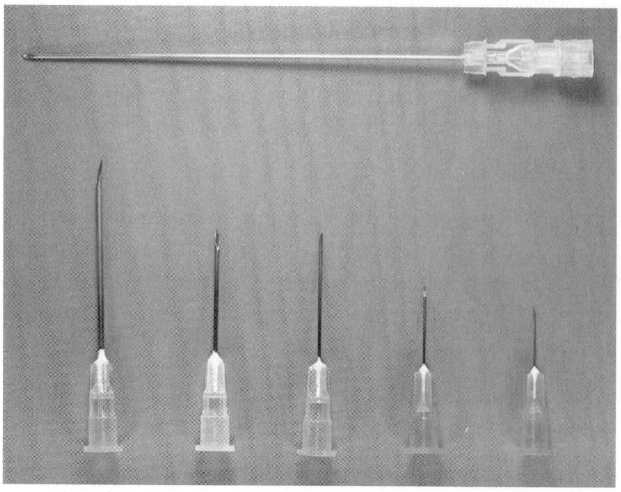

Figure 17-14. Hypodermic needles. *Top*: 20 gauge-3 ½ inch. *Left to right*: 18 gauge-1 ½ inch, 20 gauge-1 inch, 23 gauge-1 inch, 25 gauge- ⅝ inch, 27 gauge-½ inch. (Courtesy of Chistopher J. Belisle.)

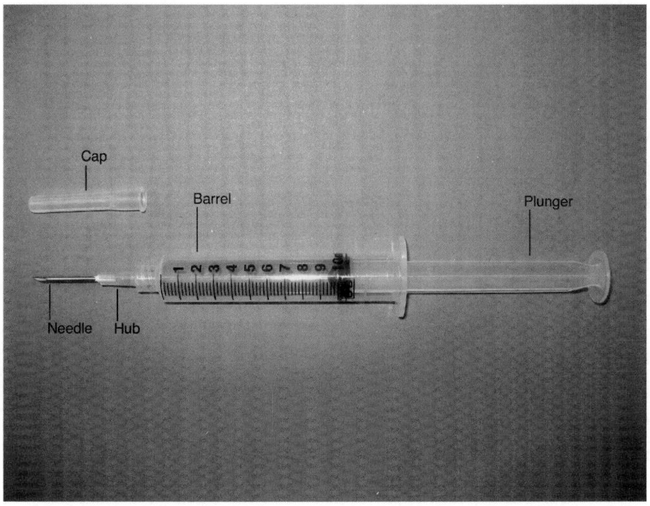

Figure 17-15. Luer-Lok syringe and needle. (Courtesy of Chistopher J. Belisle.)

B. **Syringes** are devices for injecting, withdrawing, or instilling fluids. Syringes consist of a glass or plastic barrel with a tight-fitting plunger at one end; a small opening at the other end accommodates the head of a needle (*Figure 17-15*, *Figure 17-16*).

1. The **Luer syringe**, the first syringe developed, has a universal needle attachment accommodating all needle sizes.
2. **Syringe volumes** range from 0.3 to 60 mL. Insulin syringes have unit gradations (100 units/mL) rather than volume gradations.
3. **Calibrations** are in the metric system, and vary in specificity depending on syringe size. The smaller the syringe, the smaller the measurement scale.
4. **Syringe tips** come in several types.
   a. **Luer-Lok tips** are threaded to ensure that the needle fits tightly in the syringe. Antineoplastic agents should be administered with syringes of this type.
   b. **Luer-Slip tips** are unthreaded so that the syringe and needle do not lock into place. Because of this, the needle may become dislodged.
   c. **Eccentric tips**, which are set off center, allow the needle to remain parallel to the injection site and minimize venous irritation.
   d. **Catheter tips** are used for wound irrigation and administration of enteral feedings. They are not intended for injections.

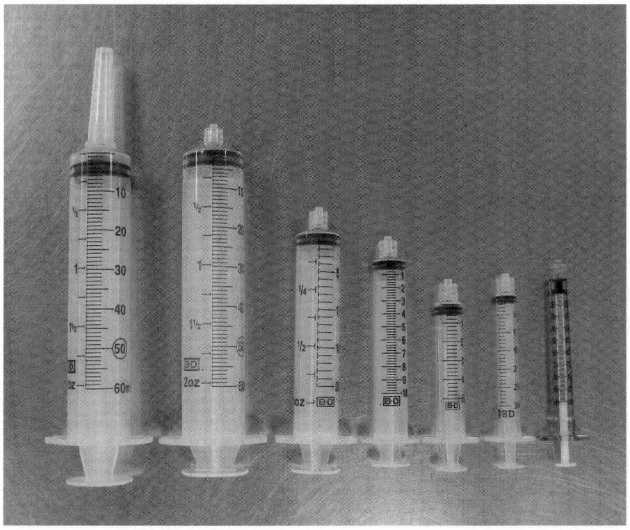

Figure 17-16. Syringes. *Left to right*: 60 mL catheter tip, 60 mL, 30 mL, 10 mL, 5 mL, 3 mL, 1 mL. (Courtesy of Chistopher J. Belisle.)

XII. INTRAVENOUS DRUG DELIVERY

A. **Injection sites**

1. **Peripheral vein injection** is preferred for drugs that do not irritate the veins, administration of isotonic solutions, and patients who require only short-term IV therapy. Generally, the dorsal forearm surface is chosen for venipuncture.
2. **Central vein injection** is preferred for administration of irritating drugs or hypertonic solutions, patients requiring long-term IV therapy, and situations in which a peripheral line cannot be maintained. Large veins in the thoracic cavity, such as the subclavian vein, are used.

B. **Infusion methods**

1. **Continuous-drip infusion** is the slow, primary-line infusion of an IV preparation to maintain a therapeutic drug level or provide fluid and electrolyte replacement.
   a. **Flow rates** must be carefully monitored. Generally, these rates are expressed as volume per unit of time (e.g., mL/hr, drops/min) and sometimes as mg/min for certain drugs.
   b. **Administration.** Drugs with a narrow therapeutic index such as oxytocin (Pitocin), heparin, and pressor agents such as norepinephrine (Levophed) and phenylephrine (Neo-Synephrine) typically are administered by this method.
2. **Intermittent infusion** allows drug administration at specific intervals (e.g., every 4 hrs) and is most often used for antibiotics.
   a. **Three different techniques** may be used.
      (1) **Direct (bolus) injection** rapidly delivers small volumes of an undiluted drug. This method is used to
         (a) Achieve an immediate effect (as in an emergency)
         (b) Administer drugs that cannot be diluted
         (c) Achieve a therapeutic serum drug level quickly
      (2) **Additive set infusion**, using a volume-control device, is appropriate for the intermittent delivery of small amounts of IV solutions or diluted medications. The fluid chamber is attached to an independent fluid supply or placed directly under the established primary IV line.
      (3) The **piggyback method** is used when a drug cannot be mixed with the primary solution. A special coupling for the primary IV tubing permits infusion of a supplementary secondary solution through the primary system. This method eliminates the need for a second venipuncture or further dilution of the supplementary preparation.
   b. In some cases, **intermittent infusion injection devices** are used. Also called scalp-vein, heparin-lock, or butterfly infusion sets, these devices permit intermittent delivery while eliminating the need for multiple venipunctures or prolonged venous access with a continuous infusion. To prevent clotting in the cannula, dilute heparin solution or NSS may be added. Benefits of intermittent infusion injection devices include the following:
      (1) This method is especially suitable for patients who do not require, or would be jeopardized by, administration of large amounts of IV fluids (e.g., those with congestive heart failure).
      (2) Because intermittent infusion injection devices do not require continuous attachment to an IV bottle or bag and pole, they permit greater patient ambulation.

C. **Pumps** and **controllers** are the electronic devices used to administer parenteral infusions when the use of gravity flow alone might lead to inaccurate dosing or risk patient safety. Pumps and controllers are used to administer parenteral nutrition, chemotherapy, cardiac medications, and blood products.

1. **Pumps** are used to deliver IV infusions with accuracy and safety.
   a. Two **types of mechanisms** are used in infusion pumps.
      (1) **Piston-cylinder mechanisms** use a piston in a cylinder or a syringe-like apparatus to pump the desired volume of fluid.
      (2) **Linear peristaltic mechanisms** use external pressure to expel the fluid out of the pumping chamber.
   b. **Types of pumps**
      (1) **Volumetric pumps** are used for intermittent infusion of medications such as antibiotics. They are also used for continuous infusion of IV fluid, parenteral nutrition, anticoagulants, and antiasthma medications.

(2) **Syringe pumps** are used to administer intermittent or continuous infusions of medications (e.g., antibiotics, opiates) in concentrated form.

(3) **Mobile infusion pumps** are small infusion devices designed for ambulatory and home patients and used for administering chemotherapy and opiate medications.

(4) **Implantable pumps** are infusion devices surgically placed under the skin to provide a continuous release of medication, typically an opiate. The reservoir in the pump is refilled by injecting the medication through a latex diaphragm in the pump.

(5) **Patient-controlled analgesic pumps** are used to administer narcotics intermittently or on demand by the patient within the patient-specific parameters, which are ordered by the physician and programmed into the pump.

(6) **Smart pumps** contain programmable "drug libraries" that reflect an institution's specific medication administration guidelines (*Figure 17-17*). These libraries can prevent an incorrect dose or administration rate entry into the pump.

c. **Benefits.** Despite their extra costs and the training required by personnel, smart pumps provide a number of important benefits. They maintain a constant, accurate flow rate and can detect infiltrations, occlusions, and air. Pumps also may decrease the amount of time a nurse spends dispensing medication. As a result, smart pumps are associated with decreased medication errors.

2. **Controllers**, unlike pumps, exert no pumping pressure on the IV fluid. Rather, they rely on gravity and control the infusion by counting drops electronically, or they infuse the fluid mechanically and electronically (e.g., volumetric controllers). In **comparison to pumps**, the following are characteristics of controllers:

a. They are less complex and generally less expensive.

b. They achieve reasonable accuracy.

c. They are very useful for uncomplicated infusion therapy but cannot be used for arterial drug infusion or for infusion into small veins.

D. **IV incompatibilities.** When two or more drugs must be administered through a single IV line or given in a single solution, an undesirable reaction can occur. Although such incompatibilities are relatively rare, their consequences can be deadly. A patient who receives a preparation in which an incompatibility has occurred could experience toxicity or an incomplete therapeutic effect.

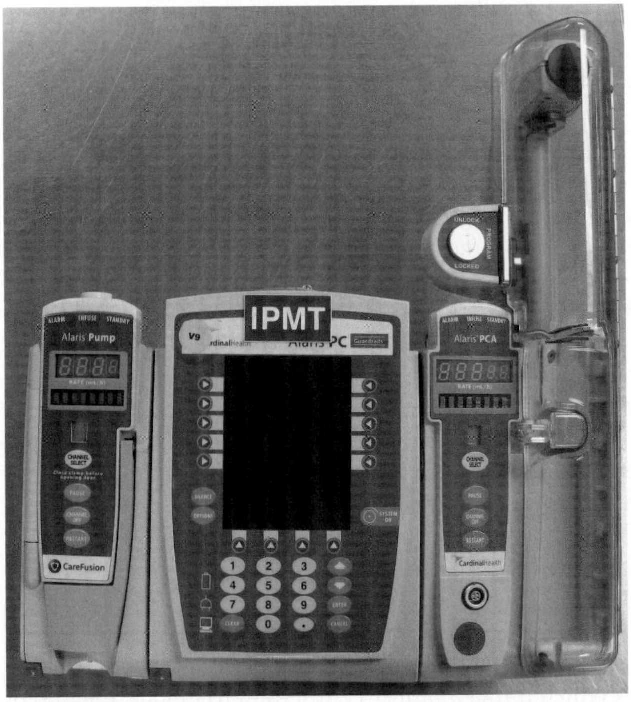

Figure 17-17. *Alaris* Smart Pump for controlled intravenous medication administration. (Courtesy of William Salkin.)

1. **Types of incompatibilities**
   a. A **physical incompatibility** occurs when a drug combination produces a visible change in the appearance of a solution. The solution should never be administered to a patient.
      (1) An **example** of physical incompatibility is the evolution of carbon dioxide when sodium bicarbonate and hydrochloric acid are admixed.
      (2) Various **types** of physical incompatibilities may occur
         (a) Visible color change or darkening
         (b) Formation of precipitate, which may result from the combination of phosphate and calcium.
   b. A **chemical incompatibility** reflects the chemical degradation of one or more of the admixed drugs, resulting in toxicity or therapeutic inactivity.
      (1) The degradation is not always visible. **Nonvisible chemical incompatibility** may be detected only by analytical methods.
      (2) Chemical incompatibility occurs in several **varieties.**
         (a) **Complexation** is a reaction between products that inactivates them. For example, the combination of calcium and tetracycline leads to formation of a complex that inactivates tetracycline.
         (b) **Oxidation** occurs when one drug loses electrons to the other, resulting in a color change and therapeutic inactivity.
         (c) **Reduction** takes place when one drug gains electrons from the other.
         (d) **Photolysis** (chemical decomposition caused by light) can lead to hydrolysis or oxidation, with resulting discoloration.
   c. A **therapeutic incompatibility** occurs when two or more drugs, IV fluids, or both are combined, and the result is a response other than that intended. An example of a therapeutic incompatibility is the reduced bactericidal activity of penicillin G when given after tetracycline. Because tetracycline is a bacteriostatic agent, it slows bacterial growth; penicillin, on the other hand, is most effective against rapidly proliferating bacteria.
2. **Factors affecting IV compatibility**
   a. **pH.** Incompatibility is more likely to occur when the components of an IV solution differ significantly in pH. This increased risk is explained by the chemical reaction between an acid and a base, which yields a salt and water; the salt may be an insoluble precipitate.
   b. **Temperature.** Generally, increased storage temperature speeds drug degradation. To preserve drug stability, drugs should be stored in a refrigerator or freezer, as appropriate.
   c. **Degree of dilution.** Generally, the more diluted the drugs are in a solution, the less chance there is for an ion interaction leading to incompatibility.
   d. **Length of time in solution.** The chance for a reaction resulting in incompatibility increases with the length of time that drugs are in contact with each other.
   e. **Order of mixing.** Drugs that are incompatible in combination, such as calcium and phosphate, should not be added consecutively when preparing an admixture of total parental nutrition (TPN). This keeps these substances from pooling, or forming a layer on the top of the IV fluid, and, therefore, decreases the chance of an incompatibility. Thorough mixing after each addition is also essential.
3. **Preventing or minimizing incompatibilities.** To reduce the chance for an incompatibility, the following steps should be taken:
   a. Each drug should be mixed thoroughly after it is added to the preparation.
   b. Solutions should be administered promptly after they are mixed to minimize the time available for a potential reaction to occur.
   c. The number of drugs mixed together in an IV solution should be kept to a minimum.
   d. If a prescription calls for unfamiliar drugs or IV fluids, compatibility references should be consulted.

E. **Hazards of parenteral drug therapy.** A wide range of problems can occur with parenteral drug administration.

1. **Physical hazards**
   a. **Phlebitis,** which is generally a minor complication, may result from vein injury or irritation. Phlebitis can be minimized or prevented through proper IV insertion technique, dilution of irritating drugs, and a decreased infusion rate.

b. **Thrombosis** is the formation of a blood clot in a vein or artery.
c. **Extravasation** may occur with administration of drugs with vesicant properties.
d. **Irritation** at the injection site can be reduced by varying the injection site and applying a moisturizing lotion to the area.
e. **Pain** from infusion is most common with peripheral IV administration of a highly concentrated preparation. Switching to central vein infusion and/or diluting the drug might alleviate the problem.
f. **Air embolism**, potentially fatal, can result from entry of air into the IV tubing.
g. **Infection**, a particular danger with central IV lines, may stem from contamination during IV line insertion or tubing changes. Infection may be local or generalized (septicemia). The infection risk can be minimized by following established protocols for the care of central lines.
h. **Allergic reactions** can result from hypersensitivity to an IV solution or additive.
i. **Central catheter misplacement** may lead to air embolism or pneumothorax. To ensure that the catheter has passed into the subclavian vein and advanced to the level of the vena cava, the placement should always be verified radiologically.
j. **Hypothermia**, possibly resulting in shock and cardiac arrest, might stem from administration of a cold IV solution. This problem can be prevented by allowing parenteral products to reach room temperature.
k. **Neurotoxicity** may be a serious complication of intrathecal or intraspinal administration of drugs containing preservatives. Preservative-free drugs should be used in these circumstances.

2. **Mechanical hazards**
   a. **Infusion pump** or **controller failure** can lead to runaway infusion, fluid overload, or incorrect dosages.
   b. **IV tubing** can become kinked, split, or cracked. It also may produce particulates, allow contamination, or interfere with the infusion.
   c. **Particulate matter** may be present in a parenteral product and can cause embolism.
   d. **Glass containers** may break, causing injury.
   e. **Rubber vial closures** may interact with the enclosed product.
3. **Therapeutic hazards**
   a. **Drug instability** may lead to therapeutic ineffectiveness.
   b. **Incompatibility** may result in toxicity or reduced therapeutic effectiveness.
   c. **Labeling errors** can cause administration of an incorrect drug or improper dosage.
   d. **Drug overdose** can be caused by runaway IV infusion, failure of an infusion pump or controller, or nursing or pharmacy errors.
   e. **Preservative and solubilizing agent toxicity** can be a serious complication, especially in children. For example, premature infants receiving parenteral products containing benzyl alcohol can develop a fatal acidotic toxic syndrome, which is referred to as the *gasping syndrome*. Rapid administration of phenytoin (Dilantin) and diazepam (Valium) both use propylene glycol as a solubilizing agent, which has been associated with cardiovascular collapse.

Study Questions

Directions: Each of the numbered items or incomplete statements in this section is followed by answers or by completions of the statement. Select the **one** lettered answer or completion that is **best** in each case.

1. Parenteral products with an osmotic pressure less than that of blood or 0.9% sodium chloride are referred to as

   (A) isotonic solutions.
   (B) hypertonic solutions.
   (C) hypotonic solutions.
   (D) iso-osmotic solutions.
   (E) neutral solutions.

2. Aseptic technique should be used in the preparation of all of the following medications with the exception of

   (A) neomycin irrigation solution.
   (B) ganciclovir (Cytovene) intraocular injection.
   (C) phytonadione (Aquamephyton) subcutaneous injection.
   (D) ampicillin (Principen) IV admixture piggyback.
   (E) bacitracin ointment.

3. Which needle has the smallest diameter?
   (A) 25 gauge, 3 ¾ inches
   (B) 24 gauge, 3 ½ inches
   (C) 22 gauge, 3 ½ inches
   (D) 20 gauge, 3 ⅜ inches
   (E) 26 gauge, 3 ⅝ inches

4. Intra-articular injection refers to injection into the
   (A) muscle mass.
   (B) subcutaneous tissue.
   (C) spinal fluid.
   (D) superficial skin layer.
   (E) joint space.

5. Advantages of the intravenous route include
   (A) ease of removal of the dose.
   (B) a depot effect.
   (C) low incidence of phlebitis.
   (D) rapid onset of action.
   (E) a localized effect.

6. A central vein, either subclavian or internal jugular, may be considered a suitable route for IV administration in which of the following situations?
   (A) When an irritating drug is given
   (B) When hypertonic drugs are given
   (C) For long-term therapy
   (D) For administering dextrose 35% as parenteral nutrition
   (E) All of the above

7. To prepare a total parenteral nutrition (TPN) that requires 10 mEq of calcium gluconate and 15 mM of potassium phosphate, the appropriate action to take would be which of the following?
   (A) Add the calcium first, add the other additives, then add the phosphate last, thoroughly mixing the solution after addition.
   (B) Add the calcium gluconate and potassium phosphate consecutively.
   (C) Do not combine the agents together but give them as a separate infusion.
   (D) None of the above.

8. Which needle gauge would be most likely used as a subcutaneous injection of epoetin?
   (A) 25 gauge, ⅝ inch
   (B) 16 gauge, 1 inch
   (C) 18 gauge, 1 ½ inches
   (D) 22 gauge, 1 ½ inches
   (E) None of the above

9. Which of the following compounded sterile products should NOT be prepared in a horizontal laminar flow hood?
   (A) Total parenteral nutrition (TPN)
   (B) Dopamine
   (C) Cisplatin (Platinol)
   (D) Nitroglycerin
   (E) Bretylium tosylate (Bretylol)

10. All of the following statements about D_5W are true EXCEPT
   (A) its pH range is 3.5 to 6.5.
   (B) it is hypertonic.
   (C) it is a 5% solution of D-glucose.
   (D) it should be used with caution in diabetic patients.
   (E) it is often used in IV admixtures.

11. All of the following are potential hazards of parenteral therapy EXCEPT
   (A) hypothermia.
   (B) phlebitis.
   (C) extravasation.
   (D) allergic reactions.
   (E) ileus.

12. Procedures for the safe handling of antineoplastic agents include all of the following EXCEPT
   (A) use of Luer-Lok syringe fittings.
   (B) wearing double-layered latex gloves.
   (C) use of negative-pressure technique when medication is being withdrawn from vials.
   (D) wearing closed-front, surgical-type gowns with cuffs.
   (E) use of horizontal laminar flow hood.

13. In preparing an intraspinal dose of bupivacaine, the best pore size filter for cold sterilization would be
   (A) 8-μm filter.
   (B) 5-μm filter.
   (C) 0.45-μm filter.
   (D) 0.22-μm filter.
   (E) None of the above.

14. Process simulation is a method of quality assurance that
   (A) evaluates the adequacy of a practitioner's aseptic technique.
   (B) requires the use of a microbial growth medium.
   (C) is carried out in a manner identical to normal sterile admixture production under routine operating conditions.
   (D) All of the above.

15. *USP* <797> was developed to
    (A) decrease microbial contamination of compounded sterile preparations.
    (B) ensure the proper use of aseptic technique during the manufacturing of sterile preparations.
    (C) prevent harm to patients, including death.
    (D) decrease unintended physical and chemical contaminates found in compounded sterile preparations.

16. When withdrawing drug solution from an ampoule, the one-way use of what kind of needle is required?
    (A) 5 micron filter needle
    (B) 25-gauge needle
    (C) 27-gauge needle
    (D) tuberculin needle

17. Proper use of sterile gloves includes which of the following:
    (A) Glove packaging should be discarded by touching only the sterile glove outerwrapper.
    (B) Sterile gloves should be donned after gowning, hand washing, and entering the ISO 5 direct compounding area.
    (C) Gloves can be placed on the hands by touching any sterile portion of the glove.
    (D) Gloves should be rinsed frequently with ethyl alcohol-based product, and changed when their integrity is compromised.

18. According to EPA regulations, the following form of pharmaceutical waste can be disposed of in a yellow container:
    (A) Nonregulated drugs
    (B) Hazardous toxic
    (C) Hazardous infectious
    (D) Trace chemotherapy

19. Low-risk compounded sterile products are prepared using the following:
    (A) Complex aseptic manipulations
    (B) Multiple pooled sterile commercial products
    (C) Sterile commercial drugs using commercial sterile devices
    (D) Nonsterile ingredients or with nonsterile devices

20. Proper preparation of the laminar airflow work bench
    (A) requires that all nonsterile supplies be removed from their outer packaging and wiped down with 70% isopropyl alcohol.
    (B) includes wiping down all surfaces by using side-to-side motions while working from the front of the work bench to the back.
    (C) does not include sterilizing the rubber stoppers of medication vials because they are sealed with a sterile safety cap.
    (D) allows the placement of larger supplies to be placed in the back of a horizontal airflow work bench.

Case Presentation

The pharmacist receives a prescription for hydromorphone (Dilaudid) injection to be compounded to a solution of 15 mg/mL. Dilaudid is commercially available in an ampoule, but the concentration is 10 mg per mL. The physician would like a more concentrated solution prepared so that 50 mL can be instilled into the titanium reservoir of a Medtronic infusion pump. The hydromorphone solution will be continuously infused, intrathecally, over approximately 30 days, for a patient with chronic back pain, uncontrolled with oral narcotics. The pharmacist checks his inventory and finds a bottle of hydromorphone powder, *USP*. He proceeds to weigh out enough powder for a 60 mL preparation. The weighing step is checked by a colleague pharmacist.

21. According to *USP* Chapter 797, this sterile preparation would be considered a
    (A) high-risk level CSP.
    (B) medium-risk level CSP.
    (C) low-risk level CSP.
    (D) None of these.

22. What would be an appropriate environment for the aseptic manipulations required for this preparation?
    (A) Pharmacy workbench or counter in ambient room air
    (B) Inside an anteroom, with ISO class 8 quality air
    (C) Inside a Barrier Isolator with ISO class 5 quality air
    (D) A horizontal laminar flow workbench, newly installed, with no certification, but manufacturer guaranteed to be ISO 5 class air quality.

23. The pharmacist begins to gather his supplies for this preparation. These should include:
    (A) Millipore 0.45 μm HV Filter with sterile water for injection.
    (B) Millipore 0.22 μm GS Filter with sodium chloride 0.9%.
    (C) Bectin-Dickinson 16-gauge, 5 micron filter needle with sodium chloride 0.9%.
    (D) Millipore AA 0.8 μm Filter with dextrose 5% in water.

24. After the solution was prepared, what would the appropriate quality assurance or double check by another pharmacist include?
    (A) Inspection of the powder and the label to ensure hydromorphone was the prepared ingredient and that the label contained a beyond use date and the 15 mg per mL concentration.
    (B) Sending a solution sample or aliquot to a microbiology lab to test for the presence of bacteria and pyrogens prior to dispensing.
    (C) Check to ensure a correct sterilizing filter was used.
    (D) Visual inspection to ensure the final aqueous solution had no visible participates.
    (E) All of the above.

Answers and Explanations

1. **The answer is C** *[see IX.B.1.b].*
Hypotonic solutions have an osmotic pressure less than that of blood (or 0.9% saline), whereas hypertonic solutions have an osmotic pressure greater than that of blood, and isotonic or iso-osmotic solutions have an osmotic pressure equal to that of blood.

2. **The answer is E** *[see II.A.4].*
Irrigation solutions, ophthalmic preparations and parenteral products, and subcutaneous and IV medications should be prepared using aseptic technique. Because bacitracin ointment is applied to the skin and does not bypass the body's protective barriers, its preparation would not be held to the same requirements.

3. **The answer is E** *[see XI.A.1].*
The gauge size refers to the outer diameter of the needle. The lower the gauge size number, the larger the needle.

4. **The answer is E** *[see VIII.I].*
Intra-articular injection refers to an injection into the joint space. This administration route generally is used for certain types of corticosteroids to reduce inflammation associated with injury or rheumatoid arthritis.

5. **The answer is D** *[see VIII.C].*
The IV route of drug administration allows for rapid onset of action and, therefore, immediate therapeutic effect. There can be no recall of the administered dose, and phlebitis or inflammation of a vein can occur. In addition, a depot effect (i.e., accumulation and storage of the drug for distribution) cannot be achieved by administering a drug intravenously. Delivering a drug intravenously results in a systemic rather than a localized effect.

6. **The answer is E** *[see XII.A.2].*
Irritating drugs, hypertonic drugs, long-term therapy, and dextrose 35% are best given by central IV administration. Peripheral vein injection is used for postoperative hydration, administration of nonirritating drugs, or isotonic solutions and for short-term IV therapy.

7. **The answer is A** *[see IX.E.4].*
Physical incompatibilities occur when two or more products are combined and produce a change in the appearance of the solution, such as the formation of a precipitate. Calcium and phosphate solutions when directly combined or added consecutively to a solution will form a white precipitate. By altering the order of mixing, they can be safely added to TPN solutions.

8. **The answer is A** *[see XI.A.1].*
Because subcutaneous injection does not require penetration through several skin layers or muscle tissue, a short needle with a narrow diameter is used. A 16- or 18-gauge needle is most commonly used in the pharmacy for preparing parenteral solutions. A 22-gauge needle would be used for intramuscular injection.

9. **The answer is C** *[III B 2 a].*
Cisplatin is an antineoplastic agent and, consequently, should be prepared only in a vertical laminar flow hood because of the potential hazard of these toxic agents to the operator.

10. **The answer is B** *[see IX.B.1.a].*
D_5W (dextrose [D-glucose] 5% in water) is acidic, its pH ranges from 3.5 to 6.5, and it is isotonic. It is often used in IV admixtures and should be used with caution in diabetic patients.

11. The answer is E *[see XII.E.1].*
Parenteral therapy is often a treatment for ileus. Hypothermia, phlebitis, extravasation, and allergic reactions can be hazards of parenteral therapy.

12. The answer is E *[see IX.D.2].*
In order to prevent drug exposure, a vertical flow laminar hood (not horizontal) should be used when an antineoplastic agent is prepared. The other precautions mentioned in the question are important safety measures for handling parenteral antineoplastics. All pharmacy and nursing personnel who handle these toxic substances should receive special training.

13. The answer is D *[see VI.D.2.c.ii].*
Because intraspinal and epidural doses of bupivacaine are frequently prepared from nonsterile powders, cold sterilization, accomplished by filtration, is a simple method of ensuring complete microbial removal. The filters listed 8 μm to 0.45 μm will remove only particulate matter. A 0.22-μm filter ensures the removal of microorganisms.

14. The answer is E *[see. V.F].*
Process simulation is one part of an overall quality assurance program. It requires duplicating sterile product preparation using a growth medium in place of actual products. It serves to evaluate the aseptic technique of the individual performing all the necessary steps of sterile product preparation.

15. The answer is C *[see I].*
Chapter <797> of the *USP* was developed to prevent harm to patients, including death. This is accomplished by following a rigorous set of guidelines, including the proper use of aseptic technique during the manufacturing of sterile preparations, and decreasing microbial and unintended physical and chemical contaminates found in compounded sterile preparations.

16. The answer is A *[see IV.J.2.a].*
Although when done properly, ampoule with opening resulting in a clean break with no glass shards, a single pass through a 5 micron filter needle or straw is still required to remove any unseen particulate matter that may be created.

17. The answer is D *[see IV.D].*
Proper use of sterile gloves includes rinsing frequently with a 62% w/w ethyl alcohol product and changing when integrity is compromised by coming in contact with nonsterile surfaces, or the glove is coughed or sneezed into.

18. The answer is D *[see IX.D.2.f.(3)].*
A color-coded system was created by the EPA to help facilities ensure safe and proper disposal of waste. Hazardous toxic, hazardous ignitable, and hazardous infectious waste should be disposed in a black container. Trace chemotherapy waste should be disposed of in a yellow container. Drain disposal waste can be flushed down the sink or sewer. Nonregulated pharmaceutical waste should be placed in a white with blue top or cream with purple top.

19. The answer is C *[see II.A.6.a.(1)].*
Low-risk CSPs are compounded from sterile commercial drugs using commercial sterile devices in an ISO class 5 located within an ISO 7 buffer area. Compounding procedures involve only transferring, measuring, and mixing manipulations using not more than three sterile products and not more than two entries into each sterile container.

20. The answer is A *[see IV.E].*
All nonsterile supplies, such as vials and infusions bags, should be removed from their outer packaging and wiped down with 70% isopropyl alcohol and lint-free cleaning cloths prior to being placed on the sterile workbench.

21. The answer is A.
The hydromorphone preparation is a high-risk level CSP because it is made from nonsterile powder.

22. The answer is C.
USP Chapter 797 requires an ISO class 5 air quality environment for this preparation. A Barrier Isolator within a clean room creates an ISO class 5 environment. Ambient room air is unacceptable for any preparation. An anteroom is generally an area of relatively high personnel and supply traffic. Although air quality may be acceptable, it does not provide an acceptable critical site of aseptic manipulations. All new laminar flow work benches should be tested for air velocity and filter integrity prior to use.

23. The answer is B.
The hydromorphone requires sterilization prior to intrathecal administration. This is best achieved with a 0.22 μm filter. Sodium chloride 0.9% is the solution most similar to the CNS fluid and would be a better choice over sterile water of dextrose 5% injection.

24. The answer is E.
Each step in sterile compounding should have an associated quality assurance double check. Inspection of the initial ingredients, review of supplies, monitoring of aseptic technique, and examination of the final product creates multiple opportunities to intercept an error and make necessary corrections. High-risk level CSPs should be used within 24 hrs in the absence of sterility testing. Given that this product will be administered over 30 days, a sterility and pyrogen test would be appropriate.

18 Parapharmaceuticals, Diagnostic Aids, and Medical Devices

JENNY A. VAN AMBURGH, TODD A. BROWN

I. AMBULATORY AIDS

A. **Canes.** These simple ambulatory aids provide balance and allow for the transfer of weight off a weakened leg.
   1. **Height.** A cane that is correctly fitted allows for maximum weight transfer without allowing the patient to lock the elbow. The correct height should provide a 25-degree angle at the elbow, or the top of the cane should come to the crease of the wrist while patient is standing erect.
   2. **Types of canes.** Canes may be made of wood or metal.
      a. **Wooden canes** come in various sizes and shapes and may be cut to the correct height for the patient.
      b. **Metal canes** are adjustable in height to fit the individual patient.
      c. **Folding canes** will fold to allow for easy transport or storage when not in use.
      d. A **quad cane** is a metal cane that has a quadrangular base with four legs. The base of the quad cane comes in two sizes. The larger base provides greater stability but is more difficult to manipulate because of the size and weight.
      e. **Seat canes** contain an area that can be folded down and used to sit on. They are useful for individuals who cannot walk long distances without resting.

B. **Crutches** may be used by patients with temporary disabilities (e.g., sprains, fractures) or by those with chronic conditions.
   1. **Use.** Crutches are used to take all the weight off an injured or weakened leg. The crutches are used in place of the leg. Crutches come in various sizes. Accessories that are used with a crutch include a tip to prevent slipping, handgrip cushion, and arm pad (for axillary crutch).
   2. **Types of crutches**
      a. An **axillary crutch**, the **most commonly used** crutch, is typically used for temporary disabilities. The top of the crutch should be 2 inches below the axilla to prevent nerve damage. The height of the handgrip should be set so that the elbow forms a 25-degree angle.
      b. A **forearm crutch** (also called a **Canadian** or **Lofstrand** crutch) remains in position by attaching to the forearm by a collar or cuff. It is commonly used by patients who need crutches on a long-term basis.
      c. A **quad crutch** is a forearm crutch with a quadrangular base that has four legs. The base is attached to the crutch with a flexible rubber mount. This allows for more stability and constant contact with the ground.
      d. A **platform crutch** contains a rectangular area in which to place the forearm. The crutch may be held by a handgrip or secured by a belt that wraps around the forearm. It is commonly used by patients who do not have enough hand strength and control for a forearm crutch.

C. **Seat lift chairs** are electric-powered chairs that raise the patient from a sitting to a standing position.

D. **Walkers** are lightweight rectangular-shaped devices that are made of metal tubing and have four widely placed legs.

1. **Use.** Walkers are used by patients who need more **support** than a cane or crutch or who have trouble with balance during ambulation. The user requires reasonably good arm, hand, and wrist function. The patient holds on to the walker and takes a step, then moves the walker and takes another step.
2. **Types of walkers.** Walkers are adjustable in height. Some walkers fold to make storage or transporting easier. Walkers can have wheels on the front legs to allow the user to move the walker by raising the back legs and rolling it instead of having to pick it up. Patients with loss of arm, wrist, or hand function on one side might use a **hemiwalker** or a **side walker**.
   a. A **hemiwalker** is similar to a standard walker except that it has one handle in the center of the walker for manipulation.
   b. A **side walker** is placed to the side of the patient instead of in front of the patient.
   c. A **reciprocal walker** contains two hinges, one on each side of the walker. This allows the user to swing each side alternately during ambulation.
   d. A **rollator** is a walker with wheels on all four legs. The movement is controlled by hand brakes.

E. **Wheelchairs.** Many different types of wheelchairs are available. The patient's disabilities, size, weight, and activities are the main considerations in wheelchair selection. The following options should be considered when selecting a wheelchair.

1. **Seat size.** The standard chair is 18 inches wide and 16 inches deep. A narrow wheelchair is 16 inches wide. Wheelchairs are available in widths up to 48 inches. The chair should be 2 inches wider than the widest part of the patient's body (usually around the buttocks or thighs). **Seat upholstery** holds the patient in the chair. Seats come in various materials to accommodate patients' needs. **Back upholstery** supports the patient's back while he or she is sitting in the chair.
2. **Weight.** Standard wheelchairs weigh 35 to 50 lb. Lightweight wheelchairs (25 to 35 lb) are available for those who are unable to manipulate a standard chair and for ease of transport.
3. **Arms** can be fixed or detachable to allow transfer on and off the chair. Half-length arms (as opposed to full length) allow the user to get closer to a table or work surface. Various types of padding and adjustments in the arm position can assist the patient in obtaining a position that is comfortable and keeping the arms on the arm rests.
4. **Tires** can be hard rubber or pneumatic (i.e., air filled) which allows the chair to transverse rougher surfaces. **Wheels** can be reinforced with spokes or can be composite based.
5. **Leg rests** can be of different sizes and are available with padding. Some have adjustable elevation to aid in healing an acute injury. **Calf rests** can be of different sizes and are available with padding. **Foot rests** can be of different sizes and are available with or without heel loops to keep the foot on the foot rest.

F. **Sports chairs** are wheelchairs that are lightweight and durable. They are designed for people who are very active.

G. **Powered wheelchairs** are designed for people who cannot wheel themselves. This type of wheelchair is powered by an electric motor and battery.

II. BATHROOM EQUIPMENT.

This equipment is used for patients who cannot get to the bathroom or for patients who need assistance using the toilet or bathtub.

A. **Elevated toilet seats** are used to increase the height at which the patient sits over the toilet. This assists patients in getting on and off the toilet. Additional support can be provided with **toilet safety rails**. These rails allow the patient to transfer weight from the feet to the hands, and they help prevent the patient from falling.

B. **Commodes** are portable toilets that are used by patients who cannot get to the bathroom. Commodes contain a frame (with or without a back rest), a seat, and a bucket. Some are adjustable in height and have arms that drop to facilitate transfer to and from the commode.

C. **Three-in-one commodes** function as a commode, elevated toilet seat, and toilet safety rails. These are beneficial for patients requiring varying assistance during recuperation.

D. **Bath benches** are seats with or without a back that fit in the bathtub and allow the patient to sit while taking a shower.

E. **Transfer benches** are placed over the outside of the bathtub. They are available with or without a back. A transfer bench assists the patient in getting into the bathtub and serves as a bath bench while the patient takes a shower.

F. **Grab bars** are bars that either attach to the wall around the bathtub or to the bathtub itself to assist patients in getting in and out of the bathtub.

III. BLOOD PRESSURE MONITORS.

Patients with hypertension use this equipment to monitor blood pressure so that appropriate therapeutic decisions can be made. A patient's blood pressure measured at home is typically 5 mm Hg lower than when measured at the office.[1] The type of monitor that is recommended should be determined by the patient's ability to use the product correctly. Items to consider when assisting a patient in the selection of a blood pressure monitor include ease of use (e.g., automatic inflation), use of the monitor with one hand (has D-ring cuff), the size of the display monitor (visually impaired patients), blood pressure cuff size, and the capability to store readings. Types of monitors include the following:

A. **Aneroid sphygmomanometer.** This type of monitor is the **accurate** and requires regular calibration. These types of monitors are portable, lightweight, and most require manual inflation of the cuff, but a separate stethoscope is not required.

B. **Electronic or digital monitor.** This type of monitor detects blood pressure by using a microphone or by oscillometric technology, which converts movement of vessels into blood pressure. This type is easier to use than an aneroid or mercury sphygmomanometer as most offer automatic inflation and deflation and there is not a need for a separate stethoscope. These models are more **expensive**, can provide inaccurate readings if the patient moves while the blood pressure is being performed, and requires frequent calibration against a provider's in-office sphygmomanometer; but they represent an alternative for patients who cannot use a sphygmomanometer. Some of these monitors come with a wrist cuff, which may be useful in overweight or obese patients for whom the regular size arm blood pressure cuff is too small. Patients with very large or very small upper arms may need to purchase a special cuff in order to obtain an accurate reading.

C. **Finger monitors.** These detect blood pressure by compressing the finger and converting blood vessel movement into blood pressure by oscillometric technology. Many environmental conditions and medications can interfere with the results of these monitors. Finger blood pressure monitors are **least accurate** and not recommended for home monitoring.

IV. HEAT AND COLD THERAPY.

For musculoskeletal disorders (e.g., sprains, strains, arthritis), treatment may include the application of heat or cold to specific areas of the body.

A. **Heat** can be applied in a dry or moist form. **Dry** heat is less effective than moist heat but is tolerated better; thus its clinical effectiveness is similar. **Moist** heat has an advantage of not causing as much perspiration and is often recommended. The application of heat produces vasodilation and muscle relaxation. Products that can deliver heat include the following:

1. A **hot water bottle**, a rubber container that is half filled with hot water. The remaining air is squeezed out of the container resulting in a flexible container that can be shaped to the area of the body for which it is being used to provide dry heat.
2. A **heating pad** is an electrically powered pad that can produce moist or dry heat. Moist heat is supplied by inserting a wet sponge in a pocket that is next to the pad. Patients should place the pad on top of the body instead of lying on the pad to prevent burning.
3. A **moist-heat pack** (also called a hydrocollator) contains silica beads, which absorb heat when placed in boiling water. The heated pack is wrapped in a towel and applied to the body to provide moist heat. A moist-heat pack must be kept moist to retain its absorbent properties. The pack should be wrapped in plastic and stored in the refrigerator or freezer.
4. A **gel pack** provides dry heat after it is heated in boiling water or in the microwave. It is reusable by repeating the heating process.

---

[1]National Heart, Lung, and Blood Institute. The seventh report of the Joint National Committee on prevention, detection, evaluation, and treatment of high blood pressure. August 2004. Available at http://www.nhlbi.nih.gov/guidelines/hypertension/jnc7full.htm.

5. **Chemical hot packs** provide dry heat by mixing chemicals from two compartments. The chemicals undergo an exothermic reaction. Some packs are reusable by reheating in boiling water or in the microwave.
6. **Paraffin baths** provide moist heat by covering the body with heated paraffin. Once the wax cools and hardens, it is removed. This method is commonly used for patients with arthritis in the hands and fingers.

B. **Cold** application is indicated mainly as acute therapy to decrease circulation to a local area and to provide pain relief. Cold is contraindicated in patients with circulatory stasis or lacerated tissue. Products that can deliver cold include the following:
1. An **ice bag** is a flexible plastic container designed to hold ice. The bag is then applied to the body.
2. A **gel pack** can be used to apply cold by freezing and then applying to the body.
3. **Chemical packs** can be used to apply cold. Chemicals from two compartments are mixed together, resulting in a chemical reaction that produces cold. These packs are used once and then disposed of.

V. DIAGNOSTIC AIDS

A. **Self-care tests** or **kits** are used as screening tests or for monitoring. Many factors can affect the accuracy of the tests. The most common factors are patients not following directions and patients having poor technique. Pharmacists should be prepared to counsel patients on the selection of a test, on the proper use, and on interpretation of results. Pharmacists should refer patients to the appropriate health care provider if necessary.

B. **Types of tests**
1. **Urine tests**
a. The **urine glucose test** detects sugar in the urine. Patients with diabetes can use this to evaluate glucose control. Blood glucose monitoring is preferred, however, because it is more accurate and gives a better description of current glycemia.
b. The **ketone test** detects the presence of ketones in the urine. This is used by patients with diabetes as an indicator of severely uncontrolled diabetes.
c. The **microalbuminuria test** detects the presence of protein in the urine (microalbuminuria). This test can be used annually by patients with diabetes to detect an early sign of kidney damage. The simple test is performed at home and mailed to the company for a professional evaluation. If the test is positive, the patient is recommended to follow up with his or her health care provider.
d. **Ovulation prediction tests** predict when ovulation occurs to increase the chance of conception. These tests detect the presence of **luteinizing hormone (LH)** in the urine. Its presence means that ovulation should occur within 20 to 48 hrs. The test is performed daily until a positive result is obtained. It is recommended to test at the same time each day between 10 A.M. and 8 P.M. and not to use the first morning urine as the LH surge typically starts in the morning. The day on which the patient begins testing depends on the length and regularity of her menstrual cycle. Patients with menstrual cycles of consistent length may need to test only for 4 days, whereas those with menstrual cycles that change in length may need to test for 8 or 9 days. False-positive results can occur if the patient is taking fertility medications (e.g., clomiphene), oral contraceptives, or hormone-replacement therapy or if the patient has polycystic ovary syndrome or impaired liver or kidney function.
e. **Pregnancy tests** detect pregnancy by the presence in the urine of **human chorionic gonadotropin (hCG)**, which is secreted after fertilization. Many pregnancy test kits can detect hCG 1 day after missed menses. False-positive results can occur if the patient takes the test too early, is taking fertility medications (e.g., hCG), or has ovarian cysts. If a patient uses a household container or a waxed cup to collect urine, it may affect the test results. Patients should be referred to the appropriate health care provider if they receive a positive result or two negative results 7 days apart and have not had menses.
f. The **urinary bacteria test** detects the presence of leukocytes and/or nitrite in the urine. The presence of nitrite is used as an indicator of a **urinary tract infection (UTI)** because the most common bacteria associated with UTIs are gram-negative bacteria, which convert nitrate to nitrite. This test is used by patients who have recurrent or chronic UTIs or many risk factors. Risk factors include previous UTIs, diabetes, urinary tract abnormalities, enlarged

prostate, and behavioral risk factors (e.g., frequent sexual activity, delayed urination, the use of spermicides or diaphragms). Because this test is not specific for bacteria, false results can occur. False positives can result from medications (e.g., phenazopyridine) the patient may be taking or from menstrual blood in the urine, depending on the test used. In addition, a false negative may be detected if the patient is taking high doses of vitamin C, adheres to a strict vegetarian diet, or has frequent urination.

g. There are various FDA-approved **urine drug tests** available for use at home. Substances that may be detected in the urine include amphetamine, methamphetamine, ecstasy, marijuana, cocaine, phencyclidine, opiates, benzodiazepine, barbiturates, methadone, tricyclic antidepressants, and oxycodone. Most urine drug tests require two steps: screening (at home—collection of urine and reviewing the results as color bands on the device) and confirmation (sending the urine sample that was collected for the home test to the drug test manufacturer's contracted laboratory; results are available in 7 to 10 business days).

2. **Blood tests**
   a. The **cholesterol test** determines a patient's total cholesterol (TC), low-density lipoprotein (LDL), high-density lipoprotein (HDL), and/or triglycerides (TGs). Some tests provide only a TC level, whereas others provide a full lipid profile (TC, LDL, HDL, and/or TGs). Some kits are a single-use test requiring the patient to apply a blood sample on a collecting card, which is mailed to a laboratory for evaluation; others can be performed and evaluated by the patient at home. Regardless of the test used, the patient places a large drop of blood on the test card or cassette. Some of the tests require the patient to fast—meaning nothing to eat or drink except water for 12 to 14 hrs before collecting the blood. These tests can be useful as screening test as well as for patients who want to monitor their therapy. Patients who tested borderline or higher for high cholesterol should be referred to the appropriate health care provider.
   b. The **blood glucose test** measures the concentration of glucose in the blood. Patients with diabetes use this information, along with diet, exercise, and medication, to keep glucose levels within a target range. Other tests are designed to be used with **blood glucose meters**, which read the test and display the actual blood glucose value. Whole blood is approximately 15% lower than plasma glucose, which is what is measured in the standard laboratory tests. Most glucometers available provide results as the "plasma equivalent," meaning they test whole blood but use an internal algorithm to calculate the plasma glucose. Patients using blood glucose tests must perform the tests properly and understand the appropriate actions to take when the resulting values are outside the desired range.
   c. Other **home blood test kits** are available that provide results at the time of testing in the home or the collected specimen is sent to a laboratory for results. These home testing kits include HIV, hepatitis C virus (HCV), glycosylated hemoglobin A1c (A1c), anemia, prostate specific antigen (PSA), and thyroid. If the specimen is mailed away for processing, the results can be obtained by calling a toll-free number.
   d. There are various **point-of-care testing (POCT)** devices that are available for use in pharmacies. Because most of them meet the Clinical Laboratory Improvements Amendments (CLIA)-waived requirements, pharmacies are able to offer these services to their patients. When selecting a POCT device for use, make sure to research the device specifications, portability, testing procedure, and cost. Examples of point-of-care tests available in selected pharmacies include electronic peak flow meters, portable spirometry, HIV rapid test, rapid *Strep* testing, coagulation analyzers, osteoporosis screening with quantitative ultrasound or peripheral dual-energy absorptiometry, and blood tests that measure A1c, fructosamine, ketones, microalbuminuria, alanine aminotransferases, and lipid profiles.
3. **Fecal occult blood tests** detect the presence of blood in the stool as a screening test for colorectal cancer. Patients drop a pad into the toilet after defecation. The pad will change color if blood is present. Patients should eat high-fiber foods during the testing period and are instructed to test three consecutive stool samples. Patients with a positive result should be referred to the appropriate health care provider. Certain conditions (gastrointestinal bleed, nosebleed, menstruation), foods (red meat), medications (nonsteroidal anti-inflammatory drugs [NSAIDs]), and toilet-bowl cleaners can produce false-positive results.

Study Questions

Directions: Each of the numbered items or incomplete statements in this section is followed by answers or by completions of the statement. Select the **one** lettered answer or completion that is **best** in each case.

1. When a patient is fitted with an axillary crutch, how far below the underarm should the top of the crutch rest?

(A) 0.5 inch
(B) 1 inch
(C) 2 inches
(D) 3 inches
(E) 4 inches

2. What angle should the elbow form when a cane is the correct height?

(A) 10 degree
(B) 25 degree
(C) 45 degree
(D) 60 degree
(E) 90 degree

3. A product that delivers moisture to the air by heating water to produce steam is called a

(A) nebulizer.
(B) humidifier.
(C) ventilator.
(D) peak flow meter.
(E) vaporizer.

4. An absorbent product designed for patients with light incontinence problems is a

(A) brief.
(B) shield.
(C) undergarment.
(D) underpad.
(E) catheter.

5. When an oral temperature is taken, the thermometer should be placed into the mouth for

(A) 1 to 2 mins.
(B) 3 to 4 mins.
(C) 5 to 6 mins.
(D) 7 to 8 mins.
(E) > 9 mins.

6. The diameter of urinary catheters is measured by which of the following scales?

(A) Leur
(B) English
(C) French
(D) gauge
(E) metric

7. A cervical collar that immobilizes the neck is called a

(A) soft cervical collar.
(B) hard cervical collar.
(C) foam cervical collar.
(D) extrication collar.
(E) rigid cervical collar.

8. Incontinence that is caused by an obstruction of the bladder is called

(A) overflow incontinence.
(B) urge incontinence.
(C) stress incontinence.
(D) functional incontinence.
(E) transient incontinence.

9. A colostomy or ileostomy could be performed for all of the following conditions *except*

(A) lower bowel obstruction.
(B) malignancy of the colon or rectum.
(C) ulcerative colitis.
(D) duodenal ulcer.
(E) Crohn disease.

10. Pregnancy test kits are designed to detect which substance?

(A) luteinizing hormone (LH)
(B) progesterone
(C) human chorionic gonadotropin (hCG)
(D) estrogen
(E) follicle-stimulating hormone

Answers and Explanations

1. **The answer is C** *[see I.B.2.a]*.
When a patient is fitted for an axillary crutch, the top of the crutch should be 2 inches below the axilla (underarm).

2. **The answer is B** *[see I.A.1]*.
When a patient is properly fitted for a cane, the elbow should form a 25-degree angle. This allows for maximum weight transfer.

3. **The answer is E** *[see X.B]*.
A vaporizer produces moisture by heating water to produce steam. A humidifier also produces moisture; however, it works by mechanically creating small water particles. A nebulizer is used to deliver liquid to the mouth and throat. A ventilator is used to assist in breathing. A peak flow meter is used to detect airway constriction.

4. **The answer is B** *[see VII.B.1]*.
Shields are pads that are placed in the underwear and held with adhesive strips. They are used for patients with light incontinence problems.

5. **The answer is B** *[see XI.A.1]*.
Oral temperature is taken by inserting the bulb of the thermometer under the tongue and sealing the lips around the thermometer for 3 to 4 mins.

6. **The answer is C** *[see XII.B]*.
The French scale is used to measure the diameter of a urinary catheter. The Leur scale is used to measure syringe tip size. The gauge scale is used to measure needle diameter. The metric scale is a general system of measurement.

7. **The answer is D** *[see VIII.D.3]*.
An extrication collar (also known as a Philadelphia collar) is used to immobilize the neck. It is commonly used in emergency situations. Soft or foam cervical collars provide mild support and remind the patient to keep the neck straight. Hard or rigid cervical collars provide moderate support but allow some movement.

8. **The answer is A** *[see VII.A.3]*.
Overflow incontinence is caused by obstruction of the bladder. Urge incontinence is caused by uncontrolled bladder contractions. Stress incontinence is caused by increases in intra-abdominal pressure. Functional incontinence is related to physical or psychological problems. Transient incontinence is caused by medications, urinary tract infections, or mental impairments.

9. **The answer is D** *[see IX.A.1–2]*.
Lower bowel obstruction, malignancy of the colon or rectum, and diverticulitis may all require a colostomy. Ulcerative colitis and Crohn disease may require an ileostomy. The treatment of a duodenal ulcer would not include a colostomy or an ileostomy.

10. **The answer is C** *[see V.B.1.d]*.
Pregnancy tests detect hCG in the urine. This is secreted after the embryo has implanted in the uterus. Ovulation-prediction tests detect LH. Progesterone, estrogen, and follicle-stimulating hormone are all involved in controlling the menstrual cycle.

19

Over-the-Counter Otic, Dental, and Ophthalmic Agents

JENNIFER D. SMITH, CONNIE LEE BARNES

I. OTIC OVER-THE-COUNTER (OTC) PRODUCTS

A. The ear can be divided into three distinct parts: the external ear, the middle ear, and the inner ear.
   1. The external ear is typically thought of as the part of the ear one can see. However, being made up of the auricle, the external auditory canal (the ear canal), and the outer surface of the tympanic membrane (the ear drum), the external ear extends much farther.
   2. The **middle ear** is an air-filled chamber that provides direct access to the inner ear and indirect access to the nose and throat by way of the eustachian tube. The middle ear houses three small bones (malleus, incus, and stapes) known as the ossicles. When sound strikes the eardrum, it vibrates, transmitting the sound vibrations to the ossicles, which in turn transmit the sound to the inner ear.
   3. The **inner ear** is a delicate structure composed of auditory and vestibular components. The auditory component (the cochlea) is responsible for hearing. The vestibular component (the semicircular canals and the vestibule) is responsible for maintaining balance and equilibrium.

B. **Common ear disorders**
   1. **Excessive/impacted cerumen** (earwax). Contrary to current social beliefs, earwax does not need to be removed with objects such as fingers, towels, and cotton-tipped applicators because these objects typically cause impaction of the earwax, rather than its removal. Instead, the external ear has a unique self-cleansing mechanism. Ear canal skin is constantly shed and removed via lateral migration from the tympanic membrane (at a rate of 2 to 3 mm per day) to the external canal, where cerumen adheres to the shed skin and other debris. Movement such as chewing moves the cerumen outward where it is removed by drying, flaking, or simply falling out. The use of hearing aids or earplugs can block this outward migration, developing earwax impaction and leading to hearing loss.
      a. The **functions** of cerumen include the following:
         (1) Lubrication of the lining of the ear canal
         (2) Temporarily repelling water
         (3) Resistance to infection owing to its acidic nature (pH = 4–5), which creates an unfavorable environment for organism survival
         (4) Trapping dust, debris, and foreign objects
      b. **Epidemiology.** Aside from impaction caused by manipulation, some patient populations are more prone to experience impacted cerumen, including patients with an overproduction of cerumen, patients with narrowed ear canals, the elderly, and patients with mental retardation.
      c. **Symptoms** of impacted cerumen include earache, itching of the ear, reflex cough, dizziness, vertigo, tinnitus, and compromised hearing.
      d. **Earwax-softening agents** may be used alone or followed by the use of an otic syringe (see I.C).
         (1) **Carbamide peroxide** 6.5% in anhydrous glycerin is the **only U.S. Food and Drug Administration (FDA) approved agent for cerumen removal**. When carbamide peroxide

makes contact with tissue enzymes, oxygen is released, producing a foaming action. This **foaming action softens impacted cerumen.**

(a) **Available agents.** Murine, Debrox, Mack's

(b) **Instructions for use.** Patients **aged 12 and older** should tilt the head sideways and instill 5 to 10 drops into the ear. The applicator tip should not be inserted into the ear canal. Patients should keep the head tilted to the side (or insert cotton) for several minutes to increase contact time with the cerumen. Repeat the process **twice daily for up to 4 days**. For children < 12 with suspected cerumen impaction, a medical provider should be consulted.

(2) Olive oil (sweet oil) is used to soften earwax and alleviate itching.

(3) Mineral oil, recommended as 2 drops in the affected ear(s) once per week, has been used to liquefy the cerumen, thus aiding in its removal.

(4) Docusate sodium given 15 mins before provider in-office irrigation has shown efficacy, but no data exist to support the superiority of docusate sodium over carbamide peroxide.

(5) Hydrogen peroxide is a component of carbamide peroxide and has weak antibacterial properties. As an otic solution, hydrogen peroxide may be diluted 1:1 with warm water and instilled in the ear to aid in cerumen softening and removal.

(6) Ear candles (coning candles), are made of paraffin-coated fabric wound into a foot-long cone that are inserted into the ear canal and lit with a match. However, no data support this dangerous process for efficacy. Furthermore, complications may include external otitis, temporary hearing loss, and burns.

e. Patients with perforated tympanic membrane, ear drainage, ear pain, or a rash in the ear should be referred to a health care provider. In the office, providers may use various devices or irrigating systems to remove impacted cerumen.

2. **Vertigo** is a loss of equilibrium in which one might describe a room as spinning. As described in I.A.3, the vestibular compartment of the inner ear is responsible for maintaining balance and equilibrium. The autonomic system may become involved if the vertigo is severe, producing dizziness, pallor, sweating, and nausea. Patients expressing symptoms of vertigo (aside from motion sickness) should be referred to a medical provider.

3. **Tinnitus** may be described by patients as a ringing, buzzing, hissing, whistling, or humming noise lasting from seconds to minutes. Tinnitus has been linked to a variety of causes, including Ménière disease, head injuries, otitis media, syphilis, temporomandibular-joint (TMJ) dysfunction, and certain medications (salicylates, nonsteroidal anti-inflammatory drugs, aminoglycosides, loop diuretics, and chemotherapeutic agents). If tinnitus is constant or severe, a medical consult is advised. Currently, there are no FDA-approved treatments for tinnitus.

4. **External otitis**, also referred to as otitis externa, is **inflammation of the external auditory canal** secondary to a bacterial or fungal infection.

a. **Cause.** External otitis, frequently referred to as swimmer's ear, is thought to be most commonly the result of **local trauma** to the external canal (e.g., cotton-tipped applicators, fingers, sharp objects) or **prolonged exposure to moisture**. Prolonged exposure to moisture (e.g., humid environment, underwater swimming, diving) promotes maceration of the thin skin lining the ear canal, allowing bacteria to penetrate and grow. Trauma to the external canal lends itself to susceptibility to damage and thus easier infiltration of microorganisms. The predominant microorganisms isolated from patients with swimmer's ear are *Pseudomonas aeruginosa* and *Staphylococcus aureus.*

b. **Symptoms.** Initial symptoms include **itching** and a sensation of **pressure/fullness in the ear**, followed by **pain**, an **otic discharge**, and a possible **decrease in hearing**. The pain may become quite intense, especially if the outer ear is touched or with movement of the jaw, such as chewing.

c. **Treatment** is with a **prescription otic antibiotic** and **corticosteroid** if bacterial in origin and otic antibiotic alone if fungal in origin, as well as discontinuation of mechanical trauma and/or swimming (until resolution of infection). Oral antibiotics are not necessary unless the infection is unresponsive to otic treatment, the patient is immunocompromised, or a middle ear infection coexists. **External otitis should not be self-treated.**

d. Prevention of external otitis is the key. Mechanical trauma to the ear by way of cotton-tipped applicators and fingers should cease immediately. Water should be removed as gently and effectively as possible after swimming or showering/bathing using a towel around the edges of the ear or a hair dryer set on low heat. It may also be beneficial to tilt the head to the side to help expel water. If reoccurrence is frequent, one might consider using molded ear plugs, but consideration should be given to the risk of impacted cerumen with the use of such devices.

5. **Water-clogged ear** may be a contributing factor to external otitis owing to tissue maceration from prolonged periods of exposure to water; however, water-clogged ear is a separate disorder. Therefore, labeling of products approved by the FDA for the treatment of water-clogged ear may not allude to its use for prevention of external otitis. The only agent FDA approved as safe and effective as an ear-drying agent is isopropyl alcohol 95% in anhydrous glycerin 5%, approved for use in **patients 12 years of age and older**. A home solution of 50/50 isopropyl alcohol and white vinegar may also be used to dry the ear. Caution must be taken not to recommend self-treatment for water-clogged ear for patients with signs of infection, discharge or bleeding from the ear, ear surgery within the previous 6 weeks, or tympanostomy tubes.
6. **Furuncles**, also known as boils, are small abscesses surrounding the base of a hair follicle in the outer portion of the external ear canal. *Staphylococcus aureus* is typically the offending organism. Furuncles are usually self-limiting and may be managed with warm compresses and a topical antibiotic.
7. **Otitis media** is a bacterial infection that is most prevalent between the ages of 3 months and 3 years, owing to the length, angle, and function of the eustachian tube in children. Symptoms include ear pain, fever, fluid discharge from the ear, and possible decreased hearing. All patients with suspected otitis media must be referred to a medical provider for evaluation and treatment.

C. **Administration of otic agents**

1. Instructions for use of otic drops
   - a. Warm the solution by holding the bottle in the hand for a few moments.
   - b. Tilt the head sideways with the affected ear upward.
   - c. Pull the earlobe up and back to straighten the canal for adults and down and back to straighten in children.
   - d. Use the other hand to squeeze the bottle of drops, carefully delivering the number of recommended drops into the ear canal. Caution should be taken not to insert the applicator into the ear canal.
   - e. Keep the head tilted sideways for several minutes or place cotton in the ear to prevent the medication from draining out. If cotton is used, it must be large enough, so as not to become lodged in the ear, and should not be left in the ear for longer than 1 hr.
   - f. Repeat the procedure on the opposite ear, if necessary.
2. **Instructions for use of an otic syringe**
   - a. Prepare a *warm* solution of plain water. Fill the otic syringe with the warm water solution.
   - b. Straighten the ear canal using the appropriate method, as noted earlier. Tilt the head over a sink or basin to catch the outflow solution.
   - c. Insert the tip of the otic syringe into ear, with the tip pointed slightly upward.
   - d. Gently squeeze the bulb of the otic syringe to allow the solution to enter the ear. Allow the solution to drain from the ear into the sink or basin. If pain or dizziness occurs, remove the syringe and consult a medical provider.
   - e. Repeat on opposite ear if necessary.

II. DENTAL OVER-THE-COUNTER PRODUCTS

A. **Dental anatomy.** Anatomically, the teeth are divided into two parts: the **crown** (above the gingival line) and the root (below the gingival line).

1. **Enamel** is the crystalline calcium salts (hydroxyapatite) that cover the crown to protect the underlying tooth structure.
2. **Dentin** is the largest part of the tooth structure, located beneath the enamel. It protects the dental pulp.
3. **Cementum** is a bonelike structure that covers the root and provides the attachment of the tooth with the periodontal ligaments.
4. **Pulp** consists of free nerve endings.

B. **Common dental problems and OTC products**

1. **Dental caries** (i.e., **cavities**) are formed by the growth and implantation of cariogenic microorganisms.

   a. **Causes**

   (1) **Bacteria** (primarily *Streptococcus mutans* and *Lactobacillaceae*) produce acids (e.g., lactic acid) that demineralize enamel. Initially, demineralized enamel appears as a white, chalky area and becomes bluish white and eventually brown or yellow.

   (2) **Diet** is another factor in the development of dental caries. Foods with a high concentration of refined sugar (i.e., sucrose) increase the risk of dental caries. Sucrose is converted by bacterial plaque into volatile acids that destroy the hydroxyapatite.

   (a) **Fructose** and **lactose** are less cariogenic than sucrose.

   (b) **Noncariogenic sugar substitutes** are xylitol, sorbitol, and aspartame.

   b. **OTC products** for dental caries include products that can alleviate the pain and sensitivity until the patient can get to the dentist. Examples of ingredients that are beneficial in this regard include lidocaine, benzocaine (e.g., Anbesol, Orajel), or an oral analgesic (e.g., aspirin, acetaminophen). FDA has issued a warning that the use of topical benzocaine is associated with a rare, but serious condition, methemoglobinemia.

2. **Plaque and calculus**

   a. **Causes**

   (1) **Plaque** is a sticky substance formed by the attachment of bacteria to the pellicle, which is a thin, acellular, glycoprotein (a mucoprotein coating that adheres to the enamel within minutes after cleaning a tooth).

   (2) **Calculus** (or **tartar**) is the substance formed when plaque is not removed within 24 hrs. The plaque begins to calcify into calculus when calcium salt precipitates from the saliva. Calculus can be removed only by a professional dental cleaning.

   b. **OTC products**

   (1) **Toothbrushes.** Soft, rounded, nylon bristles are preferred by dentists because hard bristles can irritate the gingival margins and cause the gums to recede. Manual toothbrushes vary in shape, size, design, and texture. Some toothbrushes have specially designed bristles that reach deep between teeth and along the gumline to remove stains and polish teeth and massage gums. Electric toothbrushes can benefit patients who require someone to clean their teeth for them or patients who have orthodontic appliances. Toothbrushes should be replaced when they begin to show wear or every 3 months, whichever comes first. Patients should replace their toothbrush after having an upper-respiratory infection.

   (2) **Irrigating devices** direct a high-pressure stream of water through a nozzle to the hard-to-clean areas by gently lifting the free gingiva to rinse out crevices. Two types are available: **pulsating** (i.e., intermittent low- and high-pressure water streams) and **steady** (i.e., constant and consistent water pressure), neither of which has shown superior irrigating ability.

   (a) Irrigating devices should serve as adjuncts in maintaining oral hygiene.

   (b) **Examples** include Interplak Water Jet, Hydro-Pik, and the Waterpik oral irrigator.

   c. **Dental floss** is available waxed, unwaxed, thick, thin, flavored, or unflavored. Some dental flosses are impregnated or coated with additives such as baking soda and fluoride. Also, several manufacturers are marketing floss made of materials with superior antishredding properties (e.g., Glide, Colgate Total). There are no differences among dental flosses in terms of plaque removal and prevention of gingivitis. There is no evidence of a residual wax film with the use of waxed dental floss.

   (1) The selection of dental floss depends on the characteristics of the patient, such as tooth roughness or tightness of tooth contacts (e.g., waxed floss is recommended for tight-fitting teeth because it can pass easily between the teeth without shredding).

   (2) The American Dental Association (ADA) recognizes approximately 35 brands as safe and effective including Butler, Johnson & Johnson, and Oral-B.

   d. **Dentifrices** are products that enhance the removal of stains and dental plaque by the toothbrush. These include toothpastes, antiplaque and anticalculus mouthwashes, cosmetic whiteners, desensitizing agents, disclosing agents, and dental gums.

   (1) **Toothpastes** are beneficial in decreasing the incidence of dental caries, reducing mouth odors, and enhancing personal appearance. Some toothpastes may contain the

antioxidant coenzyme Q10 (CoQ10; e.g., Perfect Smile Q10). **Ingredients** include the following:

(a) **Abrasives** are responsible for physically removing plaque and debris. Examples include silicates, sodium bicarbonate, dicalcium phosphate, sodium metaphosphate, calcium pyrophosphate, calcium carbonate, magnesium carbonate, and aluminum oxides. High-abrasive formulations are not advised for long-term use or for use by patients with exposed root surfaces.

(b) **Surfactants** are foaming agents that are incorporated into most dentifrices because their detergent action aids in removing debris. The **most frequently used** surfactants are **sodium lauryl sulfate** and **sodium dodecyl benzene sulfonate**. Sodium lauryl sulfate-containing dentifrices have been associated with an increase in the occurrence of canker sores. Dentifrices such as Oral-B Rembrandt Whitening Natural, Sensodyne, and Biotene do not contain sodium lauryl sulfate.

(c) **Humectants** prevent the preparation from drying. Examples include sorbitol, glycerin, and propylene glycol.

(d) **Suspending agents** add thickness to the product. Examples include methylcellulose, tragacanth, and karaya gum.

(e) **Flavoring agents** include sorbitol or saccharin.

(f) **Pyrophosphates** are found in tartar-control toothpastes. These products retard tartar formation; however, they form an alkaline solution that may irritate the skin. Some patients might experience a rash around the outside of the mouth. These patients should use regular toothpaste and only occasionally brush with tartar-control toothpaste (e.g., Colgate Tartar Protection with Whitening). Tartar-control toothpastes do not penetrate below the gumline, where tartar does the most damage.

(g) **Fluoride** is anticariogenic because it replaces the hydroxyl ion in hydroxyapatite with the fluoride ion to form fluorapatite on the outer surface of the enamel. Fluorapatite hardens the enamel and makes it more acid resistant. Fluoride also has demonstrated antibacterial activity.

(i) Fluoride is **most beneficial** if used from birth through **age 12 or 13** because unerupted permanent teeth are mineralizing during that time. Whether or not a patient receives fluoride depends on the concentration in his or her local drinking water (*Table 19-1*).

(ii) **Common fluoride compounds** in toothpaste include 0.24% sodium fluoride and 0.76% or 0.80% sodium monofluorophosphate (e.g., Aim, Crest, Aquafresh, Colgate). The continuous use of stannous fluoride may cause tooth discoloration.

(iii) A fluoride warning label, which recommends contacting a poison control center or seeking professional assistance if more quantity than used for brushing teeth

Table 19-1. DAILY FLUORIDE SUPPLEMENT REQUIREMENTS FOR INFANTS AND CHILDREN, BASED ON CONCENTRATION OF FLUORIDE IN DRINKING WATER

Fluoride Concentration (ppm)	Age	Fluoride Supplement Required (mg/day)
> 0.6	6 months to 3 years	0
	3–6 years	0
	6–16 years	0
0.3–0.6	6 months to 3 years	0
	3–6 years	0.25
	6–16 years	0.50
< 0.3	6 months to 3 years	0.25
	3–6 years	0.50
	6–16 years	1.00

is ingested, is required by the FDA on fluoride-containing dentifrices because the federal agency lists fluoride as a toxic substance.

(iv) The estimated toxic dose of fluoride is 5 to 10 mg/kg.

(v) Acute fluoride toxicity causes nausea, vomiting, and diarrhea.

(2) Agents with **antiplaque** potential for inclusion in dentifrices include plant extracts (sanguinarine), metal salts (zinc and stannous), phenolic compounds (triclosan), and essential oils (thymol and eucalyptol).

(a) **Triclosan** is an antimicrobial agent that has been demonstrated clinically to help prevent gingivitis, plaque, cavities, and tartar.

(i) Colgate Total contains 0.24% sodium fluoride and 0.30% triclosan and is formulated with the polymer **Gantrez**, which works to prolong the contact of triclosan with oral structures.

(ii) Therefore, Colgate Total continues to work in between brushings.

(b) Colgate Total has been accepted by the ADA as efficacious.

(3) **Anticalculous dentifrices** include the ingredients zinc chloride, zinc citrate, and 33% pyrophosphate to prevent calculus formation.

(a) The ADA does not evaluate anticalculus claims because it regards the inhibition of supragingival calculus as a nontherapeutic use.

(b) The ADA has directed that the following statement appear on all package and container labeling for accepted fluoride dentifrice products with calculus-control activity: [*Product name*] has been shown to reduce the formation of tartar above the gumline but has not been shown to have a therapeutic effect on periodontal diseases.

(4) **Cosmetic whitening agents.** The **most common ingredient** in these products that is responsible for whitening the teeth is **10% carbamide peroxide** (i.e., in Gly-Oxide, Rembrandt Professional Bleaching System) and hydrogen peroxide (i.e., in Crest Whitestrips).

(a) Carbamide peroxide is a white crystal that reacts with water to release hydrogen peroxide, which in turn liberates free oxides.

(b) Some cosmetic whiteners may contain hydrogen peroxide in gel or liquid form.

(c) Three methods of tooth bleaching exist: in-office bleaching, dentist-supported home bleaching, and OTC home bleaching.

(i) Patients should be encouraged to perform tooth bleaching only with a dentist's supervision.

(ii) Crest Extra Whitening uses a patented soft-silica technology. Owing to this technology, the product contains 50% more silica, which greatly enhances the removal of extrinsic stains without increasing abrasiveness.

(iii) Colgate Luminous also contains a silica whitening technology and fluoride.

(d) **Possible risks** associated with using whitening products include alteration of normal flora, tissue damage, tooth sensitivity, gingivitis, and potentiation of carcinogenic effects of other agents.

(e) **Antiseptics** have been used as whiteners (e.g., Gly-Oxide).

(5) **Desensitizing agents** reduce the pain in sensitive teeth caused by cold, heat, acids, sweets, or touch. These products should be nonabrasive and should not be used on a permanent basis unless directed by a dentist.

(a) Examples of **5% potassium nitrate compounds** include Colgate Sensitive, Sensodyne, Aquafresh Sensitive, and Crest Sensitivity.

(b) Dibasic sodium citrate in pluronic gel and 10% strontium chloride were classified as class III pending further evidence of effectiveness.

(6) **Disclosing agents** aid in visualizing where dental plaque has formed. These products are for occasional use only and should not be swallowed. The FDA-approved product is a vegetable dye, Food, Drug, and Cosmetic (FD&C) Red No 3. Following use, the consumer should rinse the mouth with water and then expectorate.

(7) **Mouthwashes** may contain astringents, demulcents, detergents, flavors, germicidal agents, and fluoride. They can be used for cosmetic purposes, reducing plaque, or supplementing fluoride consumption.

(a) **Cosmetic mouthwashes** freshen the breath. They are nontherapeutic and are not effective as an antiseptic agent. These mouthwashes are classified by their active ingredients, alcohol content, and appearance. The most popular products are those that contain medicinal phenol and mint. The higher the percent of alcohol, the higher the effect of the flavor within the mouth.

(b) Antiplaque mouth rinses. Mouth rinses claiming anticalculus or tartar-control activity contain the same active ingredients as anticalculus dentifrices. Cool Mint Listerine has received the ADA seal of approval.

(i) Cetylpyridinium chloride (CPC), a mouthwash ingredient, has been approved for class I for plaque and gingivitis treatment. Examples of products in this class include Cepacol, Scope, and Crest Pro-Health Rinse.

(ii) Chlorhexidine is an active ingredient in some mouthwashes. An example is Colgate PerioGard.

(iii) Staining is associated with the overuse of CPC and chlorhexidine.

(iv) Fluoridated mouthwashes are used after cleaning the teeth and should be expectorated. Nothing should be put into the mouth for 30 mins after using these mouthwashes. The ADA has approved the following products: ACT Anti-Cavity Fluoride Rinse, ACT for Kids, and Colgate Phos-Flur Rinse.

(8) Dental gums are promoted to reduce plaque, whiten teeth, possibly reduce the risk of tooth decay, and freshen breath. Chewing gum is associated with increased salivary flow, which apparently produces a beneficial buffering effect against acids in the oral cavity.

(a) Some contain baking soda as a mild abrasive cleaner and to neutralize acid.

(b) Calcium may be added to help remineralize the teeth and prevent cavities.

(c) These gums also contain xylitol, a sweetener that is less likely to cause cavities than sugar or sorbitol. Examples are Trident, Xtra Care, and Smart Mouth.

(d) These gums are not a substitute for good oral hygiene, including brushing and flossing, but may be useful for people who are unable to brush after lunch.

(e) It is not known if these products have any advantage over regular sugarless gum.

3. Gingivitis is inflammation of the gingiva. The gingiva may appear larger in size with a bluish hue caused by engorged gingival capillaries and a slow venous return.

a. Cause. Gingivitis is caused by microorganisms that eventually damage cellular and intercellular tissues. **Chronic gingivitis** may be localized or generalized. The gums readily bleed when probed or brushed, and the patient should seek dental assistance.

b. OTC products include anesthetics containing benzocaine (e.g., Orajel) to relieve the pain. FDA has issued a warning that the use of topical benzocaine is associated with a rare, but serious condition, methemoglobinemia. Mouthwashes may freshen the breath; however, it is important to consider the potential of these products to disguise and delay treatment of pathological conditions (e.g., gingivitis) before use. Also, acetaminophen (Tylenol) can be recommended. The patient should seek the advice of a dentist.

4. Periodontal disease is the result of chronic gingivitis left untreated.

a. The periodontal ligament attachment and alveolar bone support of the tooth deteriorate.

b. Risk factors include gender (men affected more than women), age (> 35 years old), smoking, lack of oral care and regular dentist visits, diabetes, hypertension, rheumatoid arthritis, and loss of anterior teeth.

c. Periodontitis may be treated with prescription products:

(1) Periostat (doxycycline hyclate, 20-mg capsules)

(2) Atridox (doxycycline hyclate 10%) in the Atrigel Delivery System.

(a) Atridox provides local antibacterial effects.

(b) Low-dose doxycycline inhibits collagenase, an enzyme that destroys connective tissue in the gums, leading to tooth loss.

5. Acute necrotizing ulcerative gingivitis (ANUG) (also called **trench mouth**) is characterized by necrosis and ulceration of the gingival surface with underlying inflammation. This condition is usually seen in teens and young adults.

a. Signs and **symptoms** of ANUG include severe pain, halitosis, bleeding, foul taste, and increased salivation.

b. The **cause** of ANUG is unknown. It is postulated that it might be associated with the overgrowth of spirochete and fusiform organisms.

c. **Risk factors** include anxiety, stress, smoking, malnutrition, and poor oral hygiene.
d. **Treatment** consists of local debridement. Also, penicillin VK (penicillin V is a derivative of penicillin G; however, it is more stable in an acidic medium and, therefore, is better absorbed from the gastrointestinal tract) or metronidazole may be used in certain cases (e.g., widespread lesions).
e. **OTC products** include acetaminophen and products with benzocaine (not eugenol because it may cause soft tissue damage). The patient should be advised to see a dentist. The use of salicylates is not recommended if the patient is predisposed to bleeding. Also, adequate nutrition, high fluid intake, and rest are essential. Rinsing the mouth with warm normal saline or 1.5% peroxide solution might be helpful for the first few days.

6. **Temporomandibular joint syndrome** is caused by an improper working relationship between the chewing muscles and the TMJ.
   a. **Signs** and **symptoms** include a dull, aching pain around the ear, headaches, neck aches, limited opening of the mouth, and a clicking or popping noise upon opening the mouth.
   b. **Risk factors** include bruxism (i.e., grinding the teeth) and occlusal (i.e., bite) abnormalities.
   c. **Treatment** consists of moist heat applied to the jaw, muscle relaxants, bite plates or occlusal splints, a diet of soft foods, correcting the occlusion, or surgery.
   d. **OTC products** that can help relieve the pain include oral analgesics (e.g., acetaminophen, ibuprofen).
7. **Teething pain.** The ADA has not accepted any product for teething pain. A **frozen teething ring** can provide symptomatic relief. Persisting pain may be treated with a local anesthetic such as benzocaine (found in Anbesol Baby and Baby Orajel). If a teething child presents with a fever, a physician should be contacted.
8. **Xerostomia** (i.e., dry mouth) is caused by improper functioning of the salivary glands (as in Sjögren syndrome and diabetes mellitus). **Artificial saliva** is available as an OTC product. The ADA has approved the following artificial saliva products: Moi-Stir, Salivart, Biotene Oral Balance.

C. **Common oral lesions and OTC products**

1. **Canker sores** (also called **recurrent aphthous ulcers or recurrent aphthous stomatitis**)
   a. The **cause** of canker sores is unknown. Studies suggest that the sores may be caused by hypersensitivity to bacteria found in the mouth or dysfunction of the immune system initiated by minor trauma or stress. This is why physicians or dentists may use prednisone or a topical steroid to reduce allergic reaction or have the patient rinse with a compounded suspension. Peridex and Listerine appear to help decrease bacteria in the mouth.
   b. **Lesions** can occur on any nonkeratinized mucosal surface in the mouth (i.e., tongue, lips) and usually appear gray to yellow with an erythematous halo of inflamed tissue surrounding the ulcer. Most lesions persist 7 to 14 days and heal without scarring.
   c. **OTC products** can control the pain of canker sores, shorten the duration of current lesions, and prevent new lesions. Products include **protectants**, **local anesthetics**, and **debriding and wound-cleansing agents.**
      (1) **Protectants** include Orabase, denture adhesives (see II.F.2), and benzoin tincture. Denture adhesives are not approved for this use by the FDA.
      (2) **Local anesthetics**, such as benzocaine or butacaine, are the **most common anesthetics** found in these OTC products.
         (a) The FDA has approved the following ingredients:
            (i) Benzocaine (5.0% to 20%)
            (ii) Benzyl alcohol (0.05% to 0.1%)
            (iii) Dyclonine (0.05% to 0.1%)
            (iv) Hexylresorcinol (0.05% to 0.1%)
            (v) Menthol (0.04% to 2.0%)
            (vi) Phenol (0.5% to 1.5%)
            (vii) Phenolate sodium (0.5% to 1.5%)
            (viii) Salicyl alcohol (1.0% to 6.0%)
         (b) Examples of OTC local anesthetics for oral use include Anbesol, Blistex, Campho-Phenique, Orajel, Zilactin-B, and Zilactin-L.
         (c) The use of products containing substantial amounts of menthol, phenol, camphor, and eugenol should be discouraged owing to their ability to irritate tissue.

(d) Aspirin should not be retained in the mouth or placed on an oral lesion in an attempt to provide relief.

(e) **Prescription products.** Amlexanox (Aphthasol) has been approved for the treatment of canker sores.

(i) It is applied four times daily after meals and at bedtime.

(ii) Advise patients to start using the product as soon as they notice symptoms and to continue until the ulcer is healed, approximately 10 days.

(f) Gelclair is indicated for local management and relief of oral pain associated with aphthous ulcers. It provides oral pain relief by acting as a protective adherent barrier over the surface of the mouth and throat.

(i) Patient should use one packet at least three times a day or as needed.

(ii) Advise patients to mix one packet with 3 tablespoons of water, swish for a minute, then expectorate. Do not eat or drink for approximately 1 hr after treatment.

(g) **Orphan Drug products. Thalidomide** is indicated for aphthous ulcer and stomatitis in severely immunocompromised patients.

(3) **Debriding and wound-cleansing agents** include 10% to 15% carbamide peroxide, 3% hydrogen peroxide, and sodium bicarbonate. The FDA considers these active ingredients to be safe and effective for debriding or wound-cleansing agents for oral health care.

2. **Cold sores/fever blisters** (also called **herpes simplex labialis**) are caused primarily by the herpes simplex virus type 1 (HSV-1). HSV-1 is contagious and is thought to be transmitted by direct contact. An outbreak may be provoked by stress, minor infection, fever, or sunlight. Cold sores usually occur on the lips and are recurrent, often arising in the same location.

a. **Presentation.** An outbreak is preceded by burning, itching, or numbness. Red papules of fluid-containing vesicles then appear, and these eventually burst and form a crust. These sores are typically self-limited and heal in 10 to 14 days without scarring.

b. **OTC products** for cold sores include products that contain softening compounds (e.g., emollient creams, petrolatum, protectants), which keep the cold sore moist to prevent it from drying and fissuring. Local anesthetics in nondrying bases (e.g., Orabase, with benzocaine) decrease pain. Highly astringent bases should be avoided. The ADA contraindicates caustic agents (e.g., phenol, silver nitrate), camphor and other counterirritants, and hydrocortisone for the treatment of cold sores. Lesions should be kept clean by gently washing with mild soap.

(1) **Docosanol 10%** cream (**Abreva**) is indicated for the treatment of cold sores. It prevents the cold sore infection from entering healthy cells. It is approved by the FDA to shorten healing time and duration of symptoms. Patients should apply the cream at the first sign of an outbreak and continue to apply the cream five times a day until the lesion is healed.

(2) **Viractin** (2% tetracaine) is used for the temporary relief of pain and itching associated with cold sores.

(3) If a **secondary infection** develops, bacitracin or Neosporin antibiotic ointments should be recommended. If necessary, the patient should consult a physician for a systemic antibiotic prescription.

(4) A lip **sunscreen** should be used for patients whose cold sores appear to be caused by sun exposure.

(5) The essential amino acid L-lysine has been used in oral doses of 300 to 1200 mg daily to accelerate recovery or suppress recurrence of cold sores. However, studies have produced conflicting data regarding L-lysine and its effect on the duration, severity, and recurrence rate of cold sores.

c. **Prescription products**

(1) **Valacyclovir (Valtrex)** is indicated for the treatment of herpes labialis.

(2) **Acyclovir cream 5% (Zovirax)** is indicated for the treatment of cold sores in adults and adolescents $>$ 12 years of age. Therapy should be initiated at the onset of sign and symptoms and applied five times per day for 4 days. Acyclovir is also available as an oral and ointment formulations.

(3) **Penciclovir cream 1% (Denavir)** is an antiviral medication for the treatment of cold sores in adults and children 12 years of age and older. Patients should apply the cream every 2 hrs while awake for 4 days, beginning at the first sign of tingling or swelling.

D. **Common oral infections and OTC products**

1. **Candidiasis** (also called **thrush**) is caused by the fungus *Candida albicans*, which is the most common opportunistic pathogen associated with oral infections. Thrush has a milky curd appearance, and affected patients should contact a physician.
2. **Oral cancer.** The most common oral cancer is **squamous cell carcinoma**, which can appear as red or white lesions, ulcerations, or tumors.
   a. **Signs** and **symptoms** include a color change in the tongue, a sore throat that does not heal, and persistent or unexplained bleeding. Patients with any of these signs should contact a physician or a dentist.
   b. **Risk factors** include smoked and smokeless tobacco as well as alcohol.
   c. **Treatment** consists of eliminating use of tobacco and alcohol in any form (e.g., alcoholic beverages, mouth rinses with alcohol). Also, treatment generally includes **wide local excision** for small lesions and **en bloc excisions** for larger lesions (in continuity with radical neck dissection if lymph nodes are involved). Radiation, alone or combined with surgery, may be appropriate. Chemotherapy may be used as palliation or as an adjunct to surgery and radiation.
   d. **OTC medications** should not be administered until after checking with a physician. For example, OTC medications used for inflammation can increase the effects of methotrexate. Chemotherapeutic agents can produce many possible side effects that require immediate medical attention (e.g., chest pain, inflammation, unusual bleeding). Some examples of side effects that usually do not require medical attention include nausea, vomiting, loss of appetite or hair, and trouble sleeping. OTC medications can be useful in these cases; however, nausea and vomiting are treated by prescription medications such as ondansetron or metoclopramide. Nonpharmacological measures, such as avoiding disturbing environmental odors and vestibular disturbances, might be helpful in minimizing nausea and vomiting.

E. **Recommended standard prophylaxis for prevention of endocarditis**

1. **Amoxicillin** 2.0 g orally 30 to 60 mins before the procedure for adults, and 50 mg/kg orally for children, is the recommended standard prophylactic regimen for all dental, oral, upper respiratory tract, and esophageal procedures.
2. For patients who are **allergic to penicillin**, the recommended **alternative oral regimens** include the following:
   a. **Clindamycin**, 600 mg for adults; 20 mg/kg for children
   b. **Cephalexin**, 2.0 g for adults; 50 mg/kg for children
   c. **Azithromycin** or **clarithromycin**, 500 mg for adults; 15 mg/kg for children, 30 to 60 mins before the procedure

F. **OTC denture products**

1. **Denture cleansers** are either **chemical** or **abrasive** in respect to their cleansing ability.
   a. **Chemical** denture cleansers include alkaline peroxide, alkaline hypochlorite, or dilute acids.
      (1) **Alkaline peroxide** is the **most commonly used** chemical denture cleanser and is available as tablets or powders. It causes oxygen to be released, which creates a cleansing effect. Alkaline peroxide does not damage the surface of acrylic resins; however, it may bleach them.
      (2) **Alkaline hypochlorite** (i.e., bleach) dissolves the matrix of plaque but has no effect on calculus. It is both bactericidal and fungicidal. A **disadvantage** of alkaline hypochlorite is that it **corrodes metal denture components**. It can also bleach acrylic resin. Therefore, it should not be used more than once a week.
   b. **Abrasive** denture cleansers are available as gel, tablet, paste, or powder (e.g., silicates, sodium bicarbonate, dicalcium phosphate, calcium carbonate).
      (1) Dentures should not be soaked in hot water because the heat could distort or warp the appliances.
      (2) The ADA accepts the following denture cleansers as safe and effective: Efferdent and Polident.
2. **Denture adherents** contain materials (e.g., karaya gum, pectin, methylcellulose) that swell, gel, and become viscous to promote adhesion, which increases the denture attachment to underlying soft tissues.
   a. **Disadvantages.** As the use of denture adherents increases, the soft tissue deteriorates. Denture adherents can also provide a medium for bacterial and fungal growth. Daily use of denture adherents is not recommended.
   b. The ADA accepts the following denture adherents as safe and effective: Fixodent, Sea-Bond, Super Poli-Grip, and Effergrip.

12. **The answer is C** *[see III.C.4]*.
Currently, there are three available ophthalmic antihistamines: ketotifen, pheniramine, and antazoline. Pheniramine and antazoline are only available in combination with the ophthalmic decongestant naphazoline. Ophthalmic antihistamines may cause burning, stinging, dry eyes, or mydriasis. Vasoconstrictors, not antihistamines, may produce rebound congestion when used in excess or for extended durations.

13. **The answer is C** *[see III.B]*.
Edetic acid is an antioxidant and benzalkonium chloride (BAK) is a preservative used in ophthalmic formulations. Zinc sulfate is the only FDA-recommended astringent. Povidone is a vehicle used in ophthalmic formulations.

14. **The answer is B** *[see II.B.2.d.(1)]*.
Sodium lauryl sulfate is used frequently as a surfactant in most dentifrices. Its detergent action aids in the removal of debris, and the foaming is usually desired by the patient. There is no evidence that surfactants possess anticaries activity or decrease periodontal disease. The FDA considers surfactants an inactive ingredient in dentifrices.

15. **The answer is D** *[see II.B.2.d.(4)]*.
Teeth-whitening agents usually contain a peroxide-based ingredient, which can penetrate the surface area of the tooth to whiten. Cosmetic agents can alter the normal flora or cause tissue irritation, gingivitis, and teeth sensitivity. Antiseptics have been used as cosmetic whiteners (e.g., Gly-Oxide) along with hydrogen peroxide (e.g., Crest Whitestrips).

16. **The answer is C** *[see II.C.1.c.(2)]*.
Local anesthetics can provide relief of canker sore pain. The most common local anesthetics found in OTC products include benzocaine and butacaine. Some examples are Anbesol, Zilactin-B, and Orajel. Aspirin should not be retained in the mouth before swallowing or placed in the area of the oral lesions because of the high risk for chemical burn with necrosis.

17. **The answer is C** *[see II.B.2.d.(5)]*.
Desensitizing agents should not be abrasive or used on a chronic basis unless directed by a dentist. The products approved by the ADA include the ingredients: 5% potassium nitrate, 10% strontium chloride, and dibasic sodium citrate 2% in pluronic gel.

18. **The answer is D (II, III)** *[see II.B.2.d.(1).D]*.
Suspending agents are products that add thickness to the dentifrices. Examples are tragacanth, karaya gum, and methylcellulose. Dicalcium phosphate is categorized as an abrasive product.

19. **The answer is C (I, II)** *[see II.C.2.a–b]*.
Cold sore treatment involves keeping the lesion moist with emollient creams, petrolatum, or protectants. Local anesthetics (e.g., benzocaine, dyclonine, salicyl alcohol) may be used. In addition, docosanol 10% cream (Abreva) and tetracaine 2% (Viractin) are available without a prescription for the treatment of cold sores. Topical counterirritants (e.g., camphor) and caustics or escharotic agents (e.g., phenol, menthol, silver nitrate) are not recommended because they may further irritate the tissue. Cold sores are usually self-limiting and heal within 10 to 14 days without scarring.

20. **The answer is D (II, III)** *[see I.B]*.
Swimmer's ear requires an otic antibiotic, which is by prescription only.

20 Over-the-Counter Dermatological Agents

LARRY N. SWANSON, RYAN S. SWANSON

I. CONTACT DERMATITIS

A. **Introduction**

1. **Types of contact dermatitis.** Contact dermatitis is one of the **most common** dermatological conditions encountered in clinical practice. It has traditionally been divided into **irritant contact dermatitis** and **allergic contact dermatitis** on the basis of the origin and immunological mechanism.
   a. **Irritant contact dermatitis** is caused by direct contact with a primary irritant. These irritants can be classified as absolute or relative primary irritants.
      (1) **Absolute primary irritants** are intrinsically damaging substances that injure, on first contact, any person's skin. Examples include strong acids, alkalis, and other industrial chemicals.
      (2) **Relative primary irritants** cause most cases of contact dermatitis seen in clinical practice. These irritants are less toxic than absolute primary irritants, and they require repeated or prolonged exposure to provoke a reaction. Examples of relative primary irritants include soaps, detergents, benzoyl peroxide, and certain plant and animal substances.
   b. **Allergic contact dermatitis.** Many plants, and almost any chemical, can cause allergic contact dermatitis. Poison ivy is a classic example of allergic contact dermatitis, which is classified as a type IV hypersensitivity reaction. This type of allergic reaction is T cell–mediated, and the following **sequence of events** must occur to provoke it:
      (1) The epidermis must come in **contact** with the hapten (i.e., the specific allergen).
      (2) The **hapten–epidermal protein complex** (i.e., the complete antigen) must form.
      (3) The antigen must **enter the lymphatic system**.
      (4) **Immunologically competent lymphoid cells**, which are selective against the antigen, must form.
      (5) On **reexposure** to the hapten, the typical, local delayed hypersensitivity reaction (i.e., contact dermatitis) occurs.
      (6) The **induction period**, during which sensitivity develops, usually requires 14 to 21 days but may take as few as 4 days or more than several weeks. **Once sensitivity is fully developed:**
         (a) Reexposure to even minute amounts of the same material elicits an eczematous response, typically with an onset of 12 hrs and a peak of 48 to 72 hrs after exposure.
         (b) Sensitivity usually persists for life.
            (i) Most contact allergens produce sensitization in only a small percentage of exposed persons.
            (ii) Allergens or substances such as poison ivy, however, produce sensitization in > 70% of the population (50% to 95% are sensitive to the poison ivy plant).
2. **General phases of contact dermatitis**
   a. **Acute stage.** Wet lesions, such as blisters or denuded and weeping skin, are evident in well-outlined patches. Also evident are erythema, edema, vesicles, and oozing.

b. **Subacute stage.** In this phase, crusts or scabs form over the previously wet lesions. Allergic contact dermatitis and irritant contact dermatitis caused by absolute primary irritants produce both the acute and subacute stages.

c. **Chronic stage.** In this phase, the lesions become dry and thickened (i.e., lichenified). Initially, dryness and fissuring are the signs. Later, erythema, lichenification, and excoriations appear. The chronic phase of contact dermatitis usually occurs more often with irritant contact dermatitis caused by relative primary irritants.

B. **Toxic plants.** Poison ivy and poison oak are the **most common causes** of allergic contact dermatitis in North America. These plants were formerly known as the *Rhus* genus, but they are now properly referred to as the *Toxicodendron* genus.

1. **Poison ivy** (*Toxicodendron radicans* and *T. rydbergii*) grows as a vine or as a bush. It is found in most parts of the United States but is especially prevalent in the northeastern part of the country. Poison ivy is often identified by its characteristic growth pattern, described by the saying, "Leaves of three, let it be."
2. **Poison oak** (*T. diversilobum*) is found in the western United States and Canada. It grows as an upright shrub or a woody vine. *T. toxicarium* is found in the eastern United States.
3. **Poison sumac** (*T. vernix*) grows in woody or swampy areas as a coarse shrub or tree and is prevalent in the eastern United States and southeastern Canada.

C. **Toxicodendron dermatitis.** For dermatitis to develop, previous sensitization (a 5- to 21-day incubation period) caused by direct contact with a sensitizing agent is required (see I.A.1.b). An oleoresin, **urushiol**, is the active sensitizing agent in poison ivy, poison oak, and poison sumac. There are slight differences in the chemical structures of the sensitizing agent in each of these plants, but the three agents cross-react.

1. **Release of the urushiol oil.** The plants must be bruised or injured to release the oleoresin. It is **present in** the **roots, stems, leaves,** and **fruit**. Urushiol may remain active on tools, toys, clothes, pets, and under fingernails if those items have had contact with the broken plants.
   a. Urushiol does not volatilize, so one cannot get dermatitis from just being near a poison ivy plant; direct contact is necessary. **Burning plants**, however, can cause droplets of oil carried by smoke to enter the respiratory system, which can cause significant respiratory distress.
   b. A cut or damaged poison ivy, poison oak, or poison sumac plant initially yields a **clear fluid** containing the oleoresin, which **turns to a black inky lacquer** on exposure to air within a few minutes. This change can be a means for confirming identification of these plants.
   c. Because the oleoresin can rapidly penetrate the skin, the affected **area must be washed with soap and water within 10 mins** after exposure to prevent the dermatitis eruption. Washing up to 30 mins after exposure is still useful in removing some of the oleoresin.
2. If an individual has been **previously sensitized**, the lesions usually occur within 6 to 48 hrs after contact with the allergen.
3. Typically, the **initial eruption** exists as small patches of erythematous papules (usually streaks). **Pruritus (itching) is the primary symptom.**
   a. Papules may progress to vesicles, which may then ooze and bleed when they are scratched. Secondary infection may then develop. Often the inflammation is severe, and a significant amount of edema occurs over the exposed area.
   b. The lesions may last from a few days to several weeks. Left untreated, the condition rarely persists longer than 2 to 3 weeks.
4. **Poison ivy dermatitis does not spread.** New lesions, however, may continue to appear for several days despite lack of further contact with the plant. This reaction may be due to the following facts:
   a. Skin that has been minimally exposed to the antigen begins to react only as the person's sensitivity heightens.
   b. Antigen is absorbed at varying rates through the skin of different parts of the body.
   c. The person inadvertently touches contaminated objects or may have residual oleoresin—for example, underneath the fingernails.
5. **Poison ivy is not contagious.** The serous fluid from the weeping vesicles are not antigenic. No one can "catch" poison ivy from another person.

D. **Treatment.** The treatment of irritant and allergic contact dermatitis focuses on therapy for the specific symptomatology.

1. A pharmacist should **refer a patient** with a poison ivy eruption to a physician if
   a. The eruption involves a large area of the body (about 25%).
   b. The eruption involves the eyes, genital area, mouth, or respiratory tract (some patients may experience respiratory difficulties if they inhale the smoke of burning poison ivy plants).
2. The **severity of the eruption** depends on
   a. The quantity of allergen that the patient has been exposed to
   b. The individual patient's sensitivity to the allergen
3. **For severe eruptions**, a patient should consult a physician, who may prescribe **systemic corticosteroids**.
   a. Systemic corticosteroids are the cornerstone of therapy. One should use sufficiently high doses to suppress this inflammation. Generally, it is recommended that prednisone be given in a dose of 60 mg/day for 5 days, then reduced to 40 mg/day for 5 days, then 20 mg/day for 5 days, then discontinued. Prepacked dosage packs of corticosteroids used over 6 days provide too low of a dose over too short period.
   b. Some blisters may be drained at their base. The skin on top of the blister should be kept intact. Draining the blister allows more topical medication to penetrate for an antipruritic effect. Baths and soaks [see I.D.4.b.(1).(b)] may be beneficial as well.
4. **For a less severe eruption**, the principal goals are to relieve the itching and inflammation and to protect the integrity of the skin.
   a. Several therapeutic classes of agents can be used **to relieve itching**.
      (1) **Oral antihistamines** (particularly H_1-receptor blockers) are perhaps the most commonly used agents for pruritus. Antihistamines act as antagonists of the H_1 receptor found on mast cells, preventing the release of histamine and the subsequent histamine-mediated allergic response. These agents are available both over-the-counter (OTC), such as diphenhydramine (Benadryl), as well as per prescription, such as hydroxyzine (Atarax). Relief from itching may also be due to the sedative effects of these agents. As such, antihistamines may be preferred in patients who have trouble sleeping due to pruritus but should be used with caution in patients who must be alert during daytime hours.
      (2) **Topical hydrocortisone** (e.g., Cortaid), which is available in concentrations up to 1%, is minimally useful for its antipruritic and anti-inflammatory effects. Patients should be cautioned against using topical hydrocortisone for more than 7 days without first consulting a physician to ensure proper diagnosis before prolonged corticosteroid use.
      (3) **Counterirritants** include camphor (0.1% to 3.0%), phenol (0.5% to 1.5%), and menthol (0.1% to 1.0%). These agents have an analgesic effect as a result of depression of cutaneous receptors. The exact antipruritic mechanism is not fully known, but a placebo effect may result from the characteristic medicinal odors of these agents.
      (4) **Astringents** are mild protein precipitants that result in contraction of tissue, which in turn decreases the local edema and inflammation.
         (a) The principal agent used is **aluminum acetate** (Burow's solution).
         (b) **Calamine** (zinc oxide with ferric oxide, which provides the pink color) may also be used. Calamine contracts tissue and helps dry the area, but the formation of the thick dried paste may not be tolerated by some people.
      (5) The application of **local anesthetics**—for example, benzocaine (5% to 20%)—may relieve itching. Relief may be of short duration (30 to 45 mins), but application of benzocaine may be especially useful at bedtime, when pruritus is most bothersome. There is some question about the frequency of the sensitizing ability of benzocaine (0.17% to 5.0%); because of this, many practitioners avoid recommending local anesthetics for contact dermatitis. Certainly, treatment should be discontinued if the rash worsens.
      (6) **Topical antihistamines**—for example, diphenhydramine (Benadryl cream or spray)—may provide relief of mild itching principally through a topical anesthetic effect rather than any antihistamine effect. Many would not recommend their use because they may also have a significant sensitizing potential, and in children with varicella infections

(in which the integrity of the skin is compromised), systemic absorption has occurred with symptoms of anticholinergic toxicity produced. Topical and oral diphenhydramine should not be used concurrently.

(7) **Zanfel** is a topical solution that claims to wash urushiol from the skin even after the oil has bonded. Little clinical evidence exists to support this claim, and the cost of the product (about $40 for a 1 oz tube) is prohibitive for many patients.

b. **Basic treatment**

(1) **Acute (weeping) lesions** (see I.A.2.a)

(a) **Wet dressings** work on the principle that water evaporating from the skin cools it and thus relieves itching. Wet dressings have an additional benefit of causing gentle debridement and cleansing of the skin.

(b) **Burow's solution** (Domeboro) in concentrations of 1:20 to 1:40 as a wet dressing or a cool bath of 15 to 30 mins for three to six times per day provides a significant antipruritic effect.

(c) **Colloidal oatmeal baths** (e.g., Aveeno) may also provide an antipruritic effect.

(d) **Topical therapy that may hinder treatment**

(i) **Local anesthetics and topical antihistamines** may sensitize.

(ii) **Calamine** may make a mess without doing much good.

(2) **Subacute dermatitis** (see I.A.2.b). **A thin layer of hydrocortisone cream or lotion (0.5% to 1%)** may be applied three to four times a day to treat subacute dermatitis. Supplemental agents, such as topical anesthetics, may be used as well.

(3) **Chronic dermatitis** (see I.A.2.c) is best treated with hydrocortisone ointment. This stage is observed more frequently in forms of contact dermatitis that involve continuous exposure to the irritant or allergen. Again, chronic use of hydrocortisone (i.e., more than 7 days) should be monitored by a physician.

E. **Prevention**

1. The best treatment for poison ivy contact dermatitis is to **prevent contact** with the offending cause. This approach involves avoiding the plant and wearing protective clothing.
2. **Barrier preparations. Bentoquatam** (Ivy Block), an organoclay, is the first poison ivy blocker approved by the U.S. Food and Drug Administration (FDA) as safe and effective for prevention of urushiol-induced dermatitis. It comes as a lotion that should be applied at least 15 mins before contact with the plant and then every 4 hrs for continued protection against urushiol. It should be applied to leave a smooth, wet, visible film on the skin. Ivy Block may be removed with soap and water. Because of its alcohol content, patients should be instructed to stay away from flame during application until the product has dried on the skin.

II. SCALY DERMATOSES

A. **Overview**

1. Scaly dermatoses are diseases affecting the outer layer of skin, known as the **epidermis**.
2. These dermatoses are also called "**hyperproliferative disorders**," as they are characterized by a greater-than-normal turnover rate of epidermal skin cells. The typical turnover rate for skin cells is 25 to 30 days, defined as the amount of time it takes to migrate from the stratum germinativum (innermost layer of the epidermis) to the stratum corneum (outermost layer of the epidermis).
3. The three primary scaly dermatoses are
   a. **Dandruff**
   b. **Seborrheic dermatitis**
   c. **Psoriasis**

B. **Etiology**

1. The exact cause for the accelerated cell turnover seen in the scaly dermatoses is unknown.
2. Patients who suffer from scaly dermatoses are found to have higher levels of ***Pityrosporum*** (a fungus that is found in the normal flora of the skin and scalp). Although there may be a link between the scaly dermatoses and elevated levels of *Pityrosporum*, it is unclear if the fungus leads to the dermatosis or if the dermatosis allows for the fungus to grow at a more rapid pace.

C. **Dandruff**

1. **Clinical presentation**
   a. Cell turnover rate is 13 to 15 days.
   b. Primarily characterized by **dry white/gray "flakes"** scattered over the **scalp**.
   c. **Scaling** and **pruritus** are the most common symptoms of dandruff.
   d. Dandruff does not appear until puberty or later and peaks in early adulthood.
   e. More severe in cooler months and less severe during summer months.
   f. Not a serious medical condition, but embarrassment to the patient is a real concern.
2. **Treatment**
   a. **Nonmedicated shampoos**
      (1) Many patients who suffer with **mild dandruff** may be able to control the condition simply by washing with a nonmedicated shampoo on a **daily basis**.
      (2) Patients should be counseled to **scrub the scalp** thoroughly while shampooing.
   b. **Medicated shampoos**
      (1) Those who suffer with more **moderate-to-severe dandruff** should be counseled to use a medicated shampoo.
      (2) Most medicated shampoos should be used at least **twice weekly** for the first **2 to 3 weeks**. Patients should then decrease to once weekly or once every other week to maintain dandruff control.
      (3) To apply medicated shampoo, thoroughly **rub shampoo into scalp and hair**. Leave on for 5 mins, then rinse and repeat. Patients may be instructed to use a scalp scrubber to ensure adequate penetration of the shampoo on the scalp.
      (4) **Cytostatic agents** work by decreasing the rate of epidermal cell turnover.
         (a) **Coal tar** (DHS Tar, Neutrogena T/Gel)
            (i) Mechanism of action is likely related to the ability of coal tar to cross-link with DNA and inhibit cell division.
            (ii) Prolonged exposure to coal tar may be carcinogenic, although patients who use coal tar only for treatment of skin conditions such as scaly dermatoses should not be at risk.
            (iii) May cause **photosensitivity** and **folliculitis**. Do not use on or near groin, anus, and axillae.
            (iv) Can **stain** clothing and bedsheets, as well as skin and hair (particularly blonde, gray, and bleached hair).
            (v) Possesses a strong, unpleasant **odor**.
            (vi) Available as shampoo, lotion, cream, ointment, foam, and soap in strengths ranging from 0.5% to 5.0%.
         (b) **Pyrithione zinc** (DermaZinc, Head & Shoulders Dry Scalp)
            (i) Cytostatic activity prevents epidermal cell growth and multiplication. Also possesses antifungal activity.
            (ii) May be applied to scalp and skin. Different concentrations are approved for different conditions. Use products with 0.3% to 2.0% concentration for brief washings, such as shampooing; use products with 0.1% to 0.25% concentration when instructing patient to apply to scalp or skin without washing off (e.g., creams and lotions).
         (c) **Selenium sulfide** (Dandrex, Selsun Blue)
            (i) Possesses cytostatic and antifungal activities.
            (ii) May cause **discoloration** of blonde, gray, and bleached hair, especially with prolonged periods of application.
            (iii) Can leave scalp unusually **oily**.
            (iv) Available as shampoo, lotion, and foam in concentrations from 1.0% (OTC) to 2.25% (via prescription).
      (5) **Keratolytic agents** work by dissolving or breaking down the outermost layer of skin, causing peeling of the stratum corneum.
         (a) **Salicylic acid** (Ionil, Salex)
            (i) Decreases skin pH, thereby increasing the movement of water into the stratum corneum, which loosens and removes epidermal cells.

(ii) Available for the treatment of scaly dermatoses at concentrations between 1.8% and 3%.

(b) **Sulfur**

(i) Exhibits antimicrobial/antifungal activity, although exact mechanism of action is unknown.

(ii) Approved as a single agent for the treatment of dandruff, but rarely marketed by itself; most commonly seen in sulfur/salicylic acid combination products (with sulfur concentrations between 2% and 5%).

(c) **Sulfur/salicylic acid combination product** (MG217 Medicated Tar-Free Shampoo, Scalpicin Maximum Strength)

(i) When used in combination, individual ingredients may not exceed FDA-approved limits for treatment of dandruff (i.e., up to 5% sulfur and 3% salicylic acid).

(ii) Sulfur can react with metals (such as copper and silver), discoloring products containing these metals.

(6) **Ketoconazole** (Nizoral A–D)

(a) A common treatment option in dandruff and seborrheic dermatitis due to its activity against *Pityrosporum* (see II.B.2).

(b) Directions for application are the same as the aforementioned, with the caveat to leave **at least 3 days** between each shampoo.

(c) Avoid use in patients < 12 years old and those who are nursing or pregnant, as safety and efficacy of ketoconazole have not been established in this population.

(d) Available as OTC-strength (1%) and prescription-strength (2%) shampoos.

c. Patients who do not experience improvement in their condition after **8 weeks** of appropriate self-treatment should be referred to their physician.

D. Seborrheic dermatitis

1. Clinical presentation

a. Cell turnover rate is 9 to 10 days.

b. Primarily characterized by **dull, greasy, yellowish-red scales**.

c. Can affect the scalp, face, ears, back, upper chest, axillae, and groin (i.e., **areas with high concentrations of oil-producing glands**).

d. As with dandruff, **scaling** and **pruritus** are most common symptoms of seborrheic dermatitis.

e. Onset is typically after puberty, affecting men more often than women.

f. More severe in cooler months and less severe during warmer months.

g. Exacerbated by **poor health and stress**.

h. Important for patients to understand that condition persists for life; there is no curative treatment.

i. Infantile seborrheic dermatitis is known as **"cradle cap."**

2. Treatment

a. **Medicated shampoos** are the cornerstone of therapy in seborrheic dermatitis.

(1) Medicated shampoos carry the same instructions for use in seborrheic dermatitis as they do for dandruff (see II.C.2.b).

(2) However, not all agents approved for treatment of dandruff have been approved for the treatment of seborrheic dermatitis. The following agents are primarily used in the treatment of seborrheic dermatitis (see II.C.2.b for a fuller discussion of these agents):

(a) Coal tar

(b) Pyrithione zinc

(c) Salicylic acid

(d) Selenium sulfide

(e) Ketoconazole

b. **Topical corticosteroids**

(1) OTC formulations of **hydrocortisone (1%)** may be used as adjunct therapy in seborrheic dermatitis.

(2) Counsel patients to use hydrocortisone on affected areas two to three times daily as needed. Hydrocortisone should not be applied to large areas of the body nor on or near the eyes.

(3) Hydrocortisone should **not be used for more than 7 days** without first consulting with the patient's physician. Treatment with a prescription-strength corticosteroid may be indicated if a patient does not fully respond to hydrocortisone.

3. **Cradle cap**
   a. Cradle cap is not a serious medical condition and generally resolves by the time the affected infant reaches 12 months.
   b. For infants with cradle cap, **shampoo the scalp frequently** with baby shampoo.
   c. In more severe cases, a small amount of emollient (such as mineral oil, baby oil, vegetable oil, or white petrolatum jelly) may be applied to the scalp to help loosen and remove crusts. Extreme caution must be taken to ensure the infant does not aspirate these emollients.
   d. A **fine-toothed comb** or **soft brush** may also be used to remove excess scales.
   e. Some cases of cradle cap may require treatment with a mild topical corticosteroid, such as hydrocortisone. This should be done only under the care of a physician, and application of a corticosteroid to an infant's face should be avoided.

E. **Psoriasis**

1. **Clinical presentation**
   a. Cell turnover rate is 3 to 4 days.
   b. Multiple forms of psoriasis exist, including plaque (80% to 90% of cases), inverse, guttate, pustular, erythrodermic, and nail psoriasis.
   c. Primarily characterized by **light pink/maroon-colored plaques covered with silvery scales.**
   d. Plaques are most commonly found on the **elbows, knees, back, scalp, and external ear canal. Fingernails and toenails** can also be affected, causing nails to appear thick and crumbling.
   e. **Itching** and **irritation** are the most common symptoms of psoriasis, although many patients may be asymptomatic.
   f. Affects men and women equally, and onset can occur at any age.
   g. As with dandruff and seborrheic dermatitis, psoriasis is less severe during warmer months.
   h. Triggered by several factors, including **infection, stress, and certain medications** (namely, nonsteroidal anti-inflammatory drugs, β-blockers, antimalarials, lithium, and withdrawal from corticosteroid therapy). **Smoking, alcohol use**, and **obesity** also increase the severity of the disease.
   i. Most cases of psoriasis are mild in severity, but death can rarely result from very severe, extensive cases. **Psoriatic arthritis** is a leading cause of morbidity.
   j. No curative treatment exists. **Remissions and exacerbations** characterize the disease course for most patients.

2. **Treatment**
   a. Only **mild cases** are indicated for self-treatment.
      (1) **Nonpharmacological measures**
         (a) Patients should be counseled to **soak in lukewarm water** several times a week and to **apply emollients** (such as petroleum jelly) to the affected areas immediately after bathing.
         (b) Overweight/obese patients should **lose weight.**
         (c) Patients who smoke should be counseled on **smoking cessation strategies.**
         (d) Alcohol consumption should be limited or avoided completely.
         (e) Patients should take measures to **reduce levels of stress** in their life if possible.
      (2) **Coal tar** and **salicylic acid** are indicated for the treatment of psoriasis, but may be preferred for those patients with psoriasis limited to the scalp area. These agents should not be applied to large areas of the body.
      (3) **Hydrocortisone** may also be effective, but its use should be limited to small areas of the body and should not be used for more than 7 days without prior prescriber approval.
   b. **Moderate-to-severe disease** (defined as affecting more than 5% to 10% of body surface area) requires physician management.
      (1) Prescription-strength **topical corticosteroids** (e.g., betamethasone, clobetasol, fluocinonide, and triamcinolone) are considered first-line agents. See *Table 20-1* for a listing of relative strengths of topical corticosteroids.
         (a) For the treatment of psoriasis, these agents are typically applied twice daily.
         (b) Systemic side effects are more likely with longer courses of therapy (i.e., > 4 weeks).

Table 20-1 RELATIVE POTENCIES OF TOPICAL CORTICOSTEROIDS

Low Potency	Medium Potency	High Potency	Very High Potency
Alclometasone (Aclovate)	Betamethasone valerate (Beta Derm, Valisone)	Betamethasone dipropionate (Diprolene)	Clobetasol (Temovate)
Desonide (DesOwen, Desonate)	Fluocinolone (Synalar)	Desoximetasone (Topicort)	Halobetasol (Ultravate)
Hydrocortisone (Cortaid, Cortizone)	Fluticasone (Cutivate) Hydrocortisone butyrate (Locoid) Hydrocortisone valerate (Westcort) Triamcinolone (Aristocort, Kenalog)	Fluocinonide (Lidex) Halcinonide (Halog) Mometasone (Elocon)	

(c) These agents are available in several vehicles, such as foams, sprays, and shampoos, to ensure maximal absorption at varying sites of application across the body.

(2) **Topical vitamin D analogs**—including calcipotriene (Dovonex) and calcitriol (Vectical)—may be used as monotherapy, although they may be more effective when used in conjunction with topical corticosteroids.

(3) Tazarotene (Tazorac) is a **topical retinoid** available as both a cream and a gel for long-term treatment of psoriasis.

(4) **Calcineurin inhibitors**—such as tacrolimus (Protopic) and pimecrolimus (Elidel)—are preferred when treating psoriasis of the face, armpits, anogenital area, or breasts, as this may avoid requiring patients to apply corticosteroids to these sensitive areas. However, these agents carry a **black box warning** due to a potential link to lymphoma and skin cancer.

(5) Various **systemic therapies** are used in the management of moderate-to-severe psoriasis.

(a) **Methotrexate** is given at low doses once a week to help manage psoriasis. It may be effective in treating psoriatic arthritis, as well. Methotrexate should be used cautiously (if at all) in patients with hepatic disease due to **hepatoxicity**. Methotrexate is classified as **FDA pregnancy category X**.

(b) **Acitretin (Soriatane)** is a synthetic retinoid (a vitamin A derivative). This agent is normally reserved for patients with severe psoriasis. Acitretin is classified as **FDA pregnancy category X**. Because studies have shown that its parent chemical, etretinate, can be detected in the body up to 2 years after discontinuing therapy, it is recommended that women of child-bearing potential who have taken acitretin not conceive for 3 years following discontinuation of the medication.

(c) **Immunosuppressive medications**—such as cyclosporine (Gengraf), azathioprine (Imuran), and hydroxyurea (Droxia)—may be used in patients with severe psoriasis when other therapies are not tolerated. Of these three agents, cyclosporine is the only one with FDA approval for treatment of psoriasis. Patients taking cyclosporine should be monitored for adverse effects, notably nephrotoxicity, hyperkalemia, and hypertension.

(d) **Biologics** are emerging as a preferred treatment option for patients with moderate-to-severe psoriasis. These agents have been shown to quickly improve psoriasis symptoms. Limits to use of these therapies include their high costs and the fact that they are administered via intramuscular (IM) or intravenous (IV) route. Biologics that have been FDA approved for psoriasis include adalimumab (Humira), alefacept (Amevive), etanercept (Enbrel), infliximab (Remicade), and ustekinumab (Stelara).

(6) **Ultraviolet radiation** (UV) has long been recognized as a safe and effective treatment for managing psoriasis. Varying types of phototherapy are available to patients. All phototherapy treatment regimens should be initiated and managed by a physician or dermatologist.

III. FUNGAL INFECTIONS

A. Overview

1. Fungal skin infections, also known as "**tineas**" or "**ringworm**" (due to its characteristic circular appearance), are some of the most commonly encountered dermatologic conditions. It is estimated that up to 20% of the American population may be infected with a tinea infection at any given time.
2. Several factors may predispose people to becoming infected with a tinea. Fungi grow best in **warm, moist environments**. Tight clothing or shoes that are worn on a repeated basis may facilitate fungal growth. Sharing public showers or pools can also promote the spread of tinea infections. Patients with diseases or conditions that suppress the body's natural immune response (such as diabetes, poor personal hygiene, malnutrition, or a compromised epithelium) are at greater risk of contracting tinea infections.
3. Nonprescription therapies usually work quite well in resolving many types of tinea infections completely.

B. Pathophysiology

1. Tinea infections are typically **superficial**. The fungi that cause tineas thrive on dead skin cells within the stratum corneum. Skin, hair, and nails may all be affected by a tinea infection.
2. The three most prevalent fungi in the United States that cause tinea infections are ***Trichophyton***, ***Microsporum***, and ***Epidermophyton***.
3. Fungi may be transmitted to an unaffected individual either through direct contact with an infected person or animal or through contact with a fomite.

C. Clinical presentation.

Tineas are categorized by the area of the body they affect.

1. **Tinea capitis** is also known as "ringworm of the **scalp**." Tinea capitis occurs more frequently in children than adults. This may be due in part to a lack of social inhibition in sharing items like brushes and combs. Epidermal gland secretions also increase at puberty and have a fungicidal effect.
2. **Tinea corporis**, or "ringworm of the **body**," is not limited to a specific area of the body. Rather, tinea corporis may take on several clinical appearances and can affect any area of the body. Often, patients with tinea corporis are infected with one or more additional tineas.
3. **Tinea cruris** is more commonly referred to as "**jock itch**." The intertriginous areas of the **groin** make it an ideal environment for fungal infections. For anatomical reasons, males are more likely to suffer from tinea cruris than females.
4. **Tinea nigra** is perhaps the least common of the tineas. It is mainly seen in people who live in humid coastal areas and may be transmitted through sand. Tinea nigra is primarily found on fingers and feet.
5. **Tinea pedis**, or "**athlete's foot**," is by far the most common tinea infection. Sports players and people who share pools or showers are at the greatest risk for contracting tinea pedis. Once present, athlete's foot is exacerbated in patients who continue to wear shoes and socks, fostering a warm and moist environment for the fungus to survive.
6. **Tinea unguium**, or **onychomycosis**, is a fungal infection of the **nails**. Toenails are more frequently affected by tinea unguium than fingernails. Onychomycosis can ultimately lead to loss of the affected nail if not treated appropriately.
7. **Tinea versicolor** is a chronic fungal infection of the skin. Tinea versicolor is caused by ***Pityrosporum*** (see II.B.2) and primarily affects people living in hot, humid climates.

D. Treatment

1. **Nonpharmacological measures**
   a. To maintain proper hygiene and to minimize the likelihood of contracting a tinea or spreading a tinea to another person, patients should **wash their body daily** with soap and water.
   b. Any contaminated towels and clothing must be **washed in hot water**.
   c. Patients with tinea infections should be counseled to **avoid sharing towels**.
   d. Allow shoes and clothing to **dry completely** before wearing them.

e. As much as possible, noninfected patients should **avoid direct contact** with and **avoid using the same showers** as people who have fungal infections.
f. If a shower must be shared, patients should be counseled to **wear shower shoes/sandals** while in the shower.

2. **Pharmacological therapies**
   a. **Nonprescription topical medications**
      (1) Only three types of tinea infections respond to self-treatment with nonprescription therapies: **tinea corporis**, **tinea cruris**, and **tinea pedis**. All other tinea infections should be referred to a physician for evaluation and treatment.
      (2) Each of the antifungals listed in the following text is applied topically for 1 to 4 weeks. These agents are generally well-tolerated, and systemic side effects are rare.
         (a) **Butenafine** (Lotrimin Ultra) is available as a 1% cream. Butenafine should only be used in patients 12 and older.
         (b) **Clotrimazole** (Desenex AF Cream, Lotrimin AF Lotion) is also sold as a 1% cream, lotion, or solution. Some patients will experience mild burning and stinging with use of clotrimazole.
         (c) **Miconazole** (Cruex Antifungal Spray Powder, Micatin Jock Itch Cream) is a 2% powder, cream, or lotion and is closely related chemically to clotrimazole.
         (d) **Terbinafine** (Lamisil AT) is available as a 1% cream, gel, or spray. Like butenafine, terbinafine should only be recommended in patients age 12 and older.
         (e) **Tolnaftate** (Tinactin) is a 1% cream, gel, or powder that has served as the OTC standard of care for fungal infections for decades (prior to many of these other products being introduced). Tolnaftate is the only active ingredient that carries FDA approval for both the treatment and prevention of athlete's foot, when used on a daily basis.
         (f) **Undecylenic acid** (Cruex Cream, Fungicure Liquid) is marketed in concentrations of 10% to 25% and comes in multiple forms, including a cream, solution, powder, and spray. Products containing undecylenic acid and its salts carry an unpleasant odor, which may be unacceptable to some patients.
   b. **Prescription treatment options.** Patients who do not respond to self-treatment with any of the OTC therapies described previously **within 1 week** should be referred to their primary care provider for evaluation. If the condition shows improvement within the first week, patients are free to continue with self-treatment.
      (1) **Topical antifungals** are available for use in patients who do not experience resolution of their tinea infection with OTC therapies or who have a tinea infection that cannot be self-treated.
         (a) **Ciclopirox** (Loprox) is available as a cream, gel, or lacquer for the treatment of tinea corporis, cruris, pedis, versicolor, and unguium.
         (b) **Econazole** (Spectazole) 1% cream is indicated for the treatment of tinea corporis, cruris, pedis, and versicolor.
      (2) More severe fungal infections require treatment with **systemic therapies**.
         (a) The **azole antifungals** [**fluconazole** (Diflucan), **itraconazole** (Sporanox), **ketoconazole** (Nizoral), **posaconazole** (Noxafil), and **voriconazole** (Vfend)] are generally well-tolerated. The azoles may cause varying degrees of hepatotoxicity, and the class is notorious for its wide spectrum of drug–drug interactions.
         (b) **Griseofulvin** (Grifulvin V) is available as both an oral tablet and suspension. Because griseofulvin increases photosensitivity, patients taking this agent should avoid prolonged exposure to the sun.
         (c) In addition to its status as an OTC topical agent, **terbinafine** (Lamisil) is also available as a prescription oral antifungal. It is considered the first-line agent for onychomycosis.

IV. ACNE

A. **Overview**

1. **Definition.** Acne vulgaris is a disorder of the pilosebaceous units, mainly of the face, chest, and back. The lesions usually start as open or closed comedones and evolve into inflammatory papules and pustules that either resolve as macules or become secondary pyoderma, which results in various sequelae.

2. **Incidence**
   a. Acne vulgaris is the **most common** skin disease of adolescence; it affects about 85% of all people between the ages of 12 and 24.
   b. It affects primarily adolescents in middle school and high school, then decreases in adulthood.
3. **Importance**
   a. Acne vulgaris is usually **self-limiting**.
   b. However, the condition is significant to adolescents because of heightened self-consciousness about appearance.
   c. A great majority of people do not consult a physician for treatment of acne; therefore, a pharmacist can play a significant role.

B. **Origins and pathophysiology**
1. The **pathogenesis** of acne vulgaris involves **three events**.
   a. **Increased sebum production**
      (1) Sebum secretion is regulated primarily by **androgens**, which are actively secreted in both sexes beginning at puberty.
      (2) One of these androgens, testosterone, is converted to **dihydrotestosterone** (**DHT**).
      (3) DHT levels induce the sebaceous glands to increase in size and activity, resulting in increased amounts of sebum.
   b. **Abnormal clumping of epithelial horny cells within the pilosebaceous unit**
      (1) Normally, keratinized horny cells are sloughed from the epithelial lining of the pilosebaceous duct in the hair follicles and are carried to the skin surface with a flow of sebum.
      (2) In the patient with acne, the keratinization process is abnormal, characterized by increased adherence and production of follicular epithelial cells. This process is called **retention hyperkeratosis**, and it results in obstruction of the outflow of the pilosebaceous unit.
   c. **Presence of *Propionibacterium acnes*** (a gram-positive anaerobe)
      (1) People with acne have skin colony counts of *P. acnes* that are significantly higher than the counts of those without acne.
      (2) *P. acnes* produces several enzymes, including lipases, that break down sebum triglycerides to short chain free fatty acids (FFAs), which are irritating, cause comedones, and result in inflammation.
2. **Sequence of acne lesion development**
   a. Mechanical blockage of a pilosebaceous duct by clumped horny cells results in a **closed comedo** (i.e., **a whitehead**).
   b. When a closed comedo develops, it can form either a papule or an **open comedo** (i.e., **a blackhead**). The **dark color** of the blackhead is attributed to a combination of melanin, oxidized lipid, and keratinocytes, **not** to **dirt**.
   c. The lesion may enlarge and fill with pus, which is then termed a pustule.
   d. In more severe cases of acne, papules may develop into nodules or cysts.
   e. The term *pimple* nonspecifically refers to whiteheads, blackheads, papules, and pustules.

C. **Clinical features**
1. **Location.** Acne vulgaris lesions usually occur on the face, neck, chest, upper back, and shoulders. Any or all types of lesions may be seen on a single patient.
2. **Symptoms.** This condition is usually asymptomatic; however, some patients may have pruritus or pain if large, tender lesions are present.
3. **Classification.** It is important to differentiate **noninflammatory** from **inflammatory** acne to determine the best treatment approach. There have been many rating or grading scales for acne severity (*Table 20-2*). **Cystic acne** is present when the follicular wall ruptures occur deeper in the dermis and nodules and cysts are seen. Because of the potential for scarring, cystic acne patients should be referred to a physician for treatment. Scarring occurs with hypertrophic ridges, keloids, or atrophic "ice pick" pits.

D. **Complicating factors.** Other factors have been implicated in the exacerbation of acne.
1. **Drugs and hormones**
   a. Many topical and systemic medications (e.g., bromides, iodides, topical coal tar products, androgens, phenytoin, progestins, lithium, corticosteroids) can be comedogenic and can make acne worse or can induce acnelike eruptions (i.e., acneiform lesions).

TABLE 20-2 ASSESSMENT OF ACNE SEVERITY

Grade of Acne	Qualitative Description	Quantitative Description
Comedonal		
I	Comedonal acne	Comedones only, < 10 on face, none on trunk, no scars; noninflammatory lesions only
	Blackheads	Open comedo; dilated hair follicle with open orifice to skin
		Dark color may be caused by oxidation of melanin or compacted epithelial cells; presence of lipids may contribute
	Whiteheads	Closed comedo; dilated hair follicle filled with keratin, sebum, and bacteria with obstructed opening to the skin
Papulopustular		
II	Papular acne	10–25 papules on face and trunk, mild scarring; inflammatory lesions < 5 mm in diameter
III[a]	Pustular acne	More than 25 pustules, moderate scarring; size similar to papules but with visible, purulent core
IV[a]	Severe/persistent pustulocystic acne	Nodules or cysts, extensive scarring; inflammatory lesions > 5 mm in diameter
	Recalcitrant severe cystic acne	Extensive nodules/cysts

[a] Some overlap with previous grade of acne.
Reprinted with permission from Foster KT, Coffey CW. Table 37-2. Acne. In: Krinsky DL, Berardi RR, Ferreri SP, et al., eds. *Handbook of Nonprescription Drugs: An Interactive Approach to Self-Care*. 17th ed. Washington, DC: American Pharmacists Association; 2012;696.

b. **Acneiform eruptions** differ from true acne lesions in that apparently no comedones form, eruptions are usually acute, and the lesions usually are all in the same stage of development.

2. **Stress** does not cause acne but may exacerbate it.
3. **Diet.** There is little evidence to support a relationship between diet and acne. Many different foods have been blamed for acne, from chocolates and sweets to shellfish to nuts and other fatty foods. Conflicting evidence exists on the effect of chocolate upon acne, making it difficult to say definitively that chocolate does or does not affect acne. Most dermatologists today make the following recommendations regarding diet:
   a. The patient should eat a well-balanced diet. As with most other diseases, and as a matter of good health, excess fats and simple carbohydrates should be avoided.
   b. The patient who insists that certain foods cause exacerbation of acne should probably avoid those foods.
4. **Physical trauma** or **irritation** can promote the rupture of plugged follicles, which can produce more inflammatory reactions. Scrubbing the face, wearing headbands, cradling the chin with the hand, and picking at the pimples can contribute to the primary inflammation process. **Gentle**, regular **washing** with soap and water can be beneficial.
5. **Cosmetics.** Some cosmetic bases and certain cosmetic ingredients are comedogenic (e.g., lanolins, petroleum bases, cocoa butter). Preparations such as cleansing creams, suntan oils, and heavy foundations should be avoided.
6. **Menstrual cycle.** Some women may notice flare-ups of acne during the premenstrual phase of the cycle. Fluctuations in the level of progesterone are the probable cause.
7. **Environmental factors.** Very humid environments or heavy sweating lead to keratin hydration, swelling, and a decrease in the size of the pilosebaceous follicle orifice, which results in duct obstruction. The sun, as well as artificial UV light, can help acne by drying and peeling the skin, but both can also aggravate acne.

E. **Treatment and care**

1. **General**
   a. Most patients can be treated successfully with either topically or systemically administered medications or both. Acne often improves when patients reach their early 20s.
   b. Even the most effective treatment programs may take several weeks to produce any clinical improvement. This aspect must be emphasized.

c. People affected with acne should avoid anything that seems to worsen the condition (e.g., cosmetics, clothing, cradling the chin with the hand).

d. The number and type of lesions should be roughly determined to assess further therapeutic responses.

e. **Self-treatment with OTC agents** is appropriate only for patients with **noninflammatory grade I acne** of mild to moderate severity.

2. **Cleansing recommendations**

a. Because many acne patients have oily skin, **gentle cleansing** two to three times daily is recommended for removing excess oil.

b. Acne lesions cannot be scrubbed away. Compulsive scrubbing may actually worsen the acne by disrupting the follicular walls and thus setting the stage for inflammation.

c. Mild facial soaps, such as Dove, Neutrogena, and Purpose, should be used to cleanse the skin.

d. Medicated soaps containing sulfur, resorcinol, or salicylic acid are of little value because the medication rinses away rather than penetrates the follicle.

e. Patients with mild comedonal acne might benefit from cleansers containing pumice, polyethylene, or aluminum oxide particles (e.g., Brasivol). However, patients with inflammatory acne or sensitive skin should avoid these products.

3. **Approaches** to treatment depend on the severity of the condition. Although acne cannot be cured, most cases can be managed successfully with topical treatment alone. Based on the pathogenesis of the condition, potential methods include

a. **Unblocking** the sebaceous duct so that the contents can be easily expelled.

b. **Decreasing** the amount of sebum that is secreted.

c. **Changing** the composition of the **sebum** to make it less irritating by decreasing the population of *P. acnes*.

4. **Nonprescription topical medications**

a. **Benzoyl peroxide** (2.5% to 10%)—for example, PanOxyl Aqua Gel—has traditionally been recognized as the most effective topical OTC agent for acne, and many OTC acne products contain it. For some time, benzoyl peroxide was considered a category III agent by the FDA, stemming from a lack of clear proof regarding its safety and efficacy. However, in 2010, benzoyl peroxide was reclassified as category I [agents that are generally recognized as safe and effective (GRASE)].

(1) **Effects.** Benzoyl peroxide has irritant, drying, peeling, comedolytic, and antibacterial effects. The clinical response shows only minimal differences among the 2.5%, 5.0%, and 10% concentrations.

(a) A **beneficial effect** should be noticed within about 2 weeks, but the usual length of a therapeutic trial is 6 to 8 weeks.

(b) As for **adverse effects**, benzoyl peroxide may cause a burning or stinging sensation, which gradually disappears. Most of the adverse effects from this agent relate to its therapeutic effect of irritating and drying the skin. For this reason, the lowest concentration available should be chosen initially. About **2.5%** of patients will **develop a contact dermatitis** with its use.

(c) The vehicle for benzoyl peroxide is also important in its overall activity. The alcohol gel vehicle tends to be more effective than the lotion or cream formulations.

(d) Benzoyl peroxide can discolor certain types of fabric or clothing material and can also bleach hair.

(2) **Mechanism of action.** Benzoyl peroxide has a dual mode of action, so it is effective against both inflammatory and noninflammatory acne.

(a) Benzoyl peroxide decomposes to release oxygen, which is lethal to the *P. acnes* anaerobe.

(b) As an irritant, it increases the turnover rate of epithelial cells, resulting in increased sloughing and promoting resolution of comedones.

(3) **Application**

(a) The affected area should be washed with mild soap and water, then gently patted dry.

(b) The product should be massaged gently into the skin, avoiding the eyes, mouth, lips, and inside of the nose.

(c) The product can be applied at night, left on for 15 to 20 mins to test sensitivity, then washed off.
(d) If no excessive irritation develops, apply once daily for the first few days.
(e) If drying, redness, or peeling does not occur in 3 days, increase application to twice daily.
(f) If patients have to use benzoyl peroxide during the day, advise them to use a sunscreen and avoid unnecessary sun exposure.

b. **Salicylic acid** (0.5% to 2.0%), an irritant keratolytic agent, results in increased turnover of the epithelial lining. Through this effect, salicylic acid probably promotes the penetration of other acne products.

c. **Sulfur** (3% to 8%), **sulfur** (3% to 8%) **combined with resorcinol** (2%), **or resorcinol monoacetate** (3%)—for example, Clearasil Adult Care Acne Treatment Cream, Acnomel
(1) Sulfur is a keratolytic agent and has antibacterial actions.
(2) Sulfur traditionally has been recognized as a less desirable product because it may be acnegenic with continued use, and it has an offensive color and odor.

d. **Resorcinol** is a keratolytic agent that has been recognized as safe and effective against acne **when the agent is combined with sulfur**.

F. **Prescription medications, both topical and systemic**, are included here for completeness and to put into perspective how OTC agents fit into acne therapy.

1. **Topical prescription agents**

a. **Tretinoin** (vitamin A acid, *trans*-retinoic acid, Retin-A) increases the turnover rate of nonadhering horny cells in the follicular canal, which results in comedo clearing and inhibits new comedo development.
(1) **Effectiveness.** Tretinoin is probably the most effective topical agent for acne, especially acne characterized by comedones. It is best used for **noninflammatory** acne. Tretinoin also may be used in combination with antibiotics or benzoyl peroxide for management of inflammatory acne.
(2) **Side effects.** Because of its irritant properties, tretinoin can cause **excessive irritation**, **erythema**, **peeling**, and increased risk for **severe sunburn**. There may be an initial exacerbation of the acne (pustular flare) at 2 to 4 weeks, but usually by 8 weeks, the patient will see marked improvement. Because this agent may cause photosensitivity, it should generally be applied at night.
(3) **Application.** The cream formulation of tretinoin, which is less irritating than the gel form, should be used initially for patients with dryer skin. The patient with very oily skin may do well initially with the gel form. The retinoids should be applied 30 mins after washing because moisture on the skin increases absorption and irritation. To minimize irritation, initially such a product can be applied every other day for 2 weeks, then daily. Other irritating substances, such as strong abrasive cleaners and astringents, should be avoided during treatment with tretinoin. Newer microsize reformulations of this agent (Retin-A Micro, Avita) are less irritating.

b. **Adapalene** (Differin) is a topical retinoid-like compound that is dosed once daily. It can be applied in the morning because of no photodegradation, and it has less potential for photosensitivity.
(1) **Effectiveness**. It appears to cause less irritation than tretinoin with equivalent efficacy. Therapeutic results should be noticed in 8 to 12 weeks. It can be used as an alternative to tretinoin in individuals with mild to moderate acne.
(2) **Side effects**. The same precautions that apply to tretinoin apply also for adapalene.

c. **Tazarotene gel and cream** (Tazorac) is a retinoid prodrug for mild to moderately severe facial acne that is applied once daily in the evening. It has similar efficacy and precautions as tretinoin, and the dose-related **adverse effects** include itching, burning, stinging, and erythema (redness). The gel form appears to be more irritating than tretinoin. A pustular flare may occur at about 10 to 14 days after this product is begun.

d. **Topical antibiotics: erythromycin** (Eryderm), **clindamycin** (Cleocin-T) and **tetracycline**. These topical antibiotics are most effective when used in combination with benzoyl peroxide or topical retinoids. Combination products containing benzoyl peroxide and erythromycin

(Benzamycin) and benzoyl peroxide and clindamycin (BenzaClin) are also available. When these antibiotics are used alone, bacterial resistance occurs rapidly. Benzoyl peroxide use in combination with these antibiotics protects against this resistance.

(1) **Mechanism of action.** The mechanism of action apparently involves suppression of the *P. acnes* organism, which in turn minimizes the inflammatory response due to the acne.

(2) **Application.** These antibiotics are applied directly to acne sites, thus minimizing serious side effects from oral administration.

(3) **Side effects.** There are **minimal** side effects to these topically applied antibiotics. **Mild burning** or **irritation** may occur. Although daily topical **clindamycin** does not produce detectable levels in the urine after 8 weeks of administration, there is a potential risk of **pseudomembranous colitis. Tetracycline** can cause a **yellow staining of the skin**.

e. **Azelaic acid** (Azelex) and **sodium sulfacetamide and sulfur** are additional topical agents that are less effective than the other topical prescription agents. These agents might be used when others are not tolerated or as adjuncts to other therapies.

2. **Systemic prescription agents**

a. **Oral antibiotics/anti-infectives** are the most effective agents against inflammatory lesions because they suppress *P. acnes*. They may be used when topical combinations are not tolerated or have failed. Oral antibiotics have an onset of action of 3 to 4 weeks. They are prescribed for daily use over 4 to 6 months and then tapered and ultimately discontinued with acne improvement. Antibiotics do not affect existing lesions, but prevent future lesions through this effect. *P. acnes* resistance to antibiotic therapy has become an increasing problem; erythromycin resistance is the most commonly reported, and minocycline resistance is reported rarely. As noted previously, concomitant administration of benzoyl peroxide may decrease the incidence of resistance.

(1) **Tetracycline** is the **most frequently used** oral antibiotic for acne. It is preferred because of its effectiveness, low toxicity, and low cost. This agent should be taken on an empty stomach; food, antacids, iron, and dairy products decrease absorption. Tetracycline also has direct anti-inflammatory effects in acne.

(a) **Initial dose** is 250 mg, two to four times daily, gradually reduced to a maintenance dose of about 250 mg per day.

(b) **Side effects.** The more common adverse effects include upset stomach, vaginal moniliasis, and photosensitivity.

(2) **Erythromycin** (E-Mycin) may be used as an alternative to tetracycline.

(a) **Initial doses** range from 500 to 2000 mg per day in divided doses. A maintenance dose ranges from 250 to 500 mg per day.

(b) **Side effects.** The primary side effect associated with erythromycin is gastrointestinal distress.

(3) **Minocycline** (Minocin) **or doxycycline** (Vibramycin). Either of these agents can be taken in doses of 50 to 200 mg per day. Because of greater lipid solubility and enhanced penetration into sebaceous follicles, these agents may be useful for refractory cases. Either can be taken if bacterial resistance is suspected to erythromycin or if intolerable gastric irritation occurs after oral tetracycline. These two agents can be taken with food. Side effects to minocycline, including dizziness or vertigo and headache, discoloration of skin and visceral tissue, and drug-induced lupus erythematosus, limit the use of this agent. Doxycycline may be photosensitizing and should be swallowed with adequate fluids to prevent esophageal ulcerations.

(4) **Trimethoprim-sulfamethoxazole** (Bactrim, Septra) has been used successfully in patients with acne resistant to erythromycin or tetracyclines. Minocycline and doxycycline are preferred over this drug combination because of its side-effect profile. **Oral clindamycin** (Cleocin) is used rarely because of the risk of pseudomembranous colitis.

b. **Oral isotretinoin** (Accutane) is a vitamin A derivative indicated for **severe nodulocystic acne**. A single course of therapy results in a long-term stable remission in $>$ 80% of patients.

(1) **Mechanism of action.** Although the exact mechanism is unknown, isotretinoin decreases sebum production and keratinization, and it reduces the population of *P. acnes*.

(2) **Dosage.** Treatment is usually begun with a daily dose of 0.5 mg/kg and increased to 1 mg/kg given in two divided doses with food for the usual duration of 20 weeks. A micronized formulation allows for lower once daily dosing with no regard to food intake.

(3) **Side effects** include

(a) **Mucocutaneous dryness.** Cheilitis (i.e., inflammation of the lips), dryness of the nasal mucosa, and facial dermatitis may occur with isotretinoin use. These effects can be treated with topical lubricants. Dryness of the eyes can also occur, so people using isotretinoin should not wear contact lenses.

(b) **Elevated serum levels.** Isotretinoin may elevate serum triglycerides and cholesterol, as well as liver enzymes.

(c) **Birth defects.** Isotretinoin is a **potent teratogen** and should not be given to pregnant women. A strict risk management program for isotretinoin use requires physicians to register patients to document negative pregnancy tests before use. Physicians who prescribe this agent and pharmacies that dispense it must be registered in an electronic FDA system.

(d) **Psychiatric effects.** There have been reports of depression, suicidal behavior, and suicide. Data are inadequate to establish a causal relationship between isotretinoin administration and depression and suicide. This information must be taken in the context that teenagers with acne may often be depressed related to their appearance.

c. **Antiandrogens and hormones**

(1) **Estrogens** can decrease sebum production through an antiandrogenic effect.

(2) Some progestin agents in oral contraceptives (e.g., norethindrone, norgestrel) have androgenic activity that can stimulate sebum secretion resulting in acne. One of the progestins, **norgestimate**, is minimally androgenic, and when it is combined with **ethinyl estradiol** as a triphasic combination oral contraceptive agent (Ortho Tri-Cyclen), it is effective in the treatment of moderate acne in some women and is FDA approved for such. **Norethindrone acetate/ethinyl estradiol** (Estrostep) is also FDA approved for acne.

(3) **Spironolactone** (**Aldactone**) is an oral antiandrogen which acts to decrease sebum production and may be used on a limited basis.

(4) **Corticosteroids.** Although corticosteroids have been implicated as causing acne, they also can be used to treat severe acne. Intralesional injections of triamcinolone and systemic corticosteroids have been used for severe inflammatory acne and severe cystic acne, respectively. Prednisone (or its equivalent) in doses of 20 mg per day or higher may be used for a short period to quickly improve acne for important events like a wedding. Topical corticosteroids are not effective.

V. DRY SKIN

A. **Overview**

1. The clinical term for dry skin is "**xerosis**."
2. The incidence of dry skin increases with age. It is estimated that over 50% of adults suffer with dry skin.
3. Dry skin occurs most often during the winter months.

B. **Pathophysiology.** Dry skin results when the stratum corneum does not retain enough water. This may result from several factors:

1. **Frequent washing and bathing** (defined as multiple times in a day)
2. **Overuse of soap** or other cleaning products that remove the skin's natural oils
3. Environments with **excessively dry air and low humidity**
4. **Inadequate fluid intake**
5. **Thinning of the epidermis** (particularly in geriatric patients)
6. Other chronic conditions, such as psoriasis, thyroid disorders, smoking, or malnutrition

C. **Clinical presentation**

1. Dry skin is most frequently characterized by **pruritus**.
2. Other signs of dry skin include a "**cracked**" **appearance to the epidermis**, **flaking or sloughing of skin cells**, and a **decrease in skin flexibility**.

D. **Treatment**

1. **Nonpharmacological measures**

a. **Bathing**

(1) Patients who suffer with dry skin should be counseled on bathing or showering for **brief periods** (3 to 5 mins) with **lukewarm** water.

(2) When bathing, patients should wash with **bath oils** (such as mineral oil), **colloidal oatmeal products** (such as Aveeno Soothing Bath Treatment Formula), or **mild cleansers** with ingredients like petrolatum and glycerin (such as Cetaphil Gentle Cleansing Bar). Many of these products will make the tub and surrounding area slippery; care must be taken when getting in and out of the bathtub while using these therapies.

(3) Immediately after stepping out of the bathtub or shower, patients should **pat themselves dry** with a soft towel (rather than rubbing all the moisture from their skin with a more aggressive drying technique).

b. Patients with dry skin should be counseled to **drink at least 64 oz of water a day** (unless preexisting medical conditions prevent them from doing so).

c. Patients who smoke should be counseled on **smoking cessation** strategies. **Caffeine and alcohol should also be avoided**, as these can exacerbate dry skin.

d. **Humidifiers** may be used to increase the moisture in the air around the patient, particularly in rooms of the house in which the patient spends lots of time (such as their bedroom).

e. **Sunscreen** should be worn whenever the patient will be outdoors.

2. **Pharmacological therapies**

a. **Emollients** (commonly referred to as **moisturizers**) soften and soothe the skin by filling the epidermis with tiny beads of oil. These products come in several different formulations, available in lotions, creams, and ointments. Emollients work best when applied to damp skin (immediately after exiting the shower, for example). Examples of emollient products include Eucerin Cream, Lubriderm Advanced Therapy Lotion, and Udderly Smooth Udder Cream. These products contain various combinations of multiple ingredients, including water, glycerin, mineral oil, and lanolin.

b. **Humectants** draw moisture into the affected area from the air and surrounding tissue. Humectants are commonly added to emollient products. Examples include glycerin, sorbitol, and propylene glycol.

c. **Keratin** is a protein that is found in the skin, hair, and nails. **Keratin-softening agents**, such as urea and lactic acid, can be found in single-ingredient products (such as Carmol 10 Lotion and Lac-Hydrin Five Lotion) or in combination with emollient products.

d. **Astringents** suppress inflammation associated with dry skin, as well as clear away the "debris" of dead skin cells. Patients should be counseled to soak a washcloth in the astringent solution and apply it to the affected area for 15 to 30 mins several times a day. Aluminum acetate (Domeboro Astringent Solution) and witch hazel are the two most commonly recommended astringents.

e. **Hydrocortisone** may be employed to treat the symptoms of inflammation and itching associated with dry skin, but it should not be used as monotherapy in the treatment of dry skin. Hydrocortisone should never be used for more than 7 days without first consulting with a physician; it is important to ensure that the patient's itching is not associated with a more serious underlying disorder.

VI. SUNLIGHT, SUNSCREENS, AND SUNTAN PRODUCTS

A. **Introduction.** Overexposure to sunlight damages skin. A suntan, which has traditionally been associated with health, is actually a response to injury. Of the three types of solar radiation, only the UV spectrum produces sunburn and suntan.

1. The **UV spectrum** ranges from 200 to 400 nanometers (nm). Natural and artificial UV light is further subdivided into three bands.

a. **UVA** (320 to 400 nm) can cause the skin to tan, and it tends to be weak in causing the skin to redden. UVA is about 1,000 times less potent than a comparable dose of UVB in causing erythema, but it is only slightly blocked out by the ozone layer and reaches the earth's surface in 10 to 100 times the amount of UVB. Some have proposed that UVA be further subdivided into UVA I (340 to 400 nm) and UVA II (320 to 340 nm). UVA I is less erythrogenic and melanogenic than UVA II or UVB. UVA II is similar in effect to UVB.

(1) **Uses.** UVA is often used in tanning booths and in psoralen plus UVA (PUVA) treatment of psoriasis.

(2) **Disadvantages.** UVA is responsible for many **photosensitivity** reactions, **photoaging**, and **photodermatoses**. UVA rays can also **penetrate deeply into the dermis** and augment the cancerous effects of UVB rays.

b. **UVB** (290 to 320 nm) **causes the usual sunburn reaction** and stimulates tanning. It has long been associated with sunlight skin damage, including the various skin cancers. It is the **most erythrogenic** and **melanogenic** of the three UV radiation bands. Small amounts of this radiation are required for normal **vitamin D synthesis** in the skin.

c. **UVC** (200 to 290 nm) does not reach the earth's surface because most of it is absorbed by the ozone layer. Artificial UVC sources (e.g., germicidal and mercury arc lamps) can emit this radiation.

2. The **visible spectrum** (400 to 770 nm) produces the "brightness" of the sun.
3. The **infrared spectrum** (770 to 1800 nm) produces the "warmth" of the sun.

B. **Sunburn and suntan**

1. **Sunburn** is generally a **superficial burn involving the epidermis**. This layer is rapidly repaired while old cells are being sloughed off in a process called **peeling**. The newly formed skin is thicker and offers protection for the lower dermal layers.

a. **Normal sequence after mild to moderate sunlight UV radiation (UVR) exposure**

(1) Erythema occurs within 20 to 30 mins as a result of oxidation of bleached melanin and dilation of dermal venules.

(2) The initial erythema rapidly fades, and true sunburn erythema begins 2 to 8 hrs after initial exposure to the sun.

(3) Dilation of the arterioles results in increased vascular permeability, localized edema, and pain, which become maximal after 14 to 20 hrs and last 24 to 72 hrs.

b. **Manifestations** range from mild (a slight reddening of the skin) to severe (formation of blisters and desquamation). If the effect is severe, the patient may experience pain, swelling, and blistering. Fever, chills, and nausea may also develop, as well as prostration, which is related to excessive synthesis and diffusion of prostaglandins.

2. **Suntan** is the result of two processes:

a. **Oxidation of melanin**, which is already present in the epidermis

b. **Stimulation of melanocytes** to produce additional melanin, which is subsequently oxidized on further exposure to sunlight

(1) With increased melanin production, the melanocytes introduce the pigment into keratin-producing cells, which gradually become darkened keratin and a full suntan in 2 to 10 days.

(2) Tanning increases tolerance to additional sunlight and reduces the likelihood of subsequent burning. However, dark skin is not totally immune to sunburn.

(3) There is little evidence to suggest that obtaining a "base tan" from a tanning booth will reduce the likelihood of sunburn.

C. **Factors affecting exposure to UVR**

1. **Time of day and season.** The greatest exposure to harmful UVB rays occurs between 10 A.M. and 4 P.M. in midsummer. UVA rays are fairly continuous throughout the day and season.
2. **Altitude.** Sunburn is more likely to occur at high altitudes. UVB intensity increases 4% with each 1,000-ft increase in altitude.
3. **Environmental factors.** Atmospheric conditions (e.g., smog, haze, smoke) may affect (i.e., decrease) the amount of UVR reaching the skin. Although direct sunlight greatly reduces the amount of UV exposure needed to produce a burn, sunburn can occur without it. For example, sunburn can also develop on a cloudy day because there is some UVR penetration through cloud layers (60% to 80%). However, the **reflection of light rays** (e.g., by snow, sand, water) greatly **increases** the amount of UV **exposure to sunlight**.
4. **Predisposing factors.** People with fair skin and light hair are at greater risk for developing sunburn and other UVR skin damage than their darker counterparts.

D. **Other reactions to sunlight (UVR) exposure**
   1. **Actinic keratosis** is a precancerous condition and may occur after many years of excessive exposure to sunlight. Typically arising during middle age or later, this disorder manifests as a sharply demarcated, roughened, or hardened growth, which may be flat or raised, and it may progress to **squamous cell carcinoma**.
   2. **Skin cancer.** Chronic overexposure to sunlight may lead to **squamous cell carcinoma**, **basal cell carcinoma**, or **malignant melanoma**.
      a. **Squamous cell carcinoma.** Lesions usually appear as thickened, rough, scaly patches, which can bleed, and most commonly develops from actinic keratosis. It accounts for about 15% of skin cancers.
      b. **Basal cell carcinoma.** This is the most common of all skin cancers and accounts for about 80% of skin cancers. It may appear as pearly or translucent bumps and originates in the basal cells.
      c. **Malignant melanoma.** Malignant melanoma originates from melanocytes and is the deadliest form of skin cancer, and its incidence has been increasing. Moles should be watched for indications of malignancy—the **ABCDs** are
         (1) Asymmetrical shape
         (2) Border irregularity
         (3) Color that is nonuniform
         (4) Diameter > 6 mm
      d. Malignant melanoma formation may be associated with intense, intermittent overexposure to the sun (sunburning).
   3. **Drug-induced photosensitivity reactions**
      a. **Types**
         (1) **Photoallergy reactions** occur when light makes a drug become antigenic or act as a hapten (i.e., a photoallergen). These reactions also require previous contact with the offending drug. Photoallergy reactions are relatively **rare** and are associated more frequently with topically applied agents than with oral medications.
            (a) **Occurrence** of these reactions is not dose related. The patient is usually cross-sensitive with chemically related compounds.
            (b) **Rashes** are most prominent on light-exposed sites (i.e., face, neck, forearms, back of hands), and they usually occur, after an incubation period of 24 to 48 hrs of combined drug and sun exposure, as an intensely pruritic eczematous dermatitis (a severe rash).
         (2) **Phototoxic reactions** occur when light alters a drug to a toxic form, which results in tissue damage that is independent of an allergic response.
            (a) **Occurrence.** These reactions are usually dose related, and the patient usually has no cross-sensitivity to other agents.
            (b) **Rashes** often appear as an exaggerated sunburn and are usually confined to areas of combined chemical and light exposure.
      b. **Implicated drugs.** Many drugs have been implicated in causing photoallergy and phototoxic reactions: thiazides, tetracyclines, phenothiazines, sulfonamides, and even sunscreens. Some drugs may produce both types of reactions.
      c. **Prevention.** Standard sunscreens do not always prevent photosensitivity reactions caused by drugs. UV light above 320 nm (i.e., UVA light) has been implicated in inducing photosensitivity reactions, so a chemical or physical sunscreen must cover this spectrum (see VI.E.2).
   4. **Photodermatoses** are skin conditions that are triggered or worsened by light within specific wavelengths. These conditions include polymorphous light eruption (PMLE), lupus erythematosus, and solar urticaria.
   5. **Photoaging** is a skin condition that is not merely an acceleration of normal aging. UVA radiation is thought to be involved. The skin appears dry, scaly, yellow, and deeply wrinkled; it is also thinner and more fragile.

E. **Sunscreen agents.** People can protect their skin from harmful UVR by avoiding exposure to sunlight and other sources of UVR, wearing protective clothing, and applying sunscreen.
   1. **Application and general information.** All exposed areas should be covered evenly and liberally (2 mg/cm^2, which requires about 1 oz of sunscreen per one total body application for an

average-size adult in a swimsuit) with sunscreen, optimally 30 mins [(2 hrs for para-aminobenzoic acid (PABA) and PABA esters)] before sun exposure to allow for penetration and binding to the skin.

a. **Substantivity.** Perspiration, swimming, sand, towels, and clothing tend to remove sunscreen and may increase the need for reapplication.
   (1) Substantivity is the ability of a sunscreen formulation to adhere to the skin while swimming or perspiring.
   (2) **Water resistant** labeling indicates that the formula retains its sun protection factor (SPF) after 40 mins of activity in the water, sweating, or perspiring.
   (3) Labeling a product as **very water resistant** indicates that the product retains SPF after 80 mins of activity in the water, sweating, or perspiring.

b. **Protection.** Sunscreen products vary widely in their ability to protect against sunburn; the SPF and UVA/UVB ray protection should be noted to determine the level of protection. Moreover, baby oil, mineral oil, olive oil, and cocoa butter are not sunscreens (but are often used to attain a tan).
   (1) **SPF** gives the consumer a guide for determining how the product will protect the skin from UV rays, principally UVB rays. An SPF of 30 blocks about 97% of the UVB rays. Scientific evidence shows a point of diminishing returns at levels > 30; any benefits that might be derived from using sunscreens with an SPF > 30 are negligible. The FDA's most recent monograph requires sunscreens with an SPF > 50 to be labeled as "SPF 50+," as clinical evidence suggests no additional UV protection above SPF 50. The American Academy of Dermatology recommends that adults and children use sunscreens with an SPF of **at least 30**.
      (a) **Definitions.** A **minimal sun protection product** has an SPF of 2 to less than 12; a **moderate sun protection product** has an SPF of 12 to less than 30; a **high sun protection product** has an SPF of 30 or more.
      (b) **Derivation.** SPF is defined as the **minimal erythema dose** (**MED**) of protected skin divided by the MED of unprotected skin. MED is the amount of solar radiation needed to produce minimal skin redness.
      (c) **Example.** A person who usually gets red after 20 mins in the sun and wants to stay in the sun for 2 hrs (120 mins) should apply a sunscreen with an SPF of 6 (120 mins $\div$ 20 mins $=$ SPF 6). An SPF 6 product should provide adequate coverage, provided it is not washed off (as from swimming) or dissolved by sweat. An SPF of 15 blocks approximately 93% of the UVB rays.
      (d) Until now, there has been **no generally accepted comparable term that measures UVA protection**, although a few have been proposed. One major concern is that people may be staying out in the sun longer when they use sunscreen products that have high SPF values. If inadequate UVA protection is provided in that product, these individuals may be exposing themselves to very high amounts of UVA, with the potential for significant overexposure to this form of UV radiation.
   (2) **Skin cancer prevention.** Sunscreen application has been shown to prevent squamous cell carcinoma, but it is not absolutely confirmed that their use prevents melanoma. In fact, some studies have found that individuals who regularly use sunscreen have a higher risk of this cancer (perhaps because they can stay out in the sun longer before burning and thus experience longer periods of sun exposure).

c. **Sensitivity.** Some people may be hypersensitive to sunscreen agents. Discontinue use if signs of irritation or a rash occur. Contact dermatitis may occur with some of these agents. If sensitive to benzocaine, procaine, sulfonamides, or thiazides, avoid PABA or PABA esters.

d. **Specific information**
   (1) Do not use these products on infants younger than 6 months of age (there is concern about absorption of these agents).
   (2) Do not use a product with an SPF < 4 on children younger than 2 years of age (there is concern that an SPF < 4 will not provide adequate protection).
   (3) Recommend sunscreen products that are broad-spectrum sunscreens (i.e., that block both UVB and UVA).

2. The two basic **types of sunscreen agents** are physical sun blocks and chemical sunscreens (*Table 20-3*).
   a. **Physical sun blocks** are opaque formulations that reflect and scatter up to 99% of light in both the UV and visible spectrums (290 to 700 nm). Examples include **titanium dioxide** and **zinc oxide**. These sun blocks are less cosmetically acceptable than chemical sunscreens because they have a greasy appearance, but they may be useful for protecting small areas (e.g., the nose). These sun blocks are also useful for photosensitization protection. Newer, more dilute versions of titanium dioxide products and microfine, transparent forms of zinc oxide are more cosmetically appealing. Red petrolatum covers a lesser spectrum (290 to 365 nm).
   b. **Chemical sunscreens** act by absorbing a specific portion of the UV light spectrum to keep it from penetrating the skin. They can be categorized on the basis of their spectra of UVR blockage and basic chemical classification. Five main groups of chemical sunscreens are available.
      (1) **PABA** and **PABA esters** primarily absorb UVB rays. Examples are *p*-aminobenzoic acid, padimate O, and glyceryl PABA.
      (2) **Cinnamates** primarily absorb UVB rays. Examples are cinoxate and octyl methoxycinnamate.
      (3) **Salicylates** primarily absorb UVB rays. Examples are ethylhexyl salicylate and homosalate.
      (4) **Benzophenones** absorb UVB rays and sometimes extend into the UVA range. Examples are oxybenzone and dioxybenzone. Because of their extension into the UVA range, they are somewhat protective against photosensitivity reactions.
      (5) **Dibenzoylmethane derivatives. Avobenzone (Parsol 1789)** or butyl methoxydibenzoylmethane, provides coverage over the entire UVA range although its absorbance decreases dramatically at 370 nm. Photosensitivity reactions from medications may not be completely prevented in the 370 to 400 nm range. In combination with other agents that cover the UVB range, reasonable protection for both the UVA and UVB ranges can be achieved. It is the only available agent that blocks UVA wavelengths up to 400 nm.
      (6) **Other chemical sunscreens. Phenylbenzimidazole sulfonic acid** does not match up with any of the classes mentioned. It covers just the UVB range 290 to 320 nm.
      (7) **Ecamsule**, an agent incorporated into a combination product (Anthelios SX) with avobenzone and octocrylene, protects against both UVA and UVB.
   c. **OTC sunscreen products.** Most sunscreen products on the market contain combinations of two or more of the classes of chemical sunscreen agents described in preceding sections. To get adequate UVA protection, choose a product with avobenzone or a product with titanium dioxide or zinc oxide.

VII. WARTS

A. Overview

1. Warts are caused by the **human papillomavirus (HPV)**.
2. It is estimated that 7% to 10% of people have some type of wart.
3. Most warts will resolve on their own in as little as 6 months to as long as 5 years.

B. Pathophysiology

1. HPV is transmitted from an infected individual to a noninfected individual via **skin-to-skin contact**. Infected skin cells that have been shed from the host's body may also transmit HPV. The virus enters the body through some type of break or tear in the epidermis. Individuals with HPV may also **autoinoculate** unaffected areas of their own body by picking or scratching at a wart and introducing viral particles into other areas with a compromised epithelium.
2. The incubation period for HPV ranges from **1 to 9 months**. The infected individual typically does not realize he or she has been infected until the wart appears.

C. Types and characteristics.
Warts are categorized by the area of the body they affect.

1. **Common warts** (verruca vulgaris) are most often seen on the hands and fingers although they can be found in nail beds and on the face. Common warts have a scaly, dome-shaped appearance.
2. **Flat warts** (verruca plana) primarily affect the hands, knees, faces, and necks of children and young adults. As implied by their name, these warts have a flat appearance and tend to be flesh-colored.

Table 20-3 FDA APPROVED SUNSCREEN INGREDIENTS[1,4–6]

Ingredient (*Brand*)	Coverage	Notes
	Chemical Sunscreens	
Benzophenones		
Dioxybenzone	UVA/UVB (260–380 nm)	Some people may have sensitivity to the benzophenones.
Oxybenzone (*Shade Sunblock* products)	UVA/UVB (270–350 nm)	
Sulisobenzone	UVA/UVB (260–375 nm)	
Cinnamates		
Cinoxate (*RV Paque*)	UVB (270–328 nm)	Cinnamates do not adhere well to the skin and need good substantivity vehicles.
Octocrylene (*Ban de Soleil SPF 8 + Color*)	UVB (250–360 nm)	
Octyl methoxycinnamate (*Hawaiian Tropic* and *Coppertone* products)	UVB (290–320 nm)	
PABA and PABA esters		
Aminobenzoic acid (PABA)	UVB (260–313 nm)	Penetrates horny layer of skin for lasting protection. Has substantivity on sweating skin but not much in water.
Padimate O (*Total Eclipse* products)	UVB (290–315 nm)	Can cause contact dermatitis and photosensitivity reactions in some people.
Salicylates		
Homosalate (*Coppertone* products, and tanning oils with low SPF)	UVB (295–315 nm)	Salicylates are weak sunscreens, but have good substantivity. They are not easily removed by sweating or swimming.
Octyl salicylate (*Sundown Sunscreen, Nivea Sun*)	UVB (280–320 nm)	
Trolamine salicylate (found in some oils with low SPF)	UVB (260–320 nm)	
Miscellaneous		
Ecamsule (*Anthelios SX*)	UVA (320–340 nm)	Approved by the FDA in 2006. Ecamsule has been marketed in Canada and Europe as *Mexoryl*.
Ensulizole	UVB (290–320 nm)	
Menthyl anthranilate (*A-Fil*)	UVA/UVB (260–380 nm)	Weak UV sunscreen with its best effectiveness in the UVA range.
Avobenzone, also known as Parsol 1789 (some Neutrogena products have *Helioplex*)	UVA (320–400 nm)	Isn't stable in light so it must be mixed with a physical sunscreen like titanium dioxide. *Helioplex* is a patented combination of oxybenzone and avobenzone with stabilizers to prevent the breakdown of avobenzone when it is exposed to light.
	Physical Sunscreens	
Red petrolatum (*RV Paque*)	UVA/UVB (290–365 nm)	These products may be comedogenic. New micronized products may be more desirable than older opaque products.
Titanium dioxide (*TI-Baby Natural*)	UVA/UVB (290–770 nm)	With a chance of systemic absorption, titanium dioxide should not be used on children younger than 6 mo or on open wounds.
Zinc oxide (*Sundown Sport Sunblock*)	UVA/UVB (290–770 nm)	

Online Continuing Education Summertime Skincare Guide for Pharmacists. *Pharmacist's Letter*. Volume 2011, Course No. 206 Self-Study Course #110206. Accessed March 21, 2012.

3. **Plantar warts** (verruca plantaris) are typically located on the soles of the feet. When positioned on a weight-bearing area of the foot, plantar warts can be especially painful. These warts may be surrounded by a thickened area of skin, making it easy to confuse plantar warts for calluses.
4. **Venereal warts** (verruca genitalia) are found on or near genitalia and the anus. In the United States, genital warts are the most common form of sexually transmitted disease (STD). Patients with venereal warts should never attempt self-treatment for their condition.

D. **Treatment**

1. **Nonpharmacological measures**
   a. Patients with warts should be counseled to minimize contact with the affected area to avoid spreading the virus to other areas of the body or to other people.
   b. Those patients that suffer with plantar warts should be counseled to wear footwear in any high traffic area. These patients should also use their own towel and bathmat when bathing.
2. **OTC treatment options**
   a. **Salicylic acid** is the only FDA-approved OTC medication for common and plantar warts in strengths ranging from 5% to 40%. Self-treatment should not exceed 12 weeks; if patients do not notice improvement by this time, they should be referred to their primary care physician. Salicylic acid is available in a collodion vehicle (Compound W Gel/Liquid) and pads (Dr. Scholl's Clear Away Discs).
   b. **Cryotherapy** may be used very cautiously in the treatment of common and plantar warts. Cryotherapy products are marketed as pressurized canisters containing dimethyl ether and propane (Wartner) or dimethyl ether, propane, and isobutane (Compound W Freeze Off). To use, apply a saturated applicator directly to the wart for 10 to 20 secs. This forms a blister under the wart that eventually causes the wart to fall off. Although most patients will experience wart resolution after a single treatment, the application may be repeated every 10 days as needed. A single wart should not be treated more than three times.
   c. **Occlusion** of the wart may be an effective OTC treatment option, as well. Duct tape is perhaps the most frequently recommended occlusive vehicle although further studies are needed to determine its true efficacy.
3. **Prescription treatment options**
   a. **Liquid nitrogen** may be applied as a form of cryotherapy under the supervision of a physician. Treatment with liquid nitrogen has a high success rate (with resolution of up to 75% of treated warts), but must be used with extreme caution. Adverse effects may include painful blistering, erythema, nerve damage, and hypopigmentation of the skin.
   b. **5-Fluorouracil (Efudex)** may be used topically for the treatment of flat warts. Treatment with 5-fluorouracil lasts from 3 to 5 weeks. The efficacy of this treatment option has yet to be determined.
   c. **Imiquimod (Aldara)** is a topical agent that is used to treat venereal warts. Imiquimod may be especially useful for those warts that are resistant to other treatments. Most patients will respond to treatment with imiquimod within a period of 4 weeks. Imiquimod is generally well-tolerated, with most adverse effects being local skin reactions. Rarely, systemic side effects may occur. Aldara is a fairly expensive treatment option.

VIII. CORNS AND CALLUSES

A. **Overview**

1. Corns and calluses are common foot disorders whose incidences increase with age.
2. Although corns and calluses are often not a serious medical concern, patients who are predisposed to having impaired blood flow to the extremities (e.g., patients with diabetes) may develop complications from untreated or improperly treated foot disorders.

B. **Pathophysiology**

1. Unlike warts, corns and calluses are not viral in origin.
2. **Friction** and/or **pressure** lead to areas of **hyperkeratosis** (thickening of the stratum corneum) on the foot.
3. Corns and calluses may result from an **uneven distribution of weight** on the feet, **ill-fitting footwear**, or **repeated mechanical rubbing of the affected area** against a shoe or other surface.

C. **Types and characteristics**
1. **Corns**
   a. **Hard corns** (known as heloma durum) appear on areas over bony protrusions, such as the tops of toes or the bottom of the foot. Hard corns possess a glossy appearance with a cone-shaped center.
   b. **Soft corns** (known as heloma molle) are found in the interdigital spaces, most often between the fourth and fifth toes. These corns have a "soft" texture that results from perspiration in the interdigital spaces. Soft corns appear thick and white and are often more painful than hard corns.
2. **Calluses** are areas of thickened skin, most commonly found on heels and the balls of the feet. Calluses are raised and yellowish-white in color, with borders that are not as clearly defined as those of corns. Because calluses are protective in nature, they are not painful when left intact.

D. **Treatment**
1. **Nonpharmacological measures**
   a. Patients with corns and calluses may be instructed to **soak the affected foot in warm water for at least 5 mins every day**. This helps to loosen dead skin. Files and pumice stones may be **used with great caution** to remove the dead skin, but care must be taken to not remove too much skin. Any tool with a sharp blade should be avoided altogether.
   b. Pads of various types, shapes, and sizes are available to help alleviate the pressure placed on corns and calluses. Foam, moleskin, and medicated pads are the most common types of padding available for the treatment of corns and calluses. Patients must be counseled that padding will only exacerbate the corn or callus if they do not also replace the offending footwear.
   c. Some patients may need to be fitted with custom-made footwear for corns or calluses that are refractory to other treatment methods. These patients should be referred to a podiatrist or other foot-care expert.
2. **Salicylic acid** (Dr. Scholl's Liquid Corn/Callus Remover, Freezone Corn and Callus Remover, Mediplast) is the only FDA-approved OTC treatment option for corns and calluses.
   a. Available in collodion and plaster vehicles in strengths ranging from **12% to 40%**.
   b. For collodion vehicles, apply 1 drop of salicylic acid to the affected area at a time until the area is completely covered. Repeat one to two times daily for up to 2 weeks.
   c. For plaster vehicles, cut the disk or pad to the size of the affected area. Leave on for 48 hrs, then remove. Repeat this process every 48 hrs for up to 2 weeks.
   d. Salicylic acid should be avoided in patients with diabetes or impaired circulation due to the potential of ulcer formation or inflammation of the affected area.

IX. PEDICULOSIS AND PEDICULICIDES

A. **Introduction.** Pediculosis is a skin infestation produced by blood-sucking lice. Lice are small, flat, wingless insects with stubby antennae and three pairs of legs that end in sharp, curved claws. **Three types of lice infest humans.**
1. *Pediculus humanus capitis* (i.e., the head louse)
2. *Pediculus humanus corporis* (i.e., the body louse)
3. *Phthirus pubis* (i.e., the pubic, or crab louse)

B. **Life cycles.** The lice that infest humans pass through similar life cycles.
1. **Location.** All lice need human warmth to survive.
   a. **Head** and **pubic lice** spend their entire cycle on the skin of the human host.
   b. **Body lice** live in clothing, coming to the skin surface only to feed.
2. **Development**
   a. Each type of louse develops from **eggs** (**nits**) that incubate for about 1 week. When the small, gray-white, tear-shaped eggs hatch, the nymphs appear.
   b. In about 3 weeks, the **nymphs** mature; then the females start to lay eggs.
   c. Each type of louse survives about 1 month as a **mature adult**. During this time, the female head louse can produce three to six eggs a day.
3. **Egg deposit**
   a. **Body lice** deposit their eggs on fibers of clothing, particularly in the seams. These lice can survive without food up to 10 days, and the eggs may remain viable for about 1 month. Daily clothing changes and boiling or ironing infested clothing can eradicate **body lice**.

b. **Head** and **pubic lice** deposit their eggs on hair strands, about ¼ inch from the skin. Adult head lice can survive on inanimate objects for about 20 hrs; head lice nits may survive up to 10 days off the body.

C. **Incidence.** The incidence of lice infestations increases each year.
1. More than 10 million cases of head lice occur each year in the United States.
2. The bulk of these cases occur between September and November, when students are back in school.
3. In outbreaks of head lice, 70% of cases occur in children younger than 12 years.
4. Infestations tend to be more common in girls, presumably because of their greater tendency to share grooming items.
5. Unlike the other two forms of lice, body lice are associated with improper hygiene and are often present in homeless people. This infestation is rare in the United States, especially when people follow proper hygiene routines.

D. **Medical problems**
1. Both adult and nymph lice are blood sucking; they feed on humans by piercing the skin and introducing a small amount of saliva (which contains an **anticoagulant**) into the feeding area. All lice types feed on blood for about 30 to 45 mins every 3 to 6 hrs.
   a. The attachment of lice to the body causes an **erythematous papule**, which may **itch**.
   b. The female louse produces a sticky **cementlike secretion** that holds the eggs in place on the hair shaft so securely that ordinary shampooing does not remove it.
2. Neither head nor crab lice transmit infections, but body lice transmit **typhus**, **relapsing fever**, and **trench fever**.
3. Lice and humans have a true **parasitic relationship**; lice depend on the human host for shelter, food, and reproductive success. Once hatched, nymphs must have access to the human host within the first 12- to 24-hr period, if they are to survive.

E. **Methods of transmission**
1. **Head lice** are most commonly **spread by head-to-head contact** with an infected person through hats, caps, scarves, pillowcases, communal combs and brushes, or clothing that is hung close together (e.g., on a coat rack).
2. **Pubic lice** are **transmitted primarily through sexual contact**, but also through shared undergarments, towels, or toilet seats.
   a. The lice affect teens and young adults most often through sexual contact.
   b. Lice frequently coexist with other sexually transmitted diseases.
   c. Scratching in the genital areas may transmit pubic lice to other hairy regions, such as the eyelashes, eyebrows, sideburns, and mustaches.

F. **Signs and symptoms**
1. **Head lice**
   a. Most patients have fewer than 10 lice.
   b. The most common sign is **head scratching**.
   c. **Skin redness around the nape** (i.e., **back**) **of the neck** and above the ears is usually seen.
   d. The lice can be identified by direct examination using wooden applicator sticks or a comb to part the hair, then looking at the hair through a magnifying glass.
   e. The lice appear as tiny brownish gray spots that are often difficult to see. The shiny, **whitish silver eggs**, which appear almost as grains of sugar, are more likely to be seen than the lice. The nits are initially **deposited** about **¼ inch from the scalp** on the hair shaft, and they may be **confused with dandruff or hairspray droplets**. Usually, hair grows at a rate of about ½ inch per month, so the duration of infestation can be assessed based on this information.
2. **Pubic lice.** The primary symptom is scratching in the genital area.
3. **Body lice.** The most common symptoms are bites and itching, which are commonly seen as vertical excoriations on the trunk area.

G. **Treatment**
1. There are **three steps** in the treatment of **head and body lice.**
   a. Treat the lice and nits with a pediculicide agent.
   b. Control the symptoms of itching to prevent secondary infection.
   c. Clean the environment of potential lice and nits.

2. **Itching.** Pharmacists should advise patients that even after the causative organism and nits have been killed, itching may persist for several days. This aspect is very important because patients may decide to use pediculicides excessively, thinking that they have been ineffective when the itching continues. **Excessive use of pediculicides may result in excessive drying, which can cause further itching.**
3. Home remedies. Because of the social stigma attached to lice infestation, some individuals may resort to harmful home remedies. Examples of such uncomfortable, ineffective, and potentially dangerous approaches that should not be used include:
   a. Shaving the head and pubic area
   b. Applying heat to the infested area with a hair dryer
   c. Soaking the head in hot water for several minutes
   d. Soaking the area of infestation with gasoline or kerosene
4. **OTC pediculicide products** are considered first-line treatments and include
   a. **Permethrin** (Nix) is a pyrethroid (i.e., a synthetic version of a pyrethrin). It is indicated for the treatment of **head lice only**.
      (1) **Mechanism of action.** Permethrin kills by **disrupting ion-transport mechanisms at the nerve membranes.** Permethrin is a synthetic mixture of chemically altered pyrethrin isomers. Because not all eggs may be killed (it takes about 4 days for the nervous system of the louse to develop) with a single application of this agent or removed with a nit comb, it may be necessary to reapply the pyrethrin product within 7 to 10 days of the first application (because the usual hatching time of the eggs is 7 to 10 days). The American Academy of Pediatrics (AAP) now recommends routine retreatment of patients with head lice, typically on day 9.
      (2) **Application.** Permethrin comes in the form of a 1% **creme rinse** and should be applied like a conventional hair conditioner after the hair has been shampooed (use a shampoo with no conditioner), rinsed, and towel dried. The hair should be thoroughly saturated with undiluted permethrin (25 to 30 mL), which should **remain on the hair for 10 mins, then rinsed.**
      (3) **Effectiveness.** A single application is generally effective in killing lice. Because the agent is retained on the hair shaft, the product provides **continuing activity for up to 14 days.** This residual effect persists regardless of normal shampooing.
         (a) Even with the residual activity, there still may be the need for retreatment in 7 to 10 days.
         (b) **Comb hair** in the previously infested area **with a fine-toothed comb** to remove dead lice and eggs.
         (c) There is, at least theoretically, the speculation that because low-level residual amounts of this agent are retained on the hair, it may be possible that when suboptimal levels are present, some lice may survive and give rise to strains that are resistant.
   b. **Pyrethrins 0.17% to 0.33% with piperonyl butoxide 2% to 4%.** This product is safe and effective for the treatment of **head** and **pubic lice**. The combination of ingredients is an example of **pharmacological synergism.**
      (1) **Pyrethrins** have a **similar mechanism of action as permethrin.** These natural insecticides are derived from a mixture of substances obtained from the flowers of the **chrysanthemum** plant.
      (2) **Piperonyl butoxide** enhances the pediculicide effect of pyrethrins by **suppressing the oxidative degradation mechanisms of the lice.** Therefore, the length of time that the pyrethrins contact the lice is increased.
      (3) **Side effects** from either agent are **uncommon.**
         (a) **Contact dermatitis** (see I) is the most frequently reported side effect.
         (b) **Allergic reactions.** Because pyrethrins are derived from a plant (chrysanthemum), they may produce hay fever (i.e., allergic rhinitis) and asthma attacks in susceptible individuals. Thus, patients who have known allergies to ragweed or chrysanthemum plants should use this product with caution.
      (4) Common **trade names** for this product include RID maximum strength Shampoo, A-200 maximum strength Shampoo.

(5) **Directions for use (shampoo)**
  (a) **Apply the product, undiluted,** to the dry hair until it is entirely wet.
  (b) Allow the product to **remain on the head for 10 mins.**
  (c) **Rinse thoroughly** with warm water.
  (d) Dry the area, preferably with a disposable cloth.
  (e) **Comb hair** in the previously infested area **with a fine-toothed comb** to remove dead lice and eggs.
  (f) Do not exceed two applications within 24 hrs. It may be necessary to reapply the shampoo in 7 to 10 days [see IX.G.4.a.(1)].

c. **OTC pediculicide treatment failure.** Treatment failure with the use of the preceding agents has been reported. Speculations as to the cause of this treatment failure include failure to follow product instructions, noncompliance with nit removal, and head lice drug resistance. Studies support the theory that there are now "super lice" that have survived exposure to pyrethrins and permethrin; resistance to pyrethrins has been better documented.

5. **Prescription products** are included here to put into perspective how the OTC agents fit into therapy.

a. **Malathion** (Ovide) is an organophosphate cholinesterase inhibitor that has been widely used as a lawn and garden insecticide. Resistance has also become an issue with this agent.
  (1) **Mechanism of action.** Sulfur atoms in the malathion bind with sulfur groups on the hair, giving a residual protective effect against reinfestation.
  (2) **Application.** Malathion is prepared as a lotion in 78% alcohol; therefore, caution should be used near an open flame or a hair dryer. The product should be sprinkled on dry hair and left for 8 to 12 hrs before rinsing. A fine-toothed comb should be used to remove the dead lice and eggs.
  (3) No systemic **adverse effects** have been reported with topical use of this medication.
    (a) The alcoholic vehicle may produce stinging and possible flammability.
    (b) Although this agent may be effective, its unpleasant odor (owing to sulfhydryl compounds), the required time of 8 to 12 hrs on the scalp, and those points noted in IX.G.5.a.(3).(a) represent the main drawbacks.
  (4) Malathion is **contraindicated in children < 24 months,** as the scalp is more permeable, possibly leading to increased absorption of the medication. Safety and efficacy in children < 6 years old have not been established.

b. **Benzyl alcohol 5%** (Ulesfia) was approved by the FDA in 2009 for the treatment of head lice in children 6 months and older.
  (1) **Mechanism of action.** Benzyl alcohol works by asphyxiating head lice. This medication is not ovicidal; thus, retreatment is necessary to kill any lice that hatched from eggs.
  (2) **Application.** Lotion should be massaged into the hair and scalp. Ensure the patient's skin and eyes are protected from any excess medication that may drip from the top of the head. Allow the lotion to remain on the head for 10 mins, then rinse the lotion from the hair and scalp. Repeat in 7 to 9 days.
  (3) The most common adverse effects associated with this medication are temporary pruritus, erythema, pyoderma, and ocular irritation.

c. **Spinosad 0.9%** (Natroba) is a topical pediculicide that was approved by the FDA in 2011 for the treatment of head lice in patients 4 years and older.
  (1) **Mechanism of action.** Spinosad is an insecticide that paralyzes and ultimately kills head lice upon ingestion of the chemical by the lice.
  (2) **Application.** Spinosad is indicated for topical application only. The suspension should be applied to dry hair and scalp. Ten minutes following application, patients should be instructed to wash their hair and scalp with warm water. Repeat in 7 days if live lice are seen at that time.
  (3) The most common adverse effects associated with this medication are localized erythema, ocular erythema, and irritation at the application site.

d. **Lindane**, or γ-benzene hexachloride, has fallen into disfavor because of the potential for toxicity and the fact that its efficacy is less than the other agents available (both prescription and OTC products). Resistance to this agent is widespread. Lindane is no longer recommended by the AAP for the treatment of head lice. Its use has been banned in California.

6. **Adjunctive therapy**

a. **Nit removal**

(1) The pediculicide products mentioned vary in their ability to kill the lice nits. To ensure successful therapy after pediculicide application, the nits should be removed with a **fine-toothed comb**. A sturdy **metal comb** (like the LiceMeister) is recommended by the National Pediculosis Association (NPA). Although some schools may have a "no nit" policy—that is, a child's hair and scalp must be free of nits before he or she is allowed to return to the classroom—missing school due to head lice is no longer endorsed by the AAP.

(2) Although various substances have been used in an effort to dislodge the nits from the hair shafts, most, if not all, have been unsuccessful. A mixture of 50% vinegar and 50% water has been recommended, but its effectiveness has been questioned. A lice egg remover containing various enzymes comes as part of a kit, but challenges have been made to its effectiveness.

b. **Treatment of other household members.** Once a lice infestation has been identified in one member of the household, all other members should be examined carefully. Everyone who is infested should be treated at the same time. Any family member that shares a bed with the infected individual should also be treated, even if live lice are not found on that family member.

c. **Adjunctive methods for controlling lice infestations**

(1) **Washable material items** such as linens, towels, hats, and clothing should be machine-washed in hot water and dried in a hot dryer to destroy lice and nits.

(2) **Nonwashable material goods** should be dry-cleaned or sealed in a plastic bag for 2 weeks.

(3) **Personal items** (e.g., combs, brushes) should be soaked in hot water (130°F) for at least 15 mins.

(4) **Furniture and household items** (e.g., carpets, chairs, couches, pillows) should be vacuumed thoroughly. OTC spray products that contain pyrethrins are no more effective than vacuuming in terms of removing the risk of reinfestation.

d. Pediculicides should not be used around the eyes. For **eyelash pubic lice infestations, petrolatum** applied five times a day has been used to supposedly "asphyxiate" lice, but this may only slow lice movement. Gentle removal with baby shampoo may be helpful.

H. **Head lice myths** are numerous. The following additional facts may reassure and inform patients and parents of patients.

1. No significant difference in incidence occurs among the various socioeconomic classes or races.
2. Hygiene and hair length are not contributing factors.
3. Head lice do not fly or jump from person to person.
4. Head lice do not carry other diseases.
5. Head lice cannot be contracted from animals, and pets are not susceptible to *Pediculus humanus capitis*.
6. The head does not have to be shaved to get rid of lice.
7. Washing hair with "brown" soap is not effective.
8. Head lice are unrelated to ticks.
9. Hair does not fall out as a consequence of infestation.
10. Head lice infestations can occur at any time of the year.

Study Questions

Directions: Each of the questions, statements, or incomplete statements can be correctly answered or completed by **one** of the suggested answers or phrases. Choose the **best** answer.

1. A woman who has not been in the sun for 4 months develops redness on her chest after lying in the sun for 20 mins. The next day, she applies a suntan lotion and develops the same degree of redness on her back in 2 hrs and 20 mins. What is the likely sun protection factor (SPF) of the lotion she is using?

(A) 14
(B) 10
(C) 12
(D) 9
(E) 7

2. Which of the following cleansing products would a pharmacist recommend for a patient with inflammatory acne?

(A) an abrasive facial sponge and soap used four times a day
(B) aluminum oxide particles used two times a day
(C) sulfur 5% soap used two times a day
(D) mild facial soap used two times a day

3. If a patient needs a second application of an over-the-counter (OTC) pyrethrin pediculicide shampoo, how many days after the first application should this be done?

(A) 4 to 5
(B) 6
(C) 7 to 10
(D) 14 to 21
(E) 15 to 17

4. All of the following treatments for personal articles infested with head lice would be effective *except*

(A) placing woolen hats in a plastic bag for 2 weeks.
(B) using an aerosol of pyrethrins with piperonyl butoxide sprayed in the air of all bathrooms.
(C) machine-washing clothes in hot water and drying them using the hot setting on the dryer.
(D) dry-cleaning woolen scarves.
(E) soaking hair brushes in hot water for 15 mins.

5. All of the following sunscreen agents or combinations of agents would likely help prevent a drug-induced photosensitivity reaction *except*

(A) titanium dioxide.
(B) octyl methoxycinnamate plus homosalate.
(C) oxybenzone and padimate O.
(D) zinc oxide.
(E) padimate O plus avobenzone.

6. All of the following would be appropriate recommendations for an adult patient in the acute stage (i.e., blistering, weeping) of poison ivy contact dermatitis *except*

(A) 60 mg per day of prednisone initially, then tapered over 15 days.
(B) Burow's solution; 1:20 wet dressing to area for 15 to 30 mins, four times per day.
(C) two soaks per day in Aveeno Bath Treatment.
(D) two applications of Ivy Block.

7. Pharmacists educating patients about acne should mention all of the following *except*

(A) eliminating all chocolate and fried foods from the diet.
(B) cleansing skin gently two to three times daily.
(C) using water-based noncomedogenic cosmetics.
(D) not squeezing acne lesions.
(E) keeping in mind that acne usually resolves by one's early 20s.

8. A 15-year-old male patient has been using benzoyl peroxide 5% cream faithfully every day for the past 2 months with no apparent side effects. All of the following can be said about this patient *except*

(A) he has been using this product for a long enough time to determine if the dose and dosage form are going to have any benefit.
(B) he should use this product no more frequently than every other day because of its irritating properties.
(C) this starting dose and dosage form are useful, especially if he has dry skin or it is wintertime.
(D) his scalp hair may look bleached if the product comes in contact with it.
(E) the product would sting if it got into his eyes.

9. All of the following descriptions match the therapeutic agent for poison ivy *except*
   - (A) calamine, phenolphthalein gives it the pink color.
   - (B) Ivy Block, useful in preventing poison ivy dermatitis.
   - (C) benzocaine, data regarding incidence of hypersensitivity are conflicting.
   - (D) hydrocortisone, useful for its antipruritic and anti-inflammatory effects.

10. All of the following statements related to sun protection are true *except* which one?
   - (A) The sun's intensity increases 20% when going from sea level to an altitude of 5000 ft.
   - (B) Water-resistant labeling on a sunscreen product indicates that it will retain its SPF after 40 mins of activity in water, sweating, or perspiring.
   - (C) Baby oil is not a sunscreen, but its application to the skin after tanning causes melanin to rise to the surface.
   - (D) Per the FDA, a product with an SPF of > 50 must now be labeled SPF "50+".
   - (E) The SPF is really only a measure of ultraviolet B (UVB) protection.

11. All of the following statements about sunscreens are correct *except* which one?
   - (A) Malignant melanoma formation may be associated with intense, intermittent overexposure to the sun (sunburning).
   - (B) Any benefits that might be derived from using sunscreens with an SPF > 30 are negligible.
   - (C) Sunscreens are best applied immediately before going out in the sun.
   - (D) Avobenzone provides sunscreen coverage for the UVA spectrum.
   - (E) Basal cell carcinoma is the most common of all skin cancers and accounts for about 80% of skin cancers.

12. All of the following statements are proper counseling point for a patient suffering with dry skin *except*?
   - (A) Avoid alcohol and caffeine, as these can exacerbate dry skin.
   - (B) Following a bath or shower, pat the skin down with a towel, leaving bits of moisture on the skin.
   - (C) Soak in a tub two to three times per week for at least 20 mins to allow for adequate water absorption into the skin.
   - (D) Avoid extremely hot baths and showers.
   - (E) Ensure adequate daily intake of water (about 8 oz glasses of water per day).

13. Dandruff is
   - (A) the result of decreased turnover of epidermal cells.
   - (B) typically not a serious medical concern.
   - (C) also known as cradle cap.
   - (D) rarely accompanied by pruritus.

14. All of the following are potential treatment options for psoriasis *except*
   - (A) salicylic acid.
   - (B) topical hydrocortisone.
   - (C) coal tar.
   - (D) ketoconazole.

15. Which of the following tinea infections is not appropriate for self-treatment and must be referred to a physician?
   - (A) Tinea nigra
   - (B) Tinea corporis
   - (C) Tinea cruris
   - (D) Tinea pedis

Answers and Explanations

1. **The answer is E** *[see VI.E.1]*.
   The SPF is the minimal erythema dose (MED) of protected skin divided by the MED of unprotected skin. Thus, 2 hrs and 20 mins (140 mins) divided by 20 mins equals an SPF of 7.

2. **The answer is D** *[see IV.E.2]*.
   For patients with inflammatory acne, the best product is a mild facial soap used two times a day. The soap should be gently rubbed into the skin with only the fingertips. Cleansing products that irritate already inflamed skin should be avoided.

3. **The answer is C** *[see IX.G.4.b.(5).(f)]*.
   Reapplication of pyrethrins with piperonyl butoxide should be within 7 to 10 days of the first application. Any lice nits that were not killed on the first application would have time to hatch and then be killed with the second application.

4. **The answer is B** *[see IX.G.4.a; IX.G.6.c]*.
   Pyrethrins with piperonyl butoxide in an aerosol form can be sprayed directly on inanimate objects (e.g., chairs, headrests) to kill head lice, but the combination should not be sprayed in the air like an aerosol deodorizer. Moreover, vacuuming the furniture would

probably be as effective as spraying it. The other selections are appropriate for personal articles infested with head lice.

5. **The answer is B** *[see VI.E.2; VI.D.3.c]*.
Octyl methoxycinnamate and homosalate protect against only UVB exposure. Because photosensitivity reactions are often associated with UVA radiation exposure, people also need sunscreen protection for this portion of the UV radiation band. The other agents listed cover at least part of both UVA and UVB spectra.

6. **The answer is D** *[see I.D.3–4; I.E.2]*.
Ivy Block is used as a barrier protectant for the prevention of poison ivy dermatitis, *not* for the treatment of an acute eruption. The other options are appropriate to recommend to someone suffering from the acute stage of poison ivy dermatitis.

7. **The answer is A** *[see IV.D.3]*.
Evidence does not show that acne definitively worsens from any particular type of food, including chocolate or fried foods. The other choices are pieces of information that the pharmacist should convey to a patient with acne.

8. **The answer is B** *[see IV.E.4.a]*.
Although the irritating properties of benzoyl peroxide might dictate applying it only every other day on initiating treatment, this patient has tolerated the agent on a daily basis for 2 months. Thus, there would be no need to decrease the application frequency. All of the other choices do apply to this patient's use of benzoyl peroxide.

9. **The answer is A** *[see I.D.4.a]*.
Ferric oxide provides the pink color of calamine. All of the other descriptions match their associated agents.

10. **The answer is C** *[see VI.C.2.; VI.E.1.a.(2); VI.E.1.b.; VI.E.1.b.(1)]*.
Baby oil is not a sunscreen, and it has no effect on melanin. SPF does measure UVB protection, and an SPF higher than 50 must be labeled SPF "50+". Water-resistant sunscreen products must retain their SPF value after 40 mins of water activity. The intensity of the sun does increase by 4% with each 1,000-ft rise in elevation.

11. **The answer is C** *[see VI.D.2; VI.E.1; VI.E.2.b; VI.E.2.b.(5)]*.
Optimally, sunscreens should be applied 1 to 2 hrs before exposure to the sun. This allows time for the product to bind to the stratum corneum, which provides better protection. The other responses are correct.

12. **The answer is C** *[see V.D.1.a–c]*.
Patients who suffer with dry skin should be counseled on bathing or showering for brief periods (3 to 5 mins) with lukewarm water.

13. **The answer is B** *[see II.A.2; II.C.1.c; II.C.1.f; II.D.1.i]*.
Dandruff is not typically a serious medical condition, but embarrassment to the patient is a real concern and must be considered when offering the patient treatment options.

14. **The answer is D** *[see II.E.2.a.(2)–(3)]*.
Ketoconazole is not an appropriate treatment option for psoriasis (the only scaly dermatosis for which ketoconazole is not indicated).

15. **The answer is A** *[see III.D.2.a.(1)]*.
Only three types of tinea infections respond to self-treatment with nonprescription therapies: tinea corporis, tinea cruris, and tinea pedis. All other tinea infections should be referred to a physician for evaluation and treatment.

21

Over-the-Counter Weight Control, Sleep, and Smoking-Cessation Aids

JENNIFER D. SMITH

I. WEIGHT CONTROL

A. Obesity is a growing epidemic in America, spanning all age groups from childhood to adulthood. The National Health and Nutrition Examination Survey (NHANES) 2007 to 2008 data revealed that at least 30% in most age groups of the U.S. population are obese. This is concerning because obesity is a health risk for several chronic disease states including, but not limited to, cardiovascular disease, stroke, type 2 diabetes, and arthritis. Consequently, this upward trend in obesity leads to growing U.S. health expenditures.

1. The U.S. Preventive Services Task Force (USPSTF) determined that the body mass index (BMI) is a reliable and valid identifier for **adults** at increased risk for morbidity and mortality owing to overweight and obesity. The BMI is calculated as either weight (in pounds) divided by height (in inches squared) multiplied by 703 or as weight (in kilograms) divided by height (in meters squared). The following guidelines relate BMI to overweight and obesity:
   a. **Overweight** is defined as a **BMI between 25 and 29.9 kg/m^2**.
   b. **Obesity** is defined as a **BMI ≥ 30 kg/m^2** and is further divided into grades: Grade 1 (BMI 30 to < 35); Grade 2 (BMI 35 to < 40); Grade 3 (BMI ≥ 40).
2. Truncal fat accumulation, measured by **waist circumference**, is a **risk factor for cardiovascular disease and other diseases** (e.g., type 2 diabetes, sleep apnea, knee osteoarthritis) regardless if the individual is considered obese. Waist circumference is **not a valid measurement in individuals with a BMI > 35 kg/m^2**. Individuals with the following waist circumferences are considered at increased risk for cardiovascular and other diseases:
   a. A waist circumference in **men > 40 inches** (102 cm)
   b. A waist circumference in **women > 35 inches** (88 cm)

B. **Management.** Diet and exercise (lifestyle modifications) are the recommended first approach to weight loss, as well as sustained weight control. Although it seems relatively simple to eat a well-balanced diet and exercise regularly, time constraints and ease of access to highly processed foods are hurdles that Americans face in the fight against the bulge.

1. **Caloric restriction.** To reduce weight (and thus BMI), energy intake should be less than the energy expended.
   a. The approximate adult energy requirements, based on actual weight, may be roughly estimated as follows. A 120-lb active woman would require approximately 1800 kcal/day to maintain her current weight.
      (1) Bedridden or sedentary individuals: 10 to 12 kcal/lb
      (2) Moderately active individuals (walking at regular pace): 13 kcal/lb

(3) Active individuals: 15 kcal/lb
(4) Very active individuals: 20 kcal/lb

b. To lose about 0.5 kg/week, a **deficit of 500 to 1000 calories (kcal) per day** must be met. A **safe rate of weight loss is considered to be 1 to 2 lb/week.**

c. Several commercially available weight loss programs (e.g., Weight Watchers, Nutrisystem, and Jenny Craig) exist today. When compared to self-help weight loss programs, some commercially available programs have shown enhanced and sustained weight loss, which may be attributable to the social support provided.

2. **Dietary fat absorption inhibitor.** Currently, the only available nonprescription agent that is FDA approved for weight loss is **orlistat**, a dietary fat absorption modifier. Dietary modifications in combination with orlistat can produce clinically modest weight loss (approximately 5% of baseline weight). Orlistat has been available in prescription form (Xenical®) since 1999, and gained FDA approval for nonprescription status in 2007 under the brand name Alli®.

a. Alli® is available for individuals 18 and older who are mildly to moderately overweight **(BMI between 25 and 28 kg/m^2)**.

b. Nonprescription dosing is **60 mg TID** (as compared to 120 mg TID for Xenical®) during or within 1 hr of each fat-containing meal. Dose-related efficacy is observed with orlistat up to 300 to 400 mg daily, but effects plateau thereafter.

c. Onset of orlistat takes approximately 2 weeks and statistically significant weight loss has been observed in obese patients after 3 months. Thus, individuals should be counseled that weight loss may not be significant with orlistat and may take several months for noticeable results.

d. The use of orlistat will result in **gastrointestinal adverse effects**, including soft or liquid stools which may be fatty or oily in appearance, increased defecation, fecal urgency, and abdominal pain. Adverse effects are directly related to the dose and inversely related to the fat content of the diet. Gastrointestinal adverse effects may lessen over time.

e. Prescription doses of orlistat have been associated with decreased absorption of vitamins A, D, E, K, and beta-carotene. However, at doses ≤ 180 mg/day given for short periods (e.g., 2 to 3 months), reduced absorption of these vitamins has not been observed. Individuals using Alli for extended periods should be counseled to take a **multivitamin once daily at bedtime**.

3. **Exercise** can decrease the appetite and increase body metabolism. Exercise adds only modestly to initial weight loss but is a key component of **sustained weight loss**.

C. **Dietary supplements.** Retail sales of weight loss supplements in the United States exceed **a billion dollars** annually. Americans have begun to seek nonprescription weight loss products for various reasons.

1. Some individuals may view dietary supplements as a quick resolution to the growing epidemic, because the obtainment of desired or reduced body weight with long-term lifestyle changes is perceived as difficult. Many advertisements of weight loss products give inflated claims, offering rapid results with little to no modification in lifestyle habits. Some people view dietary supplements as natural and, therefore, mistakenly believe they are safe to use.

2. With the implementation of the Dietary Supplement Health and Education Act of 1994, manufacturers are **not required to demonstrate product safety and efficacy before marketing** supplements. Although manufacturers of dietary supplements do not have to demonstrate product safety and efficacy, they **do have to follow good manufacturing practices**. In 2007, FDA ruled that dietary supplements must be manufactured in a manner that ensures quality and must be properly packaged and labeled as specified in the manufacturing record. Still, the lack of evidence for product safety and efficacy raises concerns for health care providers who attempt to make appropriate recommendations to patients seeking nonprescription weight loss products.

3. The U.S. Food and Drug Administration (FDA) files action against manufacturers of supplements determined unsafe, falsely labeled, labeled with misleading claims, adulterated, or misbranded.

4. The Federal Trade Commission (FTC) takes action against manufacturers providing product advertising that is misleading or makes unsubstantiated claims.

5. Numerous single- and multiple-entity products are available on the market today, each under the scrutiny of the FDA and FTC. The most commonly seen ingredients in weight loss products currently marketed, organized by purported mechanisms of action, include the following:
   a. **Increase energy expenditure**
      (1) **Ephedra.** Contains supplements that were **banned by the FDA in April 2004** owing to unreasonable risks of illness or injury when used as labeled. Products formulated with ephedrine alkaloids (ephedra, ma huang, sida cordifolia, Pinellia) were removed immediately, although, unlike other dietary supplements currently available, ephedra-containing supplements did have convincing evidence for short-term weight loss.
      (2) **Bitter orange** is an extract from the peel, flower, leaf, and fruit of the Seville orange. Typical dosage is about 1 g/day, standardized to 1.5% to 6.0% synephrine, a stimulating agent that is chemically similar to ephedrine. Currently, there are no data to support its efficacy as an agent for weight loss. If combined with other stimulants such as caffeine, bitter orange may be cardiotoxic.
      (3) **Guarana** seed contains 2.5% to 7.0% caffeine and exerts a diuretic action. Effectiveness has been demonstrated only in combination with ephedrine. Tolerance and dependence can develop with chronic use.
      (4) **Caffeine** is an FDA-approved product; efficacy of this agent for weight loss has been demonstrated only in combination with ephedrine, which has been removed from the market. Tolerance and dependence can develop with chronic use.
   b. **Modulate carbohydrate metabolism**
      (1) **Chromium**, an essential mineral, increases insulin sensitivity, lean body mass, and basal metabolic rate and decreases insulin blood levels and body fat. Chromium is used in weight loss products in the form of chromium picolinate, 200 to 400 mcg/day, with no reported significant adverse effects. Rhabdomyolysis and renal failure have been reported with the use of chromium picolinate in doses exceeding 1000 mcg/day. Although widely marketed, there have been no large, well-designed studies for the use of chromium in weight loss. Although its efficacy for weight loss remains uncertain, over 100 products marketed for weight loss contain chromium.
      (2) **Ginseng**, in the form of Panax ginseng, may improve glucose tolerance, according to preliminary data. Although ginseng is found in at least 20 commercially available weight loss products, it has no demonstrated efficacy for weight loss in humans.
   c. **Enhance satiety**
      (1) **Guar gum**, a fiber derived from the Indian cluster bean, has been deemed relatively safe in doses of 7.5 to 30.0 g/day, however, it has not demonstrated efficacy for weight loss in at least 20 clinical trials. Adverse effects include abdominal pain, flatulence, and diarrhea.
      (2) **Glucomannan** (*Amorphophallus konjac*) purportedly absorbs water in the gut, contributing to enhanced satiety and thus decreased caloric intake. Preliminary evidence has demonstrated that glucomannan (3 to 4 g/day) may be well tolerated and efficacious for weight loss. However, this agent can have a laxative effect.
      (3) **Psyllium** forms a fibrous mass with a bulk laxative effect but has not demonstrated efficacy for weight loss. Potential adverse effects are significant, including esophageal obstruction and nephrotoxicity (if seeds are crushed, chewed, or ground, a pigment may be deposited in the renal tubules). If used, patients should be instructed to not crush, chew, or grind the seeds, and adequate fluids must be consumed.
   d. **Increase fat oxidation or reduce fat synthesis**
      (1) **L-Carnitine** is synthesized in the liver, kidney, and brain. It is fundamentally important for fatty acid transport for energy production. No trials demonstrate efficacy of L-carnitine for weight loss.
      (2) **Hydroxycitric acid (HCA)** is derived from the rind of the brindle berry, a tropical fruit native to India. It is purported to inhibit mitochondrial citrate lyase, thereby suppressing acetyl coenzyme A and fatty acid synthesis. In doses of 300 to 3000 mg/day, HCA has been well tolerated, with adverse effects of headache and gastrointestinal symptoms reported. Efficacy of HCA remains questionable.

(3) **Green tea** contains a polyphenol, epigallocatechin-3-gallate, better known as **EGCG**. Each cup (8 oz) of green tea provides 10 to 80 mg of caffeine, contributing to the tea's diuretic action and central nervous system (CNS) stimulation (e.g., increased heart rate, increased blood pressure, anxiety). Green tea has demonstrated increased fat oxidation and thermogenesis but lacks data regarding efficacy in weight loss.

(4) **Vitamin B_5** has been postulated to induce weight loss; however, data are lacking to support this.

(5) **Licorice** safety and efficacy for weight loss remains unclear. Reported adverse effects of licorice include pseudoaldosteronism, hypertension, and hyperkalemia.

(6) **Conjugated linoleic acid (CLA)** is a group of *trans*-fatty acids, which is purported to alter body composition by increasing lean tissue deposition and decreasing triglyceride uptake in adipose tissue. In doses of 1.4 to 6.8 g/day, CLA may have efficacy in weight loss, especially in obese patients. Adverse effects include mild to moderate gastrointestinal symptoms. CLA may increase insulin levels and insulin resistance.

(7) Clinical trials of **pyruvate**, in doses of 6 to 44 g/day, have demonstrated weak evidence of its effectiveness for weight loss. Reported adverse effects include diarrhea and audible abdominal sounds.

(8) **Calcium** suppresses parathyroid hormone and 1,25-dihydroxyvitamin D to reduce fat synthesis and increase fat oxidation. Although some studies have linked calcium intake to weight loss, clinical trials have failed to demonstrate statistically significant results. Additionally, the Agency for Healthcare Research and Quality (AHRQ) produced an evidence report stating that clinical trials do not support weight loss due to calcium supplementation.

e. **Block dietary fat absorption. Chitosan**, a common ingredient in "fat-trapper" supplements, is derived from the exoskeleton of shellfish. In doses of 2.0 to 4.5 g/day, chitosan has not demonstrated clinically significant increases in fecal fat excretion or weight loss. Adverse effects include nausea, constipation, and flatulence. Furthermore, it is questionable if chitosan is safe in individuals with shellfish allergies.

f. **Increase water elimination. Dandelion** (*Taraxacum officinale*) seems to have a diuretic effect but has not been studied for weight loss in humans. At least 15 dietary supplements for weight loss contain dandelion.

g. **Miscellaneous. Spirulina** (blue-green algae) contains phenylalanine, an agent theorized to inhibit appetite. Spirulina was declared ineffective for weight loss in 1981 by the FDA, and no published studies have proven otherwise. At least 13 products for weight loss currently on the market contain spirulina.

II. SLEEP AIDS

A. Normal sleep and sleep requirements

1. Sleep requirements vary widely among individuals and change throughout the life cycle. The usual range of sleep time per night is 5 to 10 hrs, with an average of about 7.5 hrs. Newborns require a considerable amount of sleep time, up to 18 hrs. Adolescents typically do not become sleepy until after midnight and awaken very late in the morning (if allowed), but require a total of 9.5 hrs of sleep. The typical adult requires 7 to 8 hrs of sleep to feel adequately restored, but this time may diminish with aging.

2. **Polysomnography** is the predominant tool for characterizing sleep physiology, although guidelines from the American Sleep Disorders Association do not indicate it as useful in the diagnosis and management of patients with insomnia. Using polysomnography, researchers have identified five stages of sleep, subdivided into rapid eye movement (REM) sleep and non-REM sleep.

   a. Non-REM sleep consists of four stages. Each stage is a progression into a deeper sleep; and stages 3 and 4 are considered deep, restorative sleep. If time spent in stages 3 and 4 of sleep is diminished (as seen with aging), then sleep quality is compromised.

   b. REM sleep is considered stage 5 of sleep. Most dreaming occurs during REM sleep. If awoken while in REM sleep, dreams may be described in vivid detail.

B. Insomnia

1. **Definition.** Insomnia is defined as one or more of the following sleep-related complaints: difficulty in sleep initiation (arbitrarily defined as a delay of > 30 mins), difficulty in maintenance of sleep, shortened duration of sleep, or quality of sleep that results in adverse daytime consequences.
2. **Epidemiology.** Insomnia is the most common sleep disorder in the United States, affecting approximately 40% of the adult population. Those affected most include women, the less educated or unemployed, separated or divorced individuals, patients with chronic medical or psychiatric disorders, and substance abusers. Economic costs of insomnia are estimated to be > $90 billion annually in the United States. Direct costs include prescription and nonprescription medications, as well as visits to a health care provider. Indirect costs include absenteeism, diminished productivity, fatigue-related automobile crashes, and industrial accidents.
3. Classification of insomnia by duration.
   a. **Transient insomnia** lasts **< 1 week** and is typically the result of acute situational stress or circadian issues such as jet lag or shift work. This type of insomnia is often self-limiting.
   b. **Short-term insomnia** lasts **1 to 3 weeks** and is attributable to situational stress (e.g., acute personal loss), often related to work and family life or to medical or psychological disorders. If short-term insomnia is not managed appropriately, it may progress to chronic insomnia because individuals become increasingly anxious and frustrated about the inability to sleep. There are no established predictors to determine if short-term insomnia will continue to become chronic insomnia.
   c. **Chronic insomnia** lasts **> 3 weeks.** People with chronic insomnia need further evaluation because the condition is often the result of a medical disorder (e.g., sleep apnea, restless leg syndrome, primary insomnia), psychiatric disorder, or substance abuse. Up to 40% of chronic insomnia cases are correlated with psychiatric disorders, particularly depression.
4. Classification of insomnia based on cause.
   a. **Primary insomnia** is the main pathological condition in which a patient experiences continued insomnia in the absence of a related medical or psychiatric condition. Its pathogenesis is unknown, but the condition is treatable. Idiopathic insomnia is the inability to obtain adequate sleep, possibly stemming from a misaligned circadian rhythm. Psychophysiologic insomnia is increased wakefulness associated with the bed environment.
   b. **Secondary insomnia** is more common than primary and can be attributed to the following:
      (1) Adjustment insomnia is associated with situational stress.
      (2) Inadequate sleep hygiene is associated with lifestyle habits that reduce the amount of quality sleep, such as noise in the bedroom or the use of caffeine.
      (3) Insomnia owing to a psychiatric disorder
      (4) Insomnia owing to a medical condition, which may include restless leg syndrome, chronic pain (arthritis), migraines, or cancer
      (5) Insomnia owing to substance abuse
5. Treatment
   a. **Nonpharmacologic intervention** is inexpensive and may be effective.
      (1) Maintain a regular schedule and do not nap; avoid sleeping in late after a poor night's sleep.
      (2) Use the bed only for sleep; avoid reading or watching television in bed.
      (3) If unable to initiate sleep (or go back to sleep) within 20 mins, engage in a relaxing activity (away from bed) until drowsy, and then return to bed.
      (4) Avoid exercise within 3 to 4 hrs of bedtime.
      (5) Minimize or avoid caffeine after noon.
      (6) Minimize or avoid alcohol, tobacco, or stimulants. Many people believe alcohol to be an agent for sleep induction; however, alcohol can act as a CNS stimulant, thereby increasing nocturnal awakenings.
   b. **Nonprescription drug therapy:** It has been estimated that 40% of patients with insomnia self-medicate with either alcohol or nonprescription medications in an effort to correct the condition. The sales of single-entity nonprescription hypnotics (e.g., diphenhydramine, doxylamine) have increased since that estimate was made, but the sales of nighttime analgesics (nonprescription hypnotic plus an analgesic, typically acetaminophen) have surpassed the

single-entity products. Currently, data supporting the safety and efficacy of complementary therapy as sleep aids are lacking.

(1) **Diphenhydramine**, an ethanolamine, blocks histamine$_1$ and muscarinic receptors, thus inducing sedation. Diphenhydramine is marketed as a nighttime sleep aid as Unisom SleepGels, Compoz, and Sominex.
   (a) Diphenhydramine may be dosed for sleep induction as **25 to 50 mg/night** in patients aged 12 and older. Doses **> 50 mg show no additional benefit,** but increased adverse effects. An initial dose of 25 mg may be recommended for patients over the age of 65 with no contraindications to the agent.
   (b) **Adverse effects** of diphenhydramine are **anticholinergic,** including dry mouth, blurred vision, constipation, and urinary retention. Diphenhydramine use should be avoided in patients with glaucoma (narrow-angle), benign prostatic hypertrophy, dementia, or cardiovascular disease.
   (c) The duration of sedation from diphenhydramine is 3 to 6 hrs. However, this may be extended in elderly patients or those with delayed metabolism.
   (d) The use of diphenhydramine for the alleviation of insomnia should be **limited to 7 to 10 consecutive nights**. If used longer than recommended, decreased efficacy may be noted and REM sleep may be suppressed.
   (e) Diphenhydramine is available in combination with aspirin or acetaminophen as a **nighttime analgesic**. Data are available to support the use of these agents in combination if pain is present. However, in the absence of pain, the addition of an analgesic simply provides increased opportunities for complications and drug misadventures.

(2) **Doxylamine**, like diphenhydramine, is an ethanolamine antihistamine which induces sleep through the blockade of histamine and muscarinic receptors. Therefore, adverse effects and duration of sedation are similar to diphenhydramine. There are currently no studies demonstrating enhanced efficacy or safety of doxylamine compared to diphenhydramine.
   (a) Doxylamine is dosed as **25 mg/night**.
   (b) Doxylamine is the active ingredient in Unisom Nighttime Sleep Aid Tablets. However, it should be noted that Unisom SleepGels contain diphenhydramine.

(3) **Melatonin**, a nocturnal neurohormone secreted by the pineal gland, has a **sleep-phase-shifting effect on circadian rhythm**. Recent trials have observed effectiveness of melatonin for sleep onset in patients with misaligned circadian rhythms attributable to shift work or jet lag.
   (a) Melatonin production decreases with age, possibly attributing to sleep disorders noted in elderly patients.
   (b) Melatonin production can be decreased by tobacco, alcohol, and certain medications (nonsteroidal anti-inflammatory drugs, calcium-channel blockers, steroids, benzodiazepines, and fluoxetine).
   (c) When exogenous melatonin is **given in the early evening, the circadian phase will be advanced**. Although this may be beneficial for individuals who experience difficulty in initiating sleep, melatonin given in this manner may worsen the problem of individuals who complain of difficulty in reinitiating sleep after awakening too early.
   (d) If melatonin is **given in the morning, the circadian phase is delayed**, offering the possibility that the patient may become sleepier earlier and awaken earlier. At present, it is unclear if continued administration of exogenous melatonin will suppress endogenous production.
   (e) Melatonin may be dosed as **0.3 to 5.0 mg during the day or at night**, depending on the desired effect. A physiologic dose of melatonin is 0.1 mg, an intermediate dose is 0.3 mg, and a pharmacologic dose is 3.0 mg. **Doses > 1 mg** may improve sleep efficiency but **have not demonstrated the ability to provide quality sleep restoration** as well as the intermediate dose.
   (f) Attributable to its short half-life (30 to 50 mins), melatonin should have **minimal, if any, residual effects the following morning**.

(4) **Valerian root**, derived from *Valeriana officinalis*, is classified as generally recognized as safe (GRAS) for food use in the United States. In doses of **600 mg/day,** valerian root

is purported to induce sedation through its blockade of γ-aminobutyric acid (GABA) breakdown. Adverse reactions of valerian root include vivid dreaming. Further research is necessary to determine the safety and efficacy of valerian root as a sleep aid.

(5) **Kava**, derived from *Piper methysticum*, is one of the most common dietary supplements used in the self-management of anxiety. It is theorized that if insomnia is caused by a state of hyperarousal, then management of anxiety and nervousness will help induce the desired sleep.

(a) A typical dose of kava is **120 mg/day**.

(b) Reported adverse effects of kava are significant, including diarrhea, extrapyramidal side effects, and hepatotoxicity. A recent FDA advisory has **recommended against the use of kava because of the reports of hepatotoxicity**, including hepatitis, cirrhosis, and liver failure.

III. SMOKING CESSATION

A. **Introduction.** More than 400,000 deaths annually are attributable to diseases directly linked to cigarette smoking, including atherosclerotic vascular disease, lung cancer, and chronic obstructive pulmonary disease. It is the most preventable contributor to morbidity and mortality in the United States and yet nearly one-third of the adult population (approximately 48 million adults) continues to smoke. The resulting economic burden is startling, estimated at $50 billion annually to treat smoking-related disorders and $47 billion for the loss of wages and productivity.

B. **Physiologic effects** of nicotine involve the CNS (e.g., enhanced relaxation, improved attention) and the cardiovascular system (e.g., elevated blood pressure, tachycardia). The manifestations of smoking become more pronounced as one ages and may include any or all of the following: deepening of the voice (an untoward effect in women); a constant, hacking cough; yellowed fingernails and surrounding skin from substances found in cigarette smoke; and premature aging of the skin, most noticeable on the face.

C. **Benefits of smoking cessation** are evident for both the patient and society.

1. Patient
   a. Decreased carbon monoxide levels
   b. Restoration of olfactory and gustatory senses within days
   c. Increased self-respect, sense of accomplishment
   d. Improved lung function (up to 30%) within 2 to 3 months
   e. Reduction in the risk of coronary heart disease (50%) after 1 year. After 2 years, the risk is equivalent to individuals who never smoked.
   f. Parallel risk of stroke to that of a nonsmoker within 5 to 15 years
   g. Progressive decline in the risk of lung cancer as number of years of abstinence increases. However, the risk will never be equivalent to one who never smoked.
2. Society
   a. Decreased health care costs for treatment of diseases directly linked to smoking
   b. Decreased work absenteeism owing to smoking-related disease
   c. Cleaner environment from decreased secondhand smoke and cigarette remains (e.g., ashes or butts of cigarettes) in public places

D. **Complications of smoking cessation.** Smoking is an addiction and, therefore, not easy to give up. Nicotine withdrawal symptoms include tobacco cravings, depressed mood, insomnia, irritability, inability to concentrate, anxiety, decreased heart rate, and increased hunger. Literature suggests that when individuals stop smoking without aid, all symptoms of nicotine withdrawal resolve within 30 days, except increased hunger, which persists past the 30-day cessation period.

E. **Tailored interventions** for smoking cessation should be offered to every patient who smokes. The U.S. Public Health Service endorses an approach known as the five As, developed in 1996 by the Agency for Healthcare Policy and Research.

1. **Ask** patients if they smoke.
2. **Advise** patients who smoke to quit.
3. **Assess** the patient's willingness to quit.
4. **Assist** the patient in efforts to quit through counseling and/or pharmacologic therapy. (The combination of counseling and pharmacologic therapy has proven to be the most successful method.)

5. **Arrange** follow-up within a short time frame.
6. To assess the patient's willingness to quit, the transtheoretical model of behavior change may be a useful tool. According to this model, patients are in one of five motivational stages to change their current behavior—that is, to stop smoking.
   a. **Precontemplation.** Patient is not ready to change current behavior.
   b. **Contemplation.** Patient is considering a change in current behavior in the future but not at the present time.
   c. **Preparation.** Patient is actively considering a change in current behavior and is actively engaged in seeking more information.
   d. **Action.** Patient is actively attempting to change behavior or has changed behavior within the last 6 months.
   e. **Maintenance.** Patient has sustained changed behavior for at least 6 months.
7. For patients in the precontemplation and contemplation stages, the health care professional should still advise the patient to quit smoking and repeat the assessment at future visits. For patients in the contemplation stage, the health care professional should assist the patient by offering a referral for smoking-cessation counseling and/or pharmacologic therapy. Behavior modification works best as a multidisciplinary approach, involving the health care provider, pharmacist, nurse, and dentist.

F. **Nicotine-replacement therapy**
1. **Overview.** Nicotine-replacement therapy (NRT) is a smoking-cessation aid used to ameliorate nicotine withdrawal symptoms by providing a **nontobacco, controlled-release amount of nicotine**.
   a. Research has demonstrated that the use of NRT in individuals who smoke > 10 cigarettes a day **can double the chances of successful smoking cessation**; but it is most successful when combined with other nonpharmacologic measures, such as counseling.
   b. Currently, three available dosage forms of NRT are approved by the FDA (gum, lozenges, and patches); however, **none is effective if the patient is not mentally ready to quit**. Furthermore, NRT is **FDA approved only for smoking cessation, not cessation of smokeless tobacco** (e.g., chewing tobacco, snuff).
   c. Self-care with NRT is appropriate for individuals who smoke less than 1.5 packs of cigarettes per day. This is on the basis that each cigarette contains approximately 1 mg of nicotine. Patients smoking greater than 1.5 packs per day should be referred to a health care provider for consideration of prescription therapy for smoking cessation or should be counseled to cut back to at least 1.5 packs per day to enhance success of NRT.
2. **Safety.** Although it is recommended by the U.S. Public Health Service that all people trying to abstain from smoking should receive pharmacotherapy support, not everyone is an ideal candidate.
   a. For patients with **acute cardiovascular disease** (e.g., stroke, acute myocardial infarction, unstable angina) and **pregnant or breastfeeding women, absolute abstinence from nicotine should be recommended**. However, if the patient makes an informed decision, under the supervision of a provider, a rapidly reversible preparation is advisable (e.g., gum or lozenge).
   b. In recent studies, NRT **appears to be safe in patients with stable cardiovascular disease**. Blood pressure should be monitored closely.
   c. The sale of NRT is **restricted to those older than age 18**. Therefore, adolescents desiring smoking cessation should consult a medical provider.
   d. Patients with **asthma or depression** are instructed to consult their physician before the use of NRT. The levels of certain medications used for management of these disease states (e.g., theophylline, imipramine) may be altered by smoking cessation. The nicotine found in NRT does not alter these levels.
   e. It is recommended that patients **do not smoke while using NRT** because the purpose of NRT is to alleviate symptoms while weaning from cigarettes. Although some studies have indicated that the combination may be safe, until further research is conducted, concomitant use of NRT and cigarettes should not be seen as permissible.
   f. Patients are advised on the labeling of NRT products not to combine two forms of NRT. However, a few small studies have shown combinations of NRT to be superior to either agent

Table 21-1 RECOMMENDED SCHEDULING OF NICOTINE GUM AND LOZENGES[a]

Weeks	Dose
1–6	1 piece gum or 1 lozenge every 1–2 hrs (at least 9/day)
7–9	1 piece gum or 1 lozenge every 2–4 hrs
10–12	1 piece gum or 1 lozenge every 4–8 hrs

[a]The recommended scheduling of nicotine polacrilex gum and lozenges is identical. If nicotine is needed past the 12-week schedule, a medical provider should be consulted.

alone. Therefore, some specialists in the field do recommend combination therapy. However, until further research is conducted in the form of well-developed, large trials, combination therapy with NRT should be discouraged unless prescribed by the supervising medical provider.

3. **Available forms of NRT**
   a. **Nicotine polacrilex gum** received FDA approval for prescription sales in 1984 and nonprescription status in 1995.
      (1) **Dosing.** Sold under the trade name Nicorette Gum, this product is available in a **2-mg dose** for individuals who smoke at least 30 mins after waking in the mornings and a **4-mg dose** for those who smoke within 30 mins of waking in the morning. The typical usage is **10 pieces daily**, with a maximum recommended usage of 60 mg/day for up to 3 months. The **strength of gum purchased does not change** instead, the number of pieces used decreases over the course of treatment (*Table 21-1*).
      (2) **Chew-and-park method.** The gum should be chewed slowly, releasing a peppery, tingling sensation, at which point the gum should be "parked" between the cheek and the gum to enhance buccal absorption of the nicotine.
      (3) **Adverse effects** most commonly reported are sore jaw and mouth, mouth ulcers, and dyspepsia.
      (4) **Counseling tips**
         (a) Slowly chew the gum until a peppery, tingling sensation is felt, then park the polacrilex gum between the cheek and the gum. Once the peppery, tingling sensation disappears, begin to slowly chew the gum again until the sensation returns. The gum should be parked in a different area than before. Once the gum loses the ability to produce the peppery, tingling sensation (approximately 30 mins), discard the gum.
         (b) **Do not eat or drink for 15 mins before using nicotine gum** because it requires a basic pH for proper release and absorption of the nicotine.
         (c) **Do not use other forms of NRT or smoke** while using the gum product, unless otherwise directed by a supervising provider.
         (d) The gum may be chewed at the beginning of the first day or at least 30 mins after the last cigarette was smoked.
   b. **Nicotine lozenges**, currently sold under the trade names Nicorette Lozenges and Nicorette Mini-Lozenges, deliver nicotine into the buccal mucosa when the individual sucks on the tablet, similar to a cough drop.
      (1) **Dosing.** The lozenges, like the gum, are dosed **based on the timing of the first cigarette.** If the first cigarette is craved within 30 mins of waking, the **4-mg** lozenge should be recommended. If the first cigarette craving is after 30 mins of waking, the **2-mg** lozenge should be recommended. The **strength chosen will not change** throughout the course of cessation; instead fewer lozenges will be consumed each day during the **12-week proposed schedule** (*Table 21-1*).
      (2) **Adverse effects.** If the lozenge is consumed too quickly or swallowed (rather than dissolved) dyspepsia may be experienced. Other reported adverse effects include insomnia, nausea, hiccups, coughing, headache, and flatulence.

(3) **Counseling tips**
   (a) **Avoid chewing** or biting the lozenge. Rather suck on the lozenge slowly, moving it from side to side, until it is completely dissolved (20 to 30 mins). If accidentally swallowed, wait at least 1 hr before using another lozenge.
   (b) **Do not use other forms of NRT and do not smoke** cigarettes while using this product, unless otherwise directed by a supervising provider.
   (c) The first lozenge may be taken at the beginning of the first day or at least 30 mins after the last cigarette was smoked.
   (d) **Do not take more than 20 lozenges per day** of either the 2-mg or 4-mg dose.
   (e) **Do not eat or drink for 15 mins before using nicotine lozenge** because it requires a basic pH for proper release and absorption of the nicotine.

c. **Nicotine patches** were introduced in 1992 and acquired nonprescription status in 1996. Comparative studies of the available formulations of NRT have revealed that most individuals prefer the patch over the gum or a prescription nicotine inhaler.
   (1) Availability and dosing: Nicoderm CQ is available in three strengths: 7, 14, and 21 mg. The patch should be **tapered**, depending on the starting dose.
      (a) NicoDerm CQ 21-mg patch may be recommended to an individual who smokes > 10 cigarettes per day and then tapered as follows: 21 mg/day for 6 weeks; 14 mg/day for 2 weeks; 7 mg/day for 2 weeks.
      (b) Those who smoke < 10 cigarettes per day may begin with the NicoDerm CQ 14-mg patch and taper as follows: 14 mg/day for 6 weeks; 7 mg/day for 2 weeks.
   (2) Application: The patch must be **placed on a clean, dry, and hair-free area** of the upper body (e.g., upper arm, back) and may be worn for **16 to 24 hr/day.** Patients with early-morning cigarette cravings may require 24-hr use. However, if insomnia or vivid dreaming occurs, the patch may be removed after 16 hrs. The patch should never be placed over wounds or open areas. Use with caution in patients with severe psoriasis or eczema.
   (3) Adverse effects: The most common adverse effect of the patch is **skin irritation**, but this may be reduced by rotating the patch site.

Study Questions

Directions: Each of the questions, statements, or incomplete statements can be correctly answered or completed by **one** of the suggested answers or phrases. Choose the **best** answer.

1. All of the following statements about dietary supplements are true *except* which one?

(A) Manufacturers are not required to demonstrate product safety and efficacy before marketing supplements.
(B) Adherence to good manufacturing practices is not mandatory for manufacturers of dietary supplements.
(C) The U.S. Food and Drug Administration (FDA) files action against supplements determined unsafe.
(D) The Federal Trade Commission (FTC) takes action against manufacturers who present misleading product advertising.

2. All of the following statements about chitosan are true *except* which one?

(A) It is a common ingredient found in fat-trapper supplements.
(B) It is derived from the Indian cluster bean.
(C) Its safety is questionable for individuals with shellfish allergies.
(D) It is purported to inhibit dietary fat absorption.

3. Jane is 36 years old and wants to lose weight. Her current body mass index (BMI) is 32 kg/m^2, her waist circumference is 40 inches, and her weight is 202 lbs. She has lost a minimal amount of weight in the past using fad diets and nonprescription weight loss products but has been unable to maintain the weight loss. All of the following are true, *except*

(A) Based on her BMI, Jane is considered obese.
(B) Her waist circumference of 40 inches increases her risk for cardiovascular disease.
(C) A safe rate of weight loss for Jane would be 1 to 2 lb/week.
(D) Initiation of exercise will provide more weight loss than dietary intake changes.
(E) Her weight is a risk factor for the development of type 2 diabetes.

4. Since the sudden death of his father 2 weeks ago, Bob has been unable to sleep at night. He has difficulty going to sleep and awakens early in the morning, unable to return to sleep. Which of the following would be the correct classification of Bob's current insomnia?

(A) transient, primary insomnia
(B) short-term, primary insomnia
(C) transient, secondary insomnia
(D) short-term, secondary insomnia

5. William works the swing shift at the local manufacturing plant. Based on a recommendation from a friend at work, William would like to try melatonin to help him get to sleep faster. Which of the following is true regarding William's use of melatonin?

(A) An appropriate starting dose of melatonin is 5 mg/night.
(B) William may experience continued drowsiness the following morning owing to melatonin's long half-life.
(C) Recent trials have noted the effectiveness of melatonin in individuals participating in shift work.
(D) Tobacco use will increase endogenous melatonin production.

6. Which of the following complementary alternative medicines (CAM) is most strongly associated with hepatotoxicity, including hepatitis, cirrhosis, and liver failure?

(A) melatonin
(B) kava
(C) chitosan
(D) valerian root
(E) dandelion

7. Sylvia is 33 years old and wishes to purchase a sleep aid for her recent bout of insomnia (duration is 2 days). She has linked it to an overwhelming amount of stress she has been under lately at work, trying to meet deadlines, and her recent lack of sleep is not helping. She has no current medical conditions and takes a multivitamin daily. All of the following are true regarding Sylvia's taking diphenhydramine and doxylamine *except* which one?

(A) Sylvia may benefit from diphenhydramine 50 mg used nightly.
(B) Sylvia may use diphenhydramine for insomnia for up to 10 consecutive nights.
(C) Sylvia may benefit from doxylamine 50 mg used nightly as needed.
(D) Sylvia may experience anticholinergic side effects with the use of doxylamine.

8. Jill, a 22-year-old college student, has been encouraged by her health care provider to stop smoking. She tells her doctor that she wants to quit, but she does not want to gain weight right now or to sacrifice her grades as a result of an inability to concentrate during the day. According to the five As and the transtheoretical model of change, what is the next step Jill's health care provider should take?

(A) Jill is in the precontemplation stage of change. Her provider should reassess her willingness to quit at the next visit.
(B) Jill is in the contemplation stage of change. Her provider should reassess her willingness to quit at the next visit.
(C) Jill is in the preparation stage of change. Her provider should reassess her willingness to quit at the next visit.
(D) Jill is in the preparation stage of change. Her provider should offer her counseling and/or pharmacologic therapy for smoking cessation.

9. Zack is 55 years old and wishes to start taking nicotine lozenges to quit smoking. Which of the following is important in the recommendation and selection of nicotine lozenges?

(A) number of cigarettes smoked daily
(B) timing of his first urge for a cigarette
(C) concomitant disease states and therapies
(D) both the number of cigarettes smoked daily and concomitant disease states and therapies
(E) both the timing of his first urge for a cigarette and concomitant disease states and therapies

10. All of the following are important counseling tips for the use of nicotine replacement therapies *except* which one?
    (A) Do not eat or drink within 15 mins of chewing nicotine gum.
    (B) The initial start of nicotine replacement therapy may be 30 mins after the last cigarette.
    (C) Skin irritation associated with the use of a patch may be minimized by rotating the patch site.
    (D) Patches should be removed after 8 hrs of use if the person experiences insomnia.

11. Wendy, a 45-year-old female, is seeking advice about the use of Alli® for weight loss. Her current weight is 228 lbs and her height is 5′6″. At her last provider visit, her provider suggested she set a weight loss goal of 2 lbs per week through diet and exercise. Wendy has type 2 diabetes and hypertension, both of which are well controlled. Which of the following would be appropriate information to provide Wendy?
    (A) Orlistat may assist in modest amounts of weight loss, but noticeable results may not be evident for several months.
    (B) Orlistat is contraindicated in individuals with diabetes mellitus.
    (C) Orlistat is taken as 1 capsule three times daily 1 hr after a fat-containing meal.
    (D) Orlistat may reduce the absorption of fat-soluble vitamins, thus a multivitamin should be taken when nonprescription orlistat is initiated.

Answers and Explanations

1. **The answer is B** *[see I.C].*
Manufacturers of dietary supplements (DS) are not required to demonstrate product safety and efficacy before marketing. Previously, manufacturers of DS were not required to adhere to good manufacturing practices. However, in 2007, FDA ruled that DS must be manufactured in a manner that ensures quality and the DS must be properly packaged and labeled.

2. **The answer is B** *[see I.C.5.e].*
Derived from the exoskeleton of shellfish, chitosan is purported to block dietary fat absorption and thus is a common ingredient found in fat-trapper supplements. Because it is derived from the exoskeleton of shellfish, the safety of chitosan in individuals with shellfish allergies remains in question.

3. **The answer is D** *[see I.A.1–2; I.B.1.b–c; I.B.2].*
A BMI > 30 kg/m^2 is considered obese. Women with a waist circumference $>$ 35 inches are at increased risk of developing cardiovascular disease, as well as type 2 diabetes, sleep apnea, and osteoarthritis. If Jane's BMI had been > 35 kg/m^2, her waist circumference measurement would not be valid for determining an increased cardiovascular risk. Diet and exercise are the best approach to weight loss; however, exercise only adds a modest amount of weight loss. Decreased dietary consumption will provide the most benefit in her efforts to lose weight. A reasonable weight loss is 1 to 2 lb/week.

4. **The answer is D** *[see II.B.3–4].*
Transient insomnia is insomnia lasting $<$ 1 week, and short-term insomnia is insomnia lasting from 1 to 3 weeks. Primary insomnia is a pathological condition in which the patient experiences continued insomnia in the absence of a related medical or psychiatric condition. Secondary insomnia can be attributed to a variety of situations, especially situational stress, such as the death of a loved one.

5. **The answer is C** *[see II.B.5.b.(3)].*
Melatonin effectiveness for sleep onset has been observed in recent trials in individuals participating in shift work. However, melatonin is not FDA approved for this purpose. An initial starting dose of melatonin is 0.1 to 0.3 mg in the evening for patients desiring improved sleep onset. Doses $>$ 1 mg daily have not been able to demonstrate the quality sleep restoration seen in 0.3-mg doses. Melatonin has minimal, if any, residual effects the following morning, owing to its short half-life of 30 to 50 mins. Tobacco, alcohol, and certain medications can decrease endogenous melatonin production.

6. **The answer is B** *[see II.B.5.b.(5)].*
Kava, typically used for anxiety disorders, has been associated with hepatoxicity, including hepatitis, cirrhosis, and liver failure. An FDA advisory committee has recommended against the use of kava because of the reports of hepatotoxicity.

7. **The answer is C** *[see II.B.5.b.(1)–(2)]*.
Diphenhydramine may be dosed as 25 to 50 mg nightly for a sleep aid used for up to 7 to 10 consecutive nights. The recommended dosage for doxylamine is 25 mg nightly. Both diphenhydramine and doxylamine are ethanolamine antihistamines. Therefore, anticholinergic effects may be experienced with the use of either agent.

8. **The answer is B** *[see III.E.6]*.
Jill is in the contemplation stage, as she is considering a change in the future, but she does not feel that this is the right time to begin a smoking cessation program. Therefore, Jill's provider should reassess her willingness to quit at her next visit, when, it is hoped that Jill will be ready to quit.

9. **The answer is E** *[see III.F.3.b]*.
Dosing is based on the timing of the first urge for a cigarette, either within or after 30 mins of waking up. Concomitant disease states should be considered as well. If the patient has hypertension, he will need to be monitored more closely while using nicotine replacement therapy. If he uses certain prescription medications for asthma or depression, his medication may need to be adjusted when he stops smoking.

10. **The answer is D** *[see III.F.3.a–c]*.
Nicotine patches should be worn for 24 hrs. If the patient develops insomnia or vivid dreams from the patch, it may be removed before bed, thus allowing only 16 hrs of exposure to the nicotine. Use of the patch for only 8 hrs is not an acceptable recommendation. Patch application sites should be rotated to avoid skin irritation and patients should be counseled not to eat or drink within 15 mins of chewing the gum.

11. **The answer is A** *[see I.B.2]*.
Orlistat may alter metabolic control, necessitating a change in diabetes medication dosing regimen; however, orlistat is not contraindicated in patients with diabetes. Orlistat is dosed as 1 capsule three times daily with a fat-containing meal, but for optimal effects, it should be dosed during or within 1 hr of the meal not after the meal. It is advisable to recommend a multivitamin to individuals who will be using doses of orlistat greater than 180 mg/day or who will be using orlistat for longer than 2 to 3 months. However, at initiation of nonprescription strength orlistat (60 mg thrice daily), a multivitamin has not been observed as necessary; however, it would be advisable if the individual does continue the medication past 2 to 3 months to recommend a MVI.

22 Over-the-Counter Agents for Fever, Pain, Cough, Cold, and Allergic Rhinitis

JENNIFER D. SMITH, GERALD E. SCHUMACHER

I. ANALGESIC, ANTI-INFLAMMATORY, AND ANTIPYRETIC AGENTS.

Over-the-counter (OTC) analgesics and antipyretics relieve mild to moderate pain and reduce inflammation and fever. These agents are effective for somatic pain (e.g., musculoskeletal pain in the joints; pain from headache, myalgia, and dysmenorrhea; discomfort resulting from generalized inflammation), but they are not effective in reducing discomfort from the visceral organs (e.g., stomach, lungs, heart). Salicylates and nonsteroidal anti-inflammatory drugs (NSAIDs) reduce pain, inflammation, and fever, but acetaminophen generally is effective only for pain and fever.

A. **Pathogenesis of pain.** Intense stimulus (e.g., tissue injury) releases substances that sensitize pain receptors to mechanical, thermal, and chemical stimulation. This triggers pain receptors to send pain impulses over afferent nerve fibers to the central nervous system (CNS).
   1. **Awareness** of pain occurs in the thalamus.
   2. Pain **recognition** and **localization** occur in the cortex.
   3. **Mechanism of analgesic, anti-inflammatory, and antipyretic action.** These agents inhibit (centrally, peripherally, or both) the biosynthesis of various **prostaglandins**, substances involved in the development of pain and inflammation as well as in the regulation of body temperature.

B. **Salicylates**
   1. **Therapeutic uses**
      a. Salicylates are used to relieve mild to moderate pain and reduce inflammation and fever.
      b. Aspirin (acetylsalicylic acid), specifically, is also used to reduce the incidence of some forms of cardiovascular disease. Current evidence supports a modest reduction in the risk of strokes in women but notes less effect in men. On the other hand, evidence supports a significant reduction in the risk of myocardial infarction in men and women > 65 years but shows little effect on younger women.
      c. Men and women who have had a previous myocardial infarction, stable and unstable angina pectoris, or coronary artery bypass surgery, are candidates for aspirin use.
      d. No consensus has emerged on the prophylactic use of aspirin in healthy adults. The risks associated with aspirin use may outweigh the benefits of its widespread use.
   2. **Mechanism of action**
      a. **Analgesic and anti-inflammatory actions.** The action of aspirin results from both the acetyl and the salicylate portions of the drug. Actions of other salicylates (e.g., sodium salicylate, salicylsalicylic acid, choline salicylate) result only from the salicylate portion of the agents.

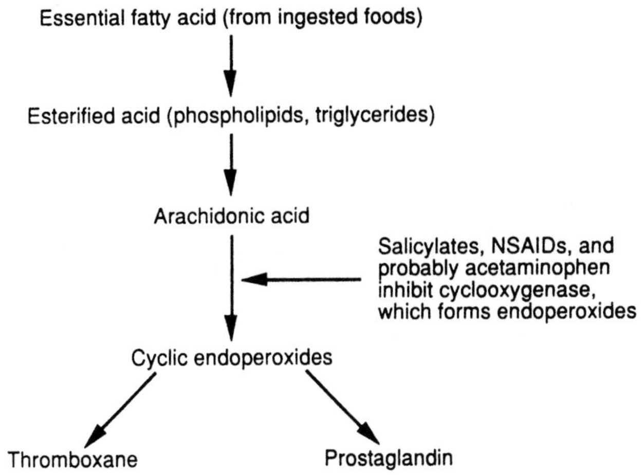

Figure 22-1. Inhibition of prostaglandin formation by aspirin, nonsteroidal anti-inflammatory drugs (NSAIDs), and acetaminophen.

(1) These drugs **inhibit cyclooxygenase,** the enzyme that is responsible for the formation of precursors of prostaglandins (PGs) and thromboxanes from arachidonic acid (*Figure 22-1*).

(2) Analgesia is produced mainly by **blocking the peripheral generation of pain impulses** mediated by prostaglandins and other chemicals. Analgesia probably secondarily involves a reduction in the awareness of pain in the CNS.

b. Antipyretic action. The principal antipyretic action occurs in the CNS. Salicylates act on the hypothalamic heat-regulating center to produce peripheral vasodilation, which results from the inhibition of prostaglandin synthesis.

c. Antiplatelet and antithrombotic actions

(1) **Antiplatelet.** Aspirin (but not other salicylates, acetaminophen, or NSAIDs) **irreversibly inhibits cyclooxygenase in platelets,** which prevents the formation of the aggregating agent thromboxane A_2.

(2) **Antithrombotic.** At low doses, aspirin inhibits thromboxane A_2 formation but has a relatively small effect on prostacyclin. This results in blocking the platelet aggregating agent thromboxane A_2 while preserving the action of the aggregation inhibitor prostacyclin (prostaglandin I_2; PGI_2).

3. Administration and dosage

a. For **analgesia** or **antipyresis in adults**, 325 to 650 mg every 4 hrs or 650 to 1000 mg every 6 hrs should be administered as needed. The maximum daily dose is 4000 mg for no longer than 10 days for pain or 3 days for fever without consulting a physician.

b. **Child dosage** depends on age. The dosages are 160 mg every 4 hrs for children 2 to 4 years of age and 400 to 480 mg every 4 hrs for children 9 to 12 years of age. Salicylates should be given for no longer than 5 days for pain, 3 days for fever, and 2 days for sore throat without consulting a physician.

c. The **antirheumatic dosage for adults** is 3600 to 4500 mg daily in divided doses.

d. For patients with **ischemic heart disease**, a 325-mg dose is given daily. Every other day is recommended for individuals with stable or unstable angina and evolving myocardial infarction. For patients without clinically apparent ischemic heart disease, the hemorrhagic complications associated with routine aspirin use may outweigh its benefit, unless individuals have established risk factors for atherosclerotic disease.

e. For patients at risk of stroke, an 81-mg dose is given daily or every other day. As described previously, the risks may outweigh the benefits.

f. **Anti-inflammatory dosages.** Although antipyretic and analgesic effects should appear within the first few doses, the anti-inflammatory effect may take 2 weeks or more to appear, even at high doses. The usual anti-inflammatory dosage of aspirin is 4000 to 6000 mg/day. The usual anti-inflammatory dosage of ibuprofen is 1200 to 3200 mg/day.

4. **Precautions**
   a. **Hypersensitivity** to aspirin occurs in up to 0.5% of the population.
      (1) Allergic reactions resulting in bronchoconstriction occur most frequently in people with **nasal polyps**.
      (2) **Cross-reactivity** with other NSAIDs occurs in > 90% of people. Cross-reactivity with acetaminophen occurs in 5% of people.
   b. **Contraindications.** Aspirin is contraindicated in patients with bleeding disorders or peptic ulcers. Also, aspirin should not be given to children or teenagers who have a viral illness, because Reye syndrome (i.e., fatty liver degeneration accompanied by encephalopathy) may occur.
   c. **Pregnancy.** Salicylates in chronic high doses are recommended with extreme caution during the last trimester of pregnancy because of
      (1) Potential bleeding problems in the mother, fetus, or neonate
      (2) Prolonging or complicating delivery
   d. **Gastrointestinal (GI) disturbances** resulting from the inhibition of the gastric prostaglandins occur in 10% to 20% of people at analgesic and antipyretic dosages. Anti-inflammatory regimens affect up to 40% of people. These effects decrease by using enteric-coated dosage forms and by taking salicylates with food or large doses of antacids. Buffered aspirin products contain insufficient buffers to counteract the adverse GI effects of aspirin.
   e. **CNS disturbances** such as tinnitus, dizziness, or headache may occur at anti-inflammatory doses in some patients.
   f. **Salicylism** (salicylate toxicity) may occur at anti-inflammatory doses. In addition to the CNS disturbances (see I.B.4.e), respiratory alkalosis, nausea, hyperthermia, confusion, and convulsions may occur.
5. **Significant interactions**
   a. Salicylates potentiate the effect of **anticoagulants** and **thrombolytic agents**.
   b. Salicylates potentiate (at anti-inflammatory doses) the effect of **hypoglycemics**.
   c. Salicylates potentiate the adverse GI reaction resulting from chronic **alcohol** or **NSAID** use.
   d. Aspirin may competitively inhibit the metabolism of **zidovudine**, resulting in potentiation of zidovudine or aspirin toxicity.
   e. **Caffeine** taken in conjunction with salicylates appears to enhance the analgesic effect.

C. **Acetaminophen**
1. **Therapeutic uses.** Acetaminophen is used to relieve mild-to-moderate pain and to reduce fever. Guidelines from the American College of Rheumatology now recommend it as first-line therapy for osteoarthritis of the knee and hip. Because it has minimal anti-inflammatory activity, it cannot be used to treat the swelling or stiffness resulting from rheumatoid arthritis.
2. **Mechanism of action.** The analgesic and antipyretic actions of acetaminophen are the same as those for aspirin (see I.B.2.a–b).
3. **Administration and dosage.** Available dosage forms are 325 mg and 500 mg. A prolonged dosage form caplet of 650 mg is also available.
   a. For **analgesia** or **antipyresis in adults**, the dosage is 500 to 1000 mg three times daily as needed. The maximum daily dose is 4000 mg for no longer than 10 days for pain or 3 days for fever without consulting a physician. For osteoarthritis, 1000 mg four times daily is recommended.
   b. For **children age 6 years or older**, 325 mg is administered every 4 to 6 hrs as needed. The maximum daily dose is 1600 mg for no longer than 5 days for pain, 3 days for fever, or 2 days for sore throat without consulting a physician.
   c. **Routine use.** Acetaminophen is routinely used in patients who are
      (1) Sensitive to the GI disturbances caused by salicylates and NSAIDs
      (2) Prone to bleeding disorders
      (3) Hypersensitive to salicylates
4. **Precautions**
   a. Patients with active alcoholism, hepatic disease, or viral hepatitis are at risk from chronic administration of acetaminophen. Toxicity is rare, but chronic daily ingestion of 5 g or more for longer than 1 month is likely to result in liver damage. Acute doses of 10 g or more are hepatotoxic.

b. Many OTC products contain acetaminophen in addition to other ingredients. It is important to counsel patients that the daily dosage limits cited in I.C.3.a–b apply to the total acetaminophen consumed from all products daily.

c. In light of both the increasingly common addition of acetaminophen to many OTC combination products and the concern for acetaminophen-induced liver toxicity, the U.S. Food and Drug Administration (FDA) is giving strong consideration to requiring prominent warning labels on all acetaminophen-containing products and reducing the adult daily dosage limit to 3250 mg. Chronic alcohol users would be recommended an even lower dose.

5. **Significant interactions.** Acetaminophen may competitively inhibit the metabolism of **zidovudine**, resulting in potentiation of zidovudine or acetaminophen toxicity.

D. **NSAIDs.** Currently, **ibuprofen** and **naproxen** are the only NSAIDs available without a prescription.

1. **Therapeutic uses.** NSAIDs are used to relieve mild-to-moderate pain and to reduce inflammation and fever. OTC drug use largely focuses on the analgesic and antipyretic indications of these agents. Maximum OTC drug dosage is generally recommended for osteoarthritis. As mentioned previously (see I.C.1), acetaminophen is recommended as initial treatment for osteoarthritis because of its safety profile, but NSAIDs are more effective for pain and inflammation. Their use is limited by greater frequency of adverse reactions (see I.D.4) than observed with acetaminophen.

2. **Mechanism of action**

a. **Analgesic and anti-inflammatory actions.** NSAIDs inhibit prostaglandin synthesis both peripherally and centrally. Like salicylates, these drugs inhibit cyclooxygenase (*Figure 22-1*). NSAIDs produce analgesia mainly by blocking the peripheral generation of pain impulses that are mediated by prostaglandins and other chemicals. Secondarily, analgesia probably involves a reduction in the awareness of pain in the CNS.

b. **Antipyretic action.** The principal antipyretic action is central. NSAIDs act on the hypothalamic heat-regulating center to produce peripheral vasodilation, which results from the inhibition of prostaglandin synthesis.

3. **Administration and dosage.** The available OTC dosage forms of ibuprofen are a 200-mg tablet and a 100-mg per 5-mL oral suspension. Naproxen sodium OTC is available as a 220-mg (200 mg of naproxen) tablet.

a. For **analgesia** or **antipyresis in adults**, the dosage of **ibuprofen** is 200 to 400 mg every 4 to 6 hrs as needed. The maximum daily dose is 1200 mg for no longer than 10 days for pain or 3 days for fever without consulting a physician. For **naproxen sodium**, the recommended dose is 220 mg every 8 to 12 hrs as needed. The maximum daily dose is 660 mg.

b. For **rheumatoid arthritis dosage in adults, ibuprofen** is recommended to a maximum daily dosage of 3200 mg (administered on a 4- to 6-hr basis), **naproxen sodium** to a daily maximum of 1100 mg (divided doses every 8 to 12 hrs).

c. **Naproxen sodium** is not recommended for children < 12 years of age. **Ibuprofen** is available as a suspension for children 2 to 11 years of age.

4. **Precautions**

a. NSAIDs are contraindicated in patients with **bleeding disorders** or **peptic ulcers**.

b. NSAIDs are recommended with extreme caution during the last trimester of **pregnancy** because of:

(1) Potential adverse effects on fetal blood flow

(2) The possibility of prolonging pregnancy

c. **GI disturbances** resulting from the inhibition of the gastric prostaglandins occur in 5% to 10% of people at analgesic and antipyretic doses. Anti-inflammatory regimens (i.e., higher doses) affect up to 20% of people. These effects decrease when NSAIDs are taken with food or large doses of antacids. Ibuprofen is often preferred to aspirin by patients because ibuprofen causes fewer GI disturbances and bleeding events.

d. **Renal toxicity** during chronic administration is a significant concern, and may occur in the form of nephrotic syndrome, hyperkalemia, or interstitial nephritis.

e. There is a growing concern about the cardiovascular toxicity of NSAIDs. Although the risk is low, ibuprofen use is more risky than naproxen.

5. **Significant interactions**
   a. NSAIDs potentiate the effect of **anticoagulants** and **thrombolytic agents**.
   b. NSAIDs potentiate (at anti-inflammatory doses) the effect of **hypoglycemics**.
   c. NSAIDs potentiate the adverse GI reactions resulting from chronic **alcohol** or **salicylate** use.
   d. **Caffeine** taken in conjunction with ibuprofen appears to enhance the analgesic effect.
   e. Hypersensitivity to **aspirin** can occur with NSAID use.
   f. OTC labeling for these agents cautions against use of combining NSAIDs.

II. THE COMMON COLD

A. **General.** The common cold is generally a mild and self-limiting viral infection of the upper respiratory tract. Rather than typical epidemiologic measures, the prevalence of the common cold is expressed as the number of incidences per individual per year. Adults typically experience two to three colds per year; preschool children typically experience five to seven colds per year. Children < 5 years old who attend daycare or have frequent interactions with a number of other children may experience as many as 12 colds per year.

B. **Etiology.** The coronaviruses, respiratory syncytial virus (RSV), and rhinoviruses are the most contributing pathogens of the common cold, and the rhinovirus is the most frequently associated pathogen. Other pathogens involved include influenza, parainfluenza, and adenoviruses.

C. **Pathogenesis.** Pathogenic events of the common cold caused by the rhinovirus begin when a small dose of virus is deposited into the nose or the eye either by direct contact or by aerosol transmission (*Figure 22.2*).
   1. Mucociliary action transports the virus to the adenoid where the virus is able to attach to the intracellular adhesion molecule (ICAM) receptors on lymphoepithelial cells. There, the

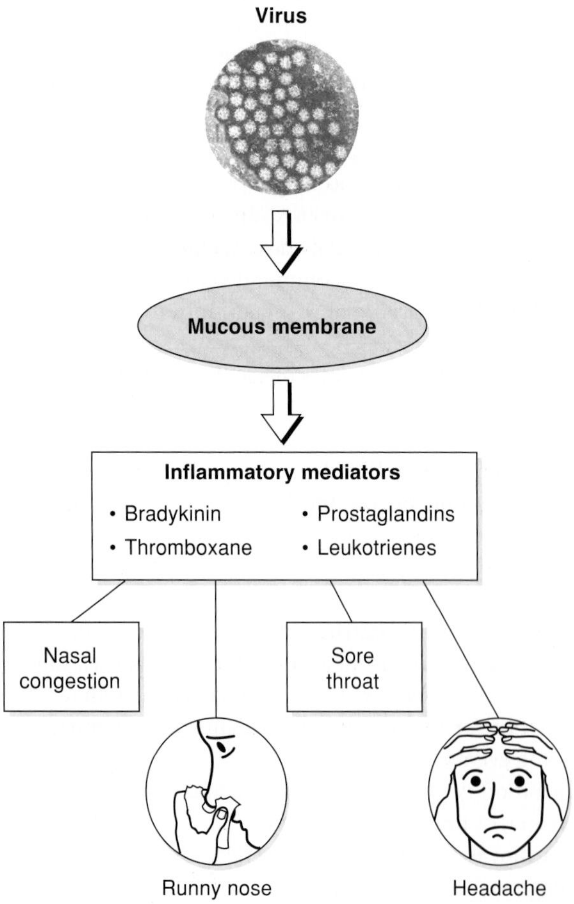

Figure 22-2. Pathogenesis of the common cold.

virus begins to replicate, triggering the release of inflammatory mediators, including histamines, kinins, certain prostaglandins, and several interleukins (e.g., interleukin 1 [IL-1], IL-6, and IL-8).

2. Within 8 to 12 hrs of viral entry into the nose or eye, the inflammatory mediators and parasympathetic nervous system reflex mechanisms lead to nasal congestion, rhinorrhea, sore throat, headache, and stimulation of cough and sneezing reflexes.

D. Symptoms

1. Once viral contact has been made, a scratchy throat may develop within 1 to 2 days.
2. A sore throat is followed by a thin, watery discharge, known as rhinorrhea, and sneezing. Within 1 to 2 days, the thin, watery discharge may become thick and purulent.
3. A dry, nonproductive cough may develop between days 3 and 5, often evolving into a productive cough.
4. The general peak of cold symptoms is 2 to 4 days, and the median duration of the common cold is 7 to 13 days.

E. Nonpharmacologic treatment includes adequate fluid intake, adequate rest, increased humidification, and/or nasal irrigation.

F. Pharmacologic treatment: Recommendations in the cough and cold aisles have changed significantly over the past few years. Previously, it was acceptable to treat the pediatric patient younger than the age of 2 for cough and cold symptoms, despite lack of data supporting this use. In 2008, an FDA public health advisory was released that nonprescription cough and cold products should not be used for individuals younger than the age of 2 due to serious and potentially life-threatening effects. In response, many manufacturers withdrew products that contained labeling for individuals younger than the age of 2, and many voluntarily relabeled their products for use in children ages 4 and older.

1. **Decongestants,** also known as sympathomimetics, are the primary treatment for nasal congestion. Decongestants are available as topical or oral delivery (*Table 22-1*).
   a. **Mechanism of action.** Both oral and topical decongestants produce vasoconstriction by stimulating α-adrenergic receptors, thereby reducing the volume of blood circulated to the nasal mucosa and decreasing mucosal edema.
   b. **Administration and dosage**
      (1) **Topical.** Available nonprescription topical decongestants include sprays (phenylephrine and oxymetazoline) and inhalers (levmetamfetamine and propylhexedrine) and are labeled for individuals ages 6 years and older.
         (a) **Phenylephrine** (topical; Neo-Synephrine): 0.25% to 1%, every 4 to 6 hrs
         (b) **Oxymetazoline** (topical; Afrin, Neo-Synephrine 12 hrs, Nostrilla, Mucinex NS, Vicks Sinex 12 hrs): 0.05%, every 10 to 12 hrs
         (c) **Levmetamfetamine** (inhaler; Vicks Vapor Inhaler):
            (i) Ages 6 to 12 years: 1 inhalation in each nostril NMT every 2 hrs
            (ii) Ages 12 years and older: 2 inhalations in each nostril NMT every 2 hrs
         (d) **Propylhexedrine** (inhaler; Benzedrex): 2 inhalations in each nostril NMT every 2 hrs
      (2) **Oral** decongestants available in the United States include pseudoephedrine and phenylephrine. Pseudoephedrine is the key ingredient in the illegal manufacturing of methamphetamine, thus the sale of pseudoephedrine has been restricted, placing it behind pharmacy counters in all states. Phenylephrine is not as easily converted into methamphetamine and thus is more readily available to consumers who are seeking relief from congestion.
         (a) **Pseudoephedrine**
            (i) Ages 2 to 5 years: 15 mg every 4 to 6 hrs; maximum dose 60 mg/24 hr
            (ii) Ages 6 to 12 years: 30 mg every 4 to 6 hrs; maximum dose 120 mg/24 hr
            (iii) Ages 12 and older: 30 to 60 mg every 4 to 6 hrs or for sustained release 120 mg every 12 hrs; maximum dose 240 mg/24 hr
         (b) **Phenylephrine**
            (i) Ages 2 to 5 years: 2.5 mg every 4 hrs
            (ii) Ages 6 to 12 years: 5 mg every 4 hrs
            (iii) Ages 12 and older: 10 mg every 4 hrs

Table 22-1 AVAILABLE TOPICAL AND ORAL DECONGESTANTS

Agent	Products	Dosing	Avoid Use In . . .	Comments/Counseling Points
		Topical Decongestants		
Oxymetazoline	Afrin; Neo-Synephrine 12 hrs; Vicks Sinex 12 hrs; Mucinex Full Force; and Mucinex Moisture Smart	2–3 sprays q10–12h	Questionable use in hypertension or receiving MAOI *May* exacerbate: hyperthyroidism, intraocular pressure, coronary heart disease, prostatic hypertrophy	Use for only 3–5 days owing to potential for rebound congestion (rhinitis medicamentosa) Oxymetazoline is long acting *Adverse effects*: cardiovascular and CNS stimulation; burning; stinging; sneezing
Phenylephrine	Neo-Synephrine	2–3 gtt q4h		
Prophylhexedrine	Benzedrex	6+ years: 2 inhalations, no more than every 2 hrs		
Levmetamfetamine	Vicks Vapor Inhaler	*6–12 years*: 1 inhalation, no more than every 2 hrs *12+ years*: 2 inhalations, no more than every 2 hrs		Lacks vasopressor effect; thus not contraindicated in patients with hypertension, thyroid disease, diabetes, narrow-angle glaucoma, or difficulty in urination owing to enlarged prostate
		Oral decongestants		
Pseudoephedrine	Sudafed	*2–6 years*: 15 mg q4–6h *6–12 years*: 30 mg q4–6h *12+ years*: 60 mg q4–6h: SR 120 mg q12h	Hypertension *May* exacerbate: hyperthyroidism, intraocular pressure, coronary heart disease, prostatic hypertrophy	Pseudoephedrine is absorbed well orally; however, phenylephrine has low oral bioavailability *Adverse effects*: cardiovascular (↑ BP, arrhythmias, tachycardia) and CNS stimulation (restlessness, insomnia, anxiety, hallucinations)
Phenylephrine	Sudafed PE	2–6 years: 2.5 mg q4h 6–12 years: 5 mg q4h 12+ years: 10 mg q4h		Concomitant use with TCA may affect BP (↑ or ↓), depending on specific decongestant

BP, blood pressure; *CNS*, central nervous system; **gtt**, drops; *MAOI*, monoamine oxidase inhibitor; *qh, every hour; TCA* tricyclic antidepressant.

c. **Precautions.** Only **under the advice of a medical provider**, and **with extreme caution** should decongestants be **recommended to patients with disease states that are sensitive to adrenergic stimulation**, including coronary heart disease, hypertension, thyroid disease, diabetes, narrow-angle glaucoma, and difficulty in urination owing to an enlarged prostate gland. Levmetamfetamine is different than the other available nasal decongestants because it lacks a vasopressor effect and, therefore, does not need to carry the warning for patients who are sensitive to adrenergic stimulation.

d. **Significant interactions.** Patients currently taking tricyclic antidepressants or monoamine oxidase inhibitors (**MAOIs**) or who are **within 2 weeks of discontinuation should avoid the use of oral and topical decongestants** owing to an increased effect on blood pressure.

e. **Counseling points**

(1) **Topical decongestants** cause localized vasoconstriction; so if used appropriately, systemic side effects should be minimal. However, given the difficulty of administration, systemic side effects are often seen with topical decongestants. *Table 22-2* provides advice for patient counseling on device selected.

(2) Patients using **topical nasal decongestants** should be cautioned to **limit use of the product to 3 to 5 days** to avoid **rhinitis medicamentosa**, a worsening of symptoms directly related to the extended use of the product. Treatment of this condition is to slowly withdraw the topical decongestant and begin oral decongestants. Topical normal saline may also be used to relieve irritated nasal passages.

(3) To avoid spread of infection, patients should be counseled not to share topical nasal decongestants with others.

(4) Topical decongestants may cause a temporary **burning or stinging sensation** when used and may also **increase nasal discharge**.

(5) Efficacy of topical decongestants may be diminished in the patient who has severely obstructed nasal passages because their use requires the ability of the medication to be delivered to the nasal mucosa.

TABLE 22-2 PATIENT COUNSELING INFORMATION FOR NASAL DECONGESTANTS

Drops	Spray (Atomizer)	Inhalers	Metered-Dose Pump (Spray)
• Blow nose • Squeeze rubber bulb on dropper and withdraw medication from bottle • Recline on bed and hang head over side (preferred) *or* tilt head back while standing or sitting • Place drops into each nostril and gently tilt head from side to side to distribute drug • Keep head tilted back for several minutes after instilling drops • Rinse dropper with hot water	• Blow nose • Remove cap from spray container • For best results, do not shake squeeze bottle • Administer one spray with head in upright position • Sniff deeply while squeezing bottle • Wait 3–5 mins, then blow nose • Administer another spray if necessary • Rinse spray tip with hot water, taking care not to allow water to enter bottle • Replace cap	• Blow nose • Warm inhaler in hand to increase volatility of medication • Remove protective cap • Inhale medicated vapor in one nostril while closing off other nostril; repeat in other nostril • Wipe inhaler clean after each use • Replace cap immediately • *Note*: Inhaler loses its potency after 2–3 months even though aroma may linger	• Blow nose • Remove protective cap • Prime metered pump by depressing several times (for first use), pointing away from face • Hold bottle with thumb at base and nozzle between first and second fingers • Insert pump gently into nose with head upright • Depress pump completely, and sniff deeply • Wait 3–5 mins, then blow nose • Administer another spray if necessary • Rinse spray tip with hot water, taking care not to allow water to enter bottle • Replace cap

(6) Once opened, **nasal inhalers should be discarded after 2 to 3 months** because the active ingredient dissipates, even when the product is tightly capped.
(7) **Pseudoephedrine may cause hypertension and palpitations.** Close monitoring should be observed in high-risk individuals.
(8) **Pseudoephedrine readily enters the CNS** and may, therefore, cause **insomnia**, restlessness, anxiety, or hallucinations. In individuals who are sensitive to this effect, the last dose should be given at least 4 to 6 hrs prior to bedtime.
(9) Notify a health care provider if symptoms worsen or do not improve within 7 days.

2. **Nasal strips** (Breathe Right) are bandagelike in appearance and function to physically open the nasal passages. Formulations include nonmedicated or with menthol.
   a. Instructions. Place the strip between the bridge and tip of the nose. As the strip attempts to resume a flattened shape, the nares are pulled into a more opened state.
   b. Uses. **Ideal in pregnancy**, **children**, and **in the elderly who take numerous medications**.
3. **Decongestion alternatives** (e.g., Coricidin HBP and its related line of products) are marketed for patients who are unable to take oral or topical nasal decongestants.
   a. Chlorpheniramine, an antihistamine, is typically the ingredient in these products.
   b. Antihistamines fail to target the primary problem: obstruction of the nasal passages.
4. **Antihistamines**
   a. **Use**
      (1) First-generation antihistamines are appropriate for the treatment of rhinorrhea, sneezing, and a nonproductive cough, but have no effect on nasal congestion. **Only first-generation antihistamines are appropriate for treatment of the common cold symptoms**. Second-generation antihistamines have preferential peripheral H_1-receptor binding, thus limiting the anticholinergic activity that is necessary to treat common cold symptoms. (*Table 22-3*).
      (2) Many providers advise against treating children for rhinorrhea and sneezing with the common cold owing to the increased risk of adverse effects. The best advice to a caregiver seeking treatment of a runny nose for a child $<$ 6 years of age is to simply let it run its course because the cold is a self-limiting viral infection.
   b. **Administration and dosing. First-generation antihistamines are not FDA approved for treatment of common cold symptoms in children younger than age 6.**
      (1) Brompheniramine (not currently available as a single-entity product)
         (a) Ages 6 to 12 years: 2 mg every 4 to 6 hrs; max dose 12 mg/24 hr
         (b) Age $>$ 12 years: 4 mg every 4 to 6 hrs; max dose 24 mg/24 hr
      (2) Chlorpheniramine (Chlor-Trimeton, Actifed)
         (a) Ages 6 to 12 years: 2 mg every 4 to 6 hrs; max dose 12 mg/24 hr
         (b) Age $>$ 12 years of age: 4 mg every 4 to 6 hrs; max dose 24 mg/24 hr
      (3) Diphenhydramine (Benadryl)
         (a) Ages 6 to 12 years: 12.5 to 25 mg every 4 to 6 hrs; max dose 150 mg/24 hr
         (b) Age $>$ 12 years: 25 to 50 mg every 4 to 6 hrs; maximum dose 300 mg/24 hr
   c. **Precautions**
      (1) **Patients with narrow-angle glaucoma and benign prostatic hypertrophy should avoid first-generation antihistamines** because the anticholinergic activities may exacerbate their condition.
      (2) Children and the elderly are most susceptible to the adverse effects of antihistamines; thus they are at increased risk of experiencing nightmares, anxiety, restlessness, unusual excitement, or irritability.
   d. **Counseling points**
      (1) Owing to **anticholinergic** properties, first-generation antihistamines may cause dry mouth (cotton mouth), blurred vision, difficulty in urination, constipation, irritability, and dizziness.
      (2) Patients taking first-generation antihistamines typically experience **sedation**, so caution should be taken driving or operating heavy machinery until one can identify how he or she will react to the ingredients. Of note, chlorpheniramine is the least sedating of the first-generation antihistamines.
      (3) Although first-generation antihistamines cause sedation in the adult patient, **children may experience paradoxical CNS stimulation**.

Table 22-3 OTC TREATMENT OF ALLERGIC RHINITIS

Agent	Product(s)	Dosing	Avoid Use In . . .	Comments/Counseling Points
Nonsedating (second-generation) antihistamine				
Loratadine	Claritin Alavert Tavist ND	*2–6 years:* 5 mg q24h *6+ years:* 10 mg q24h		No anticholinergic activity Penetrates poorly into CNS; free of sedating effects at usual doses Liver/kidney disease may need lower dosage
Cetirizine	Zyrtec	*2–5 years:* 2.5–5.0 mg qd *5+ years:* 5–10 mg qd		No anticholinergic activity May cause CNS depression Liver/kidney disease may need lower dosage
Fexofenadine	Allegra	*2–12 years:* 30 mg q12h *12+ years:* 6 mg q12h Or 180 mg q24h		Avoid concomitant administration with antacids containing aluminum and magnesium Avoid giving with fruit juices Take ER formulation on empty stomach Kidney disease may need lower dosage
Sedating (first-generation) antihistamines				
Chlorpheniramine	Chlor-Trimeton, Actifed	*2–6 years:* 1 mg q4–6h *6–12 years:* 2 mg q4–6h *12+ years:* 4 mg q4–6h	Narrow-angle glaucoma MAOI use Prostatic hypertrophy Use caution in emphysema and chronic bronchitis	Largest side effect is drowsiness, followed by typical anticholinergic side effects Children and elderly may experience paradoxical stimulation Older adults are likely to have CNS depressive side effects, including confusion and hypotension *Photosensitizing*: Advise patients to wear sunscreen and protective clothing
Diphenhydramine	Benadryl	*2–6 years:* 12.5–25 mg q4–6h *12+ years:* 25–50 mg q4–6h		

(Continued on next page)

Table 22-3 Continued.

Agent	Product(s)	Dosing	Avoid Use In . . .	Comments/Counseling Points
		Ocular antihistamines (in combination with naphazoline)		
Pheniramine	Naphcon A Opcon-A Visine-A	1–2 gtt TID–QID	Narrow-angle glaucoma: pupil dilation can cause angle-closure glaucoma	*Side effects:* burning, stinging, itching, foreign body sensation, dry eye, lid edema, and pupil dilation
Antazoline	Vasocon A	1–2 gtt TID–QID		
		Ocular Antihistamines		
Ketotifen	Zaditor	1–2 gtts BID	Narrow-angle glaucoma: pupil dilation can cause angle-closure glaucoma	*Side effects:* burning, stinging, itching, foreign body sensation, dry eye, lid edema, and pupil dilation
		Mast cell stabilizer		
Cromolyn sodium	Nasalcrom	*6+ years:* 1 spray in each nostril 3–6 times daily		Most efficacious if started before seasonal symptoms May take 3–7 days for initial response and 2–4 weeks for maximal response *Side effects:* sneezing, nasal stinging, burning Drug of choice in pregnancy for sneezing and rhinorrhea

BID, two times a day; *CNS*, central nervous system; *gtts*, drops; *MAOI*, monoamine oxidase inhibitor ; *qd*, every day; *QID*, four times a day; *TID*, three times a day.

5. **Expectorants**
   a. **Mechanism of action. Expectorants**, also known as mucolytic agents, work to loosen sputum and thin bronchial secretions by irritating the gastric mucosa and stimulating secretions of the respiratory tract. This increases the volume of the respiratory fluid and thins mucus. Therefore, it is logical to use expectorants only to **treat a productive cough**.
   b. **Administration and dosing.** The only available expectorant is **guaifenesin**, approved for patients aged 2 years and older.
      (1) **Ages** 2 to 5 years: 50 to 100 mg every 4 hrs; maximum dose 300 mg/day
      (2) **Ages** 6 to 12 years: 100 to 200 mg every 4 hrs; maximum dose 1.2 g/day
      (3) **Ages > 12 years: Extended-release tablets (Mucinex) 600 to 1200 mg every 12 hrs; Immediate-release 200 to 400 mg every 4 hrs;** maximum dose 2.4 g/day
   c. **Precautions.** Guaifenesin is generally well tolerated, but side effects may include **nausea and vomiting**, dizziness, headache, rash, or diarrhea.
   d. **Counseling tips**
      (1) For enhanced efficacy in the loosening of mucus or phlegm in the lungs, patients should **drink an ample amount of water** when taking guaifenesin.
      (2) If symptoms worsen (development of fever, rash, or unremitting headache) or no improvement is noted in 7 days, consult a medical provider.
6. **Antitussives** are recommended for a nonproductive cough.
   a. **Dextromethorphan** (DM)
      (1) **Mechanism of action.** DM is considered equipotent to codeine as a cough suppressant and works centrally in the medulla to increase the cough threshold. However, data demonstrating its efficacy as a cough suppressant are lacking.
      (2) **Administration and dosing.** Available as a dextromethorphan hydrobromide and dextromethorphan polistirex—an extended release formulation.
         (a) Patients 4 to 6 years of age: (maximum dose 30 mg/day)
            (i) DM hydrobromide: 2.5 to 5 mg every 4 hrs or 7.5 mg every 6 to 8 hrs
            (ii) DM polistirex: 15 mg every 12 hrs
         (b) Patients 6 to 12 years of age: (maximum dose 60 mg/day)
            (i) DM hydrobromide: 5 to 10 mg every 4 hrs or 15 mg every 6 to 8 hrs
            (ii) DM polistirex: 30 mg every 12 hrs
         (c) Patients > 12 years of age: (maximum dose 120 mg/day)
            (i) DM hydrobromide: 10 to 20 mg every 4 hrs or 30 mg every 6 to 8 hrs
            (ii) DM polistirex: 60 mg every 12 hrs
      (3) **Precautions**
         (a) Dextromethorphan should not be recommended for patients taking a MAOI (Nardil or Parnate) or who are within 2 weeks of discontinuation of these agents because the combination may cause serotonergic syndrome.
         (b) Adverse effects are not generally seen at typical doses, but constipation, GI upset, abdominal discomfort, and dizziness may occur.
      (4) **Counseling points**
         (a) Reports of **intentional abuse of solid dosage forms of dextromethorphan for a euphoric effect have recently increased in the adolescent population** in the United States. Although adverse effects of dextromethorphan are generally benign in recommended doses, brain damage, seizures, loss of consciousness, irregular heart beat, and death have been reported with abuse of the drug. A national campaign has been initiated to promote parental awareness of this issue.
   b. **Codeine** is a schedule C-V drug in a cough syrup, thus its sale may be restricted in some states.
      (1) **Mechanism of action.** Codeine, like dextromethorphan, works centrally in the medulla to increase the cough threshold.
      (2) **Administration and dosing** of codeine is **not recommended for children < the age of 6 years.**
         (a) Ages 6 to 12 years: 5 to 10 mg every 4 to 6 hrs; maximum dose 60 mg/day
         (b) Age > 12 years: 10 to 20 mg every 4 to 6 hrs; maximum dose 120 mg/day

(3) **Precautions**
   (a) **Adverse effects** include **drowsiness, nausea and vomiting**, excitement, abdominal discomfort, or worsening/aggravation of constipation.
   (b) An overdose of codeine may cause death from respiratory depression and cardiovascular collapse.
   (c) Caution should be used in recommending this product for patients with pulmonary disease or shortness of breath.

c. **Camphor and menthol** are the only FDA-approved topical antitussives.
(1) **Administration and dosing**
   (a) Topical ointments containing 4.7% to 5.3% camphor or 2.6% to 2.8% menthol are FDA approved for alleviation of cough. Likewise, steam inhalants containing 6.2% camphor or 3.2% menthol are approved for use in steam vaporizers.
   (b) Menthol or camphor ointment may be applied as a thick layer rubbed into the throat and chest. A warm, dry cloth may be used to cover the area. Application may be repeated up to three times daily or as directed by supervising physician.
   (c) A menthol and camphor patch may be applied to the throat or chest of patients > 2 years of age. If the patient has sensitive skin, the patch may be applied to clothing covering the throat or chest, but the patch may not adhere to some types of polyester clothing. Clothing should be left loose so that vapors reach the nose and mouth. The patch should be removed, and a new patch applied, if needed, up to three times daily.
   (d) Menthol or camphor steam inhalants may be added directly to the water (1 tablespoon per 1 quart of water) in a hot steam vaporizer, bowl, or basin. Vapors should be breathed in. This process may be repeated up to three times daily or as directed by supervising provider.
   (e) Menthol (5 to 10 mg) is also effective as an antitussive available in oral lozenges or compressed tablets. Menthol stimulates cold sensory receptors, producing a sensation of coolness and a local anesthetic effect on the respiratory passageways, thus engendering a soothing, antitussive effect.

(2) **Counseling.** Per FDA, all topical or inhalant products containing camphor or menthol must warn patients that their **use near a flame, in hot water, or in a microwave oven may cause the products to splatter and cause serious burns to the user**.

7. **Intranasal normal saline**, available in drops and sprays, may be used to moisten nasal membranes and assist in the removal of encrusted secretions.
   a. Typical use is two to three sprays in each nostril as needed. Some products may be used as a spray when held upright or as drops when held upside down.
   b. Intranasal normal saline may be **recommended** for use in all patients, including **infants** and **pregnant women**, unless directed otherwise by a physician.
8. **Local anesthetics** (e.g., benzocaine, phenol, menthol) in the form of lozenges and sprays may be useful in the alleviation of a sore throat. Mouthwashes have been recommended for use in the past; however, owing to localized action in the oral cavity, the pharyngeal wall may not be affected by these products. Because a sore throat is the initial symptom of many other illnesses, care should be taken to recommend products for sore throat alleviation only to patients who have concurrent symptoms of the common cold. **If the throat is red and inflamed, unusually painful, or has persisted for several days, the patient should be referred** to a primary care provider for further evaluation.
9. **Analgesics** are occasionally indicated in the treatment of common cold symptoms when sore throat, myalgia, and/or headache exist. Acetaminophen, ibuprofen, or naproxen sodium may be recommended, with consideration given to patient allergies, concurrent medications and disease states, and age.
10. **Combination products**
   a. Numerous products are available that contain various combinations of antihistamines, decongestants, analgesics, expectorants, and antitussives. Certain product name designations help identify the ingredients.

(1) *Nighttime* and P.M. usually signify that the product contains diphenhydramine, chlorpheniramine, or doxylamine.
(2) *Sinus* usually signifies a decongestant (e.g., pseudoephedrine, phenylephrine) and/or an analgesic (e.g., acetaminophen).
(3) *Cough* usually signifies that the product contains dextromethorphan.
(4) *Nondrowsy*, A.M., and *daytime* usually indicate that the product contains a decongestant (e.g., pseudoephedrine, phenylephrine) and typically does not contain an antihistamine.
(5) *Allergy* signifies that the product contains an antihistamine.
(6) *Cold* and *flu* indicate that the product may contain any combination of ingredients, including a decongestant, antihistamine, cough suppressant, and/or antipyretic.

b. Combination products may be useful for simplicity of dosing and adherence if patients are experiencing a variety of symptoms that can be alleviated by one product. For example, if a patient has a dry, hacking, nonproductive cough, and nasal congestion, he or she may benefit from a combination product of dextromethorphan and pseudoephedrine. However, it would be a shotgun approach to recommend a product containing an analgesic and expectorant in combination with other ingredients for this patient.

c. Disadvantages to combination products occur when previously treated symptoms resolve, but the patient continues to treat other symptoms with the same product. This adds unnecessary medication(s) to the regimen, increasing the risk of adverse events. Combination products can also be difficult to recommend when selecting the appropriate product for patients with coexisting medical conditions.

11. Complementary therapy

a. Zinc gluconate's effects on the duration or severity of the common cold have been studied. Results have been mixed, lending to what remains a controversial subject.

(1) **Mechanism of action.** Current literature describes several possible mechanisms by which zinc may exert its effect, but such means remain unclear.
(2) **Availability and dosing.** Despite its controversial use, a number of zinc products have been formulated, including tablets, capsules, chewing gums, lozenges, nasal gels, nasal sprays, and nasal swabs.
   (a) **Selected formulations should be initiated within 24 to 48 hrs of the onset of symptoms.**
   (b) Lozenges are recommended every 2 hrs for the duration of the cold.
   (c) **Nasal sprays, swabs, and gels have been withdrawn from the market due to reports of permanent anosmia associated with the products.**

b. Vitamin C. Only a small number of studies have demonstrated the ability of vitamin C (dose > 1 g/day) to reduce the frequency or severity of the common cold. The clinical significance of the results of these studies remains questionable.

c. Echinacea has been used as a popular remedy for the common cold since the late 1800s. Unfortunately, current literature does not give definitive supportive evidence for the efficacy of Echinacea in the prevention and/or treatment of the common cold.

(1) Obstacles in studying Echinacea lie in the fact that three different species of *Echinacea* exist, each with a different phytochemical composition. The composition may further be altered, depending on the part of the plant used and the time of year the plant is harvested.
(2) Current literature suggests that for Echinacea **to retain an immunostimulant effect, it should not be taken for longer than 2 to 3 weeks at a time**.

G. Exclusions to self-treatment of the common cold

1. Fever > 101.5°F
2. Chest pain
3. Shortness of breath
4. Worsening of symptoms or development of additional symptoms
5. Concurrent underlying chronic cardiopulmonary diseases
6. AIDS or chronic immunosuppressant therapy
7. Frail patients of advanced age

III. ALLERGIC RHINITIS

A. **Introduction.** Rhinitis is an inflammation of nasal membranes, characterized by the **four cardinal symptoms: nasal congestion, rhinorrhea, sneezing, and nasal itching**.

1. Risk factors for allergic rhinitis include the following:
   a. Family history of atopy
   b. Higher socioeconomic class
   c. Exposure to indoor allergens (animals and dust mites)
   d. Positive allergy skin prick test
2. Allergic rhinitis may be classified as seasonal, perennial, episodic, or occupational. Seasonal and perennial, or a combination of the two, are the most frequent classifications.
   a. Seasonal: Symptoms may occur with repetitive and predictable seasonal symptoms.
   b. Perennial: Symptoms persist throughout the year without regard to season changes.
   c. Combination: Symptoms persist throughout the year with seasonal exacerbations.

B. **Etiology.** There are five main triggers for allergic rhinitis: pollens, molds, dust mites, animal allergens, and insect allergens. These allergens trigger an immunoglobulin E (IgE) mediated immunological reaction.

1. Seasonal allergic rhinitis is typically caused by pollens and molds.
2. Perennial allergic rhinitis is typically caused by dust mites, molds, and animal allergens.

C. **Pathogenesis.** Patients become sensitized to allergens; on subsequent exposure, the allergens trigger a genetically predetermined immune response that results in the symptoms of allergic rhinitis. Allergic rhinitis may then be characterized by early- or late-phase responses.

D. **Signs and symptoms.** The presence of itchy, watery eyes, and/or nasal pruritus is what differentiates allergic rhinitis from the common cold. Because children often cannot verbalize the symptoms of allergic rhinitis, it is important to recognize these signs.

1. Repercussions of nasal pruritus include the following:
   a. **Gothic arch**, a steady upward movement of the upper lip and teeth which may result in an overbite, as a result of the "allergic salute," characterized by the constant upward rubbing of the nose with the palm of the hand.
   b. **Allergic crease**, a visible transverse line appearing between the tip and the bridge of the nose, caused by constant rubbing.
2. Ophthalmic conditions present in the individual with allergic rhinitis include allergic shiners, a darkening of the lower eyelid attributable to chronic nasal obstruction, and Morgan lines (also known as the Dennie sign), which are seen as pleats under the eyes, running parallel to the lower eyelid margins.
3. Individuals with allergic rhinitis may also experience fatigue, irritability, and malaise. Owing to these symptoms, allergic rhinitis may be a contributing factor to poor schoolwork in children afflicted by this condition.

E. **Treatment.** The primary goal in the treatment of allergic rhinitis is to control the symptoms without altering the patient's ability to function. Treatment options include environmental control, nonprescription pharmacologic treatment, and prescription treatment. This section focuses on nonprescription treatment (see *Table 22-3*).

1. The **best treatment remains avoidance of the allergen(s)**, once determined, although this is sometimes impractical. Environmental controls directed toward particular allergens can be the first initiative toward resolution of symptoms.
2. **Antihistamines**, both first and second generation, are the mainstay of treatment for allergic rhinitis.
   a. First-generation antihistamines are limited in continuous treatment of allergic rhinitis owing to their frequent dosing and related sedation. Unlike treatment of the common cold, first-generation antihistamines may be used for allergic rhinitis symptoms in patients between the ages of 2 and 5 years. These agents remain the least expensive treatment option at this time; however, this aspect must be weighed against the ability to remain alert for work and school activities.
   b. Second-generation antihistamines are advantageous because of their preferential peripheral H_1-receptor binding. This allows for minimal CNS effects, minimal sedative effects, and minimal anticholinergic activity. Three nonprescription second-generation antihistamines are currently available on the market as single-entity products or in combination with pseudoephedrine: loratadine, cetirizine, and fexofenadine. Comparison of therapeutic effectiveness

among the three products remains unclear at this time. However, in dosing comparisons, loratadine and cetirizine can be given once daily, and fexofenadine can be given once or twice daily, depending on the dose.

(1) **Administration and dosing**

(a) Loratadine (Claritin): adjust in hepatic and/or renal impairment

(i) Ages 2 to 6 years: 5 mg once daily

(ii) Ages 6 years and older: 10 mg once daily

(b) Cetirizine (Zyrtec): adjust in hepatic and/or renal impairment

(i) Ages 2 to 6 years: 2.5 to 5.0 mg once daily

(ii) Ages 6 to 12 years: 5 to 10 mg once daily

(iii) Ages 12 and older: 10 mg once daily

(c) Fexofenadine (Allegra): Available in 12 - or 24-hr dosing; adjust in renal impairment

(i) Ages 2 to 6 years: 30 mg twice daily (syrup only)

(ii) Ages 6 to 12 years: 30 mg twice daily

(iii) Ages 12 and older: 60 mg twice daily or 180 mg once daily

(2) **Drug Interactions:** Concomitant administration of **aluminum and magnesium containing antacids** (e.g., Maalox) **may decrease absorption and peak plasma concentrations of fexofenadine**. Extended release doses (once daily doses) of **fexofenadine should be taken on an empty stomach with water**. Avoid taking fexofenadine with fruit (e.g., grapefruit, orange, apple) juices because fruit juices reduce the bioavailability of fexofenadine by greater than 30%.

3. Oral decongestants are effective in relieving symptoms of nasal congestion but have no effect on other symptoms of allergic rhinitis such as rhinorrhea, pruritus, or sneezing.

a. **Because treatment of allergic rhinitis is for extended periods, oral decongestants should be used for nasal congestion rather than topical decongestants** owing to the potential for rhinitis medicamentosa.

b. The combination of a decongestant and an antihistamine has proven to be an optimal treatment regimen for allergic rhinitis.

c. Consideration must be taken into account when recommending products containing pseudoephedrine to adolescents and adults participating in sports programs, because of the "doping" effect of these agents.

4. Ocular antihistamines may be used for the treatment of ophthalmic conditions associated with allergic rhinitis.

a. Currently there are three ocular antihistamines available on the market: pheniramine, antazoline, and ketotifen. Pheniramine and antazoline are only available in combination with naphazoline (a decongestant). Ketotifen (Zaditor) became available as a nonprescription product in 2007 and is the only available ocular antihistamine that does not contain a decongestant.

b. Avoid the use of ocular antihistamines in glaucoma, as pupil dilation may cause angle-closure glaucoma.

c. Side effects may include burning, stinging, itching, foreign body sensation, dry eye, lid edema, and pupil dilation.

5. **Cromolyn sodium** (e.g., Nasalcrom) is best used as a preventive measure for the symptoms of allergic rhinitis but may also be used as treatment for all symptoms except nasal congestion. However, **maximum benefit**, when used as treatment, **will not be seen for 1 to 2 weeks**. When used for prevention, cromolyn sodium should be initiated approximately 1 week before allergen contact.

a. Cromolyn sodium has a short duration of action and, therefore, must be **dosed three to four times daily**. This frequency in dosing may result in diminished adherence.

b. Cromolyn sodium is approved for use in patients **2 years of age and older**.

c. Seek medical care if symptoms worsen or no improvement is seen within 2 weeks.

d. Adverse effects include a brief stinging or sneezing directly after administration.

F. **Exclusions to self-treatment of allergic rhinitis**

1. Symptoms of otitis media or sinusitis
2. Symptoms that suggest lower respiratory tract problems
3. History of nonallergic rhinitis

Study Questions

Directions: Each of the questions, statements, or incomplete statements can be correctly answered or completed by **one** of the suggested answers or phrases. Choose the **best** answer.

1. Which statement concerning the use of over-the-counter (OTC) analgesic agents is true?
   - **(A)** Aspirin is indicated for mild to moderate analgesia, inflammatory diseases, antipyresis, and prophylaxis for patients with ischemic heart disease.
   - **(B)** Ibuprofen is indicated for mild to moderate analgesia, reduction of fever, and prophylaxis for patients with ischemic heart disease but not for inflammatory disorders.
   - **(C)** Acetaminophen is indicated for mild to moderate analgesia but not for reduction of fever and osteoarthritis.
   - **(D)** Naproxen sodium is indicated for mild to moderate analgesia, antipyresis, and prophylaxis for patients with ischemic heart disease.

2. Which statement concerning drug interactions with over-the-counter (OTC) analgesic agents is true?
   - **(A)** Aspirin potentiates the effects of antihypertensives, cardiac glycosides, and anticoagulants.
   - **(B)** Ibuprofen potentiates the effect of zidovudine, hypoglycemics, and aminoglycosides.
   - **(C)** Acetaminophen potentiates the effect of zidovudine.
   - **(D)** For naproxen sodium, the OTC dosage recommendations are similar to the prescription dosage.

3. All of the following statements concerning contraindications with chronic use of over-the-counter (OTC) analgesic agents are correct *except* which one?
   - **(A)** Aspirin, ibuprofen, and naproxen sodium are contraindicated in patients with bleeding disorders, peptic ulcer, and the third trimester of pregnancy.
   - **(B)** Aspirin, acetaminophen, and ibuprofen are implicated in Reye syndrome.
   - **(C)** Acetaminophen is contraindicated in patients with active alcoholism, hepatic disease, or viral hepatitis.

4. Which statement concerning dosage recommendations for over-the-counter (OTC) analgesic agents is true?
   - **(A)** Aspirin for analgesia or antipyresis in adults is 325 to 650 mg every 4 hrs or 650 to 1000 mg every 6 hrs, with a maximum daily dose of 4000 mg for no longer than 10 days for pain or 3 days for fever without consulting a physician; the antirheumatic dosage for adults is 3600 to 4500 mg daily in divided doses; and patients with ischemic heart disease should take 325 mg daily or every other day.
   - **(B)** Ibuprofen for analgesia or antipyresis in adults is 300 to 600 mg every 6 to 8 hrs, with a maximum daily dose of 1800 mg for no longer than 10 days for pain or 3 days for fever without consulting a physician; the anti-inflammatory dosage for adults is 1800 to 3600 mg daily in divided doses.
   - **(C)** Acetaminophen for analgesia or antipyresis in adults is 325 mg every 8 to 2 hrs, with a maximum daily dose of 2000 mg for no longer than 10 days for pain and 3 days for fever without consulting a physician; patients with ischemic heart disease take 325 mg daily or every other day.

5. Which of the following is an inhaler ingredient deemed safe and effective for nasal congestion?
   - **(A)** oxymetazoline
   - **(B)** phenylephrine
   - **(C)** levmetamfetamine
   - **(D)** pseudoephedrine

6. A 27-year-old presents with sneezing, rhinorrhea, and nasal itching, which started 2 days ago. She feels miserable with her symptoms, which worsen when she cleans the house. Her current medications include calcium carbonate and docusate sodium. Which of the following would be the *best* recommendation for immediate symptom alleviation?
   - **(A)** chlorpheniramine
   - **(B)** pseudoephedrine
   - **(C)** topical nasal strips
   - **(D)** intranasal cromolyn

7. A 48-year-old presents with a chief complaint of a dry, hacking cough, which started yesterday. He denies fever, chills, sore throat, or congestion. His only medical condition is hypertension, which is controlled with hydrochlorothiazide (HCTZ). What would be the *best* recommendation for alleviation of his cough?
   (A) dextromethorphan
   (B) phenylephrine
   (C) fexofenadine
   (D) guaifenesin

8. Which of the following is an appropriate candidate for self-treatment with codeine for cough?
   (A) 4-year-old with nonproductive cough
   (B) 6-year-old with nonproductive cough
   (C) 15-year-old with productive cough
   (D) 22-year-old with productive cough
   (E) 92-year-old with nonproductive cough

For questions 9–10: A 42-year-old male complains of a scratchy throat, nasal congestion, and a cough that started 2 days ago. When he coughs, he brings up yellow-white phlegm. He has hypertension and dyslipidemia. Current medications include simvastatin, lisinopril, hydrochlorothiazide, carvedilol, hydralazine, isosorbide dinitrate, and amlodipine.

9. Which of the following would be the *best* recommendation for this person's cough?
   (A) codeine
   (B) dextromethorphan
   (C) diphenhydramine
   (D) guaifenesin

10. Which of the following would be the *most* appropriate recommendation for his nasal congestion?
    (A) Oral pseudoephedrine
    (B) Oral phenylephrine
    (C) Topical oxymetazoline
    (D) Topical levmetamfetamine

11. A 22-year-old female presents with sneezing, watery and itchy eyes, and a runny nose. She has no significant medical history, but she is in the midst of final exams and must remain alert. What would be the *best* recommendation for her symptoms?
    (A) Fexofenadine
    (B) Diphenhydramine
    (C) Brompheniramine
    (D) Levmetamfetamine

Answers and Explanations

1. **The answer is A** *[see I.B]*.
   Aspirin is the only analgesic agent with an approved labeling for analgesia, antipyresis, inflammation, and prophylaxis for ischemic heart disease.

2. **The answer is C** *[see I.C]*.
   Acetaminophen may competitively inhibit the metabolism of zidovudine, resulting in potentiation of zidovudine or acetaminophen toxicity. As for the other choices, OTC dosage levels are generally one-half the prescription dosage; aspirin is not commonly recognized to interact with antihypertensives or cardiac glycosides; nor is acetaminophen expected to interact with aminoglycosides.

3. **The answer is B** *[see I.B.4.b]*.
   Aspirin is the only analgesic agent associated with the development of Reye syndrome.

4. **The answer is A** *[see I.B.3; I.C.3; I.D.3]*.
   The aspirin dosage OTC recommendations are correct; the levels for acetaminophen are too low, and for ibuprofen, too high. In addition, acetaminophen does not carry an ischemic heart disease prophylaxis recommendation.

5. **The answer is C** *[see II.F.1.b.(1)]*.
   Levmetamfetamine is an inhaler ingredient that has been deemed by the FDA as safe and effective as a nasal decongestant. It is currently found in Vicks Vapor Inhaler. Oxymetazoline and phenylephrine are topical nasal decongestants found in pumps and drops but not in inhalers.

6. **The answer is A** *[see II.F.4; III.E.5]*.
   Rhinorrhea, sneezing, and nasal itching are symptoms of allergic rhinitis. Pseudoephedrine and topical nasal strips are indicated for nasal congestion, which she does not have. Both chlorpheniramine and intranasal cromolyn sodium are recommended treatments for the relief of sneezing and rhinorrhea. However, this patient needs immediate relief, and cromolyn sodium will take 1 to 2 weeks for noticeable symptom improvement.

7. **The answer is A** *[see II.F.6]*.
   The complaint is a dry, hacking cough, warranting the use of an antitussive rather than an expectorant (e.g., guaifenesin). Dextromethorphan is the only choice of antitussives provided.

8. **The answer is B** *[see II.F.6.b]*.
Codeine is appropriate for ages 6 and up for a nonproductive cough. Although a 92-year-old with a nonproductive cough fits this criteria, caution should be taken due to adverse effects associated with codeine.

9. **The answer is D** *[see II.F.5]*.
The patient is experiencing a productive cough, as noted by the yellow-white phlegm. An expectorant is the best agent for relief of a productive cough. The only available expectorant is guaifenesin, which works to loosen sputum and to thin bronchial secretions by irritating the gastric mucosa and stimulates secretions of the respiratory tract.

10. **The answer is D** *[see II.F.1.c]*.
Pseudoephedrine, phenylephrine, and oxymetazoline should be used cautiously in the patient with hypertension, particularly a patient on this many antihypertensive agents, due to stimulation of adrenergic receptors. Levmetamfetamine lacks a vasopressor effect and therefore is the least likely agent to affect his blood pressure.

11. **The answer is A** *[see III.E.2]*.
Levmetamfetamine, a nasal decongestant, would offer no benefit for the symptoms described. Although diphenhydramine and brompheniramine are first generation antihistamines, both would cause significant sedation when the patient needs to remain alert. Additionally, brompheniramine is not available as a single-ingredient product. Fexofenadine would alleviate the described symptoms without causing increased sedation.

23

Over-the-Counter Agents for Constipation, Diarrhea, Hemorrhoids, and Heartburn

JENNIFER D. SMITH

I. CONSTIPATION

A. **General information**

1. **Definition.** Constipation is defined as a decrease in the frequency of fecal elimination and is characterized by the passage of hard, dry, and sometimes painful stools. Normal stool frequency ranges from three times daily to three times per week. Patients may experience abdominal bloating, headaches, low back pain, and/or a sense of rectal fullness from incomplete evacuation of feces.
2. **Epidemiology**
   a. **Age.** Constipation is common in all age groups, however; there is a higher prevalence in people > 65 years of age.
   b. **Gender.** Women suffer from constipation more often than men.
3. **Causes.** Constipation can be caused by many factors, including the following:
   a. **Lifestyle. A diet** insufficient in fiber and/or inadequate fluid intake, **lack of exercise**, **and poor bowel habits**, such as failure to respond to the defecatory urge or hurried bowels (i.e., incomplete evacuation) can contribute to constipation.
   b. **Medications**, such as narcotic analgesics, diuretics, or anticholinergics (e.g., antidepressants, antihypertensives, antihistamines, phenothiazines, antispasmodics). In addition, nonprescription medications such as iron supplements, calcium- or aluminum-containing antacids, nonprescription nonsteroidal anti-inflammatory drugs (NSAIDs), and histamine-2 receptor antagonists (H_2RAs; i.e., ranitidine) may contribute to constipation.
   c. **Pregnancy** is a common contributor to constipation. The increased size of the uterus, hormonal changes, intake of calcium- and iron-containing prenatal vitamins, and a reduction in physical activity are all considered contributing factors.
   d. **Systemic disorders**, such as intestinal obstruction, tumor, inflammatory bowel disease, diverticulitis, hypothyroidism, hyperglycemia, irritable bowel syndrome, cerebrovascular disease, or Parkinson disease.
4. **Assessment** should include normal stool frequency, frequency and duration of the constipation, exercise routine, daily dietary fiber and fluid intake, presence of other symptoms, and current medications.

B. Treatment

1. **Nonpharmacologic**
   a. Increase intake of fluids (at least eight 8-oz servings of noncaffeinated fluids daily) and fiber (e.g., whole-grain breads and cereals, beans, prunes, peas, carrots, corn). The recommended adult intake of fiber is 20 to 35 g/day, but individuals who are consuming inadequate amounts of fiber should increase the amount of fiber intake slowly to prevent gastrointestinal distress.
   b. Increase exercise to increase and maintain bowel tone.
   c. Bowel training to increase regularity (i.e., allowing regular and adequate time for defecation).
2. **Pharmacologic** recommendations for simple constipation should begin as a **step-wise approach** with **bulk-forming laxatives** as first line, **hyperosmotic laxatives** as second line, and then **stimulant laxatives** if the previous recommendations were ineffective or intolerable. **Self-care** for the treatment of constipation should be **limited to 7 days**.
   a. **Bulk-forming laxatives** are natural or synthetic polysaccharide or cellulose derivatives that adsorb water to soften the stool and increase bulk, which stimulates peristalsis.
      (1) **Availability.** Bulk-forming agents include **psyllium** (e.g., Metamucil, Konsyl, Fiberall), **methylcellulose** (e.g., Citrucel), **calcium polycarbophil** (e.g., Konsyl Fiber caplets, FiberCon), and **wheat dextran** (e.g., Benefiber). All bulk-forming agents must be given with at least 8 oz of water to prevent choking.
      (2) **Onset of action is slow** and ranges from 12 to 24 hrs up to 72 hrs.
      (3) **Adverse effects:** Bloating, abdominal cramping, and flatulence
      (4) **Warnings and counseling points**
         (a) Bulk-forming agents should not be used if an obstructing bowel lesion, intestinal strictures, or Crohn's disease are present due to the potential to worsen the situation or result in bowel perforation. Additionally, because of the administration guidelines, bulk-forming laxatives may be inappropriate for individuals with severe fluid restrictions, such as those with heart failure or renal impairment.
         (b) Sugar-free formulations should be considered for individuals with diabetes but avoided in individuals with phenylketonuria.
         (c) The use of bulk-forming laxatives for constipation relief should be limited to 1 week; however, they can be used on a long-term basis for prevention.
   b. **Hyperosmotic laxatives** work by creating an osmotic gradient to pull water into the small and large intestines, resulting in increased peristalsis and bowel motility.
      (1) **Availability**
         (a) **Glycerin** (e.g., Fleet Glycerin Suppositories, Fleet Pedia-Lax) is only safe and effective when **used rectally**. Dosing for **ages 6 years to adult** is 2 g regular suppository or 5.4 g in liquid suppository; **ages 2 to 5 years** is 1 g regular suppository or 2.8 g in liquid suppository.
         (b) **Polyethylene glycol 3350 (e.g., Miralax, Dulcolax Balance)** is approved for self-care use in **ages 17 years and older**. It is dosed as **17 g**, stirred into 4 to 8 oz of fluid, **once daily**.
      (2) **Onset of action** varies greatly between the two nonprescription items in this class. **Glycerin** suppositories have an onset range of **15 mins to 1 hr and polyethylene glycol** has a longer onset of **1 to 3 days**.
      (3) **Adverse effects.** As expected, rectal burning may occur with glycerin products; polyethylene glycol causes adverse effects at excessive doses and can include diarrhea, nausea, bloating, cramping, and flatulence.
      (4) **Warning. Avoid** use in individuals with **kidney disease**, **irritable bowel syndrome**, during pregnancy, or while breastfeeding.
   c. **Stimulant laxatives** work by altering water and electrolyte transport by the intestines and by stimulating bowel motility (i.e., propulsive peristaltic activity). They are recommended for relief of constipation when an individual has failed or is intolerant to bulk-forming or hyperosmotic agents. However, stimulant laxatives are being used more frequently as first-line therapy for opiate-induced chronic constipation.
      (1) **Availability.** The two main classes of stimulant laxatives are anthraquinones (e.g., senna, sennosides) and diphenylmethane (e.g., bisacodyl).
         (a) **Senna** can be taken as single-entity products (e.g., Senokot, Ex-Lax, Perdiem, Fletcher's Laxative for Kids) or combined with a stool softener (e.g., Senokot-S, Peri-Colace) for relief of constipation. Senna is available as a standardized concentrate or

as sennosides, which are derived from the senna leaves. Adult dosing in solid oral formulations is 187 to 374 mg standardized concentrate and 8.6 to 17.2 mg sennosides. Senna is appropriate for self-care for pediatrics (**ages 2 and older**) and is available as a syrup, tablet, or chocolate chew.

(b) **Bisacodyl** (e.g., Dulcolax, Correctol) is available in rectal and oral formulations. Adult doses are 5 to 15 mg by mouth or 10 mg rectally once daily. Pediatric dose (**ages 6 and older**) is 5 mg orally or rectally once daily.

(2) **Onset of action.** The onset of action of the oral preparation is within 6 to 12 hrs, but the rectal preparation onset of action is quicker, within 15 to 60 mins.

(3) **Adverse effects.** All stimulant laxatives can cause **abdominal cramping**. Electrolyte and fluid deficiencies, enteric loss of protein, malabsorption, and hypokalemia are additional possible adverse effects. The suppository form may cause rectal burning.

(4) **Warnings and counseling points**

(a) Individuals with undiagnosed rectal bleeding or signs of intestinal obstruction should not use stimulant laxatives.

(b) **Cathartic colon**, which results in a poorly functioning colon, has been associated with the chronic use of stimulant laxatives. However, there is no convincing evidence that chronic use impairs the colon in structure or function. Caution should still be taken with the chronic use of stimulant laxatives due to the other associated adverse effects noted above.

(c) Sennosides may cause **discoloration of the urine** (pink/red, yellow, or brown), but this is a **harmless effect**.

(d) Tablet formulations of **bisacodyl should not be crushed or chewed** due to the enteric coating. **Milk, H_2RA** (e.g., ranitidine, cimetidine, famotidine), **and antacids may erode this enteric coating** and should be separated in dosing by at least 1 hr.

d. **Emollient laxatives**, also known as **surfactants**, work by allowing water to move more easily into the stool. This creates a softer stool, which is easier to pass. Thus, these agents are particularly useful in those who must avoid straining to pass hard stools (e.g., recent myocardial infarction, rectal surgery). Emollient laxatives have very few side effects, but they are not as effective as other laxatives.

(1) **Availability.** Emollient laxatives are salts of the surfactant **docusate**. These products contain insignificant amounts of calcium, sodium, or potassium, and there are no specific guidelines for the selection of any one product. The products include **docusate sodium** (e.g., Colace) and **docusate calcium** (e.g., Kaopectate Stool Softener). Adult dosing is 50 to 300 mg/day and dosing for children **> 2 years of age** is 50 to 150 mg/day. Each dose should be **taken with at least 8 oz of water**.

(2) **Onset of action.** Slow onset of action (24 to 72 hrs).

(3) **Adverse effects.** Diarrhea and mild abdominal cramping are possible.

(4) **Warnings.** Use should be avoided in individuals with nausea and vomiting, symptoms of appendicitis, or undetermined abdominal pain.

e. **Saline laxatives**, which include **sodium and magnesium salts**, work to **draw water into the colon**. This class of laxatives includes **magnesium citrate, magnesium hydroxide** (e.g., Milk of Magnesia, Phillips caplets), and **sodium phosphate** (e.g., Fleet's Enema).

(1) **Onset of action is 30 mins to 3 hrs** when given orally and **2 to 5 mins when given rectally**.

(2) **Side effects include abdominal cramping, excessive diuresis, nausea and vomiting, and dehydration.** As much as 20% of magnesium may be absorbed from these products, which may lead to **hypermagnesemia in patients with preexisting renal impairment**. Excessive doses of magnesium result in diarrhea.

(3) **Warnings and counseling points**

(a) The adult dose of magnesium citrate is consumption of one full bottle. Refrigeration of the product may increase palatability and help prevent crystallization.

(b) Sodium-containing salts should be **avoided in those individuals with sodium restrictions** (e.g., heart failure, edema, renal failure) and magnesium-containing products should be avoided in individuals with severe kidney disease.

(c) **Oral sodium phosphate (OSP)** products (e.g., Fleet's Phospho-Soda) have been sold for years as nonprescription products for constipation and for acute bowel evacuation.

However, the U.S. Food and Drug Administration (FDA) received numerous reports of acute phosphate nephropathy (**acute kidney injury**) associated with these products when used for acute bowel evacuation. FDA has allowed nonprescription OSP products to remain available for the treatment of constipation because acute kidney injury has not been reported at these doses. However, FDA has determined that nonprescription OSP products are not appropriate for bowel cleansing. In response, Fleet Laboratories voluntarily removed their OSP products from the market.

f. **Lubricant laxative.** Mineral oil is the only available agent in this class. It works at the colon to increase water retention in the stool.
   (1) **Availability.** Mineral oil can be given **once daily orally or rectally**. The dose for adults (age ≥ 12 years) is 15 to 45 mL orally or 118 mL rectally and for children (age 6 to 11 years) is 10 to 15 mL orally or 59 mL rectally.
   (2) **Onset of action.** 6 to 8 hrs (oral dosing) and 5 to 15 mins (rectal dosing)
   (3) **Adverse effects** include anal seepage, which can result in itching and perianal discomfort.
   (4) **Warnings and counseling points**
      (a) Mineral oil can **decrease absorption of fat-soluble vitamins** (i.e., vitamins A, D, E, and K), so it should not be used on a chronic basis.
      (b) Mineral oil should be taken on an empty stomach. Because of possible **aspiration of mineral oil into the lungs (lipid pneumonitis)**, this agent should not be taken at bedtime. Those who are elderly, debilitated, or have dysphagia are at the greatest risk of lipid pneumonitis.
      (c) Emollients (e.g., docusate) may increase the systemic absorption of mineral oil, which can lead to **hepatotoxicity**. Thus **emollient and lubricant laxatives should not be given concomitantly**.
      (d) Mineral oil is contraindicated in persons with rectal bleeding, appendicitis, or age < 6 years.

C. **Special populations**
   1. **Pediatrics.** Constipation should be expected if there is a drastic change from baseline bowel function. Nonpharmacologic methods such as increasing the amount of fluid or sugar provided or increasing the bulk content of the diet (fruit, fiber cereals, vegetables) should be tried before medications are used. If nonpharmacologic methods do not work, those < 2 years of age should be referred to a medical provider. Glycerin suppositories may be used in those > 2 years of age.
   2. **Pregnant.** Constipation in pregnancy is common and can be the result of compression of the colon by the enlarged uterus, ingestion of prenatal vitamins containing iron and calcium, and the influence of progesterone can cause bowel hypomotility. Bulk-forming agents or stool softeners are appropriate to recommend during pregnancy.
   3. **Geriatrics.** The elderly tend to be at risk for constipation due to insufficient dietary (fiber) and fluid ingestion, concurrent disease states (e.g., hypothyroidism), and/or medications (e.g., opiates, anticholinergics). A **major concern** with the geriatric population is the possible loss of fluid that can be induced by aggressive laxative treatment (e.g., enemas, high-dose saline laxatives). Hyperosmotic or stimulant laxatives may be useful for initial treatment and bulk-forming laxatives for prevention, depending on concomitant disease states.

II. DIARRHEA

A. **General information**
   1. **Definition.** Diarrhea is defined as an increase in the frequency and looseness of stools compared to one's normal bowel pattern. The overall weight and volume of the stool is increased (> 200 g or mL/day), and the water content is increased to 60% to 90%. In general, diarrhea results when the intestine is unable to absorb water from the stool, which causes excess water in the stool.
   2. **Classification.** Diarrhea can be classified based on mechanism or origin.
      a. **Classification by mechanism**
         (1) **Osmotic diarrhea** occurs when excess water is pulled into the intestinal tract. Osmotic diarrhea ceases when the patient converts to a fasting state. This may be the result of hypermagnesemia, undigested lactose or fructose, or celiac disease.

(2) **Secretory diarrhea** occurs when the intestinal wall is damaged, resulting in an increased secretion rather than absorption of electrolytes into the intestinal tract. This can occur with the ingestion of bacterial enteropathogens (e.g., *Escherichia coli, Salmonella, Shigella*).

(3) **Motility-related diarrhea** occurs when food moves through the intestines at such a rapid pace (hypermotility) that insufficient time is allowed for water and nutrient absorption. Those with diabetic neuropathy, gastric/intestinal resection, or a vagotomy are susceptible to this type of diarrhea. Medications that can also cause hypermotility include parasympathomimetic agents (e.g., metoclopramide, bethanechol), digitalis, quinidine, and antibiotics.

b. **Classification by origin**

(1) **Viral gastroenteritis** is typically caused by the **noroviruses**, which are transmitted by contaminated water or food. Other attributable viruses include rotaviruses, adenoviruses, and hepatitis A virus. Diarrhea associated with viral gastroenteritis is usually self-limiting for 2 to 3 days but may last up to 2 weeks.

(2) **Bacterial gastroenteritis** typically results from consumption of contaminated water or food. Common contributors include *E. coli, Staphylococcus aureus, Vibrio cholerae, Shigella, Salmonella, Campylobacter*, and *Clostridium difficile*. Toxin-producing bacteria affect the small intestines, resulting in a watery stool. Invasive bacteria affect the large intestines, resulting in dysentery-like stools (e.g., extreme urgency to defecate, abdominal cramping, tenesmus, fever, chills, and small-volume stools that contain blood or pus). Onset of diarrhea may range between 1 and 72 hrs, depending on the infecting bacteria. Symptoms typically subside over 3 to 5 days.

(3) **Protozoal diarrhea, caused by** *Giardia lamblia, Entamoeba histolytica*, or *Cryptosporidium*, may be described as profuse watery diarrhea, which may be accompanied by flatulence and/or abdominal pain. This type of diarrhea is self-limiting, but may persist for several weeks. Due to the extent of fluid loss over an extended duration of time, individuals with protozoal-induced diarrhea are at risk for dehydration. Self-care is inappropriate for this type of diarrhea; infected persons should be referred to a medical provider.

(4) **Diet-induced diarrhea.** Diarrhea induced by foods results from food allergies, high-fiber diets, fatty or spicy foods, large amounts of caffeine, or lactose intolerance. The best treatment is prevention by avoiding troublesome foods.

B. **Evaluation**

1. **Assessment** of the individual should include age, onset and duration of diarrhea, description of stool (i.e., frequency, consistency, volume, and presence of blood or pus), other symptoms (i.e., abdominal pain, fever, chills), aggravating or remitting factors, recent travel, and medical history.

2. **Exclusions to self-care include:**

a. **Younger than 3 years** of age or **older than 60 years** of age (with multiple medical problems), pregnant or breastfeeding patients, and patients with HIV.

b. **Blood or mucus in the stools**

c. **High fever** (> 101°F or 38°C)

d. **Dehydration or weight loss** > 5% of total body weight; signs of dehydration—dry mouth, sunken eyes, crying without tears, dry skin that is not elastic like normal skin

e. **Duration of diarrhea > 2 days**

f. **Vomiting**

C. **Treatment**

1. **Nonpharmacological.** Normal dietary intake should be recommended during bouts of diarrhea. However, fatty foods, caffeinated beverages, foods rich in simple sugars, and spicy foods should be avoided. The most important recommendation for treating acute diarrhea is to keep the individual hydrated.

a. **Fluid and electrolyte replacement.** If mild to moderate fluid loss is present, oral rehydration solution (ORS) that contains water, salt, and sugar can be recommended. This solution can be made at home by adding salt, baking soda, and sugar to water (see *Table 23-1*) or purchased ready-to-use (e.g., Pedialyte). *Table 23-2* provides recommended doses for patient age and severity of diarrhea. If fluid loss is severe (> 10% loss of body weight) and/or severe vomiting persists, then intravenous rehydration is necessary and a referral to a medical provider is most appropriate.

Table 23-1 GUIDELINES FOR ORAL-REPLACEMENT THERAPY ESTABLISHED BY THE WORLD HEALTH ORGANIZATION (WHO)

Ingredients	Dose
Sodium chloride (table salt)	90 mEq (½ teaspoon)
Potassium chloride (potassium salt)	20 mEq (¼ teaspoon)
Sodium bicarbonate (baking soda)	30 mEq (½ teaspoon)
Glucose (sugar)	20 g (2 teaspoons)
Water	Enough to make 1 L of solution

b. **Fluids to be avoided** in the dehydrated person include hypertonic fruit juices and carbonated or caffeinated beverages. These fluids may make the diarrhea worse and do not contain needed electrolytes (i.e., Na^+, K^+). Gatorade does not contain an equivalent electrolyte concentration to ORS, but may be sufficient in an individual with diarrhea who is not dehydrated.

2. **Pharmacologic. Although acute nonspecific diarrhea, including travelers' diarrhea, is typically self-limiting, antidiarrheals** may be used for symptom alleviation. Currently there are only two available nonprescription agents that the FDA has deemed to be safe and effective antidiarrheal agents: **loperamide and bismuth subsalicylate. Self-treatment of diarrhea** with these products **is limited to 2 days;** individuals experiencing longer bouts of diarrhea should be referred for medical care.
   a. **Loperamide.** Loperamide, an antiperistaltic agent, is approved as a nonprescription treatment for acute, nonspecific diarrhea, including traveler's diarrhea. **Loperamide** (e.g., Imodium A–D) provides effective control of diarrhea as quickly as 1 hr after administration.
      (1) **Availability and dosing.** Loperamide is available for **ages ≥ 6 years** in several oral formulations, including a syrup, capsule, and chewable tablet. The adult dose is 4 mg followed by 2 mg after each loose stool, not to exceed 16 mg/day. The dose for a child (ages 6 to 11 years) is also 2 mg after each loose stool, but the maximum dosage for ages 6 to 8 years is 4 mg/day, whereas the maximum dosage for ages 9 to 11 years is 6 mg/day.
      (2) **Mechanism of action.** Loperamide stimulates microopioid receptors on the circular and longitudinal musculature of the small and large intestines to normalize peristaltic intestinal movements. They slow intestinal motility and affect water and electrolyte movement through the bowel. Thus, the frequency of bowel movements is decreased, and the consistency of stools is increased.
      (3) **Adverse effects.** At recommended doses, loperamide is generally well tolerated. Side effects are infrequent and consist primarily of abdominal pain, distention, or discomfort; drowsiness, dizziness, and dry mouth.

Table 23-2 GUIDELINES FOR FLUID- AND ELECTROLYTE-REPLACEMENT THERAPY

	Dose	
Age Group	Mild (2–3 stools/day)	Moderate (4–5 stools/day)
> 5 years of age	2 L/first 4 hr, then replace ongoing losses	2–4 L/first 4 hr, then replace ongoing losses
< 5 years of age	50 mL/kg/first 4 hr, then 10 mL/kg or 1/2–1 cup per stool	100 mL/kg/4 hr, then 10 mL/kg or 1/2–1 cup per stool

(4) **Contraindications.** Loperamide should not be recommended to individuals presenting with symptoms of acute bacterial diarrhea (e.g., fever, chills, bloody diarrhea) as expulsion of the toxin is necessary. Neither should it be recommended in patients with colitis (potential for the development of toxic megacolon) nor in children < 6 years of age.

b. **Bismuth subsalicylate.** Bismuth preparations have moderate effectiveness against the prevention and treatment of traveler's diarrhea and nonspecific diarrhea, but doses required for relief are large and must be administered frequently, so these preparations may be inconvenient.

(1) **Availability and dosing.** Bismuth subsalicylate (BSS) is available without a prescription in tablet and suspension formulations. Safety and efficacy data have not been reviewed for individuals < age of 12 years and should therefore only be recommended for self-care in **individuals ≥ 12 years of age.**

(a) Chewable tablets or easy swallow caplets (e.g., Pepto-Bismol): 524 mg (two tablets) every 30 to 60 min; maximum of eight doses/day

(b) Regular strength liquid (e.g., Pepto-Bismol Original): 524 mg (30 mL) every 30 to 60 mins; maximum of eight doses/day

(c) Maximum strength liquid (e.g., Maalox Total Relief, Pepto-Bismol Maximum Strength): 1050 mg (30 mL) every hour; maximum of four doses/day

(2) **Mechanism of action.** Bismuth salts work as adsorbents but also are believed to decrease secretion of water into the bowel. It is effective and can reduce the number of stools by 50%.

(3) **Adverse effects.** BSS is relatively benign in recommended doses. The most remarkable adverse effect is **darkening of the tongue and stools** (caused by bismuth ion), which is a harmless effect occurring in > 10% of individuals ingesting BSS. In excessive doses, BSS may cause **ringing in the ears** or **neurotoxicity** (e.g., tremor, confusion, seizures, hallucinations).

(4) **Contraindications.** BSS is not appropriate to recommend to individuals with hematological diseases (e.g., hypoprothrombinemia, hemophilia), **active GI** or **peptic ulcer disease,** documented **allergies to salicylates, children < 12 years** of age or within a **6-week period following varicella vaccination,** and those **taking warfarin therapy.**

c. **Probiotics, such as lactobacillus,** are living organisms that colonize in the gastrointestinal tract to promote health benefits. Lactobacillus is not an FDA-approved agent, but it does have some data in the relief of acute, nonspecific diarrhea, not including traveler's diarrhea. However, lactobacillus can only be **recommended for maintenance of normal gastrointestinal tract function.** There are four main species used—*Lactobacillus acidophilus, L. bulgaricus, L. reuteri,* and *L. GG*—with *L. acidophilus* regarded as the more commonly used species in the United States.

(1) **Availability.** Several products containing lactobacillus are available with varying concentrations and dosing strategies. Some examples include the following:

(a) **Bacid** contains **> 500 million units of *L. acidophilus*** per capsule and is dosed as two capsules twice to four times daily for adults and children.

(b) **Culturelle** contains **10 billion units of *L. GG*** per capsule and is dosed as one capsule twice daily for adults and ½ to 1 capsule once daily for children.

(2) **Mechanism of action.** Probiotics is a means by which an **exogenous species of bacteria** is introduced into the gut to **reestablish normal gut flora.** Lactobacillus produces lactic acid, thus creating an acidic environment that is unfavorable for pathogenic microorganisms.

(3) **Adverse effects** are benign but can include **flatulence** with initiation (transient effect) and **constipation.**

(4) **Contraindications.** Lactobacillus is not appropriate in any individual with **immunosuppression or valvular heart disease** due to the risk of bacteremia, those with a **milk allergy/sensitivity** because the product is dairy based or those younger than the age of 3 years.

d. **Lactase** (e.g., Lactaid) is indicated for individuals who have insufficient amounts of lactase in the small intestine. Thus, this agent is not appropriate to treat any cause of diarrhea other than a lactase deficiency. In the body, lactose (a disaccharide present in dairy products) must be broken down to glucose and galactose to be fully digested. If the lactase enzyme is unable to break down the lactose, water is drawn into the gastrointestinal tract and results in diarrhea. The dose of lactase-containing products is one to three caplets or tablets (depending on formulation) taken with first bite of meal or drink containing lactose. Titration of doses to higher levels may be required in some patients.

III. HEMORRHOIDS

A. **General information**

1. **Definition.** Hemorrhoids are defined as abnormally large, bulging, symptomatic clusters of dilated blood vessels, supporting tissues, and overlying mucous membranes. Hemorrhoids can present in the lower rectum (internal hemorrhoids) or anus (external hemorrhoids). Simply, hemorrhoids represent downward displacement of anal cushions that contain arteriovenous anastomoses.
2. **Epidemiology.** Hemorrhoids are common, with approximately 10% to 25% of the U.S. population affected. The risk of developing hemorrhoids increases with advancing age and peaks in individuals 45 to 65 years of age. The incidence of hemorrhoids in pregnant women is higher than that of nonpregnant women of similar age. Although they are considered a minor medical problem, they may cause considerable discomfort and anxiety.

B. **Types** of hemorrhoids are determined by their anatomical position and vascular origin.

1. An **internal** hemorrhoid is an exaggerated vascular cushion with an engorged internal hemorrhoidal plexus located above the dentate line and covered with a mucous membrane.
2. An **external** hemorrhoid is a dilated vein of the inferior hemorrhoidal plexus located below the dentate line and covered with squamous epithelium.
3. A **mixed** hemorrhoid appears as a baggy swelling and exhibits simultaneous characteristics of internal and external hemorrhoids.

C. **Origin.** Although heredity may predispose a person to hemorrhoids, the exact cause is probably related to acquired factors.

1. Situations that result in **increased venous pressure** in the hemorrhoidal plexus (e.g., chronic straining during defecation; small, hard stools; prolonged sitting on the toilet; occupations that routinely require heavy lifting; pelvic tumors; pregnancy) can transform an asymptomatic hemorrhoid into a problem.
2. The hemorrhoidal veins are pushed downward during defecation or straining; with increased venous pressure, they **dilate** and **become engorged**. Over time, the **fibers** that anchor the hemorrhoidal veins to their underlying muscular coats **stretch**, which results in **prolapse**.

D. **Signs/symptoms**

1. The **most common** sign/symptom of hemorrhoids is **painless bleeding** occurring during a bowel movement. The blood is usually bright red and may be visible on the stool, on the toilet tissue, or coloring the water in the toilet.
2. **Prolapse** is the **second most common** sign/symptom of hemorrhoids. A temporary protrusion may occur during defecation, and it may need to be replaced manually. A permanently prolapsed hemorrhoid may give rise to chronic, moist soiling of the underwear. A dull, aching feeling may be heard as a complaint.
3. **Pain** is unusual unless **thrombosis** involving external tissue is present.
4. **Discomfort**, **soreness**, **pruritus**, **swelling**, **burning**, and **seepage** may also occur with hemorrhoids.

E. **Proper diagnosis is essential because other more serious conditions** may produce symptoms that mimic those of hemorrhoids and include **anal fissure** (small tear in the lining of the anus, **anal fistula** (abnormal connection between the mucosa of the rectum and the skin adjacent to the anus), **polyps** (tumor of the large intestine), or **colorectal cancer.**

F. **Treatment**

1. **Nonpharmacologic**
   a. **Avoid straining** when defecating and avoid sitting on the toilet longer than necessary.
   b. **Increase dietary fiber, water intake, and physical activity**.
   c. **Sitz baths** for 15 mins, three to four times a day, can soothe the anal mucosa. Tepid water should be used, and prolonged bathing should be avoided. Epsom salts (magnesium sulfate) added to the bath or the application of an ice pack can help reduce the swelling of an edematous or clotted hemorrhoid.
2. **Pharmacologic treatment. Nonprescription** agents are available for the treatment of burning, discomfort, inflammation, irritation, itching, pain, and swelling associated with hemorrhoids in individuals ages ≥ 12 years (*Table 23-3*). These products are simply palliative; they are not meant to cure hemorrhoids or other anorectal disease. Medical care should be sought if symptoms do

Table 23-3 GUIDE TO HEMORRHOIDAL THERAPY BASED ON APPROVED INDICATION FOR OTC ANORECTAL DRUG PRODUCTS

Therapy	Burning	Discomfort	Irritation	Itching	Pain	Soreness	Swelling
Analgesic, anesthetic, antipruritic	Yes	Yes		Yes	Yes	Yes	
Astringent	Yes	Yes	Yes	Yes			
Keratolytic		Yes		Yes			
Local anesthetic	Yes	Yes		Yes	Yes	Yes	
Protectant	Yes	Yes	Yes	Yes			
Vasoconstrictor		Yes	Yes	Yes			Yes
Hydrocortisone		Yes		Yes			Yes

not improve after 7 days of treatment or if any of the following occur: bleeding, prolapse, seepage of feces or mucus, or severe pain. Available formulations include **ointments**, **creams**, and **suppositories**. Generally, the ointment or cream dosage form is believed to be superior to a suppository, which may bypass the affected area. Some formulations are available with rectal pipes, which are most efficient when the pipe has holes. The pipe allows insertion of the medication directly in the rectum and the openings allow the ointment to cover large areas of the rectal mucosa unreachable with the finger.

a. **Local anesthetics** work by blocking nerve impulse transmission.
   (1) **Availability.** FDA-approved **agents** include **benzocaine** 20% (e.g., Americaine), **pramoxine** 1% (e.g., Pramoxine Rectal Foam), and **dibucaine** 0.25% to 1.0% (e.g., Nupercainal).
   (2) **Adverse effects.** These agents may produce a hypersensitivity reaction with burning and itching similar to that of anorectal disease. Systemic absorption is minimal unless the perianal skin is abraded. As a result of its unique chemical structure, pramoxine exhibits little cross-sensitivity compared to the other local anesthetics.
   (3) **Warnings.** Allergic reactions may occur in some patients.

b. **Vasoconstrictors** are chemicals that resemble endogenous catecholamines. These agents cause arteriole constriction in the anorectal area to reduce swelling, but the mechanism by which they relieve itching, discomfort, and irritation is unknown.
   (1) **Availability. Phenylephrine** is the only FDA-approved vasoconstrictor found in nonprescription hemorrhoidal relief agents. It is one of the active ingredients in the line of Preparation H products available in ointment, gel, suppository, and cream.
   (2) **Adverse effects.** At recommended doses, the risk of individuals receiving enough systemic absorption from hemorrhoidal vasoconstrictors to develop cardiovascular or CNS effects is minimal; however, in those with cardiovascular disease, anxiety disorders, or thyroid disease, an agent that does not contain a vasoconstrictor is a prudent recommendation.
   (3) **Warnings/contraindications.** Avoid in individuals with **cardiovascular disease, hypertension, hyperthyroidism, diabetes**, and **prostate enlargement** because of the possibility of systemic absorption.

c. **Protectants** provide a **physical barrier** between the irritated skin and stool or anal seepage, thereby relieving the itching, irritation, discomfort, and burning. Protectants are often the bases or vehicles for other agents used for anorectal disease. Products include **aluminum hydroxide gel, cocoa butter, kaolin, lanolin, hard fat, mineral oil, white petrolatum, petrolatum, glycerin** (external use only), **topical starch, cod liver oil, shark liver oil, and zinc oxide**. When protectants are incorporated into the formulation of a nonprescription product, they should make up at least 50% of the dosage unit. If two to four protectants are used, their total concentration should represent at least 50% of the whole product. Lanolin, a derivative of wool alcohol, may be allergenic to susceptible individuals.

d. **Astringents** lessen mucus and other secretions and protect underlying tissue through a local and limited protein coagulant effect. Action is limited to surface cells, but astringents provide temporary relief of itching, discomfort, irritation, and burning. Products considered to be safe and effective include calamine 5% to 25%, witch hazel 10% to 50% (external use only), and zinc oxide 5% to 25%.
e. **Keratolytics** cause desquamation and debridement of the surface cells of the epidermis, which in turn allows hemorrhoidal medications to penetrate deeper into the tissues, and thus provide temporary relief of discomfort and itching. Products considered to be safe and effective include **aluminum chlorhydroxyallantoinate** (0.2% to 2.0%) and **resorcinol** (1% to 3%). Keratolytics are reserved for external use only and resorcinol should not be used on an open wound due to the potential for a serious hypersensitivity reaction. Of note, there are currently no marketed products for hemorrhoid relief that contain these agents.
f. **Analgesics**, **anesthetics**, and **antipruritics** provide temporary relief of burning, discomfort, itching, pain, and soreness. Ingredients considered to be safe and effective for external use in the anorectal area include **menthol** (0.1% to 1.0%), **juniper tar** (1% to 5%), and **camphor** (0.1% to 3%). These agents should not be used to treat internal hemorrhoids.
g. **Corticosteroids. Hydrocortisone (0.25% to 1.0%)** is the only FDA-approved corticosteroid for anorectal disorders. Hydrocortisone causes vasoconstriction, stabilization of lysosomal membranes, and antimitotic activity, which in turn may reduce the itching, inflammation, and discomfort in the anorectal area. Hydrocortisone concentrations > 1% are available by prescription only.

IV. HEARTBURN AND DYSPEPSIA

A. General information

1. **Definition.** Heartburn (pyrosis) is a form of indigestion that occurs when contents of the stomach flow backward into the esophagus (i.e., gastroesophageal reflux). Heartburn is generally a benign physiological process that occurs in normal individuals multiple times throughout the day. However, chronic heartburn can develop into gastroesophageal reflux disease (GERD), a more severe form of reflux that involves esophageal tissue damage. Dyspepsia is frequently defined as indigestion with symptoms of bloating, fullness, and nausea. The Rome III committee, an international committee, defines dyspepsia as one or more of the following symptoms: postprandial fullness, early satiety, or epigastric pain or burning.
2. **Pathophysiology.** Heartburn is typically the result of a weakened or relaxed lower esophageal sphincter (LES). When the pressure in the stomach is enough to overcome the weak squeeze of the LES, the result is a backflow of stomach contents into the esophagus. Males or individuals older than the age of 50 years are more likely to develop heartburn. The following factors affect the tone of the LES and/or production of stomach acid:
   a. **Medications** that reduce LES tone include calcium-channel blockers (e.g., nifedipine, verapamil, diltiazem), nitrates, anticholinergic agents (e.g., tricyclic antidepressants, antihistamines), and oral contraceptives.
   b. **Foods** that reduce LES tone include chocolate, fatty foods, onions, peppermint, and garlic.
   c. **Smoking** (nicotine) reduces LES tone but can also stimulate stomach acid.
   d. **Stress** increases stomach acid.
   e. **Pregnancy and obesity** can create additional intra-abdominal pressure.
3. **Symptoms.** Heartburn typically is described as a burning sensation or pain located in the lower chest. The pain may radiate higher in the chest, into the back, and into the throat or neck. Because the pain may radiate up into the chest, heartburn may be confused with pain associated with myocardial infarction (sweating associated with severe, crushing chest pain suggests a myocardial infarction and medical attention must be sought immediately). Symptoms usually occur soon after meals and when lying down at bedtime; patients may be awakened during the night with the pain. Pain on swallowing (odynophagia) may suggest severe mucosal damage in the esophagus.
4. **Complications.** Patients with severe, uncontrolled reflux may suffer with bleeding from esophageal ulcers and pulmonary complications resulting from the aspiration of refluxed material into the upper airways and lungs. Patients who describe difficulty swallowing (i.e., dysphagia) may have an esophageal stricture, cancer, or a motility disorder.

5. **Exclusions to self-care include**
   a. Severe abdominal or back pain
   b. Unexplained weight loss
   c. Chest pain that is indistinguishable from ischemic pain
   d. Difficulty or pain on swallowing
   e. Presence or history of vomiting blood
   f. Black tarry bowel movements (if not taking iron or bismuth subsalicylate)
   g. Children < 12 years of age
   h. Possibility of being pregnant

B. **Treatment**

1. **Nonpharmacological** interventions for heartburn and dyspepsia attempt to reduce or eliminate dietary and lifestyle factors that promote reflux. Specific recommendations include the following:
   a. Elevate the head of the bed 6 to 10 inches with blocks. This position improves esophageal clearance and reduces the duration of reflux. Just propping the head up with pillows may worsen symptoms by increasing abdominal pressure.
   b. Eat evening meals at least 3 to 5 hrs before going to bed to allow adequate time for gastric emptying.
   c. Avoid foods that reduce LES tone or irritate the esophagus (e.g., tomato-based products, coffee, citrus juices, and carbonated beverages).
   d. Reduce the size of meals and avoid lying down for at least 2 hrs after meals.
   e. Stop use of tobacco products and limit alcohol intake.
   f. Lose weight if appropriate.
   g. Avoid wearing tight-fitting clothing around the abdominal area.
2. **Pharmacological.** The management of heartburn and dyspepsia may be viewed as a stepped-care approach, with antacids, nonprescription H_2RAs, and nondrug measures forming the basis for treatment. These measures may help alleviate symptoms in patients with mild to moderate heartburn and dyspepsia but cannot be expected to heal damaged esophageal mucosa or prevent complications.
   a. **Antacids.** Antacids are basic compounds that neutralize gastric acid, which increases the pH of refluxed gastric contents. As a result, the refluxed contents are not as damaging to the esophageal mucosa, and alkalinization of gastric contents increases LES tone.
      (1) **Availability and dosing.** Available antacids include **sodium bicarbonate** (e.g., Alka-Seltzer, Brioschi), **calcium carbonate** (e.g., Tums), **aluminum hydroxide** (e.g., Alternagel), and **magnesium hydroxide** (e.g., Milk of Magnesia). The adult dose is 40 to 80 mEq acid-neutralizing capacity (ANC) taken as needed for symptoms. If necessary, these doses may be titrated to a scheduled regimen, such as 40 to 80 mEq after meals and at bedtime. Patients should not take > 500 to 600 mEq ANC of antacid per day.
      (2) **Onset and duration of activity.** Antacids generally **relieve symptoms within 5 to 15 mins** of administration. Antacid suspensions generally dissolve more easily in gastric acid and therefore work quicker. In addition, sodium bicarbonate and magnesium hydroxide dissolve quickly at gastric pH and provide rapid relief; however, calcium carbonate and aluminum hydroxide dissolve slowly in stomach acid with a longer time frame for symptom relief (10 to 30 mins). The **duration of relief ranges from 1 to 3 hrs if taken 1 hr after meals** (duration of neutralization lasts only 20 to 40 mins if taken without food). Because of their short duration, patients may need to take four to five doses throughout the day for adequate symptom relief. **Antacids will not provide sustained neutralization of acid throughout the night**.
      (3) **Counseling**
         (a) Sodium bicarbonate contains 12 mEq of sodium per gram and is therefore contraindicated in patients with edema, congestive heart failure, renal failure, cirrhosis, and patients on low-salt diets.
         (b) **Calcium carbonate is the most potent** antacid ingredient but may cause constipation. **Aluminum hydroxide has the lowest neutralizing capacity** of all the antacids. Aluminum accumulation can be a problem in patients with chronic renal insufficiency.

Answers and Explanations

1. **The answer is C** *[see I.B.2].*
Glycerin and the bisacodyl suppository all produce stools in 30 mins to a few hours, whereas psyllium, a bulk-forming laxative, produces stool in 24 to 72 hrs in the same manner as a normal bolus of food or fiber.

2. **The answer is D** *[see I.B.2.d].*
These agents, known as surfactants (docusate calcium and docusate sodium), have a long onset of action (24 to 48 hrs); thus they should never be used for acute constipation but should be used mainly for patients who should not strain to pass hard stools (e.g., pregnant patients, postsurgical patients, postmyocardial infarction). Oral sodium phosphate (OSP), a saline laxative, has been associated with acute phosphate nephropathy, but not emollient laxatives.

3. **The answer is B** *[see I.B.2.a; I.B.2.c].*
Stimulant products result in a quicker, more complete, and often more violent evacuation of the bowel than do the bulk-forming agents. Bulk-forming agents are developed from complex sugars, similar to fiber, that provide bulk to increase gastrointestinal motility and water absorption into the bowel. However, patients must drink plenty of water to facilitate the absorption of water into the bowel, or they may become more constipated.

4. **The answer is C** *[see III.F.2.a.(2)].*
Because of its chemically distinct structure, pramoxine exhibits less cross-sensitivity compared to the other anesthetics and should be used in patients with a lidocaine allergy.

5. **The answer is A** *[see III.D.1].*
The most common sign/symptom of hemorrhoids is painless bleeding occurring during a bowel movement.

6. **The answer is B** *[see III.F.2.f].*
Juniper tar, menthol, and camphor are the only three agents deemed safe and effective as analgesics, anesthetics, and antipruritics by the FDA.

7. **The answer is C** *[see IV.A.5].*
Pain on swallowing often suggests severe esophageal mucosal damage, which would require prescription medications for healing. Difficulty on swallowing may indicate an esophageal stricture, cancer, or motor disorder. All of these conditions require diagnosis and treatment by a health care provider.

8. **The answer is C** *[see IV.B.1.a–g].*
Patients should be instructed to eat evening meals at least 3 hrs before going to bed. This allows sufficient time for gastric emptying, so that the volume of refluxed material will be smaller and less irritating to the esophagus.

9. **The answer is D** *[see IV.B.2.e].*
Proton pump inhibitors have an extended duration of action but a long onset of action, compared to antacids, which have a quick onset of action but a short duration of action. The combination of a H_2RA and an antacid (e.g., Pepcid Complete) allows for a quick onset of action (antacid) with an extended duration of action (H_2RA).

10. **The answer is C** *[see I.B.2.e; IV.B.2.a].*
Magnesium hydroxide (e.g., Milk of Magnesia) may be used for the symptomatic relief of heartburn, dyspepsia, and constipation. Magnesium hydroxide is most noted for its potential to cause diarrhea. Indirectly, it may provide relief from hemorrhoids if they are due to constipation but will not have a direct effect on alleviation of hemorrhoids.

24

Over-the-Counter Menstrual, Vaginal, and Contraceptive Agents

JENNIFER D. SMITH

I. MENSTRUATION AND MENSTRUAL PRODUCTS

A. **Introduction. Menstruation** is a physiological discharge of blood, endometrial cellular debris, and mucus through the vagina of a nonpregnant woman and is a result of the monthly cycling of female reproductive hormones. The menstrual cycle eliminates a mature, unfertilized egg and prepares the endometrium for the possible implantation of a fertilized egg the following month.

B. **Menstrual abnormalities**

1. **Dysmenorrhea**, which is painful menstruation, is the most common gynecologic problem in the United States.

   a. **Types**

      (1) **Primary dysmenorrhea** is pain associated with menstruation in the absence of identifiable pelvic disease. It is prompted by increased levels of prostaglandins in the menstrual fluids.

      (2) **Secondary dysmenorrhea** is associated with an underlying pelvic disorder. Possible causes include endometriosis, pelvic inflammatory disease (PID), and ovarian cysts.

   b. **Symptoms** of dysmenorrhea are primarily lower abdominal cramping and can often include nausea, vomiting, diarrhea, headache, and dizziness. Abdominal cramping usually begins at onset of menstrual flow or a few hours before onset.

   c. **Assessment.** Practitioners should **question the patient** about the following:

      (1) Current medications (including over-the-counter and herbals)

      (2) Age

      (3) Duration of dysmenorrhea

      (4) A description of the dysmenorrhea symptoms

      (5) History of pelvic disease (endometriosis, PID, ovarian cysts, infertility)

      (6) Allergy to aspirin or nonsteroidal anti-inflammatory drugs (NSAIDs)

      (7) Bleeding disorder

      (8) Exercise routine

   d. **Treatment.** Recommendation(s) should be based on the patient's assessment of the degree of pain. Pain associated with dysmenorrhea generally tapers within 2 days. Prolonged pain may be associated with an underlying problem, and patients should be referred to a physician.

      (1) **Nonpharmacologic** recommendations include rest, heat, wearing loose-fitting clothing, and exercise.

      (2) **Pharmacologic recommendations. NSAIDs** are used as the primary treatment of dysmenorrhea. Treatment with **aspirin** or **acetaminophen** can prove of benefit for the symptoms associated with primary dysmenorrhea; however, aspirin is not as potent as the other NSAIDs, and acetaminophen is not thought to prevent prostaglandin production to

a great extent although it can be helpful for treating the headache and backache that may accompany menstrual cramping. NSAID treatment provides relief for mild to moderate symptoms but will probably not help patients with severe symptoms.

(a) **Mechanism of action.** NSAIDs inhibit the synthesis and action of prostaglandins, which are responsible for the pain associated with dysmenorrhea.

(b) **Administration guidelines.** Begin therapy at the onset of pain; there is no proven value in beginning therapy in anticipation of dysmenorrhea. Acceptable recommendations include ibuprofen (e.g., Motrin, Midol Liquid Gels) 200 mg every 4 to 6 hrs (maximum 1200 mg/day) or naproxen sodium (e.g., Aleve, Pamprin All Day, Midol Extended Relief) 200 mg of naproxen every 8 to 12 hrs (maximum naproxen dose is 600 mg/day).

(c) **Adverse effects** are limited because of the brief duration of need. However, common adverse effects associated with NSAIDs include bleeding, upset stomach, abdominal pain, diarrhea, heart failure exacerbation, cardiovascular thrombic events, and dizziness. NSAIDs should be taken with food to decrease adverse gastrointestinal (GI) effects.

(d) **Warnings.** The lowest effective dose for the shortest duration needed should be recommended to lessen the potential risk for cardiovascular events. These agents are contraindicated in patients with an allergy to NSAIDs or active GI disease.

2. **Premenstrual syndrome (PMS)**

a. **Symptoms** (e.g., marked mood swings, fatigue, appetite changes, bloating, breast tenderness, irritability, feelings of depression) begin 1 to 7 days before the onset of menses.

b. **Nonpharmacological** therapy includes regular exercise, dietary modifications, and reduction of stress factors. Dietary modifications include avoiding alcohol and caffeine, which can increase irritability, and consuming a balanced diet of fruits, vegetables, and complex carbohydrates while avoiding salty foods and simple sugars (can exacerbate fluid retention). Patients experiencing symptoms abnormal to their cycle should be referred to a physician.

c. **Pharmacological treatment**

(1) **Combination products** are marketed for women (age 12 and older) with PMS symptoms. These products contain analgesics (e.g., acetaminophen, aspirin, ibuprofen, naproxen sodium), diuretics (e.g., caffeine, pamabrom), and/or an antihistamine (e.g., pyrilamine, diphenhydramine).

(a) **Diuretics** are recommended by the U.S. Food and Drug Administration (FDA) for use in eliminating water during premenstrual and menstrual periods. When **administered approximately 5 days before menses**, diuretics help relieve bloating, excess water, cramps, and tension. Included in this category are caffeine and pamabrom.

(i) **Caffeine** (e.g., Pamprin Max, Midol Complete), a **xanthine derivative**, promotes diuresis by inhibiting tubular reabsorption of sodium and chloride. The recommended dosage is 100 to 200 mg every 3 to 4 hrs. Side effects associated with caffeine use are GI disturbances and central nervous system (CNS) stimulation. Patients should be counseled to **limit the consumption of caffeine-containing foods or beverages** while taking this product.

(ii) **Pamabrom** (e.g., Aqua-ban, Midol Teen, Pamprin Cramp, Pamprin Multi-Symptom) is a theophylline derivative often used in combination with analgesics and antihistamines. The recommended dosage is 50 mg four times daily not to exceed 200 mg/day.

(b) Antihistamines, such as pyrilamine and diphenhydramine, are added to PMS products for their sedative effects although the need for sedation is questionable. At this time, there is insufficient evidence to recommend agents containing antihistamines (e.g., Pamprin Multi-Symptom, Midol Complete, Midol PM) for the alleviation of PMS symptoms.

(2) Daily **calcium supplementation** (equivalent to the recommended daily calcium intake for women of reproductive age) has been shown to reduce the emotional and physical symptoms of PMS.

(3) **Pyridoxine.** Although clinical trials do not support the efficacy of pyridoxine (vitamin B_6), it is being used for the treatment of PMS. Vitamin B_6 doses should be limited to 100 mg/day to prevent dose-associated neuropathy.

C. **Toxic shock syndrome (TSS)** is a rare but sometimes fatal illness often associated with menstruation.
1. TSS can be categorized either as menstrual or nonmenstrual, with approximately two-thirds of cases associated with menstruation. TSS is known to occur in both men and women.
2. The condition usually affects women < 30 years of age who use tampons. Women between the ages of 15 and 19 years are at the highest risk.
3. TSS is characterized by an abrupt onset (8 to 12 hrs) of flu-like symptoms (e.g., high fever, myalgia, vomiting, diarrhea). Neurologic symptoms such as headache, agitation, lethargy, seizures, and confusion can also occur.
4. TSS results from an exotoxin produced by *Staphylococcus aureus*.
5. The **primary risk factor** for TSS is the **use of tampons**, but the use of barrier contraceptives (e.g., diaphragms, cervical sponges) also increases the risk.
6. When TSS is suspected, patients should be hospitalized immediately. To lower the risk of TSS, women should use lower-absorbency tampons and alternate the use of tampons with feminine hygiene pads; however, to lower the risk to nearly zero, women should use sanitary pads instead of tampons.

II. VAGINAL PRODUCTS

A. **Vulvovaginal candidiasis**
1. **General considerations**
   a. **Occurrence.** Approximately 75% of all women will experience vulvovaginal candidiasis (VVC), also known as a yeast infection, at least once, and 50% will have a second episode. Only 5% of women experience recurrent infections (four or more infections within a 1-year period).
   b. **Cause.** *Candida albicans* is responsible for up to 92% of infections. Infections owing to *C. glabrata* are increasing.
   c. **Predisposing factors.** Antibiotics, oral contraceptives containing high-dose estrogen, pregnancy, diabetes, poor postbowel movement hygiene, and immunosuppression increase the risk for infection.
   d. **Symptoms.** Can include a thick, white, "cottage cheese-like," nonmalodorous vaginal discharge; dysuria; vaginal burning; and pruritus.
2. **Home diagnostics for VVC.** Currently, a color-keyed vaginal **pH monitor** (Vagisil) is available over-the-counter for women experiencing symptoms of VVC. VVC typically does not increase vaginal pH, but other infections such as bacterial vaginosis or *Trichomonas* may. Thus, essentially the purpose of the pH monitor is to rule out other bacterial infections and prevent erroneous treatment of an assumed yeast infection. The product is not intended to detect sexually transmitted infections.
   a. Indication. Women with symptoms of vaginal burning, itching, unpleasant odor, or unusual discharge.
   b. Use. Press wand against vaginal wall for 5 secs; compare color on the pH paper swab to the pH color chart
   c. Results. A pH of 4.5 in a symptomatic individual may be a yeast infection. A pH of 5.0 to 7.5 may indicate a different kind of vaginal infection.
   d. Counseling points
      (1) Menstrual blood can cause an elevated pH, indicating possible infection. Therefore, the test should not be performed during menstruation or for 5 days after menstruation.
      (2) Wait for 48 hrs after douching or sexual intercourse (72 hrs if a lubricant was used).
      (3) Recommended only for women with normal periods. Lack of estrogen (e.g., perimenopause or postmenopause, women who are nursing and have not restarted their period) may contribute to an elevated vaginal pH.
      (4) Symptomatic individuals with a pH of 5.0 to 7.5 should be referred for medical evaluation.
3. Exclusions to self-care
   a. First episode of symptoms
   b. Pregnant
   c. Younger than 12 years of age
   d. Systemic symptoms such as fever
   e. History of recurrent vaginal yeast infections
   f. Discharge with a fishy odor (indicates bacterial vaginosis, most often caused by anaerobic bacteria) or a thin, malodorous purulent discharge (indicates *Trichomonas* infection)

4. **Pharmacologic treatment.** Products proven safe and effective for the treatment of VVC are imidazole derivatives with antifungal activity and include tioconazole, miconazole, and clotrimazole. Each agent is available in a variety of formulations, including intravaginal creams, suppositories, ovules, and ointments.
   a. The choice of product formulation is based on patient preference. One formulation is not more effective than another.
   b. **External vaginal creams**, mainly **used to treat vulvar symptoms of pruritus**, can be used in combination with intravaginal products. Many products are available as a "combination pack" including an internal cream, ovule, or suppository and an external cream.
   c. **For most available intravaginal products, application time should be recommended as bedtime to increase vaginal mucosa contact time.** However, external creams can be used any time of day.
   d. **Products are available as 1-, 3-, or 7-day treatment plans.** Available products include Monistat (miconazole 1-, 3-, and 7-day), Vagistat (tioconazole 1-day; miconazole 3-day), and Gyne-Lotrimin (clotrimazole 3- and 7-day). Efficacy rates for these products approach 80% to 90%.
      (1) Each product must be used for the consecutive number of days outlined for the product to be effective.
      (2) The formulated products for 1- and 3-day treatments are for user convenience and should not be misinterpreted for the time to symptom resolution.
      (3) **Symptoms of VVC typically do not resolve completely for 5 to 7 days.** Thus when 1- and 3-day products are purchased, the woman should be aware that she **may still experience symptoms after she has completed the treatment** but should resolve within several days. **If symptoms are still present after 7 days, a medical provider should be consulted.**
      (4) Products for internal use may come with prefilled applicators for single use or reusable applicators. Reusable applicators should be washed with soap and water each time.
   e. **Patient counseling**
      (1) Complete the course of therapy even if symptoms improve. Symptom improvement typically will not be seen for 5 to 7 days after initiation of treatment. Seek medical treatment if symptoms have not resolved after 7 days.
      (2) Wash vaginal area with mild soap before application.
      (3) Avoid sexual intercourse during therapy.
      (4) Avoid condoms and diaphragm use for 72 hrs after therapy is completed.
      (5) Continue use during menstrual period, but tampons should not be used during VVC treatment.
      (6) Sanitary pads can be used for leakage of intravaginal products.
      (7) Side effects can include burning or irritation.
      (8) Treatment of male partners is not necessary.
   f. *Lactobacillus acidophilus*, taken by mouth or as a vaginal suppository, has inadequate data at this time to make a sound recommendation for prevention or treatment of VVC.
5. **Prevention**
   a. Dry vaginal area well with a towel after bathing.
   b. Avoid tight or damp clothing.
   c. Wear cotton underwear.
   d. Use unscented soap to avoid irritation.
   e. Avoid douching.
   f. Decrease consumption of sucrose and simple sugars.

B. **Feminine hygiene products.** There are a variety of feminine hygiene products available for cleansing and controlling odor associated with normal vaginal discharge and products available for vaginal dryness. These products are not used to treat vaginal infections.
   1. Vaginal douches (Summer's Eve) irrigate the vagina and can be used for cleansing, for soothing as an astringent, or to produce a mucolytic effect.
   2. **Vaginal lubricants** are used for **immediate relief of vaginal dryness**, which can cause pain during intercourse. Vaginal lubricants are available as oil-, water-, or silicone-based.
      a. **Oil-based** lubricants typically contain baby oil or petroleum jelly and **should not be recommended for use with latex condoms** because they can deteriorate the latex. Additionally, oil-based lubricants can harbor bacteria in the vagina and lead to infections.

b. Water-based vaginal lubricants (e.g., Astroglide, K-Y Jelly) are known to be compatible with latex condoms.

c. Silicone-based vaginal lubricants (e.g., K-Y INTRIGUE) are longer lasting than water-based lubricants and are compatible only with latex condoms.

3. **Vaginal moisturizers.** Unlike lubricants, which provide immediate relief, vaginal moisturizers (e.g., Replens, K-Y Silk-E) are for **chronic vaginal dryness**. Thus if used for intercourse, vaginal moisturizers need to be applied 2 hrs prior to allow for adequate lubrication.

III. OTC CONTRACEPTIVES

A. **Introduction.** The **efficacy** and **pregnancy rates** for various means of contraception depend greatly on the **degree of compliance**. *Table 24-1* lists ranges of pregnancy rates reported for a variety of contraceptives.

B. **Methods** of contraception that may make use of nonprescription products or devices include the following:

1. **Fertility awareness methods** make use of information concerning the menstrual cycle to determine the days when intercourse is most likely to result in a pregnancy. Calculations of the period of fertility take into account the **sperm viability** in the female reproductive tract, which is

Table 24-1 PREGNANCY RATES FOR VARIOUS MEANS OF CONTRACEPTION (%)[a]

Method of Contraception	Typical[b]	Lowest[c]
Oral contraceptives		
Combination (estrogen–progestin)	0.1–0.34	0.1
Progestin only	0.5–1.5	0.5
Mechanical/chemical		
Cervical cap[d]		
Multiparous	40	26.0
Nulliparous	20	9.0
Male condom without spermicide	12–14	3.0
Male condom with spermicide	4–6	1.8
Diaphragm[d]	20	6.0
Female condom	21	5.0
Intrauterine device	≤ 1–2	≤ 1.0–1.5
Levonorgestrel implants	≤ 1.0	≤ 1.0
Medroxyprogesterone injection	≤ 1.0	≤ 1.0
Spermicide alone	20–22	6.0
Other		
Rhythm (all types)	25	1–9
Vasectomy/tubal ligation	≤ 1	≤ 1
Withdrawal	40–50	30
No contraception	85	85

[a]During first year of continuous use.
[b]A typical couple who initiated a method that either was not always used correctly or was not used with every act of sexual intercourse, and who experienced an accidental pregnancy.
[c]The method of birth control was always used correctly with every act of sexual intercourse but the couple still experienced an accidental pregnancy.
[d]Used with spermicide.
Adapted with permission from Covington TR. *Nonprescription Drug Therapy: Guiding Patient Self-Care.* 4th ed. St. Louis, MO: Wolters Kluwer Health; 2005.

estimated to average **2 to 3 days** (up to 5 days), and the **fertile period of the ovum**, which is estimated to be **24 hr**. Recent studies indicate that conception is most likely to occur when couples have intercourse during a 6-day period ending on the day of ovulation. **Conception is highly unlikely if sexual intercourse occurs 6 or more days before ovulation or the day after ovulation.** These methods are based on reproductive anatomy and physiology and are applied according to the signs and symptoms naturally occurring in the menstrual cycle.

a. **Calendar method.** This method estimates the possible day of ovulation, based on documentation of prior menstrual cycle events. **Abstinence** should be practiced during the period around ovulation when there may be a fertilizable egg present. The calendar method is not as well-used as it once was and is not accurate for women with irregular cycles, women who are breastfeeding, or women with postponed ovulation.

b. **Temperature method.** Documentation of **basal body temperature (BBT)** can be made using a basal thermometer, which is available without a prescription.

(1) Approximately 24 hrs prior to ovulation, there is a moderate drop in basal temperature followed by a rise in temperature 24 hrs after ovulation. The rise in temperature is thought to be the result of progesterone release, which indicates the occurrence of ovulation.

(2) For this method to be successful, **abstinence** should be practiced **5 days after the onset of menses until 3 days after the drop** in basal temperature.

(3) Because the basal temperature reflects the amount of heat radiation when the body is at its metabolic low, the temperature should be taken first thing in the morning (i.e., before any activity) after at least 5 hrs of restful sleep.

(4) **The BBT** thermometer may be used **orally, vaginally, or rectally**, depending on the model selected.

(5) False changes in BBT may be caused by infection, tension, a restless night, or any type of excessive movement.

2. **Spermicidal agents** are composed of an **active spermicidal chemical**, which immobilizes or kills sperm, and an **inert base** (e.g., foam, cream, jelly, gel, tablet, or suppository), which localizes the spermicidal chemical in proximity to the cervical os. The only FDA-approved spermicidal agent is **nonoxynol-9**. However, although it is spermicidal, it is **not a microbicide and therefore cannot be used alone for protection against sexually transmitted infections.**

a. **Dosage forms. Contraceptive spermicides**, which are available in several forms, offer the greatest variety within one specific method of contraception (*Table 24-2*).

(1) **Creams, jellies, and gels** are used with a diaphragm. The concentration of spermicide is less than the necessary 8% to be employed as a single contraceptive method.

Table 24-2 SPERMICIDES[a]

Type (Product)	Comments
Film	Inserted by the female directly over the cervix; insert not less than 15 mins and not more than 3 hrs before intercourse; contraceptive protection begins 5–15 mins after insertion and remains effective no more than 3 hrs
Foam	Contraceptive protection is immediate; remains effective no more than 1 hr, additional dose is needed before any subsequent intercourse
Jellies, creams, gels	Contraceptive protection is immediate; used alone remains effective no more than 1 hr; when used with diaphragm or cap, keep diaphragm or cap in place for at least 6 hrs after last intercourse
Suppositories and tablets	Contraceptive protection begins 10–15 mins after insertion; remains effective no more than 1 hr

[a]The spermicidal agent in all listed products is nonoxynol-9.
Article adapted... Reprinted with permission from Hatcher RA. *Contraceptive Technology 1994–1996*. 16th ed. New York, NY: Irvington; 1994:180.
VCF, vaginal contraceptive film.

(2) **Foams** disperse better into the vagina and over the cervical opening but provide less lubrication than creams, jellies, and gels. They usually contain a higher concentration of spermicide (i.e., **the optimal concentration of 8% or higher**). Because of volume differences among brands, the dosage amounts vary. If vaginal or penile irritation develops, another brand should be tried.

(a) The can should be shaken vigorously 20 times before use.

(b) The foam should be inserted intravaginally about two-thirds the length of the applicator, and the contents should be discharged.

(c) Foam should be reapplied during prolonged intercourse (i.e., lasting > 1 hr) and before every subsequent act of intercourse.

(d) To ensure efficacy, the patient should wait at least 8 hrs before douching to avoid diluting the spermicide effect or "forcing" sperm into the cervix.

(3) **Suppositories and foaming tablets.** These agents are both small and convenient. Although solid at room temperature, suppositories melt at body temperature, whereas foaming tablets effervesce.

(a) The tablets should be wetted and inserted high into the vagina 10 to 15 mins before intercourse. Intercourse must occur within 1 hr or the dose must be repeated. Each repeated act of intercourse requires insertion of another tablet/suppository.

(b) To ensure efficacy, the patient should wait 6 to 8 hrs after the last act of intercourse before douching.

(4) **Film** comes as small paper-thin sheets (e.g., vaginal contraceptive film [VCF]). It is inserted on the tip of the finger into the vagina, and placed at the cervical opening 5 to 15 mins before intercourse.

(5) **Sponge.** The Today Sponge is a doughnut-shaped polyurethane device containing the spermicide nonoxynol-9. However, it may also provide contraceptive effects by serving as a mechanical barrier to the cervical entrance.

(a) The sponge should **remain in place for at least 6 hrs** and up to 30 hrs. **Contraceptive benefits are for 24 hrs**, regardless of the frequency of intercourse during this period.

(b) Increased risk of TSS with use (rare).

(c) Not recommended for use during menstruation.

(d) This method may have a higher pregnancy rate for women who have vaginally delivered a baby.

b. Side effects. Side effects are **minimal**, but may include sensation of warmth and rare allergic reactions (**contact dermatitis** with rash, stinging, itching, and swelling). If a suspected reaction occurs, one should be instructed to use another product because the issue might be the concentration of the spermicide or an additive specific to a given brand. There are no significant differences in birth defect rates between users and nonusers.

3. Male condoms are used to prevent transmission of sperm into the vagina.

a. Types. There are four different types of materials for male condoms, which include latex rubber, processed collagenous lamb cecum sheaths (lambskin), polyurethane, or polyisoprene. Condoms are labeled that they are intended to prevent HIV and other sexually transmitted infections, but caution that they do not completely eliminate the risk, particularly human papillomavirus (HPV) and herpes simplex virus (HSV).

(1) **Latex** condoms afford greater elasticity than lambskin and are more likely to remain in place on the penis.

(a) **Availability.** Various types are available (e.g., lubricated, ribbed, colored), including some with spermicide (concentration much less than that of a vaginal spermicide product). It is doubtful that spermicide-lubricated condoms offer any better protection than plain latex condoms, and they have a shorter shelf life. There is a standard size, but smaller and larger versions are available.

(b) **Concerns.** Latex rubber may cause an allergic reaction. An estimated 1% to 2% of the population is sensitized to natural rubber latex, and higher percentages are likely for those frequently exposed to latex (e.g., health care workers). The most common symptoms are genital inflammation with redness, itching, and burning. Sometimes, antioxidants or accelerators used during the manufacturing process may be the cause of the allergy.

(2) **Lambskin** condoms (e.g., Trojan NaturaLamb) are **not considered as effective as latex condoms** (and cannot be labeled as such) in preventing the transmission of STDs, including HIV. The lambskin condoms are structured to consist of membranes that reveal layers of fibers crisscrossing in various patterns. This gives the lambskin strength but also allows for an occasional pore. Therefore, lambskin **may allow HIV and hepatitis B virus**, which are smaller than sperm, to pass through.

(a) Lambskin has less elasticity than latex, and lambskin condoms may slip off the penis.

(b) Lambskin affords **greater sensitivity** than latex.

(c) Lambskin condoms are more expensive than latex condoms.

(3) A **polyurethane condom** (e.g., Avanti, Trojan Supra) is **marketed for individuals who are allergic to latex**. Some evidence exists that slippage and breakage rates may be higher than for latex condoms. In contrast to the latex condom, petroleum-based products will not degrade the polyurethane.

(4) A **polyisoprene condom** (e.g., LifeStyles Skyn) is the newest material to be **marketed for individuals who are allergic to latex**. The condom is promoted as superior to polyurethane in malleability and comfort and does protect against most sexually transmitted infections.

b. **Advantages.** The relative accessibility, ease of transport, and low cost make condoms an attractive method of contraception.

c. **Disadvantages.** Condoms are **not 100% effective** against preventing pregnancy or the spread of sexually transmitted infections. Although accessible to purchase, male condoms are, for most, **not easily transportable**. Male condoms **should not be stored in wallets, glove compartments**, etc. because of the potential for deterioration of the condom. However, a new product, Trojan2GO, provides condoms packaged as "condom cards"—packaging that is resistant to breakdown and which can be easily carried in the wallet or pocket.

d. **Use. Condoms are now packaged with detailed instructions for proper application technique and disposal.** A new condom should be used correctly each time.

e. **Counseling points**

(1) Proper lubrication can minimize the possibility of tearing and can be ensured by using either a lubricated condom or by applying a water-based lubricant to either the condom or the woman's genitalia. (*Note*: Petroleum jelly [Vaseline] should never be used because it causes deterioration of the rubber [latex] and is a poor lubricant.)

(2) Condoms should never be reused.

(3) Condoms should not be stored near excessive heat. Be sure to store condoms in a cool, dry place, out of direct sunlight. The glove compartment of a car is not a good place to store condoms. Do not store condoms in pockets, purses, or wallets for more than a few hours, unless packaging has been specifically designed for such purpose.

(4) If the condom should break or leak, spermicide foam should be immediately inserted vaginally.

(5) Do not buy or use condoms that have passed their expiration date.

(6) Condoms are **not 100% effective** against preventing pregnancy or the spread of sexually transmitted infections. If a sexually transmitted infection is suspected, contact a health care provider or public health agency.

4. The **female condom** is a **disposable nitrile sheath** that fits into the vagina, and **provides protection from pregnancy and some sexually transmitted infections**. The original female condom (FC1) was made of polyurethane, an expensive material. In 2009, FDA approved a second-generation product, the nitrile female condom **(FC2)**, which is made of **synthetic latex** and thus **less expensive** to manufacture than the FC1. Production of FC1 has ceased.

a. The sheath resembles a plastic vaginal pouch and consists of an **inner ring**, which is inserted into the vagina near the cervix much like a diaphragm, whereas the **outer ring** remains outside the vagina, covering the labia. The condom is prelubricated, and additional lubricant (oil- or water-based) may be used if needed. It may be inserted up to 8 hrs before intercourse, and can be removed at any time after ejaculation. However, the FC should be removed prior to the woman standing up to prevent semen spillage.

b. **Female condoms should not be used concurrently with a male condom** because the friction between the two condoms may **contribute to condom breakage**.

c. The FC has a **higher pregnancy failure rate than male condoms**, but does appear to protect against some sexually transmitted diseases, including HIV and cytomegalovirus. However, these data are limited, and further research is necessary to determine the extent of protection these condoms afford against sexually transmitted infections.

d. Female condoms should not be reused.

e. A main complaint with the FC1 was a "squeaking" noise with use. The FC2 has less noise associated with it, but it still can make noise during intercourse.

5. The **diaphragm** is a contraceptive device that is self-inserted into the vagina to block access of sperm to the cervix. It requires a prescription and must be used in conjunction with a nonprescription spermicide to seal off crevices between the vaginal wall and the device.

6. The **cervical cap** is a prescription rubber device smaller than a diaphragm that fits over the cervix like a thimble. It is more difficult to fit than the diaphragm.

7. **Emergency contraception (EC) is the use of a medication or device after coitus to prevent pregnancy.** Currently, the only available nonprescription agent for emergency contraception is **levonorgestrel**, but it is only available for self-care in females **ages 17 and older**.

   a. **Mechanism of action.** The exact mechanism for EC is unknown but thought to be at least two or more of the following:
      (1) inhibit or delay ovulation
      (2) prevent implantation
      (3) inhibit fertilization

   b. **Availability and dose**
      (1) **Next Choice:** contains **two tablets of levonorgestrel 0.75 mg to be taken 12 hrs apart**
      (2) **Plan B One-Step:** contains **one tablet of levonorgestrel 1.5 mg to be taken as a single dose**

   c. Timing. Levonorgestrel for EC is **most efficacious when taken within 24 hrs of intercourse but can be taken up to 72 hrs after intercourse**. Some data demonstrate efficacy up to 120 hrs (5 days) after intercourse, but if used during this time frame, women should be aware that efficacy may be diminished.

   d. Safety. When used as emergency contraception, there are **no contraindications**, given the short duration of use. Adverse effects may include nausea, vomiting, cramping, or irregular bleeding. If vomiting occurs within 2 hrs of dosing, the dose may need to be repeated.

   e. **Counseling points**
      (1) Levonorgestrel EC should not be used for ongoing contraception.
      (2) EC is not effective against the prevention of sexually transmitted infections.
      (3) Levonorgestrel EC is most efficacious if taken within 24 hrs of unprotected intercourse.
      (4) Levonorgestrel EC is ineffective once implantation has occurred.

Study Questions

Directions for questions 1–8: Each of the questions, statements, or incomplete statements in this section can be correctly answered or completed by **one** of the suggested answers or phrases. Choose the **best** answer.

1. The most common cause of vaginal yeast infections is

   (A) *Candida albicans.*
   (B) *Candida glabrata.*
   (C) *Trichomonas.*
   (D) anaerobic bacteria.

2. A female complains of vaginal burning and itching with a distinct "fishy" odor. Which of the following would be the most appropriate recommendation?

   (A) Purchase the Vagisil pH monitor.
   (B) Referral to a medical provider.
   (C) Treatment with a 1-day VVC product.
   (D) Treatment with a 7-day VVC product.

3. Which of the following would be appropriate to counsel on for a woman who is purchasing a female condom?
   - **(A)** The FC2 is superior to the male condom for pregnancy prevention.
   - **(B)** The FC2 can protect against all sexually transmitted infections.
   - **(C)** The FC2 should be used concomitantly with a male condom.
   - **(D)** The FC2 can be inserted several hours prior to intercourse.

4. When assisting a female with the purchase of a vaginal pH monitor, which of the following should be discussed?
   - **(A)** The pH monitor is not recommended in postmenopausal women.
   - **(B)** An elevated pH indicates the presence of a yeast infection.
   - **(C)** The pH of a clean-catch morning urine sample should be used.
   - **(D)** The pH monitor can detect the presence of sexually transmitted infections.

5. Which of the following would be an appropriate counseling point for a female purchasing intravaginal miconazole?
   - **(A)** Avoid treatment during menstruation.
   - **(B)** All male partners should be treated.
   - **(C)** Avoid concomitant use of external creams.
   - **(D)** Side effects can include burning or irritation.

6. All of the following statements regarding contraceptives are correct *except* which one?
   - **(A)** Using the basal temperature method, intercourse should be avoided for a full 6 days after the noted temperature transition.
   - **(B)** If a condom should break or leak, one could recommend immediate insertion of a vaginal spermicide foam.
   - **(C)** Vaginal spermicides may kill many of the causative agents of sexually transmitted diseases (STDs), but they should not be relied on alone for STD prevention.
   - **(D)** Latex condoms can be labeled for the prevention of HIV transmission.
   - **(E)** Nonoxynol-9 is a safe and effective vaginal spermicide.

7. Which of the following agents can be used alone for protection against sexually transmitted infections?
   - **(A)** Contraceptive foam
   - **(B)** Contraceptive sponge
   - **(C)** Female condom
   - **(D)** Diaphragm

8. A 17-year-old female reports breakage of a condom last night during intercourse. She has not been using oral contraception because she smokes. Which of the following would be appropriate to counsel for this patient on Plan-B One-Step?
   - **(A)** She needs a prescription to purchase Plan-B One-Step.
   - **(B)** Take one tablet now and the second tablet 12 hrs later.
   - **(C)** Take Plan B One-Step within 72 hrs of intercourse.
   - **(D)** She is not a candidate for EC because of her tobacco use.
   - **(E)** She can use this continuously for back-up contraception.

Directions for questions 9–10: Each statement in this section is most closely related to **one** of the following drug types. The drug types may be used more than once or not at all. Choose the **best** answer, **A–D**.

A Diuretics
B Salicylates
C Nonsteroidal anti-inflammatory drugs (NSAIDs)
D Narcotic analgesics

9. The primary nonprescription pharmacological treatment for pain associated with dysmenorrhea

10. Recommended by the FDA for elimination of water before and during menstruation

Answers and Explanations

1. **The answer is A** *[see II.A.1.b].*
Candida albicans remains the most common cause. Infections caused by *C. glabrata* are increasing. *Trichomonas* and anaerobic bacteria cause other types of vaginal infections.

2. **The answer is B** *[see II.A.3.f].*
The symptoms of vaginal burning and itching are consistent with VVC; however, the distinct "fishy" odor is more indicative of bacterial vaginosis, which requires prescription treatment. Although a pH monitor may show that the vaginal pH is elevated with a bacterial infection, the woman would still have to seek medical care.

3. **The answer is D** *[see III.B.4.a].*
The FC should not be used concomitantly with the male condom because of the increased risk of breakage. Its pregnancy rates are higher than the male condom; and although it does protect against some sexually transmitted infections, it does not protect against all of them. The FCs can be inserted up to 8 hrs prior to intercourse.

4. **The answer is A** *[see II.A.2].*
The vaginal pH should not change with a yeast infection but may with other vaginal infections. The sample is taken by pressing a wand against the vaginal wall, not collecting a urine sample. The monitor is not recommended for women who lack estrogen (such as postmenopausal women) or for the detection of sexually transmitted diseases.

5. **The answer is D** *[see II.A.4.e].*
Intravaginal treatment for VVC can be used during menstruation and can be used in combination with external creams. It is not necessary for male partners to be treated. Side effects can include burning or irritation.

6. **The answer is A** *[see III.B.1.b].*
Intercourse should be avoided for a full 3 days after the noted temperature transition. All of the other statements are correct.

7. **The answer is C** *[see III.B].*
The diaphragm and spermicidal agents such as the contraceptive foam or sponge can be used alone to protect against pregnancy but cannot be used alone for prevention of sexually transmitted diseases.

8. **The answer is C** *[see III.B.7].*
Plan B One-Step is most efficacious when taken within 24 hrs of intercourse but can be used up to 72 hrs after with efficacy data. It is FDA approved as a nonprescription item for individuals ages 17 and up and is a single dose tablet, as opposed to Next Choice, which is a two-step process described in answer choice B. Smoking is not a contraindication to the use of this agent.

9. **The answer is C** *[see I.B.1.d.(2)].*
NSAIDs are approved by the FDA for the treatment of primary dysmenorrhea.

10. **The answer is A** *[see I.B.2.c.(1).(a)].*
For premenstrual and menstrual relief of water retention, bloating, and tension, the FDA has approved OTC diuretics.

25 Herbal Medicines and Nutritional Supplements

TERESA M. BAILEY

I. INTRODUCTION.

Many of the drugs available on the market are derived from plants. Some of those include aspirin, atropine, belladonna, capsaicin, cascara, colchicine, digoxin, ephedrine, ergotamine, ipecac, opium, physostigmine, pilocarpine, podophyllum, psyllium, quinidine, reserpine, scopolamine, senna, paclitaxel, tubocurarine, vinblastine, and vincristine. Herb products are also derived from plants; however, these products are not considered drugs by the U.S. Food and Drug Administration (FDA).

A. **Regulations**
   1. The **Federal Food, Drug, and Cosmetic Act of 1938** mandated pharmaceutical companies to test drugs for safety before marketing.
   2. The **Kefauver–Harris Drug Amendments of 1962** mandated pharmaceutical companies to test drugs for efficacy before marketing.
   3. The **Dietary Supplement Health and Education Act of 1994** mandated the following:
      a. Dietary supplements are not drugs or food. They are intended to supplement the diet.
      b. Herbs are considered dietary supplements.
      c. Dietary supplements do not have to be standardized.
      d. The secretary of Health and Human Services may remove a supplement from the market only when it has been shown to be hazardous to health.
      e. Dietary supplements may make claims only regarding the effects on structure or function of the body. No claims regarding a particular disease or condition may be made.
      f. The following statement is required on the product label: "This product has not been evaluated by the FDA. It is not intended to diagnose, treat, cure, or prevent."
   4. **Final rule for Current Good Manufacturing Practices (CGMPs) for dietary supplements (2007)**
      a. Manufacturers are required to evaluate for identity, purity, strength, composition
   5. **German Federal Health Agency**
      a. In 1978, the German Federal Health Agency established Commission E.
      b. Commission E evaluates the safety and efficacy of herbs through clinical trials and cases published in scientific literature.
      c. There are > 380 published monographs on herbs.

B. **Herbs considered unsafe for human consumption**
   1. Carcinogenic herbs include borage, calamus, coltsfoot, comfrey, liferoot, and sassafras.
   2. Hepatotoxic herbs include chaparral, germander, kava, and liferoot.
   3. High doses of licorice for long periods may cause pseudoaldosteronism, a condition that may include headache, lethargy, sodium and water retention, hypokalemia, high blood pressure, heart failure, and cardiac arrest.
   4. Ma huang may cause myocardial infarction, strokes, or seizures.
   5. Pokeroot may be fatal in children.
   6. **Unsafe herbs according to the FDA.** In the 1990s, the FDA's Center for Food Safety and Applied Nutrition created the Special Nutritional Adverse Event Monitoring System Web site for dietary supplements. Unfortunately, by 1999 the site was no longer being updated and thus was eventually

deleted. According to the last update from that Web site, the following dietary supplements were considered unsafe by the FDA:

a. Arnica: muscle paralysis, death
b. American and European mistletoe: seizures, coma
c. Bittersweet and deadly nightshade: cardiac toxicity
d. Bloodroot: hypotension, coma
e. Broom: dehydration
f. Comfrey: cancer
g. Dutch and English tonka bean: hepatotoxicity
h. Heliotrope: hepatotoxicity
i. Horse chestnut: bleeding
j. Jimson weed: anticholinergic, hallucinations
k. Kava: hepatotoxicity
l. Lily of the valley: cardiac toxicity
m. Lobelia (nicotine): coma, death
n. Mandrake/mayapple: severe gastrointestinal symptoms
o. Morning glory: psychosis
p. Periwinkle: renal and hepatotoxicity
q. Snakeroot: reserpine derivative
r. Spindle tree: seizures
s. St. John's wort: drug interactions
t. Sweet flag: hallucinations, liver cancer
u. True jalap: purgative cathartic
v. Wahoo: seizures
w. Wormwood: seizures, paralysis
x. Yohimbe: renal failure, hypertension

II. COMMONLY USED HERBS

A. Black cohosh (*Cimicifuga racemosa*)

1. Commission E indications. Premenstrual symptoms, painful or difficult menstruation, and neurovegetative symptoms (hot flashes) caused by menopause

2. Mechanism of action

a. Black cohosh has estrogen-like effects that are exerted by an unknown mechanism, different from an estrogenic mechanism.

b. It does not appear to bind to estrogen receptors. Nor does it appear to upregulate estrogen-dependent genes.

c. It does not affect the growth of estrogen-dependent tumors in experimental animals.

3. Efficacy

a. Uncontrolled as well as double-blind, randomized, placebo-controlled clinical trials compared black cohosh to hormone therapy in perimenopausal and postmenopausal women with neurovegetative menopausal symptoms of different degrees of severity. The Kupperman menopausal index and psychiatric clinical and self-evaluation scales were significantly reduced after 3 months of treatment with black cohosh. Vaginal cytological parameters also improved in regard to estrogen stimulation. Black cohosh was shown to be superior to placebo and comparable to estriol, conjugated estrogens, and estrogen–progesterone therapy.[1]

b. Black cohosh may not be effective in premenopausal breast cancer survivors with tamoxifen-induced hot flashes.[2]

4. Contraindications/precautions

a. Pregnancy

b. Unknown if suitable for patients for whom hormone replacement therapy is contraindicated, such as estrogen-receptor-positive breast cancer

c. Commission E recommends that length of use should not exceed 6 months.

d. Use caution in liver disease, such as hepatitis and fulminant liver failure.

5. **Drug interactions**
   a. Cisplatin (Platinol) efficacy may be reduced.
   b. Theoretically, black cohosh may interact with hepatotoxic drugs such as acetaminophen (Tylenol), carbamazepine (Tegretol), and isoniazid (Nydrazid) because it is an inhibitor of cytochrome P450 3A4 (CYP3A4) and CYP2D6 isoenzymes.
   c. A case reports a patient taking atorvastatin (Lipitor) developing significantly elevated liver function enzymes after black cohosh was initiated.[3]
6. **Side effects**
   a. Occasional intestinal problems may occur, such as nausea and vomiting; weight gain is possible.
   b. Liver toxicity may occur; liver function tests should be monitored periodically.
   c. Large doses of black cohosh may cause dizziness, nausea, severe headaches, stiffness, and trembling limbs.
   d. Does not seem to increase risk of endometrial hyperplasia.
7. **Dosage.** Remifemin is a standardized product that contains 20 mg black cohosh and is taken twice daily. It is standardized to 1 mg of 27-deoxyactein per tablet.

B. **Chaste tree berry (*Vitex agnus-castus*)**
1. **Commission E indications.** Disorders of the menstrual cycle, breast swelling, and premenstrual symptoms
2. **Mechanism of action**
   a. Chaste tree berry binds to dopamine receptors and inhibits prolactin secretion.
   b. One of its ingredients, linoleic acid, binds to estrogen receptors.
   c. It increases the pituitary gland's production of luteinizing hormone and inhibits follicle-stimulating hormone (FSH).
3. **Efficacy.** One randomized, double-blind, placebo-controlled, parallel group study included 170 women with premenstrual syndrome.[4] *Vitex* was given 20 mg daily for three cycles. Self-assessment and clinical global impression significantly improved.
4. **Contraindications/precautions**
   a. Pregnancy and lactation
   b. Hormone-sensitive conditions
5. **Drug interactions**
   a. Theoretically, chaste tree berry may interact with medications that increase dopaminergic activity, such as bromocriptine (Parlodel) and levodopa.
   b. Theoretically, it may interact with medications that decrease dopaminergic activity such as the antipsychotics.
   c. Theoretically, it may interact with hormone-replacement therapy and oral contraceptives.
6. **Side effects**
   a. Mild gastrointestinal upset
   b. Skin rash
   c. Irregular menstrual bleeding
7. **Dosage.** Doses depend on the formulation. Typical dose range of chaste tree berry is 20 to 240 mg/day.

C. **Cranberry (*Vaccinium macrocarpon*)**
1. **Commission E indications.** Recurrent urinary tract infections
2. **Mechanism of action**
   a. Benzoic and quinic acids break down and form hippuric acid (bacteriostatic).
   b. Inhibition of *Escherichia coli* adherence to epithelial cells of urinary tract
3. **Efficacy**
   a. A quasi-randomized, double-blind, placebo-controlled study included 153 women who received 300 mL of cranberry juice daily for 6 months.[5] Bacteriuria with pyuria occurred less often in the cranberry group (15%) versus placebo (28%).
   b. Cranberry has not been shown to be effective for treating an active urinary tract infection.
4. **Contraindications/precautions**
   a. Nephrolithiasis
   b. Cranberry juice contains high amounts of salicylic acid and may trigger an allergic reaction in patients with an aspirin allergy or asthma.

c. Discontinue 2 weeks before surgery.
d. Ulcers, GERD

5. **Drug interactions**
   a. Increased vitamin B_{12} absorption
   b. Potential to enhance elimination of renally excreted drugs by changing urine pH
   c. Cranberry juice may interact with warfarin, increasing the international normalized ratio (INR).
   d. May inhibit cytochrome P450 2C9. Drugs that are metabolized by CYP2C9 include amitriptyline (Elavil) and diazepam (Valium).
6. **Side effects**
   a. Nausea, vomiting, diarrhea
   b. Nephrolithiasis
7. **Dosage.** Recommended dose of cranberry is 300 to 400 mg twice daily using a standardized product to include 11% to 12% quinic acid per dose. Patients may also take 8 to 16 oz 100% cranberry juice daily. Drinking lots of fluids is recommended.

D. **Dong quai (*Angelica sinensis*)**

1. **Traditional Chinese medicine indications.** Menstrual disorders, anemia, constipation, insomnia, rheumatism, neuralgia, and hypertension
2. **Mechanism of action**
   a. Dong quai is only 1:400 as active as estrogen. However, it does not appear to produce any changes to the ovaries or vaginal tissue.[6]
   b. It contains seven different coumarin derivatives: oxypeucedanin, osthole, psoralen, angelol, angelicone, bergapten, and 7-desmethylsuberosin. Many coumarins have been shown to have vasodilatory and antispasmodic effects. One of the coumarins (osthole) is a central nervous system (CNS) stimulant.
   c. It inhibits experimentally induced immunoglobulin E (IgE) titers, suggesting that components of the plant may have immunosuppressive activity.
   d. It inhibits prostaglandin E_2 (PGE_2) release and, therefore, possesses analgesic, antipyretic, and anti-inflammatory actions.
   e. It has an antiarrhythmic activity similar to quinidine.
3. **Efficacy.** A randomized, double-blind, placebo-controlled trial included 71 postmenopausal women (mean age, 52.4 years) who had FSH $<$ 30 mIU/mL with hot flashes.[7] Women received three capsules of dong quai three times daily (equivalent to 4.5 g of dong quai root daily) or placebo for 24 weeks. Dong quai did not produce estrogen-like responses in endometrial thickness or in vaginal maturation or relieve menopausal symptoms. The study is criticized for using dong quai alone because in traditional Chinese medicine, dong quai is used in combination with four or more other herbs.
4. **Contraindications/precautions**
   a. Pregnancy (uterine stimulant) and lactation
   b. Diarrhea
   c. Hemorrhagic disease; discontinue 2 weeks before surgery
   d. Hypermenorrhea
   e. Hypotension
   f. During cold or flu
   g. Allergy to parsley
   h. Breast cancer
5. **Drug interactions**
   a. Dong quai interacts with anticoagulants such as warfarin (Coumadin)
   b. Antihypertensives (hypotension)
   c. Theoretically, may interact with hormone replacement therapy and oral contraceptives.
   d. Unknown if it interacts with other cardiovascular drugs such as procainamide (Pronestyl)
6. **Side effects**
   a. Photodermatitis may occur in people collecting the plant.
   b. Burping, flatulence, and headache
   c. Safrole, found in the oil of dong quai, is carcinogenic and not recommended for ingestion.
   d. May stimulate breast cancer cells.

7. **Dosage.** A variety of doses are suggested. No standardized product is available. According to traditional Chinese medicine, dong quai alone may not be effective.

E. **Echinacea (*Echinacea purpurea, E. angustifolia*)**

1. **Commission E indications**
   a. Internal use: supportive therapy for infections of the upper respiratory tract (cold) and lower urinary tract
   b. External use: local application for the treatment of hard-to-heal superficial wounds and ulcers
2. **Mechanism of action.** Echinacea increases the body's resistance to bacteria by the following:
   a. Caffeic acid derivatives, which include cichoric acid, chlorogenic acid, and cynarin, increase phagocytosis and stimulate the production of immunopotentiating substances such as interferon, interleukins, and tumor necrosis factor.
   b. Polysaccharides, such as inulin, stimulate macrophages and inhibit hyaluronidase activity to decrease inflammation.
   c. Alkylamides, such as echinacein, have a local anesthetic effect and inhibit hyaluronidase activity to decrease inflammation.
   d. Echinacea has little or no direct bactericidal or bacteriostatic properties.
3. **Efficacy**
   a. **Treatment of common cold.** In a review of 26 controlled clinical trials evaluating echinacea's ability to strengthen the body's own defense mechanisms, it was found that 30 of 34 echinacea therapies were more effective compared to controls.[8]
   b. **Prevention of common cold.** Studies have shown that taking echinacea prophylactically to prevent the development of a cold does not seem to be effective.
4. **Contraindications/precautions**
   a. Echinacea is contraindicated in infectious and autoimmune diseases such as tuberculosis, leukosis, collagenosis, multiple sclerosis, AIDS, HIV, and lupus.
   b. Caution should be used in patients who are allergic to members of the ragweed or chrysanthemum family.
   c. The effects of echinacea in pregnancy, lactation, and children are unknown. Comparison with a control group suggested no increased risk of major malformations in 206 pregnant women.[9]
   d. Therapy should not exceed 8 weeks. Theoretically, prolonged use of echinacea may depress the immune system, possibly through overstimulation.
5. **Drug interactions**
   a. Unknown if echinacea interacts with immunosuppressants
   b. Echinacea inhibits cytochrome P450 1A2. Some drugs metabolized by CYP1A2 are caffeine (Cafcit) and theophylline.
   c. Echinacea induces and inhibits CYP3A4. Some drugs metabolized by CYP3A4 are midazolam (Versed), itraconazole (Sporanox), and fexofenadine (Allegra).
6. **Side effects**
   a. Nausea, vomiting, dizziness, tiredness
   b. Allergic reactions, acute asthma, leukopenia, and anaphylaxis
   c. May interfere with male fertility
7. **Dosage.** There are a variety of doses recommended. The most common dose is as the dried powder, 1 g or two 500-mg capsules orally three times daily. Recommended to use for 2 weeks only during a cold.

F. **Feverfew (*Tanacetum parthenium*)**

1. **Commission E indication.** Prophylaxis of migraine headaches
2. **Mechanism of action**
   a. Feverfew inhibits the release of 5-hydroxytryptamine (serotonin) from platelets, which may be the same mechanism as methysergide maleate (Sansert).
   b. It irreversibly inhibits prostaglandin synthesis through a different mechanism from that of the salicylates. It inhibits phospholipase A_2 by α-methylene butyrolactones (parthenolide and epoxyartemorin).
   c. There is an antithrombotic potential owing to a phospholipase inhibition that prevents the release of arachidonic acid.

3. **Efficacy.** An evaluation of five trials for the efficacy of feverfew in the prevention of migraines compared to placebo was conducted.[10] A variety of doses and durations were used. Some trials showed the number and severity of migraine attacks and the degree of vomiting was reduced with feverfew. The duration of attacks was unaltered. Other trials showed no benefit.
4. **Contraindications/precautions**
   a. Feverfew should be avoided in pregnancy, lactation, and children < 2 years of age.
   b. Contraindicated in individuals with allergies to chrysanthemums or ragweed.
   c. Contraindicated in patients with bleeding disorders. Discontinue 2 weeks before surgery.
5. **Drug interactions**
   a. Feverfew may interact with anticoagulants, increasing the risk of bleeding.
   b. Feverfew may inhibit the following cytochrome P450 isoenzymes: 1A2, 2C19, 2C9, and 3A4.
6. **Side effects**
   a. Gastric discomfort on oral consumption
   b. Contact dermatitis
   c. Minor ulcerations of oral mucosa, irritation of tongue, and swelling of lips may occur when fresh leaves are chewed.
   d. Palpitations
   e. Post-feverfew syndrome: Discontinuation of feverfew may produce muscle and joint stiffness and a cluster of nervous system reactions (rebound of migraines, anxiety, and insomnia).
7. **Dosage.** The usual dose of feverfew is 50 to 100 mg daily. A product containing at least 0.2% parthenolide is recommended.

G. **Fish oil**
1. **Purported uses.** Hypertension, hyperlipidemia, mental health, bipolar, psychosis, depression, anticoagulant, coronary heart disease, stroke
2. **Mechanism of action.** Fish oil contains omega-3 fatty acids, eicosapentaenoic acid (EPA) and docosahexaenoic acid (DHA). The human body cannot produce omega-3 fatty acids nor can it convert omega-6 fatty acids. Omega-3 fatty acids can form eicosanoids (prostaglandins, leukotrienes, lipoxins). Fish oil inhibits the synthesis of VLDL and triglycerides in the liver and studies have been shown to decrease triglycerides by 20% to 50% and increase HDL by 10%, but increase LDL by 0% to 45%.
3. **Efficacy.** Consuming fish oil, two servings of fatty fish per week, reduces the risk of developing primary or secondary cardiovascular disease.
4. **Contraindications/precautions.** Seafood allergy, bipolar disorder, bleeding, cardiac disease, depression, diabetes mellitus, hypertension, immunodeficiency
5. **Drug interactions**
   a. Anticoagulants/antiplatelets/thrombolytics. Increase bleeding
   b. Antihypertensives. Additive blood pressure reduction
   c. Xenical, Alli, Orlistat. Decreased fish oil absorption. Recommended to separate by 2 hrs.
6. **Side effects**
   a. Bleeding, ecchymosis (bruising), epistaxis (nosebleeds)
   b. Hypervitaminosis A, hypervitaminosis D
   c. Rash
   d. Dyspepsia, eructation (burping), nausea/vomiting, diarrhea
   e. Halitosis, dysgeusia (taste perversion)
7. **Dosage**
   a. Hypertriglyceridemia: 1 to 4 g/day orally in divided doses
   b. Hypertension: 4 g/day orally in divided doses
   c. Products providing eicosapentaenoic acid (EPA) 2.04 g and docosahexaenoic acid (DHA) 1.4 g daily are recommended.

H. **Flaxseed (*Linum usitatissimum*)**
1. **Purported uses.** Constipation, diarrhea, diabetes, menopause, hypertension, hyperlipidemia, coronary artery disease

2. **Mechanism of action**
   a. The seed coat gum of flaxseed is soluble fiber.
   b. Flaxseed contains fatty acids; of which, 55% are alpha-linolenic acid. The human body converts alpha-linolenic acid into omega-3 fatty acids, such as eicosapentaenoic (EPA) and docosahexaenoic acids (DHA).
   c. Lignans are phytoestrogens with weak estrogenic and anti-estrogenic effects.
3. **Efficacy**
   a. **Diabetes.** Flaxseed decreased A1c but did not decrease fasting blood glucose or insulin levels (Pan).
   b. **Hypercholesterolemia.** Flaxseed 40 to 50 g/day decreases LDL by 8% to 18% and decreases total cholesterol by 5% to 9%, but flaxseed does not affect HDL.
   c. **Menopause.** Flaxseed 40 g/day has been shown to significantly reduce hot flashes by about 35% and night sweats by about 44%.
4. **Contraindications/precautions.** Bleeding disorders, diabetes, gastrointestinal obstruction, and hormone-sensitive cancers
5. **Drug interactions**
   a. Anticoagulants/antiplatelets. Theoretically may have additive effects.
   b. Antidiabetic agents. Theoretically may have additive effects.
   c. Estrogens. Theoretically may have competitive effects.
   d. Flaxseed may decrease the absorption of oral drugs. It is recommended to administer medications an hour before or 2 hrs after taking flaxseed.
6. **Side effects**
   a. Soluble fiber causes bloating, flatulence, abdominal pain, diarrhea, constipation, dyspepsia, nausea.
   b. Allergic reactions
7. **Dosage**
   a. For hypercholesterolemia, baked goods (muffins or bread) containing flaxseed and ground flaxseed with 40 to 50 g of flaxseed per day
   b. For menopausal symptoms, 40 g daily of crushed flaxseed
   c. Adequate amount of fluid to prevent potential bowel obstruction

I. **Garlic (*Allium sativum*)**
1. **Commission E indications.** Supports dietary measures for the treatment of hyperlipoproteinemia and to prevent age-related changes in the blood vessels (arteriosclerosis).
2. **Mechanism of action**
   a. Garlic inhibits platelet function by interfering with thromboxane synthesis.
   b. It increases the levels of two antioxidant enzymes in the blood: catalase and glutathione peroxidase.
   c. Organic disulfides found in garlic oil inactivate the thiol enzymes such as coenzyme A (CoA) and hydroxymethylglutaryl (HMG) CoA reductase.
3. **Efficacy**
   a. In a meta-analysis of eight studies evaluating the effect on blood pressure, the overall pooled difference in change of systolic blood pressure was 7.7 mm Hg lower with garlic than with placebo; diastolic blood pressure was 5.0 mm Hg lower with garlic.[11]
   b. In a meta-analysis of five studies evaluating the effect on total serum cholesterol, patients were excluded if they were receiving lipid-lowering drugs.[12] The overall pooled total cholesterol difference between garlic and placebo was −23 mg/dL (−29 to −17).
4. **Contraindications/precautions**
   a. Caution in diabetes. Garlic may increase the release of insulin or enhance the response to insulin.
   b. Caution in pregnancy (emmenagogue and abortifacient) and lactation
   c. Caution in peptic ulcer disease and gastroesophageal reflux
   d. **Caution in bleeding disorders.** Discontinue 2 weeks before surgery
5. **Drug interactions**
   a. Anticoagulants (increased bleeding)
   b. Protease inhibitor, saquinavir (decreased efficacy)
   c. Nonnucleoside reverse transcriptase inhibitors, such as nevirapine, efavirenz (decreased efficacy)

d. Antihypertensives (hypotension)
e. Antidiabetic agents (hypoglycemia)
f. May induce the following cytochrome P450 isoenzymes: 2C9, 2C19, 3A4, 2D6, and 2E1. Caution should be used with contraceptive medications, cyclosporine, diltiazem, and verapamil (decreased efficacy).
g. Isoniazid. Decreased efficacy.

6. **Side effects.** Gastrointestinal discomfort (heartburn, flatulence), sweating, light-headedness, allergic reactions, and menorrhagia
7. **Dosage.** Between 0.6 and 1.2 g dried powder (2 to 5 mg of allicin) daily or 2 to 4 g fresh garlic
8. **Comments**
   a. Alliinase (the enzyme that converts alliin to allicin) is inactivated by acids. Enteric-coated tablets or capsules allow more absorption because they pass through the stomach and release their contents in the alkaline medium of the small intestine.
   b. Effective preparations include freeze-dried garlic power and aged garlic extract.
   c. Odorless garlic preparations may not contain the active compounds.

J. **Ginger (*Zingiber officinale*)**

1. **Commission E indications.** Dyspepsia and prophylaxis of symptoms of travel sickness
2. **Mechanism of action**
   a. Ginger promotes saliva and gastric juice secretion, which increases peristalsis and the tone of the intestinal muscle.
   b. It acts on 5-hydroxytryptamine 3 (5-HT_3) receptors in the ileum, similar to ondansetron.
   c. It inhibits thromboxane synthesis as a prostacyclin agonist.
3. **Efficacy.** A double-blind study included 36 blindfolded subjects with high susceptibility to motion sickness who were given ginger 940 mg, dimenhydrinate 100 mg, or placebo for the prevention of motion sickness induced by a tilted rotating chair. Ginger subjects remained in the chair an average of 5.5 mins, dimenhydrinate 3.5 mins, and placebo 1.5 mins. The ginger group took longer to feel sick, but once sick, the sensations of nausea and vomiting progressed at the same rate in all groups.[13]
4. **Contraindications/precautions**
   a. Bleeding disorders. Discontinue 2 weeks before surgery
   b. It is contraindicated for gallstone pain.
   c. It is recommended by the American College of Obstetricians and Gynecologists (ACOG) for use in pregnancy $<$ 17 weeks of gestation with the following cautions: Ginger is a uterine relaxant in low doses and a uterine stimulant in high doses.
   d. Diabetes (hypoglycemia)
   e. Heart conditions may worsen because ginger has positive inotropic activity.
5. **Drug interactions**
   a. Antiplatelets and anticoagulants (increased bleeding)
   b. Diabetic agents (hypoglycemia)
   c. Calcium-channel blockers (hypotension)
6. **Side effects** are dermatitis, heartburn, and diarrhea.
7. **Dosage (for travel sickness).** Daily dose is 2 to 4 g. Two 500-mg capsules taken 30 mins before travel, then one to two more capsules every 4 hrs as needed. The 1000 mg standardized extract is equivalent to
   a. 1 teaspoon fresh grated rhizome;
   b. 2 droppers liquid extract (2 mL);
   c. 2 teaspoons syrup (10 mL);
   d. 8 oz ginger ale, made with real ginger; and
   e. 4 cups ginger tea (made by steeping ½ teaspoon grated ginger for 5 to 10 mins in hot water).

K. **Ginkgo (*Ginkgo biloba*)**

1. **Commission E indications**
   a. Treatment for cerebral circulatory disturbances resulting in reduced functional capacity and vigilance (vertigo, tinnitus, weakened memory, and mood swings accompanied by anxiety)
   b. Treatment of peripheral arterial circulatory disturbance such as intermittent claudication

2. **Mechanism of action**
   a. Ginkgo contains flavonoids (quercetin, kaempferol, and isorhamnetin) and terpenoids (ginkgolides A, B, and C and bilobalide).
   b. Flavonoids provide the antioxidant activity, reduce capillary fragility, and increase the threshold of blood loss from capillaries.
   c. Ginkgolides antagonize platelet-activating factor (PAF), which induces platelet aggregation, the degranulation of neutrophils, and the production of oxygen radicals.
3. **Efficacy**
   a. In a review of the clinical and pharmacological studies on ginkgo and cerebral insufficiency, eight were found to be of good quality.[14] Seven of the trials showed positive effects of ginkgo compared to placebo. Symptoms of cerebral insufficiency evaluated were difficulties of concentration and memory, absentmindedness, confusion, lack of energy, tiredness, decreased physical performance, depression, anxiety, dizziness, tinnitus, and headaches.
   b. A randomized, double-blind, placebo-controlled study included 202 patients with either Alzheimer disease or multi-infarct dementia. These patients were given ginkgo 40 mg three times daily or placebo for 1 year. Ginkgo had a statistically significant improvement by at least two points or better on the Alzheimer Disease Assessment Scale—Cognitive (a 70-point subscale) compared to placebo (50% vs. 29%). Ginkgo showed statistically significant improvement on the Geriatric Evaluation by Relative's Rating Instrument (37% vs. 23%). There was no difference between ginkgo and placebo on the Clinical Global Impression of Change Scale.[15]
4. **Contraindications/precautions**
   a. Epilepsy. Ginkgotoxin may cause neurotoxicity and seizures.
   b. Bleeding disorders. Discontinue 2 weeks before surgery
   c. Diabetes (hypoglycemia)
   d. Infertility. Caution in difficulty conceiving.
5. **Drug interactions**
   a. Ginkgo may potentiate the bleeding properties of antiplatelets/anticoagulants.
   b. Aminoglycosides (increased ototoxicity)
   c. Thiazide (increases blood pressure)
   d. Trazodone (Desyrel) (coma)
   e. Seizure threshold lowering drugs
   f. Anticonvulsants (decreased efficacy)
   g. Antidiabetic drugs (hypoglycemia)
   h. Ginkgo may mildly affect the cytochrome P450 isoenzymes 1A2, 2C19, 2C9, 2D6, and 3A4.
6. **Side effects**
   a. Gastric disturbances, headache, dizziness, and vertigo
   b. Toxic ingestion may produce tonic–clonic seizures and loss of consciousness
   c. Spontaneous bleeding; mild to severe (intracerebral hemorrhage)
7. **Dosage.** Recommended dose is 40 mg three times daily with meals for at least 4 to 6 weeks. Standardized preparations that contain 6% terpene lactones and 24% ginkgo flavone glycosides are recommended.

L. **Asian ginseng (*Panax ginseng*, *P. quinquefolius*)**
1. **Commission E indications.** Tonic to combat feelings of lassitude and debility, lack of energy, and ability to concentrate, and during convalescence
2. **Mechanism of action**
   a. At least 28 active ingredients, known as ginsenosides, have been identified.
   b. Ginseng effects vary with extract derivative, drying method, dose, duration of treatment, and animal species that were studied. Each ginsenoside produces different pharmacological effects on the CNS, cardiovascular system, and other body systems. Different ginsenosides are capable of producing biological effects in direct opposition with those produced by others. For example, the ginsenoside Rb_1 has been shown to have a suppressive effect on the CNS, whereas Rg_1 produces a stimulatory effect.

3. **Efficacy**
   a. A randomized, double-blind, placebo-controlled, crossover study included 50 male sports teachers who performed a treadmill exercise test. Volunteers received two ginseng capsules (Geriatric Pharmaton) daily for 6 weeks or placebo. Volunteers used energy more efficiently and had greater endurance while taking ginseng.[16] However, other studies have not shown Asian ginseng to be effective.
4. **Contraindications/precautions**
   a. Pregnancy and lactation
   b. Children
   c. Avoid in patients with hypertension, emotional/psychological imbalances, headaches, heart palpitations, insomnia, asthma, inflammation, or infections with high fever.
   d. Caution should be used in patients with a history of bleeding. Discontinue 2 weeks before surgery.
   e. Diabetes (hypoglycemia)
   f. Schizophrenia
   g. Caution should be used in patients with a history of breast cancer. Ginseng may stimulate breast cancer cells.
5. **Drug interactions**
   a. Ginseng may interact with phenelzine (Nardil), producing hallucinations and psychosis.
   b. Ginseng may decrease the INR of warfarin (Coumadin).
   c. Ginseng may interact with stimulants, including caffeine (Cafcit).
   d. Ginseng may interact with oral hypoglycemic and insulin, causing hypoglycemia.
   e. It is unknown whether ginseng interacts with hormonal therapy, antihypertensives, or cardiac medications.
   f. It may inhibit cytochrome P450 2D6. Caution should be used with drugs that are metabolized via cytochrome P450 2D6, such as amitriptyline (Elavil) and fluoxetine (Prozac).
   g. It may interfere with immunosuppressants such as cyclosporine (Sandimmune) or tacrolimus (Prograf).
6. **Side effects**
   a. Nervousness, excitation, insomnia
   b. Inability to concentrate with long-term use
   c. Diffuse mammary nodularity and vaginal bleeding may be caused by ginseng's estrogen-like effect in women.
   d. Hypertension, euphoria, restlessness, nervousness, insomnia, skin eruptions, edema, and diarrhea have been reported with long-term ginseng use with an average dose of 3 g ginseng root daily.
   e. Tachyarrhythmia due to increased QT interval
7. **Dosage.** 1 to 2 g crude herb daily or 100 to 300 mg ginseng extract three times daily. Standardized products that contain at least 4% to 5% ginsenosides are recommended.

M. **Milk thistle (*Silybum marianum*)**

1. **Commission E indications.** Chronic inflammatory liver conditions and cirrhosis
2. **Mechanism of action**
   a. Silymarin is believed to be the active component in milk thistle.
   b. Silymarin stimulates the activity of RNA polymerase A and is a potent antioxidant.
   c. Silymarin alters the outer liver membrane cell structure.
3. **Efficacy.** In an evaluation of 13 trials for the efficacy of milk thistle in the treatment of alcoholic and/or hepatitis B or C virus liver diseases, milk thistle had no significant effect on overall mortality, complications of liver disease, or liver histology.[17] Liver-related mortality was significantly reduced with milk thistle when all trials were evaluated but was not significantly reduced when only high-quality trials were evaluated.
4. **Contraindications/precautions**
   a. Avoid in pregnancy
   b. Allergy to chrysanthemums/ragweed
   c. Hormone-sensitive cancers
5. **Drug interactions**
   a. Milk thistle may inhibit cytochrome P450 2C9 and 3A4.
   b. Milk thistle does not interact with indinavir (Crixivan).

6. **Side effects** include diarrhea and other gastrointestinal reactions (nausea, dyspepsia, flatulence) and allergic reactions.
7. **Dosage.** Recommended dose of milk thistle is 200 to 400 mg/day divided into three doses using a standardized product that includes 70% to 80% silymarin.

N. **Saw palmetto (*Serenoa repens*)**

1. **Commission E indications.** Treatment of micturition difficulties associated with benign prostatic hyperplasia
2. **Mechanism of action**
   a. Saw palmetto inhibits dihydrotestosterone to androgen receptors in prostate cells.
   b. It may inhibit testosterone-5-α-reductase, the enzyme responsible for the conversion of testosterone to dihydrotestosterone.
3. **Efficacy.** An evaluation of 30 studies evaluated saw palmetto in 5222 men with BPH during 4 to 60 weeks. Most of the studies compared to placebo; one study compared to finasteride, two studies compared to tamsulosin. The International Prostate Symptom Score and nocturia showed no significant difference to placebo, finasteride, or tamsulosin.[18]
4. **Contraindications/precautions**
   a. Avoid in pregnancy
   b. Avoid in children
   c. Discontinue 2 weeks before surgery
5. **Drug interactions**
   a. Theoretically, saw palmetto may interact with anticoagulants or antiplatelets.
   b. Theoretically, saw palmetto may interact with contraceptive drugs or hormone replacement therapy.
6. **Side effects**
   a. Intraoperative hemorrhage
   b. Headache
   c. Stomach upset, nausea, vomiting, diarrhea, constipation
   d. Acute hepatitis and pancreatitis
7. **Dosage.** Recommended 1 to 2 g saw palmetto or 320 mg of lipophilic extract daily, usually given 160 mg twice daily and taken with food. Products standardized to contain 90% free and 7% esterified fatty acids are recommended.

O. **St. John's wort (*Hypericum perforatum*)**

1. **Commission E indications.** In supportive treatment for anxiety and depression.
2. **Mechanism of action**
   a. **Some of the active ingredients** include hypericin, hyperin, hyperforin, melatonin, adhyperforin.
   b. Hypericin, flavonoids, and xanthones show in vitro irreversible monoamine oxidase inhibitor (MAOI) type A and B activity.
   c. St. John's wort may inhibit serotonin reuptake.
   d. St. John's wort may inhibit synaptic γ-aminobutyric acid (GABA) uptake and GABA receptor binding.
3. **Efficacy.** An evaluation of 37 trials for the efficacy of St. John's wort in the treatment of depression showed the herb may be more effective than placebo for mild-to-moderate depression.[19] St. John's wort may be as effective as other antidepressants for mild-to-moderate depression. St. John's wort may not be effective for major depression.
4. **Contraindications/precautions**
   a. Caution in fair-skinned persons when exposed to bright sunlight
   b. Caution in pregnancy (emmenagogue and abortifacient)
   c. No negative influence on general performance or the ability to drive a car or operate heavy machinery has been reported.
   d. Psychiatric conditions such as bipolar and schizophrenia may be exacerbated.
   e. Alzheimer disease. St. John's wort may induce psychosis
   f. Hypothyroidism. St. John's wort may increase thyroid-stimulating hormone.
   g. Anesthesia. St. John's wort may cause cardiovascular collapse.
   h. Surgical procedures. Discontinue 2 weeks before.
   i. Infertility. St. John's wort may inhibit oocyte fertilization and alter sperm DNA.

5. **Drug interactions**
   a. Antidepressants such as paroxetine (Paxil), sertraline (Zoloft), and nefazodone have been reported to cause serotonin syndrome when taken with St. John's wort.
   b. Antiretroviral (protease inhibitors and nonnucleoside reverse transcriptase inhibitors) levels may decrease.
   c. St. John's wort may decrease the efficacy of barbiturates.
   d. St. John's wort may increase the efficacy of clopidogrel (Plavix).
   e. Cyclosporine (Sandimmune) levels may decrease.
   f. St. John's wort may interact with other drugs metabolized through the cytochrome P450 isoenzymes 1A2, 2C9, 2C19, and 3A4.
   g. Digoxin (Lanoxin) levels may decrease.
   h. Irinotecan (Camptosar) and imatinib (Gleevec) levels may decrease.
   i. Methadone (Dolophine) levels may decrease.
   j. St. John's wort may decrease the efficacy of omeprazole (Prilosec).
   k. Oral contraceptives may have a decreased effect.
   l. St. John's wort may decrease the efficacy of HMG coenzyme reductase inhibitors (simvastatin).
   m. Tacrolimus (Prograf) levels may decrease.
   n. Theophylline levels may decrease.
   o. Triptans. Theoretically, St. John's wort may interact with the triptans.
   p. Verapamil (Calan, Covera-HS, Isoptin, Verelan) levels may decrease.
   q. St. John's wort may decrease the INR of warfarin (Coumadin).
   r. Serotonergic agents such as dextromethorphan, fenfluramine, narcotics.
   s. Anticonvulsants. Phenytoin, phenobarbital, mephenytoin.
6. **Food interactions**
   a. Older studies suggested that St. John's wort was an MAOI.[20]
   b. Newer studies suggest St. John's wort is a weak MAOI.[21]
   c. One case report published of MAOI-type food interactions such as tyramine-containing foods: cheeses, beer, wine, herring, and yeast.
7. **Side effects**
   a. Photodermatitis, allergic reactions
   b. Gastrointestinal irritations
   c. Tiredness, restlessness, sleep disturbances
   d. Elevated thyroid-stimulating hormone
   e. Elevated blood pressure
   f. Mania or hypomania
   g. May cause infertility
8. **Dosage.** Recommended 2 to 4 g daily in two to three divided doses. Standardized products containing 0.4 to 2.7 mg hypericin/day or 0.3% hypericin are recommended.

P. **Valerian (*Valeriana officinalis*)**
1. **Commission E indications.** Restlessness and nervous disturbance of sleep
2. **Mechanism of action**
   a. Several active compounds have been isolated from valerian and grouped into three categories: volatile oil, valepotriates, and alkaloids. It is believed that the sedative activity of valerian is secondary to the valepotriates.
   b. Valepotriates, valeranone 6, kessane derivatives 3a–f, valerenic acid 5a, and valerenal 5b have been reported to prolong barbiturate-induced sleeping time.
   c. Valerenic acid 5a has been shown to possess pentobarbital-like central depressant activity rather than muscle relaxant or neuroleptic effects. It has also been shown to inhibit the enzyme that triggers the breakdown of GABA.
   d. Valtrate and isovaltrate have exhibited antidepressant properties.
   e. Didrovaltrate possesses a tranquilizing ability similar to the benzodiazepines.
3. **Efficacy.** A double-blind, randomized study included eight volunteers suffering from mild insomnia who received valerian aqueous extract 450 mg or 900 mg or placebo at bedtime. Valerian 450 mg significantly improved sleep quality, sleep latency, and sleep depth compared to placebo. The 900-mg dose offered no advantage over the 450-mg dose.[22]

4. **Contraindications/precautions**
   a. Caution while driving or performing other tasks requiring alertness and coordination is recommended.
   b. Pregnancy and lactation
   c. Surgery. Valerian may have an additive effect to anesthesia.
5. **Drug interactions**
   a. CNS depressants. Valerian may potentiate the sedative effect of barbiturates, benzodiazepines, opiates, alcohol, or other sedatives.
   b. Valerian inhibits cytochrome P450 3A4.
6. **Side effects**
   a. Headaches, hangover, excitability, insomnia, uneasiness, and cardiac disturbances
   b. Hepatotoxicity
   c. Toxicity includes ataxia, decreased sensibility, hypothermia, hallucinations, and increased muscle relaxation
   d. Patients may experience a benzodiazepine-like withdrawal, so doses should be tapered down slowly.
7. **Dosage.** Dried root: 2 to 3 g/cup, one to three times daily. Standardized to contain 0.8% to 1.0% valeremic acids/dose extract: 400 to 900 mg 30 to 60 mins before bedtime.

III. OTHER DIETARY SUPPLEMENTS THAT ARE POTENTIALLY SAFE

A. **Chondroitin**
1. **Nonapproved indications.** Viscoelastic agent in ophthalmic procedures and the treatment of osteoarthritis
2. **Mechanism of action**
   a. Chondroitin is made from shark and bovine cartilage. It concentrates in cartilage where it can be used in the synthesis of new cartilaginous matrix.
   b. It increases the RNA synthesis of chondrocytes, which may increase the synthesis of proteoglycans and collagens.
   c. It may inhibit leukocyte elastase activity. Leukocyte elastase is found in high concentrations in the blood and synovial fluid of patients with rheumatic diseases.
3. **Efficacy.** A multicenter, double-blind, randomized study included 1583 patients with symptomatic knee osteoarthritis who received glucosamine 1500 mg daily, chondroitin 1200 mg daily, both glucosamine and chondroitin, celecoxib 200 mg daily, or placebo for 24 weeks. Glucosamine and chondroitin sulfate alone or in combination did not significantly reduce pain. The combination may be helpful in a subgroup of patients with moderate-to-severe knee pain.[23]
4. **Contraindications/precautions**
   a. Previous hypersensitivity to chondroitin sulfate
   b. Bleeding disorders
   c. Use caution because chondroitin is usually produced from bovine cartilage (possible transmission of mad cow disease).
   d. Pregnancy and lactation
   e. Use caution in asthma; may exacerbate asthma
5. **Drug interactions**
   a. May interact with heparin
   b. Theoretically, may interact with warfarin (Coumadin)
6. **Side effects.** Nausea, epigastric pain, and headache
7. **Dosage.** Recommended: 400 mg three times daily. Studies have shown that only 8% to 18% of oral chondroitin is absorbed.

B. **Coenzyme Q10 (ubiquinone or ubidecarenone)**
1. **Nonapproved indications.** Heart failure (HF), hypertension, stable angina, ventricular arrhythmias, cancer, heart surgery, and periodontal disease
2. **Mechanism of action**
   a. It is a naturally occurring coenzyme that has a predominant role in oxidative phosphorylation and synthesis of adenosine triphosphate (ATP), which is needed for muscle contraction and relaxation.

b. Coenzyme Q10 is an antioxidant, a membrane stabilizer, and a cofactor in many metabolic pathways.
c. It has been shown to reduce myocardial injury from ischemia and to reduce toxic myocardial damage from anthracyclines, such as doxorubicin (Adriamycin).

3. **Efficacy**
a. **Heart failure.** One randomized, double-blind, placebo-controlled, multicenter study included 641 patients with New York Heart Association class III or IV chronic congestive heart failure who were receiving conventional treatment, such as digoxin (Lanoxin), diuretics, angiotensin-converting enzyme (ACE) inhibitors, and calcium-channel blockers.[24] Patients received coenzyme Q10 2 mg/kg/day for 1 year or placebo. The number of patients requiring hospitalization secondary to congestive HF was less in the coenzyme Q10 group ($n = 73$) versus placebo ($n = 118$); significance: $p < .001$. Episodes of pulmonary edema and cardiac asthma were reduced with coenzyme Q10 ($p < .001$).
b. **Statin-induced myalgias.** Studies suggest that there is a 20% to 50% reduction in serum levels of coenzyme Q10 in hypercholesterolemic patients after a statin has been initiated. The reduction in coenzyme Q10 concentration is believed to be dose-related.[25] Several studies have evaluated the effect of coenzyme Q10 supplementation in patients taking statins. When coenzyme Q10 is given 30 to 300 mg/day, coenzyme Q10 serum concentrations significantly elevate.[25] However, a systematic review of studies showed **that exogenous coenzyme Q10 did not improve statin-induced myalgias.**[26]

4. **Contraindications/precautions**
a. Hyper and hypotension
b. Pregnancy and lactation

5. **Drug interactions**
a. HMG reductase inhibitors may lower plasma concentrations of coenzyme Q10.
b. Doxorubicin toxicity may be decreased.
c. Antihypertensives (additive effect)
d. Warfarin. Coenzyme Q10 is structurally related to vitamin K_2 so may have coagulant effects.

6. **Side effects**
a. Rash and gastrointestinal disturbances, such as nausea, anorexia, epigastric pain, and diarrhea
b. Elevations of serum aminotransferases have occurred with relatively high oral doses

7. **Dosage.** Depends on indication: 100 mg daily, up to 3000 mg daily in two to three divided doses.

C. **Glucosamine hydrochloride**

1. **Nonapproved indication.** Osteoarthritis

2. **Mechanism of action**
a. Glucosamine is usually made from shellfish and enhances cartilage proteoglycan synthesis.
b. It inhibits the deterioration of cartilage secondary to osteoarthritis.
c. It maintains an equilibrium between cartilage catabolic and anabolic processes.
d. It may have an anti-inflammatory action unlike cyclooxygenase.

3. **Efficacy.** A multicenter, double-blind, randomized study included 1583 patients with symptomatic knee osteoarthritis who received glucosamine 1500 mg daily, chondroitin 1200 mg daily, both glucosamine and chondroitin, celecoxib 200 mg daily, or placebo for 24 weeks. Glucosamine and chondroitin sulfate alone or in combination did not significantly reduce pain. The combination may be helpful in a subgroup of patients with moderate-to-severe knee pain.[23]

4. **Contraindications/precautions**
a. Hypersensitivity to glucosamine or shellfish
b. Diabetes. Glucosamine may impair insulin secretion.
c. Pregnancy and lactation
d. Asthma may be exacerbated.

5. **Drug interactions**
   a. Glucosamine may interact with antidiabetic agents.
   b. Glucosamine may induce resistance to antimitotic chemotherapy (etoposide [VePesid], doxorubicin).
   c. Theoretically, glucosamine may interact with warfarin.
6. **Side effects**
   a. Gastrointestinal side effects such as epigastric pain and tenderness, heartburn, diarrhea, and nausea
   b. CNS side effects such as drowsiness, headache, and insomnia
   c. Long-term side effects are unknown.
   d. Elevated blood glucose
7. **Dosage**. Recommended: 500 mg three times daily

D. **Melatonin**
1. **Orphan drug status.** Treatment of circadian rhythm sleep disorders in blind people who have no light perception
2. **Nonapproved indications.** Jet lag, insomnia, depression, and cancer
3. **Mechanism of action**
   a. It is a hormone made from serotonin and secreted by the pineal gland. Melatonin controls the periods of sleepiness and wakefulness. It increases GABA receptor binding.
4. **Efficacy**
   a. **Jet lag.** A randomized, placebo-controlled trial evaluated the effect of melatonin in 52 aircraft personnel. Melatonin was given either 5 mg daily 3 days before departure until 5 days after arrival (early group) or 5 mg daily upon arrival and for 3 additional days (late group). The late group had significantly less jet lag, fewer overall sleep disturbances, and a faster recovery of energy compared to the placebo group and the early group.[27]
   b. **Insomnia.** A meta-analysis on 17 randomized, double-blind, placebo-controlled trials that evaluated the sleep effect of melatonin in subjects showed that melatonin significantly decreased time to sleep onset, increased sleep efficiency, and increased total sleep duration compared to placebo.[28] Unfortunately, melatonin preparations were varied and study designs differed.
   c. **Children.** Melatonin may be effective in decreasing the time to sleep onset in children with neurodevelopmental disabilities. Melatonin does not improve total sleep time or nighttime awakenings.[29]
5. **Contraindications/precautions**
   a. Avoid in pregnancy and lactation
   b. Melatonin may aggravate depressive symptoms.
   c. Melatonin may increase the incidence of seizures.
   d. Diabetes (hyperglycemia)
   e. Hypertension (exacerbated)
   f. Caution while driving or performing other tasks requiring alertness and coordination
6. **Drug interactions**
   a. Selective serotonin reuptake inhibitors may increase melatonin serum concentrations.
   b. Other sedatives such as alcohol and benzodiazepines may exacerbate the sedative effects of melatonin.
   c. Melatonin may interfere with immunosuppressants.
   d. Antidiabetic agents may be less effective.
   e. Anticoagulants and antiplatelets (increased effect)
   f. Caffeine (theoretically, efficacy of melatonin may be decreased)
   g. Contraceptives (theoretically, efficacy of melatonin may be increased)
   h. Verapamil (increased melatonin excretion)
7. **Side effects**
   a. Side effects include drowsiness, daytime fatigue, headache, and transient depression.
   b. Long-term side effects are unknown.
8. **Dosage.** 0.3 to 5.0 mg at bedtime

IV. REFERENCES

1. Mahady GB. Black cohosh (Actaea/Cimicifuga racemosa): review of the clinical data for safety and efficacy in menopausal symptoms. *Treat Endocrinol.* 2005;4(3):177–184.
2. Jacobson JS, Troxel AB, Evans J, et al. Randomized trial of black cohosh for the treatment of hot flashes among women with a history of breast cancer. *J Clin Oncol.* 2001;19(10):2739–2745.
3. Patel NM, Derkits RM. Possible increase in liver enzymes secondary to atorvastatin and black cohosh administration. *J Pharm Prac.* 2007;20(4):341–346.
4. Schellenberg R. Treatment for the premenstrual syndrome with agnus castus fruit extract: prospective, randomised, placebo controlled study. *BMJ.* 2001;322(7279):134–137.
5. Avorn J, Monane M, Gurwitz JH, et al. Reduction of bacteriuria and pyuria after ingestion of cranberry juice. *JAMA.* 1994;271(10):751–754.
6. Murray M, Pizzorno J. *Encyclopedia of Natural Medicine.* 2nd ed. Roseville, CA: Prima Publishing; 1998.
7. Hirata JD, Swiersz LM, Zell B, et al. Does dong quai have estrogenic effects in postmenopausal women? A double-blind, placebo-controlled trial. *Fertil Steril.* 1997;68(6):981–986.
8. Melchart D, Linde K, Worku F, et al. Immunomodulation with echinacea: a systematic review of controlled clinical trials. *Phytomedicine.* 1994;1:245–254.
9. Gallo M, Sarkar M, Au W, et al. Pregnancy outcome following gestational exposure to echinacea: a prospective controlled study. *Arch Intern Med.* 2000;160(20):3141–3143.
10. Pittler MH, Ernst E. Feverfew for preventing migraine. *Cochrane Database Syst Rev.* 2004;(1): CD002286.
11. Silagy CA, Neil HA. A meta-analysis of the effect of garlic on blood pressure. J Hypertension. 1994;12(4):463–468.
12. Warshafsky S, Kamer RS, Sivak SL. Effect of garlic on total serum cholesterol. A meta-analysis. *Ann Intern Med.* 1993;119(7 pt 1):599–605.
13. Mowrey DB, Clayson DE. Motion sickness, ginger, and psychophysics. *Lancet.* 1982;1(8273): 655–657.
14. Kleijnen J, Knipschild P. Ginkgo biloba. Lancet. 1992;340:1136–1139.
15. Le Bars PL, Katz MM, Berman N, et al. A placebo-controlled, double-blind, randomized trial of an extract of Ginkgo biloba for dementia. JAMA. 1997;278(16):1327–1332.
16. Pieralisi G, Ripari P, Vecchiet L. Effects of a standardized ginseng extract combined with dimethylaminoethanol bitartrate, vitamins, minerals, and trace elements on physical performance during exercise. *Clin Ther.* 1991;13(3):373–382.
17. Rambaldi A, Jacobs BP, Iaquinto G, et al. Milk thistle for alcoholic and/or hepatitis B or C virus liver diseases. *Cochrane Database Syst Rev.* 2005;(2):CD003620.
18. Tacklind J, MacDonald R, Rutks I, et al. Serenoa repens for benign prostatic hyperplasia. *Cochrane Database Syst Rev.* 2009;(2):CD001423. doi:10.1002/14651858.CD001423.pub2
19. Linde K, Mulrow CD, Berner M, et al. St. John's wort for depression. *Cochrane Database Syst Rev.* 2005;(2):CD000448.
20. Suzuki O, Katsumata Y, Oya M, et al. Inhibition of monoamine oxidase by hypericin. *Planta Med.* 1984;50(3):272–274.
21. Müller WE, Rolli M, Schäfer C, et al. Effects of hypericum extract (LI 160) in biochemical models of antidepressant activity. *Pharmacopsychiatry.* 1997;30(suppl 2):102–107.
22. Leathwood PD, Chauffard F. Aqueous extract of valerian reduces latency to fall asleep in man. *Planta Med.* 1985;(2):144–148.
23. Clegg DO, Reda DJ, Harris CL, et al. Glucosamine, chondroitin sulfate, and the two in combination for painful knee osteoarthritis. *N Engl J Med.* 2006;354(8):795–808.
24. Morisco C, Trimarco B, Condorelli M. Effect of coenzyme Q10 therapy in patients with congestive heart failure: a long-term multicenter randomized study. *Clin Investig.* 1993;71(8 suppl):S134–S136.
25. Nawarskas JJ. HMG-CoA reductase inhibitors and coenzyme Q10. *Cardiol Rev.* 2005;13(2): 76–79.
26. Marcoff L, Thompson PD. The role of coenzyme Q10 in statin-associated myopathy: a systematic review. *J Am Coll Cardiol.* 2007;49(23):2231–2237.

27. Petrie K, Dawson AG, Thompson L, et al. A double-blind trial of melatonin as a treatment for jet lag in international cabin crew. *Biol Psychiatry*. 1993;33(7):526–530.
28. Brzezinski A, Vangel MG, Wurtman RJ, et al. Effects of exogenous melatonin on sleep: a meta-analysis. *Sleep Med Rev*. 2005;9(1):41–50.
29. Phillips L, Appleton RE. Systematic review of melatonin treatment in children with neurodevelopmental disabilities and sleep impairment. *Dev Med Child Neurol*. 2004;46(11):771–775.

Study Questions

Directions for questions: Each of the questions, statements, or incomplete statements can be correctly answered or completed by **one** of the suggested answers or phrases. Choose the **best** answer.

1. Which of the following herbs is known to cause cancer?

(A) Chaparral
(B) Comfrey
(C) Ma huang
(D) Licorice
(E) St. John's wort

2. Which of the following is a correct statement?

(A) Dietary supplements must be proven safe and effective before marketing in the United States.
(B) The following statement is optional for labeling of herbal products: "This product has not been evaluated by the FDA. It is not intended to diagnose, treat, cure, or prevent."
(C) Herbs must be standardized to be considered dietary supplements.
(D) Dietary supplement manufacturers may claim that their products affect the structure and function of the human body.
(E) Congress determines what is considered a supplement and what is considered a drug.

3. Tom would like to try echinacea to prevent cold and flu during the winter months. Which of the following statements is true about echinacea?

(A) It is contraindicated in patients allergic to parsley.
(B) It should be taken continuously only for 3 months.
(C) It is contraindicated in patients with lupus and leukosis.
(D) Prolonged use of echinacea will up regulate the immune system.
(E) Side effects include headache, rash, and dizziness.

4. Mary has a family history of heart disease and wonders if garlic would be beneficial to her. Which of the following statements is correct about garlic?

(A) Enteric-coated tablets release their contents in the stomach.
(B) Side effects include heartburn, flatulence, and sweating.
(C) The safety of garlic in pregnancy is unknown.
(D) Garlic does not interact with warfarin.

5. An 80-year-old man takes warfarin for his mechanical heart valve. He would also like to take the following herbs: Asian ginseng, feverfew, garlic, and dong quai. Which of these herbs may decrease the effectiveness of warfarin?

(A) Asian ginseng
(B) Feverfew
(C) Fish oil
(D) Garlic
(E) Dong quai

6. A 30-year-old female is 10 weeks pregnant with her second child. During her first pregnancy, she became depressed and was started on Prozac 20 mg every day. She is already beginning to notice early symptoms of depression during her second pregnancy. She would like to try St. John's wort for her depression. Which of the following statements is correct regarding St. John's wort?

(A) The safety of St. John's wort in pregnancy is unknown.
(B) St. John's wort is not helpful in treating mild depression.
(C) St. John's wort may interact with serotonin reuptake inhibitors.
(D) St. John's wort may interact with dairy products like milk and eggs.
(E) St. John's wort decreases the effects of clopidogrel (Plavix).

7. A 65-year-old is interested in taking ginkgo. Which of the following statements is correct regarding ginkgo?
   (A) There are no contraindications with ginkgo.
   (B) There is a drug–herb interaction between ginkgo and aspirin.
   (C) Toxic effects include hypertension and cardiac arrest.
   (D) There is a drug–herb interaction between ginkgo and phenelzine.
   (E) Ginkgo is contraindicated in patients with gallstone pain.

8. A 20-year-old athletic man would like to take Asian ginseng to increase his physical stamina. His girlfriend suggested that he ask a pharmacist about the safety of Asian ginseng. Which of the following statements is not correct?
   (A) Asian ginseng may interact with phenelzine, warfarin, and digoxin.
   (B) Asian ginseng should be used with caution in patients with a history of breast cancer.
   (C) Asian ginseng may interact with stimulants, including caffeine (Cafcit).
   (D) Asian ginseng should be avoided in patients with hypertension.
   (E) Asian ginseng may cause bradycardia due to increasing the QT interval.

Answers and Explanations

1. **The answer is B** *[see I.B.f]*.
   Comfrey may be carcinogenic. Chaparral may be hepatotoxic. High doses of licorice for long periods may cause pseudoaldosteronism. Ma huang may cause myocardial infarction, strokes, or seizures. St. John's wort has many drug interactions.

2. **The answer is D** *[see I.A.3.a–f]*.
   The Dietary Supplement Health and Education Act of 1994 states that dietary supplements are not considered drugs or food. Because dietary supplements are not regulated as drugs, their safety and efficacy are not mandated by the FDA. Dietary supplements are intended to supplement the diet, do not have to be standardized, may make claims regarding only the effects on structure or function of the body. The following is the correct required labeling statement: "This product has not been evaluated by the FDA. It is not intended to diagnose, treat, cure, or prevent."

3. **The answer is C** *[see II.E.1–6]*.
   Echinacea is contraindicated in infectious and autoimmune diseases such as tuberculosis, leukosis, collagenosis, multiple sclerosis, AIDS, HIV, and lupus. Caution should be used in patients who are allergic to members of the ragweed family. Therapy should not exceed 8 weeks. Theoretically, prolonged use of echinacea may depress the immune system, possibly through overstimulation. Side effects include nausea, vomiting, allergic reactions, anaphylaxis, and interference with male fertility.

4. **The answer is B** *[see II.I.1–8]*.
   Garlic should be avoided in pregnancy because it is an emmenagogue and abortifacient. It may interact with anticoagulants, increasing the risk of bleeding. Side effects include gastrointestinal discomfort (heartburn, flatulence), sweating, light-headedness, allergic reactions, and menorrhagia. Enteric-coated tablets or capsules allow more absorption because they pass through the stomach and release their contents in the alkaline medium of the small intestine.

5. **The answer is A** *[see II.L.5.b]*.
   Asian ginseng may decrease the INR of warfarin. Feverfew, fish oil, garlic, and dong quai may increase the INR of warfarin.

6. **The answer is C** *[see II.O.2–8]*.
   St. John's wort is indicated by Commission E for depression and anxiety. St. John's wort should be avoided in pregnancy because it is an emmenagogue and abortifacient. St. John's wort interacts with many medications, including serotonin reuptake inhibitors. It may interact with clopidogrel by increasing its antiplatelet effects. Food interactions may be similar to those of the MAOIs (tyramine-containing foods: cheese, beer, wine, herring, and yeast).

7. **The answer is B** *[see II.K.1–6]*.
   Contraindications and precautions for ginkgo include diabetes, epilepsy, bleeding disorders, and infertility. Ginkgo may potentiate the bleeding properties of antiplatelets. Side effects include gastric disturbances, headache, dizziness, and vertigo. Toxic ingestion may produce tonic–clonic seizures and loss of consciousness.

8. **The answer is E** *[see II.L.6.e]*.
   Asian ginseng is capable of causing tachyarrhythmias due to QT interval prolongation. Asian ginseng's contraindications include patients with hypertension. Asian ginseng may interact with phenelzine, producing hallucinations and psychosis; may decrease the INR of warfarin; and may interfere with immunosuppressants. Siberian ginseng's contraindications/precautions include hypertension. It may interact with anticoagulants and antihypertensives and may inhibit cytochrome P450 isoenzymes.

26

Clinical Pharmacokinetics and Therapeutic Drug Monitoring

GERALD E. SCHUMACHER

I. INTRODUCTION

A. **Objectives**

1. **Therapeutic drug monitoring** (TDM) in a general sense is about using serum drug concentrations (SDCs), pharmacokinetics, and pharmacodynamics to individualize and optimize patient responses to drug therapy.
2. **TDM** aims to promote optimum drug treatment by maintaining SDC within a **therapeutic range**—above, when drug-induced toxicity occurs too often; and below, when the drug is too often ineffective.

B. **Definitions**

1. Specifically, **TDM** is a practice applied to a small group of drugs in which there is a direct relation between SDCs and pharmacological response as well as a narrow range of concentrations that are effective and safe and for which SDCs are used in conjunction with other measures of clinical observation to assess patient status.
2. **Clinical pharmacokinetics**, a term often used interchangeably with TDM, is more generally the application of pharmacokinetic principles for the rational design of an individualized dosage regimen.
3. For definitions of the terms used and the concepts applicable in basic and clinical pharmacokinetics, see Chapter 5 on pharmacokinetics.

C. **Rationale and reasons**

1. **The rationale** for TDM makes three assumptions.
   a. Measuring patient SDC provides an opportunity to adjust for variations in patient pharmacokinetics by individualizing drug dosage.
   b. The SDC is a better predictor of patient response than dose.
   c. There is a good relation between SDCs and pharmacological response.
2. **Reasons for measuring SDC**
   a. Drug levels are used in conjunction with other clinical data to assist practitioners in determining how a patient is responding.
   b. Drug levels provide a basis for **individualizing** patient dosage regimens.
   c. Drug levels assist in determining if a change in **patient-specific** pharmacokinetics has occurred during a course of treatment, whether as a result of a change in physiological state, a change in diet, or addition of other drugs.
   d. Assuring **drug compliance** is often cited as a reason for measuring SDC, but it is unreliable for this purpose. In truth, a noncompliant patient may outwit practitioners by manipulating preappointment behavior to induce an SDC that is nonreflective of the patient's drug-taking behavior.

II. APPLYING CLINICAL PHARMACOKINETICS IN TDM

A. What the practitioner controls and does not control in TDM

1. *Figure 26-1* shows the relation between dose rate of drug administered, pharmacokinetic variables, SDC, and pharmacological response.
2. Note that the only variables that the practitioner controls are the amount of drug administered and how often it is given. These variables may be manipulated to compensate for the patient's pharmacokinetic and pharmacodynamic variables (i.e., bioavailability, clearance, steady-state SDC, pharmacological response), which the practitioner does not control, to achieve some designated SDC that yields a pharmacological response usually observed within the drug's commonly accepted therapeutic SDC range.

B. The concept of therapeutic range

1. For many drugs, a specific serum concentration range can be designated for each drug that maximizes effectiveness and minimizes toxicity. The range of SDC is called the **therapeutic range** for the drug.
2. The notion of a therapeutic range is more a **probabilistic concept** than an absolute entity. It is probable that most patients will show effective and safe responses within the therapeutic range. However, a minority of patients will need SDC above or below the upper or lower limits, respectively, of the therapeutic range to achieve an effective response. Similarly, a minority of patients will not show toxicity at SDCs modestly above the therapeutic range, whereas others will show toxicity below the therapeutic range.
3. Therefore, TDM is about **individualizing** patient dosage regimens to achieve SDC within patient-specific therapeutic ranges for a drug. More often than not, a patient-specific range will fall within the generally stated therapeutic range.

C. The concept of population pharmacokinetic values

1. **A population pharmacokinetic value or parameter** refers to the mean (average) value noted for a given cohort of people (e.g., adults 20 to 60 years of age, patients with a defined range of renal impairment). Usually, this population value is normalized on a weight basis (e.g., amikacin volume of distribution in normal adults of 0.25 L/kg). When a population parameter is stated without defining the target population, it usually refers to adults; further, when the value also is not normalized (e.g., volume of distribution of amikacin of 15 to 20 L), it usually refers to adults of average weight (approximately 60 to 80 kg).
2. Hardly anyone is average. Individual values of the population studied are summed to determine a mean value that is then reported as the **population value**. Individualizing patient dosage regimens takes this into account by adjusting observed patient-specific values and responses to expected population measures.
3. So the practitioner starts the determination of a patient-specific dosage regimen by assuming that the patient behaves like the average member of his or her population with respect to pharmacokinetics, serum level, and expected response and uses population pharmacokinetic parameters to calculate the dosage regimen needed to meet the desired SDC objective.
4. If the patient is responding appropriately after administering the dosage regimen until steady state is reached based on using population values, then no adjustment in regimen is necessary.
5. If, however, the starting assumption of using average values turns out to be incorrect because the patient's response is either subtherapeutic or toxic due to patient-specific pharmacokinetic and/or pharmacodynamic values that are atypical for the population, the practitioner's only option (except for changing the drug) is to manipulate the practitioner-controlled input variables, **dose and frequency**, to bring the pharmacological response within the desired range.

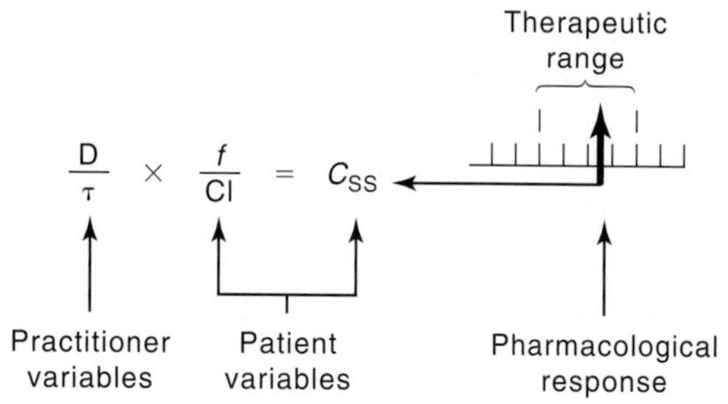

Figure 26-1. Pharmacokinetic factors influencing serum drug concentration and pharmacological response. *f*, bioavailability; *Cl*, clearance; C_{ss}, steady-state serum drug concentration; *D*, dose; *τ*, frequency of administration of dose.

D. Timing of SDC measurements

1. SDCs are sometimes measured **early in a course of therapy**, before steady state is reached, to determine patient-specific pharmacokinetic parameters, rather than relying on population values.
2. More commonly, SDCs are measured **during a steady-state dosage interval** (τ_{ss}) because the objective is to determine if the SDC is within a desired therapeutic range—a range that has previously been determined almost invariably during τ_{ss}.
3. Because SDCs are most commonly measured at steady state and referenced to values obtained at steady state, it is necessary to wait after starting drug administration until at least three to four assumed half-life ($t_{½}$) values (88% to 94% of reaching full steady state) so that SDC will be measured during a period when steady state may be assumed, for clinical purposes, to have been reached or approximated (e.g., approximately 90% of steady state or greater; so for an assumed $t_{½}$ of 6 hrs, wait 18 to 24 hrs after initiating drug treatment to measure SDC).
4. If there are no changes in patient response, there is usually **no need to take subsequent daily SDC measurements**, once an appropriate SDC has been achieved. Only if something occurs that may be expected to alter the patient's pharmacokinetic values (e.g., coadministration of another potentially modifying drug, change in physiological state) are frequent measurements necessary.
5. If a steady-state SDC (**C_{ss}**) is used appropriately to relate a patient's C_{ss} to a population or patient-specific therapeutic range, then it is important to note when during the steady-state dosage interval (τ_{ss}) the C_{ss} was measured in studies determining the therapeutic range. In other words, is the therapeutic range the practitioner is using as a basis for individualizing regimens based on C_{ss} measured **early** (apparent **$C_{max,ss}$**), near the **midpoint** (apparent **$C_{avg,ss}$**), or near the end (apparent **$C_{min,ss}$**) of τ_{ss}?
6. **Errors** in interpretation occur when C_{ss} for a patient is measured at a time during τ_{ss} that is markedly different than the time used for establishing the therapeutic range (e.g., measuring C_{ss} in a patient 1 hr after giving a dose on an every 12-hrs regimen when the C_{ss} for the referenced therapeutic range was actually taken at the end of τ_{ss} [**$C_{min,ss}$**]).
7. Errors in timing of C_{ss} are of greater concern for drugs with a short $t_{½}$ than for drugs with a long $t_{½}$. C_{ss} fluctuation during τ_{ss} is much greater in the former than the latter case.

III. TDM DRUGS AND COMMON CHARACTERISTICS

A. TDM drugs

1. Drugs for which TDM is commonly used are noted in *Table 26-1*, along with the population therapeutic range.
2. Drugs for which TDM is infrequently used in general situations but perhaps more commonly used by specialty practitioners or clinics are noted in *Table 26-2*.

B. Common characteristics of TDM drugs. Drugs that qualify for TDM have, as a minimum, the following characteristics in common:

1. SDC is the most practical intermediate end point to be used when there is no clearly observable therapeutic or toxic end point.
2. SDC is a reasonable proxy for drug concentration at the site of action.

Table 26-1 DRUGS OFTEN MONITORED USING SERUM DRUG CONCENTRATIONS

Drug	Therapeutic Range for C_{ss}
Amikacin	$C_{max,ss}{}^{a} = 20–30\ \mu g/mL$; $C_{min,ss} < 10\ \mu g/mL$
Cyclosporine	Varies with transplanted organ, time after transplant, time of sampling during dosage interval, and method of analysis
Digoxin	$0.8–2.0^{b}$ ng/mL
Gentamicin	$C_{max,ss}{}^{a} = 5–10\ \mu g/mL$; $C_{min,ss} < 2\ \mu g/mL$
Phenytoin	10–20 μg/mL
Tobramycin	$C_{max,ss}{}^{a} = 5–50\ \mu g/mL$; $C_{min,ss} = 2\ \mu g/mL$
Vancomycin	$C_{max,ss}{}^{a} = 30–50\ \mu g/mL$; $C_{min,ss} = 5–10\ \mu g/mL$

[a]End of 30- to 60-min infusion.
[b]Levels for atrial fibrillation often exceed 2 ng/mL.

Table 26-2 DRUGS MONITORED USING SERUM DRUG CONCENTRATIONS IN SPECIALTY SITUATIONS

Carbamazepine
Indinavin
Lithium
Methotrexate
Mycophenolate
Serolimus
Tacrolimus

3. The range of therapeutic and safe serum concentrations is narrow.
4. There is no predictable dose–response relation.
5. The pharmacological effect observed persists for a relatively long time. Acute, short, or intermittent effects are not well regulated by using serum drug levels.
6. A drug assay is available that is accurate, precise, specific, rapid, and relatively inexpensive.

IV. EQUATIONS FREQUENTLY USED IN TDM

A. **Linear pharmacokinetic drug clearance—normal renal function.** Linear clearance assumes that a **proportional** change in dose leads to the same **proportional** change in SDC. It also assumes that $t_{½}$ and drug clearance remain **constant** as the dose changes. See IV.D for an example of using some of the following equations.

1. **Estimating drug clearance (Cl)**

$$\text{Cl} = \frac{V}{1.4t_{½}} \quad (1)$$

where V is the apparent volume of distribution of drug.

2. **Maximum concentration ($C_{\text{max,ss}}$)** during τ_{ss}, when absorption is assumed to be much faster than elimination.

$$C_{\text{max,ss}} = \frac{(S)(f)(\text{dose}/V)}{1 - 10^{-0.3(\tau/t_{½})}} \quad (2)$$

where S is the fraction of the dosage form that is the active moiety and f is the bioavailability.

3. **Minimum concentration ($C_{\text{min,ss}}$)** during τ_{ss}, when absorption is assumed to be much faster than elimination.

$$C_{\text{min,ss}} = (C_{\text{max,ss}})\,[10^{-0.3(\tau/t_{½})}] \quad (3)$$

4. **Average concentration resulting from intermittent administration ($C_{\text{avg,ss}}$)** during τ_{ss}

$$C_{\text{avg,ss}} = \frac{(S)(f)(\text{dose}/\tau)}{\text{Cl}} \quad (4)$$

where dose/τ is the amount of drug administered during each selected unit of time (e.g., hours, minutes).

5. **Steady-state concentration resulting from continuous administration ($C_{\text{inf,ss}}$).** For the same dose rate (dose/τ), ($C_{\text{avg,ss}}$) for intermittent administration **is the same as** ($C_{\text{inf,ss}}$) for continuous administration.

$$C_{\text{inf,ss}} = \frac{(S)(f)(\text{dose}/t_{\text{inf}})}{\text{Cl}} \quad (5)$$

B. **Linear pharmacokinetic drug clearance—impaired renal function**

1. **Estimating creatinine clearance from serum creatinine** when serum creatinine is assumed to be stable, not changing daily, and weight is expressed by the patient's total weight, unless total weight is equal to or more than 20% of ideal (lean) body weight, in which case ideal weight should be used in the calculation.

$$Cl_{\text{cr}}\ (\text{mL/min, males}) = \frac{(140 - \text{age})(\text{weight})}{(Cr_s)(72)} \quad (6)$$

where Cr_s denotes serum creatinine in mg/dL and weight expressed in kg. The female value is 85% of the estimated male value in (6).

2. **Estimating prolonged drug $t_{1/2}$ or reduced drug Cl associated with reduced Cl_{cr}**

$$\frac{(\mathrm{Cl})_{ri}}{(\mathrm{Cl})_{n}} = \frac{(t_{1/2})_{n}}{(t_{1/2})_{ri}} = 1 - F + F[(Cl_{cr})_{ri}/(Cl_{cr})_{n}] \quad (7)$$

where *ri* and *n* denote the renal impaired and normal conditions, respectively; *F* is the fraction of drug administered that is eliminated unchanged (unmetabolized); and Cl_{cr} represents creatinine clearance in mL/min. Important *F* values for some common TDM drugs are: aminoglycosides = 0.98, digoxin = 0.8, and vancomycin = 0.95.

3. **Using $C_{avg,ss}$ as a target** so that $C_{avg,ss}$ in the renal-impaired patient is maintained the same as $C_{avg,ss}$ in normals.

$$\frac{(\mathrm{dose}/\tau)_{ri}}{(\mathrm{dose}/\tau)_{n}} = \frac{\mathrm{dose}_{ri} \times \tau_{n}}{\mathrm{dose}_{n} \times \tau_{ri}} = 1 - F + F\,[(Cl_{cr})_{ri}/(Cl_{cr})_{n}] \quad (8)$$

4. **Using $C_{max,ss}$ as a target** so that $C_{max,ss}$ in the renal impaired is maintained the same as $C_{max,ss}$ in normals.

$$\text{dose per } \tau_{ri} = (\mathrm{dose}_{L})\,[1 - 10^{-0.3(\tau_{ri}/t_{1/2ri})}] \quad (9)$$

where dose_L is a loading dose intended to achieve the same $C_{max,ss}$ in the renal impaired as in the normal patient.

C. **Nonlinear pharmacokinetic drug clearance—normal renal function. Nonlinear** clearance assumes that a proportional change in dose leads to a **disproportional** change in SDC. It also assumes that $t_{1/2}$ and Cl **change** as the dose changes and also as the amount of drug in the body from a given dose changes. Drugs exhibiting nonlinear clearance present a much greater challenge than linear clearance drugs because the assumptions in the latter case of proportional changes in dose yielding same proportional changes in C_{ss} and constant Cl and $t_{1/2}$ do not apply for nonlinear drugs. For nonlinear drugs, increases in dose lead to increases in $t_{1/2}$, decreases in Cl, and changes in C_{ss} that are excessive compared to the proportionate change in dose.

1. **Estimating drug clearance**

$$Cl = \frac{V_{max}}{K_m + C_{avg,ss}} \quad (10)$$

where V_{max} is the maximum amount of drug that can be eliminated per unit of time (e.g., day) and K_m is the drug serum concentration at which the rate of elimination is 50% of V_{max}.

2. **Estimating $C_{avg,ss}$ resulting from a given dose/τ**

$$C_{avg,ss} = \frac{(K_m)(S)(f)(\mathrm{dose}/\tau)}{V_{max} - (S)(f)(\mathrm{dose}/\tau)} \quad (11)$$

3. **Estimating dose/τ needed for a desired $C_{avg,ss}$**

$$\mathrm{dose}/\tau = \frac{(V_{max})(C_{avg,ss})}{(K_m + C_{avg,ss})(S)(f)} \quad (12)$$

D. **An example of applying some of the previous equations to developing and modifying dosage regimens**

1. A common dosage regimen for intravenous (IV) gentamicin is 1.7 mg/kg every 8 hrs (as a 30-min infusion). Regimens are usually adjusted to achieve $C_{max,ss}$ and $C_{min,ss}$ within 5 to 10 mcg/mL and less than 2 mcg/mL, respectively. Does the preceding regimen meet the target concentration objectives in normal patients? Assume the following population parameters in normals: $Cl = 0.09$ L/kg/hr, $t_{1/2} = 2.5$ hrs, $V = 0.25$ L/kg. For IV administration, $f = 1$, and $S = 1$ for the dosage form (label amount represents the actual amount of gentamicin).

2. **In normals**, using equations (2) and (3).

$$C_{max,ss} = \frac{(1)(1)(1.7\text{ mg/kg})/(0.25\text{ L/kg})}{1 - 10^{-0.3\,(8\text{ hr}/2.5\text{ hr})}} = 7.6\text{ mcg/mL}$$

$$C_{min,ss} = 7.6\text{ mcg/mL} \times 10^{-0.3\,(8\text{ hr}/2.5\text{ hr})} = 0.8\text{ mcg/mL}$$

These values fall within the target concentration ranges for the average patient with normal renal function.

3. **In the renal impaired,** what should be done to modify the preceding regimen for a patient who is 60 years old, 70 kg, male, with a Cr_s of 2.5 mg/dL? In this patient, if the preceding regimen were used, the prolonged $t_{½}$ would yield $C_{max,ss}$ = 15.2 mcg/mL and $C_{min,ss}$ = 8.4 mcg/mL, values clearly above the target concentration ranges.
   a. Using equation (6) for estimating Cl_{cr} in this patient.

$$Cl_{cr} = \frac{(140 - 60 \text{ yrs})(70 \text{ kg})}{(2.5 \text{ mg/dL})(72)} = 31 \text{ mL/min}$$

   b. Then using equation (7) for estimating $t_{½}$ in this patient, assuming F = 0.98 and $(Cl_{cr})_n$ = 120 mL/min.

$$\frac{(2.5 \text{ hrs})}{(t_{½})_{ri}} = 1 - 0.98 + 0.98\,(31/120) = 0.27(t_{½})_{ri} = 9.3 \text{ hrs}$$

   c. Then, using equation (9), first determine a loading dose (D_L) to achieve the same $C_{max,ss}$ of approximately 8 mcg/mL as estimated in IV.D.2 for a patient with normal renal function:

$$D_L = (C_{max,ss})(V)/(S)(f)$$

$$D_L = (8 \text{ mcg/mL})(0.25 \text{ L/kg})/(1)(1) = 2 \text{ mg/kg}$$

   Next, determine fraction of drug lost during τ, assuming a τ_{ri} of 24 hrs, and using the $(t_{½})_{ri}$ of 9.3 hrs estimated in IV.D.3.b.

$$\text{Fraction lost} = 1 - 10^{-0.3(\tau/t_{½})} = 1 - 10^{-0.3(24/9.3)} = 0.84$$

   Lastly, calculate D per τ_{ri}:

$$\text{D per } \tau_{ri} = (D_L)[1 - 10^{-0.3(\tau/t_{½})}]$$

$$= (2 \text{ mg/kg})(0.84) = 1.7 \text{ mg/kg}$$

   Thus, a D_L of 2 mg/kg followed by 1.7 mg/kg every 24 hrs is expected to maintain levels in this patient similar to that in normals.

V. EFFECT OF PHYSIOLOGICAL ALTERATIONS ON PHARMACOKINETIC VARIABLES

A. General considerations. It is apparent from *Figure 26-1* and the equations in section IV that any changes in pharmacokinetic variables result in changes in C_{ss} and perhaps pharmacodynamic outcomes. This may necessitate changes in D/τ compared to normals. For renal impairment, **quantitative** estimates of resulting changes in Cl and $t_{½}$, compared to normal values, are available using the equations in section IV. For hepatic, cardiac, pulmonary, and other impairments potentially inducing changes in normal pharmacokinetic variables, only **qualitative** estimates are possible.

B. Renal impairment, when marked, reduces drug clearance for drugs primarily dependent on the kidney for elimination. As noted in the equations in section IV.B, physiological markers like serum creatinine and creatinine clearance are used to estimate the changes in Cl and $t_{½}$ resulting from reductions in Cr_s and Cl_{cr}.

C. Hepatic impairment exerts a complex influence on drug pharmacokinetics. Two processes may be altered: blood flow rate in delivering drug to the liver and the capacity of enzymes to metabolize the drug. In general terms, moderate to severe hepatic impairment is expected to slow overall Cl and prolong $t_{½}$ for drugs highly dependent on the liver for elimination.

D. Cardiac impairment, when substantial, decreases hepatic and renal clearances, reduces volume of distribution, and may slow absorption for some drugs. The effect of compromised perfusion is most critical for drugs that are both highly dependent on the liver for clearance and efficiently metabolized by the liver in normal patients.

E. Aging results in reductions in renal (consistently) and hepatic (inconsistently) clearances. The clearance of drugs primarily dependent on the kidney declines by nearly 50% and the half-life nearly doubles over a 40- to 50-year period from young adulthood. On the other hand, some drugs primarily dependent on the liver for clearance show no age-related changes, whereas others do. Changes with age in absorption, volume of distribution, and serum protein binding of drugs show no consistent pattern.

F. From a clinical viewpoint, serum **protein binding** of drugs becomes an important issue in TDM for drugs bound more than 80% to serum proteins. Because hepatic and renal clearances, volume of distribution, and pharmacological response are mediated by the free (unbound) form of the drug in serum, interpatient variations in protein binding not only result in variations in pharmacokinetics in normals, but loss of serum proteins during renal and hepatic impairments may also result in modified drug clearance and pharmacological response.

VI. USING TEST PERFORMANCE CHARACTERISTICS IN TDM

A. **Rationale and reasons**

1. In TDM, the SDC functions like a diagnostic test to assist in classifying patient status.
2. On the one hand, the patient's SDC may be used, in conjunction with a population SDC cutoff value measure for the drug, which acts as a separator, to classify the patient as a member of either drug-induced toxic (patient SDC > upper cutoff value) or therapeutic (within therapeutic range) subpopulations.
3. Alternately, the patient's SDC may classify the patient as part of the therapeutic or subtherapeutic (SDC < lower cutoff value) subpopulations.
4. Although classifying patients in subpopulations is the most common use of SDC in TDM, a more informed application of SDC is to use the result to modify the clinician's probability of patient status. This is the use of SDC as part of a Bayesian approach to diagnostic test interpretation.

B. **Test performance characteristics.** Test performance indices are not perfect classifiers of patient status and should never be used as the sole measure for determining how the patient is reacting to the drug. A number of test performance indices characterize the accuracy of a diagnostic test to accurately classify patients as toxic, therapeutic, or subtherapeutic. Four of these indices are most useful in interpreting SDC.

1. **Positive predictive value (PPV)**
   a. **Comparing drug-induced toxic versus nontoxic patients (using upper SDC cutoff level).** PPV denotes the proportion of patients with a **positive test** (patient SDC > upper cutoff SDC) who are in a drug-induced **toxic** condition. So, the value of PPV represents the probability of a positive test being accurate in classifying the patient as toxic.
   b. **Comparing therapeutic versus subtherapeutic patients (using lower SDC cutoff level).** PPV denotes the proportion of patients with a **positive test** (patient SDC > lower cutoff SDC) who are **responding appropriately**. So, the value of PPV in this case represents the probability of a positive test being accurate in classifying the patient as therapeutic.
2. **Negative predictive value (NPV)**
   a. **Comparing drug-induced toxic versus nontoxic patients (using upper SDC cutoff level).** NPV denotes the proportion of patients with a **negative test** (patient SDC < upper cutoff SDC) who are **not** manifesting drug-induced **toxicity**. So, the value of NPV represents the probability of a negative test being accurate in classifying the patient as nontoxic.
   b. **Comparing therapeutic versus subtherapeutic patients (using lower SDC cutoff level).** NPV denotes the proportion of patients with a **negative test** (patient SDC < lower cutoff SDC) who are **subtherapeutic**. So, the value of NPV in this case represents the probability of a negative test being accurate in classifying the patient as subtherapeutic.
3. **Positive likelihood ratio (PLR).** In defining conditions as + or − (as in + = toxic and − = negative or + = therapeutic and − = subtherapeutic), **PLR** is the probability that a + **patient** has a + **test** divided by the probability that a − **patient** has a + **test** (e.g., the probability that a **toxic** patient has an SDC > cutoff divided by the probability that a **nontoxic** patient has an SDC > cutoff). The **higher** the **PLR,** the **more** discriminating the test.
4. **Negative likelihood ratio (NLR).** NLR is the probability that a + **patient** has a − **test** divided by the probability that a − **patient** has a − **test**. The **lower** the **NLR**, the **more** discriminating the test.
5. **Illustrating the use of PPV, NPV, PLR, and NLR.** For digoxin, using a test upper cutoff of 2 ng/mL, PPV is 0.59, NPV is 0.95, PLR is 7, and NLR is 0.2.
   a. **For PPV**, this means that the proportion of patients with a positive test result (SDC > upper cutoff) who truly have digoxin-induced toxicity is 59%. For an individual patient with SDC > cutoff, the probability of toxicity is 0.59.

b. **For NPV**, this means that the proportion of patients with a negative test result (SDC < upper cutoff) who truly are nontoxic is 95%. For an individual patient with SDC < cutoff, the probability of nontoxicity is 0.95.
c. **For PLR**, digoxin-induced toxic patients will have a positive test result seven times more often than do nontoxic patients.
d. **For NLR**, digoxin-induced toxic patients will have a negative test result 20% as often as will nontoxic patients.
e. These results suggest that a negative digoxin test result rules out toxicity (0.95) about 1.6 times (0.95/0.59) as effectively as a positive test rules in digoxin-induced toxicity (0.59). A positive test appears to be unreliable as an indicator of digoxin-induced toxicity, but a negative test appears to be highly predictive of nontoxicity. Furthermore, the PLR suggests that a positive SDC test is six times more likely to come from a digoxin-induced toxic than a nontoxic patient. On the other hand, the NLR implies that it is one-fifth as likely (0.2) that a negative test comes from a digoxin-induced toxic compared to a nontoxic patient.
f. Knowledge of test performance characteristics of SDC measures provides the practitioner with an index of the usefulness of the SDC in categorizing patients.

C. **Using a Bayesian approach.** Using SDC in conjunction with likelihood ratio information enhances the application of the SDC in decision making. A Bayesian approach to probability revision allows the practitioner to make a pretest assessment of patient status, order a diagnostic test, and use the probability information contained in the test result to revise the assessment of status.

1. The relation between pretest, test, and posttest assessment is shown in the following equation:

$$\text{(pretest odds)(likelihood ratio)} = \text{(posttest odds)} \qquad \textbf{(13)}$$

where pretest refers to the pretest odds of the condition being present prior to obtaining the patient's SDC and posttest refers to the posttest odds of the condition being present after learning the SDC.

2. **Odds** are defined as + results divided by − results (+/−). **Probability** is defined as + results divided by total results (+/total, where total is the sum of + and − results).
3. Odds are converted to probability as follows:

$$\text{Probability} = \text{odds}/(1 + \text{odds}) \qquad \textbf{(14)}$$

4. Probability is converted to odds as follows:

$$\text{Odds} = \text{probability}/(1 - \text{probability}) \qquad \textbf{(15)}$$

5. An example of applying a Bayesian approach to modifying the probability of patient status. Using the digoxin test performance characteristics noted in VI.B.5:
   a. Assume that a practitioner assesses by visual inspection that the probability of digoxin-induced toxicity in a patient is 0.25 (the pretest probability). She orders a serum digoxin concentration (SDC), and uses the measurement to revise her assessment of digoxin-induced toxicity in the patient (the posttest probability).
   b. Further assume that the test performance characteristics for the SDC are: PLR = 7 and NLR = 0.2.
   c. Using equations (13), (14), and (15), a pretest probability of 0.25 is the same as pretest odds of toxicity of ⅓ [0.25/(1 − 0.25)], using equation (15).
   d. If the SDC test for the patient comes back positive (SDC > 2 ng/mL), then PLR = 7 is used to revise the odds of toxicity. If the SDC test is negative (SDC ≤ 2 ng/mL), then NLR = 0.2 is used.
   e. Assume the patient's **SDC** = 2.4 ng/mL, then using equation (13) yields (⅓)(7) = 2.3. So, the posttest odds of toxicity are 2.3/1. Converting these odds to probability using equation (14): [2.3/(1 + 2.3)] = 0.71. The **posttest probability of toxicity is 0.71**. The pretest probability of 0.25 has nearly tripled (0.71/0.25) using the SDC as feedback.
   f. **Assume instead that the patient's** SDC = **1.4 ng/mL**; then using equation (13) yields (⅓)(0.2) = 0.07. So, the posttest odds of toxicity are 0.07/1. Converting these odds to probability using equation (14): [0.07/(1 + 0.07)] = ~0.07. **The posttest probability of toxicity is 0.07**.
   g. Although a positive SDC test nearly tripled the probability of toxicity earlier, a negative test cuts the probability to less than ⅓ of its pretest value. This demonstrates the usefulness of using SDC in combination with practitioner assessment as a guide to quantifying the probability of patient status.

VII. SUMMARY

A. TDM applies to a small number of drugs with a narrow range of effective and safe SDC wherein optimum drug treatment is promoted by maintaining SDC within a population or patient-specific therapeutic range, above which drug-induced toxicity occurs too often and below which the drug is too often ineffective.

B. A practitioner initiates drug treatment using a dose rate that assumes that the patient shows mean population values for the pharmacokinetic variables, even though it is expected that few patients will ever possess the mean value being used. If the resulting C_{ss} and/or pharmacological response is other than expected and the patient becomes at risk for subtherapeutic or drug-induced toxicity, it is likely due to the interpatient variability in pharmacokinetic values and pharmacodynamic response that characterizes the need for TDM; therefore, the dose rate is modified to produce a patient-specific C_{ss} that represents the best tradeoff of effectiveness and toxicity.

C. Timing of sampling of SDC is critical to reduce errors in interpretation of the measurement. SDC should be sampled at steady state, after postabsorption and postdistribution equilibrium is achieved, and a time during τ_{ss} that matches the time at which the therapeutic range was established.

D. The choice of $C_{max,ss}$, $C_{min,ss}$, $C_{avg,ss}$, or $C_{inf,ss}$ to estimate dosage regimens depends on the therapeutic range objective and, in the latter case, intravenous rather than intermittent administration.

E. For the renal-impaired patient, the dosage reduction factor is calculated to achieve, depending on the therapeutic range objective, a $C_{max,ss}$ or $C_{avg,ss}$ in the renal-impaired patient that is similar to that desired if the patient had normal renal function.

F. The SDC measure is more than a number used to relate the patient's value to a population therapeutic range. The SDC is a form of diagnostic test used: (1) to assist in classifying patient status and (2) as feedback to revise practitioner estimates of patient status. Therefore, it is important to know the predictive values and likelihood ratios of SDC tests.

Study Questions

Directions: Each of the numbered items or incomplete statements in this section is followed by answers or by completions of the statement. Select the one lettered answer or completion that is **best** in each case.

1. Define therapeutic drug monitoring. What is meant by the term TDM?
   (A) The use of drug serum concentration measurements for drugs in which there is (1) a correlation between serum concentration and response and (2) a narrow range of effective and safe concentrations, to assess patient status as an adjunct to clinical observation
   (B) The use of drug serum concentration measurements to determine population values for a drug's half-life value
   (C) The use of drug serum concentration measurements to assess the accuracy of the drug concentration assay
   (D) Observing the effects of drugs in human
   (E) Using drug serum concentration measurements to differentiate effective from ineffective drugs

2. The therapeutic range for digoxin is often stated as 0.8 to 2.0 ng/mL. What does this mean?
   (A) Fifty percent of people taking digoxin show a safe and effective response when the serum drug concentration is between 0.8 and 2.0 ng/mL.
   (B) Most people achieve the desired response to digoxin with minimum adverse effects when the serum digoxin concentration is maintained between 0.8 and 2.0 ng/mL. Fewer patients are managed effectively at < 0.8 ng/mL, but some may respond quite appropriately at lower levels. The frequency of adverse effects increases as the level increases above the upper limit of the therapeutic range, but a few patients are managed effectively without adversity above the range.
   (C) Twenty-five percent of people show an effective response to digoxin at < 0.8 ng/mL, and 75% show an effective response at 2.0 ng/mL.
   (D) Twice daily administration of digoxin, but not three times daily, requires that serum drug concentrations stay within 0.8 to 2.0 ng/mL.
   (E) Digoxin serum drug concentrations outside of the 0.8 to 2.0 ng/mL range are ineffective and/or unsafe.

3. Assume that for digoxin, the therapeutic range is cited as $C_{avg,ss} = 0.8$ to 2.0 ng/mL. If the patient is assumed to have an estimated digoxin $t_{½}$ of 48 hrs, how long would you wait to take a serum digoxin concentration measurement, and when during τ would you schedule it?
   - **(A)** 28 days, then 3 to 4 hrs after the dose is administered
   - **(B)** 14 days, then 6 to 8 hrs after the dose is administered
   - **(C)** 7 days, then 10 to 14 hrs after the dose is administered
   - **(D)** 3 days, then 1 to 2 hrs after the dose is administered
   - **(E)** 1 day, then 18 to 22 hrs after the dose is administered

4. Differentiate linear from nonlinear drug clearance. What is the effect on TDM?
   - **(A)** Linear drug clearance is first order, the Cl and $t_{½}$ are independent of drug dosage, and proportional changes in dose result in the same proportional changes in C_{ss}. Nonlinear drug clearance is zero order, Cl and $t_{½}$ change as dose changes (or as the amount of drug in the body changes), and proportional changes in dose yield disproportionate changes in C_{ss}.
   - **(B)** Linear drug clearance presents fewer serum concentration peaks and troughs during the dosage interval than does nonlinear drug clearance.
   - **(C)** Linear drug clearance is zero order, the Cl and $t_{½}$ are dependent on drug dosage, and proportional changes in dose do not result in the same proportional changes in C_{ss}. Nonlinear drug clearance is first order, and equations are not available to predict drug serum concentration from the dose rate.
   - **(D)** Drugs with linear clearance have shorter $t_{½}$ values than drugs with nonlinear clearance.
   - **(E)** Drugs with linear clearance are administered less often than drugs with nonlinear clearance.

5. What is the positive predictive value of a diagnostic test?
   - **(A)** The fraction of patients with a positive outcome who have a positive test result.
   - **(B)** Being more than 50% correct in predicting success or failure upon using a drug regimen.
   - **(C)** The fraction of patients who achieve a successful response in using a drug.
   - **(D)** The fraction of patients with a positive test result who turn out to have a positive outcome.
   - **(E)** The probability that knowledge of a drug serum concentration results in a successful response to treatment.

6. A 70-year-old, 80-kg male with serum creatinine of 3 mg/dL is scheduled to start tobramycin therapy. What regimen is recommended to achieve $C_{max,ss}$ within 5 to 10 mcg/mL (use the midpoint of 7.5 mcg/mL for the calculation) and $C_{min,ss} < 2$ mcg/mL. Try an every 24-hr regimen to start and, if unsuccessful in achieving the target concentration goals, alter τ and recalculate. Assume in normals the following values: $t_{½} = 2.5$ hrs, $V = 0.25$ L/kg, $F = 0.98$, $S = 1$, $f = 1$, $Cl_{cr} = 120$ mL/min
   - **(A)** A loading dose of 1.8 to 2.0 mg/kg followed by 1.0 mg/kg every day
   - **(B)** A loading dose of 1.8 to 2.0 mg/kg followed by 1.5 mg/kg every day
   - **(C)** 2.0 mg/kg every day
   - **(D)** 1.0 mg/kg every day
   - **(E)** 0.5 mg/kg every day

Answers and Explanations

1. **The answer is A** *[see I.B.1]*.

2. **The answer is B** *[see II.B]*.

3. **The answer is C** *[see II.D.3]*.
If the patient's estimated $t_{½}$ is 48 hrs, 90% of steady state is expected to be achieved between 3 and 4 $t_{½}$ intervals or 6 to 8 days in this case. For clinical purposes, we choose 90% attainment of steady state as the minimum time to estimate drug accumulation. A level drawn at 7 days seems reasonable. Once a τ_{ss} has been selected, the time for scheduling a level should correspond with the reference time for the therapeutic range. In this case, $C_{avg,ss}$ was cited as the reference time, so a measurement scheduled for sometime near the midpoint of τ_{ss} (around 12 hrs) is reasonable.

4. **The answer is A** *[see IV.A–C]*.
This presents challenges in TDM because for linear drugs, the clinician can expect a change in C_{ss} proportional to a change in dose, but for nonlinear drugs, this is not true.

5. **The answer is D** *[see VII.B]*.
The positive predictive value of a diagnostic test is an index of how effective the test is in classifying patients correctly. For example, using a C_{ss} measure for a given drug, knowing that the positive predictive value is 0.8, given a group of patients with a C_{ss} above the test cutoff value, 80% of the patients will be accurately classified as having a positive outcome. If the test is being used to classify toxic versus nontoxic patients, 80% of the patients with C_{ss} above the test cutoff will experience drug-induced toxicity. If, instead, the test is being used to classify effective versus subeffective response in patients, 80% of the patients with C_{ss} above the test cutoff will experience effective response.

6. **The answer is B** *[see IV.D.3]*.
Using the equation for estimating Cl_{cr} in this patient from IV.B.1:

$$Cl_{cr} = (140 - 70 \text{ yrs})(80 \text{ kg})/(3 \text{ mg/dL})(72)$$
$$= 26 \text{ mL/min}$$

Then, using the equation for estimating $t_{½}$ in this patient from IV.B.2:

$$\frac{(2.5 \text{ hrs})}{(t_{½})_{ri}} = 1 - 0.98 + 0.98\ (26/120)$$
$$= 0.23(t_{½})_{ri} = 10.9 \text{ hrs}$$

Then, using equation [IV.D.3.c], first determine a loading dose (D_L) to achieve the desired $C_{max,ss}$ of 7.5 mcg/mL:

$$D_L = (C_{max,ss})(V)/(S)(f)$$

$$D_L = (7.5 \text{ mcg/mL})(0.25 \text{ L/kg})/(1)(1) = 1.9 \text{ mg/kg}$$

Then, determine fraction of drug lost during τ, assuming a τ_{ri} of 24 hrs, and using the $(t_{½})_{ri}$ of 10.9 hrs estimated earlier using the equation in IV.D.3.c:

$$\text{fraction lost} = 1 - 10^{-0.3(24/10.9)} = 0.78$$

$$\text{fraction left} = 10^{-0.3(24/10.9)} = 0.22$$

Lastly, calculate D per τ_{ri}:

$$\text{D per } \tau_{ri} = (D_L)(\text{fraction lost per } \tau_{ri})$$
$$= (1.9 \text{ mg/kg})(0.78) = 1.5 \text{ mg/kg}$$

This dose of 1.5 mg/kg every 24 hrs is based on achieving an estimated $C_{max,ss}$ = 7.5 mcg/mL, as noted earlier. To check the estimated $C_{min,ss}$ use equation (3) in [4.A.3]:

$$C_{min,ss} = (C_{max,ss})\ [10^{-0.3(\tau/t_{½})}]$$
$$= (7.5)\ [10-^{0.3(24/10.9)}] = 1.6 \text{ mcg/mL}$$

Thus, a D_L of 1.9 mg/kg followed by 1.5 mg/kg every 24 hrs is expected to attain the desired $C_{max,ss}$ and $C_{min,ss}$ levels in this patient. Of course, many estimates were made along the way (Cl_{cr}, $t_{½}$, V), so if the patient's $C_{max,ss}$ and $C_{min,ss}$ vary from what has been expected from the calculations, it is likely because of the estimates being at variance with the actual value(s) in the patient.

by the higher density of capillaries in skeletal muscle during infancy, which increases blood circulation.

(2) Intramuscular administration of drugs is generally discouraged in the pediatric population because of the pain associated with the injection and the risk of nerve damage from inadvertent injection into nerve tissue.

(3) This route is generally reserved for the administration of vitamin K where it produces a longer lasting depot-like effect to prevent hemorrhagic disease of the newborn, vaccines, and occasionally antibiotics when intravenous access is not available. If it is used, the volume should not exceed 0.5 mL for infants and younger children and 1.0 mL for older children.

d. **Rectal administration.** Absorption by this route is fairly reliable, even for preterm neonates. Administration may be complicated in infants; however, by the increased number of pulsatile contractions in the rectum compared to adults, making expulsion of a suppository more likely.

e. **Pulmonary administration.** Inhalation of medications is increasingly being used in infants and older children to avoid systemic exposure. Although developmental changes in the pulmonary vasculature and respiratory mechanics likely alter the pharmacokinetics of drugs given by inhalation, little is known about the effects of growth and maturation on this route of drug administration.

3. **Drug distribution.** Growth and maturation affect many of the factors that determine drug distribution. Body water content, fat stores, plasma protein concentrations, organ size and perfusion, hemodynamic stability, tissue perfusion, acid–base balance, and cell membrane permeability all undergo significant changes from infancy to adolescence.

a. **Body water and fat content.** Total body water content decreases with increasing age. This is primarily the result of a larger extracellular body water content in neonates and young infants that decreases with age. Approximately 80% of a newborn's body weight is water. By 1 year of age, this value declines to 60%, similar to that of an adult. Highly water-soluble compounds, such as gentamicin (Garamycin), have a larger volume of distribution in neonates than in older children. As a result, larger milligram per kilogram doses are often needed to achieve desired therapeutic concentrations. Conversely, body fat increases with age from 1% to 2% in a preterm neonate to 10% to 15% in a term neonate and 20% to 25% in a 1-year-old. Lipophilic drugs, such as diazepam (Valium), have a smaller volume of distribution in infants than in older children and adults.

b. **Protein binding.** Acidic drugs bind to **albumin**, whereas basic substances bind primarily to **α_1-acid glycoprotein** (AGP). The quantity of total plasma proteins, including both of these substances, is reduced in neonates and young infants. In addition, the serum albumin of newborns may have a reduced binding affinity. These two factors result in an increase in the free fraction of many drugs (*Table 27-2*). The increase in the free fraction may result in enhanced pharmacological activity for a given dose. **The relative decrease in serum proteins may also produce increased competition by drugs and endogenous substances, such as bilirubin, for binding sites.** Drugs that are highly bound to albumin, such as the sulfonamides, may displace bilirubin from its binding sites and allow deposition in the brain, referred to as kernicterus. As a result, these drugs are contraindicated in the first 2 months of life.

Table 27-2 PROTEIN-BOUND DRUGS WITH A HIGH FREE FRACTION IN NEONATES

Ampicillin (Principen)	Penicillin G (Pfizerpen)
Digoxin (Lanoxin)	Phenobarbital
Diazepam (Valium)	Phenytoin (Dilantin)
Lidocaine (Xylocaine)	Propranolol (Inderal)
Morphine (Duramorph)	Theophylline
Nafcillin (Nallpen)	

4. **Metabolism.** The most significant research in developmental pharmacology during the past decade has come in the area of drug metabolism. **Developmental changes have been identified for many phase I** (oxidation, reduction, hydroxylation, and hydrolysis) and **phase II** (conjugation) **reactions.** The maturation of metabolic function results in the need for age-related dosage alterations for many common therapies and may explain the increased risk for drug toxicity in infants and young children.
   a. The activity of **phase I enzymes, such as the cytochrome P450 (CYP) enzymes, changes significantly during maturation.** Activity of the primary isoenzyme present during the prenatal period, CYP3A7, declines rapidly after birth. This enzyme exists in barely measurable quantities in adults. It may appear early in fetal life to detoxify dehydroepiandrosterone and retinoic acid that are transferred across the placenta from maternal circulation. At birth, CYP2E1 and CYP2D6 levels begin to rise. Enzymes associated with the metabolism of many common drugs, including CYP3A4, CYP2C9, and CYP2C19, appear within the first weeks of life, but their levels increase slowly. The last of the enzymes to develop, CYP1A2, is present by 1 to 3 months of life. The activity of these enzymes does not appear to increase in a direct linear manner with age but varies over time. By 3 to 5 years of age, most patients have CYP isoenzyme activity levels similar to that of adults.
      (1) The altered pharmacokinetic profiles of drugs in children may, in large part, be explained by these developmental changes in the CYP enzyme system. One of the most well-studied enzymes is **CYP1A2.** This enzyme is nearly nonexistent in fetal liver cells, and activity is minimal in neonates. As a result, the rate of metabolism of caffeine in the neonate is slow, resulting in an elimination half-life of 40 to 70 hrs. Enzyme activity increases by 4 to 6 months of age. Within the first year of life it exceeds adult values, producing a caffeine half-life of approximately 5 hrs. Infants receiving caffeine (Cafcit) for apnea of prematurity or chronic lung disease must have periodic adjustments in their dose to account for these changes in metabolism and maintain therapeutic serum concentrations.
      (2) **Genetic polymorphism** also plays a significant role in determining metabolic function in children. Recent studies with atomoxetine (Strattera) have shown that children with reduced CYP2D6 function (i.e., poor metabolizers) had greater improvement in their attention deficit hyperactivity disorder (ADHD) symptoms than children who were extensive metabolizers, using a standard weight-based dose. The poor metabolizers also had an increased incidence of adverse effects as a result of having higher atomoxetine serum concentrations.
      (3) **Alcohol dehydrogenase** activity is only 3% to 4% of adult values at birth and does not achieve adult values until approximately 5 years of age. Because of this, newborns have a reduced ability to detoxify benzyl alcohol, a preservative found in many injectable products. Newborns exposed repeatedly to these products will accumulate benzyl alcohol, which may lead to a potentially fatal condition referred to as "gasping syndrome," with metabolic acidosis, respiratory failure, seizures, and cardiovascular collapse. Because of this risk, it is recommended that neonates receive preservative-free products or those containing alternative preservatives.
   b. **Phase II reactions** (conjugation with glycine, glucuronide, or sulfate to form more water-soluble compounds) also undergo considerable change during early childhood.
      (1) Uridine 5′-diphosphate glucuronosyltransferase (UGT) enzyme activity is minimal at birth. As a result, **glucuronidation is decreased in neonates**, compared with older children and adults. The rate of glucuronidation increases with increasing patient age. This can be seen in the decreasing half-life of morphine (Duramorph) during the first year of life, which mirrors the maturation of UGT2B7 function. The average half-life in a preterm neonate is 10 to 20 hrs, compared to 4 to 13 hrs in a neonate, 5 to 10 hrs in infants between 1 and 3 months of age, and 1 to 8 hrs in older infants and young children.
      (2) Unlike glucuronidation, **sulfation develops in utero and is well developed in the neonate.** Several of the sulfotransferases are present during gestation, where they metabolize hormones and catecholamines. The variation in the function of these two phase II reactions can be seen with the developmental changes in acetaminophen (Tylenol) metabolism. In early infancy, acetaminophen is converted primarily through formation of sulfate conjugates; but with increasing age, glucuronidation becomes the predominate form of metabolism.

c. Although most of the recent research into pediatric drug metabolism has focused on the development of enzyme function in neonates, several new studies highlight additional changes in metabolic function during adolescence. For example, lopinavir (marketed with ritonavir as Kaletra) pharmacokinetics undergoes significant age and gender-related changes at the time of puberty. Lopinavir clearance increases by more than 30% in boys after age 12, compared to minimal changes in clearance in girls after the onset of puberty.

5. **Elimination.** Development of renal function is a complex and dynamic process. Nephrons begin forming as early as the ninth week of gestation and are complete by 36 weeks. Although the functional units of the kidneys are present, their capacity is significantly reduced at birth. Glomerular filtration rate in neonates is approximately half that of adults. Values are further reduced in preterm neonates. Glomerular filtration rate increases rapidly during the first 2 weeks of life and typically reaches adult values by 8 to 12 months of age. Tubular secretion rate is also reduced at birth to approximately 20% of adult capacity but matures by 12 months of age.
   a. **Immature renal function results in significant alterations in the elimination of many drugs.** Pharmacokinetic studies for several drugs, including the aminoglycosides, digoxin (Lanoxin), and vancomycin (Vancocin), have shown a direct correlation between clearance and patient age. Prolongation of the half-life should be anticipated for all renally eliminated drugs administered to neonates and is most pronounced in preterm neonates.
   b. **To account for the reduced ability of a neonate to eliminate these drugs, longer dosing intervals are often required.** Failure to account for the reduction in renal function may result in drug accumulation and toxicity. Dosage adjustment is typically based on urine output, with values greater than 1 mL/kg/hr indicating adequate renal function. Although a trend towards increasing serum creatinine over a period of time may indicate worsening renal function, calculation of creatinine clearance is not routinely used to determine drug dosing in pediatrics. Creatinine values in neonates may be falsely elevated during the perinatal period due to transfer of maternal creatinine across the placenta, whereas values in older infants and young children may be low due to limited muscle mass and provide misleading assurance that renal function is adequate. As a result, the equations used for determining creatinine clearance, such as Cockcroft–Gault or Modification of Diet in Renal Disease (MDRD), are not considered appropriate for use in infants and children.

C. **Pharmacodynamic considerations.** Unlike the rapidly accelerating knowledge of the pharmacokinetic changes associated with development, less is known of the pharmacodynamic changes associated with maturation. Preliminary investigations of warfarin (Coumadin) pharmacodynamics have demonstrated a relationship between greater anticoagulant response and increasing patient age. Studies have suggested that neonates may have lower numbers of β-adrenergic receptors, reduced binding affinity, or conformational changes of the receptor binding site, which might explain their decreased responsiveness to dopamine and epinephrine for the treatment of hypotension. Future research in age-related pharmacodynamic changes is needed to optimize the safe and effective use of drugs in infants and children.

D. **Pediatric drug administration and monitoring.** Drug administration, including the selection of agent and dose as well as the preparation of the dose and therapeutic drug monitoring, is complicated in the pediatric population. Pharmacists caring for children must not only be knowledgeable about the changes in pharmacokinetics and pharmacodynamics described previously, but must also be able to use this information in the assessment of the appropriateness of a medication order or prescription. In addition, they should understand the need to carefully check all dosage calculations and be able to alter available dosage formulations when necessary to tailor them for infants and young children.

1. **Accurate dosage calculations are critical in the care of infants and children.** Pharmacists should use pediatric dosing information available in general drug references or pediatric-specific references such as *The Pediatric Dosage Handbook* (Lexi-Comp), the *Harriet Lane Handbook* (Mosby), or *Neofax* (Thomson Reuters). To account for differences in pharmacokinetic parameters, most pediatric doses are based on body weight. In the case of some drugs, such as chemotherapy, doses are based on body surface area (BSA). This value can be determined from the patient's height and weight, using either a nomogram or the following equation:

$$\text{BSA (m}^2\text{)} = \frac{\text{height (cm)} \times \text{weight (kg)}}{3600}$$

There is no absolute rule for when adolescent patients should start to be dosed as adults. In general, adult dosing guidelines may be used in patients weighing more than 40 to 50 kg or when the calculated weight-based pediatric dose exceeds the standard adult dose.

2. **The need to calculate pediatric doses introduces a greater risk for dosage errors.** Dosing errors have been found to be more common in medication orders for children than in any other patient population. Studies suggest a medication error rate of 5% to 15% in pediatric inpatients, with the greatest number of errors occurring during the ordering process. The need to calculate individual doses, along with potential decimal errors and transcription errors, increases the potential for mistakes. In addition, there is often a wide range of patient ages and weights within a single hospital or clinic. It is not uncommon to have patient doses vary by 10-fold, as an infant weighing 5 kg and an adolescent weighing 50 kg may be cared for by the same health care providers. Pharmacists practicing in a neonatal intensive care unit may have extremely low birth weight patients weighing as little as 0.5 kg alongside large infants with congenital or birth-related complications weighing 5 kg. All calculations should be double-checked, and orders outside of the normal pediatric dosage range verified with the prescriber. Computerized physician order entry (CPOE) with embedded clinical decision support and dose-checking software reduces the potential for errors but does not replace the need for order review by a trained pharmacist.
3. **Dosage formulations may need to be altered to make them useful for infants and children.** Because young children cannot typically swallow tablets and capsules, these solid dosage formulations must often be converted to oral solutions or suspensions. Several compounding resources, including *Extemporaneous Formulations for Pediatric, Geriatric and Special Needs Patients* (American Society of Health-System Pharmacists) and *Pediatric Drug Formulations* (Harvey Whitney Books), are available to provide pharmacists with formulations that have been tested to ensure drug stability. With coaching, most children can learn to swallow solid dosage forms between 6 and 8 years of age.
4. **Medications must be stored appropriately and doses measured accurately.** Families should be given complete instructions for the storage, use, and disposal of all medications for children. This should include instructions on the accurate measurement of oral liquids. Oral syringes are preferred for infants, but oral dosing spoons and cups may be used for older children. Written information, ideally targeted to the pediatric patient population as in *The Pediatric Medication Education Text* (American College of Clinical Pharmacy), is a useful adjunct to oral communication and allows families to provide detailed instructions to extended family members, preschool and school personnel, babysitters, and other care providers. Safe storage of all household medications should be stressed with all families as a part of good poison prevention practices.
5. **Intravenous (IV) medications may be prepared as more concentrated solutions because of the limits on fluid administration to infants and young children.** Although a typical adult may receive up to 4 to 5 L of IV fluids per day, the total daily fluid requirements for a preterm neonate may be as little as 20 to 50 mL. As a result of these limitations, medication volumes are typically minimized in order to allow more of the daily total to be used to provide either enteral or parenteral nutrition. Special equipment, such as syringe pumps and microbore tubing, is used to ensure accurate delivery of drugs in small fluid volumes. Currently available syringe pumps can deliver volumes as small as 0.1 mL over 1 hr. Smart pump technology, which incorporates dose checking and the ability to set dosing limits, has significantly reduced the frequency of IV medication errors in hospitalized pediatric patients. Microbore IV tubing is used to minimize the amount of dead space between the delivery device and the patient, further improving the accuracy of drug delivery. Pharmacists must also be capable of assessing literature on the compatibility with drugs and IV fluids because pediatric patients often have limited IV access, so that multiple solutions may need to be infused through the same IV site.

E. **Therapeutic drug monitoring** is often essential to optimizing drug therapy in infants and children. For most drugs, including aminoglycosides, antiepileptics, cyclosporine, methotrexate, tacrolimus, and vancomycin, the therapeutic ranges developed for and used in adults are also appropriate for monitoring pediatric patients. A potential complication in interpreting serum drug concentrations is the **presence of endogenous substances**, which may cross-react with analytical drug assays. This has been demonstrated for digoxin (Lanoxin) in neonates and infants, for whom endogenous digoxin-like reactive substances (EDLRS) may produce falsely elevated serum digoxin concentrations. Standard assay techniques can be modified to exclude EDLRS as a complicating factor.

F. **Pharmacists should also be aware of differences in adverse drug reactions between children and adults.** Most of the adverse reaction information available in drug product labeling or cited in pharmacy references has been obtained from clinical trials in adults. As several studies have demonstrated, the adverse reaction profile in children may be significantly different from that observed in older subjects. For example, severe dermatologic reactions to lamotrigine (Lamictal), including Stevens–Johnson syndrome, were infrequent during premarketing phase III clinical trials. When the drug was introduced into the market in the United States and began to be used in children off-label, a higher rate of dermatologic reactions was reported in children. Subsequent research revealed the incidence of severe dermatologic reactions to be 0.8% in children compared to 0.3% in adults. A reduction in the pediatric starting dose, along with recommendations for a more gradual dose escalation, has reduced the number of severe reactions. There are also adverse effects known to occur primarily in children due to pharmacokinetic differences. Valproic acid-induced hepatotoxicity has been reported most frequently in children less than 2 years of age, likely related to their reduced ability to eliminate the toxic 4-en-valproate metabolite. Other examples of drug reactions that occur more often in children than adults include the development of Reye syndrome, a derangement of cellular mitochondrial function resulting in liver failure following aspirin use, and the higher incidence of renal dysfunction with nonsteroidal anti-inflammatory drugs used during the first 6 months of life. Differences such as these further highlight the need for more clinical research in children.

G. In addition, **pharmacists should take an active role in promoting medication adherence (compliance) in children.** Several studies have shown adherence rates in pediatric patients to be 30% to 70%. It is surprising that some of the poorest adherence rates have been associated with chronic diseases such as asthma, epilepsy, and diabetes and in children requiring immunosuppressive therapy after organ transplantation. As in adults, counseling about medication adherence should include efforts to identify and overcome barriers to therapy, education about the importance of medical management, and programs to incorporate medication regimens into normal daily tasks. When working with families of younger children, pharmacists should also explore problems with dosage formulation (such as taste or texture aversion) and dosing frequency. Medications with once or twice daily dosing avoid the need for administration at school or day care and have been shown to increase adherence. In older children and adolescents, pharmacists should be aware of their growing need for autonomy and work with the patient and his or her family to foster the goal of self-care. Most children can begin to take an active role in their medication preparation and administration by the age of 12, although the age at which they can assume responsibility for their treatment varies considerably. As part of an interdisciplinary health care team, pharmacists can serve a vital role in improving medication adherence, reducing the likelihood of treatment failure and supporting a lifelong commitment to a healthy lifestyle among their pediatric patients.

Study Questions

Directions for questions 1–14: Each of the questions, statements, or incomplete statements in this section can be correctly answered or completed by **one** of the suggested answers or phrases. Choose the **best** answer.

For questions 1–4: AH is a 1.2-kg female born prematurely at 30 weeks of gestational age. Her mother had an infection with a fever at the time of delivery. AH was admitted to the neonatal intensive care unit for presumed sepsis and placed on empiric antibiotic therapy with ampicillin (50 mg/kg IV every 12 hrs) and gentamicin (2.5 mg/kg IV every 8 hrs).

1. Which of the following variables will *most* likely be used to calculate doses for AH's antibiotics?

(A) Height
(B) Hepatic function
(C) Weight
(D) Age
(E) Serum creatinine

2. After the administration of four doses of gentamicin, a serum concentration obtained 5 mins before the next dose was 2.5 mcg/mL. Which of the following answers best describes the pharmacokinetic differences observed in premature neonates (compared to older children and adults) that might explain this value?
   (A) Larger volume of distribution, longer half-life
   (B) Larger volume of distribution, shorter half-life
   (C) Smaller volume of distribution, longer half-life
   (D) Smaller volume of distribution, shorter half-life
   (E) Similar volume of distribution, shorter half-life

3. Ampicillin may exhibit pharmacokinetic differences in AH because of its protein binding characteristics. Which of the following answers best describes the effect of AH's age on ampicillin protein binding?
   (A) Increased protein binding, resulting in a greater free fraction
   (B) Increased protein binding, resulting in a reduced free fraction
   (C) Decreased protein binding, resulting in a greater free fraction
   (D) Decreased protein binding, resulting in a reduced free fraction
   (E) Decreased protein binding, resulting in no significant change in free fraction

4. As the pharmacist providing services for the neonatal intensive care unit, you evaluate medication orders and make recommendations to the medical team. Which of the following would be the *most* appropriate recommendation for AH's care?
   (A) Change to oral antibiotics for better absorption.
   (B) Double-check the calculations to avoid decimal errors.
   (C) Dilute the gentamicin with a larger volume of IV fluids to make it easier to measure.
   (D) Use a pediatric-specific therapeutic range for monitoring gentamicin.
   (E) Change to sulfamethoxazole and trimethoprim (Bactrim) for single-agent antibacterial coverage.

5. Although the total body water content of an adult accounts for approximately 60% of body weight, the total body water content of a healthy newborn is
   (A) 40%.
   (B) 50%.
   (C) 70%.
   (D) 80%.
   (E) 90%.

6. Administration of a sulfonamide antibiotic may displace bilirubin from binding sites on which of the following substances, leading to passage of bilirubin into the brain and the development of kernicterus?
   (A) α_1-acid glycoprotein
   (B) albumin
   (C) β-adrenergic receptors
   (D) uridine 5′-diphosphate glucuronosyltransferase
   (E) sulfotransferase

7. Caffeine administered to neonates for the treatment of apnea of prematurity undergoes metabolism through which of the following cytochrome P450 enzymes, also the last major drug-metabolizing enzyme to develop after birth?
   (A) CYP1A2
   (B) CYP2C19
   (C) CYP2D6
   (D) CYP3A4
   (E) CYP3A7

8. Both glomerular filtration and tubular secretion rates are reduced in infants compared to adults. Which list of drugs is the *most* likely to have prolonged clearance during infancy because of immature renal function alone?
   (A) Amikacin, caffeine, and retinoic acid
   (B) Acetaminophen, atomoxetine, and retinoic acid
   (C) Acetaminophen, benzyl alcohol, and vancomycin
   (D) Amikacin, gentamicin, and vancomycin
   (E) Atomoxetine, lopinavir, and vancomycin

9. As a pharmacy manager in a children's hospital, you are responsible for implementing new technologies that have the potential to reduce medication errors in children. Which of the following has the *most* potential to reduce the largest number of errors?
   (A) Bar-code scanning
   (B) CPOE with dose-checking software
   (C) Inventory management systems
   (D) Smart pump technology
   (E) Standard IV concentrations

10. You are counseling the grandmother of a 3-year-old boy who has a prescription for amoxicillin/clavulanate (Augmentin) to treat uncomplicated otitis media. Which of the following issues would be *least* likely to affect medication adherence (compliance)?
    (A) Lack of education about the medication
    (B) Cost
    (C) Dosing interval (frequency)
    (D) Taste
    (E) Autonomy

Answers and Explanations

1. **The answer is C** *[see I.D.1].*
Most pediatric doses are based on body weight. This single variable incorporates growth and maturation while allowing a simple calculation for dose. Height is often difficult to measure accurately in children, and the calculation of body surface area is typically reserved for those drugs with narrow therapeutic indices, such as chemotherapy.

2. **The answer is A** *[see I.B.3.a; I.B.5].*
Aminoglycosides such as gentamicin exhibit a larger volume of distribution in neonates because of their larger body water content. Neonates also typically have a longer elimination half-life as the result of having reduced renal function during the first 6 months of life.

3. **The answer is C** *[see I.B.3.b; Table 27-2].*
Neonates have both a reduced quantity of plasma proteins as well as a reduction in the affinity of albumin to bind to other substances. As a result, the free fraction of many drugs, including ampicillin, is increased.

4. **The answer is B** *[see I.D; I.E].*
All pediatric orders should be carefully checked for calculation errors. Errors are more common in the pediatric population as the result of weight-based dosing and the need for mathematical calculations. The use of the oral route would not be advisable in this patient because of the potential reduced drug absorption. Likewise, the dilution of the dose with more IV fluid or the use of a sulfa drug would not be appropriate for this patient's age. Finally, the therapeutic range for gentamicin is the same in pediatric patients as in adults.

5. **The answer is D** *[see I.B.3.a].*
A healthy newborn will have total body water content approximately 80% of his or her body weight. The higher total body water content is the result of larger extracellular body water content. This value will decrease over the first year of life to reach adult values by 1 year of age.

6. **The answer is B** *[see I.B.3.b; I.B.4.b].*
Like bilirubin, sulfonamides and other acidic drugs bind to albumin in human serum. In contrast, basic substances bind to α_1-acid glycoprotein. Uridine 5′-diphosphate glucuronosyltransferase and sulfotransferase are metabolic enzymes involved in conjugation.

7. **The answer is A** *[see I.B.4.a].*
Caffeine is metabolized via CYP1A2 to demethylated xanthines: paraxanthine, theobromine, and theophylline. CYP1A2 is the last of the major drug-metabolizing enzymes to develop during infancy, reaching peak enzymatic activity by 4 to 6 months of life. The pharmacokinetic profile of caffeine during infancy has been extensively studied, with initial publications dating to the 1970s.

8. **The answer is D** *[see I.B.4–5].*
The aminoglycosides (amikacin, gentamicin, and tobramycin) and vancomycin are examples of drugs that undergo renal elimination and as a result have prolonged clearance in infants. Acetaminophen, atomoxetine, caffeine, lopinavir, and retinoic acid are metabolized. Their clearance is more heavily influenced by hepatic enzymatic activity than by glomerular filtration or tubular secretion rates.

9. **The answer is B** *[see I. D].*
Mistakes made during ordering account for the largest percentage of pediatric medication errors. The need to calculate the appropriate weight-based dose places the prescriber at risk for mathematical errors, including decimal errors resulting in 10-fold variations in dose. Dose-checking software, a common feature of the CPOE systems of many hospitals and many retail pharmacies, has been shown in several studies to significantly reduce prescriber errors. The other methods, although all associated with reductions in medication error rates, have produced less dramatic results.

10. **The answer is E** *[see I.G].*
Although the other options are all important aspects of counseling to enhance medication adherence in children, autonomy (the ability to provide self-care or give medications independently) would not be a consideration for a 3-year-old child. Autonomy becomes a much more critical issue in determining adherence in adolescence.

Geriatrics

28

ALAN H. MUTNICK

I. DRUG USE IN GERIATRIC PATIENTS.

In 2000, more than 12% of the American population was > 65 years of age, representing more than 35 million Americans, while consuming approximately 30% of all health care costs. It is estimated that three out of every four elderly people are taking prescription medications. Anticipated total drug usage, including nonprescription medications, reveals that 50% of all drugs used in the United States are used by the geriatric population.

A. **Adverse drug reactions.** Geriatric patients are at increased risk for drug-induced adverse effects. Incidence of adverse drug reactions (ADRs) in patients older than 65 years is two to three times greater compared to younger patients. The risk is five times higher in people approaching age 90. One in five of all elderly patients experience an ADR. In some patients, these are overlooked because they mimic the characteristics of other diseases.

1. Factors that are responsible for the higher prevalence of ADRs in the geriatric population include polypharmacy, multiple disease states, altered pharmacokinetic disposition among the elderly (reduced drug elimination, increased sensitivity to drug effects, etc.), poor relationship with health care providers, increasing severity of illness, and poor patient compliance and supervision.
   a. Studies have shown that > 35% of geriatric patients living in the community use six or more medications; approximately one-half of patients residing in long-term care facilities use five or more medications. People 65 years and older use approximately 40% of the drugs prescribed and 50% of the over-the-counter (OTC) medications taken.
   b. Patients taking multiple medications have a greater chance of experiencing ADRs owing to drug–drug interactions and the potential for overlap or synergy between adverse effect profiles.
   c. Patients with multiple disease states are at higher risk for having a drug–disease state interaction.
   d. In addition to the aforementioned risk factors for developing an ADR, it is difficult to predict how geriatric patients will respond to any given medication owing to altered pharmacokinetic and pharmacodynamic profiles.
   e. Another issue complicating geriatric drug therapy is adherence. Factors that have been shown to increase nonadherence include poor relationships with health care providers, lower socioeconomic status, living alone, polypharmacy, complicated drug regimens, and multiple comorbidities. As many as 60% of geriatric patients do not take their medications as prescribed and may self-medicate as often as once a week. If patients are hospitalized, their prescribed drug doses may represent a significant overdosage or underdosage, which could cause unintended effects.
   f. Elderly patients can have diseases that make adhering to drug therapy difficult. Conditions that affect vision, such as macular degeneration or cataract formation, can make reading prescription labels and medication instructions troublesome. Hearing loss can prevent patients from understanding and health care professionals from effectively communicating medication information and patient instructions. Arthritis can add to the difficulty of opening medication bottles. In these instances, providing patients with medication or "pill" boxes and written medication lists may limit potential barriers to patient adherence. Recognizing these factors, pharmacists can increase adherence in elderly patients.

C. Pharmacodynamics

1. Geriatric patients can be more or less responsive to certain drugs compared to younger patients. Reasons for this may include altered receptor sensitivity, receptor number, or receptor response. Studies have shown that elderly patients may show a diminished response to β-blockers and β-agonists.
2. In contrast, geriatric patients have an exaggerated response to anticholinergic drugs—drugs affecting the CNS such as narcotics, analgesics, benzodiazepines, and warfarin. Elderly patients should be monitored carefully when taking these medications. Initiation of any of these therapies should be at lower doses than recommended for younger patients. Avoidance of these drugs may not be possible, but if better alternatives exist, they should be used first.

D. Drug therapy considerations

1. Drug therapy in geriatric patients is an involved process and can be very complex because of age-related changes in pharmacokinetics and pharmacodynamics.
2. Additionally, a lack of clinical trials designed to evaluate the safety and efficacy of drug therapy in the elderly population increases the problem.
3. The higher incidence of adverse effects in geriatric patients may be in part the result of the complexity of drug therapy and the relative lack of clinical trials in this population. *Table 28-2* lists several drugs and doses that should be avoided in the elderly owing to higher risks of adverse effects and/or lack of efficacy.
4. Owing to alterations in gait, balance, and mobility, falls and consequent adverse events are frequent occurrences in geriatric patients.
   a. The high prevalence of osteoporosis in the elderly results in an increased incidence of fractures. Complications associated with fractures, particularly hip fractures, are significant causes of morbidity and mortality.
   b. Medications causing orthostatic hypotension, drowsiness, dizziness, blurred vision, or confusion have the potential to cause or worsen postural instability and increase falls in the elderly.
   c. It is well established that many psychoactive agents, especially long-acting benzodiazepines, are associated with an increased risk of falls in the elderly. If a benzodiazepine must be prescribed, low-dose lorazepam (Ativan®) or oxazepam (Serax®) are better choices because of the lack of active metabolites and their metabolism involves phase II hepatic reactions only.
5. Geriatric patients tend to be sensitive to medications that possess anticholinergic effects. Dry mouth, urinary retention, blurred vision, constipation, tachycardia, memory impairment, and confusion are typical anticholinergic adverse effects associated with several classes of drugs (*Table 28-3*). These agents can also induce delirium in some people.
   a. When possible, drugs with anticholinergic effects should be avoided in the elderly. In those instances when this is not an option, the least anticholinergic agent should be chosen and initiated at the lowest effective dose. For example, if a tricyclic antidepressant is needed, desipramine (Norpramin®) and nortriptyline (Pamelor®) possess less anticholinergic activity than amitriptyline (Elavil®) and imipramine (Tofranil®) and therefore would be better initial therapeutic options.
   b. Frequent monitoring for and patient and family education on signs and symptoms of possible anticholinergic adverse effects is always warranted when these drugs are prescribed in the elderly.

E. General principles. To aid clinicians in providing appropriate geriatric drug therapy, some general principles have been developed.

1. Start with a low dose, and titrate the medication dose slowly.
2. Owing to reduced renal and hepatic function, the half-lives of many drugs are prolonged in the elderly. Selection of agents should involve consideration of the specific pharmacokinetics of each drug in the geriatric population.
3. Rapid dose escalations prevent attainment of the optimal therapeutic response because a steady-state concentration of the drug is not reached and increases the risks of developing an ADR.
4. The fewest number of drugs should always be used to treat patients.
5. Always evaluate possible drug toxicity. Geriatric patients can have atypical presentations of ADRs, which may manifest as CNS changes (e.g., altered mental status).
6. Review concomitant medications and diseases to evaluate the possible interactions with new drugs.
7. Reassess the need for each medication on a regular basis.

Table 28-2 TARGET DRUGS AND DOSES TO AVOID IN GERIATRIC PATIENTS

Drug	Comments
	Analgesics
Pentazocine (Talwin)	Avoid; safer and more effective alternatives
Meperidine (Demerol)	Avoid; safer and more effective alternatives
	Antidepressants
Amitriptyline (Elavil)	Avoid; anticholinergic adverse effects, increased risk of falls, and QT prolongation; use nortriptyline or desipramine as alternatives
Amitriptyline, perphenazine (Triavil)	Avoid; use separate antidepressant and antipsychotic agents in appropriate geriatric doses as necessary
Doxepin (Sinequan)	Avoid; safer and more effective alternatives
	Antiemetics
Trimethobenzamide (Tigan)	Avoid; more effective alternatives available
	Antihistamines
Sedating OTC agents, cold preparations	Avoid; potent anticholinergic effects
Hydroxyzine (Atarax)	Avoid; potent anticholinergic effects
Cyproheptadine (Periactin)	Avoid; potent anticholinergic effects
Chlorpheniramine (Chlor-Trimeton)	Avoid; potent anticholinergic effects
	Antihypertensives
Hydrochlorothiazide (HydroDIURIL)	Doses > 25 mg/day should be avoided
Methyldopa (Aldomet)	Avoid; safer alternatives
Propranolol (Inderal)	Lipophilic nonselective β-blocker with increased potential for adverse effects; avoid; use a cardioselective β-blocker instead
Reserpine	Avoid; risk of adverse effects (e.g., sedation, depression)
	Antipsychotics
Haloperidol (Haldol)	Avoid unless indicated for psychotic disorder; use in small doses (1 mg); risk of sudden death in higher doses
Thioridazine (Mellaril)	Avoid unless indicated for psychotic disorder
	Antispasmodics
Belladonna	Avoid long-term use; anticholinergic adverse effects
Dicyclomine (Bentyl)	Avoid long-term use; anticholinergic adverse effects
Hyoscyamine (Pyridium)	Avoid long-term use; anticholinergic adverse effects

(Continued on next page)

Table 28-2 Continued.

Drug	Comments
	Decongestants
Oxymetazoline (Afrin)	Daily use for > 3 days should be avoided
Phenylephrine (Neo-Synephrine)	Daily use for > 3 days should be avoided
Pseudoephedrine (Sudafed)	Avoid; anticholinergic effects and potential to raise blood pressure
	H2 antagonists
Cimetidine (Tagamet)	Avoid; adverse CNS effects
	Hypoglycemic agents
Chlorpropamide (Diabinese)	Avoid; long half-life can cause prolonged hypoglycemic episodes and can induce SIADH
	Muscle relaxants
Carisoprodol (Soma)	Risk of adverse events greater than potential benefits; all use should be avoided
Cyclobenzaprine (Flexeril)	Risks of adverse events greater than potential benefits
Methocarbamol (Robaxin)	Risks of adverse events greater than potential benefits
Orphenadrine (Norflex)	Risks of adverse events greater than potential benefits
	NSAIDs
Indomethacin (Indocin)	Avoid; CNS adverse effects; use alternative NSAID
Noncyclooxygenase selective NSAIDs	Avoid long-term use of naproxen, oxaprozin and piroxicam; increased risks of adverse effects
	Platelet inhibitors
Dipyridamole (Persantine)	Avoid; lack of efficacy and adverse effects (orthostatic hypotension) at high doses; aspirin is safer and more effective
	Sedative hypnotics
Long-acting benzodiazepines	Avoid; accumulation and increased risk of falls, sedation, and delirium
Chlordiazepoxide (Librium)	
Diazepam (Valium)	
Flurazepam (Dalmane)	
Short-acting benzodiazepines	Nightly use should be avoided; increased risk of falls, daytime sedation, and delirium
Alprazolam (Xanax)	
Oxazepam (Serax)	
Triazolam (Halcion)	
Meprobamate (Miltown)	All use should be avoided
Barbiturates	All use should be avoided; safer alternatives exist

CNS, central nervous system; *NSAIDs*, nonsteroidal anti-inflammatory drugs; *OTC*, over-the-counter; *SIADH*, syndrome of inappropriate antidiuretic hormone secretion. Modified with permission from Fick DM, Cooper JW, Wade WE, et al. Updating the Beers criteria for potentially inappropriate medication use in older adults. *Arch Intern Med.* 2003;163:2716–2724.

Table 28-3 DRUGS AND DRUG CLASSES POSSESSING ANTICHOLINERGIC EFFECTS

Antidiarrheal agents	Propantheline (Pro-Banthine)
Diphenoxylate/atropine (Lomotil)	Oxybutynin (XL formulation has fewer effects) (Ditropan)
Antiemetics/antivertigo agents	Tolterodine (Detrol)
Meclizine (Antivert)	Class Ia antiarrhythmic agents
Scopolamine (Transderm scopolamine)	Disopyramide (Norpace)
Trimethobenzamide (Tigan)	Quinidine
Promethazine (Phenergan)	Parkinson's agents
Prochlorperazine (Compazine)	Amantadine (Symmetrel)
Antihistamines, sedating types	Benztropine (Cogentin)
Antipsychotic agents	Procyclidine (Kemadrin)
Antispasmodics	Trihexyphenidyl-Artane
Belladonna alkaloids	Skeletal muscle relaxants
Chlordiazepoxide/clidinium-Librax	Cyclobenzaprine (Flexeril)
Dicyclomine (Bentyl)	Orphenadrine (Norflex)
Hyoscyamine (Pyridium)	Tricyclic antidepressants

Study Questions

Directions for questions 1–14: Each of the questions, statements, or incomplete statements in this section can be correctly answered or completed by **one** of the suggested answers or phrases. Choose the **best** answer.

1. Which of the following medications due to its lack of active metabolites and dependency on phase II hepatic reactions is least likely to cause a fall in a geriatric patient?
   - **(A)** amitriptyline (Elavil®)
   - **(B)** haloperidol (Haldol®)
   - **(C)** benztropine (Cogentin®)
   - **(D)** diazepam (Valium®)
   - **(E)** oxazepam (Serax®)

2. Which of the following drugs would be expected to cause anticholinergic adverse effects in the elderly?
   - **(A)** diazepam (Valium®)
   - **(B)** ciprofloxacin (Cipro®)
   - **(C)** tolterodine (Detrol®)
   - **(D)** propranolol (Inderal®)
   - **(E)** cimetidine (Tagamet®)

3. Which of the following antihypertensive agents should be avoided in elderly patients?
   - **(A)** amlodipine (Norvasc®) 5 mg every day
   - **(B)** atenolol (Tenormin®) 25 mg every day
   - **(C)** benazepril (Lotensin®) 10 mg every day
   - **(D)** hydrochlorothiazide (HydroDIURIL®) 25 mg every day
   - **(E)** methyldopa (Aldomet®) 250 mg three times a day

4. Which of the following benzodiazepines is expected to cause the *least* amount of adverse effects in the elderly?
   - **(A)** chlordiazepoxide (Librium®)
   - **(B)** diazepam (Valium®)
   - **(C)** flurazepam (Dalmane®)
   - **(D)** lorazepam (Ativan®)
   - **(E)** temazepam (Restoril®)

5. Which of the following factors is associated with an increased risk of noncompliance in the elderly?
   - **(A)** Polypharmacy
   - **(B)** Hypertension
   - **(C)** Living with a spouse in an isolated environment
   - **(D)** Expensive medications
   - **(E)** Good relationship with physician

Directions for questions 6-7: The questions and incomplete statements in this section can be correctly answered or completed by **one or more** of the suggested answers. Choose the answer, **A–E.**

A if **I only** is correct
B if **III only** is correct
C if **I and II** are correct
D if **II and III** are correct
E if **I, II, and III** are correct

6. Which of the following pharmacokinetic parameters is most likely to affect the manner in which a drug will affect a geriatric patient?

I. Drug absorption
II. Phase I reactions within the liver
III. Drug distribution

7. Which of the following statements regarding renal excretion in the geriatric patient is correct?

I. All renally eliminated drugs should be monitored for the need for dose reductions in order to reduce potential toxicity.
II. Cockcroft–Gault formula provides a good estimation of creatinine clearance in most patient populations.
III. Serum creatinine is a very sensitive indicator of renal function in the elderly.

8. Patient AM is a 60-year-old obese Caucasian male who is about to be started on several renally eliminated drugs for various diseases he has been diagnosed with. Patient is 5′9″, weighs 220 lb, and has a serum creatinine of 2.0 mg/dL. What is Mr. AM's calculated creatinine clearance?

(A) 56 mL/min
(B) 128 mL/min
(C) 47 mL/min
(D) 109 mL/min
(E) 100 mL/min

Answers and Explanations

1. The answer is E *[see I.D.4.b–c and I.B.4.b].*
Medications that can cause orthostatic hypotension, drowsiness, dizziness, blurred vision, or confusion have the potential to cause falls in geriatric patients. Psychoactive agents such as haloperidol along with long-acting benzodiazepines such as diazepam are associated with an increased risk of falls in the elderly. Additionally, agents that have high anticholinergic effects can cause blurred vision while also being capable of inducing delirium (amitriptyline [Elavil®]; benztropine [Cogentin®]). However, oxazepam is a short-acting benzodiazepine dependent on phase II reactions for metabolism, which are not affected by advancing age, and would be a suitable alternative in the elderly patient.

2. The answer is C *[see I.D.5.a; Table 28-3].*
Tricyclic antidepressants, antispasmodics, antiemetics, and Parkinson's agents represent the largest group of drugs possessing anticholinergic activity, which have the potential for inducing significant negative effects in the elderly. Blurred vision, urinary retention, constipation, dry mouth, tachycardia, and memory impairment are a few of the significant side effects associated with their use in the elderly. Tolterodine, an antispasmodic, works by antagonizing acetylcholine receptors, which aids patients with an overactive bladder. However, this anticholinergic effect can pose substantial problems in elderly patients due to the side effects associated with its use.

3. The answer is E *[see I; Table 28-2].*
The use of methyldopa should be avoided in elderly patients owing to risk of CNS adverse effects and hypotension. Hydrochlorothiazide should be avoided in elderly patient when doses are expected to exceed 25 mg per day.

4. The answer is D *[see I.B.4.a–b and I.D.4.c; Table 28-2].*
Chlordiazepoxide, diazepam, and flurazepam should be avoided in elderly patients owing to active metabolites and long-elimination half-lives. Lorazepam represents the safest alternative because of a relatively short half-life, absence of active metabolites, and it is dependent on phase II hepatic metabolism, which is minimally affected with aging while being devoid of phase I hepatic metabolism.

5. The answer is A *[see I.A.1.e].*
Lower socioeconomic status, living alone, polypharmacy, complicated drug regimens, poor relationships with health care providers, and multiple disease states are all risk factors for noncompliance in the geriatric population.

6. **The answer is D; II and III are correct** *[see I.B.1–4].*
Phase I reactions (oxidation, reduction, and hydrolysis) can be reduced in the elderly, and several therapeutic classes such as benzodiazepines and select analgesics represent situations in which changes in hepatic metabolism may be important due to a prolongation of plasma half-lives with a resultant drug accumulation. Drug absorption has been shown to be altered in the elderly; however, the level of alterations has not yet been shown to affect the extent of absorption being reduced. Phase II reactions in the liver are represented by glucuronidation, acetylation, and sulfation and have not yet been shown to require therapeutic adjustments while dosing such agents.

7. **The answer is C; I and II are correct** *[see I.B.3.a–d].*
The disposition of drugs administered to patients, which are eliminated renally, is the best documented age-related change, which occurs in the elderly. The need to monitor such agents and adjust their doses based on elimination characteristics will help reduce added accumulation and the tendency for toxicity in those with declining renal function. The elderly are predisposed to such effects as renal function is reduced with advancing age. The Cockcroft–Gault formula is a useful tool for estimating most patients' creatinine clearance, when given a serum creatinine; however, it must be recognized that it provides merely an estimate and might not reflect exact renal function is all patient populations. The serum creatinine is used as an indirect measurement for renal function primarily due to its relationship to creatinine clearance and glomerular filtration rate. However, in the elderly due to reduced levels of muscle and consequent reductions in the degree of creatinine produced, normal levels of serum creatinine do not translate into normal levels of renal function.

8. **The answer is A** *[see I.B.3.d].*

$$\text{Creatinine Clearance (mL/min)} = \frac{(140 - \text{age}) \times (\text{weight kg})}{72 \times \text{serum creatinine (mg/dL)}}$$

$$\text{Creatinine Clearance (mL/min)} = \frac{(140 - 60) \times (100\text{ kg})}{72 \times \text{serum creatinine (2.0 mg/dL)}}$$

$$\text{Creatinine Clearance (mL/min)} = \frac{(80) \times (100\text{ kg})}{72 \times (2.0\text{ mg/dL})}$$

$$\text{Creatinine Clearance (mL/min)} = \frac{8000}{144}$$

$$\text{Creatinine Clearance (mL/min)} = 55.6\text{ mL/min} = 56$$

travels through the tube into the uterus. The blastocyst contains numerous types of relatively undifferentiated tissues that will ultimately become the fetus, the placenta, and the fetal membranes. Superficial implantation in the endometrium occurs within the first 5 days. During the second week, differentiation begins and the placenta has started to form. During these weeks, there is an "all or none" phenomenon. With no placenta to transfer substances to the blastocyst, there is no susceptibility to teratogens. Exposure to environmental agents during this time will have either little or no effect on the embryo or will destroy most cells, leading to pregnancy termination.

2. **Weeks 3 to 8.** It is during this time that the placenta becomes fully functional and organogenesis occurs. This is the most critical period of development, when the embryo is most susceptible to teratogens. All major organ systems develop structurally during these weeks. All are completely formed by the end of the ninth week, with the exception of the central nervous system (CNS). Major congenital anomalies, such as cardiac abnormalities, spina bifida, and limb defects occur during this time.
3. **Weeks 9 to 38 (the fetal period).** At the ninth week, the embryo is referred to as a fetus. Development during this time is primarily functional, with overall growth occurring throughout. The fetus may be at risk during exposure to potentially fetotoxic drugs or viruses. Exposure to a drug is generally not associated with major congenital malformations; however, minor congenital anomalies and functional defects may occur during this time.

B. **Placental transfer of drugs.** The placenta is the functional unit between the fetal and the maternal blood supply. There is no mixing of the two systems, but exchange of nutrients, oxygen, and waste products occurs primarily via passive diffusion. This process is driven by the concentration gradient between the two systems. There are a few substances that are actively transported across the placenta (e.g., amino acids); drugs that are structurally similar to these compounds will also be transported by this mechanism.

1. **Placental metabolism.** The placenta produces several pregnancy-related hormones that are mainly secreted into the maternal circulation. Some of the other substances produced by the placenta are enzymes that metabolize drugs. A common example of this is prednisone metabolism, so that very little steroid reaches the fetus.
2. **Factors affecting placental drug transfer.** For a drug to cause a teratogenic or pharmacological effect in the embryo or fetus, it must cross from the maternal circulation to the fetal circulation or tissues. Generally, the principles that apply to drug transfer across any lipid membrane can be applied to placental transfer of a drug. Most substances administered for therapeutic purposes have, by design, the ability to cross the placenta to the fetus. The critical factor is whether the rate and extent of transfer are sufficient to cause significant drug concentrations in the fetus. There are many factors that affect the rate and extent of placental drug transfer.
   a. **Molecular weight.** Low-molecular-weight drugs (< 500 Da) diffuse freely across the placenta. Drugs of a higher molecular weight (500 to 1000 Da) cross less easily. Drugs composed of very large molecules (e.g., heparin) do not cross the placental membranes.
   b. **Drug pK$_a$.** Weakly acidic and weakly basic drugs tend to rapidly diffuse across the placental membranes. Ionized compounds do not cross the placenta.
   c. **Lipid solubility.** Moderately lipid-soluble drugs easily diffuse across the placental membranes. It is important to note that many drugs have been formulated for oral administration and are designed for optimal lipid membrane transfer.
   d. **Drug absorption.** During pregnancy, gastric tone and motility are decreased, which results in delayed gastrointestinal emptying time. This typically does not affect drug absorption. However, nausea and vomiting, which are most common in the first trimester but may continue throughout pregnancy, may affect absorption.
   e. **Drug distribution.** The volume of distribution increases significantly during pregnancy and increases with advancing gestational age. The alteration in volume of distribution is the result of an increased plasma volume. Total body fluid (intravascular and extravascular volume) increases, as does adipose tissue. The placenta itself may also be a site for distribution. Hydrophilic drugs will have a higher volume of distribution leading to lower peak levels. Plasma concentrations of drugs that are widely distributed are usually lower than those with a small volume of distribution. Therefore, less drug is available to cross the placenta.
   f. **Plasma protein binding.** Placental transfer of a highly plasma-protein-bound drug is less likely because only the free drug crosses the placenta. During pregnancy, a reduction in the levels of

two major drug-binding proteins—albumin and AGP—is observed. A dilutional effect occurs with albumin and other protein concentrations, which can increase the free fraction of drugs.

g. **Physical characteristics of the placenta.** As a pregnancy progresses, the placental membranes become progressively thinner, resulting in a decrease in diffusion distance. The placenta also expands, causing a greater surface area for the transfer of substances.

h. **Maternal pharmacokinetic changes.** The dramatic increase in blood volume that occurs primarily during the first 30 weeks of pregnancy enhances blood flow through the kidneys and liver. Drugs that are excreted renally will experience a more rapid clearance, which could decrease the overall exposure time of the drug to the placenta. Metabolism of some drugs is increased, whereas others decrease; cytochrome P450 system enzymes 2D6, 2C9, and 3A4 increase in activity, whereas 1A2 and 2C19 are inhibited.

i. **Drug half-life.** Drugs that remain in circulation longer have a higher likelihood of placental passage due to the prolonged exposure.

3. **Teratogenic drugs**

a. Teratogens are defined as agents that increase the risk of or cause a congenital anomaly to occur. These defects can be structural, functional, or behavioral in nature. Women may blame a specific exposure during their pregnancy as the cause of a fetal anomaly; however, the defect may have no known cause, as is the case in 3% of all births in the United States.

b. It may take years of exposures to actually link a specific drug to certain defects. Animal studies can only suggest potential problems in humans but are often the only source of information regarding safety of agents during early pregnancy. The dose that animals often receive exceeds the normal human dose, which diminishes the applicability of these data to humans.

c. The fetus is unable to metabolize or eliminate drugs as quickly as the mother. Some substances may be excreted into the amniotic fluid and then resorbed in the fetal intestines after the fluid is swallowed. Therefore, some drugs may have a longer exposure time in the fetus, whereas others are eliminated more rapidly.

d. Because fetal organ systems develop at different times, specific teratogenic effects depend mainly on the point of gestation when the drug was ingested.

e. The teratogenic rate of substances indicates how frequently anomalies occur and over what exposure period. For example, one of the most potent known teratogens, thalidomide, had a teratogenic rate of 20% with a single exposure, yet only one-third of women who ingested the drug gave birth to affected infants. Other agents may increase the rate of specific defects over the general population, but the absolute incidence may be extremely low.

f. The FDA developed a classification system that groups drugs according to the degree of their potential risk during pregnancy.[1]

(1) **Category A.** Adequate, well-controlled studies in pregnant women have not shown an increased risk of fetal abnormalities.

(2) **Category B.** Animal studies have revealed no evidence of harm to the fetus; however, there are no adequate and well-controlled studies in pregnant women. Or animal studies have shown an adverse effect, but adequate and well-controlled studies in pregnant women have failed to demonstrate a risk to the fetus.

(3) **Category C.** Animal studies have shown an adverse effect, and there are no adequate and well-controlled studies in pregnant women. Or no animal studies have been conducted, and there are no adequate and well-controlled studies in pregnant women.

(4) **Category D.** Studies—adequate, well-controlled, or observational—in pregnant women have demonstrated a risk to the fetus. However, the benefits of therapy may outweigh the potential risk.

(5) **Category X.** Studies—adequate, well-controlled, or observational—in animals or pregnant women have demonstrated positive evidence of fetal abnormalities. The use of the product is contraindicated in women who are or may become pregnant.

g. **Problems with the current system.** The current system was created in 1979 and has not been revised since its inception. With many agents there is a paucity of human data, despite the

[1]Federal Register, June 26, 1979;44(124):37434–37467.

fact the drug may carry a category B rating. Most newly marketed agents will be placed in category C, amid other agents with little data in humans or animals. This is the most difficult category to assess. Although there may be case reports of drug exposures, these tend to bias information toward fetal risk; most publish only outcomes with potential drug-related effects. Few drugs will ever be assigned a category A status because large, randomized, well-controlled trials are rarely conducted in pregnant women.

h. Examples of teratogenic agents

(1) **Vitamin A derivatives.** Drugs such as isotretinoin (Accutane) and etretinate (Tegison) are potent teratogens in humans. These agents should be discontinued several months before pregnancy.

(2) **Warfarin** (Coumadin) is most teratogenic in the first trimester (weeks 6 to 9), but can also cause malformations during the second and third trimesters as well. Early exposure is associated with a pattern of defects known as fetal warfarin syndrome. These defects can include hypoplasia of the nose and extremities, congenital heart disease, and seizures. CNS abnormalities are increased with later use. Heparins may be an appropriate substitute when anticoagulation is necessary; however, they are not as effective for preventing thrombosis in women with artificial heart valves.

(3) **Androgenic agents** can cause virilization of female fetuses, creating ambiguous genitalia. Finasteride (Propecia) can cause genital abnormalities in male offspring. Estrogen and progestins, fortunately, do not have this effect. Many women continue to take birth control pills during the first month or two after conception until the pregnancy is discovered.

(4) **Ethanol.** Alcohol consumed in large amounts for prolonged periods during pregnancy (> 4 to 5 drinks per day) is known to cause fetal alcohol syndrome (FAS). Features of FAS include growth restriction, craniofacial dysmorphology, and CNS malfunctions, along with various other abnormalities. At least 30% of women who abuse alcohol will deliver an infant affected by FAS. Moderate alcohol consumption (2 drinks per day) can also lead to similar defects, although usually not the complete syndrome. Even though the most problematic time is during the first 2 months of pregnancy, moderate drinking during the second trimester is associated with an increased rate of spontaneous abortions.

(5) **Antineoplastics.** Many agents in this class are associated with fetal anomalies after first trimester chemotherapy administration. Growth restriction often occurs regardless of the timing of exposure. Owing to the mechanism of action of these agents, many are embryocidal.

(6) **Anticonvulsants.** Drugs such as phenytoin (Dilantin), valproic acid (Depakene), and carbamazepine (Tegretol) have all been associated with fetal anomalies. However, maternal benefit from these agents often outweighs the risk to the fetus. Anticonvulsants should not be stopped during pregnancy, but if appropriate, they should be discontinued several months before fertilization. Valproic acid and carbamazepine can increase the risk of neural tube defects; women taking these agents should receive folic acid supplementation starting before conception. Toxic epoxide radicals are thought to be the mechanism of teratogenicity with several of these agents. Genetic alterations in the epoxide hydrolase enzyme activity can reduce or increase the severity of abnormalities.

(7) **Infections.** Viral infections, such as rubella, cytomegalovirus, parvovirus, coxsackie, and varicella can be associated with growth restriction, congenital anomalies, premature delivery, and potential embryo toxicity or fetal demise. Nearly all maternal infections have been thought to cause growth restriction.

(8) **Cigarette smoking.** Cigarettes contain many toxic and carcinogenic compounds in addition to nicotine. Nicotine is a potent vasoconstricting agent capable of reducing uterine blood flow and increasing uterine vascular resistance. Smoking not only increases the risk of a growth-restricted fetus but also increases the risk of spontaneous abortions, premature delivery, placental abruption, and premature rupture of the membranes. Small increases in defects of the heart, limbs and feet, skull, urinary system, abdomen, intestines, and muscles have also been associated with cigarettes. Smoking may also alter the effects of other substances, perhaps enhancing toxicity of both agents.

4. **Other problematic therapies.** Some agents given during pregnancy may result in pharmacological effects that are not necessarily toxic, yet need to be considered when medications are given during the later weeks of pregnancy.
   a. **CNS depression** may occur with barbiturates, tranquilizers, antidepressants, and narcotics. Also, anesthetics and other agents commonly given during labor may cause significant CNS and respiratory depression in newborns (e.g., magnesium sulfate or opioid analgesics).
   b. **Neonatal bleeding.** Maternal ingestion of agents such as nonsteroidal anti-inflammatory drugs (NSAIDs) and anticoagulants at therapeutic doses near term may cause bleeding problems in the newborn.
   c. **Drug withdrawal.** Habitual maternal use of barbiturates, narcotics, benzodiazepines, alcohol, and other substances of abuse may lead to withdrawal symptoms in newborns.
   d. **Constriction of the ductus arteriosus.** Maternal use of NSAIDs in the third trimester may cause the ductus arteriosus to close prematurely and could result in pulmonary hypertension in the newborn.

IV. DRUG EXCRETION IN BREAST MILK.

Today, more than 60% of women choose to breastfeed their infants. Of these women, 90% to 95% receive a medication during the first postpartum week, most commonly for pain control after delivery. It is important to understand the principles of drug excretion in breast milk and specific information on the various medications to minimize risks from drug effects in the nursing infant.

A. **Transfer of drugs from plasma to breast milk.** Drug transfer into breast milk is governed by many of the same principles that influence human placental drug transfer.
   1. Most drugs cross into breast milk via passive diffusion along a concentration gradient formed by the un-ionized drug content on each side of the membrane.
   2. Breast milk contents change throughout a feeding. Colostrum, the very first milk produced, is much higher in protein than mature milk and the fat content is minimal. Mature milk consists of foremilk at the beginning of a feeding and hindmilk at the end. The protein and fat content increase throughout the nursing session. Therefore drugs that partition into more lipid solutions will have the highest concentration in hindmilk.
   3. A milk to plasma ratio can be determined for specific agents when both blood and milk concentrations are known. Most drugs have a ratio < 1; lower numbers indicate that less drug crosses into breast milk. Because the milk to plasma ratio may change within a feeding, the average breast milk concentration is usually used, if available.
   4. It is possible to calculate the dose an infant receives if the breast milk concentration is known. A typical infant drinks 150 mL/kg/day. Multiplying the average concentration by the breast milk volume consumed will give the total daily exposure. It is important to remember that this drug must now be ingested by the infant, so the bioavailability of the drug is critical to calculate the actual daily dose. Doses $< 10\%$ of the maternal dose on a milligram per kilogram per day basis are preferable.
   5. Some medications are not absorbed orally but may pass into breast milk when administered intravenously to the mother. Although the drug may not enter the infant's blood, it may have effects on the gastrointestinal tract. For example, the bioavailability of gentamicin is negligible; however, it may cause diarrhea or sterilize the bowel.

B. **Drug factors.** The drug and its environment influence the rate and extent of drug passage into the breast milk.
   1. **Molecular weight.** Drugs weighing < 200 Da cross into milk easily. Larger molecules can dissolve in the lipid membrane or pass through small pores. Large molecules, such as insulin, do not cross into breast milk.
   2. **pH gradient.** Human milk is more acidic than plasma.
      a. Weak acids may diffuse across the membrane and remain un-ionized, allowing for passage back into the plasma. Lower amounts of these drugs will cross than those that are weak bases.
      b. Weak bases may diffuse into the breast milk and ionize, which causes drug trapping. This creates higher levels of drug in the breast milk; these drugs will have a milk to plasma ratio > 1. This effect though is not usually clinically significant, especially when the maternal serum concentration is very low.

3. **Drug pK_a.** Only the un-ionized form of a drug is able to pass through the lipid membrane.
4. **Plasma protein binding.** The free fraction of a drug is available to pass into the breast milk. In general, drugs with high plasma-protein-binding properties tend to remain in the plasma and pass into the milk in low concentrations. Milk proteins and lipids also may bind drugs when they are created in the mammary glands; this may represent another route of entry, rather than passive diffusion.
5. **Lipid solubility.** Lipid solubility is necessary for a drug to pass into the breast milk. Highly lipid-soluble drugs (e.g., diazepam [Valium]) may pass into the breast milk in relatively high amounts and, therefore, may present a significant dose of drug to the nursing infant.
6. **Equilibration.** Some drugs may rapidly equilibrate between maternal plasma and breast milk. These agents will diffuse across the membrane as the drug concentration changes in the maternal system. Other agents may never reach equilibrium between milk and plasma. These drugs tend to slowly diffuse into breast milk and will respond gradually to changes in maternal concentrations.

C. **Maternal factors.** Maternal pharmacology plays a significant role in the rate and extent of drug passage into breast milk. The extent of plasma protein binding and changes in the mother's ability to metabolize or eliminate the drug influence the amount of drug that is available to pass into the breast milk. Equally important are the maternal dose of the drug, the dosing schedule or frequency, and the route of administration.

D. **Drugs affecting hormonal influence of breast milk production.** The primary hormone responsible for controlling breast milk production is prolactin. A decrease in milk production may result in diminished weight gain in the nursing infant, the need for supplementation, or premature cessation of breastfeeding.

1. **Drugs that decrease serum prolactin levels.** Drugs such as bromocriptine have been used to suppress lactation in women who choose not to breastfeed. This practice has long been abandoned because myocardial infarctions, seizures, and stroke were attributed to its use. Other drugs include
   a. ergot alkaloids
   b. L-dopa
2. **Drugs that increase serum prolactin levels.** Metoclopramide (Reglan) has been useful therapeutically to enhance milk production. The following drugs are known to increase serum prolactin levels, but they are not used for this purpose. These drugs include
   a. methyldopa (Aldomet)
   b. haloperidol (Haldol)
   c. phenothiazines

E. **Factors to assess.** In assessing the safety of an agent during breastfeeding, several considerations should be addressed.

1. Inherent toxicity of the drug
2. Drug safety data in infants
3. Amount of drug ingested
4. Duration of therapy
5. Age of the infant or degree of prematurity
6. Drug pharmacokinetics in the mother and child

F. **Factors to minimize drug exposure to the infant.** One of the goals when using medications in the breastfeeding mother is to maintain a natural, uninterrupted pattern of nursing. In many instances, it may be possible to withhold a drug when it is not essential or delay therapy until after weaning. Other factors include

1. **Medication selection.** When a specific product is being selected, it is important to choose the agent that is distributed into the milk the least, if possible.
   a. Other desirable characteristics include a short half-life, inactive metabolites, and high protein binding.
   b. In addition, it is desirable to select agents with lower plasma concentrations, which may involve an alternative route of administration.
   c. Single doses may be preferable to a longer therapy course if the agent is contraindicated in breastfeeding. This can allow for the mother to pump and discard her milk for a defined time, often 12 to 24 hrs, rather than discontinue breastfeeding altogether.

2. **Maternal dose relative to infant feeding.** One of the goals of drug dosing in lactating women is minimal infant exposure to the drug. It is desirable to adjust the dosing and nursing schedules so that a drug dose is administered at the time of or immediately after the infant's feeding. Medications should be dosed before the infant's longest sleep.

G. **Examples of drugs that readily enter breast milk.** These agents should be used with caution in nursing mothers.
   1. **Narcotics, barbiturates, and benzodiazepines.** CNS active agents, such as diazepam, may have a hypnotic effect on the nursing infant. These effects are related to the maternal dose. Alcohol consumption may have a similar effect.
   2. **Antidepressants and antipsychotics.** These classes of drugs appear to pass into the breast milk; however, no serious adverse effects have been reported. The long-term behavioral effects of chronic exposure to these drugs on developing newborns are unknown.
   3. **Anticholinergic compounds.** These drugs may result in adverse CNS effects in the infant and may reduce milk volume in the mother. Dicyclomine (Bentyl) is contraindicated in nursing mothers because it may result in neonatal apnea.

V. INCONTINENCE

A. **Definition.** Incontinence is defined as an inability to control urine or feces elimination. There are four major types of urinary incontinence: stress, urge (overactive bladder), overflow, and mixed (stress and urge incontinence).

B. **Epidemiology.** The reported incidence of urinary incontinence varies widely, ranging from 10% to 35% in women. Incontinence becomes more common as women age but is not a normal part of aging.

C. **Cause.** Gender, age, hormonal status, birthing trauma, and genetic differences in connective tissue all contribute to the development of incontinence.

D. **Diagnosis** is made with a voiding diary (frequency of urination, leakage of urine, symptoms during urination such as pain or discomfort, or the need to strain or splint to urinate), a physical examination, surgical and obstetric history, medication history, mental status examination in the elderly, and a urinalysis. Special diagnostic procedures, such as a cystourethrogram, can be performed if the initial diagnosis and treatment is ineffective.

E. **Stress urinary incontinence** (SUI) involves the involuntary loss of urine during physical activity that increases the intra-abdominal pressure (e.g., coughing, sneezing). This is usually caused by urethral underactivity, decreased tone of the urethral sphincter, or hypersensitivity of the bladder neck.
   1. **Treatment** of SUI usually involves
      a. **Behavioral therapy.** Bladder retraining involves voiding on a schedule, usually hourly to start. Once this is managed without leakage, the time between voids is increased by 15-min intervals, until the elapsed time between voids is between 2 and 4 hrs. Pelvic floor muscle strengthening, known as Kegel exercises, can reduce incontinence by up to 50%.
      b. **Weight loss** of 5% to 10% can dramatically improve symptoms especially in the postpartum period when stress incontinence is a common problem.
      c. **Fluid restriction** to less than 2L daily.
      d. **Drug therapy**
         (1) **Vaginal estrogen** improves tone and blood supply of the urethral sphincter muscles increasing urethral closure pressure and increasing mucosal thickness, thus improving functioning.
         (2) **Alpha-adrenergic agents** induce muscle contraction in the bladder neck and urethra, increasing outlet resistance. Pseudoephedrine (Sudafed) is the remaining agent in this class.
         (3) **Duloxetine** (Cymbalta) which has a direct effect on the urethra (enhancing closure) via peripheral adrenergic activation (40 to 80 mg daily).
         (4) **Imipramine** (Tofranil), a tricyclic antidepressant, decreases bladder contractility and increases outlet resistance. Doses of 75 mg once daily and 25 mg three times daily have been successful in studies.
      e. **Surgical options.** Colposuspension elevates the bladder neck and the urethra, restoring the urethrovesical junction; sling procedures elevate the urethra and increase urethral

compression; or tension-free tape reduces urethral mobility or produces a kink in the urethra during increases in intra-abdominal pressure.

F. **Urge incontinence** is described by the sudden sense of needing to urinate followed by the loss of urine. This involuntary contraction of the bladder or bladder overactivity is known as detrusor instability. The detrusor is the muscle located in the bladder wall; relaxation allows bladder to expand. Another common symptom is frequent urination during the day and night.

1. **Treatment** of urge incontinence involves

a. **Behavioral therapy.** Bladder retraining entails initially voiding every 1 to 1.5 hrs even if leakage or the urge to void occurs before this time, eventually increasing the interval by 30 mins until 3 to 4 hrs elapses between voids. Also, avoiding foods that may irritate the bladder such as caffeine, carbonation, acidic foods, and spicy foods is helpful.

b. **Drug therapy**

(1) **Anticholinergic agents** act on muscarinic receptors to decrease contractility. However, these agents have the potential to cause significant side effects, especially in the elderly. Extended-release formulations usually have lower anticholinergic effects.

(a) **oxybutynin** (Ditropan, Ditropan XL, Oxytrol), 2.5 mg to 5.0 mg two to four times daily, 5 mg to 30 mg daily extended-release, 3.9 mg patch twice weekly.

(b) **tolterodine** (Detrol, Detrol LA), 2 mg twice daily or 4 mg daily extended-release. The dose should be decreased by 50% in women taking CYP3A4 inhibitors.

(c) **trospium** (Sanctura), 20 mg twice daily, adjusted to 20 mg daily in renal impairment or elderly women ($>$ 75 years).

(d) **darifenacin** (Enablex), 7.5 to 15 mg daily, women with moderate hepatic impairment or taking CYP3A4 inhibitors should not receive more than 7.5 mg daily.

(e) **solifenacin** (VESIcare), 5 to 10 mg daily with 5 mg daily recommended in women with renal impairment, moderate hepatic impairment, or in those taking CYP3A4 inhibitors.

(2) **Flavoxate** (Urispas) is a urinary antispasmodic that can be helpful. Doses range from 100 to 200 mg three to four times daily.

c. **Surgery.** Augmentation cystoplasty uses intestinal segments to improve the storage function of the bladder.

G. **Overflow incontinence** is a constant loss of urine or inadequate bladder emptying. This type of incontinence is not common in women. Women with neurological impairment who may not feel the urge to void are predisposed to this type of incontinence because of bladder overdistention. A post-void residual, measuring the urine volume remaining in the bladder after urination, can make this diagnosis. A blockage in the urethra can also cause overflow incontinence.

1. **Treatment**

a. **Behavioral therapy.** Voiding or self-catheterization should occur at specific intervals to prevent overdistention. In severe cases of neurological impairment (such as significant dementia), the patient may require incontinence pads or long-term catheterization.

b. **Drug therapy.** Tamsulosin (Flomax) may be helpful by relaxing striated and smooth muscle, decreasing urethral resistance, and relieving symptoms. Initial doses should be 0.4 mg daily with a maximum of 0.8 mg daily. It is important to note that some women receiving alpha-adrenergic blocking agents for hypertension develop incontinence.

c. **Surgery.** Surgery may be required if a urethral blockage is the cause of incontinence.

VI. MENOPAUSE

A. **Definition.** Menopause is defined as the irreversible cessation of the reproductive cycle and menses after the ovaries permanently fail to respond to gonadotropins. Removal of the ovaries (oophorectomy) in premenopausal women and premature ovarian failure also will lead to menopausal symptoms. Menopause occurs naturally around age 51, but often occurs earlier in smokers due to increased estrogen metabolism in these women.

B. **Symptoms.** Symptoms of menopause are due to the lack of estrogen. They include vasomotor instability (hot flushes), atrophic changes of the vagina and urethra/bladder (symptoms of burning, itching, bleeding, dyspareunia/painful intercourse, or incontinence), and a menopausal syndrome (sleep disturbances and mood swings).

Table 29-2 EFFICACY OF NONHORMONAL THERAPY ON HOT FLASHES

Therapy	Initial Dose	Study Results, % Decrease in Hot Flashes
Venlafaxine (Effexor)	75 mg XL daily	61% vs. 27% with placebo
Paroxetine (Paxil)	10 mg daily	50%–51% vs. 16% with placebo
Fluoxetine (Prozac)	20 mg daily	50% vs. 36% with placebo
Gabapentin (Neurontin)	300 mg TID	41% vs. 29% with placebo
Clonidine (Catapres)	0.5 mg PO BID or 0.1 mg/day TD weekly	37% vs. 20% with placebo 80% vs. 36% with placebo
Methyldopa (Aldomet)	250 mg BID	Visual analog scale improvement

PO, by mouth; *TID*, three times daily; *BID*, twice daily; *TD*, transdermal; *XL*, extended release.

C. **Treatment**
1. **Lifestyle changes.** Recommendations include lowering the core body temperature by dressing in layers, consuming cold food and beverages, and using cooling techniques, such as a fan or cold towels placed on the back of the neck.
2. **Hormone therapy.** Hormone therapy has become controversial in recent years but can be helpful in very symptomatic women. The lowest dose for the shortest duration is the current recommendation. Estrogen decreases the risk of colon cancer and decreases the risk of noninsulin dependent diabetes. However, combined hormone therapy can increase the risk for breast cancer, whereas estrogen alone does not appear to have this effect. Estrogen also increases cardiovascular risks and thromboses.
3. **Nonhormonal therapy.** Many other therapies have been studied for the treatment of vasomotor symptoms (*Table 29-2*).
4. **Herbal therapies/phytoestrogens.** Many therapies have been studied, but few agents have been shown to be more effective than placebo.
   a. **Black cohosh** possibly decreases hot flashes, but therapy should be limited to 6 months or less. Black cohosh can increase the density of breast tissue, making mammograms more difficult to interpret.
   b. **Red clover** has a small decrease in frequency of hot flushes over placebo.
   c. **Soy** has not been shown to be beneficial in many studies.
   d. **Other herbs.** Other herbs studied or recommended by some for hot flashes include ginseng, dong quai, damiana, licorice, motherwort, fennel, and evening primrose oil.

VII. OSTEOPOROSIS

A. **Definition.** Osteoporosis can be defined as an imbalance of osteoblast and osteoclast activity. Osteoblasts form bone, whereas osteoclasts break down bone (resorption). Receptor activator of nuclear factor kappa-B (RANK) and osteoprotegerin (OPG) are proteins that are intimately involved with bone remodeling. RANK is key for the differentiation and activation of osteoclasts. OPG has the opposite effect, blocking the effects of RANK by binding to the RANK ligand. The ultimate result of OPG is to decrease the activity of osteoclasts, thus preventing bone resorption.

B. **Epidemiology.** In 2009, approximately 13% of the American population was > 65 years of age, representing nearly 38 million Americans. The risk of a fracture doubles every 7 to 8 years in women older than the age of 50. Nonmodifiable risk factors for osteoporosis include female sex, age, low body mass index, small frame, family history of osteoporosis, menopausal status, and ethnicity/race. In an observational study, osteoporosis was diagnosed in different ethnicities. Women with highest risk to lowest rate of osteoporosis were Native Americans > Asians > Hispanics > Caucasians > African Americans. Risk factors that can be modified include alcohol intake > 3 servings per day, low activity level, smoking, and estrogen deficiency.

C. **Diagnosis.** Routine health care should include measuring height; vertebral fractures will shorten stature and having one vertebral fracture increases the risk for more. Screening for osteoporosis should be done in women 60 to 64 years with one major risk factor and all women > 65 years, women with a low trauma fracture, women who have lost > 0.5 inch of height within 1 year or > 1.5 inches overall, and to monitor therapy. The World Health Organization developed the Fracture Risk Assessment tool (FRAX) to evaluate a woman's risk of having a hip or any major osteoporotic fracture over the next 10 years. It takes into account family history and many risk factors. It is only indicated in women > 50 years who have not started any drug therapy for osteoporosis. Peripheral bone mineral density scans can be done at community health screenings using heel ultrasonography on the nondominant foot. These screenings can help identify women who need further screening with a dual energy x-ray absorptiometry (DXA) scan. The DXA scan is the gold standard and bone mineral density (BMD) is measured at the hip and spine. The results generate a T score; a score of −1 to −2.5 indicates low bone mass/osteopenia and a score ≤ −2.5 makes the diagnosis of osteoporosis. A DXA scan should not be performed more frequently than every 1 to 2 years.

D. **Therapy**

1. **Lifestyle changes** are important to increase bone mass. Adolescent and young women need to build bone early in life. A healthy lifestyle incorporates weight bearing exercises such as walking and isometric exercises such as weight lifting, not smoking, and limiting alcohol and caffeine intake. Sunlight converts vitamin D into an active form in the skin, but adequate exposure is difficult for most women to achieve. Using suntan lotion negates the effect of sunlight and only more equatorial areas of the world have enough direct sunlight during the winter months.
2. **Calcium and vitamin D.** Adequate calcium ingestion may not occur with dietary intake and supplementation is often recommended. Vitamin D has been shown in studies to decrease the number of falls, thus reducing the number of fractures. The recommended intake of calcium according to the National Osteoporosis Foundation (NOF) is 1200 mg with 800 to 1000 international units of vitamin D for women older than age 50. Calcium therapy taken without vitamin D might increase the risk of myocardial infarctions.
3. **Bisphosphonates** are selected as first line in many women (*Table 29-3*). They are effective in reducing fractures in the hip and spine, working to decrease osteoclast activity. Oral dosing is complicated by their poor absorption when taken within 1 hr of a meal or beverage. They also require the woman to remain upright after dosing to prevent esophageal irritation and erosion. They can cause unusual side effects, such as jaw necrosis and atypical fractures of the femur. They are generally contraindicated in women with a creatinine clearance less than 30 mL/min. The duration of therapy is not completely established, although 5 years is recommended by some experts.
4. **Hormone therapy.** Estrogens inhibit bone resorption and promote bone formation. They reduce fractures in the hip, spine, and nonvertebral locations. Bone mass is maintained with conjugated equine estrogen doses of 0.3 mg daily. The higher the estrogen dose, the higher the increase in BMD; however, the lowest dose of estrogen should be used in naturally postmenopausal women to control vasomotor symptoms.
5. **Selective estrogen receptor modulators** (SERMs). Raloxifene (Evista) increases BMD spine and hip and reduces vertebral fractures. Raloxifene is helpful in women also needing protection against breast cancer, but the agent can cause menopausal symptoms in women due to its estrogen antagonism in selective tissues. The dose for prevention and treatment of osteoporosis is 60 mg daily.

Table 29-3 BISPHOSPHONATES FOR OSTEOPOROSIS TREATMENT AND PREVENTION

Bisphosphonate	Treatment Dose	Prophylaxis Dose	Fracture Reduction
Alendronate (Fosamax)	10 mg daily PO or 70 mg PO weekly	5.0 mg PO daily or 35 mg PO weekly	50% H, V, NV
Risedronate (Actonel)	5.0 mg PO daily or 35 mg PO weekly or 150 mg PO monthly	Same as treatment regimens	35%–45% V, NV
Ibandronate (Boniva)	2.5 mg PO daily or 150 mg PO monthly or 3.0 mg IV monthly	Same as treatment regimens	50% V
Zoledronic Acid (Reclast)	5.0 mg IV yearly	5.0 mg IV every other year	51% H, 70% V

H, hip fracture; *V*, vertebral (spine) fracture; *NV*, nonvertebral fracture; *PO*, by mouth; *IV*, intravenous.

Table 29-4 EFFICACY OF VARIOUS OSTEOPOROSIS MEDICATIONS

Therapy	↓ Hip Fx	↓ Spine Fx	↓ Nonspine Fx	↑ BMD
Estrogen	34%	35%		5%[a]
Raloxifene		40%		
Bisphosphonates	40%	60%		3.3%–4.8%
Calcitonin		33%		1%
Teriparatide	35%	65%	35%	5%
Denosumab	40%	68%	20%	5%

Fx, fracture; *BMD*, bone mineral density.
[a] with 1.25 mg daily conjugated equine estrogens.

6. **Calcitonin.** Calcitonin (Miacalcin) works on osteoclasts to inhibit bone resorption. It helps maintain a normal calcium level in serum and increases bone stores. Calcitonin is helpful with the pain associated with vertebral fractures. It is most commonly administered intranasally but is also available in an injectable formulation for subcutaneous or intramuscular administration. Parenteral doses are 100 mcg every other day, whereas the intranasal is 200 mcg daily in alternating nostrils.
7. **Teriparatide.** Teriparatide (Forteo) is recombinant human parathyroid hormone that is administered subcutaneously daily (20 mcg). It stimulates osteoblast activity, increases gastric absorption and renal reabsorption of calcium, increases BMD in the hip and spine, and prevents vertebral fractures. It is not considered first line due to cost and a lack of long-term data. It must be kept refrigerated, making this therapy more difficult for some women.
8. **Denosumab.** Denosumab (Prolia) is a monoclonal antibody that binds to the RANK ligand, inhibiting osteoclast formation and activity. Essentially, it works like OPG. It is effective at reducing fractures of the hip, spine, and nonvertebral sites. Denosumab is a subcutaneous injection of 60 mg given every 6 months. It is indicated in women who have failed or are intolerant to other osteoporosis therapies (*Table 29-4*).

Study Questions

Directions for questions 1–8: Each of the questions, statements, or incomplete statements in these sections can be correctly answered or completed by **one** of the suggested answers or phrases. Choose the **best** answer.

1. A 23-year-old woman was diagnosed with significant PMS in her teens, now presents with persistent irritation with her significant other resulting in frequent arguments. Possible therapies for her include all of the following *except*
   (A) sertraline 100 mg days 14 to 28.
   (B) paroxetine 30 mg daily.
   (C) venlafaxine XR 75 mg daily.
   (D) clonazepam 1 mg twice daily.
   (E) citalopram 20 mg daily.

2. The best therapy for an obese woman with PCOS to improve menstrual regularity will be
   (A) spironolactone.
   (B) metformin.
   (C) weight loss.
   (D) pioglitazone.

3. Which of the following therapies enhances osteoblast activity?
   (A) Calcium and vitamin D
   (B) Calcitonin
   (C) Denosumab
   (D) Teriparatide
   (E) Risedronate

4. Which of the following medications is safe to use in the third trimester of pregnancy?
   (A) Acetaminophen
   (B) Nonsteroidal anti-inflammatory drugs
   (C) Warfarin
   (D) OxyContin
   (E) Aspirin

5. Placental transfer of a drug is affected by all of the following characteristics *except*
   (A) molecular weight.
   (B) fetal gender.
   (C) gestational age.
   (D) lipid solubility of the drug.
   (E) plasma protein binding.

6. When selecting a benzodiazepine product for a woman who has chronic panic disorder, all of the following drug properties are desirable for breastfeeding her 8-month-old infant who was born at term *except*
   (A) hepatic metabolism to inactive metabolites.
   (B) a short half-life.
   (C) a rapid onset of action.
   (D) high lipid solubility.

7. Drug safety in pregnancy of a specific agent can be assessed best by
   (A) the FDA classification system, especially category C drugs.
   (B) case reports.
   (C) physician knowledge.
   (D) databases such as REPROTOX.

8. The primary difference between PMS and PMDD is
   (A) PMS has an earlier onset of symptoms.
   (B) PMS is more debilitating.
   (C) PMDD can be treated with antidepressants.
   (D) PMDD is more common.

Directions for questions 9–12: The questions and incomplete statements in this section can be correctly answered or completed by **one or more** of the suggested answers. Choose the answer, **A–E.**

(A) if **I only** is correct
(B) if **III only** is correct
(C) if **I and II** are correct
(D) if **II and III** are correct
(E) if **I, II, and III** are correct

9. The definition of polycystic ovarian syndrome includes
   I. hyperandrogenism
   II. diabetes
   III. obesity

10. Therapy for stress urinary incontinence can include
   I. oxybutynin
   II. tamsulosin
   III. imipramine

11. Behavioral therapy and bladder retraining is most helpful in which types of incontinence?
   I. stress incontinence
   II. urge incontinence
   III. overflow incontinence

12. According to the principles of drug excretion into the breast milk, which combination of the following properties would result in the *highest* drug concentration in breast milk?
   I. low molecular weight, moderately lipophilic
   II. low plasma protein bound, weakly basic
   III. highly plasma protein bound, weakly acidic

13. Following principles of teratogenicity, drug exposure during which of the following times could cause fetal abnormalities?
   I. first 2 weeks of gestation
   II. weeks 3 to 8 of gestation
   III. the fetal period

Answers and Explanations

1. **The answer is D** *[see I.D.6 and Table 29-1].*
Clonazepam can be used in premenstrual dysphoric syndrome but should be limited to women who have anxiety as the most prevalent symptom. That is not the case for this woman. All of the remaining agents are appropriate for PMDD. Luteal phase dosing has been studied and may not be as effective as daily therapy.

2. **The answer is C** *[see II.E.1.3-5].*
Weight loss of 5% to 10% can restore cycle regularity in more than 50% of women. Weight loss and an appropriate diet will also decrease insulin and androgen levels. Spironolactone is helpful for hirsutism but not cycle regularity. Metformin and thiazolidinediones have both been used to improve ovulation and thus cycle regularity. Metformin can also reduce the risk of diabetes development; however, weight loss in the long run will provide the most benefit to the patient.

3. **The answer is D** *[see VII.D.2-8].*
Teriparatide increases bone mass by stimulating osteoblast activity. Estrogens also stimulate osteoblast activity, but other therapies work by inhibiting osteoclast activity. Denosumab involves the RANK ligand, which then inhibits osteoclast activity.

4. **The answer is A** *[see III.B.3.e.(1)–(2);III.B.4.a–d].*
Acetaminophen is a safe and effective analgesic that can be used in therapeutic doses during pregnancy. NSAIDs may interfere with the onset or progress of labor when used in the third trimester. NSAIDs and warfarin, when used near delivery, may cause bleeding problems in the newborn infant. In addition, warfarin use in the third trimester may be associated with fetal CNS abnormalities. OxyContin use in the third trimester may induce neonatal withdrawal following delivery.

5. **The answer is B** *[see III.B.2].*
Fetal gender does not affect placental transfer of a drug. The molecular weight and the lipid solubility of a drug greatly influence its ability to cross the placental membranes. Plasma protein binding affects the amount of free drug available to cross the placenta. Gestational age influences the volume of distribution of the drug as well as the thickness of the placental membranes.

6. **The answer is D** *[see IV.B.5; IV.F.1.a].*
When any drug is used by a nursing mother, it is desirable to have the least amount of active drug available in the maternal circulation to diffuse into the breast milk. A rapidly acting (for maternal onset of action), rapidly eliminated (i.e., short half-life) drug with inactive metabolites is optimal. If the drug is highly lipid soluble, it is more likely to pass into breast milk.

7. **The answer is D** *[see III.B.3.f].*
The FDA classification system does not assess risk well in category C drugs. Category A and to some extent category B drugs have been shown to be safest in pregnancy. Case reports of pregnancy exposures tend to bias data toward adverse outcomes. The best source of information is from available databases, such as REPROTOX or Teris, or with published books such as Brigg's *Drugs in Pregnancy and Lactation.*

8. **The answer is C** *[see I.A].*
PMDD is more debilitating than PMS, usually due to major depression that can accompany the other symptoms. Several antidepressants are available for treatment of PMDD. The onset of symptoms varies with both conditions. PMS is much more common than PMDD.

9. **The answer is A (I)** *[see II.A,B].*
The definition of polycystic ovarian syndrome includes hyperandrogenism and hyperinsulinemia. Insulin resistance is common and diabetes can result, but these conditions are not part of the diagnosis. Only half of the women with PCOS are obese.

10. **The answer is B (III)** *[see V.E.1.d.(4)].*
Imipramine is helpful to paralyze the bladder, leading to decreased contractility. Oxybutynin is an anticholinergic agent indicated for urge incontinence. The use of this agent can be helpful in mixed incontinence. Tamsulosin is helpful in some cases of overflow incontinence and this agent can certainly worsen stress incontinence.

11. **The answer is E (I, II, III)** *[see V.E.1.a; V.F.1.a; V.G.1.a].*
Bladder retraining and behavioral therapy is helpful for all types of incontinence. The type of bladder retraining depends on the type of incontinence although the concepts are similar between stress and urge incontinence. Overflow incontinence bladder also involves voiding at regular intervals, but they are typically not as frequent as those involved with the other types of incontinence.

12. **The answer is C (I, II)** *[see IV.B.1–5].*
High-molecular-weight substances are less likely to pass into breast milk because of their size. Drugs that are highly plasma protein bound may reach the breast milk only in small amounts, because a large portion of the drug is bound to the maternal plasma proteins and, therefore, only a small amount is free to diffuse into breast milk. A low molecular weight, moderately lipophilic drug passes easily into breast milk. A drug that has a low degree of plasma protein binding has a significant amount of drug free to diffuse into breast milk. A weakly basic drug may ionize after reaching the breast milk and therefore remain trapped in the milk.

13. **The answer is D (II, III)** *[see III.A.1–3].*
During first 2 weeks after fertilization, the embryo is impervious to teratogens. Any exposure during this time will have either no effect or the embryo will be destroyed. During the remaining weeks of the pregnancy, teratogens may exert effects on the fetus. Teratogenic effects are not always structural in nature; they can be functional or behavioral. Therefore, exposures during the fetal period can also be problematic.

30 Clinical Laboratory Tests

D. BYRON MAY

I. GENERAL PRINCIPLES

A. **Laboratory tests** are performed for multiple purposes, including to discover a disease, confirm or differentiate a diagnosis, stage or classify a disease, and monitor effectiveness of therapy.

B. **Laboratory tests are classified as screening or diagnostic.** Screening tests are used in patients with no signs or symptoms of a disease (e.g., serum cholesterol for assessing cardiovascular disease risk). Diagnostic tests are done in patients with signs and symptoms of disease or with an abnormal screening test.

C. **Monitoring drug therapy**

1. **Laboratory test results** are used to investigate potential problems with a patient's anatomy or physiology. Pharmacists usually monitor laboratory tests to
   a. **Assess the therapeutic and adverse effects of a drug** (e.g., monitoring the serum uric acid level after allopurinol is administered, checking for increased liver function test values after administration of isoniazid)
   b. **Determine the proper drug dose** (e.g., assessment of the serum creatinine or creatinine clearance value before use of a renally excreted drug)
   c. **Assess the need for additional or alternate drug therapy** (e.g., assessment of white blood cell count after an antibiotic is administered)
   d. **Prevent test misinterpretation resulting from drug interference** (e.g., determination of a false-positive result for a urine glucose test after cephalosporin administration)
2. These tests can be **expensive**, and requests for them must be balanced against potential benefits for patients and how the laboratory test will affect your decision regarding therapy. Generally, lab tests should be ordered only if the results will affect the decisions about the management of the patient.

D. **Definition of normal values**

1. **Normal laboratory test results** fall within a predetermined range of values, and **abnormal values** fall outside that range. The normal range of a laboratory test is usually determined by applying statistical methods to results from a representative sample of the general population. Usually, the mean $\pm$ 2 standard deviations is taken as the normal range.
   a. **Normal limits may be defined somewhat arbitrarily**; thus, values outside the normal range may not necessarily indicate disease or the need for treatment (e.g., asymptomatic hyperuricemia).
   b. Many factors (e.g., age, sex, time since last meal) must be taken into account when evaluating test results.
   c. **Normal values also vary among institutions** and may depend on the method used to perform the test.
   d. The goal is *not* to make all laboratory values normal; resist urges to do something in a clinically stable patient.
   e. Attempts have been made in recent years to standardize the presentation of laboratory data by using the International System of Units (SI units). Controversy surrounds this issue in the United States, and resistance to adopt this system continues. The SI unit of measure is a method of reporting clinical laboratory data in a standard metric format. The basic unit of mass for the SI is the mole. The mole is not influenced by the addition of excess weight of salt or ester formulations. Technically and pharmacologically, the mole is more meaningful than the gram because each physiological reaction occurs on a molecular level.

Efforts to implement the SI system began in the 1970s, resulting in the adoption of full SI-transition policies by a few major medical and pharmaceutical journals in the 1980s. Reluctance to use this system by many clinicians in the United States has forced changes in the policies by some journals to report both conventional and SI units or to report the conversion factor between the two systems. It is still controversial which method should be used to report clinical laboratory values. There are arguments for and against the universal conversion to the SI system. Readers should be aware that some journals report SI and/or conventional units in their text. Particular attention should be paid to the units associated with a reported laboratory value, and access to a conversion table may be necessary to avoid confusion in the interpretation of the data. When appropriate, both conventional and SI units will be reported in this chapter.

2. **Laboratory error** must always be considered when **test results do not correlate with expected results for a given patient**. If necessary, the test should be repeated. Common sources of laboratory error include spoiled specimens, incomplete specimens, specimens taken at the wrong time, faulty reagents, technical errors, incorrect procedures, and failure to take diet or medication into account.
3. During hospital admission or routine physical examination, a **battery of tests** is usually given to augment the history and physical examination. Basic tests may include an electrocardiogram (ECG), a chest x-ray, a sequential multiple analyzer **(SMA) profile**, **electrolyte tests (e.g., Chemistry or Basic Metabolic Panel [BMP])**, **a complete blood count** (**CBC**), and **urinalysis**.

E. **Quantitative tests, qualitative tests, and analytical performance**

1. Tests with normal values reported in ranges (i.e., 3.5 to 5.0 mEq/L) are called **quantitative**.
2. Tests with **positive (+)** or **negative (−)** outcomes are called **qualitative**.
3. Those with varying degrees of positivity (e.g., 1+, 2+, 3+ glucose in the urine) are termed **semiquantitative**.
4. The quality of a quantitative assay is measured in terms of **accuracy** (accuracy is defined as the extent to which the mean measurement is close to the true value). **Precision** refers to the reproducibility of the assay.

II. HEMATOLOGICAL TESTS.

Blood contains three types of formed elements: red blood cells (RBCs), white blood cells (WBCs), and platelets (*Figure 30-1*). A CBC typically includes RBC count, total WBC count, hemoglobin (Hb), hematocrit (Hct), RBC indices (mean cell volume [MCV], mean cell Hb [MCH], mean cell Hb concentration [MCHC]), reticulocyte count, and platelet count.

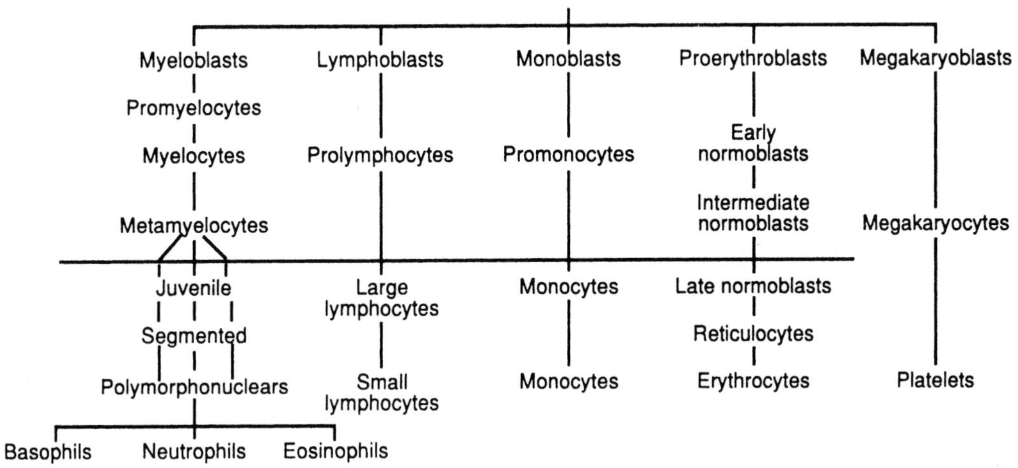

Figure 30-1. Derivation of blood elements from stem cells. Cells located below the *horizontal* line are found in normal peripheral blood, with the exception of the late normoblasts.

Table 30-2 EXAMPLES OF CHANGES IN TOTAL WHITE BLOOD CELL (WBC) COUNT AND WBC DIFFERENTIAL IN RESPONSE TO BACTERIAL INFECTION

	WBC Count	
Cell Type	**Normal**	**With Bacterial Infection**
Total WBCs	8,000 (100%)	15,500 (100%)
Neutrophils		
Polymorphonuclear leukocytes	60%	82%
Bands	3%	6%
Lymphocytes	30%	10%
Monocytes	4%	1%
Eosinophils	2%	1%
Basophils	1%	0%

(2) **Neutrophilic leukocytosis.** This describes a response to an appropriate stimulus in which the total neutrophil count increases, often with an increase in the percentage of immature cells (**a shift to the left**). This may represent a systemic bacterial infection, such as pneumonia (*Table 30-2*).

(a) **Certain viruses** (e.g., chickenpox, herpes zoster), some **rickettsial diseases** (e.g., Rocky Mountain spotted fever), some **fungi**, and **stress** (e.g., physical exercise, acute hemorrhage or hemolysis, acute emotional stress) may also cause this response.

(b) Other causes include **inflammatory diseases** (e.g., acute rheumatic fever, rheumatoid arthritis, acute gout), **hypersensitivity reactions to drugs**, **tissue necrosis** (e.g., from myocardial infarction, burns, certain cancers), **metabolic disorders** (e.g., uremia, diabetic ketoacidosis), **myelogenous leukemia**, and **use of certain drugs** (e.g., epinephrine, lithium).

(3) **Neutropenia**, a decreased number of neutrophils, may occur with an **overwhelming infection of any type** (bone marrow is unable to keep up with the demand). It may also occur with **certain viral infections** (e.g., mumps, measles), with **idiosyncratic drug reactions**, and as a result of chemotherapy. Neutropenia is defined as an absolute neutrophil count (ANC) of < 1000 cells/mm^3. Some define absolute neutropenia as an ANC of < 500 cells/mm^3. The ANC is calculated by multiplying the percent of neutrophils by the total WBC count:

$$\text{WBC} = 4000/\text{mm}^3$$
$$\text{neutrophils} = 60\%$$
$$\text{ANC} = 4000 \times 0.6 = 2400 \text{ cells/mm}^3$$

b. **Basophils** stain deeply with blue basic dye. Their function in the circulation is not clearly understood; in the tissues, they are referred to as **mast cells**.

(1) **Basophilia**, an increased number of basophils, may occur with chronic myelogenous leukemia (CML) as well as other conditions.

(2) A decrease in basophils is generally not apparent because of the small numbers of these cells in the blood.

c. **Eosinophils** stain deep red with acid dye and are classically associated with immune reactions. **Eosinophilia**, an increased number of eosinophils, may occur with such conditions as **acute allergic reactions** (e.g., **asthma**, **hay fever**, **drug allergy**) and **parasitic infestations** (e.g., trichinosis, amebiasis).

d. **Lymphocytes** play a dominant role in immunological activity and appear to produce antibodies. They are classified as B lymphocytes or T lymphocytes; T lymphocytes are further divided into helper-inducer cells (T_H4 cells) and suppressor cells (T_H8 cells).

(1) **Lymphocytosis**, an increased number of lymphocytes, usually accompanies a normal or decreased total WBC count and is most commonly caused by **viral infection**.

(2) **Lymphopenia**, a decreased number of lymphocytes, may result from **severe debilitating illness**, **immunodeficiency**, or from **AIDS**, which has a propensity to attack T_H4 cells.

(3) **Atypical lymphocytes** (i.e., T lymphocytes in a state of immune activation) are classically associated with **infectious mononucleosis**.

e. **Monocytes** are phagocytic cells. **Monocytosis**, an increased number of monocytes, may occur with **tuberculosis (TB)**, **subacute bacterial endocarditis**, and during the recovery phase of some **acute infections**.

C. **Platelets (thrombocytes).** These are the smallest formed elements in the blood, and they are involved in **blood clotting** and vital to the formation of a hemostatic plug after vascular injury.

1. **Normal values for a platelet count** are 150,000 to 300,000/mm^3 (1.5 to 3.0 $\times$ 10^{11}/L).
2. **Thrombocytopenia**, a decreased platelet count, can occur with a variety of conditions, such as idiopathic thrombocytopenic purpura or, occasionally, from such drugs as quinidine and sulfonamides.
   a. Thrombocytopenia is **moderate** when the platelet count is $<$ 100,000/mm^3.
   b. Thrombocytopenia is **severe** when the platelet count is $<$ 50,000/mm^3.

III. COMMON SERUM ENZYME TESTS.

Small amounts of enzymes (catalysts) circulate in the blood at all times and are released into the blood in larger quantities when tissue damage occurs. Thus, serum enzyme levels can be used to **aid in the diagnosis of certain diseases**.

A. **Creatine kinase (CK)**

1. Creatine kinase—formerly known as creatine phosphokinase (CPK)—is found primarily in heart muscle, skeletal muscle, and brain tissue.
2. CK levels are used primarily to **aid in the diagnosis of acute myocardial** (*Figure 30-2*) **or skeletal muscle damage**. However, vigorous exercise, a fall, or deep intramuscular injections can cause significant increases in CK levels.
3. The **isoenzymes** of CK—**CK-MM**, found in skeletal muscle; **CK-BB**, found in brain tissue; and **CK-MB**, found in heart muscle—can be used to differentiate the source of damage.
   a. Normally, serum CK levels are virtually all the **CK-MM isoenzyme**.
   b. Increase in **CK-MB** levels provides a sensitive indicator of myocardial necrosis.

B. **Lactate dehydrogenase (LDH)**

1. LDH catalyzes the interconversion of lactate and pyruvate and represents a group of enzymes present in almost all metabolizing cells.

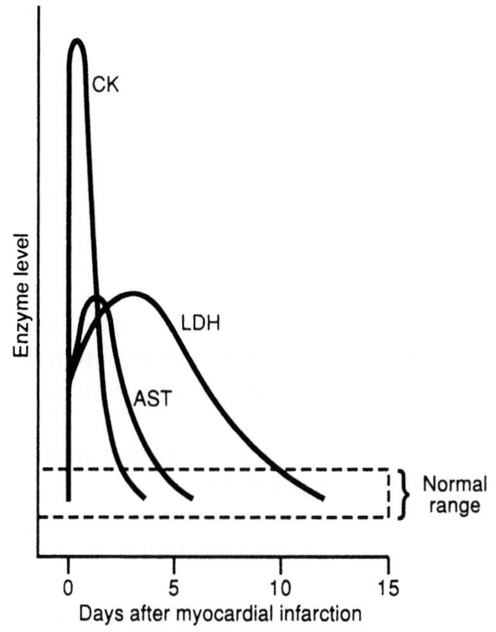

Figure 30-2. The increase of serum creatine kinase (*CK*), lactate dehydrogenase (*LDH*), and aspartate aminotransferase (*AST*) levels after a myocardial infarction.

2. Five individual **isoenzymes** make up the total LDH serum level.
   a. **LDH_1** and **LDH_2** appear primarily in the heart.
   b. **LDH_3** appears primarily in the lungs.
   c. **LDH_4** and **LDH_5** appear primarily in the liver and skeletal muscles.
3. The distribution pattern of LDH isoenzymes may aid in diagnosing myocardial infarction, hepatic disease, and lung disease.

C. **Alkaline phosphatase (ALP)**
1. ALP is produced primarily in the **liver** and **bones**.
2. Serum ALP levels are **particularly sensitive to partial or mild biliary obstruction**—either extrahepatic (e.g., caused by a stone in the bile duct) or intrahepatic, both of which cause levels to increase.
3. **Increased osteoblastic activity**, as occurs in Paget disease, hyperparathyroidism, osteomalacia, and others, also increases serum ALP levels.

D. **Aspartate aminotransferase (AST)**
1. Aspartate aminotransferase—formerly known as **serum glutamic-oxaloacetic transaminase (SGOT)**—is found in a number of organs, primarily in heart and liver tissues and, to a lesser extent, in skeletal muscle, kidney tissue, and pancreatic tissue.
2. **Damage to the heart** (e.g., from **myocardial infarction**) results in increased AST levels about 8 hrs after injury (*Figure 30-2*).
   a. Levels are **increased markedly** with **acute hepatitis**; they are **increased mildly** with **cirrhosis** and a **fatty liver**.
   b. Levels are also **increased** with **passive congestion of the liver**, such as occurs in congestive heart failure (CHF).

E. **Alanine aminotransferase (ALT)**
1. Alanine aminotransferase—formerly known as **serum glutamic-pyruvic transaminase (SGPT)**—is found in the liver, with lesser amounts in the heart, skeletal muscles, and kidney.
2. Although ALT values are **relatively specific for liver cell damage**, ALT is **less sensitive than AST**, and extensive or severe liver damage is necessary before abnormally increased levels are produced.
3. ALT also **increases less consistently and less markedly than AST after an acute myocardial infarction**.

F. **Cardiac troponins (I, T, and C)**
1. Troponins are a relatively new method to identify myocardial cell injury and thus assist in the diagnosis of acute myocardial infarction. These troponins may possess superior specificity in situations in which false-positive elevations of CK-MB are likely.
2. Troponin T is found in cardiac and skeletal muscle, troponin I is found only in cardiac muscle, and troponin C is present in two isoforms found in skeletal and cardiac muscle. Troponin T has shown prognostic value in unstable angina and in detecting minor myocardial cell injury with greater sensitivity than CK-MB.
3. The normal value for troponin T is < 0.1 ng/mL and I is < 1.5 ng/mL.

IV. LIVER FUNCTION TESTS

A. **Liver enzymes**
1. **Levels of certain enzymes** (e.g., LDH, ALP, AST, ALT) **increase with liver dysfunction** (see III).
2. These **enzyme tests indicate only that the liver has been damaged**. They do not assess the liver's ability to function. Other tests provide indications of liver dysfunction.

B. **Serum bilirubin**
1. Bilirubin, a breakdown product of Hb, is the **predominant pigment in bile**. Effective bilirubin conjugation and excretion depend on **hepatobiliary function** and on the **rate of RBC turnover**.
2. Serum bilirubin levels are reported as **total bilirubin** (conjugated and unconjugated) and as **direct bilirubin** (conjugated only).
   a. Bilirubin is released by Hb breakdown and is bound to albumin as water-insoluble **indirect bilirubin** (unconjugated bilirubin), which is not filtered by the glomerulus.
   b. **Unconjugated bilirubin** travels to the liver, where it is separated from albumin, conjugated with diglucuronide, and then actively secreted into the bile as **conjugated bilirubin** (direct bilirubin), which is filtered by the glomerulus (*Figure 30-3*).
3. **Normal values of total serum bilirubin** are 0.1 to 1.0 mg/dL (2 to 18 mmol/L); of **direct bilirubin**, 0.0 to 0.2 mg/dL (0 to 4 mmol/L).

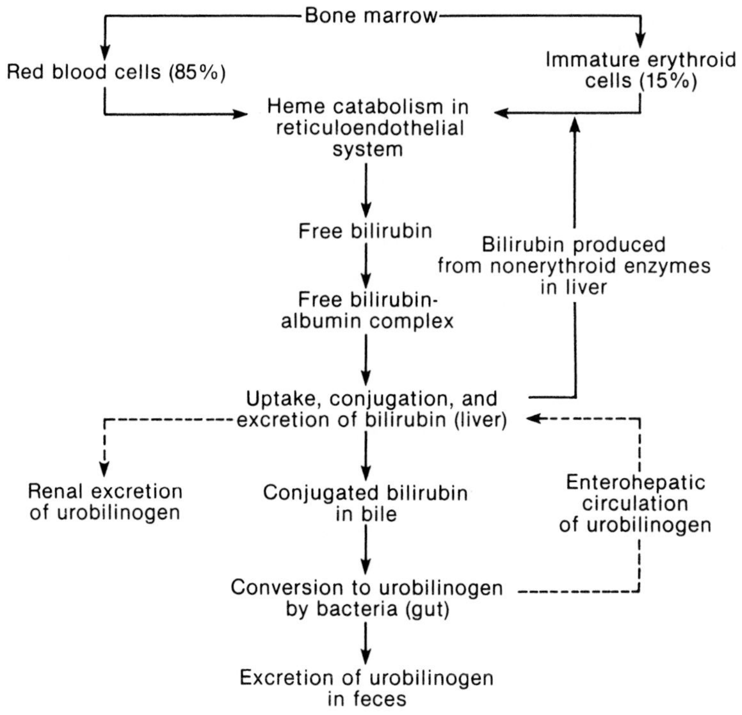

Figure 30-3. Bilirubin metabolism.

4. **An increase in serum bilirubin** results in **jaundice** from bilirubin deposition in the tissues. There are three major causes of increased serum bilirubin.
   a. **Hemolysis** increases total bilirubin; direct bilirubin (conjugated) is usually normal or slightly increased. Urine color is normal, and no bilirubin is found in the urine.
   b. **Biliary obstruction**, which may be intrahepatic (as with a chlorpromazine reaction) or extrahepatic (as with a biliary stone), increases total bilirubin and direct bilirubin; intrahepatic cholestasis (e.g., from chlorpromazine) may increase direct bilirubin as well. Urine color is dark, and bilirubin is present in the urine.
   c. **Liver cell necrosis**, as occurs in viral hepatitis, may cause an increase in both direct bilirubin (because inflammation causes some bile sinusoid blockage) and indirect bilirubin (because the liver's ability to conjugate is altered). Urine color is dark, and bilirubin is present in the urine.

C. **Serum proteins**
1. **Primary serum proteins** measured are **albumin** and the **globulins** (i.e., α, β, γ).
   a. **Albumin** (4 to 6 g/dL) maintains serum oncotic pressure and serves as a transport agent. Because it is primarily manufactured by the liver, liver disease can decrease albumin levels. Albumin can also be used to assess nutritional status.
   b. **Globulin** (23 to 35 g/L) relates to the total measurement of immunoglobins (antibodies) found in the serum and function as transport agents and play a role in certain immunological mechanisms. A decrease in albumin levels usually results in a compensatory increase in globulin production.
2. **Normal values** for total serum protein levels are 6 to 8 g/dL (60 to 80 g/L).

V. URINALYSIS.

Composed of chemical and microscopic tests of the urine used to provide basic information regarding renal function, urinary tract disease, and the presence of certain systemic diseases. Components of a standard urinalysis include physical (color, turbidity, odor, specific gravity, and osmolality), chemical (pH, Hb, glucose, protein, glucose, ketone, leukocyte esterase, nitrites, bilirubin) and microscopic examination (RBC, WBC, epithelial cells, casts, bacteria).

A. **Appearance.** Normal urine is **clear** and ranges in color from **pale yellow to deep gold. Changes in color** can result from drugs, diet, or disease.
1. A **red color** may indicate, among other things, the presence of blood or phenolphthalein (a laxative).

2. A **brownish yellow color** may indicate the presence of conjugated bilirubin.
3. **Other shades of red, orange, or brown** may be caused by ingestion of various drugs (e.g., rifampin).

B. pH
1. **Normal pH** ranges from 4.5 to 9.0 but is typically **acidic** (around 6.0).
2. **Alkaline pH** may indicate such conditions as alkalosis, a **Proteus** infection, or acetazolamide use. It may also reflect changes caused by leaving the urine sample at room temperature.

C. Specific gravity
1. **Normal range** for specific gravity is 1.003 to 1.035; it is usually between 1.010 and 1.025.
2. Specific gravity is influenced by the number and nature of solute particles in the urine.
   a. **Increased specific gravity** may occur with such conditions as diabetes mellitus (excess glucose in the urine) or nephrosis (excess protein in the urine).
   b. **Decreased specific gravity** may occur with diabetes insipidus, which decreases urine concentration.
   c. **Specific gravity, fixed at 1.010** (the same as plasma), occurs when the kidneys lose their power to concentrate or dilute.

D. Protein
1. **Normal values** for urine protein are 50 to 80 mg per 24 hr because the glomerular membrane prevents most protein molecules in the blood from entering the urine.
2. **Proteinuria** occurs with many conditions (e.g., renal disease, bladder infection, venous congestion, fever).
   a. The presence of a **specific protein** can help identify a specific disease state (e.g., Bence Jones protein may indicate multiple myeloma).
   b. Most often, the protein in urine is **albumin**. Albuminuria may indicate abnormal glomerular permeability.

E. Glucose
1. The normal **renal threshold** for glucose is a blood glucose level of about 180 mg/dL; **glucose does not normally appear in urine** as detected by popular testing methods.
2. **Glycosuria** usually indicates diabetes mellitus (DM). There are certain less common causes (e.g., a lowered renal threshold for glucose).

F. Ketones
1. Ketones **do not normally appear in urine**. They are excreted when the body has used available glucose stores and begins to metabolize fat stores.
2. The **three ketone bodies** are **β-hydroxybutyric acid** (80%), **acetoacetic acid** (about 20%), and acetone (a small percentage). Some commercial tests (e.g., Ames products) measure only acetoacetic acid, but usually all three are excreted in parallel proportions.
3. **Ketonuria** usually indicates uncontrolled DM, but it may also occur with starvation and with zero- or low-carbohydrate diets.

G. **Evaluation. Microscopic examination** of centrifuged urine sediment normally reveals 0 to 1 RBC, 0 to 4 WBCs, and only an occasional cast per high-power field (HPF).
1. **Hematuria** (i.e., the presence of RBCs) may indicate such conditions as trauma, a tumor, or a systemic bleeding disorder. In women, a significant number of **squamous cells** suggests vaginal contamination (menstruation).
2. **Casts** (i.e., protein conglomerations outlining the shape of the renal tubules in which they were formed) may or may not be significant. Excessive numbers of certain types of casts indicate renal disease.
3. **Crystals**, which are pH dependent, may occur normally in acid or alkaline urine. **Uric acid crystals** may form in acid urine; **phosphate crystals** may form in alkaline urine.
4. **Bacteria** do not normally appear in urine. The finding of 50 or more bacteria per HPF may indicate a urinary tract infection (UTI); smaller values may indicate urethral contamination.

VI. COMMON RENAL FUNCTION TESTS

A. Introduction
1. Renal function may be assessed by measuring **blood urea nitrogen (BUN)** and **serum creatinine**. Renal function decreases with age, which must be taken into account when interpreting test values.
   a. These tests primarily evaluate glomerular function by assessing the **glomerular filtration rate (GFR)**.

b. In many **renal diseases**, urea and creatinine accumulate in the blood because they are not excreted properly.
c. These tests also aid in determining **drug dosage** for drugs excreted through the kidneys.

2. **Azotemia** describes excessive retention of nitrogenous waste products (BUN and creatinine) in the blood. The clinical syndrome resulting from decreased renal function and azotemia is called **uremia.**
   a. **Renal azotemia** results from renal disease, such as glomerulonephritis and chronic pyelonephritis.
   b. **Prerenal azotemia** results from such conditions as severe dehydration, hemorrhagic shock, and excessive protein intake.
   c. **Postrenal azotemia** results from such conditions as ureteral or urethral stones or tumors and prostatic obstructions.
3. **Clearance**—a theoretical concept defined as the volume of plasma from which a measured amount of substance can be completely eliminated, or cleared, into the urine per unit time—can be used to estimate glomerular function.

B. BUN

1. **Urea**, an end product of protein metabolism, is produced in the liver. From there, it travels through the blood and is excreted by the kidneys. Urea is **filtered at the glomerulus**, where the tubules reabsorb approximately 40%. Thus, under normal conditions, **urea clearance** is about 60% of the true GFR.
2. **Normal values for BUN** range from 8 mg/dL to 18 mg/dL (3.0 to 6.5 mmol/L).
   a. **Decreased BUN levels** occur with **significant liver disease.**
   b. **Increased BUN levels** may indicate **renal disease.** However, factors other than glomerular function (e.g., protein intake, reduced renal blood flow, blood in the gastrointestinal tract) readily affect BUN levels, sometimes making interpretation of results difficult.

C. Serum creatinine

1. Creatinine (CR), the metabolic breakdown product of muscle creatine phosphate, has a relatively constant level of daily production. Blood levels vary little in a given individual.
2. Creatinine is **excreted** by glomerular filtration and tubular secretion. **Creatinine clearance** parallels the GFR within a range of $\pm$ 10% and is a **more sensitive indicator of renal damage than BUN levels** because renal impairment is almost the only cause of an increase in the serum creatinine level.
3. **Normal values for serum creatinine** range from 0.6 to 1.2 mg/dL (50 to 110 mmol/L).
   a. Values vary with the **amount of muscle mass**—a value of 1.2 mg/dL in a muscular athlete may represent normal renal function, whereas the same value in a small, sedentary person with little muscle mass may indicate significant renal impairment.
   b. Generally, the **serum creatinine value doubles with each 50% decrease in GFR.** For example, if a patient's normal serum creatinine is 1 mg/dL, 1 mg/dL represents 100% renal function, 2 mg/dL represents 50% function, and 4 mg/dL represents 25% function.

D. Creatinine clearance

1. Creatinine clearance, which represents the **rate at which creatinine is removed from the blood by the kidneys**, roughly approximates the GFR.
   a. The value is given in units of milliliters per minute, representing the volume of blood cleared of creatinine by the kidney per minute.
   b. **Normal values** for men range from 75 to 125 mL/min.
2. Calculation requires knowledge of **urinary creatinine excretion** (usually over 24 hrs) and concurrent **serum creatinine levels. Creatinine clearance is calculated** as follows:

$$Cl_{\mathrm{CR}} = \frac{C_{\mathrm{u}}V}{C_{\mathrm{CR}}}$$

   where Cl_{CR} is the creatinine clearance in milliliters per minute, C_{U} is the concentration of creatinine in the urine, V is the volume of urine (in milliliters per minute of urine formed over the collection period), and C_{CR} is the serum creatinine concentration.
3. Suppose the serum creatinine concentration is 1 mg/dL, and 1440 mL of urine was collected in 24 hrs (1440 mins) for a urine volume of 1 mL/min. The urine contains 100 mg/dL of creatinine. Creatinine clearance is calculated as:

$$\frac{100\ \mathrm{mg/mL} \times 1\ \mathrm{mL/min}}{1\ \mathrm{mg/dL}} = 100\ \mathrm{mL/min}$$

4. Incomplete bladder emptying and other problems may interfere with obtaining an accurate timed urine specimen. Thus, **estimations of creatinine clearance** may be necessary. These estimations require only a serum creatinine value. One estimation uses the method of **Cockcroft and Gault**, which is based on body weight, age, and gender.
   a. This formula provides an **estimated value**, calculated for **males** as:

$$Cl_{CR} = \frac{[140 - \text{age (in years)}] \times \text{body weight (in kg)}}{72 \times C_{CR}\ \text{(in mg/dL)}}$$

   b. For **females**, use 0.85 of the value calculated for males.
   c. **Example:** A 20-year-old man weighing 72 kg has a C_{CR} of 1.0 mg/dL; thus

$$C_{CR} = \frac{(140 - 20\ \text{years}) \times 72\ \text{kg}}{72 \times 1\ \text{mg/dL}} = 120\ \text{mL/min}$$

5. **Determination of GFR.** The modified diet in renal disease (MDRD) equation is considered a more accurate measurement of GFR than other equations used to estimate renal function (e.g., Cockcroft–Gault) in patients with *reduced* GFR and is used in staging renal disease. Patients must have a serum creatinine concentration.
   a. The MDRD equation for **males** is as follows:

$$\text{GFR} = 186\ (\text{Pcr})^{-1.154} \times \text{age}^{-0.203}$$

   where Pcr is serum creatinine. For **females**, multiply the result by 0.742; for **African Americans**, multiply by 1.210.
   b. The MDRD has been validated in Caucasians, patients with diabetic kidney disease, kidney transplant recipients, and African Americans and Asians with nondiabetic kidney disease.
   c. The MDRD equation has *not* been validated in patients < 18 years of age, pregnant women, patients > 70 years of age, other ethnic groups, patients with normal kidney function who are at an increased risk for chronic kidney disease, and patients with normal renal function.
   d. Many institutions are routinely reporting an MDRD-derived GFR estimation for patients as a routine component of a blood chemistry study. This value should be used to assist the clinician in staging a patient's degree of renal dysfunction and is not a substitute for creatinine clearance as estimated by the Cockcroft and Gault equation, which should be used for drug dosing in renal impairment. The MDRD estimate has not been evaluated for the purpose of drug dosing.

VII. ELECTROLYTES

A. Sodium (Na)

1. Sodium is the major cation of the **extracellular** fluid. Sodium, along with chloride (Cl), potassium (K), and water, is important in the regulation of osmotic pressure and water balance between intracellular and extracellular fluids. **Normal values** are 135 to 147 mEq/L or mmol/L.
2. The sodium concentration is defined as the ratio of sodium to water, not the absolute amounts of either. Laboratory tests for sodium are used mainly to detect disturbances in water balance and body osmolality. The kidneys are the major organs of sodium and water balance.
3. An increase in sodium concentration (**hypernatremia**) may indicate impaired sodium excretion or dehydration. A decrease in sodium concentration (hyponatremia) may reflect overhydration, abnormal sodium loss, or decreased sodium intake.
4. Patients with kidney, heart, or pulmonary disease may have difficulty with sodium and water balance. In adults, changes in sodium concentrations most often reflect changes in water balance, not salt imbalances. Therefore, sodium concentration is often used as an indicator of fluid status, rather than salt imbalance.
5. Control of sodium by the body is accomplished mainly through the hormones aldosterone and antidiuretic hormone (ADH).
   a. ADH is released from the pituitary gland in response to signals from the hypothalamus. ADH's presence in the distal tubules and collecting ducts of the kidney causes them to become more permeable to the reabsorption of water; therefore, concentrating urine.

b. Aldosterone affects the distal tubular reabsorption of sodium as opposed to water. Aldosterone is released from the adrenal cortex in response to low sodium, high potassium, low blood volume, and angiotensin II. Aldosterone causes the spilling of potassium from the distal tubules into the urine in exchange for sodium reabsorption.

6. **Hyponatremia** is usually related to total body depletion of sodium—as in mineralocorticoid deficiencies, sodium-wasting renal disease, replacement of fluid loss with nonsaline solutions, gastrointestinal (GI) losses, renal losses, or loss of sodium through the skin—or to dilution of serum sodium—as in cirrhosis, CHF, nephrosis, renal failure, excess water intake, or syndrome of inappropriate antidiuretic hormone (SIADH) secretion.

7. **Hypernatremia** usually results from a loss of free water or hypotonic fluid or through excessive sodium intake. Free water loss is most often associated with diabetes insipidus, but fluid loss can be via the GI tract, renal, skin, or respiratory systems. Excess sodium intake can occur through the administration of hypertonic intravenous (IV) solutions, mineralocorticoid excess, excessive sodium ingestion, or after administration of drugs high in sodium content (e.g., ticarcillin, sodium bicarbonate [HCO^{-3}]).

B. Potassium (K)

1. Potassium is the most abundant **intracellular** cation (intracellular fluid potassium averages 141 mEq/L). Approximately 3500 mEq of potassium is contained in the body of a 70-kg adult. Only 10% of the body's potassium is extracellular. Normal values are 3.5 to 5.0 mEq/L or mmol/L.

2. The serum potassium concentration is not an adequate measure of the total body potassium because most of the body's potassium is intracellular. Fortunately, the clinical signs and symptoms of potassium deficiency—malaise, confusion, dizziness, electrocardiogram (ECG) changes, muscle weakness, and pain—correlate well with serum concentrations. The serum potassium concentration is buffered by the body and may be "normal" despite total body potassium loss. Potassium depletion causes a shift of intracellular potassium to the extracellular fluid to maintain potassium concentrations. There is approximately a 100 mEq total body potassium deficit when the serum potassium concentration decreases by 0.3 mEq/L. This may result in misinterpretation of serum potassium concentrations as they relate to total body potassium.

3. The role or function of potassium is in the maintenance of proper electrical conduction in cardiac and skeletal muscles (muscle and nerve excitability); it exerts an influence on the body's water balance (intracellular volume) and plays a role in acid–base equilibrium.

4. Potassium is regulated by
   a. Kidneys (renal function)
   b. Aldosterone
   c. Arterial pH
   d. Insulin
   e. Potassium intake
   f. Sodium delivery to distal tubules

5. **Hypokalemia** can occur. The kidneys are responsible for approximately 90% of the daily potassium loss. Other losses occur mainly through the GI system. Even in states of no potassium intake, the kidneys still excrete up to 20 mEq of potassium daily. Therefore, prolonged periods of potassium deprivation can result in hypokalemia. Hypokalemia can also result from potassium loss through vomiting or diarrhea, nasogastric suction, laxative abuse, and by diuretic use (mannitol, thiazides, or loop diuretics). Excessive mineralocorticoid activity and glucosuria can also result in hypokalemia. Potassium can be shifted into cells with alkalemia and after administration of glucose and insulin.

6. **Hyperkalemia** most commonly results from decreased renal elimination, excessive intake, or from cellular breakdown (tissue damage, hemolysis, burns, infections). Metabolic acidosis may also result in a shift of potassium extracellularly as hydrogen ions move into cells and are exchanged for potassium and sodium ions. As a general guideline, for every 0.1 unit, pH change from 7.4, the potassium concentration will change by about 0.6 mEq/L. If a patient has a pH of 7.1 and a measured potassium of 4.5 mEq/L, the actual potassium concentration would be

$$0.3 \text{ (units less than 7.4)} \times 0.6 = 1.8$$
$$\text{Potassium concentration} = 4.5 - 1.8 = 2.7 \text{ mEq/L}$$

Correction of the acidosis in this situation will result in a dramatic decrease in potassium unless supplementation is instituted.

C. Chloride (Cl)

1. Chloride is the major anion of the extracellular fluid and is important in the maintenance of acid–base balance. Alterations in the serum chloride concentration are rarely a primary indicator of major medical problems. Chloride itself is not of primary diagnostic significance. It is usually measured to confirm the serum sodium concentration. The relationship among sodium, chloride, and HCO^{-3} is described by the following:

$$Cl^{-} + HCO^{-3} + R = Na^{+}$$

where R is the anion gap. The **normal value** for Cl is 95 to 105 mEq/L or mmol/L.

2. **Hypochloremia** is a decreased chloride concentration, and it is often accompanied by metabolic alkalosis or acidosis caused by organic or other acids. Other causes include chronic renal failure, adrenal insufficiency, fasting, prolonged diarrhea, severe vomiting, and diuretic therapy.
3. **Hyperchloremia** is an increased chloride concentration that may indicate hyperchloremic metabolic acidosis. Hyperchloremia in the absence of metabolic acidosis is unusual because chloride retention is often accompanied by sodium and water retention. Other causes include acute renal failure, dehydration, and excess chloride administration.

D. Bicarbonate (HCO^{-3})/carbon dioxide (CO_2) content

1. The carbon dioxide (CO_2) content represents the sum of the bicarbonate (HCO^{-3}) concentration and the concentration of CO_2 dissolved in the serum. The HCO^{-3}/CO_2 system is the most important buffering system to maintain pH within physiological limits. Most disturbances of acid–base balance can be considered in terms of this system. Normal values are 22 to 28 mEq/L or mmol/L.
2. The relationship among this system is defined as follows:

$$HCO^{-3} + H^{+} \times H_2CO_3 \times H_2O + CO_2$$

(bicarbonate ions bind hydrogen ions to form carbonic acid). Clinically, the serum HCO^{-3} concentration is measured because acid–base balance can be inferred if the patient has normal pulmonary function.

3. **Hypobicarbonatemia** is usually caused by metabolic acidosis, renal failure, hyperventilation, severe diarrhea, drainage of intestinal fluid, and by drugs such as acetazolamide. Toxicity caused by salicylates, methanol, and ethylene glycol can also decrease the HCO^{-3} level.
4. **Hyperbicarbonatemia** is usually caused by alkalosis, hypoventilation, pulmonary disease, persistent vomiting, excess HCO^{-3} intake with poor renal function, and diuretics.

VIII. MINERALS

A. Calcium (Ca)

1. Calcium plays an important role in nerve impulse transmission, muscle contraction, pancreatic insulin release, and hydrogen ion release from the stomach, as a cofactor for some enzyme reactions and blood coagulation and, most important, bone and tooth structural integrity. Normal total calcium values are 8.8 to 10.3 mg/dL or 2.20 to 2.56 mmol/L.
2. The total calcium content of normal adults is 20 to 25 g/kg of fat-free tissue, and about 44% of this calcium is in the body skeleton. Approximately 1% of skeletal calcium is freely exchangeable with that of the extracellular fluid. The reservoir of calcium in bones maintains the concentration of calcium in the plasma constant. About 40% of the calcium in the extracellular fluid is bound to plasma proteins (especially albumin), 5% to 15% is complexed with phosphate and citrate, and 45% to 55% is in the unbound, ionized form. Most laboratories measure the total calcium concentration; however, it is the free, ionized calcium that is important physiologically. Ionized calcium levels may be obtained from the laboratory. Clinically, the most important determinant of ionized calcium is the amount of serum protein (albumin) available for binding. The normal serum calcium range is for a serum albumin of 4.0 g/dL. A good approximation is that for every 1.0 g/dL decrease in albumin, 0.8 g/dL should be added to the calcium laboratory result. Doing this corrects the total plasma concentration to reflect the additional amount of free (active) calcium.
3. **Hypocalcemia** usually implies a deficiency in either the production or response to parathyroid hormone (PTH) or vitamin D. PTH abnormalities include hypoparathyroidism, pseudohypoparathyroidism, or hypomagnesemia. Vitamin D abnormalities can be caused by decreased

nutritional intake, decreased absorption of vitamin D, a decrease in production, or an increase in metabolism. Administration of loop diuretics causing diuresis can also decrease serum calcium.

4. **Hypercalcemia** is an increased calcium concentration, and it is usually associated with malignancy or metastatic diseases. Other causes include hyperparathyroidism, Paget disease, milk-alkali syndrome, granulomatous disorders, thiazide diuretics, excessive calcium intake, or vitamin D intoxication.

B. **Phosphate (PO_4)**

1. Phosphate is a major intracellular anion and is the source of phosphate for adenosine triphosphate (ATP) and phospholipid synthesis. Serum calcium and PO_4 are influenced by many of the same factors. It is useful to consider calcium and PO_4 together when interpreting lab results. Normal PO_4 values are 2.5 to 5.0 mg/dL or 0.80 to 1.60 mmol/L.
2. **Hyperphosphatemia** and **hypophosphatemia** can occur. The extracellular fluid concentration of phosphate is influenced by PTH, intestinal absorption, renal function, nutrition, and bone metabolism. Hyperphosphatemia is usually caused by renal insufficiency, although increased vitamin D or phosphate intake, hypoparathyroidism, and hyperthyroidism are also causes. Hypophosphatemia can occur in malnutrition, especially when anabolism is induced, after administration of aluminum-containing antacids or calcium acetate, in chronic alcoholics, and in septic patients. Hyperparathyroidism and insufficient vitamin D intake can also induce hypophosphatemia.

C. **Magnesium (Mg)**

1. Magnesium is the second most abundant intracellular and extracellular cation. It is an activator of numerous enzyme systems that control carbohydrate, fat and electrolyte metabolism, protein synthesis, nerve conduction, muscular contractility, as well as membrane transport and integrity. Normal values are 1.6 to 2.4 mEq/L or 0.80 to 1.20 mmol/L.
2. **Hypomagnesemia** and **hypermagnesemia** can occur. **Hypomagnesemia** is found more often than hypermagnesemia. Depletion of magnesium usually results from excessive loss from the GI tract or the kidneys. Depletion can occur from either poor intestinal absorption or excessive GI fluid loss. Signs and symptoms include weakness, muscle fasciculations with tremor, tetany, and increased reflexes. Decreased intracardiac magnesium may manifest as an increased QT interval with an increased risk of arrhythmia. **Hypermagnesemia** is most commonly caused by increased magnesium intake in the setting of renal insufficiency. Other causes include excess magnesium intake, hepatitis, and Addison disease. Signs and symptoms of hypermagnesemia include bradycardia, flushing, sweating, nausea and vomiting, decreased calcium level, decreased deep-tendon reflexes, flaccid paralysis, increased pulse rate and QRS intervals, respiratory distress, and asystole.

Study Questions

Directions for questions 1–16: Each of the questions, statements, or incomplete statements in this section can be correctly answered or completed by **one** of the suggested answers or phrases. Choose the **best** answer.

1. Hematological testing of a patient with AIDS is most likely to show which of the following abnormalities?

    (A) basophilia
    (B) eosinophilia
    (C) lymphopenia
    (D) reticulocytosis
    (E) agranulocytosis

2. Hematological studies are most likely to show a low reticulocyte count in a patient who has which of the following abnormalities?

    (A) aplastic anemia secondary to cancer chemotherapy
    (B) acute hemolytic anemia secondary to quinidine treatment
    (C) severe bleeding secondary to an automobile accident
    (D) iron-deficiency anemia 1 week after treatment with ferrous sulfate
    (E) megaloblastic anemia owing to folate deficiency 1 week after treatment with folic acid

3. All of the following findings on a routine urinalysis would be considered normal *except* which one?
   (A) pH: 6.5
   (B) glucose: negative
   (C) ketones: negative
   (D) white blood cells (WBCs): 3 per high-power field (HPF), no casts
   (E) red blood cells (RBCs): 5 per HPF

4. A 12-year-old boy is treated for otitis media with cefaclor (Ceclor). On the seventh day of therapy, he spikes a fever and develops an urticarial rash on his trunk. Which of the following laboratory tests could best confirm the physician's suspicion of a hypersensitivity (allergic) reaction?
   (A) complete blood count (CBC) and differential
   (B) serum hemoglobin (Hb) and reticulocyte count
   (C) liver function test profile
   (D) lactate dehydrogenase (LDH) isoenzyme profile
   (E) red blood cell (RBC) count and serum bilirubin

5. An increased hematocrit (Hct) is a likely finding in all of the following individuals *except* which one?
   (A) a man who has just returned from a 3-week skiing trip in the Colorado Rockies
   (B) a woman who has polycythemia vera
   (C) a hospitalized patient who mistakenly received 5 L of intravenous (IV) dextrose 5% in water (D_5W) over the last 24 hrs
   (D) a man who has been rescued from the Arizona desert after spending 4 days without water
   (E) a woman who has chronic obstructive pulmonary disease

6. A 29-year-old white man is seen in the emergency room. His white blood cell (WBC) count is 14,200 with 80% polys. All of the following conditions could normally produce these laboratory findings *except* which one?
   (A) a localized bacterial infection on the tip of the index finger
   (B) acute bacterial pneumonia caused by *Streptococcus pneumoniae*
   (C) a heart attack
   (D) a gunshot wound to the abdomen with a loss of 2 pints of blood
   (E) an attack of gout

7. A 52-year-old male construction worker who drinks "fairly heavily" when he gets off work is seen in the emergency room with, among other abnormal laboratory results, an increased creatine kinase (CK) level. All of the following circumstances could explain this increase *except* which one?
   (A) He fell against the bumper of his car in a drunken stupor and bruised his right side.
   (B) He is showing evidence of some liver damage owing to the heavy alcohol intake.
   (C) He has experienced a heart attack.
   (D) He received an intramuscular (IM) injection a few hours before the blood sample was drawn.
   (E) He pulled a muscle that day when lifting a heavy concrete slab.

8. A 45-year-old man with jaundice has spillage of bilirubin into his urine. All of the following statements could apply to this patient *except* which one?
   (A) His total bilirubin is increased.
   (B) His direct bilirubin is increased.
   (C) He may have viral hepatitis.
   (D) He may have hemolytic anemia.
   (E) He may have cholestatic hepatitis.

For questions 9–11: A 70-year-old black man weighing 154 lbs complains of chronic fatigue. Several laboratory tests were performed with the following results:

blood urea nitrogen (BUN) 15 mg/dL
aspartate aminotransferase (AST) within normal limits
white blood cell (WBC) count 7500/mm^3
red blood cell (RBC) count 4 million/mm^3
hematocrit (Hct) 29%
hemoglobin (Hb) 9 g/dL

9. This patient's mean cell hemoglobin concentration (MCHC) is
   (A) 27.5.
   (B) 28.9.
   (C) 31.0.
   (D) 33.5.
   (E) 35.4.

10. His mean cell volume (MCV) is
   (A) 61.3.
   (B) 72.5.
   (C) 77.5.
   (D) 90.2.
   (E) 93.5.

11. From the data provided and from the calculations in questions 9 and 10, this patient is best described as
    (A) normal except for a slightly increased blood urea nitrogen (BUN).
    (B) having normochromic, microcytic anemia.
    (C) having sickle-cell anemia.
    (D) having hypochromic, normocytic anemia.
    (E) having folic acid deficiency.

12. All of the following statements about sodium (Na) are true *except* which one?
    (A) The normal range for sodium is 135 to 147 mEq/L.
    (B) Sodium is the major cation of the extracellular fluid, and the laboratory test is used mainly to detect disturbances in water balance.
    (C) Hyponatremia usually results from the total body depletion of sodium or through a dilutional effect.
    (D) Control of the sodium concentration is mainly through regulation of arterial pH.

13. A 53-year-old woman with diabetes mellitus is seen in the emergency room. Her blood glucose is 673 mg/dL and ketones are present in her blood. A diagnosis of diabetic ketoacidosis (DKA) is made. Other important laboratory values are potassium of 4.8 mEq/L, 4+ glucose in urine, and an arterial pH of 7.1. All of the following statements apply to this patient *except* which one?
    (A) Her potassium value is normal; therefore, no potassium supplementation is likely to be necessary.
    (B) Her potassium value should be corrected owing to her acidosis; a corrected potassium would be 3.0 mEq/L.
    (C) Potassium supplementation should be instituted because her total body potassium is depleted.
    (D) Factors affecting potassium in this patient include glycosuria and arterial pH.

14. A 50-year-old man presents with bicarbonate of 18 mEq/L. All of the following could be a cause of his low bicarbonate level *except*
    (A) metabolic acidosis.
    (B) salicylate toxicity.
    (C) diuretic therapy.
    (D) diarrhea.

15. All of the following statements about calcium (Ca) and phosphorus (PO_4) are true *except* which one?
    (A) An alcoholic with a serum albumin of 2.0 g/dL and a serum total calcium of 8.0 mg/dL has a corrected total calcium of 9.6 mg/dL.
    (B) Calcium and PO_4 levels should be interpreted together because many of the same factors influence both minerals.
    (C) Metastatic cancer often induces a decrease in serum calcium levels.
    (D) A patient with renal failure may present with hypocalcemia and hyperphosphatemia.

16. All of the following are important functions of magnesium (Mg) *except*
    (A) nerve conduction.
    (B) phospholipid synthesis.
    (C) muscle contractility.
    (D) carbohydrate, fat, and electrolyte metabolism.

Directions for questions 17–19: The questions and incomplete statements in this section can be correctly answered or completed by **one or more** of the suggested answers. Choose the answer, **A–E**.

A if **I only** is correct
B if **III only** is correct
C if **I and II** are correct
D if **II and III** are correct
E if **I, II, and III** are correct

17. Factors likely to cause an increase in the blood urea nitrogen (BUN) level include
    I. intramuscular (IM) injection of diazepam (Valium).
    II. severe liver disease.
    III. chronic kidney disease.

18. A patient who undergoes serum enzyme testing is found to have an increased aspartate aminotransferase (AST) level. Possible underlying causes of this abnormality include
    I. methyldopa-induced hepatitis.
    II. congestive heart failure (CHF).
    III. pneumonia.

19. Serum enzyme tests that may aid in the diagnosis of myocardial infarction include
    I. alkaline phosphatase.
    II. creatine kinase (CK).
    III. lactate dehydrogenase (LDH).

Answers and Explanations

1. **The answer is C** *[see II.B.2.d.(2)].*
Valuable diagnostic information can be obtained through quantitative and qualitative testing of the cells of the blood. A finding of lymphopenia (i.e., decreased number of lymphocytes) suggests an attack on the immune system or some underlying immunodeficiency. AIDS attacks the T_H4 population of lymphocytes and thus may result in lymphopenia.

2. **The answer is A** *[see II.A.5].*
The reticulocyte count measures the amount of circulating immature RBCs, which provides information about bone marrow function. A low reticulocyte count is a likely finding in a patient with aplastic anemia—a disorder characterized by a deficiency of all cellular elements of the blood owing to a lack of hematopoietic stem cells in bone marrow. A variety of drugs (e.g., those used in anticancer therapy) and other agents produce marrow aplasia. A high reticulocyte count would likely be found in a patient with hemolytic anemia or acute blood loss or in a patient who has been treated for an iron, vitamin B_{12}, or folate deficiency.

3. **The answer is E** *[see V.B; V.E–G].*
Microscopic examination of the urine sediment normally shows < 1 RBC and from 0 to 4 WBCs per HPF. Other normal findings on urinalysis include an acid pH (i.e., around 6) and an absence of glucose and ketones.

4. **The answer is A** *[see II.B.2.c].*
An allergic drug reaction will usually produce an increase in the eosinophil count (eosinophilia). This could be determined by ordering a WBC differential.

5. **The answer is C** *[see II.A.2].*
Overhydration with an excess infusion of D_5W produces a low Hct. The other situations described in the question result in increases of the Hct.

6. **The answer is A** *[see II.B.2.a].*
The patient has leukocytosis with an increased neutrophil count (neutrophilia). A localized infection does not normally result in an increase in the total leukocyte count or neutrophil count. The other situations given in the question can produce a neutrophilic leukocytosis.

7. **The answer is B** *[see III.A].*
Because CK is not present in the liver, alcoholic liver damage would not result in an increase in the level of this enzyme. CK is present primarily in cardiac and skeletal muscle. The other situations described in the question could all result in the release of increased amounts of CK into the bloodstream.

8. **The answer is D** *[see IV.B].*
The patient with jaundice (deposition of bilirubin in the skin) usually has an increase in the total bilirubin serum level. Spillage of bilirubin into the urine requires an increased level of direct bilirubin, which is likely with viral hepatitis or cholestatic hepatitis. In hemolytic anemia, direct bilirubin is not usually increased, and therefore, there would be no spillage of bilirubin into the urine.

9. **The answer is C** *[see II.A.4.c].*

10. **The answer is B** *[see II.A.4.a].*

11. **The answer is B** *[see II.A.4; VI.B.2].*
The MCHC is calculated as follows:

$$\text{MCHC} = \frac{\text{Hb} \times 100}{\text{Hct}} = \frac{9 \times 100}{29} = 31.0$$

The mean cell volume (MCV) is calculated as follows:

$$\text{MCV} = \frac{\text{Hct (\%)} \times 10}{\text{RBC (millions)}} = \frac{29 \times 10}{4} = 72.5$$

The patient described in the question is anemic because his Hb is 9 (normal: 14 to 18). The anemia is normochromic because the patient's MCHC of 31 is normal (normal range: 31 to 37), but the anemia is microcytic because the patient's MCV is 72.5 (normal: 80 to 100). The patient's BUN, 15 mg/dL, is within the normal range of 10 to 20 mg/dL.

12. **The answer is D** *[see VII.A.1; VII.A.5–7].*
Sodium, the major extracellular cation, is measured mainly to assist in the determination of fluid status and water balance. Regulation of sodium is mainly through the kidneys via ADH and aldosterone.

13. **The answer is A** *[see VII.B.2; VII.B.4; VII.B.6].*
A "normal" potassium level in the setting of metabolic acidosis, especially in a patient with DKA, should be treated appropriately. If the serum potassium level is corrected for the patient's acidosis, the corrected level is 3.0 mEq/L. This corresponds to depletion in total body potassium stores. Once the acidosis and hyperglycemia begin to correct with appropriate treatment, potassium levels will decrease precipitously unless supplementation is begun. It is important to recognize that a laboratory value in the "normal" range may not actually be normal, especially when potassium is involved.

14. **The answer is C** *[see VII.D.3–4].*
Low HCO^{-3} is usually found in patients with acidosis or renal failure and after hyperventilation or severe diarrhea. In general, disturbances in acid–base balance cause alteration in the serum HCO^{-3} or CO_2 content. Diuretic therapy can cause an alkalosis and an increase in HCO^{-3}.

15. The answer is C *[see VIII.A.2–4; VII.B.2]*.
Malignancy or other metastatic diseases are most often associated with hypercalcemia, not hypocalcemia. Ionized calcium is the free active form, and this level is increased in the setting of a low albumin. Therefore, the total calcium level must be adjusted to account for increased ionized calcium in this setting. Both minerals are influenced by many of the same factors and thus are often interpreted together. Renal function is one such factor whereby a decrease in renal function (i.e., renal failure) can result in a low level of calcium and a high level of PO_4.

16. The answer is B *[see VIII.C.1]*.
Magnesium is the second most abundant intracellular and extracellular cation. It is an activator of numerous enzyme systems that control carbohydrate, fat, and electrolyte metabolism; protein synthesis; nerve conduction; muscular contractility; and membrane transport and integrity. PO_4, on the other hand, is important for ATP and phospholipid synthesis.

17. The answer is B (III) *[see VI.B.2]*.
Chronic kidney disease can cause an increase in the BUN level; a heavy protein diet and bleeding into the GI tract are other factors that can produce this finding. Severe liver disease can prevent the formation of urea and, therefore, is likely to cause a decrease in the BUN level. Although an IM injection of diazepam (Valium) may cause an increase in the serum CK or AST level, it would have no effect on the BUN.

18. The answer is C (I, II) *[see III.D]*.
A lung infection, such as pneumonia, normally would not cause an increase in the release of AST, an enzyme primarily found in the liver and heart. In acute hepatitis, a marked increase of AST is a likely finding. AST levels also can be increased with passive congestion of the liver, as occurs in CHF.

19. The answer is D (II, III) *[see III.A–C]*.
Usually, the CK, ALT, AST, and LDH enzyme levels are increased after a myocardial infarction. Alkaline phosphatase is not present in cardiac tissue and, therefore, would not be useful in the diagnosis of a myocardial infarction.

31

Coronary Artery Disease

ALAN H. MUTNICK

I. INTRODUCTION

A. **Definition. Coronary artery disease (CAD)** is a general term that refers to several diseases other than atherosclerosis, which causes a narrowing of the major epicardial coronary arteries. **Ischemic heart disease (IHD)** is a form of heart disease with primary manifestations that result from myocardial ischemia owing to atherosclerotic CAD. This term encompasses a spectrum of conditions, ranging from the asymptomatic preclinical phase to acute myocardial infarction and sudden cardiac death and is used throughout this chapter.

B. **Incidence**

1. IHD continues to be the most common chronic life-threatening illness in the United States (231.1 to 297.9 deaths per 100,000); cancer is the second leading cause of death (159.1 to 228.1 deaths per 100,000). It currently affects 11 million citizens in the United States, and it has been estimated that if all forms of major CAD were eliminated, life expectancy would increase by almost 7 years to our current population.
2. Each year, more than 5 million patients present to emergency rooms with chest discomfort and related symptoms, and approximately 1.5 million are hospitalized for acute coronary syndromes. Each year in the United States, more than 1 million patients suffer an acute myocardial infarction (MI).

C. **Economics.** Based on models evaluating the costs associated with the treatment of Medicare patients with common IHD-related diagnosis, it has been estimated that the direct costs of hospitalization are > $15 billion yearly, with an additional $4.5 billion yearly in diagnostic procedures.

D. **Clinical guidelines.** Owing to the clinical, humanistic, and economic effect that IHD has in the United States, evidence-based practice guidelines have evolved based on the differences in the diagnosis and management of IHD. The author has relied heavily on the use of those guidelines to ensure the most up-to-date recommendations based on the clinical literature. ***However, the author has chosen to limit the treatment options to those within a class I benefit; (Benefit >>> Risk) with the associated level of evidence rather than providing each recommendation for all four classes (I, IIa, IIb, III).*** Guidelines that are pertinent to daily pharmacy practice include the following:

1. Fraker TD Jr, Fihn SD, 2002 Chronic Stable Angina Writing Committee, et al. 2007 chronic angina focused update of the ACC/AHA 2002 guidelines for the management of patients with chronic stable angina: a report of the American College of Cardiology/American Heart Association Task Force on Practice Guidelines Writing Group to develop the focused update of the 2002 guidelines for the management of patients with chronic stable angina. *J Am Coll Cardiol.* 2007;50(23): 2264–2274. http://content.onlinejacc.org/cgi/reprint/50/23/2264.pdf
2. Anderson JL, Adams CD, Antman EM, et al. ACC/AHA 2007 guidelines for the management of patients with unstable angina/non–ST-elevation myocardial infarction: a report of the American College of Cardiology/American Heart Association Task Force on Practice Guidelines (Writing Committee to Revise the 2002 Guidelines for the Management of Patients With Unstable Angina/Non–ST-Elevation Myocardial Infarction) developed in collaboration with the American College

of Emergency Physicians, the Society for Cardiovascular Angiography and Interventions, and the Society of Thoracic Surgeons endorsed by the American Association of Cardiovascular and Pulmonary Rehabilitation and the Society for Academic Emergency Medicine. *J Am Coll Cardiol.* 2007;50(7):e1–e157. http://content.onlinejacc.org/cgi/reprint/50/7/e1.pdf

3. Wright RS, Anderson JL, Adams CD, et al. 2011 ACCF/AHA focused update incorporated into the ACC/AHA 2007 of the guidelines for the management of patients with unstable angina/non–ST-elevation myocardial infarction: a report of the American College of Cardiology Foundation/American Heart Association Task Force on Practice Guidelines developed in collaboration with the American Academy of Family Physicians, Society for Cardiovascular Angiography and Interventions, and the Society of Thoracic Surgeons. *J Am Coll Cardiol.* 2011;57(19):e215–e367. http://content.onlinejacc.org/cgi/reprint/57/19/e215.pdf
4. Antman EM, Anbe DT, Armstrong PW, et al. ACC/AHA guidelines for the management of patients with ST-elevation myocardial infarction—executive summary. A report of the American College of Cardiology/American Heart Association Task Force on Practice Guidelines (Writing Committee to revise the 1999 guidelines for the management of patients with acute myocardial infarction). *J Am Coll Cardiol.* 2004;44(3):671–719. http://content.onlinejacc.org/cgi/reprint/44/3/671.pdf
5. Canadian Cardiovascular Society, American Academy of Family Physicians, American College of Cardiology, et al. 2007 focused update of the ACC/AHA 2004 guidelines for the management of patients with ST-elevation myocardial infarction: a report of the American College of Cardiology/American Heart Association Task Force on Practice Guidelines. *J Am Coll Cardiol.* 2008;51(2):210–247. http://content.onlinejacc.org/cgi/reprint/51/2/210.pdf
6. Kushner FG, Hand M, Smith SC Jr, et al. 2009 focused updates: ACC/AHA guidelines for the management of patients with ST-elevation myocardial infarction (updating the 2004 guideline and 2007 focused update) and ACC/AHA/SCAI guidelines on percutaneous coronary intervention (updating the 2005 guideline and 2007 focused update): a report of the American College of Cardiology Foundation/American Heart Association Task Force on Practice Guidelines. *J Am Coll Cardiol.* 2009;54(23):2205–2241. http://content.onlinejacc.org/cgi/reprint/54/23/2205.pdf
7. National Cholesterol Education Program (NCEP). *Third report of the National Cholesterol Education Program (NCEP) Expert Panel: Detection, evaluation, and treatment of high blood cholesterol in adults (Adult Treatment Panel III). Final Report.* NIH Publication No. 02-5215. Bethesda, MD: National Institutes of Health; 2002. Available at http://www.nhlbi.nih.gov/guidelines/cholesterol/atp3_rpt.htm

E. Manifestations

1. **Angina pectoris**, an episodic, reversible oxygen insufficiency, is the most common form of IHD (see II).
2. The term **acute ischemic (coronary) syndromes** describes a group of clinical symptoms representing acute myocardial ischemia. The clinical symptoms include acute myocardial infarction, which includes either ST-segment elevation (STEMI) or non–ST-segment elevation (NSTEMI), and unstable angina (UA) (see III).

F. Etiology. The processes, singly or in combination, that produce IHD include decreased blood flow to the myocardium, increased oxygen demand, and decreased oxygenation of the blood. Generally, significant IHD is defined via angiography as a stenosis that is ≥ 70% of the diameter of at least one major coronary artery segment or 50% of the diameter of the left main coronary artery.

1. **Decreased blood flow** (*Figure 31-1*)
   a. **Atherosclerosis**, with or without coronary thrombosis, is the most common cause of IHD. In this condition, the coronary arteries are progressively narrowed by smooth muscle cell proliferation and the accumulation of lipid deposits (plaque) along the inner lining (intima) of the arteries.
   b. **Coronary artery spasm**, a sustained contraction of one or more coronary arteries, can occur spontaneously or be induced by irritation (e.g., by coronary catheter or intimal hemorrhage), exposure to the cold, and ergot-derivative drugs. One long-term study demonstrated that coronary spasm was most often associated with an atypical chest pain syndrome and cigarette smoking. These spasms can cause Prinzmetal angina and even MI. Variant angina (Prinzmetal angina) is a form of unstable angina that usually occurs spontaneously, is characterized by transient ST-segment elevation, and most commonly resolves without progression to MI.

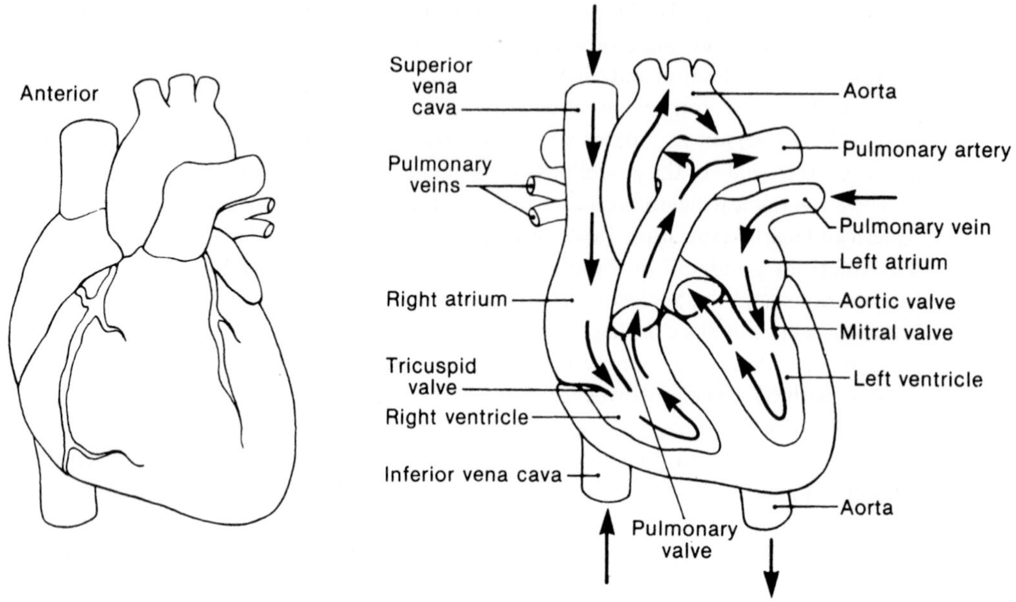

Figure 31-1. Oxygen and other nutrients are borne to the myocardium through the two major coronary arteries (the left and right) and their tributaries. The hemodynamic consequences of ischemic heart disease depend on which of the coronary vessels are involved and what part of the myocardium those vessels supply.

c. **Traumatic injury**, whether blunt or penetrating, can interfere with myocardial blood supply (e.g., the impact of a steering wheel on the chest causing a myocardial contusion in which the capillaries hemorrhage).

d. **Embolic events**, even in otherwise normal coronary vessels, can abruptly restrict the oxygen supply to the myocardium.

2. **Increased oxygen demand usually in the presence of a fixed restricted oxygen supply** can occur with exertion (e.g., exercise, shoveling snow) and emotional stress as well as under circumstances external to the coronary arterial bed, which increases sympathetic stimulation and heart rate. Some factors affecting cardiac workload and therefore myocardial oxygen supply and demand are listed in *Table 31-1*.

a. **Diastole.** Under normal circumstances, almost all of the oxygen is removed (during diastole) from the arterial blood as it passes through the heart. Thus, little remains to be extracted if oxygen demand increases. To increase the coronary oxygen supply, blood flow has to increase. The normal response mechanism is for the blood vessels, particularly the coronary arteries, to dilate, thereby increasing blood flow.

b. **Systole.** The two phases of systole—contraction and ejection—strongly influence oxygen demand.

(1) The **contractile (inotropic) state of the heart** influences the amount of oxygen it requires to perform.

Table 31-1 FACTORS AFFECTING CARDIAC PARAMETERS THAT CONTROL MYOCARDIAL OXYGEN DEMAND

Factor	Heart Rate	Blood Pressure	Ejection Time	Ventricular Volume	Inotropic Effect
Exercise	Increase	Increase	Decrease	Increase or decrease	Increase
Cold	Increase	Increase	—	—	—
Smoking	Increase	Increase	Increase	—	Increase
Nitroglycerin	Increase	Decrease	Decrease	Decrease	Increase
β-Blockers	Decrease	Decrease	Increase	Increase	Decrease

(2) **Increases in systolic wall tension**, influenced by left ventricular volume and systolic pressure, increase oxygen demand.

(3) **Lengthening of ejection time** (i.e., the duration of systolic wall tension per cardiac cycle) also increases oxygen demand.

(4) **Changes in heart rate** influence oxygen consumption by changing the ejection time.

3. **Reduced blood oxygenation.** The oxygen-carrying capacity of the blood may be reduced, as occurs in various forms of anemia or hypoxemia.

G. **Risk factors** for IHD and goals for secondary prevention have been updated with the recently released Guidelines for the Management of Patients with ST-Elevation Myocardial Infarction and are provided in *Table 31-2*.

H. **Therapeutic considerations.** Because most IHD occurs secondary to atherosclerosis, which is a long-term, cumulative process, medical efforts focus on reducing risk factors through individual patient education and media campaigns. Once manifestations occur, treatment addresses their specific variables.

II. ANGINA PECTORIS

A. **Definition.** The term **angina pectoris** is applied to varying forms of transient chest discomfort that are attributable to insufficient myocardial oxygen.

1. Angina is a clinical syndrome characterized by discomfort in the chest, jaw, shoulder, back, and arms, which is usually aggravated by exertion or stress and relieved by nitroglycerin.
2. Angina can occur in patients with valvular heart disease, uncontrolled hypertension, as well as in noncardiac organ systems such as the chest wall, esophagus, or lungs.

B. **Common causes.** Atherosclerotic lesions that produce a narrowing of the coronary arteries are the major cause of angina. However, tachycardia, anemia, hyperthyroidism, hypotension, and arterial hypoxemia can all cause an oxygen imbalance.

C. **Types**

1. **Stable (classic) angina**

a. In this most common form, has a more predictable pattern, which is brought on by exertion, emotional stress, or a heavy meal, which is usually relieved by rest, nitroglycerin, or both.

b. Five components are usually considered: quality, location, and duration of pain; factors provoking pain; and factors that relieve pain.

c. Pain has been referred to as "squeezing," "grip-like," "pressure-like," "suffocating," and "heavy" and is usually referred to as a discomfort rather than "pain."

d. The anginal episode typically lasts for "minutes" and is usually substernal but has a tendency to radiate to the neck, jaw, epigastrium, or arms.

e. Characteristically, the discomfort builds to a peak, radiating to the jaw, neck, shoulder, and arms, and then subsides without residual sensation. Angina is normally related to physical exertion, and the discomfort usually subsides quickly (i.e., in 3 to 5 mins) with rest; if precipitated by emotional stress, the episode tends to last longer (i.e., about 10 mins).

f. Stable angina is characteristically the result of a fixed obstruction in a coronary artery.

2. **Unstable angina.** (See also III.)

a. In many patients who experience unstable angina, symptoms will be caused by significant coronary artery disease. Angina is considered unstable and requires further evaluation if patients experience

(1) Rest angina, which usually is prolonged $>$ 20 mins occurring within a week of presentation

(2) Severe new-onset angina refers to angina of at least Canadian Cardiovascular Society Classification (CCSC) to class III severity, with onset within 2 months of initial presentation

(3) Increasing angina refers to previously diagnosed angina that is distinctly more frequent, longer in duration, or lower in threshold

(4) Decreased response to rest or nitroglycerin

b. Unstable angina predicts a higher short-term risk, represents a progressive clinical entity, may signal incipient MI, is referred to as an acute coronary syndrome, and should be reported promptly to a physician.

Table 31-2 RISK FACTORS FOR ISCHEMIC HEART DISEASE AND GUIDELINES FOR THEIR MODIFICATION, WHEN APPLICABLE

I. Risk factors: Not necessarily modifiable

Family history of ischemic heart disease

Age and gender (i.e., prevalence is higher among men than among premenopausal women and increases for both genders with age)

Chronic stress or type A personality (i.e., aggressive, ambitious, chronically impatient, competitive)

Gout

II. Secondary preventive goals: As recommended in the 2007 smoking-complete cessation, no exposure to environmental tobacco smoke. *Class 1 recommendation

Status of tobacco use should be asked about at every visit.

Every tobacco user and family members who smoke should be advised to quit at every visit.

The tobacco user's willingness to quit should be assessed.

The tobacco user should be assisted by counseling and developing a plan for quitting.

Follow-up, referral to special programs, or pharmacotherapy (including nicotine replacement and pharmacological treatment) should be arranged.

Exposure to environmental tobacco smoke at work and home should be avoided.

Blood pressure control: Blood pressure should be reduced to less than 140/90 mm Hg or less than 130/90 mm Hg if chronic kidney disease or diabetes mellitus. *Class 1 recommendation

Initiate or maintain lifestyle modification (weight control, increased physical activity, alcohol moderation, decreased sodium intake, and increased emphasis on consumption of fresh fruits, vegetables, and low-fat dairy products).

Add blood pressure medication, as tolerated, treating initially with β-adrenoreceptor blockers and/or ACE inhibitors.

The addition of other blood pressure lowering drugs such as thiazides as needed to achieve the goal blood pressure.

Blood lipid management: Low density lipoprotein-cholesterol (LDL-C) levels should be less than 100 mg/dL. (If triglycerides are greater than or equal to 200 mg/dL, total cholesterol minus high density lipoprotein cholesterol (HDL-C) should be less than 130 mg/dL.) *Class I recommendation

Initiate dietary therapy in all patients; which includes reducing intake of saturated fats (< 7% of total calories), trans fatty acids, and cholesterol (< 200 mg/day).

The addition of plant stanol/sterols (2 g/day) and/or viscous fiber (> 10 g/day) to further lower LDL-C.

Promotion of daily physical activity and weight management.

It may be reasonable to encourage the increase in the consumption of omega-3 fatty acids in the form of fish or in capsule form (1 g/d) for risk reduction.

A fasting lipid profile should be assessed in all patients and within 24 hrs of hospitalization for those with an acute cardiovascular or coronary event.

Physical activity: Participate in 30 mins of physical activity 7 days a week. *Class 1 recommendation

It is recommended that all patients have a risk assessment with a physical activity history and/or an exercise test to guide prescription.

All patients should be encouraged to participate in 30 to 60 mins of moderate-intensity aerobic activity, (i.e., brisk walking) on most, preferably all, days of the week, supplemented by an increase in daily lifestyle activities (e.g., walking breaks at work, gardening, household work).

Advise medically supervised programs for high-risk patients (e.g., recent acute coronary syndrome or revascularization, heart failure).

Weight management: Body mass index (BMI) of 18.5 to 24.9 kg/m^2 with waist circumference of less than 35 inches (women) and less than 40 inches (men). *Class 1 recommendation

Assessment of body mass index and/or waist circumference on each visit and consistently.

Encourage weight maintenance/reduction through an appropriate balance of physical activity, caloric intake, and formal behavioral programs when indicated to maintain/achieve a body mass index between 18.5 and 24.9 kg/m^2.

The initial goal of weight loss therapy should be to reduce body weight by approximately 10% from baseline.

With success, further weight loss can be attempted if indicated.

If waist circumference is greater than or equal to 35 inches in women and greater than or equal to 40 inches in men, it is useful to initiate lifestyle changes and consider treatment strategies for metabolic syndrome as indicated.

(Continued on next page)

Table 31-2 Continued.

Diabetes management: Achieve a glycosylated hemoglobin (HbA1c) level of less than 7% *Class 1 recommendation

It is recommended to initiate lifestyle and pharmacotherapy to achieve near-normal levels of HbA1c.

Aggressive modification of other risk factors such as physical activity, weight management, blood pressure control, and cholesterol management, as recommended above is beneficial.

Coordination of diabetic care with patient's primary care physician or endocrinologist is beneficial.

*Class I recommendation: The benefits of the intervention/treatment are much greater than the risk, and the procedure/treatment should be performed.
ACE, angiotensin-converting enzyme.

3. **Angina decubitus (nocturnal angina)**
   - **a.** This angina occurs in the recumbent position and is not specifically related to either rest or exertion.
   - **b.** Gravitational forces shift fluids within the body with a resultant increase in ventricular volume, which increases oxygen needs and produces angina decubitus, and which may indicate cardiac decompensation.
   - **c.** Diuretics alone or in combination effectively reduce left ventricular volume and may aid the patient.
   - **d.** Nitrates such as nitroglycerin may relieve the paroxysmal nocturnal dyspnea (PND) associated with angina decubitus by reducing preload, owing to venous pooling, and improving left ventricular dysfunction.
   - **e.** PND refers to a condition where fluid accumulation in the lungs, normally due to gravitational forces when one is in the recumbent position, makes it very difficult for a patient to breath. Some have referred to this as "cardiac asthma," as the patient is unable to breath and it gets progressively worse. Sleeping with several additional pillows might allow gravity to work on the added fluid in the lungs, with a resultant decrease in symptoms. However, the underlying cause needs to be corrected or the PND will remain.
4. **Prinzmetal angina (vasospastic or variant angina)**
   - **a.** Coronary artery spasm that reduces blood flow precipitates this angina. The spasm may be superimposed on a coronary artery that already has a fixed obstruction owing to thrombi or plaque formation.
   - **b.** It usually occurs at rest (i.e., pain may disrupt sleep) rather than with exertion or emotional stress, and usually resolves without progression to an acute MI. However, if the attack is prolonged, MI, life-threatening ventricular arrhythmias, and sudden cardiac death can occur.
   - **c.** Characteristically, an electrocardiogram (EKG/ECG) taken during an attack reveals a transient ST-segment elevation, which returns toward normal after the acute attack. The gold standard for identifying Prinzmetal angina is the use of coronary angiography with the administration of agents capable of inducing vasospasm, such as ergot alkaloids.
   - **d.** Calcium-channel blockers, rather than β-blockers, are most effective for this form of angina. Nitroglycerin may not provide relief, depending on the cause of vasospasm.

D. Physical examination is usually not revealing, especially between attacks. However, the patient's history, risk factors, and full description of attacks—precipitation pattern, intensity, duration, relieving factors—usually prove diagnostic.

E. Diagnostic test results

1. The **EKG/ECG** is normal in 50% or more of patients with stable angina pectoris, and a normal resting EKG/ECG does not exclude severe IHD. However, an EKG/ECG with evidence of left ventricular hypertrophy or ST-T-wave changes consistent with myocardial ischemia favors the diagnosis of angina pectoris. The presence of Q waves from a previous MI makes the diagnosis of IHD very likely. An EKG/ECG obtained during chest pain is abnormal in 50% of patients with angina who have a normal resting EKG/ECG. The ST segment can be either elevated or depressed.
2. **Stress testing (exercise EKG/ECG)** is a well-established procedure, which aids the diagnosis in patients who have normal resting EKGs/ECGs. The most commonly used definition for a positive test is a ≥ 1-mm ST-segment depression or elevation for ≥ 60 to 80 msec either during or after

exercise. Exercise stress testing is preferable to other variations of the stress test (pharmacological) in patients who are able to exercise.

3. **Pharmacological stress testing** is performed in suspected IHD patients when they are not able to perform more than moderate exercise due to various reasons (i.e., severe arthritis, prior injury, reduced exercise tolerance as a result of debilitating illnesses, etc.), or in patients who are unable to increase the heart rate.
   a. Intravenous dipyridamole (Persantine®; coronary vasodilation), adenosine (Adenocard®; coronary vasodilation) by inhibiting cellular uptake and degradation of adenosine increase coronary blood flow, and high-dose dobutamine (Dobutrex®; 20 to 40 mcg/kg/min) increase oxygen demand through increased heart rate, systolic blood pressure, and myocardial contractility causing an increase in myocardial blood flow are all able to induce detectable cardiac ischemia in conjunction with EKG/ECG testing.
   b. Side effects occur for each of the agents and include **dipyridamole** (angina, 18% to 42%; arrhythmias, 2%; headache, 5% to 23%; dizziness, 5% to 21%; nausea, 8% to 12%; and flushing, 3%), **adenosine** (chest pain, 57%; headache, 35%; flushing, 25%; shortness of breath, 15%; and first-degree atrioventricular [AV] heart block, 18%), **dobutamine** (premature ventricular beats, 15%; premature atrial beats, 8%; supraventricular tachycardia and nonsustained ventricular tachycardia, 3% to 4%; nausea, 8%; anxiety, 6%; headache, 4%; and tremor, 4%).
4. **Stress perfusion imaging** with thallium-201 or more recently, technetium-99m (^{99m}Tc) (sestamibi [Cardiolite®] or tetrafosmin [Myoview®]), can diagnose multivessel disease, localized ischemia, and may be able to determine myocardial viability. Coronary arteriography and cardiac catheterization are very specific and sensitive but are also invasive, expensive, and risky (the mortality rate is 1% to 2%); therefore, they must be used judiciously when trying to confirm suspected angina and to differentiate its origin.
5. Various drugs can have an effect on the EKG/ECG and should be considered before, during, and after an exercise test is carried out. Examples include
   a. Digoxin (Lanoxin®) produces abnormal exercise-induced ST depression in 25% to 40% of apparently healthy, normal subjects without ischemia.
   b. β-Adrenergic blockers may delay the development of an abnormal EKG/ECG if patients receive them before or during a stress test. If possible, therapy should be slowly withheld from the patient at least four to five half-lives before the exercise testing. If it is not possible to withdraw therapy, the clinician needs to recognize that the test might be less reliable.
   c. Antihypertensives such as vasodilators can alter the stress test by altering the normal hemodynamic response of blood pressure. In addition, short-term use of nitrates can attenuate angina and ST-segment changes associated with myocardial ischemia.

F. **Treatment goals**
1. To prevent MI and death, thereby increasing a patient's quality of life
2. To reduce symptoms of angina and occurrence of ischemia, which should improve a patient's quality of life
3. To remove or reduce **risk factors**
4. The management of angina pectoris includes therapies aimed at reversing cardiac risk factors.
   a. **Hyperlipidemia**, if present, should be treated. Reducing cholesterol and low-density lipoprotein (LDL) is associated with a reduced risk of cardiovascular disease and incidence of ischemic cardiac events, as demonstrated by several recent studies using β-hydroxy-β-methylglutaryl-coenzyme A (HMG-CoA) reductase inhibitors. The NCEP has published guidelines for treatment of high blood cholesterol (Adult Treatment Panel III), and a fourth set of guidelines is currently being developed with a publication date in 2012.
      (1) Total cholesterol is no longer the primary target of treatment; LDL cholesterol is now the primary target.
      (2) Current recommendations include the completion of a lipoprotein profile—total cholesterol, LDL cholesterol, high-density lipoprotein (HDL) cholesterol, and triglycerides—as the preferred initial test, rather than screening for total cholesterol and HDL alone. Additionally, the ATP-3 guidelines identify LDL cholesterol < 100 mg/dL as optimal and raises categorical low HDL cholesterol from < 35 mg/dL to < 40 mg/dL because the latter is a better measure of a depressed HDL.

Finally, the ATP-3 lowered the triglyceride classification cutpoints to give more attention to moderate elevations.

(3) Persons are categorized into one of four levels of risk to identify group-specific treatment modalities: (1) *high-risk*, established IHD or IHD risk equivalents (diabetes, noncoronary forms of atherosclerotic disease); (2) *moderately high-risk*, multiple (more than two) risk factors and a calculated 10-year risk of 10% to 20%; (3) *moderate risk*, multiple (more than two) risk factors and a calculated 10-year risk of 10%; and (4) *lower risk*, zero to one risk factor.

(4) All individuals with IHD or IHD risk equivalents have been called "high risk," and the treatment goals is to have LDL-cholesterol (LDL-C) levels < 100 mg/dL. Other recommendations are as follows:

(a) If baseline LDL-C is < 100 mg/dL (goal of treatment), patients with IHD should be given instructions on diet and exercise and have levels monitored annually; although the guidelines suggest an optional goal of obtaining an LDL-C of < 70 mg/dL.

(b) If baseline LDL-C is ≥ 100 mg/dL, an LDL-lowering drug should be started along with therapeutic lifestyle changes (TLCs). Lifestyle-related risk factors include things such as obesity, physical inactivity, elevated triglyceride, low-HDL-C, or metabolic syndrome.

(c) Adult Treatment Panel III did not mandate LDL-lowering drugs for patients with baseline LDL-C levels between 100 and 129 mg/dL, but suggested intensifying lifestyle and the optional use of drug therapies to lower LDL to < 100 mg/dL. However, if the patient had elevated triglycerides or low high-density lipoprotein cholesterol (HDL-C), a drug should be started that targets these abnormalities—for example, nicotinic acid or fibric acid if the patient has elevated triglycerides (> 200 mg/dL) or low HDL levels (< 40 mg/dL). If triglycerides are ≥ 500 mg/dL, consider fibrate or niacin before LDL-lowering therapy.

(5) For moderately high-risk patients, the recommended LDL-C goal is < 130 mg/dL, but a goal of < 100 mg/dL is an optional goal, based on recent clinical trial evidence. In addition, a recommendation to initiate TLCs when the patient has an LDL-C ≥ 130 mg/dL.

(6) For moderate risk patients, the recommended LDL-C goal is < 130 mg/dL. In addition, a recommendation to initiate TLC when the patient has an LDL-C ≥ 160 mg/dL.

(7) For lower risk patients, the recommended LDL-C goal is < 160 mg/dL, but again, a recommendation to initiate TLC for those patients with an LDL ≥ 190 mg/dL.

(8) The **metabolic syndrome** is closely linked to insulin resistance, when the normal actions of insulin are impaired. Excess body fat and physical inactivity promote the development of the syndrome; however, some individuals may be predisposed genetically. Patients with three or more of the following characteristics are referred to as having the metabolic syndrome and should be treated accordingly: abdominal obesity, triglycerides > 150 mg/dL, HDL levels of < 40 mg/dL for men and < 50 mg/dL for women, blood pressure readings ≥ 130/85 mm Hg, and a fasting serum glucose level ≥ 110 mg/dL.

(9) **Increased interest in triglycerides** due to a long-standing association between elevated triglyceride levels and cardiovascular disease. The continuing rise since 1976 of triglyceride levels in concert with the growing incidence of obesity, type 2 diabetes mellitus, and insulin resistance has occurred at a time when LDL-C levels have continued to decrease. This ongoing concern has resulted in a recent scientific statement from the American Heart Association with the intent to update clinicians on the continued role that triglycerides play in cardiovascular disease. (Available through the Internet at: **http://circ.ahajournals.org/cgi/reprint/123/20/2292?maxtoshow=&hits=10&RESULTFORMAT=&fulltext=triglycerides&searchid=1&FIRSTINDEX=0&volume=123&issue=20&resourcetype=HWCIT**)

G. Individual drug classes

1. Bile acid-binding resins

a. Mechanism of action. These insoluble, nonabsorbable, anion-exchange resins bind bile acids within the intestines and prevent them from being reabsorbed. Bile acids are synthesized from cholesterol.

b. **Indications.** These agents have been shown to be safe and effective in lowering LDL-C, especially in patients with modestly elevated levels, in primary prevention, in young adult men, and in postmenopausal women. They are effective in combination with other agents.

c. **Currently available agents** include the following:

(1) Cholestyramine (Questran®): 4 to 24 g by mouth in two daily doses

(2) Colestipol (Colestid®): 2 to 16 g by mouth in one to four daily doses

(3) Colesevelam (Welchol®): six to seven tablets (625 mg/tablet) by mouth in one daily dose

d. **Precautions and monitoring effects**

(1) These resins are taken just before meals and present palatability problems in patients.

(2) Gastrointestinal (GI) intolerance, especially constipation, flatulence, and dyspepsia are frequent.

(3) Absorption of many other drugs can be affected. Other drugs should be taken 1 hr before or 4 to 6 hrs after resins.

2. **Statins or HMG-CoA reductase inhibitors**

a. **Mechanism of action.** These agents inhibit the enzyme HMG-CoA, resulting in a reduction in cholesterol production.

b. **Indications.** These agents are effective in lowering LDL levels while increasing HDL levels and lowering triglyceride levels. They are primarily used to lower LDL cholesterol levels and are generally considered to be the most effective of the lipid lowering agents.

c. **Currently available agents** include the following:

(1) Atorvastatin (Lipitor®): 10 to 80 mg by mouth daily

(2) Fluvastatin (Lescol®): 20 to 80 mg by mouth in one to two doses

(3) Lovastatin (Mevacor®, various): 10 to 80 mg by mouth in the evening

(4) Pitavastatin (Livalo®): 1 to 4 mg by mouth daily

(5) Pravastatin (Pravachol®): 10 to 80 mg by mouth daily

(6) Rosuvastatin (Crestor®): 5 to 40 mg by mouth daily

(7) Simvastatin (Zocor®, various): 5 to 80 mg by mouth in the evening

(a) **Recent FDA alert on dosing limitations for products containing simvastatin:** Simvastatin 80 mg is limited to patients that have been taking this dose for > 12 consecutive months without evidence of myopathy and are not currently taking or beginning to take a simvastatin dose-limiting or contraindicated interacting medication.

d. **Precautions and monitoring effects**

(1) GI adverse effects are less frequently seen than with other classes of agents. Headache and dyspepsia frequently occur and should be evaluated, then followed up in 6 to 8 weeks, and then at each follow-up visit thereafter.

(2) These agents can elevate liver function tests—alanine aminotransferase (ALT) and aspartate aminotransferase (AST), which requires initial evaluation, then after approximately 12 weeks of therapy, then annually thereafter.

(3) Although the incidence of myopathy is believed to be low (0.08%) for lovastatin and simvastatin, elevations of creatine kinase (CK) > 10 times the upper limit of normal have been reported with pravastatin, with similar potential for the other members of the group. Cerivastatin (Baycol) was voluntarily removed from the market owing to the reported deaths of 31 patients from rhabdomyolysis while receiving the drug alone or in combination with gemfibrozil (Lopid). Consequently, routine monitoring is necessary in all patients as follows:

(a) Evaluate muscle symptoms and check CK before starting therapy, evaluate in 6 to 12 weeks after starting therapy, and then at each follow-up visit.

(b) Patients presenting with muscle soreness, tenderness, or pain should have a CK measurement on presentation to minimize the development of myopathies.

(c) Concurrent therapy with other agents, including cyclosporine, macrolide antibiotics, azole antifungals, niacin, fibrates, or nefazodone, may increase the risk.

3. **Fibric acid derivatives**

a. **Mechanism of action.** These agents are presumed to inhibit cholesterol synthesis and lower LDL-C and bile acids. They are most effective in lowering triglyceride levels by reducing the concentration of very-low-density lipoproteins (VLDL). In some patients, they modestly lower LDL-C and raise HDL-C.

b. **Precautions and monitoring effects**
   (1) GI effects are the most commonly experienced adverse effect.
   (2) These agents can elevate liver function tests; routine monitoring should be carried out.
   (3) Use with statins can lead to elevated CK, and monitoring is necessary to identify myopathies or rhabdomyolysis.

c. **Currently available agents** include the following:
   (1) Fenofibrate (Tricor®, various): 145 to 160 mg by mouth daily
   (2) Gemfibrozil (Lopid®, various): 600 mg by mouth twice daily

4. **Niacin**

a. **Mechanism of action.** Numerous studies have demonstrated the role of niacin in the lowering of LDL-C and triglycerides through various mechanisms such as participation in tissue respiration oxidation–reduction reactions, which decreases hepatic LDL and VLDL production; inhibition of adipose tissue lipolysis; decreased hepatic triglyceride esterification; and increases in lipoprotein lipase activity. *Table 31-3* presents several agents and their effects on lipoproteins.

b. **Indications.** Niacin is valuable in treating patients with elevated total cholesterol and low LDL-C levels. It works primarily by reducing the production of VLDL in the liver and has been shown to lower LDL-C and triglycerides while also increasing HDL-C. It is used in combination therapy.

c. **Currently available agents** include the following:
   (1) Niacin controlled-release (Niaspan®): 1000 to 2000 mg by mouth at bedtime
   (2) Niacin controlled-release (Slo-Niacin®): 1 to 2 g by mouth at bedtime
   (3) Niacin immediate-release (Niacor®,Various): 1500 to 3000 mg by mouth two to three times daily

d. **Precautions**
   (1) Adverse GI effects are experienced with the use of niacin.
   (2) Patients may experience flushing and itchy skin, which may be reduced with the administration of 325 mg aspirin about 30 mins before the dose.
   (3) Cases of severe liver toxicity have been reported. Liver function tests should be performed in patients receiving this drug.

Table 31-3 SELECTED AGENTS AND THEIR EFFECTS ON LIPOPROTEINS

Class/Agent	Lipid/Lipoprotein Effects	Daily Dose	Adverse Drug Effects
HMG-CoA reductase inhibitors (statins)	LDL: 18%–55% reduction HDL: 5%–15% increase TG: 7%–30% reduction	Lovastatin: 10–80 mg Pravastatin: 20–40 mg Simvastatin: 5–80 mg Fluvastatin: 20–80 mg Atorvastatin: 10–80 mg Rosuvastatin: 5–40 mg	Myopathy, increased liver enzymes
Bile acid sequestrants	LDL: 15%–30% reduction HDL: 3%–5% increase TG: No change or increase	Cholestyramine: 4–16 g Colestipol: 5–20 g Colesevelam: 2.6–3.8 g	GI distress, constipation, decreased absorption of other drugs
Nicotinic acid	LDL: 5%–25% reduction HDL: 15%–35% increase TG: 20%–50% reduction	Immediate-release: 1.5–3.0 g Extended-release: 1–2 g Sustained-release: 1–2 g	Flushing, hyperglycemia, hyperuricemia (or gout), upper GI distress, hepatotoxicity
Fibric acids	LDL: 5%–20% reduction HDL: 10%–20% increase TG: 20%–50% reduction	Gemfibrozil: 600 mg twice daily Fenofibrate: 145–160 mg Clofibrate: 1000 mg twice daily	Dyspepsia, gallstones, myopathy, unexplained non-CHD deaths in WHO study

CHD, coronary heart disease; *GI*, gastrointestinal; *HDL*, high-density lipoprotein; *HMG-CoA*, β-hydroxy-β-methylglutaryl-coenzyme A; *LDL*, low-density lipoprotein; *TG*, triglycerides; *WHO*, World Health Organization. Adapted from Grundy SM, Becher D, Clark LT, et al. Third Report of the National Cholesterol Education Program (NCEP): detection, evaluation, and treatment of high blood cholesterol in adults (Adult Treatment Panel III) [NIH Publication No. 01-3670]. Washington, DC: U.S. Department of Health and Human Services; May 2001. Available at http://www.nhlbi.nih.gov/guidelines/cholesterol/atp3xsum.pdf.

5. **Ezetimibe (Zetia®)**
   a. **Mechanism of action.** Works by selectively inhibiting the intestinal absorption of cholesterol and related phytosterols, with a resultant decrease in intestinal cholesterol delivered to the liver, decreased hepatic cholesterol stores, and an increase in the clearance of cholesterol from the blood. Ezetimibe has demonstrated the ability to reduce total cholesterol, LDL-C, apolipoprotein B, and triglyceride levels while increasing HDL levels in patients with hypercholesterolemia.
   b. **Indications.** Ezetimibe as adjunctive therapy along with dietary measures, alone in patients with primary heterozygous familial and nonfamilial hypercholesterolemia, or in combination with the HMG-CoA reductase inhibitors in homozygous familial hypercholesterolemia.
   c. **Dose.** Normal dosing recommendations are a 10-mg dose given once daily.
   d. **Precautions.** As monotherapy, studies to date have not revealed significant side effects above those seen with placebo administration. However, when used in combination with HMG-CoA reductase inhibitors, reports have described an increased incidence (approximately 1.4%) in the elevation of liver transaminase levels (three times the upper limit of normal) as compared to the incidence of 0.4% with HMG-CoA agents used alone.
6. **Combination products**
   a. Ezetimibe/simvastatin (Vytorin®) uses the individual class properties of the HMG-CoA reductase inhibitors (simvastatin) to reduce cholesterol production with the absorption-inhibiting properties of ezetimibe to target cholesterol with two differing mechanisms, which might aid in improving patient compliance.
      (1) Available product is supplied as 10/10, 10/20, 10/40, 10/80 combinations of ezetimibe and simvastatin, respectively, and the daily recommended dose is one tablet by mouth every evening.
      (2) Side effects reflect the additive side effect properties of ezetimibe and simvastatin and warrant consideration when occurring during therapy. **Recent FDA alert on dosing limitations for products containing simvastatin:** Simvastatin 80 mg is limited to patients that have been taking this dose for > 12 consecutive months without evidence of myopathy and are not currently taking or beginning to take a simvastatin dose-limiting or contraindicated interacting medication.
   b. Lovastatin/niacin (Advicor®) is a product that incorporates the actions of the HMG-CoA reductase inhibitor lovastatin with an extended-release niacin component into a single product, using differing mechanisms, which might aid in improving patient compliance.
      (1) Available product is supplied as 20/500, 20/750, 20/1000, 40/1000 immediate-release tablet combinations of lovastatin and niacin, respectively. The recommended daily dose is one to two tablets by mouth at bedtime.
      (2) Side effects reflect the additive side effect properties for both lovastatin and niacin and warrant consideration during therapy.
   c. Amlodipine/atorvastatin (Caduet®) is a combination product that incorporates the actions of the dihydropyridine calcium-channel blocker amlodipine with the lipid-lowering properties of the HMG-CoA reductase inhibitor atorvastatin. The calcium-channel blocker offers no benefit for lipid lowering but represents a potentially beneficial product for a patient with coexisting disease states, such as IHD and hypertension, for which the use of a calcium-channel blocker would be warranted.
      (1) Available product is supplied as 2.5/10, 2.5/20, 2.5/40, 5/10, 5/20, 5/40, 5/80, 10/10, 10/20, /10/40, and 10/80; which consist of amlodipine and atorvastatin, respectively, in an immediate-release dosage form. The recommended daily dose is one to two tablets by mouth at bedtime.
      (2) Side effects reflect the additive side effect properties for both amlodipine and atorvastatin and warrant consideration during therapy.
   d. Simvastatin/niacin (Simcor®) is a product that incorporates the actions of the HMG-CoA reductase inhibitor simvastatin with an extended-release niacin component into a single product, using differing mechanisms, which might aid in improving patient compliance.
      (1) Available product is supplied as 500/20, 500/40, 750/20, 1000/20, 1000/40 which consist of extended-release niacin and simvastatin, respectively, in an immediate-release dosage form. The recommended daily dose is one to two tablets by mouth at bedtime.

(2) Side effects reflect the additive side effect properties for both niacin and simvastatin and warrant consideration during therapy. **Recent FDA alert on dosing limitations for products containing simvastatin:** Simvastatin 80 mg is limited to patients that have been taking this dose for > 12 consecutive months without evidence of myopathy and are not currently taking or beginning to take a simvastatin dose-limiting or contraindicated interacting medication.

e. Omega-3-acid ethyl esters (Lovaza®) is the first FDA-approved omega-3 fatty acid, which is indicated for patients with elevated levels of triglycerides (> 500 mg/dL).

(1) Mechanism of action. Although not entirely worked out yet, may work by one of several mechanisms, including an increased hepatic beta-oxidation, a reduction in the hepatic synthesis of triglycerides, or an increase in plasma lipoprotein lipase activity.

(2) Available product is supplied as a 1-g capsule; the recommended daily dose is four capsules by mouth daily in one to two doses.

(3) Side effects that have been reported include burping, infection, flu-like symptoms, upset stomach, change in one's sense of taste, back pain, and rash.

f. Hypertension. Treatment of hypertension according to the Joint National Conference VII guidelines has received a class I recommendation based on data from multiple randomized clinical trials with large numbers of patients (A, high) and should be controlled. Class I recommendations are based on evidence or general agreement that a given procedure or treatment is useful and effective (see Chapter 33).

g. Smoking should be stopped if at all possible and has received a class I recommendation based on data derived from a limited number of randomized trials with small numbers of patients (B, intermediate).

(1) Transdermal use of nicotine-containing patches has become one strategy for aiding the cessation of smoking. Products such as Nicotrol®, NicoDerm®, and others are available in varying strengths both as prescription and over-the-counter treatments, in order to wean patients off the use of cigarettes over an 8- to 12-week period, using descending doses.

(2) Nicotine gum (oral nicotine polacrilex chewing pieces) is available in 2- or 4-mg pieces as an over-the-counter product. Nicorette® is usually used for 3 months to aid in cessation of smoking.

(3) Bupropion is a prescription antidepressant, which is also marketed under the brand name of Zyban® as an aid to smoking cessation.

(4) Varenicline (Chantix®) is an approved product, which works as a partial neuronal α_4-β_2 nicotinic receptor agonist in the brain to reduce the craving for nicotine. Therapy is started with a dose of 0.5 mg by mouth daily for 3 days, followed by 0.5 mg tablets twice daily for 4 days, then 1 mg twice daily thereafter for 12 weeks, which can be given for an additional 12 weeks if successful.

h. Obesity should be reduced through diet and an appropriate exercise program in patients with hypertension, hyperlipidemia, or diabetes mellitus and has received a class I recommendation based on expert consensus as the primary basis (C, low).

H. Therapeutic agents

1. Recent evidence-based guidelines have provided recommendations for the treatment of patients with chronic stable angina. (See I.D.1; Fraker et al.). Recommendations use the following levels of rankings:

Ranking Based on Size of Treatment Effect	Assessment of Benefit Versus Risk	Recommended Action
Class I	Benefit >>> risk	Treatment should be used
Class IIa	Benefit >> risk	Reasonable to use treatment
Class IIb	Benefit ≥ risk	Treatment may be considered
Class III	No benefit; potentially harmful	No proven benefit; even harmful

Estimate of Certainty for Treatment Effect	Extent of Populations Studied	Types of Trials Used
Level A	Multiple populations evaluated	Data derived from multiple trials/ meta-analyses
Level B	Limited populations evaluated	Data derived from a single trial or nonrandomized study
Level C	Very limited populations evaluated	Consensus opinion of experts or case reports

2. **Nitrates (e.g., nitroglycerin)**
   a. **Mechanism of action**
      (1) The primary value of nitrates is venous dilation, which reduces left ventricular volume (preload) and myocardial wall tension, decreasing oxygen requirements (demand).
      (2) Nitrates may also reduce arteriolar resistance, helping reduce afterload, which decreases myocardial oxygen demand.
      (3) By reducing pressure in cardiac tissues, nitrates also facilitate collateral circulation, which increases blood distribution to ischemic areas.
      (4) Pharmacological effects have been shown to improve exercise tolerance, prolong the time to onset of angina, and the appearance of ST-segment depression during exercise testing.
   b. **Indications**
      (1) Acute attacks of angina pectoris can be managed with sublingual, transmucosal (Nitrolingual® spray or Nitrostat® sublingual tablets), or intravenous delivery.
      (2) Indications include the prevention of anticipated attacks, using tablets (oral or buccal) or transdermal paste or patches. Sublingual nitrates (Nitrostat®) can be used before eating, sexual activity, or a known stressful event.
      (3) Nitrates are used in treatment of stable angina. They may not be effective as a single agent for treatment of Prinzmetal angina, although some studies have shown nitrates to prevent or reverse vasospasm at varying doses. Intravenous nitroglycerin is used in the immediate treatment of unstable angina and is used for long-term therapeutic relief.
      (4) Nitrates used in combination with β-adrenergic blockers have been shown to be more effective than nitrates or β-adrenergic blockers used alone.
   c. **Choice of preparation** should be based on onset of action, duration of action, and patient compliance and preference because all nitrates have the same mechanism of action.
   d. **Precautions and monitoring effects**
      (1) To maximize the therapeutic effect, patients should thoroughly understand the use of their specific dosage forms (e.g., sublingual tablets, transdermal patches or pastes, tablets, capsules).
      (2) Blood pressure and heart rate should be monitored because all nitrates can increase heart rate while lowering blood pressure.
      (3) Preload reduction can be assessed through reduction of pulmonary symptoms such as shortness of breath, paroxysmal nocturnal dyspnea, or dyspnea.
      (4) Nitrate-induced headaches are the most common side effect.
         (a) Patients should be warned of the nature, suddenness, and potential strength of these headaches to minimize the anxiety that might otherwise occur.
         (b) Compliance can be enhanced if the patient understands that the effect is transient and that the headaches usually disappear with continued therapy.
         (c) Acetaminophen ingested 15 to 30 mins before nitrate administration may prevent the headache.
   e. **Effective therapy** should result in fewer anginal attacks without inducing significant adverse effects (e.g., postural hypotension, hypoxia). If maximal doses are reached and the patient still experiences attacks, additional agents should be administered.
   f. **Nitrate tolerance** is a major problem with the long-term use of nitroglycerin and long-acting nitrates. Several agents such as ACE inhibitors (sulfhydryl-containing drugs), acetylcysteine, and diuretics have been shown to reverse nitrate tolerance by increasing the availability of

sulfhydryl radicals. However, practical considerations suggest that less frequent administration (8 to 12 hrs of nitrate-free intervals) is effective without introducing additional agents.

3. **β-Adrenergic blockers.** Based on the 2007 Focused Guidelines for Patients With Chronic Stable Angina, a class 1a recommendation states that it is beneficial to start and continue β-blocker therapy indefinitely in all patients who have had MI, acute coronary syndrome, or left ventricular dysfunction with or without heart failure symptoms, unless contraindicated.
   a. **Mechanism of action.** β-Blockers reduce oxygen demand, both at rest and during exertion, by decreasing the heart rate and myocardial contractility, which also decreases arterial blood pressure.
   b. **Indications**
      (1) These agents reduce the frequency and severity of exertional angina that is not controlled by nitrates.
      (2) Nitrates have been combined with calcium antagonists, when slow-release dihydropyridines (e.g., felodipine [Plendil®], amlodipine [Norvasc®]) are preferred over diltiazem (Cardizem®) or verapamil (Calan®). If patients need to receive a β-adrenergic blocker along with verapamil or diltiazem owing to the added effects, they have the potential to induce bradycardia, AV heart block, and fatigue.
   c. **Precautions and monitoring effects**
      (1) Doses should be increased until the anginal episodes have been reduced or until unacceptable side effects occur.
      (2) β-Blockers should be avoided in Prinzmetal angina (caused by coronary vasospasm) because they increase coronary resistance and may induce vasospasm.
      (3) Asthma is a relative contraindication because all β-blockers increase airway resistance and have the potential to induce bronchospasm in susceptible patients.
      (4) Patients with diabetes and others predisposed to hypoglycemia should be warned that β-blockers mask tachycardia, which is a key sign of developing hypoglycemia.
      (5) Patients should be monitored for excessive negative inotropic effects. Findings such as fatigue, shortness of breath, edema, and paroxysmal nocturnal dyspnea may signal developing cardiac decompensation, which also increases the metabolic demands of the heart.
      (6) Sudden cessation of β-blocker therapy may trigger a withdrawal syndrome that can exacerbate anginal attacks (especially in patients with IHD) or cause MI.
   d. **Choice of preparations.** All β-blockers are likely to be equally effective for stable (exertional) angina. For further review of β-adrenergic blockers, see Chapter 33-Hypertension. For a list of β-adrenergic blockers, see Table 33-4, and for complete descriptions for each β-adrenergic blocker, see Chapter 33: III.B.3.a.

4. **Calcium-channel blockers**
   a. **Mechanism of action.** Two actions are most pertinent in the treatment of angina.
      (1) These agents prevent and reverse coronary spasm by inhibiting calcium influx into vascular smooth muscle and myocardial muscle. This results in increased blood flow, which enhances myocardial oxygen supply.
      (2) Calcium-channel blockers decrease coronary vascular resistance and increase coronary blood flow, resulting in increased oxygen supply.
      (3) Calcium-channel blockers decrease systemic vascular resistance and arterial pressure; in addition, they decrease inotropic effects, resulting in decreased myocardial oxygen demand.
   b. **Indications**
      (1) Calcium-channel blockers are used in stable (exertional) angina that is not controlled by nitrates and β-blockers and in patients for whom β-blocker therapy is inadvisable. Combination therapy—with nitrates, β-blockers, or both—may be most effective.
      (2) These agents, alone or with a nitrate, are particularly valuable in the treatment of Prinzmetal angina. They are considered the drug of choice in treatment of angina at rest.
   c. **Individual agents**
      (1) **Diltiazem (Cardizem®) and verapamil (Calan®)**
         (a) These drugs produce negative inotropic effects, and patients must be monitored closely for signs of developing cardiac decompensation (i.e., fatigue, shortness of breath, edema, paroxysmal nocturnal dyspnea). When coadministered with β-blockers or other agents that produce negative inotropic effects (e.g., disopyramide [Norpace®], quinidine Various, procainamide [Pronestyl®], flecainide [Tambocor®]), the negative effects are additive.

Table 31-4 SELECTED AGENTS AND THEIR DOSES IN THE TREATMENT OF CORONARY ARTERY DISEASE

Class/Agent	Dose/Dosage Schedule	Comments
	Nitrates	
Nitroglycerin sublingual tablets (Nitrostat®)	0.3–0.6 mg up to 1.5 mg	Short-term effects: 1–7 mins
Nitroglycerin spray (Nitrolingual®)	0.4 mg as needed	Similar to sublingual tablets
Nitroglycerin transdermal (Nitro-Dur®)	0.2–0.8 mg/hr every 12 hrs	Remove patch for 8–12 hrs to reduce tolerance
Nitroglycerin intravenous infusion (Various)	5–200 mcg/min	Short acting requiring continuous infusion and monitoring
Isosorbide mononitrate (Imdur®, Monoket®)	10–40 mg daily in two doses	Also available as extended-release product for single daily dosing
Isosorbide dinitrate SL	2.5–10 mg SL every 2–3 hrs	For acute angina attacks
Isosorbide dinitrate oral tablets (Various)	5–80 mg, two to three times daily	Longer acting up to 8 hrs
Isosorbide dinitrate slow-release tablets (Dilatrate-SR®)	40 mg once or twice daily	Duration of activity up to 8 hrs
	β-Adrenergic blockers	
Propranolol (Inderal®)	20–80 mg twice daily	Possesses both β_1- and β_2-blocker effects
Metoprolol (Lopressor®)	50–200 mg twice daily	Possesses β_1-blocker effects
Atenolol (Tenormin®)	50–200 mg/day	Possesses β_1-blocker effects
Nadolol (Corgard®)	40–80 mg/day	Possesses both β_1- and β_2-blocker effects
Timolol	10 mg twice daily	Possesses both β_1- and β_2-blocker effects
Acebutolol (Sectral®)	200–600 mg twice daily	Possesses β_1-blocker effects
Betaxolol (Kerlone®)	10–20 mg/day	Possesses β_1-blocker effects
Bisoprolol (Zebeta®)	10 mg/day	Possesses β_1-blocker effects
Esmolol (intravenous) (Brevibloc®)	50–300 mcg/kg/min	Possesses β_1-blocker effects
Labetalol (Trandate®, Various)	200–600 mg twice daily	Possesses both α_1-, β_1-, and β_2-blocker effects
Pindolol (Various)	2.5–7.5 mg three times daily	Possesses both β_1- and β_2-blocker effects
Carvedilol (Coreg®)	25 mg twice daily	Possesses both α_1- β_1-, and β_2-blocker effects
Penbutolol (Levatol®)		Possesses both β_1- and β_2-blocker effects
	Calcium-channel blockers	
Dihydropyridine derivatives		
Nifedipine (Procardia®)	Immediate-release; 30–90 mg daily	Short duration of action of 4–6 hrs
Amlodipine (Norvasc®, Various)	5–10 mg once daily	Long duration of action
Felodipine (Plendil®)	5–10 mg once daily	Long duration of action
Isradipine (Dynacirc®)	2.5–10 mg twice daily	Intermediate duration of action
Nicardipine (Cardene®)	20–40 mg three times daily	Short duration of action
Nisoldipine (Sular®)	20–40 mg once daily	Short duration of action

Table 31-4 Continued.

Class/Agent	Dose/Dosage Schedule	Comments
	Miscellaneous	
Diltiazem (Cardizem®)	Immediate-release: 30–80 mg four times daily	Short duration of action; important consideration necessary owing to hypotension, bradycardia, and edema
	Slow-release: 120–320 mg once daily	Long duration of action; important consideration necessary owing to hypotension, bradycardia, and edema
Verapamil (Calan®)	Immediate-release: 80–160 mg three times daily	Short duration of action; important consideration necessary owing to hypotension, bradycardia, edema, myocardial depression, and heart failure
	Slow-release: 120–480 mg once daily	Long duration of action; important consideration necessary owing to hypotension, bradycardia, edema, myocardial depression, and heart failure

(b) Patients should be monitored for signs of developing bradyarrhythmias and heart block because these agents have negative chronotropic effects.

(c) Verapamil (Calan®) frequently causes constipation that must be treated as needed to prevent straining at stool, which could cause an increased oxygen demand (Valsalva maneuver). Verapamil is not recommended in patients with sick sinus syndromes, AV nodal disease, or heart failure (HF).

(2) **Nifedipine (Procardia®)**

(a) This calcium-channel blocker is believed to possess the greatest degree of negative inotropic effects compared to the newer second-generation members of this group, amlodipine (Norvasc®) and felodipine (Plendil®). Nifedipine 10 mg (chewed or swallowed) has been used to treat Prinzmetal angina or refractory spasm in patients who are not hypotensive. Controversy still exists about the use of short-acting, rapid-release agents such as nifedipine in patients with IHD.

(b) Because nifedipine increases the heart rate somewhat, it can produce tachycardia, which would increase oxygen demand. Coadministration of a β-blocker should prevent reflex tachycardia.

(c) Its potent peripheral dilatory effects can decrease coronary perfusion and produce excessive hypotension, which can aggravate myocardial ischemia.

(d) Dizziness, light-headedness, and lower extremity edema are the most common adverse effects, but these tend to disappear with time or dose adjustment.

(3) **Amlodipine (Norvasc®), clevidipine (Cleviprex®), felodipine (Plendil®), isradipine (Dynacirc®), nicardipine (Cardene®), and nisoldipine (Sular®)** are second-generation dihydropyridine derivative, calcium-channel blockers. They have been used effectively as once- or twice-a-day agents owing to their long activity. Because of the potent negative inotropic effects of these agents, they are not recommended in patients with HF (amlodipine has been shown to have less negative potential in HF than other members of the class). Clevidipine is available in the injectable form only and is administered as a continuous slow IV infusion.

5. **Antiplatelet agents**

a. Aspirin. Based on the 2007 Focused Guidelines for Patients With Chronic Stable Angina, a class Ia recommendation states that aspirin should be started at 75 to 162 mg/day and continued indefinitely in all patients unless contraindicated.

b. Ticlopidine (Ticlid®) is a thienopyridine derivative that inhibits platelet aggregation induced by adenosine diphosphate. However, unlike aspirin, it has not been shown to decrease adverse cardiovascular events in patients with stable angina and has been associated with thrombotic thrombocytopenic purpura on an infrequent basis.

c. **Clopidogrel (Plavix®)** is also a thienopyridine derivative related to ticlopidine, but it possesses antithrombotic effects that are greater than those of ticlopidine. Clopidogrel is a therapeutic option in those angina patients who cannot take aspirin because of contraindications. Doses of 75 mg daily are recommended to prevent the development of acute coronary syndromes.
   (1) Recently there has been added concern regarding the interaction which takes place when patients receiving clopidogrel are also given one of the proton pump inhibitors (PPIs), such as omeprazole (Nexium®). The American College of Cardiology Foundation, in conjunction with the American College of Gastroenterology and the American Heart Association, has issued a consensus document regarding the concomitant use of PPIs and thienopyridines, specifically clopidogrel. The following highlighted recommendations are discussed within the consensus statement as they relate to the combinations of clopidogrel and PPIs:
      (a) PPIs are appropriate in patients with multiple risk factors for GI bleeding who are also receiving antiplatelet therapy (e.g., clopidogrel).
      (b) Although pharmacokinetic and pharmacodynamic studies have demonstrated varying effects of PPIs on the extent of clopidogrel metabolic conversion to the active metabolite, no evidence has established clinically meaningful differences in outcomes.
      (c) A clinically significant interaction cannot be excluded in subgroups who are poor metabolizers of clopidogrel.
      (d) Until solid evidence exists to support staggering PPIs with clopidogrel, the dosing of PPIs should not be altered.

d. Based on the 2007 Focused Guidelines for Patients With Chronic Stable Angina, a class Ib recommendation states that the use of warfarin in conjunction with aspirin and/or clopidogrel is associated with an increased risk of bleeding and should be monitored closely.

6. **ACE inhibitors.** Based on the 2007 Focused Guidelines for Patients With Chronic Stable Angina, the following recommendations have been made for ACE inhibitors.
   a. Class 1a recommendation states that ACE inhibitors should be started and continued indefinitely in all patients with left ventricular ejection fraction ≤ 40% and in those with hypertension, diabetes, or chronic kidney disease unless contraindicated.
   b. Class Ib recommendation that ACE inhibitors should be started and continued indefinitely in patients who are not lower risk (lower risk defined as those with normal left ventricular ejection fraction in whom cardiovascular risk factors are well controlled and revascularization has been performed), unless contraindicated.
   c. Class IIa recommendation that it is reasonable to use ACE inhibitors among lower risk patients with mildly reduced or normal left ventricular ejection fraction in whom cardiovascular risk factors are well controlled and revascularization has been performed.
   d. Current guidelines do not suggest which agent to use, and it is anticipated that ongoing trials with additional agents will provide additional information regarding dosing regimens and potential differences that might exist among the class of drugs.

7. **Angiotensin receptor blockers (ARBs).** Based on the 2007 Focused Guidelines for Patients With Chronic Stable Angina, three new recommendations have been made for the use of ARBs in patients with chronic stable angina.
   a. Class Ia recommendation that ARBs are recommended for patients who have hypertension, have indications for but are intolerant of ACE inhibitors, have heart failure, or have had a myocardial infarction with left ventricular ejection fraction ≤ 40%.
   b. Class IIb recommendation that ARBs may be considered in combination with ACE inhibitors for heart failure due to left ventricular systolic dysfunction.
   c. Class Ia recommendation that aldosterone blockade is recommended for use in post-MI patients without significant renal dysfunction or hyperkalemia who are already receiving therapeutic doses of an ACE inhibitor and a β-blocker, have a left ventricular ejection fraction ≤ 40%, and have either diabetes or heart failure.

8. **Chelation therapy.** Based on the 2007 Focused Guidelines for Patients With Chronic Stable Angina, a class IIIc recommendation stated that chelation therapy (intravenous infusions of ethylenediaminetetraacetic acid or EDTA) is not recommended for the treatment of chronic angina or arteriosclerotic cardiovascular disease and may be harmful because of its potential to cause hypocalcemia.

III. ACUTE CORONARY SYNDROME (ACS)

A. **Definition.** ACS is a relatively new term that has been introduced into the medical literature to describe any pattern of clinical symptoms that reflects the development of acute MI (*Figure 31-2*). This category includes the symptoms related to STEMI, NSTEMI, and unstable angina.

B. **Incidence.** It has been estimated that nearly 8 million patients seen in emergency departments each year in the United States are seen for chest pain, and that up to 5 million of these patients are admitted to the hospital. More than 1.5 million of the patients admitted to the hospital are admitted with an ACS (330,000 with STEMI, and 1.24 million with UA and NSTEMI).

C. Classification of patients presenting with presumed ACS is critical to the appropriate determination of prognosis as well as clinical interventions. In ACS owing to STEMI and NSTEMI, a portion of the cardiac muscle suffers a severe and prolonged restriction of oxygenated coronary blood. In most patients, the cause is an occlusive or near-occlusive thrombus overlying or adjacent to a ruptured atherosclerotic plaque. This results in cellular ischemia, tissue injury, and tissue necrosis. About 1.5 million people suffer an acute myocardial infarction (AMI) each year. UA is believed to indicate an impending AMI, and the goal of treatment is to prevent the development of the AMI.

1. **STEMI.** A condition that requires immediate reperfusion therapy, if possible, through either thrombolysis or percutaneous coronary intervention (PCI).
   a. The introduction of thrombolysis or PCI for the management of STEMI has demonstrated ability to remove the offending thrombus from the affected coronary artery.
   b. Damage to the myocardial tissue is not routinely reversible, as in the case of angina pectoris, owing to potential death of myocardial tissue if reperfusion does not take place early enough.
2. **UA and NSTEMI.** Similar conditions for which there is no evidence showing the benefit to patients of reperfusion therapy. Specific guidelines have been developed for the diagnosis and management of these conditions. Up to 25% of patients who have both NSTEMI and elevated cardiac enzymes eventually develop Q-wave MI; the remaining patients develop non–Q-wave MI. Patients with UA carry a 10% to 20% risk of progression to an MI if untreated; treatment has been shown to reduce the risk to 5% to 7%.

D. **Diagnosis.** The EKG/ECG is at the center of the decision pathway for the evaluation and management of patients with ACS and is confirmed with serial cardiac markers in > 90% of patients presenting with significant ST-segment elevation. Patients who present without ST-segment elevation

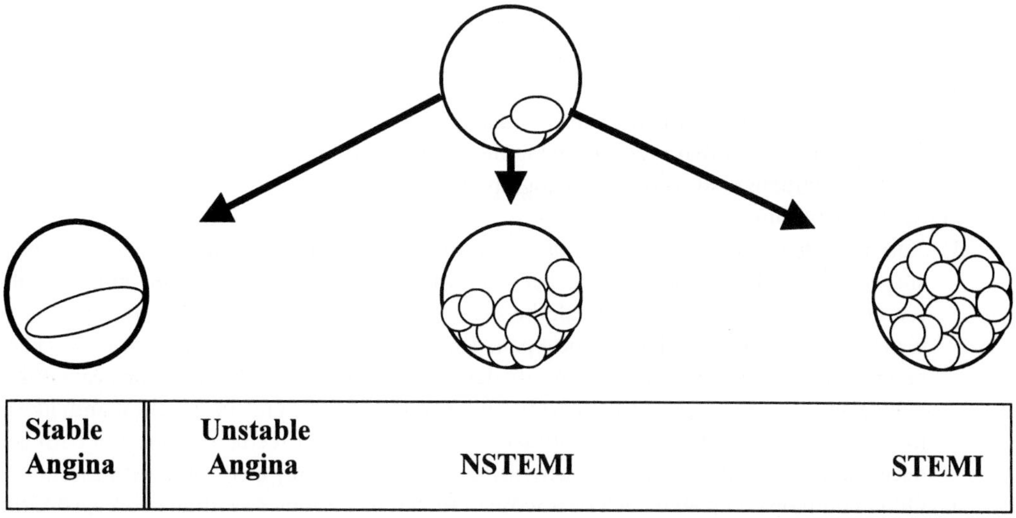

Figure 31-2. Evolutionary progression of ACSs. As atherosclerosis (most common cause of ischemic heart disease) advances, the reduction in myocardial perfusion results in the development of the ACS owing to unstable angina, NSTEMI, or STEMI. The thrombi, which form in unstable angina, NSTEMI, and STEMI, are rich in both fibrin and platelets. Adapted from Vanscoy G. Integrating new fibrinolytic findings into AMI reperfusion and combination therapy: 2002 and beyond. Paper presented at the meeting of the Delaware Valley Chapter of the Pennsylvania Society of Health-Systems Pharmacists; March 7, 2002. *STEMI*, ST-segment elevation; *NSTEMI*, non–ST-segment elevation.

are considered to have either UA or NSTEMI; the final diagnosis is made later, after the presence or absence of serial cardiac markers is determined.

1. **Diagnostic test results.** The development of an ACS is a life-threatening emergency; diagnosis is presumed—and treatment is instituted—based on the patient's complaints and the results of an immediate 12-lead EKG/ECG. Laboratory tests and further diagnostic tests can rule out or provide confirmation and help identify the locale and extent of myocardial damage.
2. **Serial 12-lead EKG.** Abnormalities may be absent or inconclusive during the first few hours after presentation of the ACS and may not aid the diagnosis in about 15% of the cases. When present, characteristic findings show progressive changes.
   a. First, ST-segment elevation (injury current) appears in the leads, reflecting the injured area. Peaked upright or inverted T waves usually indicate acute myocardial injury, the early stages of a transmural Q-wave MI. Persistent ST depression may also indicate a non–Q-wave MI.
   b. Q waves developing (indicating necrosis) is generally diagnostic of an MI but can be seen in other conditions.
   c. Unequivocal diagnosis can be made only in the presence of all three abnormalities. However, the manifestations depend on the area of injury. For example, in non–Q-wave infarction, only ST-segment depression may appear.
   d. The most serious arrhythmic complication of an AMI is ventricular fibrillation, which may occur without warning.
   e. Ventricular premature beats (VPBs) are the most commonly encountered arrhythmias and may require treatment.
3. **Cardiac enzymes**
   a. **Creatine kinase–heart muscle** (CK-MB) is first elevated 3 to 12 hrs after the onset of pain, peaks in 24 hrs, and returns to baseline in 48 to 72 hrs. Other conditions elevate the CK-MB enzyme but do not demonstrate the typical pattern of rise and fall as seen in an MI. Until recently, CK-MB had been the principal serum cardiac marker used in the evaluation of ACS.
   b. **Cardiac troponin I** (cTnI) and **cardiac troponin T** (cTnT) are even more sensitive than CK-MB. They represent a powerful tool for risk stratification and have greater sensitivity and specificity than CK-MB. However, they do provide a low sensitivity in the early phases of an MI ($<$ 6 hrs after symptom onset) and require repeat measurements at 12 to 16 hrs, if negative. Levels increase 3 to 12 hrs after the onset of pain, peak at 24 to 48 hrs, and return to baseline over 5 to 14 days.
   c. **Lactate dehydrogenase** (LDH) is followed for its characteristic patterns of rise and fall. The ratio of LDH_1:LDH_2 is helpful in diagnosing an MI. LDH assays are being replaced by cTnT assays.
4. **Cardiac imaging.** As cardiac enzyme assays improve, the use of noninvasive cardiac imaging techniques are not indicated for initial diagnosis of an MI. Tests include ^{99m}Tc-pyrophosphate scintigraphy, myocardial perfusion imaging, radionucleotide ventriculography, two-dimensional echocardiography, and coronary angiography.

E. Signs and symptoms

1. Recent evidence-based clinical guidelines indicate a class I recommendation for patients with suspected ACS with chest discomfort at rest for longer than 20 mins; hemodynamic instability or recent syncope or presyncope should be strongly considered for immediate referral to an emergency department or specialized chest pain unit. The foremost characteristic of ACS is persistent, severe chest pain or pressure, commonly described as crushing, squeezing, or heavy (likened to having an elephant sitting on the chest). The pain generally begins in the chest and, like angina, may radiate to the left arm, the abdomen, back, neck, jaw, or teeth. The onset of pain generally occurs at rest or with normal daily activities; it is not commonly associated with exertion.
2. Other common complaints include a sense of impending doom, sweating, nausea, vomiting, and difficulty breathing. In some patients, fainting and sudden death may be the initial presentation of ACS.
3. Observable findings include extreme anxiety, restless, agitated behavior, and ashen pallor.
4. Some patients, particularly those with diabetes or the elderly, may experience only mild or indigestion-like pain or a clinically silent MI, which may only manifest in worsening heart failure, loss of consciousness, acute confusion, dyspnea, a sudden drop in blood pressure, or a lethal arrhythmia.

F. Overall treatment goals in ACS

1. To relieve chest pain and anxiety
2. To reduce cardiac workload and stabilize cardiac rhythm
3. To prevent/reduce myocardial damage by limiting the area affected and preserving pump function
4. To prevent or arrest complications, such as lethal arrhythmias, AMI, HF, or sudden death
5. To reopen (or reperfuse) closed coronary vessels with thrombolytic drugs and/or PCI

G. Treatment of UA and NSTEMI

1. Anti-ischemic therapy
   a. Current evidence-based clinical guidelines indicate class I recommendations for the following therapeutic interventions in patients with UA or NSTEMI:
      (1) Bed rest with continuous EKG/ECG monitoring for ischemia and arrhythmia detection in patients with ongoing rest pain.
      (2) Patients with UA/NSTEMI with ongoing ischemic discomfort should receive SL nitroglycerin (NTG) 0.4 mg every 5 min $\times$ 3 doses, after which time reassess for potential need for intravenous nitroglycerin. Intravenous NTG is indicated in the first 48 hrs in patients with UA/NSTEMI for treatment of persistent ischemia, heart failure, or hypertension.
      (3) Supplemental oxygen for patients with cyanosis or respiratory distress and continued need for supplemental oxygen in the presence of hypoxemia.
      (4) Aspirin in doses of 162 to 325 mg (chewable) should be given to patients with UA/NSTEMI as soon as possible, if the patient has not already taken.
      (5) An oral β-adrenergic blocker should be administered within the first 24 hrs to all patients without contraindications. Intravenous β-adrenergic blockers should only be used for specific indications and not as routine therapy.
      (6) In patients with continuing or frequently recurring ischemia when β-adrenergic blockers are contraindicated, a nondihydropyridine calcium antagonist (i.e., diltiazem or verapamil) is recommended as initial therapy in the absence of severe left ventricular dysfunction or other contraindications. In patients presenting with left ventricular dysfunction, current evidence shows that these agents might worsen the clinical status.
      (7) An ACE inhibitor should be administered orally within the first 24 hrs to patients with pulmonary congestion or left ventricular ejection fraction $\leq$ 40% in the absence of hypotension (systolic blood pressure less than 100 mm Hg or less than 30 mm Hg below baseline) or known contraindications. An ARB may be used for ACE inhibitor–intolerant patients.
2. **Therapeutic agents.** *Table 31-4* lists selected agents and dosing regimens.
   a. **Nitrates (e.g., nitroglycerin).** (See II.H.)
   b. **Morphine.** Guidelines for UA/NSTEMI and STEMI from 2007 have stated that morphine is considered a class I recommendation in patients with STEMI; however, in UA/NSTEMI patients, it might increase the rate of adverse events and has been downgraded from a class I recommendation to a class IIa. In the absence of contraindications, morphine sulfate can be administered to patients if there is uncontrolled ischemic pain despite the use of NTG provided additional therapy to treat the underlying ischemia.
      (1) **Mechanism of action.** Morphine causes venous pooling and reduces preload, cardiac workload, and oxygen consumption. Morphine should be administered intravenously, starting with 2 mg and titrating at 5- to 15-min intervals until the pain is relieved or toxicity becomes evident.
      (2) **Indications.** Morphine sulfate is a reasonable choice for myocardial pain and anxiety in doses of 1 to 5 mg IV every 5 to 30 mins as needed, based on level of patient pain and blood pressure.
      (3) **Precautions and monitoring effects**
         (a) Because morphine increases peripheral vasodilation and decreases peripheral resistance, it can produce orthostatic hypotension and fainting.
         (b) Patients should be monitored for hypotension and signs of respiratory depression.
         (c) Morphine has a vagomimetic effect that can produce bradyarrhythmias. If EKG/ECG monitoring reveals excess bradycardia, it should be reversed by administering atropine (0.5 to 1.0 mg).
         (d) Nausea and vomiting may occur (about 20% incidence), especially with initial doses, and patients must be protected against aspiration of stomach contents.

(e) Severe constipation is a potential problem with ongoing morphine administration. The patient may need to use a Valsalva maneuver while straining at the stool, which can produce bradycardia or can overload the cardiac system and trigger cardiac arrest. Docusate (100 mg twice daily) is a useful prophylactic.

c. **Oxygen** is considered a class I recommendation for anti-ischemic therapy, and should be administered to patients with an arterial saturation less than 90%, respiratory distress, or other high-risk features for hypoxemia. The use of pulse oximetry is useful for the continuous measurements of oxygen saturation. Mild hypoxemia is common in AMI patients. Increasing the oxygen content of the blood, thus improving oxygenation of the myocardium, is a top priority as continuing hypoxia rapidly increases myocardial damage.

d. **Thrombolytic agents (fibrinolytics)** have not demonstrated beneficial clinical outcomes in the absence of STEMI. Studies carried out to date have failed to show benefit with using thrombolytics in UA versus standard therapy to prevent MI. In addition, thrombolytic agents actually increased the risk of MI in such patients. Therefore, based on current evidence-based guidelines, thrombolytic agents are not recommended in the management of ACS without ST-segment elevation.

3. **Antiplatelet and anticoagulation therapy.** *Table 31-5* lists selected agents and dosing regimens.

a. Current evidence-based clinical guidelines indicate class I recommendations for the following therapeutic interventions in patients with UA or NSTEMI:

(1) Antiplatelet therapy should be initiated promptly. Aspirin should be administered as soon as possible after presentation and continued indefinitely.

(2) Clopidogrel (Plavix®) (loading dose, 300 to 600 mg; followed by maintenance dose, 75 mg by mouth daily) should be administered to hospitalized patients who are unable to take aspirin because of hypersensitivity or major GI intolerance.

(3) In hospitalized patients for whom an early noninterventional approach is planned, clopidogrel should be added to aspirin and anticoagulants as soon as possible on admission and administered for at least 1 month and ideally up to 1 year.

(4) The usefulness of glycoprotein IIb/IIIa receptor antagonists as part of a preparatory strategy for patients with STEMI before their arrival in the cardiac catheterization laboratory for PCI is uncertain; and received a class IIb, level b recommendation.

(5) In patients for whom a PCI is planned, an additional antiplatelet agent should be added to aspirin as follows prior to the planned PCI: i) clopidogrel should be given in a dose of 300 to 600 mg, or prasugrel (Effient®), 60 mg OR; ii) an intravenous glycoprotein IIb/IIIa inhibitor (GP IIb/IIIa) preferably tirofiban or eptifibatide should be added to the previous aspirin therapy. Abciximab (ReoPro®) is indicated only if there is no appreciable delay to angiography, and PCI is likely to be performed; otherwise, IV eptifibatide or tirofiban is the preferred choice of GP IIb/IIIa inhibitor. Patients should continue receiving clopidogrel in doses of 75 mg daily or prasugrel, 10 mg daily for 12 months after the PCI.

(6) In patients taking clopidogrel or prasugrel in whom elective coronary artery bypass grafting (CABG) is planned, the drugs should be withheld for 5 and 7 days, respectively.

(7) Anticoagulant therapy should be added to antiplatelet therapy in UA/NSTEMI patients as soon as possible after presentation. For patients in whom an invasive strategy is selected, regimens with established efficacy with a high level of evidence include enoxaparin and heparin. The most recent focused guidelines add that for patients in whom a conservative strategy is selected, regimens using either enoxaparin (Lovenox®) or heparin or fondaparinux (Arixtra®) can be used. In patients in whom a conservative strategy is selected and who have an increased risk of bleeding, fondaparinux is preferable.

(8) A platelet glycoprotein IIb/IIIa antagonist or clopidogrel should be administered, in addition to aspirin and heparin, to patients for whom catheterization and PCI are planned. The agent may also be administered just before PCI.

H. STEMI

1. Of the more than 1.68 million patients admitted to hospitals with ACS each year, more than 500,000 of them will be diagnosed with STEMI. Approximately 90% of those diagnosed with STEMI will have complete occlusion of the infarct-related artery by a thrombus.

Table 31-5 SELECT ANTIPLATELET/ANTICOAGULANT AGENTS USED IN THE TREATMENT OF STEMI PATIENTS

Class/Agent	Dosing Regimen	Level of Evidence (Guidelines)
	Oral antiplatelets/anticoagulants	
Aspirin*	**For acute STEMI patients:**	
	162 mg should be chewed by patients who have not taken aspirin before presentation with STEMI.	Class I
	For all post-PCI STEMI stented patients:	
	1. 162–325 mg daily for at least 1 month after bare-metal stent implantation, 3 months after sirolimus-eluting stent, and 6 months after paclitaxel-eluting stent, and then indefinitely at doses of 75–132 mg daily.	Class IIa
	2. In patients where there is concern of bleeding, 75–162 mg (lower dose) aspirin is reasonable during the initial period after stent implantation.	Class IIa
Clopidogrel (Plavix)	1. 75 mg orally daily added to ASA in STEMI patients.	Class I-Post-STEMI patients
	2. Treatment should be at least 14 days.	Class I-Post-STEMI patients
	3. Loading dose of 300 mg orally (patients < 75 years who receive fibrinolytic therapy or who do not receive reperfusion therapy)	Class IIa-Post-STEMI patients
	4. 75 mg orally per day, long-term maintenance therapy (e.g., 1 year) (regardless of whether they undergo reperfusion with fibrinolytic therapy).	Class IIa-Post-STEMI patients
	For all post-PCI STEMI stented patients:	
	5. Receive a drug-eluting stent (DES), clopidogrel 75 mg daily should be given for at least 12 months if patients are not at high risk of bleeding.	Class I
	6. Receive a bare metal stent (BMS), clopidogrel should be given for a minimum of 1 month and ideally up to 12 months (unless the patient is at increased risk of bleeding; then it should be given for a minimum of 2 weeks).	Class I
	7. For patients taking clopidogrel for whom CABG is planned, if possible, the drug should be withheld for at least 5 days, and preferably for 7, unless the urgency for revascularization outweighs the risks of bleeding.	Class I
Warfarin	1. Managing warfarin to INR = 2.0 to 3.0 in post-STEMI patients. Use of warfarin in conjunction with aspirin and/or clopidogrel is associated with increased risk of bleeding and should be monitored closely.	Class I-Post-STEMI patients
	2. In patients requiring warfarin, clopidogrel, and aspirin therapy, an INR of 2.0 to 2.5 is recommended with low-dose aspirin (75–81 mg) and a 75 mg dose of clopidogrel.	
	Parenteral antiplatelets/anticoagulants	
Heparin (UFH)	1. Bolus of 60 U/kg, maximum 4000 U IV followed by an initial infusion 12 U/kg/hr, (maximum of 1000 U/hr) in patient at high risk for systemic emboli (large or anterior MI, atrial fibrillation, previous embolus, known LV thrombus, or cardiogenic shock.	Class I-Post-STEMI
	2. IV or SQ UFH or with subcutaneous LMWH for at least 48 hrs. In patients whose clinical condition necessitates prolonged bed rest and/or minimized activities, it is reasonable that treatment be continued until the patient is ambulatory.	Class IIa-Post-STEMI and not undergoing reperfusion, and no contraindications.

(Continued on next page)

Table 31-5 Continued.

Class/Agent	Dosing Regimen	Level of Evidence (Guidelines)
	3. SQ UFH, 7,500 units–12,500 units twice daily for prophylaxis for deep venous thrombosis (DVT) until completely ambulatory, may be useful, but the effectiveness of such a strategy is not well established in the contemporary era of routine aspirin use and early mobilization.	Class IIb
	For STEMI patients receiving PCI:	
	4. Bolus of 70–100 U/kg, and maintenance to target 1.5–2.0 times aPTT, if no GP IIb/IIIa previously given. However, if a GP IIb/ IIIa has been given previously, 50–70 U/kg bolus, and maintenance to target, as above.	Class I
Enoxaparin (Lovenox)	**Patients undergoing reperfusion with fibrinolytics:**	
	For patients younger than 75 years of age:	
	1. 30 mg intravenous bolus, followed in 15 mins by 1.0 mg/kg SQ every 12 hrs (serum creatinine < 2.5 mg/dL in men and 2.0 mg/dL in women).	Class I-Post-STEMI
	For patients ≥ 75 years of age,	
	2. 0.75 mg/kg SQ every 12 hrs. (No loading dose). Maintenance doses with enoxaparin should continue for the duration of the index hospitalization, up to 8 days. Regardless of age, if the creatinine clearance (using the Cockcroft-Gault formula) during the course of treatment is estimated to be less than 30 mL/min, the subcutaneous regzimen is 1.0 mg/kg every 24 hrs.	Class I-Post-STEMI
Fondaparinux (Arixtra)	**Patients undergoing reperfusion with fibrinolytics:**	
	1. 2.5 mg IV, followed by 2.5 mg SQ once daily. (serum creatinine is less than 3.0 mg/dL)	Class I-Post-STEMI
	2. Maintenance doses with fondaparinux should be continued for the duration of the index hospitalization, up to 8 days.	Class I-Post-STEMI
Bivalirudin (Angiomax)	**Patients undergoing PCI:**	
	1. Initial IV bolus dose of 0.75 mg/kg, followed by 1.75 mg/kg/hr infusion for the duration of the procedure.	Class I-Post-STEMI
Abciximab (ReoPro)	0.25 mg/kg IV bolus followed by infusion of 0.125 mcg/kg/min for 12–24 hrs	Class IIa, for use in addition to aspirin and heparin in STEMI patients for whom catheterization and PCI are planned just before PCI. Class III, in STEMI patients for whom PCI is not planned.
Eptifibatide (Integrilin)	180 mcg/kg IV bolus followed by infusion of 2.0 mcg/kg/min for 72–96 hrs.	Class I, for use in addition to aspirin and heparin in STEMI patients for whom catheterization and PCI are planned, and in patients just before PCI. Class IIa, in addition to aspirin and a LMWH or UFH in STEMI patients without continuing ischemia who have no other high-risk features and for whom PCI is not planned. Class IIb, in addition to aspirin and a LMWH or UFH in STEMI patients without continuing ischemia who have no other high-risk features and for whom PCI is not planned.
Tirofiban (Aggrestat)	0.4 mcg/kg/min for 30 mins followed by infusion of 0.1 mcg/kg/min for 48–96 hrs.	

*Assuming no aspirin resistance, allergy, or increased risk of bleeding.
aPTT, activated partial thromboplastin time; CABG, coronary artery bypass graft; *GP*, glycoprotein; *INR*, international normalized ratio; IV, intravenous; *LMWH*, low-molecular-weight-heparin; PCI, percutaneous coronary intervention; *SQ*, subcutaneously. *STEMI*, ST-segment elevation; *UFH*, unfractionated heparin

2. When the lesion ruptures, it triggers the release of adenosine diphosphate (ADP), serotonins, and thromboxane A_2, which leads to platelet aggregation and the formation of the primary clot. Thromboplastin, released from the injured vessel initiates the clotting cascade, and the resulting fibrin traps red blood cells (RBCs), platelets, and plasma protein to form an intraluminal thrombus. The subsequent clot dissolution is caused by the conversion of plasminogen to plasmin, which is mediated by plasminogen activators.
3. According to updated management guidelines (see I.D.6.), all patients with STEMI should receive either primary PCI within 90 mins of first medical contact (class Ia recommendation) or fibrinolytic therapy within 30 mins of hospital presentation if they cannot be transferred to a PCI center and undergo PCI within 90 mins of first medical contact, unless fibrinolytic therapy is contraindicated (class Ib recommendation).
4. It is beyond the realm of this text to expand on the clinical implications for primary PCI, facilitated PCI, and rescue PCI, as described in the 2009 Focused Updates: ACC/AHA Guidelines for the Management of Patients With ST-Elevation Myocardial Infarction (Updating the 2004 Guideline and 2007 Focused Update) and ACC/AHA/SCAI Guidelines on Percutaneous Coronary Intervention (Updating the 2005 Guideline and 2007 Focused Update). Consequently, the review will focus strictly on the pharmacologic agents recommended for use in the STEMI patient population, which include fibrinolytics, analgesics, anticoagulants, thienopyridines, antiplatelets, ACE inhibitors, ARBs, and β-adrenergic receptor blockers as either primary treatment or secondary preventive and long-term management, as discussed in the guidelines.
   a. **Fibrinolytics.** Administration of thrombolytic agents causes the thrombus clot to be lysed when administered early after symptom onset ($<$ 6 to 12 hrs) and to restore blood flow. The conversion of plasminogen to plasmin promotes fibrinolysis and breakdown of the clot.
      (1) **Indications**
         (a) Thrombolytic agents were used in patients with STEMI with chest pain $<$ 6 to 12 hrs. Successful early reperfusion has been shown to reduce infarct size, improve ventricular function, and improve mortality. However, benefits may be seen in patients using thrombolytic therapy as late as 12 hrs after pain starts. Therapy of choice when PCI is not available.
         (b) Intravenous administration of a recombinant tissue-plasminogen activator (t-PA) such as alteplase (Activase®), a recombinant plasminogen activator (r-PA) such as reteplase (Retavase®), or tenecteplase (Tnkase®), may restore blood flow in an occluded artery if administered within 12 hrs of an AMI, although $<$ 6 hrs is optimal. The goal of treatment of STEMI patients is to initiate thrombolytic therapy within 30 to 60 mins of arrival in an emergency room.
            (i) t-PA is relatively fibrin specific and is able to lyse clots without depleting fibrinogen, and Tnkase has a greater fibrin specificity.
            (ii) Most studies have shown that each agent, when used early, can reopen (reperfuse) occluded coronary arteries and reduce mortality by up to 30% from STEMI. However, considerations such as ease of use, market availability, onset of action, incidence of bleed, and cost are important factors in determining which agent to use for a given hospital and patient.
      (2) **Individual agents**
         (a) **Alteplase (Activase®)**
            (i) **Absolute contraindications** to t-PA include active internal bleeding; recent cerebrovascular accident (CVA); intracranial neoplasm; aneurysm; pregnancy; arteriovenous malformations; recent (within 2 months) intracranial surgery, spinal surgery, or trauma; and severe uncontrolled hypertension, bleeding diathesis, or hemorrhagic ophthalmic conditions.
            (ii) A **front-loaded regimen**—an accelerated infusion that consists of a total dose of 100 mg or less that is given over 1.5 hr—may be more beneficial. The initial dose of 15 mg is given as an IV bolus, 1 to 2 mins, while an infusion is begun to
               (a) Infuse t-PA at the rate of 0.75 mg/kg over 30 mins (not to exceed 50 mg)
               (b) Followed by t-PA infused at 0.5 mg/kg over 60 mins (not to exceed 35 mg)
            (iii) An alternate dosing regimen is based on the patient's weight.
               (a) **Dosage for patients > 65 kg.** A total of 100 mg of t-PA is generally administered to all patients who weigh > 65 kg over a 3-hr period. Although many

regimens have been used, generally speaking, 6 to 10 mg of t-PA is given as an IV bolus over 1 to 2 mins, followed by the remaining infusion rates over the next 3 hrs: a 54- to 60-mg IV infusion over the first hour, a 20-mg IV infusion over the second hour, and a 20-mg IV infusion over the third hour.

(b) **Dosage for patients < 65 kg.** A dose of 1.25 mg/kg is given over a 3-hr period, with 10% of the total dose given initially as a bolus dose over 1 to 2 mins.

(b) **Reteplase (Retavase®)**

(i) **Absolute contraindications** to reteplase are similar to those for t-PA, although additional cautionary statements are given for patients with severely impaired renal function or liver function.

(ii) **Dosing** is initiated with the intravenous administration of 10 units over a 2-min period, and then repeated after 30 mins, if there are no complications.

(c) **Tenecteplase (Tnkase®)**

(i) **Absolute contraindications** to tenecteplase are similar to those for t-PA and r-PA with the following addition: use with caution in patients recently receiving a glycoprotein IIb/IIIa agent, pregnant patients, elderly patients, patients with endocarditis, and patients with severe liver disease.

(ii) Tenecteplase is approved for use in acute treatment of STEMI at doses of 30 to 50 mg (based on the patient's weight) as a single IV bolus over 10 to 15 secs. Rapid rate of administration, fibrin specificity, fewer bleeding complications compared to t-PA, and superiority over t-PA in late-treated patients make tenecteplase a likely candidate to replace t-PA as the agent of choice in STEMI.

(3) **Adjunctive fibrinolysis therapy.** The 2007 Focused Guidelines for ST-segment elevated MI discuss the use of analgesia, β-adrenergic receptor blockers, anticoagulants, and thienopyridines in STEMI patients based on the quality of available literature for their use.

(a) Analgesia

(i) Morphine sulfate in doses of 2 to 4 mg IV in increments of 2 to 8 mg IV, repeated in 5- to 15-min intervals, is the analgesic of choice for the management of pain due to STEMI (class Ic).

(ii) Patients taking NSAIDs with the exception of aspirin, before being treated for STEMI should stop taking them due to increased risk of mortality, reinfarction, hypertension, heart failure, and myocardial rupture associated with their use (class Ic).

(b) **Aspirin** administered (160 to 325 mg) during acute thrombolytic therapy has been shown to affect thrombolysis positively by preventing platelet aggregation and has reduced postinfarct mortality. Doses of aspirin, 75 to 162 mg daily have been recommended for long-term use at hospital discharge. Other agents include ticlopidine (Ticlid®) and clopidogrel (Plavix®) for those unable to take aspirin.

(c) **β-Adrenergic blockers**

(i) It is recommended to initiate and/or continue β-blocker therapy indefinitely in all MI, acute coronary, or left ventricular dysfunction patients with or without signs of heart failure, unless contraindicated.

(ii) Patients who may initially present with contraindications to receiving β-blockers during the initial 24 hrs of their STEMI should be reevaluated for receiving such therapy as a secondary preventive measure (class Ic).

(iii) Patients with moderate or severe left ventricular failure should receive β-blocker therapy as a secondary preventive measure but with a gradual dose escalation titration (class Ib).

(iv) It is reasonable to administer an IV β-blocker to a STEMI patient at the time of presentation if they have hypertension and do not have any of the aforementioned contraindications to receiving them (class IIa).

(d) **Anticoagulants**

(i) Patients who undergo reperfusion with fibrinolytics should receive anticoagulant therapy for at least 48 hrs and ideally throughout the hospitalization, up to 8 days (class Ic).

(ii) Patients who receive anticoagulants for more than 48 hrs should receive an agent other than unfractionated heparin (UFH) due to the increased risk of heparin-induced thrombocytopenia with its prolonged use (class Ia).

(iii) Anticoagulant regimens with established efficacy in STEMI include:

— **UFH.** Initial IV bolus of 60 units/kg (maximum 4000 units) followed by an IV infusion of 12 units/kg/hr (maximum of 1000 units/hr) initially. The dose should be adjusted to maintain an activated partial thromboplastin time (aPTT) of 1.5 to 2 times control (class Ic).

— **Enoxaparin (Lovenox®).** An initial 30 mg IV bolus, followed in 15 mins by a subcutaneous injection of 1 mg/kg every 12 hrs (assuming serum creatinine is less than 2.5 mg/dL in men, 2.0 mg/dL in women in patients younger than 75 years of age). For patients 75 years of age and older, the IV bolus dose is eliminated, and the patient is given a subcutaneous dose of 0.75 mg/kg every 12 hrs. CAUTION: In all patients, if the creatinine clearance is estimated to be less than 30 mL/min, the dosing regimen should be changed to 1 mg/kg every 24 hrs. The current guidelines recommend the use of maintenance dosing of enoxaparin for the duration of hospitalization, up to a maximum of 8 days (class Ia).

— **Fondaparinux (Arixtra®).** An initial dose of 2.5 mg intravenously and subsequent subcutaneous injections of 2.5 mg given once daily (assuming serum creatinine is less than 3.0 mg/dL). The current guidelines, as in the case of enoxaparin, recommend the use of maintenance dosing of fondaparinux for the duration of hospitalization, up to a maximum of 8 days (class Ib).

(iv) Anticoagulants have also been shown to be effective in STEMI patients prior to undergoing PCI, with the following dosing recommendations:

— **UFH.** For prior treatment, administer additional boluses of UFH as needed to support the procedure, but take into account whether other agents such as GP IIb/IIIa receptor antagonists (class Ic). Bivalirudin (Angiomax®) can also be used in patients previously treated with UFH (class Ic).

— **Enoxaparin (Lovenox®).** For prior treatment, if the last subcutaneous dose of enoxaparin was given within the previous 8 hrs, no additional drug is needed; however, if the last dose was administered 8 to 12 hrs earlier, an intravenous dose of 0.3 mg/kg should be given (class Ib).

— **Bivalirudin (Angiomax®).** With the most recent national guidelines updated for STEMI/PCI, bivalirudin received a class I, level b recommendation as useful supportive measure for primary PCI with or without prior treatment with UFH. Bivalirudin has also received a class IIa, level b recommendation in STEMI patients undergoing PCI who are at a high risk of bleeding due to its relatively low risk of bleeding compared to other anticoagulants.

(v) Anticoagulants (non-UFH regimens) have also been recommended for patients with STEMI who do not undergo reperfusion therapy for the duration of the initial hospitalization (class IIa). Dosing regimens that can be used include enoxaparin or fondaparinux in the same dosing regimens as in those patients receiving fibrinolytic (see iv previously).

(e) Thienopyridines

(i) Clopidogrel (Plavix®) should be added to aspirin in STEMI patients regardless of whether they undergo reperfusion with fibrinolytics or do not receive reperfusion (class Ib). Doses of 75 mg by mouth daily should be administered. Treatment should continue for at least 14 days (class Ib).

(ii) Prasugrel (Effient®) 60 mg should be given as soon as possible prior to PCI, if clopidogrel is not being used (class Ib). Prasugrel should be given in those patients not receiving clopidogrel within 1 hr of PCI (class Ib).

(iii) Patients receiving clopidogrel (Plavix®) or prasugrel (Effient®) who are planning on undergoing CABG should discontinue therapy 5 to 7 days prior to the surgery, respectively, unless the urgency of the procedure outweighs the risks of excess bleeding (class Ic).

(iv) For patients younger than 75 years receiving fibrinolytic therapy or not receiving reperfusion therapy, it is reasonable to administer an oral clopidogrel loading dose of 300 mg. (No data are available to guide decision making regarding an oral loading dose in patients ≥ 75 years of age.) (class IIa).

(v) Long-term maintenance therapy (e.g., 1 year) with clopidogrel (75 mg/day orally) can be useful in STEMI patients regardless of whether they undergo reperfusion with fibrinolytic therapy or do not receive reperfusion therapy (class IIa).

(vi) Patients who have received a stent, i.e., bare-metal or drug eluting during PCI for ACS, should continue to receive maintenance therapy of clopidogrel (Plavix®) or prasugrel (Effient®), 75 mg or 10 mg, respectively, by mouth daily for at least 12 months (class Ib).

(4) Secondary prevention and long-term management: *Table 31-2* provides a combination of risk factors as well as disease-based recommendations, which have been incorporated into the 2007 Focused Guidelines for STEMI patients. Additionally, the guidelines include recommendations made for select pharmacologic agents that include aspirin, clopidogrel, warfarin, ACE inhibitors, angiotensin receptor blockers, aldosterone blockade, and β-blockers, and influenza vaccination.

(a) Aspirin

(i) All post-PCI STEMI patients receiving a stent (bare-metal, sirolimus, paclitaxel) without contraindications to aspirin should receive aspirin 162 to 325 mg daily for 1 to 6 months depending on the type of stent used. After the initial 1 to 6 months, a maintenance dose of aspirin should be continued at a dose of 75 to 162 mg daily, indefinitely (class Ib).

(ii) In those patients where there is concern for a high risk of bleeding, doses of aspirin 75 mg to 162 mg daily are reasonable during the initial period and after stent implantation (class IIa).

(b) Warfarin (Coumadin®)

(i) Managing warfarin to an INR = 2.0 to 3.0 in post-STEMI patients when clinically indicated (e.g., atrial fibrillation, left ventricular thrombus, and paroxysmal or chronic atrial fibrillation or flutter) is recommended (class Ia).

(ii) Use of warfarin in conjunction with aspirin and/or clopidogrel is associated with increased risk of bleeding and should be monitored closely (class Ib).

(iii) For patients requiring warfarin, clopidogrel, and aspirin therapy, an INR of 2 to 2.5 is recommended with low-dose aspirin (75 to 81 mg) and a 75 mg dose of clopidogrel (class Ic).

(c) ACE inhibitors (see Hypertension Chapter; *Table 33-4* for listing of available agents)

(i) ACE inhibitors should be started and continued indefinitely in all patients recovering from STEMI with LVEF ≤ 40% and in those patients with hypertension, diabetes, or chronic kidney disease, unless contraindicated (class Ia).

(ii) ACE inhibitors should be started and continued indefinitely in patients recovering from STEMI who are not lower risk (lower risk defined as those with normal LVEF in whom cardiovascular risk factors are well controlled and revascularization has been performed), unless contraindicated (class Ib).

(d) ARBs (see Hypertension Chapter; *Table 33-4* for listing of available agents)

(i) ARBs are recommended in patients who are intolerant of ACE inhibitors and have had an STEMI with LVEF ≤ 40% or have heart failure (class Ia).

(ii) ARB therapy is beneficial in other patients who are ACE inhibitor–intolerant and have hypertension (class Ib).

(e) Aldosterone-blocking agents (Spironolactone [Aldactone®], Eplerenone [Inspra®])

(i) Use of aldosterone blockade in post-STEMI patients without significant renal dysfunction or hyperkalemia is recommended in patients who are already receiving therapeutic doses of an ACE inhibitor and β-blocker, have an LVEF of ≤ 40% and have either diabetes or heart failure (class Ia).

(f) β-Adrenergic blockers

(i) It is beneficial to start and continue β-blocker therapy indefinitely in all patients who have had an STEMI, ACS, or left ventricular dysfunction with or without heart failure symptoms, unless contraindicated (class Ia).

(g) Influenza vaccine (Fluvirin®, FluMist®)

(i) Patients with cardiovascular disease should have an annual influenza vaccination (class Ib).

I. Complications. MI potentiates many complications; the most common of these include the following:

1. **Lethal arrhythmias.** See Chapter 32-Arrhythmias for a detailed discussion.
2. **Heart failure.** See Chapter 34-Heart Failure for a detailed discussion.
   - **a.** Left ventricular failure causes pulmonary congestion. Diuretics, especially furosemide (Lasix®), help reduce the congestion.
   - **b.** ACE inhibitors, β-adrenergic blockers, angiotensin receptor blockers, and direct-acting aldosterone antagonists play a key role in the treatment of heart failure.
3. **Cardiogenic shock**
   - **a.** In this life-threatening complication, cardiac output is decreased, and pulmonary artery and pulmonary capillary wedge pressures are increased. This typically occurs when the area of infarction exceeds 40% of muscle mass and compensatory mechanisms only strain the already compromised myocardium.
   - **b.** Vasopressors: for example, norepinephrine (Levophed®), epinephrine (Adrenalin®), dopamine (Various) in high doses, and vasopressin (Pitressin®) enhance blood pressure through β-adrenergic stimulation and V1 receptors within smooth muscle (vasopressin) and may be indicated, as per Advanced Cardiac Life Support (ACLS) protocol.
   - **c.** Inotropic drugs—for example, epinephrine, dopamine (middle doses), dobutamine (Dobutrex®), isoproterenol (Isuprel®), and digoxin (Lanoxin®)—are rapidly acting agents used to increase myocardial contractility and improve cardiac output.
   - **d.** Vasodilators—for example, nitroprusside (Nipride®)—reduce preload, lower pulmonary capillary wedge pressure by dilating veins, and reduce afterload by decreasing resistance to left ventricular ejection.
   - **e.** Additional treatment may include invasive procedures such as intra-aortic balloon pumping.

Study Questions

Directions for questions 1–16: Each of the questions, statements, or incomplete statements in this section can be correctly answered or completed by **one** of the suggested answers or phrases. Choose the **best** answer.

1. Exertion-induced angina, which is relieved by rest, nitroglycerin, or both, is referred to as

(A) Prinzmetal angina.
(B) unstable angina.
(C) stable angina.
(D) variant angina.
(E) preinfarction angina.

2. Myocardial oxygen demand is increased by all of the following factors *except*

(A) exercise.
(B) smoking.
(C) cold temperatures.
(D) isoproterenol.
(E) metoprolol.

3. Which of the following agents used in Prinzmetal angina has spasmolytic actions, which increase coronary blood supply?

(A) nitroglycerin
(B) diltiazem
(C) timolol
(D) isosorbide mononitrate
(E) propranolol

4. The development of ischemic pain occurs when the demand for oxygen exceeds the supply. Determinants of oxygen demand include all of the following choices *except* which one?

(A) contractile state of the heart
(B) myocardial ejection time
(C) left ventricular volume
(D) right atrial pressure
(E) systolic pressure

5. Myopathy is an adverse effect of all the following agents *except*

(A) lovastatin.
(B) simvastatin.
(C) pravastatin.
(D) gemfibrozil.
(E) colestipol.

Directions for question 6 : The question can be correctly answered by one or more of the suggested answers. Choose the answer, **A–E**.

(A) if **I only** is correct
(B) if **III only** is correct
(C) if **I and II** are correct
(D) if **II and III** are correct
(E) if **I, II, and III** are correct

6. Which of the following is considered a component of acute coronary syndrome (ACS)?

I. unstable angina
II. non–ST-segment elevated myocardial infarction (NSTEMI)
III. ST-segment elevated myocardial infarction (STEMI)

Directions for questions 7–11: Each of the following descriptions is most closely related to one of the following drugs. The descriptions may be used more than once or not at all. Choose the **best** answer, **A–E.**

(A) Inhibition of intestinal absorption of cholesterol
(B) Lowering of low-density lipoproteins (LDLs), triglycerides, and increased high-density lipoprotein (HDL) along with potential anti-inflammatory effects
(C) Recommendations for this agent have been substantially expanded beyond an alternative for aspirin-intolerant patients due to recent trials demonstrating its benefit in select ACS patients.
(D) Recommended for ACS patients who cannot tolerate aspirin
(E) Recommended over unfractionated heparin (UFH) as an anticoagulant in patients with unstable angina (UA) or NSTEMI

7. tirofiban (Aggrastat®)

8. enoxaparin (Lovenox®)

9. simvastatin (Various)

10. clopidogrel (Plavix®)

11. ezetimibe (Zetia®)

Answers and Explanations

1. The answer is C *[see II.C.1.a–f].*
Classic, or stable, angina refers to the syndrome in which physical activity or emotional excess causes chest discomfort, which may spread to the arms, legs, neck, and so forth. This type of angina is relieved promptly (within 1 to 10 mins) with rest, nitroglycerin, or both.

2. The answer is E *[see II.H.3.a; Table 31-1].*
Owing to the β-adrenergic blocking effects of metoprolol (e.g., decreased heart rate, decreased blood pressure, decreased inotropic effect), there is a net decrease in myocardial oxygen demand. This is the direct opposite of the effects seen with the β-agonist isoproterenol. Exercise, cigarette smoking, and exposure to cold temperatures have all been shown to increase myocardial oxygen demand.

3. The answer is B *[see II.4.d and II.H.4.c].*
Calcium-channel blocking agents such as diltiazem have been shown to be capable of reversing spasm and, therefore, increasing coronary blood flow in Prinzmetal angina. The calcium-channel blockers have proven benefit in the treatment of Prinzmetal angina, a syndrome believed due more to a spastic event than to a fixed coronary occlusion. β-adrenergic blockers such as timolol and propranolol (Inderal®) are not indicated in the treatment of Prinzmetal angina, and nitrates such as nitroglycerin and isosorbide mononitrate are not the primary agents indicated and in many cases do not have any effect.

4. **The answer is D** *[see I.F.2.B.(1)–(4)]*.
As with most muscles in the body, the contractile force of the heart dictates the amount of oxygen that the heart needs to perform efficiently. Consequently, as contractility decreases, the oxygen needs of the heart increase. As contractility continues to decrease, the volume of fluid in the left ventricle increases owing to poor muscle performance and increasing tension within the ventricle, resulting in additional oxygen requirements. As the amount of tension within the ventricle increases per cardiac cycle, there is again an added requirement for oxygen by the heart muscle.

5. **The answer is E** *[see II.G.2.d.(3); II.G.3.c.(2)]*.
Myopathy is an adverse effect of all the HMG-CoA reductase inhibitors (lovastatin, simvastatin, pravastatin, atorvastatin, fluvastatin, and rosuvastatin), and the combination of the fibric acid derivatives (gemfibrozil, fenofibrate, and clofibrate) has been shown to increase the creatine kinase levels and predispose patients to myopathies and rhabdomyolysis.

6. **The answer is E (I, II, III)** *[see I.E.2]*.
During recent years, there has been an attempt to link the various clinical symptoms of IHD into key categories, based on the presentation and symptoms at the time of evaluation. ACS refers to those situations that reflect an acute ischemic event and includes UA, NSTEMI, and STEMI. Clinical guidelines have incorporated treatment modalities based on these three presentations. UA and NSTEMI have similar recommended therapies, and STEMI has different treatment guidelines. Stable angina is not considered one of the ACS but represents the starting point for the progression of atherosclerosis, resulting in IHD.

7. **The answer is C** *[see III.G.3.a.(5)]*.
Tirofiban is an antiplatelet that is referred to as a glycoprotein IIb/III, a receptor antagonist. This class of drugs works to prevent platelet aggregation by inhibiting the interaction between the primary binding site of platelets and has been shown to be effective in the prevention of thrombosis.

8. **The answer is E** *[see III.G.3.a.(7) and III.H.4.a.(3).(d).(iii); Table 31-5]*.
Enoxaparin is an example of a low-molecular-weight heparin (LMWH). As a group, the major advantage of these drugs over the more traditional heparin is that they exhibit a more predictable anticoagulant response. Owing to their lower molecular weight and decreased binding to plasma proteins, they have better bioavailability than heparin. In addition, their decrease in plasma protein binding and binding to the endothelium results in half-lives that are two to four times longer than that of heparin. Current clinical practice guidelines recommend enoxaparin over heparin in patients with UA or NSTEMI, unless CABG is planned within 24 hrs.

9. **The answer is B** *[see II.G.2.c.(7)]*.
Simvastatin is one of the currently available HMG-CoA reductase inhibitors that have been shown to significantly reduce LDL levels and nonfatal MI or CHD (30% to 40% reduction). Recent studies have demonstrated that inflammation may be an important mechanism involved in ACS and that statins might exert an important anti-inflammatory effect within coronary arteries (independent of their cholesterol-lowering effects).

10. **The answer is D** *[see II.H.5.c]*.
The most recently introduced guidelines for the treatment of ACS has incorporated recent trials, which have shown the value of clopidogrel in various patient populations with ACS. Besides being used in those who are unable to take or tolerate aspirin, it is included as "add-on" therapy for patients receiving aspirin who suffer from ACS.

11. **The answer is A** *[see II.G.5.a]*.
Ezetimibe reduces cholesterol levels via a different mechanism of action than previous agents. By selectively blocking the intestinal absorption of cholesterol, it is able to stop one of the major pathways responsible for increasing available cholesterol within the body. Ezetimibe has demonstrated the ability to reduce total cholesterol, LDL, apolipoprotein B, and triglyceride levels while increasing HDL levels in patients with hypercholesterolemia. Simvastatin has recently been incorporated into a combination product with ezetimibe (Vytorin), which uses the individual class properties of the HMG-CoA reductase inhibitors (simvastatin) to reduce cholesterol production with the absorption-inhibiting properties of ezetimibe to target cholesterol with two different mechanisms, which might also aid in improving patient compliance with taking the medication.

32 Cardiac Arrhythmias

ALAN H. MUTNICK

I. INTRODUCTION.

Sudden death from cardiac causes in the United States has been estimated to occur in the range of 300,000 to 350,000 cases annually. Depending on the definition, sudden cardiac death could be classified as low as 13% of all natural deaths up to approximately 50% of all deaths from cardiovascular causes occurring shortly after onset (instantaneous to 1 hr), with the majority of sudden deaths being caused by acute ventricular tachyarrhythmias. These incidence reports might appear to create greater need for the knowledge necessary to appropriately use antiarrhythmics for this high-risk patient population. However, previously conducted studies have cast doubt on the true place of antiarrhythmics in the treatment and prevention of cardiac arrhythmias. Studies such as the Cardiac Arrhythmia Suppression Trial (CAST) have demonstrated that certain classes of antiarrhythmics increased mortality in patients treated with antiarrhythmics as compared to placebo. Since the release of the data from the CAST trial, subsequent studies have confirmed the finding that certain antiarrhythmics do possess "proarrhythmic" effects when used injudiciously. Consequently, the use of trial and error to determine antiarrhythmic therapy has given way to an era of outcome-based antiarrhythmic drug decision making. By understanding the causes of arrhythmias and being aware of drug–drug and drug–target interactions, we are more likely to understand the key considerations to maximize therapeutic strategies while minimizing drug-induced toxicities.

A. **Definition.** Cardiac arrhythmias are deviations from the normal heartbeat pattern. They include **abnormalities of impulse formation**, such as heart rate, rhythm, or site of impulse origin and **conduction disturbances**, which disrupt the normal sequence of atrial and ventricular activation.

B. **Electrophysiology**

1. **Conduction system**

   a. **Two electrical sequences** that cause the heart chambers to fill with blood and contract are initiated by the conduction system of the heart.

      (1) **Impulse formation**, the first sequence, takes place when an electrical impulse is generated automatically.

      (2) **Impulse transmission**, the second sequence, occurs once the impulse has been generated, signaling the heart to contract.

   b. **Four main structures** composed of tissue that can generate or conduct electrical impulses make up the conduction system of the heart.

      (1) The **sinoatrial (SA) node** in the wall of the right atrium contains cells that spontaneously initiate an action potential. Serving as the main pacemaker of the heart, the SA node initiates 60 to 100 beats/min.

         (a) Impulses generated by the SA node trigger atrial contraction.

         (b) Impulses travel through internodal tracts—the anterior tract, middle tract, posterior tract, and anterior interatrial tract (*Figure 32-1*).

      (2) At the **atrioventricular (AV) node** situated in the lower interatrial septum, the impulses are delayed briefly to permit completion of atrial contraction before ventricular contraction begins.

      (3) At the **bundle of His**—muscle fibers arising from the AV junction—impulses travel along the left and right bundle branches, located on either side of the intraventricular septum.

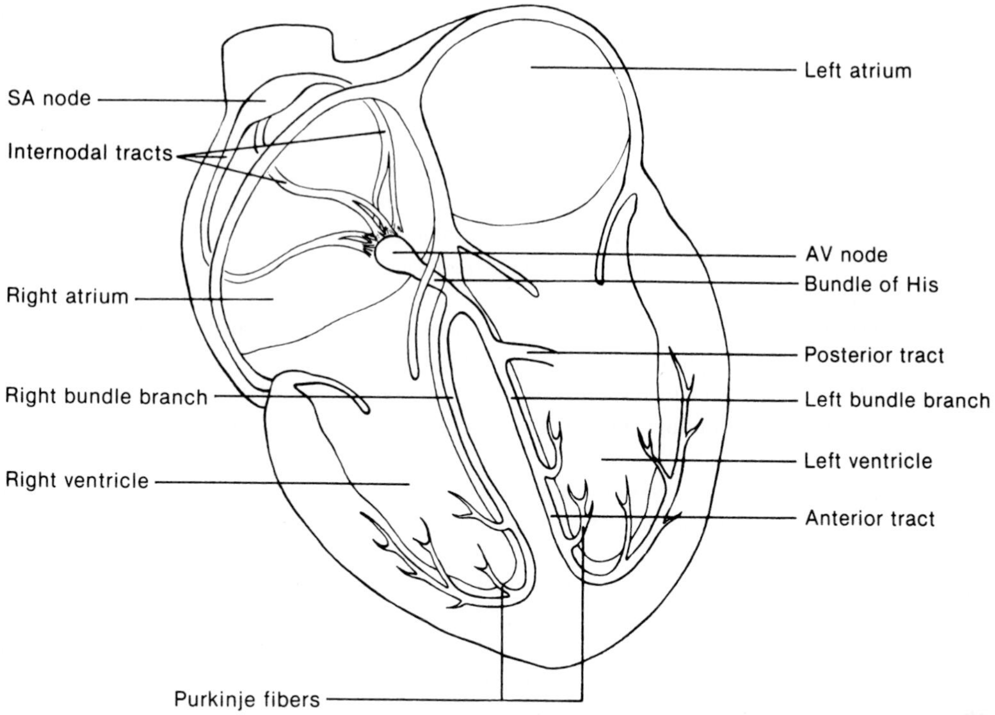

Figure 32-1. Electrical pathways of the heart. *AV*, atrioventricular; *SA*, sinoatrial.

(4) The impulses reach the **Purkinje fibers**, a diffuse network extending from the bundle branches and ending in the ventricular endocardial surfaces. Ventricular contraction then occurs.

c. **Latent pacemakers.** The AV junction, bundle of His, and Purkinje fibers are latent pacemakers; they contain cells capable of generating impulses. However, these regions have a slower firing rate than the SA node. Consequently, the SA node predominates except when it is depressed or injured, which is known as **overdrive suppression**.

2. **Myocardial action potential.** Before cardiac contraction can take place, cardiac cells must depolarize and repolarize.

a. **Depolarization** and **repolarization** result from changes in the electrical potential across the cell membrane, caused by the exchange of sodium and potassium ions.

b. **Action potential**, which reflects this electrical activity, has five phases (*Figure 32-2*).

(1) **Phase 0 (rapid depolarization)** takes place as sodium ions enter the cell through fast channels; the cell membrane's electrical charge changes from negative to positive.

(2) **Phase 1 (early rapid repolarization).** As fast sodium channels close and potassium ions leave the cell, the cell rapidly repolarizes (i.e., returns to resting potential).

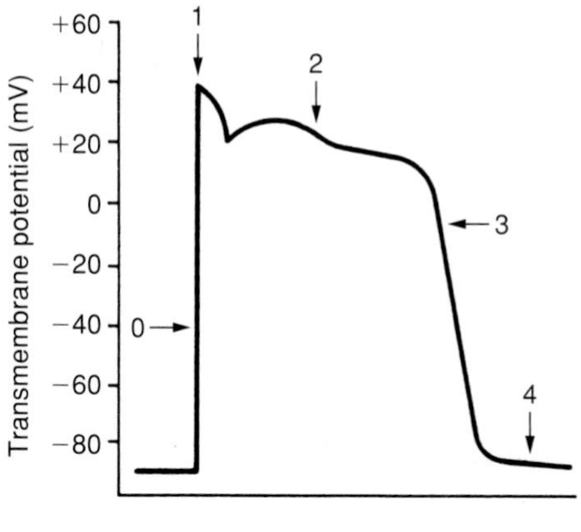

Figure 32-2. Myocardial action potential curve. This curve represents ventricular depolarization–repolarization. Phases: *0*, rapid depolarization; *1*, early rapid repolarization; *2*, plateau; *3*, final rapid repolarization; *4*, slow depolarization.

(3) **Phase 2 (plateau).** Calcium ions enter the cell through slow channels while potassium ions exit. As the cell membrane's electrical activity temporarily stabilizes, the action potential reaches a plateau (represented by the notch at the beginning of this phase in *Figure 32-2*).

(4) **Phase 3 (final rapid repolarization).** Potassium ions are pumped out of the cell as the cell rapidly completes repolarization and resumes its initial negativity.

(5) **Phase 4 (slow depolarization).** The cell returns to its resting state with potassium ions inside the cell and sodium and calcium ions outside.

c. During both depolarization and repolarization, a cell's ability to initiate an action potential varies.

(1) The cell cannot respond to any stimulus during the **absolute refractory period** (beginning during phase 1 and ending at the start of phase 3).

(2) A cell's ability to respond to stimuli increases as repolarization continues. During the **relative refractory period**, which occurs during phase 3, the cell can respond to a strong stimulus.

(3) When the cell has been completely repolarized, it can again respond fully to stimuli.

d. Cells in different cardiac regions depolarize at different speeds, depending on whether fast or slow channels predominate.

(1) Sodium flows through fast channels; calcium flows through slow channels.

(2) Where fast channels dominate (e.g., in cardiac muscle cells), depolarization occurs quickly. Where slow channels dominate (e.g., in the electrical cells of the SA node and AV junction), depolarization occurs slowly.

3. Electrocardiography. The electrical activity occurring during depolarization–repolarization can be transmitted through electrodes attached to the body and transformed by an **electrocardiograph (EKG/ECG) machine** into a series of waveforms (EKG/ECG waveform). *Figure 32-3* shows a normal EKG/ECG waveform.

a. The **P wave** reflects atrial depolarization.

b. The **PR interval** represents the spread of the impulse from the atria through the Purkinje fibers.

c. The **QRS complex** reflects ventricular depolarization (phase 0).

d. The **ST segment** represents phase 2 of the action potential—the absolute refractory period (part of ventricular repolarization).

e. The **T wave** shows phase 3 of the action potential—ventricular repolarization.

C. Classification. Arrhythmias generally are classified by origin (i.e., supraventricular or ventricular).

1. Supraventricular arrhythmias stem from enhanced automaticity of the SA node (or another pacemaker region, above the bundle of His or ventricular tissue) or from reentry conduction.

2. Ventricular arrhythmias occur below the bundle of His, when an ectopic (abnormal) pacemaker triggers a ventricular contraction before the SA node fires (e.g., from a conduction disturbance or ventricular irritability).

3. Special note

a. Torsades de pointes (TdP; French for "twisting of the points") has received increased attention during recent years as a major proarrhythmic event, which has been reported with antiarrhythmic drug therapy. It is defined as a polymorphic ventricular tachycardia with a twisting QRS complex morphology, which sometimes occurs with drugs that prolong ventricular repolarization (QT interval widening). Although initial reports of TdP centered around antiarrhythmic drugs (quinidine), today, more than 50 drugs, both antiarrhythmic agents and other

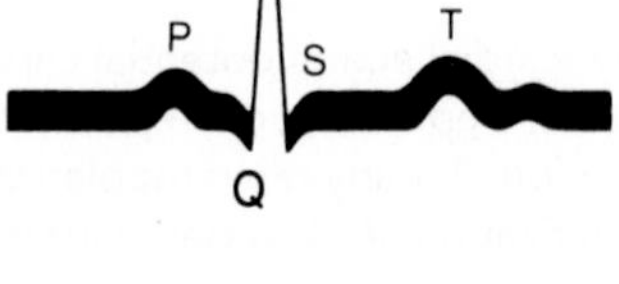

Figure 32-3. Normal EKG/ECG waveform.

classes of drugs, such as antibiotics, have been shown to affect the duration of the QT interval and have been associated with this arrhythmia.

b. A Web site devoted to providing education and research on drug-induced arrhythmias, especially those due to prolongation of the QT interval on the electrocardiogram (EKG/ECG), is available. The site, http://www.torsades.org/medical-pros/drug-lists/drug-lists.htm, is currently maintained by Dr. Raymond Woosley.

c. Dr. Woosley and colleagues have established the International Registry for Drug-Induced Arrhythmias, to which one can submit a suspected "drug-induced arrhythmia event." The registry also provides a list of drugs reported to prolong the QT interval or cause TdP (http://www.Torsades.org). Four drug lists have been created based on the relative risk of inducing TdP or a prolonged QT interval.

d. It is beyond the intention of this chapter to provide a comprehensive listing, as done on Dr. Woosley's Web site. However, the four categories of drug lists include the following with select examples:

(1) **List 1: Drugs that are generally accepted by authorities to carry a risk of causing TdP**; that is, amiodarone (Cordarone®), chlorpromazine (Thorazine®), clarithromycin (Biaxin®), disopyramide (Norpace®), dofetilide (Tikosyn®), erythromycin (Erythrocin®), haloperidol (Haldol®), ibutilide (Corvert®), methadone (Dolophine®), moxifloxacin (Avelox®), pentamidine (NebuPent®), pimozide (Orap®), procainamide (Various), quinidine (Quinaglute®), sotalol (Betapace®), and thioridazine (Mellaril®).

(2) **List 2: Drugs that in some reports have been associated with TdP and/or QT prolongation but at this time lack substantial evidence for causing TdP**; that is, amantadine (Symmetrel®), azithromycin (Zithromax®), clozapine (Clozaril®), dolasetron (Anzemet®), dronedarone (Multaq®), escitalopram (Lexapro®), felbamate (Felbatol®), flecainide (Tambocor®), foscarnet (Foscavir®), fosphenytoin (Cerebyx®), granisetron (Kytril®), isradipine (DynaCirc®), levofloxacin (Levaquin®), nicardipine (Cardene®), ondansetron (Zofran®), quetiapine (Seroquel®), risperidone (Risperdal®), sunitinib (Sutent®), tacrolimus (Prograf®), venlafaxine (Effexor®), voriconazole (Vfend®), and ziprasidone (Geodon®).

(3) **List 3: Drugs with a conditional risk of TdP—drugs that carry a risk of TdP and/or QT prolongation under certain conditions, such as patients with long QT syndrome, drug overdose, or coadministration of interacting drugs**; that is, amitriptyline (Elavil®), ciprofloxacin (Cipro®), citalopram (Celexa®), clomipramine (Anafranil®), desipramine (Norpramin®), diphenhydramine (Benadryl®), doxepin (Silenor®), fluconazole (Diflucan®), fluoxetine (Prozac®), galantamine (Razadyne®), imipramine (Tofranil®), itraconazole (Sporanox®), ketoconazole (Nizoral®), nortriptyline (Pamelor®), paroxetine (Paxil®), ritonavir (Norvir®), sertraline (Zoloft®), solifenacin (VESIcare®), trazodone (Desyrel®), trimethoprim-sulfamethoxazole (Bactrim), trimipramine (Surmontil).

(4) **List 4: Drugs to be avoided for use in patients with diagnoses or suspected congenital long QT syndrome.** (Drugs on Lists 1, 2, and 3 would also be included here.) That is, albuterol (Ventolin®), amphetamine (Adderall®), dobutamine (Dobutrex®), dopamine (Intropin®), isoproterenol (Isuprel®), lapatinib (Tykerb®), levalbuterol (Xopenex®), and vardenafil (Levitra®).

D. Causes

1. Precipitating causes. Arrhythmias result from various conditions, including

a. Heart disease—infection, coronary artery disease (CAD), valvular heart disease, rheumatic heart disease, ischemic heart disease

b. Myocardial infarction (MI)

c. Systemic hypertension

d. Hyperkalemia/hypokalemia

e. Chronic obstructive pulmonary disease (COPD)—emphysema, bronchitis

f. Thyroid disorders

g. Drug therapy (both antiarrhythmic and nonantiarrhythmic drugs)

h. Toxic doses of cardioactive drugs (e.g., digitalis preparations)

i. Increased sympathetic tone

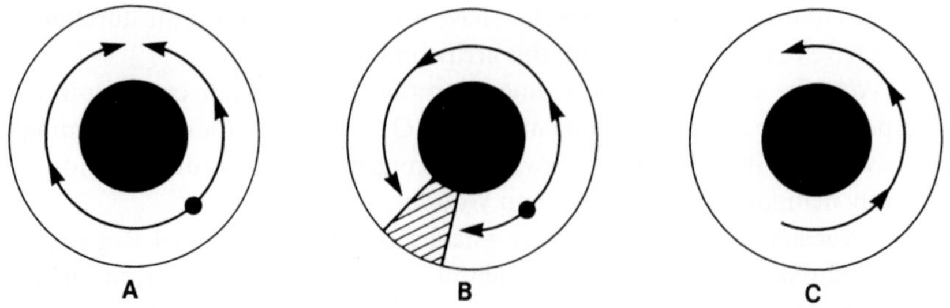

Figure 32-4. Reentry arrhythmias. **A.** Two waves of excitation going in opposite directions. **B.** A unidirectional wave of excitation. **C.** Reexcitation of tissue in a slow conduction area.

j. Decreased parasympathetic tone
k. Vagal stimulation (e.g., straining at stool)
l. Increased oxygen demand (e.g., from stress, exercise, fever)
m. Metabolic disturbances
n. Cor pulmonale

2. **Mechanisms of arrhythmias.** Abnormal impulse formation, abnormal impulse conduction, or a combination of both may give rise to arrhythmias.
   a. **Abnormal impulse formation** may stem from
      (1) Depressed automaticity, as in escape beats and bradycardia
      (2) Increased automaticity, as in premature beats, tachycardia, and extrasystole
      (3) Depolarization and triggered activity, leading to sustained ectopic firing
   b. **Abnormal impulse conduction** results from
      (1) A conduction block or delay
      (2) **Reentry** occurs when an impulse is rerouted through certain regions in which it has already traveled. Thus, the impulse depolarizes the same tissue more than once, producing an additional impulse (*Figures 32-4* and *32-5*). Reentry sites include the SA and AV nodes as well as various accessory pathways in the atria and ventricles (*Figure 32-6*). For reentry to occur, the following conditions must exist:
         (a) Markedly shortened refractoriness or a slow conduction area that allows an adequate delay so that depolarization recurs.
         (b) Unidirectional conduction

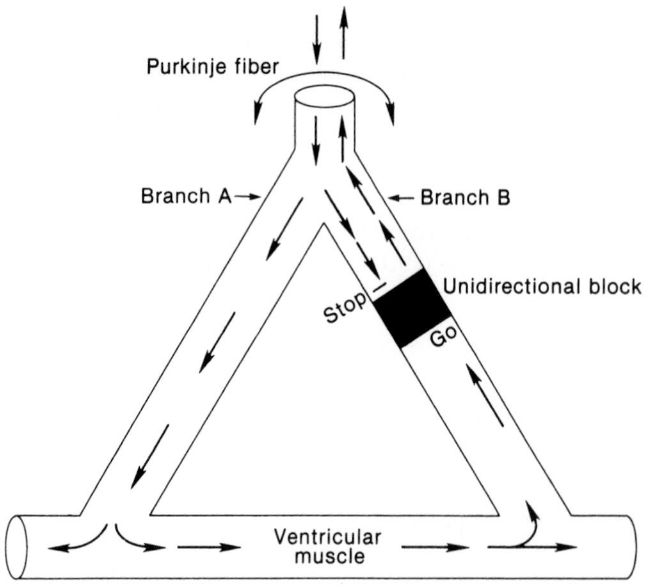

Figure 32-5. Ventricular reentry: a branched Purkinje fiber joining ventricular muscle. The *dark area* represents the site of a unidirectional block. In this depolarization region, the impulse heading toward the atrioventricular node continues upward, whereas the impulse traveling toward the muscle is blocked. Because retrograde conduction in *branch B* is slow, cells in *branch A* have time to recover and respond to the reentrant impulse.

3. **Administration and dosage**
   a. **Quinidine (Various)** is administered orally, usually in three to four daily doses of 200 to 400 mg as a rapid-release sulfate salt (83% quinidine). However, sustained-release products in the form of a gluconate (62% quinidine) salt in doses of 324 to 648 mg, which corresponds to 300 to 600 mg of the sulfate salt, may be given every 12 hrs. (In special circumstances, it has been given intravenously or intramuscularly with caution.) To achieve an effective plasma concentration rapidly, a loading dose of 600 to 1000 mg may be administered in doses of 200 mg every 2 hrs to a maximum of 1000 mg, or a 5 to 8 mg/kg intravenous infusion can be given at a rate of 0.3 mg/kg/min.
   b. **Procainamide (Various)** is available for intravenous or intramuscular use.
      (1) For **acute therapy**, intravenous administration is preferred.
         (a) Intermittent intravenous administration calls for the administration of an intravenous dose of 3 to 6 mg/kg infusion (up to 100 mg) over 2 to 4 mins, repeated every 5 to 10 mins until the arrhythmia is abolished, side effects occur, or 1 g has been given. The usual effective dose is 500 to 1000 mg.
         (b) Rapid intravenous administration calls for infusion of 1.0 to 1.5 g at a rate of 20 to 50 mg/min.
         (c) Once the arrhythmia is terminated, 1.5 to 5.0 mg/min is given as a continuous infusion.
      (2) For **long-term therapy**, oral administration with procainamide is no longer available in the United States.
   c. **Disopyramide (Norpace®, Norpace CR®)** is available in oral form.
      (1) Usually, 300 to 400 mg is given as a loading dose to attain an effective plasma level rapidly.
      (2) For maintenance therapy, doses of 400 to 800 mg/day are given in four doses every 6 hrs (nonsustained-release capsule) or in two doses every 12 hrs (sustained-release capsule).
   d. **Lidocaine (Xylocaine®)** may be administered intravenously or intramuscularly.
      (1) An intravenous loading dose rapidly achieves a therapeutic plasma level.
         (a) Initially, 1 to 1.5 mg/kg (100 mg) is administered.
         (b) A second injection of half the initial dose may be required 5 mins later, up to a maximum of 300 mg.
      (2) Continuous intravenous infusion of 2 to 4 mg/min produces an effective plasma level in 7 to 10 hrs.
      (3) In an emergency, an intramuscular injection rapidly achieves an effective plasma level. The usual dosage is 300 to 400 mg injected into the deltoid muscle.
   e. **Mexiletine (Various)** is administered orally and should be initiated in the hospital setting.
      (1) A loading dose of 400 mg followed by maintenance dosage in 8 hrs.
      (2) If this fails to control the arrhythmia, the dosage may be increased to 400 mg every 8 hrs. (Alternatively, doses may be given every 12 hrs.)
      (3) Normal maintenance doses are 200 to 300 mg every 8 hrs.
   f. **Flecainide (Tambocor®)** is administered orally and should be initiated in the hospital setting.
      (1) Initial dosage is 50 mg every 12 hrs, and the dosage may be increased in twice-daily increments of 50 mg every 4 days to a maximum of 300 mg/day.
      (2) The usual maintenance dose is 100 mg every 12 hrs.
   g. **Propafenone (Rythmol®, Rythmol SR®)** is administered orally and should be initiated in the hospital setting.
      (1) Initial dosage is 150 mg every 8 hrs and can be increased every 3 to 4 days to the desired therapeutic effect or side effects.
      (2) The usual maintenance dose is 150 to 200 mg every 8 hrs (Rythmol®) or every 12 hrs (Rythmol SR®) up to a maximum of 900 mg/day.
4. **Precautions and monitoring effects. Note:** Proarrhythmia (the ability to cause an arrhythmia) is the most important risk associated with the use of antiarrhythmic drug therapy. Bradyarrhythmias and ventricular tachyarrhythmias, such as TdP, can occur. These often take place during the initiation of antiarrhythmic drug treatment and should be considered

when decision makers choose between outpatient and inpatient initiation of antiarrhythmic therapy.

a. Quinidine (Various)

- **(1)** This drug is contraindicated in patients with
  - **(a)** Complete AV block unless a ventricular pacemaker is in place.
  - **(b)** Marked prolongation of the QT interval or prolonged QT syndrome because ventricular tachyarrhythmia (TdP) may arise, resulting in quinidine syncope (i.e., syncope or sudden death).
- **(2)** An increase of 50% or more in the duration of the QRS complex necessitates dosage reduction.
- **(3)** Quinidine has a narrow therapeutic index. Therapeutic serum levels are in the range of 2 to 6 μg/mL, depending on the specificity of the assay. Toxicity may cause acute cardiac effects, such as pronounced slowing of conduction in all heart regions; this, in turn, may lead to SA block or arrest, ventricular tachycardia, or asystole.
- **(4)** The EKG/ECG should be monitored during quinidine therapy to detect signs of cardiotoxicity. To counteract quinidine-induced ventricular tachyarrhythmias, catecholamines, glucagon, or sodium lactate may be given.
- **(5)** In patients receiving quinidine for atrial tachyarrhythmias, vagolytic effects may increase impulse conduction at the AV node, resulting in an accelerated ventricular response. To prevent this, agents that slow AV nodal conduction (e.g., verapamil, digoxin) may be administered.
- **(6)** The dosage should be reduced in elderly patients (> 60 years old) and in patients with hepatic dysfunction or congestive heart failure (CHF).
- **(7)** Embolism may occur on restoration of normal sinus rhythm after prolonged atrial fibrillation. To prevent or minimize this complication, anticoagulants may be administered before quinidine therapy begins.
- **(8)** Quinidine may cause cinchonism at high serum concentrations, manifested by tinnitus, hearing loss, blurred vision, and gastrointestinal (GI) disturbances. In severe cases, nausea, vomiting, diarrhea, headache, confusion, delirium, photophobia, diplopia, and psychosis may occur.
- **(9)** GI reactions are the most common adverse reactions to quinidine. About 30% of patients experience diarrhea; nausea and vomiting may also occur. Arising almost immediately after the first dose, these symptoms sometimes warrant discontinuing the drug. However, aluminum hydroxide or use of the polygalacturonate salt may reverse this.
- **(10)** Hypersensitivity reactions include anaphylaxis, thrombocytopenia, respiratory distress, and vascular collapse.

b. Procainamide (Various)

- **(1)** This drug is contraindicated in patients with hypersensitivity to procaine and related drugs, myasthenia gravis, second- or third-degree AV block with no pacemaker, a history of procainamide-induced systemic lupus erythematosus (SLE), prolonged QT syndrome, or TdP.
- **(2)** An increase of 50% or more in the duration of the QRS complex necessitates dosage reduction.
- **(3)** Procainamide has a narrow therapeutic index. Therapeutic serum levels are reported in the range of 4 to 10 μg/mL. *N*-acetyl procainamide (NAPA) levels of 15 to 25 μg/mL are considered therapeutic. The active metabolite, NAPA, possesses differing pharmacological cardiovascular effects, and serum levels need to be evaluated independently of procainamide. Toxicity may cause acute cardiac effects (e.g., pronounced slowing of conduction in all heart regions), which, in turn, may lead to SA block or arrest, ventricular tachycardia, or asystole.
- **(4)** High serum procainamide levels may induce ventricular arrhythmias (e.g., PVCs, ventricular tachycardia, or fibrillation). The EKG/ECG should be monitored continuously to detect these problems. Catecholamines, glucagon, or sodium lactate may be administered to counteract these arrhythmias.

(5) Hypotension may occur with rapid intravenous administration.
(6) GI effects are less common than with quinidine therapy.
(7) Hypersensitivity reactions are the most severe adverse effects of procainamide. These reactions include drug fever, agranulocytosis, and an SLE-like syndrome.
   (a) An SLE-like syndrome is manifested by fatigue, arthralgia, myalgia, and low-grade fever.
   (b) Antinuclear antibody titer is positive in 50% to 80% of patients receiving procainamide. However, only 20% to 30% of these patients develop symptoms of the SLE-like syndrome.
   (c) Drug discontinuation usually is necessary when symptomatic SLE-like syndrome occurs.
(8) The dosage should be reduced and given over 6 hrs to patients with renal or hepatic impairment, as the drug half-life is increased in these patients.
(9) Lower doses may be needed in patients with CHF to adjust for the lower volume of distribution.
(10) Embolism may occur on restoration of normal sinus rhythm after prolonged atrial fibrillation. An anticoagulant is frequently administered before procainamide therapy begins to prevent this complication.

c. Disopyramide (Norpace®)
(1) This drug may cause marked hemodynamic compromise and ventricular dysfunction. It is contraindicated in patients with cardiogenic shock or second- or third-degree AV block with no pacemaker.
(2) Disopyramide should be avoided or used with extreme caution in patients with heart failure (HF). It should also be used cautiously in patients with urinary tract disorders, myasthenia gravis, and renal or hepatic dysfunction.
(3) In patients receiving this drug for atrial tachyarrhythmias, vagolytic effects may increase impulse conduction at the AV node, resulting in an accelerated ventricular response. To prevent this, agents that slow AV nodal conduction (e.g., verapamil, digoxin) may be given.
(4) Anticholinergic effects of this drug include dry mouth, constipation, urinary hesitancy or retention, and blurred vision.
(5) Therapeutic plasma levels range from 2 to 4 μg/mL.

d. Lidocaine (Xylocaine®)
(1) This drug may cause hemodynamic compromise in patients with severe cardiac dysfunction. Generally, however, it has few untoward cardiovascular effects.
(2) Lidocaine should be used cautiously and in reduced dosage in patients with CHF or renal or hepatic impairment.
(3) Central nervous system (CNS) reactions are the most pronounced adverse effects of lidocaine. These reactions may range from lightheadedness and restlessness to confusion, tremors, stupor, and convulsions.
(4) Tinnitus, blurred vision, and anaphylaxis have been reported.
(5) Plasma lidocaine levels of 1.5 to 6.5 μg/mL are therapeutic.
(6) Lidocaine's metabolites—glycinexylidide and monoethylglycinexylidide—may have neurotoxic as well as antiarrhythmic effects.

e. Mexiletine (Various)
(1) This drug is contraindicated in patients with cardiogenic shock or second- or third-degree AV block with no pacemaker.
(2) Tremor is an early sign of mexiletine toxicity. Dizziness, ataxia, and nystagmus indicate an increasing plasma drug concentration.
(3) Hypotension, bradycardia, and widened QRS complexes may develop during mexiletine therapy.
(4) Adverse GI effects include nausea and vomiting.
(5) Therapeutic serum levels range from 0.50 to 2.0 μg/mL.

f. Flecainide (Tambocor®)
(1) This drug is contraindicated in patients with cardiogenic shock or second- or third-degree AV block with no pacemaker.

(2) The EKG/ECG should be monitored during flecainide therapy because this drug may exacerbate existing arrhythmias or precipitate new ones. Flecainide was shown in the CAST study to increase mortality in patients with asymptomatic ventricular arrhythmias and, therefore, should be reserved for patients with life-threatening ventricular arrhythmias that are refractory to other drugs.
(3) This drug has a significant negative inotropic effect and may bring on or worsen CHF and cardiomyopathy.
(4) Adverse CNS effects (e.g., dizziness, headache, tremor) and GI effects (e.g., nausea, abdominal pain) may occur.
(5) Blurred vision and dyspnea have been reported.
(6) Therapeutic serum levels recommended for flecainide are between 0.2 and 1.0 μg/mL.

g. **Propafenone (Rythmol®)**
(1) This drug, such as other antiarrhythmic agents, may cause new or worsened arrhythmias. Such proarrhythmic properties range from an increased frequency of PVCs to the development of severe ventricular tachycardia, ventricular fibrillation, and TdP. This proarrhythmic effect has been under discussion for the class Ic agents; thus, when used, these agents should be monitored closely. The findings from the CAST study must be weighed against the benefits of using these agents for treating significant ventricular arrhythmias.
(2) Dizziness is a side effect that has been reported in as many as 10% to 15% of patients taking the drug.
(3) Other associated side effects include vomiting, a metallic bitter taste in the mouth, constipation, headache, and new or worsening CHF and asthma.
(4) Therapeutic serum levels recommended for propafenone are between 0.06 and 1.0 μg/mL.

5. **Significant interactions**

a. **Quinidine**
(1) Quinidine may increase serum levels of **digoxin** and increase the effects of **digitalis** on the heart, with a resultant increase in toxicity.
(2) Severe orthostatic hypotension may occur with concomitant administration of **vasodilators** (e.g., **nitroglycerin**).
(3) **Phenytoin**, **rifampin (Rifadin®)**, and **barbiturates** may antagonize quinidine activity and reduce its therapeutic efficacy.
(4) **Nifedipine (Procardia®)** may reduce plasma quinidine levels.
(5) **Antacids**, **sodium bicarbonate**, and **sodium acetazolamide (Diamox®)** may increase plasma quinidine levels, possibly resulting in toxicity.
(6) Quinidine may produce additive hypoprothrombinemic effects with **coumarin** anticoagulants.

b. **Amiodarone (Cordarone®)** and **cimetidine (Tagamet®)** may increase plasma procainamide levels, possibly leading to drug toxicity.

c. **Phenytoin** accelerates disopyramide metabolism, possibly reducing its therapeutic efficacy.

d. **Lidocaine**
(1) **Phenytoin** may increase the cardiodepressant effects of lidocaine.
(2) **β-Blockers** (class II antiarrhythmics) may reduce lidocaine metabolism, possibly leading to drug toxicity.

e. **Mexiletine (Various). Phenobarbital**, **rifampin (Rifadin®)**, and **phenytoin (Dilantin®)** reduce plasma mexiletine levels and may decrease therapeutic efficacy.

B. **Class II antiarrhythmics**

1. **Indications.** These drugs—**β-adrenergic blockers**—among the drugs in this class indicated for the treatment of select arrhythmias are propranolol (Inderal®), esmolol (Brevibloc®), and acebutolol (Sectral®) are approved for antiarrhythmic use.

a. **Propranolol (Inderal®)** may be given to
(1) Control supraventricular arrhythmias (e.g., atrial fibrillation or flutter, paroxysmal supraventricular tachycardia [PSVTs])
(2) Treat tachyarrhythmias caused by catecholamine stimulation (e.g., in hyperthyroidism, during anesthesia)
(3) Suppress severe ventricular arrhythmias in **prolonged QT syndrome**
(4) Treat digitalis-induced ventricular arrhythmias

(5) Terminate certain ventricular arrhythmias (e.g., PVCs in patients without structural heart disease)

(6) In the most recently completed guidelines, the intravenous administration of β-adrenergic blockers was given a class I recommendation with a "B" level of evidence to slow the ventricular response to atrial fibrillation in acute setting, with cautious considerations to those with hypotension or HF.

b. **Esmolol (Brevibloc®)** is used to treat supraventricular tachycardias; it possesses a very short (9 mins) half-life, and has been used to control the ventricular response to atrial fibrillation or flutter during or after surgery.

c. **Acebutolol (Sectral®)** has been used in the management of ventricular arrhythmias; although not specifically listed within the recent guidelines, like esmolol and propranolol, the β-adrenergic blockers were given a class I ranking for ventricular control in patients with atrial fibrillation.

2. **Mechanism of action.** Class II antiarrhythmics reduce sympathetic stimulation of the heart, decreasing impulse conduction through the AV node and lengthening the refractory period. Additionally, this class of antiarrhythmics slows the sinus rhythm without significantly changing the QT or QRS intervals, resulting in a reduced heart rate and a decrease in myocardial oxygen demand.

3. **Administration and dosage**

a. **Propranolol (Inderal®)** may be given intravenously or orally when used as an antiarrhythmic.

(1) Emergency therapy calls for slow intravenous administration of 1 to 3 mg diluted in 50 mL dextrose 5% in water or normal saline solution. This dose is infused slowly (no faster than 1 mg/min). A second dose of 1 to 3 mg may be given 2 mins later.

(2) For oral therapy, 10 to 80 mg/day is given in three to four doses. (However, 1000 mg or more may be required for resistant ventricular arrhythmias.)

b. **Esmolol (Brevibloc®)** is given intravenously. A loading dose of 500 mcg/kg/min is infused over 1 min, followed by a 4-min maintenance infusion of 50 mcg/kg/min. If a satisfactory response is not achieved within 5 mins, the loading dose is repeated and followed by a maintenance infusion of 100 mcg/kg/min.

c. **Acebutolol (Sectral®)** is given orally. An oral dose of 400 mg is given by mouth daily up to a maximum of 1200 mg/day for the treatment of ventricular arrhythmias.

4. **Precautions and monitoring effects**

a. **Propranolol (Inderal®)**

(1) This drug is contraindicated in patients with sinus bradycardia, second- or third-degree AV block, cardiogenic shock, severe HF, or asthma.

(2) The β-blocking effects of this drug may lead to marked hypotension, exacerbation of HF and left ventricular failure, or cardiac arrest.

(3) Blood pressure, heart rate, and the EKG/ECG should be monitored during intravenous infusion.

(4) Embolism may occur upon restoration of normal sinus rhythm after sustained atrial fibrillation. An anticoagulant may be given before propranolol therapy begins to prevent this complication.

(5) Propranolol may depress AV node conduction and ventricular pacemaker activity, resulting in AV block or asystole.

(6) This drug may mask the signs and symptoms of hypoglycemia. It also may mask signs of shock.

(7) Fatigue, lethargy, increased airway resistance, and skin rash have been reported.

(8) Nausea, vomiting, and diarrhea may occur.

(9) Sudden withdrawal of propranolol may lead to acute MI, arrhythmias, or angina in cardiac patients. Drug therapy is discontinued by tapering the dose over 4 to 7 days.

b. **Esmolol (Brevibloc®)**

(1) This drug is contraindicated in patients with severe CHF or sinus bradycardia.

(2) Hypotension occurs in approximately 30% of patients receiving esmolol. This effect can be reversed by reducing the dosage or stopping the infusion.

(3) This drug is for short-term use only and should be replaced by a long-acting antiarrhythmic once the patient's heart stabilizes.

(4) Dizziness, headache, fatigue, and agitation may occur.

(5) Other adverse effects include nausea, vomiting, and bronchospasm.

c. **Acebutolol (Sectral®)**
   (1) Similar contraindications as other β-blockers; heart block, uncompensated HF, sick sinus syndrome.
   (2) Major monitoring parameters for patients include serum creatinine level, heart rate, and blood pressure.
   (3) Therapy should not be rapidly discontinued but rather gradually over 10 to 14 days. Abrupt discontinuation in cardiac patients may exacerbate an angina attack or a more significant acute coronary syndrome.

5. **Significant interactions**
   a. **Propranolol (Inderal®)**
      (1) Severe vasoconstriction may occur with concomitant **epinephrine** administration.
      (2) **Digitalis** preparations can cause excessive bradycardia.
      (3) **Calcium-channel blockers**—for example, **diltiazem (Cardizem®)** and **verapamil (Calan®)**—and other negative **inotropic** and **chronotropic drugs**—such as **disopyramide (Norpace®)** and **quinidine**—add to the myocardial depressant effects of propranolol.
   b. **Esmolol (Brevibloc®). Morphine (MS Contin®)** may raise plasma esmolol levels.

C. **Class III antiarrhythmics**

1. **Indications**
   a. **Amiodarone (Cordarone®)** is given to control malignant ventricular arrhythmias and is recommended within the advance cardiac life support (ACLS) guidelines, has been given a class I recommendation for victims with ventricular tachyarrhythmia during a cardiac arrest, for attempting a stable rhythm after further defibrillations. A "B" level of evidence has been documented. Unlike most other antiarrhythmics, with the exception of the β-adrenergic blockers, amiodarone has been shown to reduce arrhythmic deaths in patients after an MI. Additionally, amiodarone received a class IIa recommendation for patients with sustained ventricular tachycardia that is hemodynamically unstable and refractory to conversion with countershock or procainamide or other agents. Amiodarone has also received a class I rating for intravenous administration to control the heart rate in atrial fibrillation and HF patients who do not have an accessory pathway.
   b. **Sotalol (Betapace®)** is used to treat supraventricular and ventricular tachyarrhythmias. Sotalol antagonizes both β_1- and β_2-adrenergic receptors but also prolongs the phase 3 action potential. It is this property that distinguishes it from other β-adrenergic blockers and is the reason why it is classified as a class III antiarrhythmic agent rather than a class II agent (β-adrenergic blocker).
   c. **Ibutilide (Corvert®)** is used in the conversion of atrial fibrillation and flutter of recent onset (duration $<$ 30 days). In the most recent guidelines provided for the treatment of atrial fibrillation, ibutilide received along with dofetilide, a class I recommendation with "A" level of evidence for its use in the pharmacologic cardioversion of atrial fibrillation.
   d. **Dofetilide (Tikosyn®)** is available in the United States under restricted access in the treatment of atrial fibrillation/flutter. As mentioned earlier, within the most recent guidelines provided for the treatment of atrial fibrillation, dofetilide received, along with ibutilide, a class I recommendation with "A" level of evidence for its use in the pharmacological cardioversion of atrial fibrillation.

2. **Mechanism of action.** Class III antiarrhythmic drugs primarily work on the potassium channels of the action potential and prolong the refractory period and action potential; they have no effect on myocardial contractility or conduction time.

3. **Administration and dosage**
   a. **Amiodarone (Cordarone®).** Available for both oral and intravenous use and should only be initiated in the hospital setting. Amiodarone has been incorporated into the ACLS guidelines and recommended by the expert panel members as the first-choice antiarrhythmic for shock-refractory ventricular fibrillation/ventricular tachycardia.
      (1) It is available for oral use; 800 to 1600 mg every 12 hrs is given for 7 to 14 days, then 200 to 400 mg daily thereafter.
      (2) Oral treatment is used to suppress ventricular and supraventricular arrhythmias but can take days or weeks to take effect. Oral doses of 100 to 600 mg/day (usually 300 to 400 mg/day) for maintenance therapy in ventricular tachycardia and 100 to 200 mg/day for maintenance therapy for supraventricular tachycardias are given.

(3) Intravenous formulation is available for treatment and prophylaxis of recurrent ventricular fibrillation or hemodynamically unstable ventricular tachycardia in refractory patients.

(4) The intravenous form is rapidly distributed throughout the body. Recommended doses include a rapid loading infusion of 150 mg over 10 mins, followed by a slow infusion of 1.0 mg/min for 6 hrs (360 mg), and then a maintenance infusion of 0.5 mg/min for the remainder of the 24-hr period. Patients usually receive 2 to 4 days of infusions before conversion to oral form. However, a maintenance infusion can be continued for 2 to 3 weeks.

b. Sotalol (Betapace®) is available commercially as an oral tablet, and therapy should be initiated within the hospital setting. Normal dosing of 80 mg twice daily initially and increasing doses at 2- to 3-day intervals to a maximum dose of 640 mg/day, given in two to three doses throughout the day.

c. Ibutilide (Corvert®) is available only for injection in a 0.1-mg/mL, 10-mL vial. Normal doses for the conversion of recent-onset atrial fibrillation to normal sinus rhythm is a dose of 1 mg (0.01 mg/kg for those < 60 kg) over 10 mins, with a repeat dose in 10 mins if the arrhythmia does not end.

d. Dofetilide (Tikosyn®) is available only for oral administration in 0.125-, 0.25-, and 0.5-mg capsules under the trade name of Tikosyn and should only be initiated in a hospital setting with trained personnel and the equipment necessary to provide continuous cardiac monitoring during initiation of therapy.

(1) A normal dose for the conversion of recent-onset atrial fibrillation to normal sinus rhythm is 0.5 mg twice daily for patients with creatinine clearance values > 60 mL/min; doses are reduced 50% (0.25 mg) for those with creatinine clearance values of 40 to 60 mL/min, and doses are reduced an additional 50% (0.125 mg) for those with creatinine clearance values of 20 to 40 mL/min.

(2) Maintenance therapy is based on the EKG/ECG, with doses being reduced with QTc prolongation exceeding 15% of the baseline value. Any patient developing a QTc interval exceeding 500 msec should have therapy discontinued immediately.

(3) Dofetilide should not be given to those with creatinine clearance values < 20 mL/min.

4. Precautions and monitoring effects

a. Amiodarone (Cordarone®)

(1) Life-threatening pulmonary toxicity may occur during amiodarone therapy, especially in patients receiving > 400 mg/day. Baseline as well as routine pulmonary function tests reveal relevant pulmonary changes.

(2) Most patients develop corneal microdeposits 1 to 4 months after amiodarone therapy begins. However, this reaction rarely causes visual disturbance, but the patient should be monitored with routine ophthalmological examinations.

(3) Blood pressure and heart rate and rhythm should be monitored for hypotension and bradyarrhythmias.

(4) Patients should be monitored routinely for the possible development of hepatic dysfunction, thyroid disorders (e.g., hyperthyroidism, hypothyroidism), and photosensitivity.

(5) CNS reactions include fatigue, malaise, peripheral neuropathy, and extrapyramidal effects.

(6) Nausea and vomiting have been reported.

(7) This drug has an extremely long half-life (up to 60 days). Therapeutic response may be delayed for weeks after oral therapy begins; adverse reactions may persist up to 4 months after therapy ends.

b. Sotalol (Betapace®)

(1) Side effects of this drug are directly related to β-blockade and prolongation of repolarization.

(2) Transient hypotension, bradycardia, myocardial depression (negative inotropic effect), and bronchospasm have all been associated with this drug.

(3) This drug carries all the contraindications associated with other β-blockers along with those owing to its electrophysiologic properties.

c. Ibutilide (Corvert®)

(1) Infusion should be discontinued as soon as the atrial arrhythmia is terminated or if sustained or nonsustained ventricular arrhythmia or marked QT prolongation is documented.

(2) Continuous EKG/ECG monitoring is required for at least 4 hrs after discontinuing the infusion or until the QT interval returns to baseline.

d. **Dofetilide (Tikosyn®)**

(1) Patients need to be monitored closely for the subsequent development of ventricular arrhythmias with increasing doses of dofetilide or with declining renal status. In clinical trials, ventricular tachycardias, including TdP, are the most frequently occurring arrhythmias due to dofetilide.

(2) Hypokalemia and those situations that might cause hypotension will predispose a patient to prolongation of the QT interval, which could put a dofetilide patient at risk for toxic arrhythmias.

5. **Significant interactions**

a. **Amiodarone (Cordarone®)**

(1) Amiodarone may increase the plasma levels of **quinidine**, **procainamide**, **diltiazem**, **digitalis**, and **flecainide**.

(2) It may increase the pharmacological effect of **β-blockers**, **calcium-channel blockers**, and **warfarin**.

(3) **Special note:** Amiodarone has been reported to have numerous drug–drug interactions among all categories of drugs. To avoid the development of a significant drug–drug interaction, a thorough patient medication profile should be carried out for each patient having amiodarone therapy initiated, as well as each time a patient currently receiving amiodarone is given an additional drug.

b. **Sotalol (Betapace®)**

(1) Sotalol must be used cautiously in those patients receiving agents with cardiac-depressant properties.

(2) Agents such as sotalol that prolong the QT interval may induce malignant arrhythmias when used in combination with other class Ia antiarrhythmics, especially in the presence of low potassium levels.

c. **Ibutilide (Corvert®)** should be avoided with other agents that prolong repolarization or within 4 hrs of administration.

d. **Dofetilide (Tikosyn®)** should be avoided in patients who have hypokalemia or preexisting QT prolongation.

D. **Class IV antiarrhythmics**

1. **Indications**

a. **Calcium-channel blockers** (e.g., verapamil [Calan®]; diltiazem [Cardizem®]) are used mainly to treat and prevent supraventricular arrhythmias.

(1) They are first-line agents for the suppression of PSVTs stemming from AV nodal reentry.

(2) They can rapidly control the ventricular response to atrial flutter and fibrillation.

b. Other calcium-channel blockers available include amlodipine (Norvasc®), clevidipine (Cleviprex®), felodipine (Plendil®), isradipine (DynaCirc®), nicardipine (Cardene®), nifedipine (Procardia®), nimodipine (Nimotop®), and nisoldipine (Sular®), but these agents have primarily been used in the treatment of angina pectoris and hypertension and will not be discussed further in this section.

2. **Mechanism of action.** Class IV antiarrhythmics are calcium-channel blockers. They decrease conduction through those areas of the heart dependent on slow calcium channels, which include the SA and AV nodes.

3. **Administration and dosage**

a. To control atrial arrhythmias, verapamil usually is administered intravenously. A dose of 2.5 to 10 mg is given over at least 2 mins and may be repeated in 30 mins, if necessary. A 5 to 10 mg/hr continuous intravenous infusion has also been used in treating arrhythmias.

b. To prevent PSVTs, verapamil may be given orally in four daily doses of 80 to 120 mg each.

c. To control atrial arrhythmias, diltiazem usually is administered intravenously. A dose of 20 mg (0.25 mg/kg) is given over 2 mins. If an adequate response is not obtained, a second dose of 25 mg (0.35 mg/kg) is administered after 15 mins. A 5 to 15 mg/hr intravenous continuous infusion has also been used in treating arrhythmias.

4. **Precautions and monitoring effects**

a. Verapamil and diltiazem are contraindicated in patients with AV block; left ventricular dysfunction; severe hypotension; concomitant, intravenous β-blockers; and atrial fibrillation with an accessory AV pathway.

b. These drugs must be used cautiously in patients with CHF, sick sinus syndrome, MI, and hepatic or renal impairment.

c. Because of the negative chronotropic effect, verapamil and diltiazem must be used cautiously in patients who have slow heart rates or who are receiving digitalis glycosides.

d. The EKG/ECG (especially the respiratory rate (RR) interval) should be monitored during therapy.

e. Patients > 60 years old should receive reduced dosages and slower injection rates.

f. Constipation and nausea have been reported with verapamil.

5. Significant interactions

a. Concomitant administration of **β-blockers** or **disopyramide** may precipitate HF.

b. **Quinidine** may increase the risk of calcium-channel blocker–induced hypotension.

c. Verapamil may increase serum **digoxin** concentrations, and diltiazem may do the same to a lesser extent.

d. **Rifampin** may enhance the metabolism of calcium-channel blockers, with a resultant decrease in pharmacological effect.

e. Verapamil and diltiazem may inhibit **theophylline** metabolism and may require reductions in theophylline dosage.

f. Diltiazem and verapamil inhibit the metabolism of **cyclosporine (Gengraf®)** and may require reductions in cyclosporine dosages.

E. Unclassified antiarrhythmics

1. Atropine (Various)

a. Indications. Atropine is therapeutic for symptomatic sinus bradycardia and junctional rhythm.

b. Mechanism of action. An anticholinergic, atropine blocks vagal effects on the SA node, promoting conduction through the AV node and increasing the heart rate.

c. Administration and dosage. For antiarrhythmic use, atropine is administered in a dose of 0.4 to 1.0 mg by intravenous push; the dose is given every 5 mins to a maximum of 2.0 mg.

d. Precautions and monitoring effects

(1) Thirst and dry mouth are the most common adverse effects of atropine.

(2) CNS reactions (e.g., restlessness, headache, disorientation, dizziness) may occur with doses over 5 mg.

(3) Tachycardia and ophthalmic disturbances (e.g., mydriasis, blurred vision, photophobia) may occur with doses of 1 mg or more.

(4) Initial doses may induce a reflex bradycardia owing to incomplete suppression of vagal impulses.

2. Adenosine (Adenocard®)

a. Indications. Adenosine is indicated for the conversion of acute supraventricular tachycardia (SVT) to normal sinus rhythm.

b. Mechanism of action. Adenosine is a naturally occurring nucleoside, which is normally present in all cells of the body. It has been shown to

(1) slow conduction through the AV node,

(2) interrupt reentry pathways through the AV node, and

(3) restore normal sinus rhythm in patients with PSVTs.

c. Administration and dosage. For antiarrhythmic effects, adenosine is given as a rapid bolus intravenous injection in a 6-mg dose over 1 to 2 secs. If the first dose does not eliminate the arrhythmia within 1 to 2 mins, the dose should be increased to 12 mg and again given as a rapid intravenous dose. An additional 12-mg dose may be repeated if necessary.

d. Precautions and monitoring effects

(1) The effects of adenosine are antagonized by methylxanthines, such as caffeine and theophylline. Theophylline has been successfully used for treating adenosine-induced side effects, such as hypotension, sweating, and palpitations. If side effects are encountered, aggressive therapy is not required because of the ultrashort half-life of the drug (10 secs or less).

(2) The main side effect associated with adenosine use in up to 18% of patients is facial flushing, but this effect is normally very short-lived.

(3) Other side effects associated with adenosine use include shortness of breath, chest pressure, nausea, headache, and a metallic taste.

e. **Additional use.** Adenosine has been used as an adjunctive agent in patients undergoing various types of pharmacological stress testing (e.g., thallium). In this situation, adenosine is given as a continuous infusion over a period of 4 to 6 mins and is able to provide a form of exercise tolerance test in patients not able to exert themselves owing to age, fatigue, and various other physical handicaps.

3. **Magnesium sulfate (Various)**
   a. **Indications.** Previous national guidelines have recommended magnesium for the treatment of drug-induced long QT syndrome. In the most recent ACLS guidelines, published in 2010, magnesium received a class IIb rating with a "class B" level of evidence, for its use *strictly* in patients presenting with TdP associated with a long QT interval. Additionally, magnesium has been used in the treatment of arrhythmias (ventricular tachycardia/fibrillation, due to hypomagnesemia).
   b. **Mechanism of action.** Acts on the myocardium by slowing the rate of impulse formation at the SA node and therefore slows down conduction. Magnesium is also necessary in the exchange of calcium, sodium, and potassium in and out of cells, which in the case of TdP might lower the amplitude of the early after depolarizations.
   c. **Administration and dosage.** For the treatment of TdP, 1 to 6 g over several minutes, occasionally followed by approximately 3 to 20 mg/min by IV infusion for 5 to 48 hrs, depending on response and serum magnesium concentrations.
      (1) Alternatively, for TdP associated with cardiac (pulseless) arrest, 1 to 2 g in 10 mL 5% dextrose injection over 5 to 20 mins.
      (2) Alternatively, for TdP in a patient with pulses, give a loading dose of 1 to 2 g (8 to 16 mEq) in 50 to 100 mL 5% dextrose injection over 5 to 60 mins.
      (3) **Intraosseous** TdP associated with cardiac (pulseless) arrest, 1 to 2 g in 10 mL 5% dextrose injection over 5 to 20 mins.
   d. **Precautions and monitoring effects**
      (1) Routine monitoring of magnesium levels, in order to prevent hypermagnesemia, while also monitoring calcium levels and phosphorus levels, which can be reduced when administering IV magnesium.

4. **Digoxin (Lanoxin®)**
   a. **Indications.** Recent guidelines recommend that digoxin is effective in stable, narrow-complex regular tachycardias if rhythm remains uncontrolled or unconverted by adenosine or vagal maneuvers or if SVT is recurrent. Additionally, digoxin has been shown effective to control the ventricular rate in patients with atrial fibrillation or atrial flutter.
   b. **Mechanism of action.** As a cardiac glycoside, digoxin has positive inotropic effects; however, for rhythm control digoxin relies on its "parasympathomimetic properties," which slow conduction through the AV node and decrease impulses going through to the ventricles.
   c. **Administration and dosage.** Digoxin can be given as 8 to 12 mcg/kg with half of that being given over 5 mins, and the remaining 50% given in two doses at 4 and 8 hrs later.
   d. **Precautions and monitoring effects**
      (1) The onset of action is slow and depending on the circumstances might not be acceptable for acute arrhythmias.
      (2) Long-term use of digoxin will expose the patient to numerous monitoring requirements, including renal function, drug–drug interactions, and fluid and electrolyte monitoring, in order to minimize likelihood of adverse drug reactions.

5. **Dronedarone (Multaq®)**
   a. The newest antiarrhythmic, which was a major focal point for recently updated guidelines for the treatment of atrial fibrillation, and which has not yet been formally added into the current Vaughan Williams classification.
   b. Within the updated guidelines, dronedarone (Multaq®) received a class IIa rating with a "class B" level of evidence, to decrease the need for hospitalization for cardiovascular events in patients with paroxysmal atrial fibrillation or after conversion of persistent atrial fibrillation. Additionally, it was felt that dronedarone could be initiated during outpatient therapy. However, within the same guidelines, dronedarone was also given a class III for use in class IV HF or patients who have had an episode of decompensated HF in the past 4 weeks, especially with depressed left ventricular function (ejection fraction $< 35\%$).

c. Dronedarone (Multaq®) is available and is doses as 400 mg by mouth twice daily in the prevention of atrial fibrillation and/or flutter.
d. Dronedarone (Multaq®), similar to amiodarone, there are numerous drug–drug interactions with dronedarone; consequently, each newly added therapy should be evaluated in order to identify the potential impact when starting, as well as when ending each therapy.

Study Questions

Directions: Each of the questions, statements, or incomplete statements can be correctly answered or completed by **one** of the suggested answers or phrases. Choose the **best** answer.

1. Strong anticholinergic effects limit the antiarrhythmic use of

(A) quinidine (Various).
(B) procainamide (Various).
(C) mexiletine (Various).
(D) flecainide (Tambocor®).
(E) disopyramide (Norpace®).

2. A pronounced slowing of phase 0 of the myocardial action potential results in a prolongation of either atrial depolarization, causing a prolonged P wave on the electrocardiogram (EKG/ECG), or ventricular depolarization, causing a prolonged QRS complex characterized by which class of antiarrhythmics?

(A) Class I
(B) Class II
(C) Class III
(D) Class IV
(E) Class V

3. Which of the following class III antiarrhythmics has been reported as "carrying a risk for" causing torsades de pointes?

(A) lidocaine (Xylocaine®)
(B) amiodarone (Cordarone®)
(C) quinidine (Various)
(D) flecainide (Tambocor®)
(E) diltiazem (Cardizem®)

4. A patient receiving a class I antiarrhythmic agent complains of GI symptoms, including nausea, vomiting, and occasional diarrhea after taking a dose. The patient is most likely receiving

(A) lidocaine (Xylocaine®).
(B) procainamide (Various).
(C) quinidine (Various).
(D) flecainide (Tambocor®).
(E) propranolol (Inderal®).

5. Class III antiarrhythmics have which of the following effects to the cardiac cell's action potential?

(A) Slow the rate of rise for phase 0 of depolarization.
(B) Delay the fast-channel conductance of sodium ions.
(C) Prolong phases 2 and 3 of repolarization.
(D) Inhibit the slow-channel conductance of calcium ions.
(E) Prolong the refractory period of the action potential.

6. Which of the following drugs is a class IV antiarrhythmic that is primarily indicated for the treatment of supraventricular tachyarrhythmias?

(A) ibutilide (Corvert®)
(B) mexiletine (Various)
(C) diltiazem (Cardizem®)
(D) procainamide (Various)
(E) propranolol (Inderal®)

7. Relatively new antiarrhythmic agent, which has not yet been formally added into the Vaughan Williams classification table but received a class IIa rating with a class B level of evidence to decrease the need for hospitalization in patients with paroxysmal atrial fibrillation or after conversion of persistent atrial fibrillation. Which of the following agents is best described by the above statements?

(A) aliskiren (Tekturna®)
(B) inamrinone (Various)
(C) dronedarone (Multaq®)
(D) amiodarone (Cordarone®)
(E) dofetilide (Tikosyn®)

8. Which of the following drugs is a class III antiarrhythmic agent that is effective in the acute management of atrial fibrillation or atrial flutter of recent onset?

(A) propranolol (Inderal®)
(B) ibutilide (Corvert®)
(C) metoprolol (Lopressor®)
(D) disopyramide (Norpace®)
(E) diltiazem (Cardizem®)

9. All of the following problems represent concerns when patients are started on amiodarone *except*
   (A) extremely long $t_{½}$.
   (B) need for multiple daily doses.
   (C) development of hyperthyroidism or hypothyroidism.
   (D) development of liver toxicity.
   (E) interactions with numerous other drugs.

10. Based on the criteria used for recent national guidelines used within the cardiology arena, which of the following recommendations would most likely result in the use of a selected antiarrhythmic therapy for a patient with atrial fibrillation?
   (A) Class I; level C
   (B) Class I; level A
   (C) Class IIa; level B
   (D) Class III; level A
   (E) Class IIb; level A

Answers and Explanations

1. **The answer is E** *[see II.A.4.c.(4)].*
Disopyramide has anticholinergic actions about one-tenth the potency of atropine. Effects include dry mouth, constipation, urinary retention, and blurred vision. Therefore, it cannot be used in patients with glaucoma or with conditions causing urinary retention. Moreover, disopyramide has a negative inotropic effect and must, therefore, be used with great caution, if at all, in patients with preexisting ventricular failure.

2. **The answer is A** *[see I.B.2 and II.A].*
The class I antiarrhythmics (fast-channel blockers) slow impulse conduction by depressing the flow of sodium ions into cells during phase 0 of the action potential.

3. **The answer is B** *[see I.C.3.d; Table 32-1].*
Torsades de pointes is a form of ventricular tachyarrhythmia characterized by electrocardiographic changes, which include a markedly prolonged QT interval. This potentially fatal reaction has now been reported for both antiarrhythmics and nonantiarrhythmics. Antiarrhythmics, which have been reported to cause torsades de pointes, include amiodarone, disopyramide, dofetilide, flecainide, ibutilide, procainamide, quinidine, and sotalol. Of the agents listed, only amiodarone is a class III antiarrhythmic.

4. **The answer is C** *[see II.A.4.a].*
The patient's complaints are typical of many patients receiving quinidine as an antiarrhythmic. GI side effects are the major ones associated with quinidine administration, with diarrhea being reported in up to 30% of patients receiving the drug. These GI side effects are different from those associated with high serum concentrations of quinidine, where tinnitus, hearing loss, and blurred vision are added to the GI symptoms in a syndrome referred to as cinchonism.

5. **The answer is E** *[see II.C.2].*
Class III antiarrhythmic agents work primarily on the potassium channels of the action potential and prolong the refractory period and action potential. Class Ia agents slow the rate of rise for phase 0 depolarization, as well as slowing fast-channel conduction of sodium and phases 2 and 3 of repolarization. Class IV agents (verapamil, diltiazem) inhibit the slow-channel conductance of calcium ions.

6. **The answer is C** *[see II.D.2].*
Of the agents listed, diltiazem is a calcium-channel blocker and represents the class IV antiarrhythmics. Diltiazem has been used for its direct-acting effects on impulse conduction throughout the heart. Diltiazem is used to treat and prevent supraventricular arrhythmias. Ibutilide is a class III agent, procainamide is a class Ia drug, mexiletine is a class Ib agent, and propranolol, a β-adrenergic blocker, is class II. Mexiletine, quinidine, and propranolol are all also effective for supraventricular arrhythmias, and ibutilide is indicated for the treatment of atrial fibrillation/flutter of recent onset.

7. **The answer is C** *[see II.E.5.a–d].*
Dronedarone (Multaq®) is the newest of the currently available antiarrhythmic agents and has yet to be included within the Vaughan Williams antiarrhythmic classification table. It also was the primary subject for a recently focused guidelines update for the treatment of patients with atrial tachyarrhythmias. Aliskiren (Tekturna®) is a relatively new agent referred to as a direct renin antagonist, which is available for the treatment of hypertension. Inamrinone (Various) is referred to as a phosphodiesterase inhibitor, which has been used for its positive inotropic actions in the treatment of heart failure. Amiodarone (Cordarone®) and dofetilide (Tikosyn®) are both considered class III Vaughan Williams antiarrhythmic agents.

8. The answer is B *[see II.C.1.d]*.

Dofetilide, ibutilide, amiodarone, and sotalol are class III antiarrhythmic agents. Class III agents prolong the refractory period and myocardial action potential and are used to treat ventricular arrhythmias. However, dofetilide and ibutilide are approved as class III agents indicated for the conversion from atrial fibrillation and flutter of recent onset to normal sinus rhythm. Propranolol, along with other β-blockers, is a class II antiarrhythmic; metoprolol is not routinely used in the treatment of arrhythmias; and disopyramide and diltiazem are class Ia and class IV antiarrhythmics, respectively.

9. The answer is B *[see II.C.3.a; II.C.4.a; II.C.5.a]*.

Amiodarone is a class III antiarrhythmic agent and acts by prolonging repolarization of cardiac cells. Amiodarone can be given either orally or parenterally and is often dosed as a once-a-day or twice-a-day maintenance dosage. Due to an extremely long elimination half-life, therapeutic response may be delayed for weeks. Therefore, an initial loading phase is often advisable. This requires hospitalization with close monitoring for desired effects, untoward reactions, and adjustments in dosage. Amiodarone has numerous drug–drug interactions with both other antiarrhythmic agents, as well as other nonarrhythmic agents. During therapy with amiodarone, patients may develop hypothyroidism or hyperthyroidism, pulmonary disorders (black box warning), hepatic dysfunction (black box warning), and various other unwanted effects.

10. The answer is B *[see I.H.1–2]*.

Recent national guidelines within the cardiology societies have used a scoring system, which includes two elements: one provides a recommendation based on benefit to risk where a class I recommendation has the greatest benefit compared to risk, as compared to class III where the risk may be equal to or worse than the risk; and a second element evaluates the degree of populations studied, where level A has been studied in numerous populations with well-controlled clinical trials, as compared to level C with very limited populations studied and reliance on opinion and case reports. A class I level A recommendation would be the best one would find, to help justify the use of a specific treatment or intervention, based on the cardiology guidelines criteria.

33 Hypertension

ALAN H. MUTNICK

I. GENERAL CONSIDERATIONS

A. **Definition. Hypertension** is blood pressure elevated enough to perfuse tissues and organs. Elevated systemic blood pressure is usually defined as a systolic reading ≥ 140 mm Hg and a diastolic reading ≥ 90 mm Hg (≥ 140/90 mm Hg). The "Seventh Report of the Joint National Committee on Detection, Evaluation, and Treatment of High Blood Pressure" (JNC-7) added a "prehypertension" category that includes individuals with systolic blood pressure readings of 120 to 139 mm Hg or diastolic blood pressure readings of 80 to 89 mm Hg; this category is now included in contemporary management strategies.

   1. It has been 7 years since the most recent set of national guidelines referred to as JNC-7; however, currently the National Heart, Lung, and Blood Institute is leading the development of an integrated set of cardiovascular risk reduction guidelines for adults using state-of-the-art methodology.
   2. The integrated approach will include updates for Cholesterol Guideline Update (ATP IV), Hypertension Guideline Update (JNC-8), and Obesity Guideline Update (Obesity-2) Integrated Cardiovascular Risk Reduction Guideline. The current timeline calls for the release of JNC-8 for public review and comment during the fall of 2011 and the release of the final update during the spring of 2012.
   3. The majority of this chapter will focus on the current guidelines, as described within the JNC-7 guidelines. However, the recently released 2011 Consensus document on the treatment of hypertension in the elderly has been added and can be viewed in their entirety with the following citation:
      a. Aronow WS, Fleg JL, Pepine CJ, et al. ACCF/AHA 2011 expert consensus document on hypertension in the elderly: a report of the American College of Cardiology Foundation Task Force on Clinical Expert Consensus Documents. *Circulation*. 2011;123(21):2434–2506.

B. **Classification** of hypertension is shown in *Table 33-1*. The table reflects the recommendations of the JNC-7.

C. The **relationship between elevated blood pressure and cardiovascular disease** was addressed in the JNC-7, which formalizes the fact that the higher the blood pressure, the greater the chance of a myocardial infarction (MI), heart failure (HF), stroke, or kidney disease. *Table 33-2* provides cardiovascular risk factors and/or lifestyle factors that affect the prognosis and treatment of hypertension and the various types of target-organ damage associated with hypertension.

D. **Incidence. Hypertension is the most common cardiovascular disorder.** Approximately 43 million Americans have blood pressure measurements > 140/90 mm Hg. This number translates to almost 25% of the adult population. The incidence increases with age—that is, 60% to 71% of people > 60 years of age have hypertension, according to data obtained from the Third National Health and Nutrition Examination Survey (NHANES III).

   1. **Primary (or essential) hypertension**, in which no specific cause can be identified, constitutes > 90% of all cases of systemic hypertension. The average age of onset is about 35 years.
   2. **Secondary hypertension**, resulting from an identifiable cause, such as renal disease or adrenal hyperfunction, accounts for the remaining 2% to 5% of cases of systemic hypertension. This type usually develops between the ages of 30 and 50.

Table 33-1 CLASSIFICATION OF HYPERTENSION FOR ADULTS ≥18 YEARS OF AGE

				Management		
					Initial Drug Therapy	
Classification	**Systolic (mm Hg)[a]**		**Diastolic (mm Hg)[a]**	**Lifestyle Modification**	**Without Compelling Indication**	**With Compelling Indications**
Normal	< 120	and	< 80	Encourage		
Prehypertension	120–139	or	80–89	Yes	No antihypertensive drug indicated, unless presence of a compelling indication[b] requiring use of drug therapy	Drug(s) for compelling indications
Stage 1 hypertension	140–159	or	90–99	Yes	Thiazide-type diuretics for most; may consider ACE inhibitor, ARB, β-blocker, CCB, or combination	Drug(s) for compelling indications; other antihypertensive drugs (diuretics, ACE inhibitor, ARB, β-blocker, CCB) as needed
Stage 2 hypertension	≥ 160	or	≥ 100	Yes	Two-drug combination for most (usually thiazide-type diuretic and ACE inhibitor, ARB, β-blocker, or CCB)	Drug(s) for compelling indications; other antihypertensive drugs (diuretics, ACE inhibitor, ARB, β-blocker, CCB) as needed

[a]Treatment is determined by the patient's highest blood pressure category.
[b]Selected drug therapies have been identified from clinical trials to possess positive clinical outcomes for specific clinical situations and represent compelling indication for their use. Compelling indications (and drug therapies): heart failure (diuretics, β-blockers, ACE inhibitors, ARB, aldosterone antagonists), postmyocardial infarction (β-blockers, ACE inhibitors, and aldosterone antagonists), high coronary disease risk (diuretic, β-blocker, ACE inhibitors, CCB), diabetes (diuretic, β-blockers, ACE inhibitors, ARB, CCB), chronic kidney disease (ACE inhibitors, ARB), and recurrent stroke prevention (diuretic, ACE inhibitors).
Based on Joint National Committee on Detection, Evaluation, and Treatment of High Blood Pressure. The seventh report of the Joint National Committee on Detection, Evaluation, and Treatment of High Blood Pressure: the JNC-7 report.
ACE, angiotensin-converting enzyme; *ARB*, angiotensin-receptor blocker; *CCB*, calcium-channel blocker.

Table 33-2 CARDIOVASCULAR AND/OR LIFESTYLE RISK FACTORS FOR CONSIDERATION IN THE MANAGEMENT OF HYPERTENSION

Hypertension
Cigarette smoking
Obesity (BMI ≥ 30)
Physical inactivity
Dyslipidemia (as a component of the metabolic syndrome)
Diabetes mellitus (as a component of the metabolic syndrome)
Microalbuminuria or estimated glomerular filtration rate < 60 mL/min
Age (> 55 years for men; > 65 years for women)
Family history of premature cardiovascular disease (men < 55 years; women < 65 years)

BMI, body mass index (calculated as weight in kilograms divided by the square of height in meters).
Based on Joint National Committee on Detection, Evaluation, and Treatment of High Blood Pressure. The seventh report of the Joint National Committee on Detection, Evaluation, and Treatment of High Blood Pressure: the JNC-7 report.

E. Physiology

Blood pressure = (stroke volume × heart rate) × total peripheral vascular resistance (TPR)

Altering any of the factors on the right side of the blood pressure equation results in a change in blood pressure, as shown in *Figure 33-1*.

1. **Sympathetic nervous system. Baroreceptors** (pressure receptors) in the carotids and aortic arch respond to changes in blood pressure and influence arteriolar dilation and arteriolar constriction. When stimulated to constrict, the contractile force strengthens, increasing the heart rate and augmenting peripheral resistance, thus increasing cardiac output. If pressure remains elevated, the baroreceptors reset at the higher levels and sustains the hypertension. Little evidence to date suggests that epinephrine and norepinephrine, two major neurotransmitters of the sympathetic nervous system, have a clear role in the cause of hypertension. However, many of the drugs used to treat hypertension lower blood pressure by blocking the sympathetic nervous system.
2. **Renin–angiotensin–aldosterone system.** Sympathetic stimulation, renal artery hypotension, and decreased sodium delivery to the distal tubules stimulate the release of renin by the kidney (juxtaglomerular apparatus of the kidney). Renin (an enzyme) reacts with a circulating substrate, angiotensinogen, to produce angiotensin I (a weak vasoconstrictor). Within the pulmonary

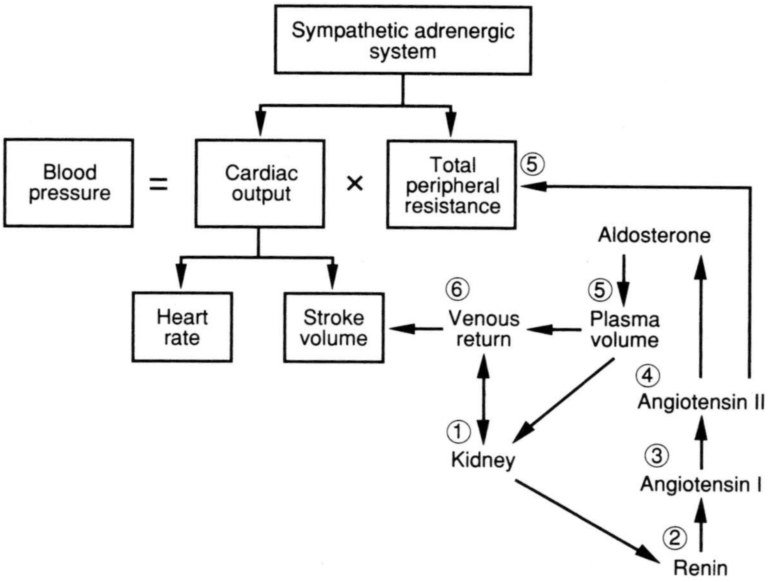

Figure 33-1. Blood pressure regulation: the determinants of blood pressure as they relate to cardiac output and total peripheral resistance. Angiotensin II, a potent vasopressor, not only increases total peripheral resistance but also, by stimulating aldosterone release, leads to an increase in plasma volume, venous return, stroke volume, and ultimately an increase in cardiac output.

endothelium is another enzyme, referred to as angiotensin-converting enzyme (ACE), which is able to hydrolyze the decapeptide angiotensin I to form the octapeptide angiotensin II (a potent natural vasoconstrictor). Angiotensin II has several important functions in the regulation of fluid volume.

a. It stimulates the release of aldosterone from the adrenal gland (zona glomerulosa), which results in increased sodium reabsorption, fluid volume, and blood pressure.

b. It constricts resistance vessels, which increases peripheral vascular resistance and arterial pressure.

c. It stimulates the release of vasopressin or antidiuretic hormone (ADH) from the posterior pituitary gland, which acts within the kidneys to increase fluid retention.

d. It stimulates cardiac hypertrophy and vascular hypertrophy.

e. It facilitates norepinephrine release from sympathetic nerve endings and inhibits norepinephrine reuptake by nerve endings, which enhances sympathetic function.

3. Mosaic theory centers around the fact that multiple factors, rather than one factor alone, are responsible for sustaining hypertension. The interactions among the sympathetic nervous system, renin–angiotensin–aldosterone system, and potential defects in sodium transport within and outside the cell may all play a role in long-term hypertension. Additional factors contributing to the development include genetics, endothelial dysfunction, and neurovascular anomalies. Other vasoactive substances that are involved in the maintenance of normal blood pressure have also been identified; these include nitric oxide (vasodilating factor), endothelin (vasoconstrictor peptide), bradykinin (potent vasodilator inactivated by ACE), and atrial natriuretic peptide (naturally occurring diuretic).

4. Fluid volume regulation. Increased fluid volume increases venous system distention and venous return, affecting cardiac output and tissue perfusion. These changes **alter vascular resistance**, increasing the blood pressure.

F. Complications. Untreated systemic hypertension, regardless of cause, results in inflammation and necrosis of the arterioles, narrowing of the blood vessels, and restriction of the blood flow to major body organs (*Table 33-3*). When blood flow is severely compromised, target-organ damage ensues.

1. Cardiac effects

a. Left ventricular hypertrophy (cardiac remodeling) compensates for the increased cardiac workload. Signs and symptoms of heart failure occur, and the increased oxygen requirements of the enlarged heart may produce angina pectoris.

b. Hypertension can be caused by accelerated atherosclerosis. Atheromatous lesions in the coronary arteries lead to decreased blood flow, resulting in angina pectoris. MI and sudden death may ensue.

2. Renal effects

a. Decreased blood flow leads to an increase in renin–aldosterone secretion, which heightens the reabsorption of sodium and water and increases blood volume.

b. Accelerated atherosclerosis decreases the oxygen supply, leading to renal parenchymal damage with decreased filtration capability and to azotemia. The atherosclerosis also decreases blood flow to the renal arterioles, leading to nephrosclerosis and, ultimately, renal failure (acute as well as chronic).

3. Cerebral effects. Decreased blood flow, decreased oxygen supply, and weakened blood vessel walls lead to transient ischemic attacks, cerebral thromboses, and the development of aneurysms with hemorrhage. There are alterations in mobility, weakness and paralysis, and memory deficits.

4. Retinal effects. Decreased blood flow with retinal vascular sclerosis and increased arteriolar pressure with the appearance of exudates and hemorrhage result in visual defects (e.g., blurred vision, spots, blindness).

II. SECONDARY HYPERTENSION

A. Clinical evaluation. Because most patients presenting with high blood pressure have primary rather than secondary hypertension, extensive screening is unwarranted. A thorough history and physical examination followed by an evaluation of common laboratory tests should rule out most causes of secondary hypertension. Patient age (primary hypertension is normally seen between 30 and 55 years of age), sudden onset of worsening of hypertension, and blood pressure elevations not responding to

Table 33-3 TARGET-ORGAN DAMAGE ASSOCIATED WITH HYPERTENSION

Organ/System and Findings	Basis of Findings
Cardiovascular	
Blood pressure persistently ≥ 140 mm Hg systolic and/or ≥ 90 mm Hg diastolic	Constricted arterioles, causing abnormal resistance to blood flow
Angina pain	Insufficient blood flow to coronary vasculature
Left ventricular hypertrophy/dyspnea on exertion	Heart failure
Edema of extremities	Decrease in blood supply
Neurological	
Severe occipital headaches with nausea and vomiting, drowsiness, anxiety, and mental impairment	Vessel damage within brain characteristic of dizziness, severe mental impairment, hypertension, resulting in transient ischemic attacks or strokes
Renal	
Polyuria, nocturia, and diminished ability to concentrate urine; protein and red blood cells in urine; elevated serum creatinine	Arteriolar nephrosclerosis (hardening of arterioles within kidney)
Ocular	
Retinal hemorrhage and exudates	Damage to arterioles that supply retina
Peripheral vascular	Absence of pulses in extremities with or without intermittent claudication; development of aneurysm

Based on Joint National Committee on Detection, Evaluation, and Treatment of High Blood Pressure. The seventh report of the Joint National Committee on Detection, Evaluation, and Treatment of High Blood Pressure: the JNC-7 report.

treatment are findings consistent with secondary hypertension. If a secondary cause is not found, the patient is considered to have essential (primary) hypertension.

1. A patient's **history** and **other physical findings** suggest an underlying cause of hypertension. These include the following:
   a. Weight gain, moon face, truncal obesity, osteoporosis, purple striae, hirsutism, hypokalemia, diabetes, and increased plasma cortisol may signal Cushing syndrome.
   b. Weight loss, episodic flushing, diaphoresis, increased urinary catecholamines, headaches, intermittent hypertension, tremors, and palpitations suggest pheochromocytoma.
   c. Steroid or estrogen intake, including oral contraceptives, nonsteroidal anti-inflammatory drugs (NSAIDs), nasal decongestants, tricyclic antidepressants, appetite suppressants, cyclosporine, erythropoietin, and monoamine oxidase (MAO) inhibitors suggests drug-induced hypertension.
   d. Repeated urinary tract infections, elevated serum creatinine levels, nocturia, hematuria, and pain on urinating may signify renal involvement (e.g., chronic kidney disease).
   e. Abdominal bruits, recent onset, and accelerated hypertension indicate renal artery stenosis (e.g., renovascular disease).
   f. Muscle cramps, weakness, excess urination, and isolated hypokalemia may suggest primary aldosteronism.
   g. Sleep apnea, coarctation of the aorta, thyroid disease, and parathyroid disease have been included by the JNC-7 as additional secondary causes of hypertension.

2. **Laboratory findings**
   a. Blood urea nitrogen (BUN) and creatinine elevations suggest renal disease.
   b. Increased urinary excretion of catecholamine or its metabolites (e.g., vanillylmandelic acid, metanephrine) confirms pheochromocytoma.
   c. Serum potassium evaluation revealing hypokalemia suggests primary aldosteronism or Cushing syndrome.
3. **Diagnostic tests**
   a. Renal arteriography, ultrasound, or renal venography may show evidence of renal artery stenosis.
   b. Electrocardiography (ECG) may reveal left ventricular hypertrophy or ischemia.

B. **Cause**
1. **Primary aldosteronism.** Hypersecretion of aldosterone by the adrenal cortex increases distal tubular sodium retention, expanding the blood volume, which increases total peripheral resistance.
2. **Pheochromocytoma.** A tumor of the adrenal medulla stimulates hypersecretion of epinephrine and norepinephrine, which results in increased total peripheral resistance.
3. **Renal artery stenosis.** Decreased renal tissue perfusion activates the renin–angiotensin–aldosterone system (see I.E.2).

C. **Treatment.** Secondary hypertension requires treatment of the underlying cause (e.g., surgical intervention accompanied by supplementary control of hypertensive effects; see III.B).

III. ESSENTIAL (PRIMARY) HYPERTENSION

A. **Clinical evaluation** requires a thorough history and physical examination followed by a careful-analysis of common laboratory test results.
1. **Objectives**
   a. To rule out uncommon secondary causes of hypertension
   b. To determine the presence and extent of target-organ damage
   c. To determine the presence of other cardiovascular risk factors in addition to high blood pressure
   d. To reduce morbidity and mortality through multiple strategies that reduce blood pressure through lifestyle modifications with or without pharmacological treatment with minimal side effects
2. **Predisposing factors**
   a. **Family history** of essential hypertension, stroke, and premature cardiac disease.
   b. **Patient history** of intermittent elevations in blood pressure.
   c. **Racial predisposition.** Hypertension is more common among African Americans than Whites.
   d. **Obesity.** Weight reduction has been shown to reduce blood pressure in a large proportion of hypertensive patients who are $>$ 10% above ideal body weight.
   e. **Smoking**, resulting in vasoconstriction and activation of the sympathetic nervous system, is a major risk factor for cardiovascular disease.
   f. Stress
   g. High dietary intake of saturated fats or sodium
   h. Sedentary lifestyle
   i. Diabetes mellitus
   j. Hyperlipidemia
   k. Major risk factors according to the JNC-7 include smoking, diabetes mellitus, age ($>$ 55 for men; $>$ 65 for women), family history of cardiovascular disease, and dyslipidemia.
   l. Target-organ damage/clinical cardiovascular disease according to the JNC-7 includes heart disease (e.g., left ventricular hypertrophy, angina, prior MI, heart failure), stroke or transient ischemic attacks, nephropathy, peripheral artery disease, and retinopathy.
3. **Physical findings**
   a. Serial blood pressure readings $\geq$ 140/90 mm Hg should be obtained on at least two occasions before specific therapy is begun, unless the initial blood pressure levels are markedly elevated (i.e., $>$ 210 mm Hg systolic; $>$ 120 mm Hg diastolic, or both) or are associated with target-organ damage. A single elevated reading is an insufficient basis for a diagnosis.

b. Essential hypertension usually does not become clinically evident—other than through serial blood pressure elevations—until vascular changes affect the heart, brain, kidneys, or ocular fundi.

c. Examination of the ocular fundi is valuable; their condition can indicate the duration and severity of the hypertension.

(1) **Early stages.** Hard, shiny deposits; tiny hemorrhages; and elevated arterial blood pressure occur.

(2) **Late stages.** Cotton-wool patches, exudates, retinal edema, papilledema caused by ischemia and capillary insufficiency, hemorrhages, and microaneurysms become evident.

4. Untreated hypertension increases the likelihood of the development of numerous organ problems, which include left ventricular failure, MI, renal failure, cerebral hemorrhage or infarction, and severe changes in the retina of the eye.

B. Treatment (*Tables 33-4* and *33-5*, *Figure 33-2*)

1. **General principles.** Treatment primarily aims to lower blood pressure toward "normal" with minimal side effects and to prevent or reverse organ damage. Currently, there is no cure for primary hypertension. Treating systolic and diastolic blood pressures to targets that are < 140/90 mm Hg is associated with a decrease in cardiovascular complications. For patients with hypertension who have diabetes or renal disease, the blood pressure goal recommended by the JNC-7 is 130/80 mm Hg.

a. **Candidates for treatment**

(1) All patients with a diastolic pressure of > 90 mm Hg, a systolic pressure of > 140 mm Hg, or a combination of both should receive antihypertensive drug therapy.

(2) For those patients with a diastolic pressure of 80 to 89 mm Hg or a systolic pressure of 120 to 139 mm Hg (prehypertension), no drug treatment is indicated unless the patient has a compelling indication. However, lifestyle modifications, such as weight reduction, dietary sodium reduction, increased physical activity, and moderation of alcohol consumption, should be initiated.

b. **Nonspecific measures.** Before initiating antihypertensive drug therapy, patients are encouraged to eliminate or minimize controllable risk factors (see III.A.2).

c. **Pharmacological treatment.** The recommendations of the JNC-7 suggest that recent clinical trials have demonstrated that most hypertensive patients will require two or more antihypertensive drugs.

(1) Thiazide diuretics should be the initial choice of therapy because they have demonstrated a reduction in morbidity and mortality when used as initial monotherapy. They have been shown to lower morbidity and mortality rates, have shown adequate long-term safety data, and have demonstrated patient tolerability.

(2) Thiazide diuretics should be considered initial agents for treatment unless there are compelling indications for other medications.

(3) Agents such as ACE inhibitors, angiotensin-receptor blockers, β-blockers, and calcium-channel blockers have all been recommended for patients who cannot receive a thiazide diuretic or in combination with a thiazide diuretic for adequate control of blood pressure. This may include the use of ACE inhibitors in hypertensive patients having systolic dysfunction after a MI, a diabetic nephropathy patient who might benefit from an ACE inhibitor in combination with a diuretic, or a patient with HF.

d. **Monitoring guidelines.** Specific monitoring guidelines for the various drug categories are outlined in III.B.2–7.

(1) Blood pressure should be monitored routinely to determine the therapeutic response and to encourage patient compliance.

(2) Clinicians must be alert to indications of adverse drug effects. Many patients do not link side effects to drug therapy or are embarrassed to discuss them, especially effects related to sexual function or effects that appear late in therapy.

e. **Patient compliance**

(1) Because hypertension is usually a symptomless disease, how the patient "feels" does not reflect the blood pressure level. In fact, the patient may actually report "feeling normal" with an elevated blood pressure and "abnormal" during a hypotensive episode because of the light-headedness associated with a sudden drop in blood pressure. Because essential hypertension requires a lifelong drug regimen, it is extremely difficult but necessary to impress on patients the need for compliance with their therapeutic regimen.

Table 33-4 COMMON ANTIHYPERTENSIVE DRUGS

I. Diuretics

- **A.** Thiazide diuretics
  - Chlorothiazide (Diuril®)
  - Chlorthalidone (Various)
  - Hydrochlorothiazide (Microzide®)
  - Indapamide (Various)
  - Methyclothiazide (Various)
  - Metolazone (Zaroxolyn®)
- **B.** Loop diuretics
  - Bumetanide (Various)
  - Ethacrynic acid (Edecrin®)
  - Furosemide (Lasix®)
  - Torsemide (Demadex®)
- **C.** Potassium-sparing diuretics
  - Amiloride (Various)
  - Eplerenone (Inspra®)
  - Spironolactone (Aldactone®)
  - Triamterene (Dyrenium®)

II. Vasodilators (direct acting)

- Hydralazine (Various)
- Minoxidil (Various)
- Nitroprusside (Nitropress®)

III. Angiotensin-converting enzyme (ACE) inhibitors

- Benazepril (Lotensin®)
- Captopril (Capoten®)
- Enalapril (Vasotec®)
- Enalaprilat (IV) (Various)
- Fosinopril (Various)
- Lisinopril (Prinivil®, Zestril®)
- Moexipril (Univasc®)
- Perindopril (Aceon®)
- Quinapril (Accupril®)
- Ramipril (Altace®)
- Trandolapril (Mavik®)

IV. Angiotensin II receptor antagonists

- Azilsartan (Edarbi®)
- Candesartan cilexetil (Atacand®)
- Eprosartan (Teveten®)
- Irbesartan (Avapro®)
- Losartan (Cozaar®)
- Olmesartan (Benicar®)
- Telmisartan (Micardis®)
- Valsartan (Diovan®)

V. Renin inhibitors

- Aliskiren (Tekturna®)

VI. Sympatholytics

- **A.** β-Adrenergic blocking agents
  - Acebutolol (Sectral®)
  - Atenolol (Tenormin®)
  - Betaxolol (Kerlone®)
  - Bisoprolol (Zebeta®)
  - Carvedilol (Coreg®)
  - Esmolol (Various - IV)
  - Labetalol (Trandate®)
  - Metoprolol (Lopressor®, Toprol XL®)
  - Nadolol (Corgard®)
  - Nebivolol (Bystolic®)
  - Penbutolol (Levatol®)
  - Pindolol (Various)
  - Propranolol (Inderal®)
  - Timolol (Various)
- **B.** Centrally acting α-agonists
  - Clonidine (Catapres®)
  - Guanabenz (Various)
  - Guanfacine (Tenex®)
  - Methyldopa (Various)
- **C.** Postganglionic adrenergic neuron blockers
  - Reserpine (Various)
- **D.** α-Adrenergic blocking agents
  - Doxazosin (Cardura®)
  - Prazosin (Minipress®)
  - Terazosin (Hytrin®)
- **E.** Calcium-channel blockers
  1. Benzodiazepine derivatives
     - Diltiazem (Cardizem®)
  2. Diphenylalkylamine derivatives
     - Verapamil (Calan®)
  3. Dihydropyridines
     - Amlodipine (Norvasc®)
     - Clevidipine (Cleviprex®)
     - Felodipine (Plendil®)
     - Isradipine (DynaCirc CR®)
     - Nicardipine (Cardene®)
     - Nifedipine (Procardia XL, Adalat CC®)
     - Nisoldipine (Sular®)

Table 33-5 COMMON COMBINATION PRODUCTS FOR HYPERTENSION

I. Diuretics
- Hydrochlorothiazide—spironolactone (Aldactazide®)
- Hydrochlorothiazide—triamterene (Dyazide®)
- Hydrochlorothiazide—amiloride (Various)

II. Diuretics—β-adrenergic blockers
- Bendroflumethiazide—nadolol (Corzide®)
- Chlorthalidone—atenolol (Tenoretic®)
- Hydrochlorothiazide—propranolol (Inderide®)
- Hydrochlorothiazide—metoprolol (Lopressor HCT®)
- Hydrochlorothiazide—bisoprolol (Ziac®)

III. Diuretics—angiotensin-converting enzyme (ACE) inhibitors
- Hydrochlorothiazide—captopril (Capozide®)
- Hydrochlorothiazide—benazepril (Lotensin HCT®)
- Hydrochlorothiazide—lisinopril (Prinzide®, Zestoretic®)
- Hydrochlorothiazide—enalapril (Vaseretic®)
- Hydrochlorothiazide—fosinopril (Various)
- Hydrochlorothiazide—moexipril (Uniretic®)
- Hydrochlorothiazide—quinapril (Accuretic®)

IV. Diuretics—angiotensin II receptor antagonists
- Hydrochlorothiazide—losartan (Hyzaar®)
- Hydrochlorothiazide—irbesartan (Avalide®)
- Hydrochlorothiazide—valsartan (Diovan HCT®)
- Hydrochlorothiazide—telmisartan (Micardis HCT®)
- Hydrochlorothiazide—candesartan (Atacand HCT®)
- Hydrochlorothiazide—eprosartan (Teveten HCT®)
- Hydrochlorothiazide—olmesartan (Benicar HCT®)

V. Angiotensin-converting enzyme (ACE) inhibitors—calcium-channel blockers
- Enalapril—felodipine (Lexxel®)
- Trandolapril—verapamil (Tarka®)
- Benazepril—amlodipine (Lotrel®)

VI. Angiotensin II receptor antagonists—calcium-channel blockers
- Olmesartan—amlodipine (Azor®)
- Valsartan—amlodipine (Exforge®)
- Telmisartan—amlodipine (Twynsta®)

VII. Triple products
- Amlodipine/Valsartan/Hydrochlorothiazide (Exforge HCT®)
- Amlodipine/Olmesartan/Hydrochlorothiazide (Tribenzor®)
- Aliskiren/Amlodipine/Hydrochlorothiazide (Amturnide®)

VIII. Other
- Hydrochlorothiazide—hydralazine (Hydra-zide®)
- Hydrochlorothiazide—methyldopa (Various)
- Amlodipine—atorvastatin (Caduet®)
- Clonidine—chlorthalidone (Clorpres®)
- Hydralazine—isosorbide dinitrate (BiDil®)
- Aliskiren—valsartan (Valturna®)
- Aliskiren—amlodipine (Tekamlo®)
- Aliskiren—hydrochlorothiazide (Tekturna HCT®)

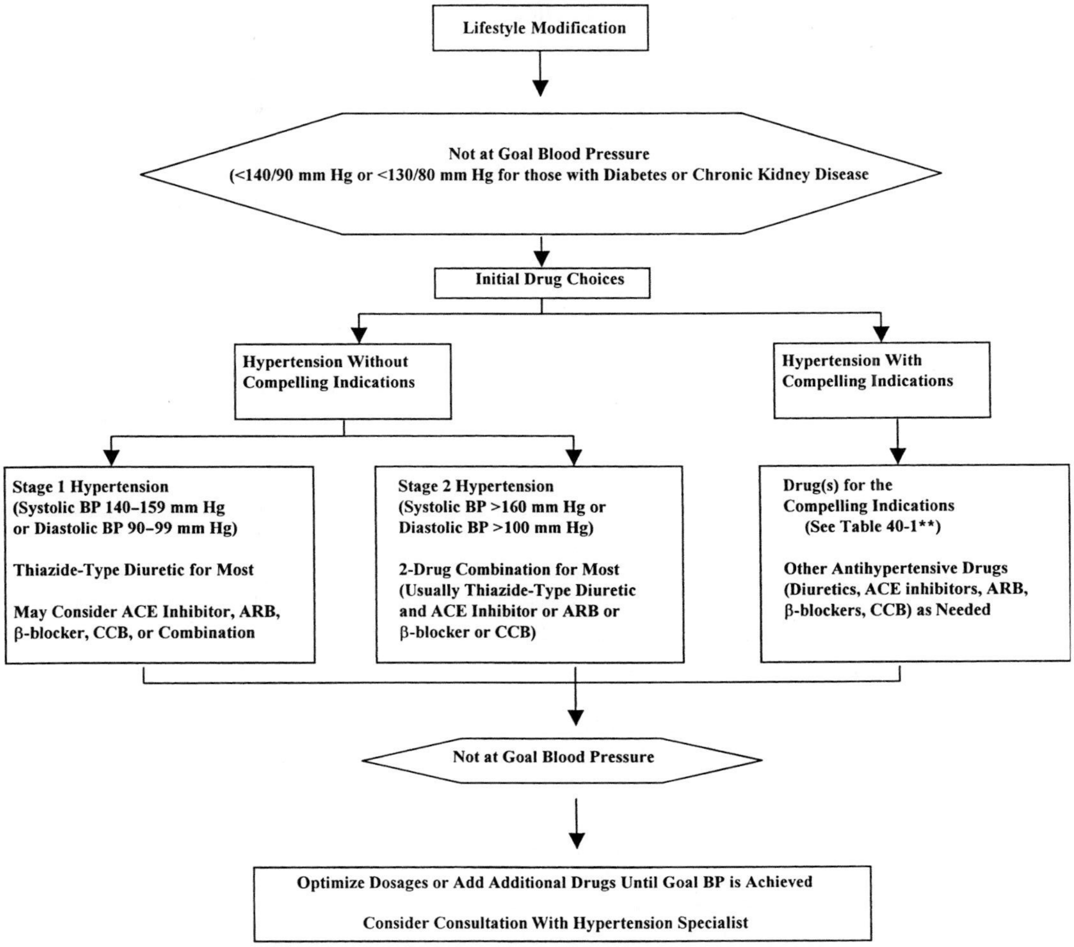

Figure 33-2. Algorithm for the treatment of hypertension. *ACE*, angiotensin-converting enzyme; *ARB*, angiotensin-receptor blocker; *BP*, blood pressure; *CCB*, calcium-channel blocker. [Based on the recommendations from the Seventh Report of the Joint National Committee on Detection, Evaluation, and Treatment of High Blood Pressure (JNC-7).]

(2) Recognizing the seriousness of the consequences of noncompliance is key. Patients should be told that prolonged, untreated hypertension, known as the "silent killer," can affect the heart, brain, kidneys, and ocular fundi.

2. **Diuretics**

a. **Thiazide diuretics** and their derivatives are currently recommended as initial therapy for hypertension. JNC-7 recommends initiating therapy with a low dose (12.5 mg of hydrochlorothiazide [Microzide®]), increasing the dose if necessary, and not exceeding a dose of 50 mg of hydrochlorothiazide or its equivalent.

(1) **Actions.** Antihypertensive effects are produced by directly dilating the arterioles and reducing the total fluid volume. Thiazide diuretics increase the following:

(a) Urinary excretion of sodium and water by inhibiting sodium and chloride reabsorption in the distal convoluted (renal) tubules

(b) Urinary excretion of potassium and, to a lesser extent, bicarbonate

(c) The effectiveness of other antihypertensive agents by preventing reexpansion of extracellular and plasma volumes

(2) **Significant interactions. NSAIDs**, such as the now common over-the-counter forms of ibuprofen (Advil®, Motrin®), interact to diminish the antihypertensive effects of the thiazide diuretics.

(3) **Precautions and monitoring effects**
   (a) Potassium ion (K^+) depletion may require supplementation, increased dietary intake, or the use of a potassium-sparing diuretic, such as spironolactone (Aldactone®).
   (b) Uric acid retention may occur; this is potentially significant in patients who are predisposed to gout and related disorders.
   (c) Blood glucose levels may increase, which may be significant in patients with diabetes.
   (d) Calcium levels may increase because of the potential for retaining calcium ions.
   (e) Patients with known allergies to sulfa-type drugs should be questioned to determine the significance of the allergy.
   (f) Other common effects include fatigue, headache, palpitations, rash, vertigo, and transitory impotence.
   (g) Hyperlipidemia, including **hypertriglyceridemia**, hypercholesterolemia, increased low-density lipoprotein (LDL) cholesterol, and decreased high-density lipoprotein (HDL) cholesterol, must be evaluated routinely to prevent an added risk for coronary artery disease.
   (h) Fluid losses must be evaluated and monitored to prevent dehydration, postural hypotension, and even hypovolemic shock.
   (i) Alterations in fluids and electrolytes (e.g., hypokalemia, hypomagnesemia, hypercalcemia) may predispose patients to cardiac irritability, with a resultant increase in cardiac arrhythmias. ECG is performed routinely to detect and prevent the development of life-threatening arrhythmias.

(4) **Usual effective doses**
   (a) **Chlorothiazide (Diuril®):** 250 to 500 mg daily or twice daily
   (b) **Chlorthalidone (Various®):** 12.5 to 25 mg daily
   (c) **Hydrochlorothiazide (HydroDIURIL®):** 12.5 to 50 mg daily
   (d) **Indapamide (Various):** 1.25 to 5.0 mg daily
   (e) **Methyclothiazide (Various):** 2.5 to 5.0 mg daily
   (f) **Metolazone (Zaroxolyn®):** 2.5 to 5.0 mg daily

b. **Loop (high-ceiling) diuretics**

(1) **Indications.** These agents are indicated when patients are unable to tolerate thiazides, experience a loss of thiazide effectiveness, or have impaired renal function (clearance < 30 mL/min).

(2) **Actions.** Furosemide (Lasix®), ethacrynic acid (Edecrin®), bumetanide (Various), and torsemide (Demadex®) act primarily in the ascending loop of Henle; hence, they are called "loop" diuretics. By acting within the loop of Henle, they decrease sodium reabsorption. Their action is more intense but of shorter duration (1 to 4 hrs) than that of the thiazides; loss of patent exclusivity has resulted in an increase in the availability of generic products, which had reduced the coasts associated with their usage.

(3) **Significant interactions.** As with the thiazides, the antihypertensive effect of loop diuretics may be diminished by **NSAIDs**.

(4) **Precautions and monitoring effects.** Loop diuretics have the same effects as thiazides (see III.B.2.a), in addition to the following:
   (a) Loop diuretics have a complex influence on renal hemodynamics; thus, patients must be monitored closely for signs of hypovolemia.
   (b) Because these agents should be used cautiously in patients with episodic or chronic renal impairment, BUN and serum creatinine levels should be checked routinely.
   (c) Transient deafness has been reported. If the patient is taking a potentially ototoxic drug (e.g., an aminoglycoside antibiotic), another class of diuretic (e.g., a thiazide diuretic) should be substituted.

(5) **Usual effective doses**
   (a) **Bumetanide (Various):** 0.5 to 2.0 mg daily
   (b) **Ethacrynic acid (Edecrin®):** 25 to 100 mg daily
   (c) **Furosemide (Lasix®):** 20 to 80 mg daily
   (d) **Torsemide (Demadex®):** 2.5 to 10 mg daily

c. Potassium-sparing diuretics

(1) **Indications.** The diuretics in this group—spironolactone (Aldactone®), amiloride (Various), and triamterene (Dyrenium®)—are indicated for patients in whom potassium loss is significant and supplementation is not feasible. These agents are often used in combination with a thiazide diuretic because they potentiate the effects of the thiazide while minimizing potassium loss. **Spironolactone (Aldactone®)** is particularly useful in patients with hyperaldosteronism, as it has direct antagonistic effects on aldosterone (aldosterone-receptor blocker). **Eplerenone** (Inspra®), is another aldosterone-receptor blocker recently approved by the U.S. Food and Drug Administration (FDA) that, similar to spironolactone, blocks aldosterone binding at the mineralocorticoid receptor. Both of these agents have been used in hypertension and have an increased level of use in the treatment of HF (see Chapter 34).

(2) **Actions.** Potassium-sparing diuretics achieve their diuretic effects differently and less potently than the thiazides and loop diuretics. Their most pertinent shared feature is that they promote potassium retention.

(3) **Significant interactions.** Coadministration with **ACE inhibitors** or **potassium supplements** significantly increases the risk of hyperkalemia.

(4) **Precautions and monitoring effects**

(a) Potassium-sparing diuretics should be avoided in patients with acute renal failure and used with caution in patients with impaired renal function (monitor serum creatinine) because they can retain potassium.

(b) **Triamterene (Dyrenium®)** should not be used in patients with a history of kidney stones or hepatic disease.

(c) **Hyperkalemia** is a major risk, requiring routine monitoring of serum electrolytes. BUN and serum creatinine levels should be checked routinely to signal incipient excess potassium retention and impaired renal function.

(5) **Usual effective doses**

(a) **Amiloride (Various):** 5 to 10 mg daily

(b) **Spironolactone (Aldactone®):** 25 to 100 mg daily and 400 mg daily to treat hyperaldosteronism

(c) **Triamterene (Dyrenium®):** 50 to 100 mg daily

(d) **Eplerenone (Inspra®):** 50 to 100 mg daily

d. Combination products. A growing number of products are available as combination products and can be found within *Table 33-5*.

3. Sympatholytics

a. β-Adrenergic blockers

(1) **Indications.** β-Blockers are particularly effective in patients with rapid resting heart rates (i.e., atrial fibrillation, paroxysmal supraventricular tachycardia) or for those compelling indications, such as heart failure, post-MI, high coronary disease risk, and diabetes mellitus, as described within the JNC-7 report.

(2) **Actions.** Proposed mechanisms of action include the following:

(a) Stimulation of renin secretion is blocked.

(b) Cardiac contractility is decreased, thus diminishing cardiac output.

(c) Sympathetic output is decreased centrally.

(d) Reduction in heart rate decreases cardiac output.

(e) β-Blocker action may combine all of the above mechanisms.

(3) **Epidemiology.** Young (< 45 years) whites with high cardiac output, high heart rate, and normal vascular resistance respond best to β-blocker therapy.

(4) **Precautions and monitoring effects**

(a) Patients must be monitored for signs and symptoms of **cardiac decompensation** (i.e., reduction in cardiac output) owing to the fact that decreased myocardial contractility can trigger compensatory mechanisms, leading to HF (see Chapter 34).

(b) ECGs should be monitored routinely because all β-blockers can decrease electrical conduction within the heart and cause bradyarrhythmias.

(c) Relative cardioselectivity is dose dependent and is lost as dosages are increased. **No β-blocker is totally safe in patients with bronchospastic disease**—that is asthma and chronic obstructive pulmonary disease (COPD).

(d) Abrupt stoppage of a β-blocker in cardiac patients puts the patient at risk for a **withdrawal syndrome** that may produce
   (i) exacerbated anginal attacks,
   (ii) myocardial infarction, and
   (iii) a life-threatening rebound of blood pressure to levels exceeding pretreatment readings.
(e) β-Blocker therapy should be used with caution in patients with the following conditions:
   (i) **Diabetes mellitus.** β-Blockers can mask hypoglycemic symptoms, such as tachycardia.
   (ii) **Raynaud phenomenon or peripheral vascular disease.** Vasoconstriction can occur and, in predisposed patients, might result in a clinically significant problem.
   (iii) **Neurological disorders.** Several β-blockers enter the central nervous system (CNS), potentiating related side effects (e.g., fatigue, lethargy, poor memory, weakness, or mental depression).
(f) Impotence and decreased libido may result in reduced patient compliance.

(5) **Significant interactions.** β-Adrenergic blockers interact with numerous agents, requiring cautious selection, administration, and monitoring.

(6) **β-Blocker terms**
(a) **Relative cardioselective activity.** Relative to propranolol (Inderal®), β-blockers have a greater tendency to occupy the β_1-receptor in the heart, rather than the β_2-receptors in the lungs.
(b) **Intrinsic sympathomimetic activity.** These agents have the ability to release catecholamines and to maintain a satisfactory heart rate. Intrinsic sympathomimetic activity may also prevent bronchoconstriction and other direct β-blocking actions.

(7) **Specific agents**
(a) **Propranolol (Inderal®)** was the first β-adrenergic blocking agent shown to block both β_1- and β_2-receptors. The **usual daily dose range** is 40 to 160 mg. It is available both as a rapid-acting product and a long-acting product (Inderal-LA®); the usual daily dose range is 60 to 180 mg.
(b) **Metoprolol (Lopressor®)** was the first β-adrenergic blocking agent to show relative cardioselective blocking activity, with relatively less blockade of the β_2-receptors in the lung when compared to propranolol. The **usual daily dose** is 50 to 100 mg. A sustained-release form of the drug is now available, as the succinate salt (Toprol XL®), which requires less frequent dosing (daily vs. once or twice daily for immediate-release metoprolol).
(c) **Nadolol (Corgard®)** was the first β-adrenergic blocking agent that allowed once-daily dosing. It blocks both β_1- and β_2-receptors, similar to propranolol. The **usual daily dose** is 40 to 120 mg.
(d) **Atenolol (Tenormin®)** was the first β-adrenergic blocking agent to combine once-daily dosing (nadolol) with relative cardioselective blocking activity (metoprolol). The **usual daily dose** is 25 to 100 mg.
(e) **Timolol (Various)** was the first β-adrenergic blocking agent shown to be effective after an acute MI to prevent sudden death. It blocks both β_1- and β_2-receptors. The **usual daily dose** is 20 to 40 mg.
(f) **Pindolol (Various)** was the first β-adrenergic blocking agent shown to have high intrinsic sympathomimetic activity. The **usual daily dose** is 10 to 40 mg.
(g) **Labetalol (Trandate®)** was the first β-adrenergic blocking agent shown to possess both α- and β-adrenergic blocking activity. The **usual daily dose** is 200 to 800 mg. Labetalol is also effective for treating hypertensive crisis (*Table 33-6*).
(h) **Acebutolol (Sectral®)** was the first β-adrenergic blocking agent that combined efficacy with once-daily dosing (nadolol), possessing intrinsic sympathomimetic activity (pindolol) and having relative cardioselective blocking activity (metoprolol). The **usual daily dose** is 200 to 800 mg.
(i) **Esmolol (Brevibloc®)** was the first β-adrenergic blocking agent to have an ultrashort duration of action. This agent is not used routinely in treating hypertension owing to its duration of action and the need for intravenous administration. However, it has

Table 33-6 RAPID-ACTING PARENTERAL ANTIHYPERTENSIVE AGENTS FOR HYPERTENSIVE CRISIS

Drug	Dose/Route	Onset of Action	Duration of Action	Comments
Vasodilators				
Sodium nitroprusside (Nitropress®)	0.3–10 mg/kg/min as IV infusion	0.5–1 mins	1–2 mins	Immediate effect, very short duration; nausea, vomiting, muscle twitching, sweating, thiocyanate and cyanide intoxication
Nicardipine hydrochloride (Various)	5–15 mg/hr IV	< 5–15 mins	1–4 hrs	Intermediate onset and duration; tachycardia may occur, headache, flushing, local phlebitis
Fenoldopam mesylate (Corlopam®)	0.1–0.3 mcg/kg/min as IV infusion	< 5 mins	30 mins	Intermediate onset and duration; action on dopamine D_1-receptors (dilation of renal/mesenteric vessels might be preferred over nitroprusside for long-term or with renal dysfunction; tachycardia, headache, nausea, flushing
Nitroglycerin (Various)	5–200 mcg/min (0.3–6.0 mg/hr) as IV infusion	2–5 mins	3–5 mins	Useful in coronary artery disease; headache, vomiting, methemoglobinemia, tolerance with prolonged use
Enalaprilat (Various)	0.625–1.25 mg every 6 hrs IV	15–30 mins	4–6 hrs	Useful in HF, but avoid in renal impairment; precipitous fall in blood pressure in high-renin states
Hydralazine (Various)	10–20 mg IV/IM	10–20 mins	3–8 hrs	Afterload reduction through arteriole dilation resulting in increased cardiac output; tachycardia, flushing headache, vomiting, aggravation of preexisting angina
Clevidipine (Cleviprex®)	1–21 mg/hr	2–4 mins	5–15 mins	A fit nausea, fever caution with lipid disorder
Adrenergic inhibitors				
Labetalol hydrochloride (Various)	40–80 mg IV bolus every 10 mins, or 0.5–2.0 mg/min IV infusion	5–10 mins	3–6 hrs	Contraindicated in HF, bronchospastic patients, or bradycardia; predictable hypotensive effect; vomiting, scalp tingling, burning in throat, heart block, orthostatic hypotension
Esmolol (Brevibloc®)	250–500 mcg/kg/min for 2 mins, then 50–100 mcg/kg/min for 4 mins; may repeat if needed	1–2 mins	10–20 mins	β-Adrenergic blocker with ultra-short duration of effect; primary use in perioperative situation owing to short duration and quick onset; hypotension, nausea
Phentolamine (OraVerse®)	5–15 mg IV	1–2 mins	3–10 mins	α-Adrenergic blocker causing peripheral dilation; tachycardia, flushing, headache

HF, heart failure; *IM*, intramuscular; *IV*, intravenous.

been used for hypertension and or tachycardia during and after surgical procedures. The **usual dose** is 150 to 300 mcg/kg/min up to 300 mcg/kg/min intravenously.

(j) **Betaxolol (Kerlone®)** is a β-adrenergic blocker that possesses relative cardioselective blocking activity similar to metoprolol but has a half-life that allows for once-daily dosing. The **usual daily dose** is 5 to 20 mg.

(k) **Penbutolol (Levatol®)** is a β-adrenergic blocking agent that has weak intrinsic sympathomimetic activity like pindolol and allows for once-daily dosing. The **usual daily dose** is 10 to 20 mg.

(l) **Bisoprolol (Zebeta®)** is a β-adrenergic blocking agent that is cardioselective and has no intrinsic sympathomimetic activity. It allows for once-daily dosing, and the **usual daily dose** is 2.5 to 10 mg.

(m) **Carvedilol (Coreg®)** is a β-adrenergic blocking agent that has β-blocking properties as well as α-blocking properties, with a resultant vasodilation. The drug is administered twice daily with a starting dose of 6.25 mg titrated at 7- to 14-day intervals to a dose of 25 mg twice daily. **Usual daily doses** are 12.5 to 50 mg daily.

(n) **Nebivolol (Bystolic®)** is a β-adrenergic blocking agent that has cardioselective β_1 blocking tendencies, similar to several other agents in the class. Initial reports also suggest that nebivolol has vasodilatory properties through its release of nitric oxide. Nebivolol is administered in a single daily dose of 5 mg with dose titration required based on therapeutic response.

b. **Peripheral α_1-adrenergic blockers**—for example, prazosin (Minipress®), terazosin (Hytrin®), and doxazosin (Cardura®)

(1) **Indications.** This group of drugs is available for hypertensive patients who have not responded to initial antihypertensive therapy.

(2) **Actions.** The α_1-blockers (indirect vasodilators) block the peripheral postsynaptic α_1-adrenergic receptor, causing vasodilation of both arteries and veins. Also, the incidence of reflex tachycardia is lower with these agents than with the vasodilator hydralazine (Various). These hemodynamic changes reverse the abnormalities in hypertension and preserve organ perfusion. Recent studies have also shown that these agents have no adverse effect on serum lipids and other cardiac risk factors.

(3) **Precautions and monitoring effects**

(a) **First-dose phenomenon.** A syncopal episode may occur within 30 to 90 mins of the first dose; similarly associated are postural hypotension, nausea, dizziness, headache, palpitations, and sweating. To minimize these effects, the first dose should be limited to a small dose (1 mg) and administered just before bedtime.

(b) Additional adverse effects include diarrhea, weight gain, peripheral edema, dry mouth, urinary urgency, constipation, and priapism. Doxazosin (Cardura®) in doses of 2 to 8 mg/day was one of the treatment arms in the recent Antihypertensive and Lipid-Lowering Treatment to Prevent Heart Attack Trial (ALLHAT), and the treatment was discontinued prematurely owing to an apparent 25% increase in the incidence of combined cardiovascular disease outcomes than patients in the control group receiving the diuretic chlorthalidone. The added risk for HF, stroke, and coronary heart disease were the major outcomes affected in the doxazosin arm.

(4) **The average daily doses are**

(a) **Prazosin (Minipress®):** 2 to 20 mg

(b) **Terazosin (Hytrin®):** 1 to 20 mg

(c) **Doxazosin (Cardura®):** 1 to 16 mg

c. **Centrally active α-agonists** have been used in the past as alternatives to initial antihypertensives, but their use in mild-to-moderate hypertension has been reduced primarily owing to other available agents. They act primarily within the CNS on α_2-receptors to decrease sympathetic outflow to the cardiovascular system.

(1) **Methyldopa (Various)**

(a) **Actions.** Methyldopa decreases total peripheral resistance through the aforementioned mechanism while having little effect on cardiac output or heart rate (except in older patients).

(b) **Precautions and monitoring effects**

(i) Common untoward effects include orthostatic hypotension, fluid accumulation (in the absence of a diuretic), and rebound hypertension on abrupt withdrawal. Sedation is a common finding upon initiating therapy and when increasing doses; however, the sedative effect usually decreases with continued therapy.

(ii) Fever and other flu-like symptoms occasionally occur and may represent hepatic dysfunction, which should be monitored by liver function tests.

(iii) A positive Coombs test develops in 25% of patients with chronic use (> 6 months). Less than 1% of these patients develop a hemolytic anemia. (Red blood cells, hemoglobin, and blood count indices should be checked.) The anemia is reversible by discontinuing the drug.

(iv) Other effects include dry mouth, subtly decreased mental activity, sleep disturbances, depression, impotence, and lactation in either gender.

(c) The **usual daily dose** is 250 mg to 1 g

(2) **Clonidine (Catapres®)**

(a) **Indications.** Clonidine is effective in patients with renal impairment, although they may require a reduced dose or a longer dosing interval.

(b) **Actions.** Clonidine stimulates α_2-receptors centrally, decreasing vasomotor tone and heart rate.

(c) **Precautions and monitoring effects**

(i) Intravenous administration causes an initial paradoxical increase in pressure (diastolic and systolic) that is followed by a prolonged drop. As with methyldopa, abrupt withdrawal can cause rebound hypertension.

(ii) Sedation and dry mouth are common but usually disappear with continued therapy.

(iii) Clonidine has a tendency to cause or worsen depression, and it heightens the depressant effects of alcohol and other sedating substances.

(d) The **usual daily dose** is 0.1 to 0.8 mg divided in two doses.

(e) Patient compliance is a major issue for most hypertensive patients. The recently released once-weekly patch (Catapres-TTS®), which provides 0.1 to 0.3 mg per 24 hrs, may improve compliance.

(3) **Guanabenz (Various)** and **guanfacine (Tenex®)**

(a) **Indications.** These agents are recommended as adjunctive therapy with other antihypertensives for additive effects when initial therapy has failed.

(b) **Actions.** Guanabenz and guanfacine are centrally active α_2-agonists that have actions similar to clonidine.

(c) **Precautions and monitoring effects.** These agents should be used cautiously with other sedating medications and in patients with severe coronary insufficiency, recent MI, cerebrovascular accident (CVA), and hepatic or renal disease. Side effects include sedation, dry mouth, dizziness, and reduced heart rate.

(d) The **usual daily doses** are 4 to 8 mg in two doses for guanabenz and 1 to 3 mg in one dose for guanfacine.

d. Postganglionic adrenergic neuron blockers. This class of antihypertensive drugs is best avoided unless it is necessary to treat severe refractory hypertension that is unresponsive to all other medications because agents in this class are poorly tolerated by most patients.

(1) **Reserpine (Various)**

(a) **General considerations.** Because of the high incidence of adverse effects, other agents are usually chosen first. When used, reserpine is given in low doses and in conjunction with other antihypertensive agents. Reserpine in very low doses (0.05 mg) combined with a diuretic, such as chlorothiazide (50 to 100 mg), may be an alternative to traditional doses of 0.05 to 0.25 mg/day.

(b) **Actions.** Reserpine acts centrally, as well as peripherally, by depleting catecholamine stores in the brain and in the peripheral adrenergic system.

(c) **Precautions and monitoring effects**

(i) A history of depression is a contraindication for reserpine. Even low doses, such as 0.25 mg/day, can trigger a range of psychic responses, from nightmares to suicide attempts. Drug-induced depression may linger for months after the last dose.

(ii) Peptic ulcer is also a contraindication for using reserpine. Even a single dose tends to increase gastric acid secretion.

(iii) Common adverse effects include drowsiness, dizziness, weakness, lethargy, memory impairment, sleep disturbances, and weight gain. Nasal congestion is also common but may decrease with continued therapy.

(d) The **usual daily dose** of **reserpine** is 0.1 to 0.25 mg.

4. **ACE inhibitors**

a. **General considerations.** The ACE inhibitors—benazepril (Lotensin®), captopril (Capoten®), enalapril (Vasotec®), enalaprilat (Various-IV), fosinopril (Various), lisinopril (Zestril®), moexipril (Univasc®), perindopril (Aceon®), quinapril (Accupril®), ramipril (Altace®), and trandolapril (Mavik®)—are a rapidly growing group of drugs.

b. **Indications.** Previous guidelines used ACE inhibitors as first-line alternatives for treating hypertension in patients unable to tolerate thiazides or β-blockers. However, JNC-7 recommendations have identified specific patient populations that have compelling indications—such as diabetes mellitus, post-MI, high coronary disease risk, chronic kidney disease, and recurrent stroke prevention—for which the ACE inhibitors are indicated in the treatment of hypertension or prehypertension. This has been primarily because of studies documenting their clinical efficacy, as well as minimal effect on patients' abilities to maintain normal function.

c. **Actions**

(1) These agents inhibit the conversion of angiotensin I (a weak vasoconstrictor) to angiotensin II (a potent vasoconstrictor), which decreases the availability of angiotensin II.

(2) ACE inhibitors indirectly inhibit fluid volume increases when interfering with angiotensin II by inhibiting angiotensin II–stimulated release of aldosterone, which promotes sodium and water retention. The net effect appears to be a decrease in fluid volume, along with peripheral vasodilation.

d. **Significant interactions**

(1) The antihypertensive effect of ACE inhibitors may be diminished by **NSAIDs** (e.g., over-the-counter forms of ibuprofen).

(2) Potassium-sparing diuretics increase serum potassium levels when used with ACE inhibitors, and potassium levels need to be closely monitored in these patients.

e. **Precautions and monitoring effects**

(1) Neutropenia is rare but serious; there is an increased incidence in patients with renal insufficiency or autoimmune disease.

(2) Proteinuria occurs, particularly in patients with a history of renal disease. Urinary proteins should be monitored regularly.

(3) Serum potassium levels should be monitored regularly for hyperkalemia. The mechanism of action tends to increase potassium levels somewhat. Patients with renal impairment are at increased risk.

(4) Renal insufficiency can occur in patients with predisposing factors, such as renal stenosis, and when ACE inhibitors are administered with thiazide diuretics. Renal function should be monitored (e.g., through monitoring levels of serum creatinine and BUN).

(5) A dry cough may occur but disappears within a few days after the ACE inhibitor is discontinued. All ACE inhibitors have the potential to cause this side effect, but switching to an alternative agent may improve the symptoms.

(6) Other untoward effects include rashes, an altered sense of taste (dysgeusia), vertigo, headache, fatigue, first-dose hypotension, and minor gastrointestinal disturbances.

f. **Specific agents**

(1) **Captopril (Capoten®).** The original ACE inhibitor is given initially as a 12.5 to 25 mg dose three times daily and is increased to a **usual daily dose** of 25 to 100 mg in two or three doses. Initial dose is usually lower if patient is on diuretics to avoid initial hypotensive response.

(2) **Enalapril (Vasotec®)** is a prodrug, which is rapidly converted to its active metabolite, enalaprilat. Initial doses are 5 mg daily, with a **usual daily dose** of 5 to 40 mg in one to two doses. In addition, the enalaprilat form (Various) of the drug has been used effectively for treating acute hypertensive crisis (*Table 33-6*).

(3) **Lisinopril (Zestril®)** is a long-acting analog of enalapril, given initially as a 5 to 10 mg daily dose and adjusted to a **usual daily dose** of 10 to 40 mg in one dose.

(4) Benazepril (Lotensin), fosinopril (Various), moexipril (Univasc), perindopril (Aceon), quinapril (Accupril), ramipril (Altace), and trandolapril (Mavik) have as their major benefit a longer duration of action, which in many patients may result in once-daily dosing and improved compliance. **Average daily doses** for these agents are
   - (a) **Benazepril (Lotensin®):** 10 to 40 mg in one to two doses
   - (b) **Fosinopril (Various):** 10 to 40 mg in one dose
   - (c) **Moexipril (Univasc®):** 7.5 to 30 mg in one dose
   - (d) **Perindopril (Aceon®):** 4 to 8 mg in one to two doses
   - (e) **Quinapril (Accupril®):** 10 to 80 mg in one dose
   - (f) **Ramipril (Altace®):** 2.5 to 20 mg in one dose
   - (g) **Trandolapril (Mavik®):** 1 to 4 mg in one dose

(5) Further study of these agents continues, and their use in other cardiovascular, as well as noncardiovascular diseases continues to expand.

5. Angiotensin II type I receptor antagonists

a. Indications. This class of drugs has been one of the fastest growing groups of drugs for the treatment of hypertension. Currently, eight agents are available: azilsartan (Edarbi®), candesartan cilexetil (Atacand®), eprosartan (Teveten®), irbesartan (Avapro®), losartan (Cozaar®), olmesartan (Benicar®), telmisartan (Micardis®), and valsartan (Diovan®).

b. Actions. This class of drugs works by blocking the binding of angiotensin II to the angiotensin II receptors. By blocking the receptor site, these agents inhibit the vasoconstrictor effects of angiotensin II while also preventing the release of aldosterone from the adrenal glands. These two properties of angiotensin II have been shown to be important causes for developing hypertension. Clinically, angiotensin receptor blockers appear to be equally effective for the treatment of hypertension as ACE inhibitors.

c. Precautions and monitoring effects

(1) Similar to ACE inhibitors, increases in serum potassium levels can occur, especially in patients receiving potassium-sparing diuretics. When used alone, hyperkalemia has not been reported to be severe enough to require stopping its use. However, as in patients receiving ACE inhibitors, potassium levels need to be monitored closely in those with compromised renal function.

(2) Renal function is an important consideration for patients receiving angiotensin receptor blockers (ARBs). Similar to ACE inhibitors, declining renal function or acute renal failure will result in elevated serum potassium levels, owing to the kidneys inability to excrete potassium. BUN and serum creatinine levels should be monitored to prevent the development of hyperkalemia.

d. Dosage guidelines for the available agents are as follows:

(1) **Candesartan cilexetil (Atacand):** 8 to 32 mg in one to two doses
(2) **Eprosartan (Teveten):** 400 to 800 mg in one to two doses
(3) **Irbesartan (Avapro):** 150 to 300 mg in one dose
(4) **Losartan (Cozaar):** 25 to 100 mg in one to two doses
(5) **Olmesartan (Benicar):** 20 to 40 mg in one dose
(6) **Telmisartan (Micardis):** 20 to 80 mg in one dose
(7) **Valsartan (Diovan):** 80 to 320 mg in one to two doses
(8) **Azilsartan (Edarbi):** 80 mg daily in one dose

e. Current status

(1) Many authorities believe that in the treatment of hypertension, there do not appear to be significant differences between ACE inhibitors and ARBs.

(2) Familiarity and cost might well provide the basis of the selection of one agent over another at this time.

(3) ARBs have found use in special hypertensive populations with compelling indications, such as diabetes mellitus, HF, and chronic kidney disease, especially in patients who cannot tolerate an ACE inhibitor.

6. **Calcium-channel blockers**
   a. **Indications.** The calcium-channel blockers are considered alternative drugs for the initial treatment of hypertension in select patient populations that are unable to take β-adrenergic receptor blockers, such as patients with a high coronary disease risk or diabetes mellitus who also have bronchospastic disease or Raynaud disease. Currently, nine agents—amlodipine (Norvasc®), clevidipine (Cleviprex®), diltiazem (Cardizem®), felodipine (Plendil®), isradipine (DynaCirc CR®), nicardipine (Cardene SR®), nifedipine (Procardia XL®), nisoldipine (Sular®), and verapamil (Calan®)—are available.
   b. **Actions**
      (1) Calcium-channel blockers inhibit the influx of calcium through slow channels in vascular smooth muscle and cause relaxation. Low-renin hypertensive, black, and elderly patients respond well to these agents.
      (2) Although the calcium-channel blockers share a similar mechanism of action, each agent produces different degrees of systemic and coronary arterial vasodilation, sinoatrial (SA) and atrioventricular (AV) nodal depression, and a decrease in myocardial contractility.
   c. **Significant interactions. β-Adrenergic blockers**, when used with calcium-channel blockers, may have an additive effect on inducing HF and bradycardia. Electrical conduction to the AV node may be further depressed when patients are given agents such as verapamil (Calan®) or diltiazem (Cardizem®) along with β-blockers.
   d. **Precautions and monitoring effects**
      (1) Diltiazem (Cardizem®) and verapamil (Calan®) must be used with extreme caution or not at all in patients with conductive disturbances involving the SA or AV node, such as second- or third-degree AV block, sick sinus syndrome, and digitalis toxicity.
      (2) Nifedipine (Procardia®) use has been associated with flushing, headache, and peripheral edema; the patient may find these troublesome and thus may become noncompliant. Using the sustained-release product, Procardia® once daily has been shown to effectively reduce these effects.
      (3) Verapamil use has been associated with a significant degree of constipation, which must be treated to prevent stool straining and noncompliance.
   e. **Specific agents**
      (1) **Diltiazem (Cardizem®).** Availability of extended-release products (Cardizem CD®, Cardizem-LA®, Dilacor XR®, Tiazac®) has reduced the frequency of daily doses in the treatment of hypertension. A single daily dose of 120 to 540 mg is effective for treating mild-to-moderate hypertension. Diltiazem already has proven efficacy as an antiarrhythmic and an antianginal agent.
      (2) **Nifedipine (Procardia®).** The release of once-daily sustained-release preparations (Procardia XL®, Adalat CC®) has made this agent effective as a once-daily therapy for long-term treatment of hypertension. A previously reported long list of side effects has been reduced with the sustained-release product at a single daily dose of 30 to 90 mg. Immediate-release nifedipine has been reported to cause ischemic events, and the current recommendation is to avoid its use if at all possible.
      (3) **Verapamil (Calan®).** This drug is similar to diltiazem in its actions (though with more potent effects on electrical conduction depression). Sustained-release products (Calan SR®, Isoptin SR®, Covera-HS®, Verelan PM®) at doses of 120 to 480 mg daily have been shown to be efficacious for long-term management of mild-to-moderate hypertension, whereas side effects such as dizziness, constipation, and hypotension are reduced.
      (4) Amlodipine (Norvasc®), clevidipine (Cleviprex®), isradipine (DynaCirc®), felodipine (Plendil®), nicardipine (Cardene SR®), and nisoldipine (Sular®) are second-generation calcium-channel blockers. These agents have been developed to produce more selective effects on specific target tissues than the first-generation agents: diltiazem, nifedipine,

and verapamil. These agents are chemically similar to nifedipine and are referred to as dihydropyridine derivatives. The daily dose ranges are

(a) **Amlodipine (Norvasc®):** 2.5 to 10 mg in one dose
(b) **Isradipine (DynaCirc®):** 2.5 to 10 mg in one to two doses
(c) **Felodipine (Plendil®):** 2.5 to 20 mg in one dose
(d) **Nicardipine (Cardene SR®):** 60 to 120 mg as an extended-release product twice daily
(e) **Nisoldipine (Sular®):** 10 to 40 mg in one dose
(f) **Clevidipine (Cleviprex®):** Intravenous administration only; as 1 to 2 mg/hr, doubled at 90-second intervals up to target blood pressure goal.

7. **Vasodilators.** These drugs are used as second-line agents in patient's refractory to initial therapy with diuretics, β-blockers, ACE inhibitors, ARBs, or calcium-channel blockers. Vasodilators directly relax peripheral vascular smooth muscle—arterial, venous, or both. The direct vasodilators should not be used alone owing to increases in plasma renin activity, cardiac output, and heart rate.

a. **Hydralazine (Various)**

(1) **Actions.** Hydralazine directly relaxes arterioles, decreasing systemic vascular resistance. It is also used intravenously or intramuscularly in managing hypertensive crisis.

(2) **Precautions and monitoring effects**

(a) Because hydralazine triggers compensatory reactions that counteract its antihypertensive effects, it is most useful when combined with a β-blocker, central α-agonist, or diuretic as a latter-step agent.
(b) Reflex tachycardia is common and should be considered before initiating therapy.
(c) Hydralazine may induce angina, especially in patients with coronary artery disease and those not receiving a β-blocker.
(d) Drug-induced systemic lupus erythematosus (SLE) may occur.
(i) Baseline and serial complete blood counts (CBCs) with antinuclear antibody titers should be followed routinely to detect SLE.
(ii) Slow acetylators of this drug have an increased incidence of SLE. Their risk may be reduced by administering doses of < 200 mg/day.
(iii) Fatigue, malaise, low-grade fever, and joint aches may signal SLE.
(e) Other adverse effects may include headache, peripheral neuropathy, nausea, vomiting, fluid retention, and postural hypotension.

(3) The **usual daily dose** is 25 to 100 mg.

b. **Minoxidil (Various)**

(1) **Actions.** A more potent vasodilator than hydralazine, minoxidil relaxes arteriolar smooth muscle directly, decreasing peripheral resistance. It also decreases renal vascular resistance while preserving renal blood flow. Effective in most patients, minoxidil is commonly used to treat patients with severe hypertension that has been refractory to conventional drug regimens.

(2) **Precautions and monitoring effects**

(a) Peripheral dilation results in a reflex activation of the sympathetic nervous system and an increase in heart rate, cardiac output, and renin secretion.
(b) Because this agent promotes sodium and water retention, particularly in the presence of renal impairment, patients should be monitored for fluid accumulation and signs of cardiac decompensation. Administering minoxidil along with a sympatholytic agent and a potent diuretic (e.g., furosemide) minimizes increased sympathetic stimulation and fluid retention.
(c) Hypertrichosis (i.e., excessive hair growth) is a common side effect, particularly if the drug is continued for > 4 weeks.

(3) The **usual daily dose** is 2.5 to 80 mg.

c. **Nitroprusside (Nitropress)**

(1) **Actions.** A direct-acting peripheral dilator, this agent has potent effects on both the arterial and venous systems. It is usually used only in short-term emergency treatment of acute hypertensive crisis, when a rapid effect is required. Onset of action is almost instantaneous and is maximal in 1 to 2 mins. Nitroprusside is administered intravenously with continuous blood pressure monitoring.

(2) **Precautions and monitoring effects.** To prevent acute hypotensive episodes, initial doses should be very low, followed by slow titration upward until the desired effect is achieved.

(a) Once the solution is prepared, it should be protected from light. Color changes are a signal that replacement is needed.

(b) Thiocyanate toxicity may develop with long-term treatment—particularly in patients with reduced renal activity—but can be treated with hemodialysis. Symptoms may include fatigue, anorexia, disorientation, nausea, psychotic behavior, or muscle spasms.

(c) Cyanide toxicity can occur (rarely) with long-term, high-dose administration. It may present as altered consciousness, convulsions, tachypnea, or even coma.

(3) The **usual dose** is 0.3 to 10 mcg/kg/min as a continuous intravenous infusion.

8. **Renin Inhibitors**

a. **Indications.** Aliskiren (Tekturna®) is the first of this new class of drugs recently approved by the FDA for the treatment of hypertension.

b. **Actions.** Unlike ACE inhibitors and ARBs, which act during the later stages of the renin-angiotensin system to reduce angiotensin II (see I.E.2-*Figure 33-1*), aliskiren works directly on the enzyme renin, to reduce the eventual production of angiotensin II.

c. **Aliskiren (Tekturna®)** is available in 150 and 300 mg tablets. The usual starting dose is 150 mg daily, and for those who do not respond the dose can be increased to 300 mg daily. Doses greater than 300 mg have not been shown to offer additional blood pressure lowering effects.

d. **Aliskiren** has already been incorporated into four combination products for the treatment of hypertension, once a patient has been stabilized on a therapeutic regimen.

(1) **Aliskiren/valsartan (Valturna®)** 150/160 and 300/320, respectively

(2) **Aliskiren/amlodipine (Tekamlo®)** 150/5, 150/10; and 300/5, 300/10, respectively

(3) **Aliskiren/hydrochlorothiazide (Tekturna HCT®)** 150/12.5, 150/25; and 300/12.5, 300/25, respectively

(4) **Aliskiren/amlodipine/hydrochlorothiazide (Amturnide®)**
Aliskiren 150 mg, amlodipine 5 mg, and hydrochlorothiazide 12.5 mg
Aliskiren 300 mg, amlodipine 5 mg, and hydrochlorothiazide 12.5 mg
Aliskiren 300 mg, amlodipine 5 mg, and hydrochlorothiazide 25 mg
Aliskiren 300 mg, amlodipine 10 mg, and hydrochlorothiazide 12.5 mg
Aliskiren 300 mg, amlodipine 10 mg, and hydrochlorothiazide 25 mg

e. **Significant interactions.** Furosemide serum levels have been reported to be reduced significantly when administered in patients receiving aliskiren. This might result in a diminished pharmacologic effect from furosemide.

f. **Precautions and monitoring effects**
Unlike the ACE inhibitors and ARBs, which have the potential to increase serum potassium levels, patients receiving aliskiren have not shown significant increases in potassium as compared to patients studies receiving placebo. However, in a population of diabetic patients receiving both ACE inhibitors or ARBs in combination with aliskiren, close monitoring of serum electrolytes and renal function is required due to an increased frequency of elevated serum potassium levels.

IV. HYPERTENSIVE EMERGENCIES

A. **Definition.** A hypertensive emergency is a severe elevation of blood pressure (i.e., > 180 mm Hg systolic or > 110 mm Hg diastolic) that demands reduction—either immediate (within minutes) or prompt (within hours) to prevent or limit target-organ damage.

1. Conditions requiring immediate reduction include hypertensive encephalopathy, acute left ventricular failure with pulmonary edema, eclampsia, dissecting aortic aneurysm, acute MI, stroke, and intracranial hemorrhage.

2. Conditions requiring prompt reduction include malignant or accelerated hypertension.

B. Treatment

1. The **reduction in blood pressure must be gradual** (e.g., a 20% to 25% decrease in mean arterial pressure over the first hour) rather than precipitous to avoid compromising perfusion of critical organs, particularly cerebral perfusion.
2. **Specific agents** used in hypertensive crisis are shown in *Table 33-6*.

V. PRINCIPLES OF HYPERTENSION TREATMENT IN THE ELDERLY.

Drug therapy for the elderly has been recommended in the past but with a greater degree of concern due to alterations in end organ functions, changes in drug distribution and elimination, and impact which declining blood pressure has in this patient population. A recent expert consensus document supported by the American College of Cardiology Foundation Task Force on Clinical Expert Consensus Documents was completed in April of 2011, and forms the basis for the brief overview to conclude this chapter. (See I.A.3.a.)

A. General principles for drug therapy in the elderly

1. Initial therapy should be started with a low dose and gradually increased, if needed to the maximal tolerated dose. If the drug is not tolerated as doses are increased toward target, a second drug from a different class should be substituted for the initial drug.
2. If the initial therapy does not achieve the targeted goal, a second agent from a different class should be added and the initial agent should be continued provided the initial drug was well tolerated.
3. If the target blood pressure goal is not achieved after reaching the full dose for the second agent, a third agent from yet another class should be added.
4. For the initiation of therapy, if the blood pressure is greater than 20/10 mm Hg above the targeted goal, therapy should be initiated with two antihypertensive agents.

B. Selection of special drug classes in the elderly

1. Thiazide diuretics
   - **a.** Thiazide diuretics, hydrochlorothiazide (Microzide®) and chlorthalidone (Various), have been recommended for initiating therapy in the elderly.
   - **b.** Despite the various age-related changes, which can be exacerbated with diuretic usage, the consensus of experts felt that the initial reductions in intravascular volume, peripheral vascular resistance, and blood pressure offset them and are usually well tolerated in the elderly.
   - **c.** Therapeutic drug monitoring, routine monitoring of fluid and electrolyte status in order to prevent the development of orthostatic hypotension (depletion of sodium and water), arrhythmias (hypokalemia, hypomagnesemia, and hyponatremia), hyperuricemia, glucose intolerance, and dyslipidemia, which can all be exacerbated by thiazide diuretics.
2. Nonthiazide diuretics
   - **a.** Indapamide (Various) is a sulfonamide diuretic used in the treatment of hypertension, which does not increase uric acid levels but has been associated with increases in blood glucose levels, as well as potassium-independent prolongation of the QT interval. It also needs to be used carefully in patients also receiving lithium.
   - **b.** Loop diuretics described by the consensus group included furosemide (Lasix®), bumetanide (Various), and torsemide (Demadex®) have shown value in treating hypertension in patients with HF or chronic kidney disease. Fluid and electrolytes must be monitored for increases in glucose, as well as hypokalemia and hyponatremia.
   - **c.** Potassium-retaining diuretics have also been included in the consensus document and include the mineralocorticoid antagonists spironolactone (Aldactone®) and eplerenone (Inspra®), as well as the sodium transport channel antagonists, amiloride (Various) and triamterene (Dyrenium®). These agents are generally used in combination with other agents.
3. β-adrenergic blockers
   - **a.** Have not demonstrated convincing value in elderly being treated for hypertension. Although many feel they have a role, especially when added to a diuretic.
   - **b.** The consensus group recommended their use in elderly hypertensive patients with coronary artery disease, HF, select arrhythmias, migraine headaches, and senile tremor.

4. Calcium-channel blockers
   a. A wide array of effects on heart muscle, SA and AV nodal function, peripheral arteries, and coronary circulation provide them with a positive recommendation by the consensus group.
   b. Clinical trials have shown the group of agents to be safe and efficacious in the elderly with hypertension.
   c. Due to the numerous clinical applications for the calcium-channel blockers, the consensus group recommended their use in elderly hypertensive patients with the comorbid conditions that include angina and supraventricular arrhythmias.
   d. The group added concern for the primary adverse effects of the largest group of calcium-channel blockers, the dihydropyridines as being due to peripheral dilation, which include edema, headache, postural hypotension, which could result in added risks of falls in the elderly.
   e. Final review from the consensus document results in the conclusions that the short-acting rapid-release dihydropyridines, that is, nifedipine (Procardia®), must be avoided, as should verapamil (Calan®) and diltiazem (Cardizem®) in those patients predisposed to heart block, and the need to avoid the first generation calcium-channel blockers, verapamil (Calan®), diltiazem (Cardizem®), and nifedipine (Procardia®) in patients with left ventricular dysfunction. This leaves the second generation dihydropyridine derivatives, as described earlier in this chapter.
5. Angiotensin-converting enzyme inhibitors (ACEIs) and ARBs
   a. ACEIs are considered first-line therapy in the elderly hypertensive patient with HF due to their ability to reduce morbidity and mortality in patients with HF. They have also been shown to retard the progression of diabetic renal disease and hypertensive nephrosclerosis.
   b. Main adverse effects associated with ACEIs include hypotension, chronic dry cough, and, rarely, angioedema or rash. Renal failure can develop in those with renal artery stenosis, and hyperkalemia can occur in patients taking potassium supplements, as well as those with renal insufficiency. Rarely, neutropenia or agranulocytosis can occur; close monitoring is suggested during the first months of therapy.
   c. Serum creatinine and potassium levels should be monitored for both classes of drugs in order to prevent the development of hyperkalemia due to the potential for increased potassium retention as well as reduced renal function.
   d. The consensus experts recommended the use of ARBs as first-line therapy in elderly hypertensive patients with diabetes mellitus and an alternative in elderly hypertensives with heart failure who cannot tolerate the ACEIs.
6. Direct acting renin inhibitors
   a. Aliskiren (Tekturna®) is the first of the direct acting renin inhibitors, and the consensus experts felt that it has similar effectiveness to ARBs and ACEIs for lowering blood pressure, without the dose-related increase in adverse events in the elderly.
   b. Combination therapy with hydrochlorothiazide (Microzide®), ramipril (Altace®), or amlodipine (Norvasc®) causes a greater reduction in blood pressure than when either agent is used alone. Data in combination with β-blockers is lacking, only a very limited amount of data are available in black hypertensive patients, and there is no data on the use of aliskiren (Tekturna®) in patients with glomerular filtration rates less than 30 mL/min/1.73 m^2.
   c. Aliskiren appears to be well tolerated in patients older than 75 years of age, including those with renal disease.
7. Miscellaneous agents
   a. Vasodilator agents such as hydralazine (Various) and minoxidil (Various) have demonstrated unfavorable side effects (i.e., tachycardia, fluid accumulation, atrial arrhythmias) and are therefore not included as initial therapy for the elderly. They have been suggested only as part of a combination regimen.
   b. Centrally acting agents such as clonidine (Catapres®) are less than ideal in the elderly due to their sedative properties and ability to induce bradycardias. Additionally, the sudden abruption in usage leads to increased blood pressure and heart rate, which could pose added dangers in the elderly population.
   c. Combination therapy provides an opportunity to maximize efficacy while reducing adverse events, enhanced convenience, and patient compliance.

Study Questions

Directions for questions 1–6: Each of the questions, statements, or incomplete statements in this section can be correctly answered or completed by **one** of the suggested answers or phrases. Choose the **best** answer.

1. Which of the following agents represents an angiotensin II receptor antagonist (ARB)?
   - **(A)** trandolapril (Mavik®)
   - **(B)** carvedilol (Coreg®)
   - **(C)** irbesartan (Avapro®)
   - **(D)** moexipril (Univasc®)
   - **(E)** nimodipine (Various)

2. Reflex tachycardia, headache, and postural hypotension are adverse effects that limit the use of which of the following antihypertensive agents?
   - **(A)** prazosin (Minipress®)
   - **(B)** captopril (Capoten®)
   - **(C)** methyldopa (Various)
   - **(D)** guanabenz (Various)
   - **(E)** hydralazine (Various)

3. A 65-year-old man presents with stage I hypertension. He has diabetes mellitus and chronic kidney disease and is intolerant to lisinopril. Which of the following agents would be an appropriate selection for initial treatment in this patient based on the guidelines from the "Seventh Report of the Joint National Committee on Detection, Evaluation, and Treatment of High Blood Pressure" (JNC-7)?
   - **(A)** chlorothiazide (Various)
   - **(B)** propranolol (Inderal®)
   - **(C)** nitroprusside (Nitropress®)
   - **(D)** candesartan (Atacand®)
   - **(E)** clonidine (Catapres®)

4. A patient with stage I hypertension who has bronchospastic airway disease and who is noncompliant would be best treated with which of the following β-blocking agents?
   - **(A)** timolol (Various)
   - **(B)** penbutolol (Levatol®)
   - **(C)** esmolol (Brevibloc®)
   - **(D)** acebutolol (Sectral®)
   - **(E)** propranolol (Inderal®)

5. Long-standing hypertension leads to tissue damage in all of the following organs *except* the
   - **(A)** heart.
   - **(B)** lungs.
   - **(C)** kidneys.
   - **(D)** brain.
   - **(E)** eyes.

6. According to the "Seventh Report of the Joint National Committee on Detection, Evaluation, and Treatment of High Blood Pressure" (JNC-7), which of the following agents is suitable as initial therapy for treating stage I hypertension (assuming no compelling indications for another type of drug)?
   - **(A)** chlorothiazide (Various)
   - **(B)** labetalol (Trandate®)
   - **(C)** atenolol (Tenormin®)
   - **(D)** propranolol (Inderal®)
   - **(E)** bisoprolol (Zebeta®)

Directions for questions 7–9: The questions and incomplete statements in this section can be correctly answered or completed by **one or more** of the suggested answers. Choose the answer, **A–E**.

- A if **I only** is correct
- B if **III only** is correct
- C if **I and II** are correct
- D if **II and III** are correct
- E if **I, II, and III** are correct

7. A patient treated with a spironolactone (Aldactone®) should be monitored regularly for altered plasma levels of
   - **I.** potassium.
   - **II.** serum creatinine.
   - **III.** blood urea nitrogen (BUN).

8. Before antihypertensive therapy begins, secondary causes of hypertension should be ruled out. Laboratory findings that suggest an underlying cause of hypertension include
   - **I.** a decreased serum potassium level.
   - **II.** an increased urinary catecholamine level.
   - **III.** an increased blood cortisol level.

9. In an otherwise healthy adult with stage I hypertension, appropriate initial antihypertensive therapy would be
   - **I.** chlorthalidone (Various)
   - **II.** metoprolol (Lopressor®)
   - **III.** bisoprolol (Zebeta®)

Directions for questions 10–14: Each list of adverse effects in this section is most closely associated with **one** of the following antihypertensive agents. The agents may be used more than once or not at all. Choose the **best** answer, **A–E.**

(A) clonidine (Catapres®)
(B) olmesartan (Benicar®)
(C) nitroprusside (Nitropress®)
(D) prazosin (Minipress®)
(E) propranolol (Inderal®)

10. Thiocyanate intoxication, hypotension, and convulsions

11. Bradycardia, bronchospasm, and cardiac decompensation

12. Angioedema, cough, and hyperkalemia

13. Rebound hypertension, dry mouth, and drowsiness

14. First-dose syncope, postural hypotension, and palpitations

Directions for questions 15–19: Each description listed in this section is most closely associated with **one** of the following β-adrenergic blocking agents. The agents may be used more than once or not at all. Choose the **best** answer, **A–E.**

(A) esmolol (Brevibloc®)
(B) labetalol (Trandate®)
(C) bisoprolol (Zebeta®)
(D) nadolol (Corgard®)
(E) pindolol (Visken®)

15. A β-blocker with intrinsic sympathomimetic activity

16. A β-blocker that also blocks α-adrenergic receptors

17. A β-blocker with an ultrashort duration of action

18. A β-blocker with a long duration of action and nonselective blocking activity

19. A β-blocker with relative cardioselective blocking activity

Answers and Explanations

1. The answer is C *[see III.B.5.a].*
Irbesartan is one of the relatively new classes of drugs used in the treatment of hypertension referred to as an angiotensin II receptor antagonist, which blocks the production of angiotensin II and consequently its effects as a powerful vasoconstrictor and stimulant for aldosterone release. Trandolapril and moexipril are ACE inhibitors; carvedilol is a β-adrenergic blocking agent; and nimodipine is a calcium-channel blocker used in the treatment of subarachnoid hemorrhage.

2. The answer is E *[see III.B.7.a].*
Hydralazine is a vasodilator that works by directly relaxing arterioles, thereby reducing peripheral vascular resistance. Its effectiveness as an antihypertensive agent is compromised; however, by the compensatory reactions it triggers (e.g., reflex tachycardia) and by its other adverse effects (e.g., headache, postural hypotension, nausea, palpitations). Fortunately, the unwanted effects of hydralazine are minimized when it is used in combination with a diuretic agent and a β-blocker. Hydralazine is most effective as a supplemental antihypertensive drug in combination with first-line therapy.

3. The answer is D *[see III.B.5.e.(3)].*
Candesartan, an angiotensin II receptor blocker, which acts by blocking the binding of angiotensin II to the angiotensin II receptors. By blocking the receptor site, this class of drugs inhibits the vasoconstrictor effects of angiotensin II and prevents the release of aldosterone owing to angiotensin II from the adrenal glands. JNC-7 guidelines call for the use of diuretics in the initial treatment of hypertension, unless the patient has compelling indications that have been shown to benefit from the use of specific classes of drugs. This patient has diabetes and chronic kidney disease and is unable to tolerate the ACE inhibitor lisinopril; therefore, an ARB would be an acceptable alternative for this patient rather than a β-blocker (propranolol) or diuretic (chlorothiazide). Nitroprusside is normally used in the treatment of hypertensive emergencies as an intravenous infusion, and clonidine is not considered initial treatment for hypertension.

4. **The answer is D** *[see III.B.3.a.(7).(a)–(n)]*.
The β-adrenergic blocking agents continue to demonstrate effectiveness in the treatment of hypertension. A major feature of some of these agents is their relative selectivity for β_1-receptors (in the heart) rather than for β_2-receptors (in the lung), which provides advantages in the treatment of certain patients (e.g., those with bronchospastic airway or COPD). Of the β-blockers listed, acebutolol is less likely than the rest to block β_2-receptors because of its relative cardioselective-blocking activity. Acebutolol also has a long duration of action, which could be helpful in the noncompliant patient by requiring fewer doses per day. Penbutolol has weak intrinsic sympathomimetic activity like pindolol but lacks relative cardioselectivity, despite its long duration of action. Esmolol by nature of its continuous intravenous infusion would not lend itself to chronic ambulatory therapy. Timolol is a long-acting β-blocker and lacks the relative cardioselective properties that acebutolol possesses.

5. **The answer is B** *[see I.F; Table 33-3]*.
Left untreated, hypertension can be lethal because of its progressively destructive effects on major organs, such as the heart, kidneys, and brain. The eyes also suffer damage; the lungs, however, do not. End-organ damage caused by hypertension includes left ventricular hypertrophy, heart failure, angina pectoris, myocardial infarction, renal insufficiency caused by atherosclerotic lesions, nephrosclerosis, cerebral aneurysm and hemorrhage, retinal hemorrhage, and papilledema.

6. **The answer is A** *[see III.B.2.a]*.
Thiazide diuretics are considered the first-line treatment choice for hypertension and should be used alone or in combination with other antihypertensives, if necessary. β-Blockers such as labetalol, atenolol, bisoprolol, and propranolol are no longer considered initial agents for treating hypertension unless there is a compelling reason for their use. β-Blockers have shown positive clinical outcomes in patients with heart failure, post-MI, high coronary disease risk, and diabetes (compelling indications) and would be acceptable options for patients presenting with prehypertension or hypertension with a compelling indication.

7. **The answer is E (I, II, III)** *[see III.B.2.c.(4)]*.
Spironolactone is a direct-acting aldosterone-receptor blocker and decreases its effects on sodium and water retention. However, a benefit of spironolactone is its potassium-sparing effect, through the exchange of sodium for potassium in the kidney. Patients with reduced renal function and acute renal failure (evidenced by elevations in serum creatinine) lose their ability to excrete potassium, and this needs to be monitored when patients are started on spironolactone. BUN and creatinine are good indirect indicators of renal function.

8. **The answer is E (I, II, III)** *[see II.A.2]*.
Low serum potassium levels in a hypertensive patient suggest primary aldosteronism. Elevated urinary catecholamines suggest a pheochromocytoma; other signs and symptoms of this tumor include weight loss, episodic flushing, and sweating. Elevated serum cortisol levels suggest Cushing syndrome; the patient is also likely to have a round (moon) face and truncal obesity. Secondary hypertension requires treatment of the underlying cause; supplementary antihypertensive drug therapy may also be needed.

9. **The answer is A (I)** *[see III.B.2.a]*.
Thiazide diuretics such as chlorthalidone are now considered, based on the JNC-7, first-line therapy for hypertension, barring any compelling indications, such as heart failure, diabetes, chronic kidney disease, or post-MI, when other antihypertensive agents would be indicated. β-Adrenergic blockers, such as metoprolol and bisoprolol, are no longer indicated as initial antihypertensive agents for treating hypertension.

10. **The answer is C** *[see III.B.7.c.(2)]*.

11. **The answer is E** *[see III.B.3.a.(4)]*.

12. **The answer is B** *[see III.B.5.c.(2)]*.

13. **The answer is A** *[see III.B.3.c.(2).(c)]*.

14. **The answer is D** *[see III.B.3.b.(3).(a)]*.
The goal of treatment in hypertension is to lower blood pressure toward normal with minimal side effects. All antihypertensive drugs can cause adverse effects. The primary purpose of the JNC-7 guidelines is to acknowledge the long-term benefits of diuretics in the treatment of hypertension.

15. **The answer is E** *[see III.B.3.a.(7).(f)]*.

16. **The answer is B** *[see III.B.3.a.(7).(g)]*.

17. **The answer is A** *[see III.B.3.a.(7).(i)]*.

18. **The answer is D** *[see III.B.3.a.(7).(c)]*.

19. **The answer is C** *[see III.B.3.a.(7).(l)]*.
The β-adrenergic blocking agents are valuable for managing hypertension and are used as initial antihypertensives. The β-blockers are sympathetic antagonists. They act by blocking various receptors of the sympathetic nervous system. They differ in their selectivity for these sympathetic receptors. For example, β_1-blockers have relative cardioselective activity—that is, they block β_1-receptors (in the heart) rather than β_2-receptors (in bronchial smooth muscle) and, therefore, are highly useful antihypertensive agents. Intrinsic sympathomimetic activity also appears to reduce the problem of bronchoconstriction; moreover, drugs with this property can also maintain a satisfactory heart rate.

34 Heart Failure

ALAN H. MUTNICK

I. INTRODUCTION

A. **Definition. Heart failure (HF)** is a complex clinical syndrome that can result from any cardiac disorder that impairs the ability of the ventricle to deliver adequate quantities of blood to the metabolizing tissues during normal activity or at rest. The condition in the past has been referred to as "congestive heart failure," owing to the **edematous state** commonly produced by the fluid backup resulting in shortness of breath, fatigue, limitation of exercise tolerance, and fluid retention. Fluid retention may lead to pulmonary and peripheral edema. More recently, because all patients do not necessarily present with fluid overload at the initial or follow-up evaluations, the term "heart failure" is used to more adequately reflect the clinical syndrome.

B. **Mortality rate.** Approximately 300,000 patients die as a result of the direct or indirect consequences of HF each year, and the number of deaths owing to HF (primary or secondary causes) has increased steadily, despite treatment advances. The risk of death is 5% to 10% annually in patients with mild symptoms and is as high as 30% to 40% in patients with advanced disease manifestations.

C. **Incidence of HF.** HF is a common medical condition that affects almost 5 million people in the United States, with more than 500,000 new cases diagnosed each year. Between 1.5% and 2.0% of the population has HF, and the incidence increases to 6% to 10% in patients older than age 65. HF makes up 20% of all hospitalizations in patients older than 65 years of age. HF is the only major cardiovascular disorder that is increasing in incidence and prevalence. During the last 10 years, there has been a dramatic increase in the number of hospitalizations, primarily owing to HF (810,000 in 1990 to more than 1 million, currently). The reasons for the increased numbers of hospital admissions include the aging of the population in the United States and improved treatment results obtained for myocardial infarction, coronary artery bypass surgery, and stenting.

D. **Cost of HF.** The total costs (direct and indirect) for the treatment of HF in the United States during 2005 were approximately \$27.9 billion. Currently in the United States, more than \$2.9 billion is spent annually on drugs used in the treatment of HF.

E. **Causes**

1. Although the disease occurs most commonly among the elderly (80% of patients hospitalized with HF are older than 65 years of age), it may appear at any age as a consequence of underlying cardiovascular disease.
2. There currently is no single diagnostic test for HF, and the clinical diagnosis is normally based on patient history and physical examination.
3. HF should not be considered an independent diagnosis because it is superimposed on an underlying cause.
   a. Coronary artery disease (CAD) is the cause of HF in about two-thirds of patients with left ventricular systolic dysfunction.
   b. The remaining third of patients have a nonischemic cause of systolic dysfunction owing to other causes of myocardial stress, which include trauma, disease, or other abnormal states (e.g., pulmonary embolism, infection, anemia, pregnancy, drug use or abuse, fluid overload, arrhythmia, valvular heart disease, cardiomyopathies, congenital heart disease).
4. The New York Heart Association (NYHA) developed a classification system still used today to quantify the functional limitations of HF patients. The NYHA classes are as follows:
   a. Class I. Degree of effort necessary to elicit HF symptoms equals those that would **limit normal individuals**.

b. Class II. Degree of effort necessary to elicit HF symptoms occurs with **ordinary exertion**.
c. Class III. Degree of effort necessary to elicit HF symptoms occurs with **less-than-ordinary exertion**.
d. Class IV. Degree of effort necessary to elicit HF symptoms occurs while **at rest**.

5. A criticism of the NYHA classification is its dependence on subjective assessments by the clinical practitioner, which changes frequently and might not accurately reflect different treatment options based on the degree of symptoms. Consequently, more recently, the "American College of Cardiology/American Heart Association (ACC/AHA) Guidelines for the Evaluation and Management of Chronic Heart Failure" offered new classification scheme that depicts HF as an evolving clinical entity and details a progression based on risk factors and structural changes, which may be asymptomatic or symptomatic. Within this classification, specific treatments can be targeted at each stage to affect morbidity and mortality (*Table 34-1*). The introduction of the four stages of HF are not intended to replace the NYHA classification but rather to complement it.

F. **Forms of HF.** As mentioned, HF is a complex syndrome and has been described in various ways. The cardinal manifestations of HF are dyspnea and fatigue, which may limit exercise tolerance, result in fluid retention, and lead to pulmonary congestion and peripheral edema. However, the following sections provide several ways that have been used to describe the pathophysiology and the symptomatology involved in the condition. Although the terms *low output* versus *high output* and *left sided* versus *right sided* are not routinely used in the clinical setting, their use here is to help convey important educational aspects of HF and are presented only for the purpose of simplifying the discussion of the pathophysiology and symptomatology.

1. **Low-output versus high-output failure**
   a. If metabolic demands are within normal limits but the heart is unable to meet them, the failure is designated **low output** (the most common type).
   b. If metabolic demands increase (e.g., hyperthyroidism, anemia) and the heart is unable to meet them, the failure is designated **high output**. Compared to low-output failure, correction of the underlying cause of high-output failure is paramount as the initial treatment modality.

Table 34-1 STAGES OF HEART FAILURE (HF) BASED ON EVOLUTION AND PROGRESSION OF CLINICAL FINDINGS

Stage	Description	Examples
A	Patients at high risk of developing HF because of the presence of conditions that are strongly associated with the condition; such patients have no identified structural or functional abnormalities of the pericardium, myocardium, or cardiac valves and have never shown signs or symptoms of HF	Hypertension, atherosclerotic disease, diabetes mellitus, obesity, metabolic syndrome, history of cardiotoxic drug therapy or alcohol abuse, personal history of rheumatic fever, family history of cardiomyopathy
B	Patients who have developed structural heart disease that is strongly associated with the development of HF but who have never shown signs or symptoms condition	Left ventricular remodeling, including left ventricular hypertrophy or low ejection fraction; asymptomatic valvular disease of the previous myocardial infarction
C	Patients who have current or prior symptoms of HF associated with underlying structural heart disease	Known structural heart disease, dyspnea, or fatigue; reduced exercise tolerance
D	Patients with refractory HF who require specialized interventions	Patients with marked symptoms at rest despite maximal medical therapy (are frequently hospitalized for HF and cannot be safely discharged from the hospital, patients in the hospital awaiting heart transplantation, patients at home receiving continuous intravenous support for symptom relief or being supported with a mechanical circulatory assist device, patients in a hospice setting for the management of HF)

Adapted from Hunt SA, Abraham WT, Chin MH, et al. 2009 focused update incorporated into the ACC/AHA 2005 guidelines for the diagnosis and management of heart failure in adults: a report of the American College of Cardiology Foundation/American Heart Association Task Force on Practice Guidelines. *J Am Coll Cardiol.* 2009;53:e1– e90.

Table 34-2 SUBSTANCES THAT MAY EXACERBATE HEART FAILURE

Promote Sodium Retention	Produce Osmotic Effect	Decrease Contractility
Androgens	Albumin	Antiarrhythmic agents (e.g., disopyramide, flecainide, quinidine)
Corticosteroids	Glucose	β-Adrenergic blockers
Diazoxide	Mannitol	Select calcium-channel blockers (e.g., diltiazem, nifedipine, verapamil)
Estrogens	Saline	Direct cardiotoxins (e.g., doxorubicin, ethanol, cocaine, amphetamines)
Licorice	Urea	Tricyclic antidepressants
Lithium carbonate		
NSAIDs		

NSAIDs, nonsteroidal anti-inflammatory drugs.

3. During recent years, several sets of guidelines have been developed for the treatment of HF. Most recently, a panel of leading physicians and researchers in the field of HF provided recommendations. See within the following citations:
   Hunt SA, Abraham WT, Chin MH, et al. 2009 focused update incorporated into the ACC/AHA 2005 guidelines for the diagnosis and management of heart failure in adults: a report of the American College of Cardiology Foundation/American Heart Association Task Force on Practice Guidelines. Developed in collaboration with the International Society for Heart and Lung Transplantation. *J Am Coll Cardiol.* 2009;53(15):e1–e90.
   Jessup M, Abraham WT, Casey DE, et al. Writing on behalf of the 2005 Guideline Update for the Diagnosis and Management of Chronic Heart Failure in the Adult Writing Committee. 2009 focused update: ACCF/AHA guidelines for the diagnosis and management of heart failure in adults: a report of the American College of Cardiology/American Heart Association Task Force on Practice Guidelines. *J Am Coll Cardiol.* 2009;53:1343–1382.
4. These guidelines represent the most up-to-date standards for the prevention, diagnosis, and treatment of HF (*Table 34-3*).
   a. The guidelines focus on four stages in the development of HF: stages A and B include patients "**at risk**" for HF, and stages C and D include patients who have developed HF. Each of the four stages of HF is associated with select treatment strategies and recommendations, which will be included in the following sections.
   b. Treatment of patients with refractory end-stage HF (stage D) should include the primary therapeutic agents that are used for stages A, B, and C. However, lack of an acceptable response will require specialized nonpharmacologic modalities, such as mechanical circulatory support, transplantation, and end-of-life care for those exhibiting no benefit.
   c. Ranking recommendations

Ranking Based on Size of Treatment Effect	Assessment of Benefit versus Risk	Recommended Action
Class I	Benefit >>> risk	Treatment should be used
Class IIa	Benefit >> risk	Reasonable to use treatment
Class IIb	Benefit ≥ risk	Treatment may be considered
Class III	No benefit; potentially harmful	No proven benefit; even harmful

Estimate of Certainty for Treatment Effect	Extent of Populations Studied	Types of Trials Utilized
Level A	Multiple populations evaluated	Data derived from multiple trials/meta-analyses
Level B	Limited populations evaluated	Data derived from a single trial or nonrandomized study
Level C	Very limited populations evaluated	Consensus opinion of experts or case reports

Table 34-3 APPROACH TO HEART FAILURE (HF)[a]

	At Risk for Heart Failure		Heart Failure	
	Stage A	**Stage B**	**Stage C**	**Stage D**
Patients	Patients at high risk of developing HF because of presence of conditions that are strongly associated with development of condition; such patients have no identified structural or functional abnormalities of the pericardium, myocardium, or cardiac valves, and have never shown signs or symptoms of HF.	Patients who have developed structural heart disease that is strongly associated with development of HF but who have never shown signs or symptoms of the condition.	Patients who have structural heart disease with current or prior symptoms of HF.	Patients with refractory HF who require specialized interventions.
Goals	Treat hypertension. Encourage smoking cessation. Treat lipid disorders. Encourage regular exercise Discourage alcohol intake, illicit drug use. Control metabolic syndrome.	Same as stage A	Same as stages A and B Dietary salt restriction	Same as stages A, B, and C Decision concerning appropriate level of care OPTIONS • Compassionate end-of-life care • Extraordinary measures ◦ Heart transplant ◦ Chronic inotropes ◦ Permanent mechanical support ◦ Experimental surgery or drugs
Drugs	• ACEIs or ARBs in appropriate patients with high risk diabetes, atherosclerotic vascular disease, etc.	• ACEIs or ARBs in appropriate patients • β-blockers in appropriate patients	• Diuretics for fluid retention • ACEIs • β-Blockers DRUGS IN SELECT PATIENTS • Aldosterone antagonists • ARBs • Digitalis • Hydralazine/nitrates	
Devices in select patients		• Implantable defibrillators	• Biventricular pacing • Implantable defibrillators	

[a]The guidelines listed here are definitive , based here are definitive, based on available evidence, and are not intended to reflect the entire set of guidelines with less-than-substancial evidence. Adapted from Hunt SA, Abraham WT, Chin MH, et al 2009 focused update incorporated into the ACC/AHA 2005 guidelines for the diagnosis and management of heart failure in adults: a report of the American College of Cardiology Foundation/American Heart Association Task Force on Practice Guildelines.
J Am Coll Cardiol. 2009;53:e1–e90.
ACEIs, angiotensin-converting enzyme inhibitors; *ARB*, angiotensin II receptor blockers.

II. PATHOPHYSIOLOGY. HF and decreased cardiac output trigger a complex scheme of compensatory mechanisms designed to normalize cardiac output (cardiac output = stroke volume × heart rate). The principal manifestation of progression in cardiac dysfunction is a change in the geometry of the left ventricle, resulting in ventricular dilation and hypertrophy, with a resultant increase in a more spherical shape—referred to as *cardiac remodeling*. This results in increases in ventricular wall tension, depression in mechanical performance, and retention of normal cardiac fluid, which worsen the remodeling process.

A. **Compensation.** These mechanisms are shown in *Figure 34-2*.
   1. **Sympathetic responses.** Inadequate cardiac output stimulates reflex (norepinephrine and epinephrine) activation of the sympathetic nervous system and an increase in circulating catecholamines. The heart rate increases, and blood flow is redistributed to ensure perfusion of the most vital organs (the brain and the heart).
   2. **Hormonal stimulation.** The redistribution of blood flow results in reduced renal perfusion, which decreases the glomerular filtration rate (GFR). Reduction in GFR results in
      a. sodium and water retention and
      b. activation of the renin–angiotensin–aldosterone system, which further enhances sodium retention and thus volume expansion.
   3. **Concentric cardiac hypertrophy** describes a mechanism that thickens cardiac walls, providing larger contractile cells and diminishing the capacity of the cavity in an attempt to precipitate expulsion at lower volumes (See above-Pathophysiology-*cardiac remodeling*).
   4. **Frank–Starling mechanism.** The premise of this response is that increased fiber dilation heightens the contractile force, which then increases the energy released.
      a. Within physiological limits, the heart pumps all the blood it receives without allowing excessive accumulation within the veins or cardiac chambers.
      b. As blood volume increases, the various cardiac chambers dilate (stretch) and enlarge in an attempt to accommodate the excess fluid.
      c. As these stretched muscles contract, the contractile force increases in proportion to their distention. Then the extended fibers snap back (as a rubber band would), expelling the extra fluid into the arteries.
      d. Additional evidence suggests that the release of cytokines (e.g., tumor necrosis factor) occurs in concert with elevated levels of circulating norepinephrine, angiotensin II, aldosterone, endothelin, and vasopressin, which may all play a role in adversely affecting the heart structure, resulting in depressed performance.

B. **Decompensation.** Over time, the compensatory mechanisms become exhausted and increasingly ineffective, entering a vicious spiral of decompensation in which the mechanisms surpass their limits and become self-defeating—as they work harder, they only exhaust the system's capacity to respond.
   1. As the strain continues, total peripheral resistance and afterload increase, thereby decreasing the percentage of blood ejected per unit of time. Afterload is determined by the amount of contractile force needed to overcome intraventricular pressure and eject the blood.
      a. **Afterload** is the tension in ventricular muscles during contraction. In the left ventricle, this tension is determined by the amount of force needed to overcome pressure in the aorta. Afterload (also known as intraventricular systolic pressure) is sometimes used to describe the amount of force needed in the right ventricle to overcome pressure in the pulmonary artery.
      b. **Preload** is the force exerted on the ventricular muscle at the end of diastole, which determines the degree of muscle fiber stretch. This concept is also known as ventricular end-diastolic pressure. Preload is a key factor in contractility because the more these muscles are stretched in diastole, the more powerfully they contract in systole.
   2. As the fluid volume expands, so do the demands on an already exhausted pump, allowing increased volume to remain in the ventricle.
   3. The resulting fluid backup (from the left ventricle into the lungs; from the right ventricle into peripheral circulation) produces the signs and symptoms of HF.

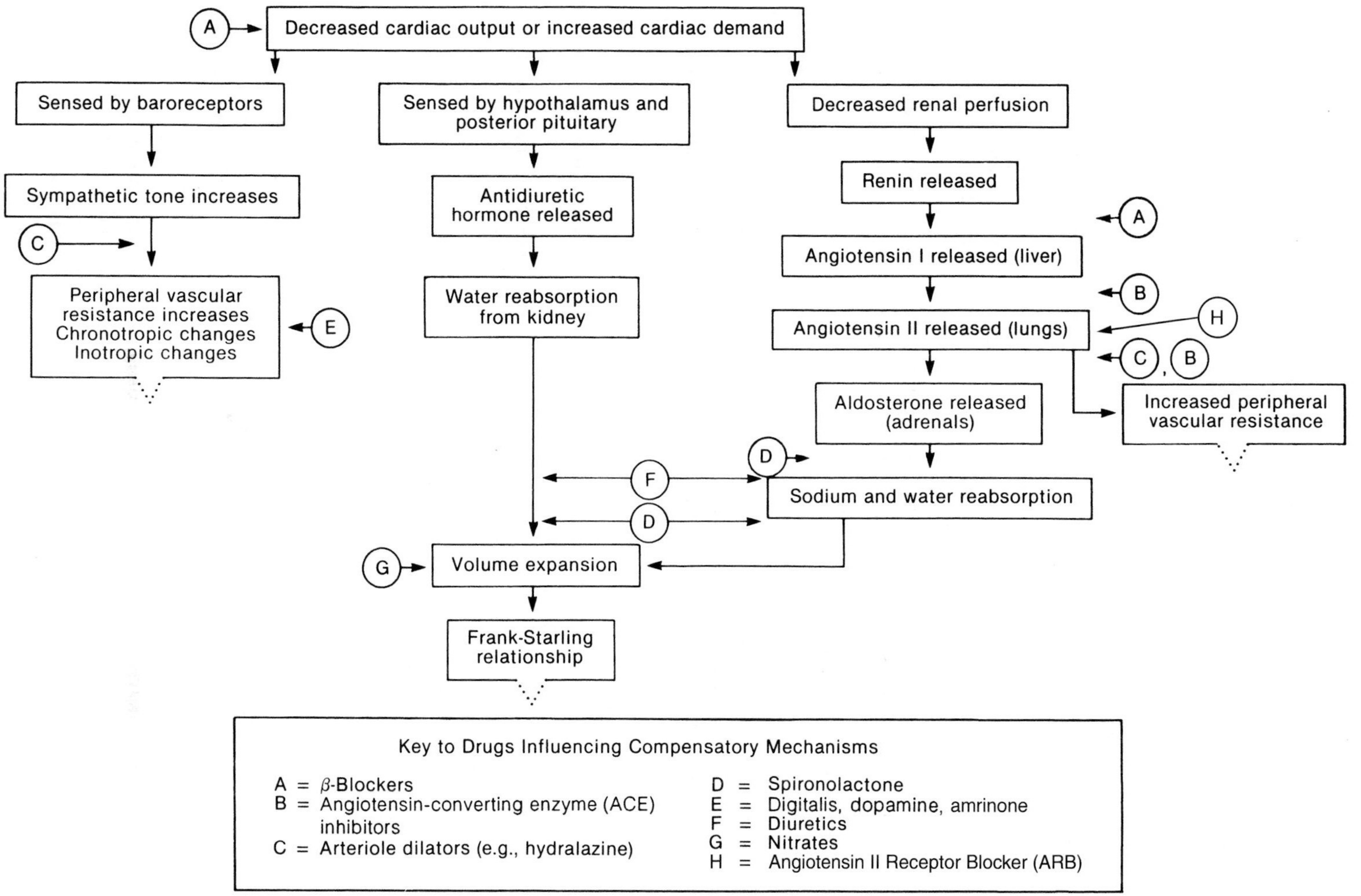
A
Decreased cardiac output or increased cardiac demand
Sensed by baroreceptors
Sympathetic tone increases
C
Peripheral vascular resistance increases Chronotropic changes Inotropic changes
E
Sensed by hypothalamus and posterior pituitary
Antidiuretic hormone released
Water reabsorption from kidney
F
D
G
Volume expansion
Frank-Starling relationship
Decreased renal perfusion
Renin released
A
Angiotensin I released (liver)
B
Angiotensin II released (lungs)
H
C, B
Increased peripheral vascular resistance
Aldosterone released (adrenals)
D
Sodium and water reabsorption
Key to Drugs Influencing Compensatory Mechanisms
A = β-Blockers
B = Angiotensin-converting enzyme (ACE) inhibitors
C = Arteriole dilators (e.g., hydralazine)
D = Spironolactone
E = Digitalis, dopamine, amrinone
F = Diuretics
G = Nitrates
H = Angiotensin II Receptor Blocker (ARB)

Figure 34-2. Compensatory mechanisms in heart failure.

III. CLINICAL EVALUATION. Assessment of fluid status and LVEF (*Table 34-3*).

A. **Fluid accumulation behind the left ventricle**

1. **Signs and symptoms**
   a. Dyspnea
      (1) As HF progresses, the amount of effort required to trigger **exertional dyspnea** lessens.
      (2) **Both paroxysmal nocturnal dyspnea** and **orthopnea** result from volume pooling in the recumbent position and can be relieved by propping up the patient with pillows or having the patient sit upright. (Orthopnea is often gauged by the number of pillows the patient needs to sleep comfortably.)
   b. Dry, wheezing cough
   c. Exertional fatigue and weakness
   d. Nocturia. Edematous fluids that accumulate during the day migrate from dependent areas when the patient is in a recumbent position and renal perfusion increases.
2. **Physical findings**
   a. Rales (or crackles) indicate the movement of air through fluid-filled passages.
   b. Tachycardia is an early compensatory response detected through an increased pulse rate.
   c. S_3 ventricular gallop is a vibration produced by rapid filling of the left ventricle early in diastole.
   d. S_4 atrial gallop is a vibration produced by increased resistance to sudden, forceful ejection of atrial blood in late diastole; it does not vary with inspiration in left-sided failure and is more common in diastolic dysfunction.
3. **Diagnostic test results**
   a. Cardiomegaly (heart enlargement), left ventricular hypertrophy, and pulmonary congestion may be evidenced by chest radiograph, electrocardiogram (ECG), and reduction in left ventricular function via echocardiography and radionuclide ventriculography.
   b. Arm-to-tongue circulation time is prolonged.
   c. Transudative pleural effusion may be suggested by radiograph and confirmed by analysis of aspirated pleural fluid.

B. **Fluid accumulation behind the right side of the heart**

1. **Signs and symptoms**
   a. Complaints by the patient of tightness and swelling (e.g., "My ring is too tight," "My skin feels too tight") suggest edema.
   b. Nausea, vomiting, anorexia, bloating, or abdominal pain on exertion may reflect hepatic and visceral engorgement, resulting from venous pressure elevation.
2. **Physical findings**
   a. JVD reflects increased venous pressure and is a cardinal sign of HF.
   b. S_3 ventricular gallop (see III.A.2.c).
   c. S_4 atrial gallop intensifies on inspiration in right-sided failure.
   d. Hepatomegaly (a tender, enlarged liver) is revealed when pushing on the edge of the liver results in a fluid reflux into the jugular veins, causing bulging (positive hepatojugular reflux).
   e. Bilateral leg edema is an early sign of right-sided HF; pitting ankle edema signals more advanced HF. However, edema is common to many disorders, and a pattern of associated findings, such as concurrent neck vein distention, is required for differential diagnosis.
3. **Laboratory findings. Elevated levels of hepatic enzymes**—for example, alanine aminotransferase (ALT)—reflect hepatic congestion.
4. **Evaluation of natriuretic peptides.** A class IIa recommendation that was given for the measurement of natriuretic peptides (brain natriuretic peptide [BNP] and N-terminal prohormone of BNP [NT-proBNP]) can be useful in the evaluation of patients presenting in the urgent care setting in whom the diagnosis of HF is uncertain. Elevated levels of BNP have been associated with a reduction in the LVEF, as well as in left ventricular hypertrophy, acute myocardial infarction, and ischemia, although they are not specific for HF and can occur in patients with obstructive lung disease and pulmonary emboli. The guidelines suggest that elevated levels of BNP tend to occur more in HF patients with low ejection fractions as compared to those with normal ejection fractions. In conclusion, elevated levels of natriuretic peptides may be helpful in adding weight

to a diagnosis of HF but should not be used as the sole evidence in making a diagnosis of HF or for eliminating a diagnosis of HF.

IV. THERAPY

A. **Bed rest**

1. **Advantages**
   a. Bed rest decreases metabolic needs, which reduces cardiac workload.
   b. Reduced workload, in turn, reduces pulse rate and dyspnea.
   c. Bed rest also helps decrease excess fluid volume by promoting diuresis.
2. **Disadvantages.** Physical activity (except during acute decompensation) should be encouraged to avoid physical deconditioning and exercise intolerance. The risk of venous stasis increases with bed rest and can result in thromboembolism. Antiembolism stockings help minimize this risk, as do passive or active leg exercises, when the patient's condition permits.
3. **Progressive ambulation** should follow adequate bed rest.

B. **Dietary controls**

1. **Consuming small but frequent meals** (four to six daily) that are low in calories and residue provide nourishment without unduly increasing metabolic demands.
2. **Moderate sodium restriction** along with daily measurements of weight help maximize the lowest and safest doses of diuretics, a primary tool in reducing central volume in HF.
   a. Renal function should be evaluated to assess sodium conservation if severe sodium restriction is contemplated.
   b. Moderate sodium restriction (2 to 4 g of dietary sodium/day) can be achieved with relative ease by limiting the addition of salt during cooking and at the table.
   c. The patient should be advised about medications and common products that contain sodium and cautioned about their use (e.g., antacids, sodium bicarbonate or baking soda, commercial diet food products, water softeners). *Table 34-2* lists other substances that promote sodium retention.

C. **Drug-related considerations.** Therapeutic interventions might improve cardiac performance in the following ways:

1. Drugs may increase the cardiac ejection fraction by directly stimulating cardiac contractility.
   a. The use of positive inotropic agents can produce immediate benefits; however, the long-term benefit has not been appreciated and in some cases may actually increase morbidity and mortality.
   b. The most recent national guidelines provide a class IIb recommendation with a level C level of evidence for intravenous inotropic drugs, such as dopamine, dobutamine, or milrinone, in patients presenting with documented several systolic dysfunction, low blood pressure, and evidence of low cardiac output, with or without congestion, in order to maintain systemic perfusion and preserve end-organ performance.
2. Drugs may increase the ejection fraction by decreasing the impedance to ejection through relaxation of peripheral blood vessels.
   a. The use of vasodilators, such as nitroprusside, nitroglycerin, and nesiritide, may produce short-term benefit but do not necessarily produce clinical benefits in the long-term.
   b. The most recent national guidelines provide a class IIa recommendation with a level C level of evidence for hospitalized patients with HF who are fluid overloaded in the absence of hypotension, where such agents are added to diuretic therapy or in those patients who have not responded adequately to diuretic therapy.
   c. Hydralazine (Various), an arteriole dilator with afterload reducing properties, has received a class I recommendation with a level A level of evidence in the updated national guidelines, in combination with isosorbide dinitrate to standard medical (i.e., ACEIs, ARBs, β-adrenergic blockers) regimens, to improve outcomes in African Americans with NYHA III or IV HF.
3. Drugs may improve the ejection fraction by affecting the cardiac remodeling process. Neurohormonal antagonists such as ACEIs, β-adrenergic receptor blockers, ARBs, and vasodilator-growth inhibitors, such as nitrates, may not produce immediate benefits, but long-term use might improve clinical status and decrease future cardiac events.
4. ACEIs, ARBs, diuretics, and β-adrenergic blockers usually form the basic core of treatment for HF.

D. ACEIs

1. Recent guidelines recommend the use of ACEIs in many types of patients with HF owing to left ventricular systolic dysfunction unless the patients have a contraindication to their use or have demonstrated intolerance to their use.
   a. ACEIs received a class IIa recommendation with a level A level of evidence for prevention of HF in patients at risk, **stage A**, who have atherosclerotic vascular disease, diabetes mellitus, or hypertension with associated cardiovascular risk factors.
   b. ACEIs received a class I recommendation with a level A level of evidence for use in all patients with a recent or remote history of MI, **stage B**, regardless of ejection fraction or presence of HF, and a class I recommendation with a level A level of evidence for use in patients with a reduced ejection fraction and no symptoms of HF, even if they have not experienced an MI.
   c. ACEIs received a class I recommendation with a level A level of evidence for use in all patients with current or prior symptoms of HF (**stage C**), and reduced LVEF, unless contraindicated.
   d. ACEIs did not receive a recommendation for use in HF patients with **stage D** due to the need for special procedures, such as transplantation, implantable pumps, etc.
   e. ACEIs did receive a class IIb recommendation with a level C level of evidence for use in HF patients with normal LVEFs.
2. Relative contraindications include history of intolerance or adverse reactions, serum potassium > 5.5 mEq/L, serum creatinine levels > 3 mg/dL, symptomatic hypotension, severe renal artery stenosis, and pregnancy.
3. ACEIs have been shown to reduce symptoms, improve clinical status, enhance the overall quality of life, and reduce death, as well as the risk of death or hospitalization in mild, moderate, and severe HF patients with or without CAD.
4. They inhibit the enzyme responsible for the conversion of angiotensin I (a weak vasoconstrictor) to angiotensin II (a potent vasoconstrictor). This action significantly decreases total peripheral resistance, which aids in reducing afterload.
5. Inhibiting the production of angiotensin II interferes with stimulation of aldosterone release, thus indirectly reducing retention of sodium and water, which decreases venous return and preload.
6. In patients with a history of fluid retention or who present with fluid retention, a diuretic can be added to an ACEI.
7. ACEIs are indicated for the long-term management of chronic HF and are generally recommended in combination with a β-adrenergic blocker and diuretic.
8. All ACEIs that have been studied in the treatment of HF have shown benefit. The selection of agent and dose should be based on currently available large-scale studies in which target doses of ACEIs—captopril (Capoten®), enalapril (Vasotec®), lisinopril (Zestril®), perindopril (Aceon®), ramipril (Altace®), and trandolapril (Mavik®)—are different from those used to treat hypertension. *Table 34-4* provides a comparative review of ACEIs currently used in the treatment of HF.
9. Common side effects to be monitored include hypotension (patients should be well hydrated before initiation of ACEIs), dizziness, reduced renal function (increased serum creatinine of 0.5 mg/dL or more requires reassessment), cough, and potassium retention (if potassium levels are high without supplementation, discontinue the ACEI for several days and then try to restart at lower dose).
10. Angioedema is a life-threatening side effect of ACEIs that has been reported to occur in $< 1\%$ of patients. It has been reported to occur at a more frequent rate in black patients, and the suspicion of the reaction would justify the avoidance of ACEIs in such patients.

E. ARBs

1. This class of drugs is now considered a reasonable alternative to the use of ACEIs for similar usage in HF patients.
2. Currently available agents include azilsartan (Edarbi®), candesartan cilexetil (Atacand®), eprosartan (Teveten®), irbesartan (Avapro®), losartan (Cozaar®), olmesartan (Benicar®), telmisartan (Micardis®), and valsartan (Diovan®); and initial studies on several of the agents have shown potential benefits for treating HF.
3. Current guidelines suggest that ACEIs should be preferred over the ARBs. However, ARBs may be used in patients who initially responded to ACEIs and/or are intolerant to ACEIs.

Table 34-4 COMPARATIVE DOSES OF SELECT AGENTS USED IN THE TREATMENT OF HEART FAILURE (HF)

Drug	Initial Daily Dose(s)	Maximal Total Daily Dose
Loop diuretics		
Bumetanide (Various)	0.5–1.0 mg once or twice	10 mg
Furosemide (Lasix®)	20–40 mg once or twice	600 mg
Torsemide (Demadex®)	10–20 mg once	200 mg
Thiazide diuretics		
Chlorthalidone (various)	12.5–25 mg once	200 mg
Chlorothiazide (Diuril®)	250–500 mg once or twice	2000 mg
Hydrochlorothiazide (Microzide®)	25 mg once or twice	200 mg
Indapamide (Various)	2.5 mg once	5 mg
Metolazone (Zaroxolyn®)	2.5 mg once	20 mg
Potassium-sparing diuretics		
Amiloride (Midamor®)	5 mg once	20 mg
Spironolactone (Aldactone®)	12.5–25 mg once	50 mg
Triamterene (Dyrenium®)	50–75 mg twice	300 mg
ACEIs		
Benazepril (Lotensin®)	5 mg daily	20 mg daily
Captopril (Capoten®)	6.25 mg three times	450 mg
Enalapril (Vasotec®)	2.5 mg twice	40 mg
Fosinopril (Monopril®)	5–10 mg once	80 mg
Lisinopril (Zestril®)	2.5–5.0 mg once	40 mg
Moexipril (Univasc®)	Not indicated in HF	
Perindopril (Aceon®)	2 mg once	32 mg
Quinapril (Accupril®)	5 mg twice	40 mg
Ramipril (Altace®)	1.25–2.5 mg once	10 mg
Trandolapril (Mavik®)	1 mg once	4 mg
Angiotensin II receptor blockers		
Candesartan (Atacand®)	4–8 mg once	32 mg
Losartan (Cozaar®)	25–50 mg once	100 mg
Valsartan (Diovan®)	20–40 mg twice	320 mg
Aldosterone antagonists		
Spironolactone (Aldactone®)	12.5 mg once	50 mg
Eplerenone (Inspra®)	25 mg once	50 mg
β-Adrenergic receptor blockers		
Bisoprolol (Zebeta®)	1.25 mg once	10 mg
Carvedilol (Coreg®)	3.125 mg twice	50 mg; 100 mg for patients > 85 kg
Metoprolol succinate (Toprol XL®) (extended-release)	12.5–25 mg once	200 mg

F. **β-Adrenergic blocking agents**

1. Unlike ACEIs, which strictly work by blocking the effects of the renin–angiotensin system, β-adrenergic blockers interfere with the sympathetic nervous system—that is, norepinephrine-induced peripheral vasoconstriction, norepinephrine-induced sodium excretion by the kidney, norepinephrine-induced cardiac hypertrophy, norepinephrine-induced arrhythmia generation, norepinephrine-induced hypokalemia, or norepinephrine-induced cell death (apoptosis) through increased stress owing to norepinephrine stimulation.
2. β-Adrenergic blockers, specifically bisoprolol (Zebeta), sustained-release metoprolol (Toprol XL), and carvedilol (Coreg), have been shown to decrease the risk of death or hospitalization, as well as improve the clinical status of HF patients (*Table 34-4*).
3. β-Adrenergic blockers have been shown to be beneficial in select stages of patients with HF as a result of left ventricular dysfunction, unless they have a contraindication to their use or are unable to tolerate their effects owing to hypotension, bradycardia, bronchospasm, and the like.
   a. β-Adrenergic blockers received a class I with a level A level of evidence in the most recent national guidelines for patients with a recent or remote history of MI regardless of ejection fraction or presence of HF (**stage B**) or in all patients without a history of MI who have a reduced LVEF with no HF symptoms.
   b. β-Adrenergic blockers received a class I with a level A level of evidence in the most recent national guidelines for one of the three agents (i.e., bisoprolol [Zebeta®], carvedilol [Coreg®], and sustained-release metoprolol succinate [Toprol XL®] for all stable HF patients with current or prior symptoms of HF and reduced LVEF, unless contraindicated (**stage C**).
4. β-Adrenergic blockers are generally used in conjunction with diuretics, ACEIs, or ARBs. β-Adrenergic blockers should not be taken without diuretics in patients with a current or recent history of fluid retention to avoid its development and to maintain sodium balance.
5. Side effects of β-adrenergic blockers may occur during the early days of therapy but do not generally prevent their long-term use; and progression of the disease may be reduced, even if symptoms of the disease have not responded to β-adrenergic blocker therapy. Therapy should be initiated with low doses and titrated upward slowly as tolerated.
6. Patients should be monitored for signs of fluid retention by having patients weigh themselves daily and report any significant increases, which might warrant increases in diuretic doses or reductions in the dose of the β-adrenergic blocker. In addition, fatigue, hypotension, bradycardia, and heart block are reported side effects that should be monitored to ensure appropriate attention and management.
7. Studies support the use of β-adrenergic blockers in patients with stage C HF—and not in the acute management of patients, as in an intensive care unit (ICU). Patients should have no or minimal evidence of fluid retention and have no recent evidence for the use of an intravenous inotropic agent. In addition, β-adrenergic blockers should be considered in patients who develop HF post–MI if they are able to tolerate the negative inotropic effects.
8. Initiation of β-adrenergic blockers should not be undertaken until the patient is stable without fluid overload or hypotension and is on concomitant medications, which include diuretics and/or ACEIs or ARBs.
9. Patient education is an important aspect for initiating β-adrenergic blockers therapy, and patients need to be informed that they might not see positive effects for several months after obtaining the target dosage of the agent.

G. **Diuretics**

1. The most recently updated national guidelines provide a class I recommendation with a level C level of evidence for the use of diuretics in patients with current or prior symptoms of HF and reduced LVEF who have evidence of fluid retention (**stage C**). Diuretics are generally best used in conjunction with an ACEI, ARB, and/or β-adrenergic blocker.
2. Diuretics have been shown to cause a reduction in jugular venous pressures, pulmonary congestion, peripheral edema, and body weight in short-term studies and have been shown to improve cardiac function and exercise tolerance in intermediate-term studies.
3. The goal of diuretic therapy is to reduce and eventually eliminate signs and symptoms of fluid retention as assessed by JVD, peripheral edema, or both. Slow titration upward in doses may be necessary to minimize hypotension and should be continued until fluid retention is eliminated.

4. Body weight is an effective method of monitoring fluid losses and is best done on a daily basis by the patient.
5. Patients who experience diuretic resistance or tolerance to their effects might need intravenous administration, a combination of two agents with differing mechanisms (furosemide [Lasix®] and metolazone [Zaroxolyn®]) or the addition of agents, such as dopamine or dobutamine, which increase renal blood flow. Furthermore, evaluation of patient drug profiles may identify the addition of sodium-retaining agents, such as nonsteroidal anti-inflammatory drugs (NSAIDs).
6. All diuretics increase urine volume and sodium excretion but differ in their pharmacological properties.
7. **Select diuretic classes**
   a. **Thiazide diuretics** include chlorothiazide (Diuril®), hydrochlorothiazide (Microzide®), chlorthalidone (Various), and indapamide (Various). They are effective and commonly used in HF, specifically in patients with hypertension, but they deplete potassium stores in the process. These agents are relatively weak because they are able to increase the fractional excretion of sodium to only 5% to 10% of the filtered load. However, they have been shown to lose their effectiveness in HF patients with moderately impaired renal function (creatinine clearance < 30 mL/min).
   b. **Loop diuretics** include furosemide (Lasix®), ethacrynic acid (Edecrin®), bumetanide (Various), and torsemide (Demadex®) and have become the preferred diuretics. They have the ability to increase sodium excretion to 20% to 25% of the filtered load and to maintain their efficacy until renal function is severely impaired (creatinine clearance < 5 mL/min) plus have the added advantage of reducing venous return independent of diuresis. In addition, furosemide's action is more intense, making it useful as a rapid-acting intravenous agent in reversing acute pulmonary edema, owing to its direct dilating effects on pulmonary vasculature (see *Table 34-4* for dosage).
   c. **Potassium-sparing diuretics** include amiloride (Midamor®), spironolactone (Aldactone®), and triamterene (Dyrenium®) and may help avoid the incidence of hypokalemia. However, they also possess a weaker diuretic effect than the other diuretics. As the number of HF patients receiving ACEIs or ARBs continues to increase, fewer patients may require supplemental potassium therapy.
8. **Aldosterone antagonists.** Spironolactone (Aldactone®) is a potassium-sparing diuretic but was the first aldosterone antagonist available for clinical use in the United States, when it had been shown to have direct blocking effects on the actions of aldosterone. Results from a large study, the Randomized Aldactone Evaluation Study (RALES), revealed that the addition of low doses (12.5 to 25 mg daily) of spironolactone to patients with class IV symptoms (NYHA) taking ACEIs reduced the risk of death and hospitalization.
   a. Current national guidelines provide a class I recommendation with a level C level of evidence that spironolactone (Aldactone®) be considered in patients with **stage C** HF—as add-on therapy to ACEIs or ARBs and a β-adrenergic blocker—who can be closely monitored for changes in renal function and potassium levels in those patients where previous therapy was not effective in resolving congestion.
   b. Patients receiving spironolactone should have serum potassium levels evaluated and reduced to < 5.0 mEq/L along with a serum creatinine level < 2.5 mg/dL before initiation of therapy. Potassium levels should be routinely monitored to prevent the subsequent development of hyperkalemia.
   c. Eplerenone (Inspra®) was the second aldosterone receptor antagonist introduced and is currently indicated in the treatment of hypertension and in post-MI patients with HF. It has not yet been formalized into the current national guidelines as spironolactone (Aldactone®) has been.

H. **Vasodilators**
1. The current national guidelines provide a class IIa and a level C for the use of vasodilators in hospitalized patients with evidence of severely symptomatic fluid overload in the absence of systemic hypotension, when added to diuretics and/or in those who do not respond to diuretics alone.
2. These agents include nitroprusside (Nitropress®), nitroglycerin (Various), and nesiritide (Natrecor®)
3. Individual agents
   a. **Nitroprusside** (**Nitropress®**) is administered intravenously in doses of 0.3 to 10 mcg/kg/min as a continuous infusion in order to provide potent dilation of both arteries and veins, with a resultant decrease in preload and afterload. It has a very short onset of action and very short duration of action. Nitroprusside is capable of causing a substantial fall in blood pressure and usually will

require intensive invasive monitoring to prevent large fluctuations in clinical outcomes. Long-term use is capable of causing thiocyanate toxicity, primarily in those with reduced renal function.

b. Nesiritide (Natrecor®) has been shown to effectively reduce left ventricular filling pressures, but the outcomes on cardiac output, urinary output, and sodium output have had varying results. An important adverse effect on the kidney has been reported resulting in the need for closer monitoring.

(1) Nesiritide (Natrecor®) is a recombinant form of human BNP, which is a naturally occurring hormone secreted by the ventricles. It is the first of this drug class to become available for human use in the United States.

(2) Nesiritide is approved for the intravenous treatment of patients with acutely decompensated HF associated with shortness of breath at rest or with minimal activity.

(3) Nesiritide binds to natriuretic peptide receptors in blood vessels, resulting in increased production of cyclic guanosine monophosphate (cGMP) in target tissues, which mediates vasodilation. In HF, nesiritide reduces pulmonary capillary wedge pressure and systemic vascular resistance.

(4) Initial treatment involves a bolus dose of 2.0 mcg/kg followed by a continuous intravenous infusion of 0.01 mcg/kg/min to a maximum dose of 0.03 mcg/kg/min.

(5) Monitoring for hypotension, elevated serum creatinine, headache, nausea, and dizziness is the key to successful use. Concomitant use of ACEIs may increase the risk of symptomatic hypotension (systolic blood pressure < 90 mm Hg and syncope).

(6) Nesiritide has been shown to improve symptoms in the setting of acute HF, but the effect on morbidity and mortality has not yet been proven. At this point in time, owing to lack of pivotal studies demonstrating its benefit, nesiritide's use as intermittent or continuous outpatient treatment is not recommended.

c. Nitrates. Venous dilation by nitrates increases venous pooling, which decreases preload.

(1) Their arterial effects seem to result in decreased afterload with continued therapy.

(2) Nitrates are available in many forms and doses. Because individual reactions to these agents vary widely, dosages have to be adjusted; but, in general, they are higher for HF than for angina. *Table 34-5* provides examples of nitrate doses that have been used in HF.

d. Hydralazine (Various). This arteriole dilator decreases afterload and increases cardiac output in patients with HF. As mentioned next, it is also used in combination with nitrates in select patient populations with HF.

e. Combination therapy. Hydralazine has been used with isosorbide dinitrate (Isordil) to reduce afterload (or with nitroglycerin to reduce preload) for treating chronic HF.

(1) As mentioned previously, hydralazine received a class I recommendation with a level A level of evidence in the updated national guidelines, in combination with isosorbide dinitrate to standard medical (i.e., ACEIs, ARBs, β-adrenergic blockers) regimens, in order to improve outcomes in African Americans with NYHA III or IV HF.

(2) The combination has also received a class IIa recommendation with a level B level of evidence, for adding to patients with reduced LVEF who are already receiving ACEIs and β-adrenergic blockers for symptomatic HF and who have persistent symptoms.

Table 34-5 EXAMPLES OF NITRATES THAT HAVE BEEN USED IN HEART FAILURE

Form of Nitrate	Typical Dose	Dosing Interval
Intravenous nitroglycerin (Various)	5–200 mcg/min	Continuous infusion
Nitroglycerin buccal tablets (Nitrostat®)	1–3 mg	4–6 hrs
Nitroglycerin capsules (sustained release) (Various)	6.5–19.5 mg	4–6 hrs
Nitroglycerin ointment (Nitro-Bid®)	1–3 inches	4–6 hrs
Sublingual nitroglycerin (Various)	0.4 mg	1–2 hrs
Oral isosorbide dinitrate (Various)	10–60 mg	4–6 hrs
Sublingual isosorbide dinitrate (Various)	5–10 mg	4 hrs

(3) The combination of these two agents—hydralazine and isosorbide dinitrate (BiDil®), 37.5 mg/20 mg tablets respectively, should not be used as initial therapy over ACEIs, ARBs, or β-adrenergic blockers but could be considered in patients who have persistent symptoms despite the use of these agents.

(4) Suggested dosing regimens include hydralazine (various) 50 to 100 mg four times daily and isosorbide dinitrate (Isordil Titradose®) 10 to 40 mg three times daily.

I. Digitalis glycosides

1. Digitalis, specifically digoxin (Lanoxin®), continues to play a role in the treatment of HF, but ongoing evaluations have altered its place in the long-term management of HF. In the most recent national guidelines provided, digoxin (Lanoxin®) received a class IIa recommendation with a level B level of evidence, as beneficial in patients with current or prior symptoms.
2. Digitalis also received a class IIb recommendation with a level C level of evidence for its lack of proven usefulness to minimize symptoms of HF in patients with HF and normal LVEF.
3. Digoxin (Lanoxin®) received a class IIa recommendation with a level A level of evidence to control the ventricular rate in HF patients with atrial fibrillation.
4. **Therapeutic effects**
   a. **Positive inotropic effects** were previously felt to provide most of the benefits through increased cardiac output, decreased cardiac filling pressure, decreased venous and capillary pressure, increased renal blood flow, and decreased heart size.
   b. Recent evidence suggests that digitalis acts by furthering the activation of neurohormonal systems rather than as a positive inotropic agent. This results in deactivation of renin–angiotensin–aldosterone compensation, which promotes diuresis, reduces fluid volume, decreases renal sodium reabsorption, and diminishes edema.
   c. **Negative chronotropic effects** occur from the effect of digitalis on the sinoatrial (SA) node when given in doses that produce high total body stores (e.g., 15 to 18 mcg/kg). This effect is likely to be beneficial to control the ventricular rate in HF patients with atrial fibrillation.
5. **Choice of agent.** All of the digitalis glycosides have similar properties; however, digoxin is the most commonly used preparation in the United States.
   a. Digoxin is available in tablet, injection, elixir, and capsule forms.
   b. Calculation of doses must factor in the differences in systemic availability among these forms. For example, digoxin solution in capsules is more bioavailable than digoxin tablets; therefore, 0.125-mg tablets are equivalent to 0.1-mg capsules. In the majority of patients, the dosage of digoxin should be the equivalent of 0.125 to 0.25 mg daily of the tablet formulation.
6. **Dosage and administration.** The range between therapeutic and toxic doses is extremely narrow. There is no magic threshold level for digoxin therapy, but serum concentrations of 0.8 to 1.0 ng/mL have been associated with therapeutic response and minimal toxicity.
7. **Precautions and monitoring effects**
   a. Decreased potassium levels favor digoxin binding to cardiac cells and increase its effect, thus increasing the likelihood of digitalis toxicity. This antagonism is particularly significant for the HF patient who is receiving a diuretic (many of which decrease potassium levels). Conversely, increased potassium levels decrease digoxin binding and decrease its effect. This is likely in patients taking potassium or an ACEI or ARB (which increase potassium reabsorption).
   b. **Calcium** ions act synergistically with digoxin, and increased levels increase the force of myocardial contraction. At excessive levels, arrhythmias and systolic standstill can develop.
   c. **Magnesium** levels are inversely related to digoxin activity. As magnesium levels decrease, the predisposition to toxicity increases and, within reason, vice versa.
   d. **Serum digoxin levels**
      (1) In cardiac glycoside therapy, the patient's clinical state is the most practical barometer of a successful regimen. However, should questions arise about compliance, absorption, or a drug–drug interaction, serum digoxin levels may be helpful.
      (2) After oral ingestion of digoxin, serum levels rise rapidly, then drop sharply as the drug enters the myocardium and other tissues. Therefore, a meaningful evaluation requires a determination of the relationship between serum digoxin levels and myocardial tissue levels.
      (3) The most meaningful results are obtained if serum samples are taken after steady state has been reached and 6 to 8 hrs after an oral dose (3 to 4 hrs after an intravenous dose).

e. **Renal function studies.** Because the kidney is the primary metabolic route for **digoxin**, renal function studies, such as serum creatinine levels, aid the evaluation of elimination kinetics for digoxin.

8. Digitalis toxicity is a fairly common occurrence because of the narrow therapeutic range and can be fatal in a significant percentage of patients experiencing a toxic reaction. Patients should be routinely monitored for drug–drug interactions that might exist for patients receiving digitalis therapy.
   a. **Signs of toxicity** include the following:
      (1) Anorexia, a common and early sign
      (2) Fatigue, headache, and malaise
      (3) Nausea and vomiting
      (4) Mental confusion and disorientation
      (5) Alterations in visual perception (e.g., blurring, yellowing, a halo effect)
      (6) Cardiac effects:
         (a) Premature ventricular contractions and ventricular tachycardia and fibrillation
         (b) SA and atrioventricular (AV) block
         (c) Atrial tachycardia with AV block
   b. **Treatment of toxicity**
      (1) Digitalis is discontinued immediately, as is any potassium-depleting diuretic.
      (2) If the patient is hypokalemic, potassium supplements are administered and serum levels are monitored to avoid hyperkalemia through overcompensation. However, potassium supplements are contraindicated in a patient with severe AV block.
      (3) Arrhythmias may be treated with lidocaine (Xylocaine®) (usually a 100-mg bolus, followed by infusion at 2 to 4 mg/min) or phenytoin (Dilantin®) (as a slow intravenous infusion of 25 to 50 mg/min, to a maximum of 1 g).
      (4) Cholestyramine (Questran®) has been used effectively in an acute digoxin overdose by binding to digitalis, and which may help prevent absorption and reabsorption of digitalis in the bile.
      (5) Patients with very high serum digoxin levels (such as those resulting from a suicidal overdose) may benefit from the use of purified digoxin-specific Fab fragment antibodies (DigiFab). One vial (40 mg) will bind 0.5 mg of digitalis. The dosage is calculated based on the estimated total body store of digitalis.

J. **Calcium-channel blockers**
1. Owing to the lack of evidence supporting efficacy, calcium-channel blockers should not be used for the treatment of HF. Current guidelines provides a class III recommendation with a level C level of evidence, and states that "Calcium-channel blockers with negative inotropic effects may be harmful in asymptomatic patients with low LVEF and no symptoms of HF after an MI."

K. **Inotropic agents**
1. Have been used in the emergency treatment of patients with HF. However, long-term oral therapy with these agents has not improved symptoms or clinical status and has been reported to increase mortality, especially in patients with advanced HF.
2. The current national guidelines provide a class IIb recommendation with a level C level of evidence for the use of intravenous inotropic drugs, such as dopamine (Various), dobutamine (Various), or milrinone (Various), as reasonable treatments for patients presenting to the hospital with documented severe systolic dysfunction, low blood pressure, and evidence of low cardiac output, with or without congestion, in order to maintain system perfusion and preserve end-organ performance.
3. The current national guidelines also provide a class III recommendation with a level B level of evidence for the use of parenteral inotropic agents in normotensive patients in the hospitalized setting, with acute decompensated HF without evidence of decreased organ perfusion.
4. Current national guidelines provide a class IIb recommendation with a level C for the use of continuous intravenous infusions of positive inotropic agents for palliation of symptoms in patients with refractory end-stage HF—**stage D**.
5. Current national guidelines provide a class III recommendation with a level A level of evidence and states that the "routine intermittent infusions of vasoactive and positive inotropic agents are not recommended for patients with refractory end-stage HF—**stage D**."
   a. Dopamine (Various) continuous intravenous infusions
      (1) **Low doses** of 2 to 5 mcg/kg/min stimulate specific dopamine receptors within the kidney to increase renal blood flow, and thus increase urine output.

(2) **Moderate doses** of 5 to 10 mcg/kg/min increase cardiac output (positive inotropic effect) in HF patients.

(3) **High doses**

(a) As doses are raised above 10 mcg/kg/min, α-adrenergic stimulation occurs peripherally, resulting in increased total peripheral resistance and pulmonary pressures.

(b) When the infusion exceeds 8 to 9 mcg/kg/min, the patient should be monitored for tachycardia. If the infusion is slowed or interrupted, the adverse effect should disappear because dopamine has a very short half-life in plasma.

b. Dobutamine (Various) continuous intravenous infusions

(1) Patients who are unresponsive to, or adversely affected by, dopamine may benefit from dobutamine in doses of 5 to 20 mcg/kg/min.

(2) Although dobutamine resembles dopamine chemically, its actions differ somewhat. For example, dobutamine does not directly affect renal receptors and, therefore, does not act as a renal vasodilator. It increases urinary output only through increased cardiac output.

(3) Serious arrhythmias are a potential occurrence, although less likely to occur than with dopamine. Slowing or interrupting the infusion usually reverses this effect, as it does for dopamine.

(4) Dobutamine and dopamine have been used together to treat cardiogenic shock, but similar use in HF has yet to be accepted.

c. Inamrinone (Various) continuous intravenous infusion is referred to as nonglycoside, nonsympathomimetic, inotropic agents.

(1) A bipyridine derivative, inamrinone has both a positive inotropic effect and a vasodilating effect.

(2) By inhibiting phosphodiesterase located specifically in the cardiac cells, it increases the amount of cyclic adenosine monophosphate (cAMP).

(3) Inamrinone has been used in patients with HF that have been refractory to treatment with other inotropic agents.

(4) Effective regimens have used loading intravenous infusions of 0.75 mg/kg over 2 to 3 mins followed by maintenance infusions of 5 to 10 mg/kg/min.

(5) **Precautions and monitoring effects**

(a) Inamrinone is unstable in dextrose solutions and should be added to saline solutions instead. Because of fluid balance concerns, this can be a potential problem in patients with HF.

(b) Because of the peripheral dilating properties, patients should be monitored for hypotension.

(c) Thrombocytopenia has occurred and is dose dependent and asymptomatic.

(d) Ventricular rates may increase in patients with atrial flutter or fibrillation.

d. Milrinone (Various) continuous intravenous infusion is similar to inamrinone. It possesses both inotropic and vasodilatory properties.

(1) This agent has been used as short-term management to treat patients with HF.

(2) Most milrinone patients in clinical trials have also been receiving digoxin and diuretics.

(3) Effective dosing regimens have used a loading dose of 50 mcg/kg administered slowly over 10 mins intravenously, followed by maintenance doses of 0.375 mcg/kg/min by continuous infusion, based on the clinical status of the patient.

(4) **Precautions and monitoring effects**

(a) Renal impairment significantly prolongs the elimination rate of milrinone, and infusions need to be reduced accordingly.

(b) Monitoring is necessary for the potential arrhythmias occurring in HF, which may be increased by drugs such as milrinone and other inotropic agents.

(c) Blood pressure and heart rate should be monitored when administering milrinone, owing to its vasodilatory effects and its potential to induce arrhythmias.

(d) Additional side effects include mild-to-moderate headache, tremor, and thrombocytopenia.

L. Patient education

1. Patients should be made aware of the importance of taking their medications exactly as prescribed and should be advised to watch for signs of toxicity.

2. Patients should be educated on the need for lifestyle modifications that will have a positive effect on reducing HF development and reducing HF symptoms, including daily weight monitoring,

Table 35-3 HEPARIN DOSAGE ADJUSTMENT PROTOCOL[a]

Patient's aPTT (sec)[b]	Repeat Bolus Dose (units)	Stop Infusion (min)	Change Rate of Infusion (mL/hr)[c] [units/24 hrs]	Timing of Next aPPT
< 50	5000	0	+3 [2880]	6 hrs
50–59	0	0	+3 [2880]	6 hrs
60–85[d]	0	0	0	Next morning
86–95	0	0	−2 [−1920]	Next morning
96–120	0	30	−2 [−1920]	6 hrs
> 120	0	60	−4 [−3840]	6 hrs

[a]Starting dose of 5000 units intravenous IV bolus followed by 32,000 units/24 hrs as a continuous infusion. First aPTT performed 6 hrs after the bolus injection; dosage adjustments are made according to protocol and the aPTT is repeated as indicated in the far-right column.
[b]The normal range for aPTT with Dade Actin FS reagent is 27–35 secs; the range may vary, depending on the sensitivity of the reagent.
[c]Concentration of heparin equal to 40 units/mL.
[d]A therapeutic range of 60–85 secs is equivalent to a heparin level of 0.2–0.4 units/mL by whole blood protamine titration or 0.3–0.7 units/mL as a plasma antifactor Xa level. The therapeutic range varies with the responsiveness of the aPTT reagent to heparin.
aPTT, activated partial thromboplastin time.
Used with permission: Cone Health Clinical References-Anticoagulation Protocol.

b. Traditionally, it was taught that for many aPTT reagents, a therapeutic effect was achieved with an **aPTT ratio of 1.5 to 2.5**.

c. However, because aPTT reagents may vary in their sensitivity, it is **inappropriate to use the same aPTT ratio (i.e., 1.5 to 2.5) for all reagents**. The therapeutic range for each aPTT reagent should be calibrated to be equivalent to a heparin level of 0.2 to 0.4 units/mL by whole blood (protamine titration) or to an **antifactor Xa level (i.e., plasma heparin level) of 0.3 to 0.7 units/mL collected at the sixth hour for UFH**.

B. Oral anticoagulants—warfarin

1. Indications

a. Warfarin is proven effective in the
  (1) primary and secondary prevention of VTED;
  (2) prevention of systemic arterial embolism in patients with tissue and mechanical prosthetic heart valves or atrial fibrillation;
  (3) prevention of acute myocardial infarction (MI) in patients with peripheral arterial disease; and
  (4) prevention of stroke, recurrent infarction, and death in patients with acute MI.

b. Warfarin may also be used in patients with valvular heart disease to prevent systemic arterial embolism, although its effectiveness has never been demonstrated by a randomized clinical trial.

2. Mechanism of action

a. Oral anticoagulants (e.g., warfarin) are vitamin K antagonists, producing their anticoagulant effect by **interfering with the cyclic interconversion of vitamin K and its 2-, 3-epoxide (vitamin K epoxide)**.

b. Inhibition of this process leads to the depletion of vitamin K_{H2} and **results in the production of hemostatically defective, vitamin K–dependent coagulant proteins or clotting factors (prothrombin or factors II, VII, IX, and X)**.

c. These vitamin K–dependent coagulant proteins or clotting factors (factors VII, IX, X, and II, respectively) decline over 6 to 96 hrs.

3. Pharmacokinetics

a. Warfarin is a **racemic mixture** of roughly equal amounts of two optically active isomers: the **R and S forms**.

b. Warfarin is rapidly absorbed from the gastrointestinal tract and reaches maximal blood concentrations in healthy volunteers in 90 mins.

c. **Dose response** to warfarin is influenced by
  (1) Pharmacokinetic factors (i.e., differences in absorption and metabolic clearance)
  (2) Pharmacodynamic factors (i.e., differences in the hemostatic response to given concentrations of warfarin)
  (3) Technical factors—for example, inaccuracies in prothrombin time (PT) and international normalized ratio (INR) testing and reporting

Table 35-4 FACTORS THAT MAY POTENTIATE OR INHIBIT WARFARIN EFFECTS

Factor	Potentiate Anticoagulant Effect	Inhibit Anticoagulant Effect
Drugs	Phenylbutazone Metronidazole Sulfinpyrazone Trimethoprim-sulfamethoxazole Disulfiram Amiodarone Erythromycin Anabolic steroids Clofibrate Cimetidine Omeprazole Thyroxine Ketoconazole Isoniazid Fluconazole Piroxicam Tamoxifen Quinidine Vitamin E (large doses) Phenytoin Penicillin	Cholestyramine Barbiturates Rifampin Griseofulvin Carbamazepine
Other	Low vitamin K intake Reduced vitamin K absorption Liver disease Hypermetabolic states (e.g., thyrotoxicosis) Alcohol (chronic use)	High vitamin K intake Alcohol (acute use)

Used with permission: Cone Health Clinical References-Anticoagulation Protocol.

(4) Patient-specific factors—for example, diet (increased intake of green, leafy vegetables), poor patient compliance (missed doses, self-medication, alcohol consumption) and poor communication between patient and physician (undisclosed use of drugs that may interact with warfarin) (*Table 35-4*).

4. Administration and dosage

a. **Warfarin**, a coumarin compound, is the most widely used oral anticoagulant in North America. Although it is primarily **administered orally**, an injectable preparation is available in the United States.

b. Commence oral anticoagulant therapy in the inpatient setting with the **anticipated daily maintenance dose of warfarin**, which can be variable.

c. **The initial dose of warfarin therapy can be flexible** (*Table 35-5*).

(1) Patient-specific parameters used to determine the initial dose of warfarin include the patient's weight (e.g., obesity, concurrent use of interacting drugs known to inhibit the anticoagulant effect of warfarin and the desired rapid anticoagulant effect).

(2) Based on these patient-specific parameters, some clinicians may use a larger initial dose of warfarin (e.g., 7.5 to 10 mg), which should not be misconstrued as a loading dose. For patients sufficiently healthy to be treated as outpatients—specific to VTE treatment—the suggestion is to commence warfarin therapy with 10 mg daily for the first 2 days, followed by dosing based upon the INR response.

d. The initial dose of warfarin should be **overlapped with UFH, LMWH, or a pentasaccharide** for a minimum of **5** days for treating established embolic disease to 7 days (*Table 35-1*).

Table 35-5 PRACTICAL ORAL ANTICOAGULATION DOSING

Day	Rapid Anticoagulation	Anticoagulation[a]
1	5–10 mg	5 mg
2	5–10 mg	5 mg
3	2.5–7.5 mg (adjust based on INR)[b]	5 mg (adjust based on INR)[b]

[a]Rapid anticoagulation is not required or there is a risk of bleeding.
[b]Adjust dosage based on INR until the INR is stable and therapeutic.
INR, international normalized ratio.
Used with permission: Cone Health Clinical References-Anticoagulation Protocol.

e. The **duration of warfarin therapy** depends on each patient's indication(s) for use (*Table 35-6*).

f. **Reversal of warfarin effects** may be necessary owing to an elevated INR or bleeding complications associated with oral anticoagulant therapy (*Table 35-7*).

5. **Monitoring warfarin therapy.** PT and INR monitoring are usually to be performed at baseline and daily when commencing warfarin in the inpatient acute care setting. Commencing warfarin in the outpatient setting after establishing a baseline INR may see the subsequent INR determinations being performed based upon well-established protocols specific to the outpatient setting. In either setting (inpatient or outpatient), INRs will be performed daily on commencing oral anticoagulant therapy (e.g., warfarin), until such time that the INR has been found to be therapeutic.

a. Laboratory monitoring is performed by measuring the **PT** for calculation of the INR.

(1) The PT is **responsive to suppression of three** of the four vitamin K–dependent procoagulant **clotting factors** (**prothrombin** or **factors II**, **VII**, and **X**).

(2) The common commercial PT reagents vary markedly in their responsiveness to coumarin-induced reduction in clotting factors; therefore, PT results reported using different reagents are not interchangeable among laboratories.

b. The problem of variability in responsiveness of PT reagents has been overcome by the introduction of a standardized test known as the **INR**.

(1) The INR is equal to:

$$\text{INR} = \left(\frac{\text{patient PT}}{\text{mean laboratory control PT}}\right)^{ISI}$$

where ISI (international sensitivity index) is a measure of the responsiveness of a given thromboplastin to reduction of the vitamin K–dependent coagulation factors. The **lower the ISI**, the **more responsive the reagent** and the closer the derived INR will be to the observed PT ratio.

(2) Current recommendations suggest two levels of therapeutic intensity: a less-intense range corresponding to an INR of 2.0 to 3.0, and a more-intense range corresponding to an INR of 2.5 to 3.5. The range corresponds to the indication (*Table 35-8*).

Table 35-6 DURATION OF WARFARIN THERAPY[a]

Duration	Indications
3–6 months	First event with reversible[b] or time-limited risk factor
≥ 6 months	Idiopathic venous thromboembolism, first event
12 months to lifetime	First event[c] with cancer (until resolved), anticardiolipin antibody, antithrombin deficiency
	Recurrent event, idiopathic or with thrombophilia

[a]See Table 43-4 for factors that may influence warfarin effects. All recommendations are subject to modification by individual characteristics, including patient preference, age, comorbidity, and likelihood of recurrence.
[b]Reversible or time-limited risk factors: surgery, trauma, immobilization, estrogen use.
[c]Proper duration of therapy is unclear in first event with homozygous factor V Leiden, homocystinemia, deficiency of protein C or S or multiple thrombophilias, and in recurrent events with reversible risk factors.
Used with permission: Cone Health Clinical References-Anticoagulation Protocol.

Table 35-7 GUIDELINES FOR REVERSAL OF WARFARIN EFFECTS

Clinical Situation	Guidelines
INR > therapeutic range but < 5.0; no clinically significant bleeding, rapid reversal not indicated for reasons of surgical intervention	
INR significantly above therapeutic range	Lower the dose or omit the next dose; resume warfarin therapy at a lower dose when the INR approaches desired range.
INR minimally above therapeutic range	Dose reduction may not be necessary.
INR > 5.0 but < 9.0; no clinically significant bleeding	
No additional risk factors for bleeding	Omit the next dose or two of warfarin; monitor INR more frequently; resume warfarin therapy at a lower dose when the INR is in therapeutic range.
Increased risk of bleeding	Omit the next dose of warfarin; give vitamin K_1 (1.0–2.5 mg orally).
More rapid reversal needed before urgent surgery or dental extraction	Give vitamin K_1 (2–4 mg orally); closely monitor INR; repeat dose of vitamin K_1 if INR not substantially reduced by 24–48 hrs.
INR > 9.0; no clinically significant bleeding	Give vitamin K_1 (3–5 mg orally); closely monitor INR; repeat dose of vitamin K_1 if INR not substantially reduced by 24–48 hrs.
INR > 20.0; serious bleeding, major warfarin overdose requiring very rapid reversal of anticoagulant effect	Give vitamin K_1 (10 mg by slow intravenous infusion) with fresh frozen plasma transfusion or prothrombin complex concentrate, depending on urgency; vitamin K_1 injections may be needed every 12 hrs.
Life-threatening bleeding, serious warfarin overdose	Give prothrombin complex concentrate with vitamin K_1 (10 mg by slow intravenous infusion); repeat if necessary, depending on INR.
Continuing warfarin therapy indicated after high doses of vitamin K_1	Give heparin until the effects of vitamin K_1 have been reversed and patient is responsive to warfarin.

INR, international normalized ratio.
Used with permission: Cone Health Clinical References-Anticoagulation Protocol.

(3) Once the desired therapeutic INR has been achieved for 2 consecutive days (e.g., for concomitant heparin plus warfarin overlap therapy), follow-up INR monitoring can be performed according to the following protocol:
- **(a)** Week 1: monitor INR two or three times
- **(b)** Week 2: monitor INR two times
- **(c)** Weeks 3 to 6: monitor INR once a week

Table 35-8 RECOMMENDED THERAPEUTIC GOAL AND RANGE FOR ORAL ANTICOAGULANT THERAPY

	INR	
Indication	**Goal**	**Range**
Prophylaxis of venous thrombosis (high-risk surgery)	2.5	2.0–3.0
Treatment of venous thrombosis	2.5	2.0–3.0
Treatment of pulmonary embolism	2.5	2.0–3.0
Prevention of systemic embolism	2.5	2.0–3.0
Tissue heart valves	2.5	2.0–3.0
Anterior myocardial infarction (to prevent systemic embolism)	2.5	2.0–3.0
Anterior myocardial infarction (to prevent recurrent infarction)	3.0	2.5–3.5
Valvular heart disease	2.5	2.0–3.0
Atrial fibrillation	2.5	2.0–3.0
Mechanical prosthetic valves (high risk)	3.0	2.5–3.5

INR, international normalized ratio.
Used with permission: Cone Health Clinical References-Anticoagulation Protocol.

(d) Weeks 7 to 14: monitor INR once every 2 weeks
(e) Week 15 to end of therapy: monitor INR once every 4 weeks (if INR dose responsiveness remains stable; if dose adjustment is necessary, a more frequent monitoring schedule is employed until stable dose responsiveness is achieved)

c. Upon commencing oral anticoagulant therapy, **prolongation of the PT/INR** does not occur until depletion of the vitamin K–dependent procoagulant clotting factors occurs. This delay is **variable over 2 to 4 days**. During this delay, if active venous thrombosis is present, either UFH, LMWH, or a synthetic pentasaccharide is concomitantly commenced to adequately anticoagulate the patient while awaiting the therapeutic effect of warfarin.

C. Low-molecular-weight heparin

1. **Indications**
   a. LMWH indications vary by manufacturer.
   b. Each of the LMWHs has been evaluated in a large number of randomized clinical trials and has been proven to be safe and efficacious for **the prevention and treatment of VTE**.
   c. To date, different LMWHs have been evaluated for their role in
      (1) prevention of venous thrombosis,
      (2) treatment of VTED, and
      (3) management of unstable angina pectoris/non–Q-wave MI.
2. **Chemistry.** LMWHs are fragments of standard commercial-grade heparin produced by either chemical or enzymatic depolymerization. LMWHs are approximately one-third the size of heparin. Like **heparin**, which has a **mean molecular weight of 15,000 Da** (range 3000 to 30,000 Da), **LMWHs** are heterogeneous in size with a **mean molecular weight of 4000 to 5000 Da** (range 1000 to 10,000 Da).
3. Mechanism of action
   a. LMWHs achieve their **major anticoagulant effect by binding to antithrombin** through a unique pentasaccharide sequence that enhances the ability of antithrombin **to inactivate factor IIa (thrombin) and factor Xa**.
      (1) Heparin and **LMWHs catalyze the inactivation of factor IIa (thrombin) by binding to antithrombin through the unique pentasaccharide sequence and to thrombin to form a ternary complex**. A minimum chain length of 18 saccharides (including the pentasaccharide sequence) is required for ternary complex formation.
         (a) Virtually, all heparin molecules contain at least 18 saccharide units.
         (b) Only 20% to 50% of the different LMWHs contain fragments with 18 or more saccharide units.
         (c) Therefore, **compared with heparin, which has an anti-factor Xa to anti-factor IIa binding affinity ratio of approximately 1:1**, the various commercial **LMWHs have an antifactor Xa to antifactor IIa binding affinity ratio varying from 2:1 up to 4:1**, depending on their molecular size distribution (*Table 35-9*).
      (2) In contrast, inactivation of factor Xa by antithrombin does not require binding of the heparin molecules to the clotting enzyme. Therefore, inactivation of factor Xa is achieved by small molecular weight heparin fragments provided that they contain the high-affinity pentasaccharide.

Table 35-9 PHARMACOKINETIC AND PHARMACODYNAMIC PARAMETERS OF DIFFERENT LOW-MOLECULAR-WEIGHT HEPARINS (LMWHS)

LMWH	Brand Name	Average Molecular Weight	Bioavailability	Half-Life	Xa:IIa Binding-Affinity Ratio
Dalteparin	Fragmin	6000 Da	87%	3–5 hrs	2.7:1
Enoxaparin	Lovenox	4500 Da	92%	4.5 hrs	3.8:1
Tinzaparin	Innohep	6500 Da	87%	3.9 hrs	2.8:1

b. The **antithrombotic and hemorrhagic effects** of heparin have been compared with LMWHs in a variety of **experimental animal models**.
   (1) When compared on a gravimetric basis, **LMWHs are said to cause decreased** potential for **hemorrhagic episodes**.
   (2) These differences in the relative antithrombotic to hemorrhagic ratios among these polysaccharides could be explained by the observation that **LMWHs have less inhibitory effects on platelet function** and vascular permeability.

4. **Pharmacokinetics.** The plasma recoveries and pharmacokinetics of LMWHs differ from heparin because of differences in the binding properties of the two sulfated polysaccharides to plasma proteins and endothelial cells.
   a. LMWHs bind much less avidly to heparin-binding proteins than heparin; a property that contributes to the superior bioavailability of LMWHs at low doses and their more predictable anticoagulation effect.
   b. LMWHs do not bind to endothelial cells in culture; a property that could account for their longer plasma half-life and their dose-independent clearance. Principally, the renal route clears LMWHs; therefore, the biologic half-life of LMWHs is increased in patients with renal failure.

5. **Administration and dosage**
   a. Dosing of LMWHs is **disease state** and **product specific**; different doses are administered based on the indication for use and the manufacturer of the specific LMWH. *Table 35-10* shows manufacturer's suggested, U.S. Food and Drug Administration (FDA) approved dosing for specific indications.

D. **Synthetic pentasaccharide**

1. **Indications**
   a. **Synthetic pentasaccharide** (fondaparinux [Arixtra]) is indicated for
      (1) thromboprophylaxis against DVT/PE after
         (a) hip fracture surgery
         (b) hip fracture surgery, extended prophylaxis
         (c) knee replacement surgery
         (d) hip replacement surgery
         (e) abdominal surgery
      (2) treatment of
         (a) acute DVT
         (b) acute PE

2. **Chemistry.** Synthetic pentasaccharide is a selective **factor Xa inhibitor**. The molecular weight of the synthetic pentasaccharide product is 1728 Da.

3. **Mechanism of action**
   a. The antithrombotic activity of fondaparinux is the result of antithrombin-mediated selective inhibition of factor Xa. Neutralization of factor Xa interrupts the blood coagulation cascade and thus inhibits thrombin formation and thrombus development.
   b. Fondaparinux does not inactivate thrombin (activated factor II) and has no known effect on platelet function.

4. **Pharmacokinetics**
   a. After subcutaneous administration, the drug is completely bioavailable, and steady-state peak plasma levels are achieved in approximately 3 hrs after administration of the dose.
   b. The elimination half-life is 17 to 21 hrs, enabling once daily dosing.
   c. The drug does not seem to be metabolized, appears in the urine in active form, and is renally eliminated.

5. **Administration and dosage**
   a. Fondaparinux must not be administered intramuscularly.
   b. **For prophylaxis against VTE,** the drug should not be used in patients with body weight < 50 kg because the incidence of major bleeding was found to double in this patient population during clinical trials.
   c. **For prophylaxis against VTE,** a usual **dose of 2.5 mg subcutaneously once daily for 5 to 9 days** is recommended for **all prophylaxis indications**. The initial dose should be started 6 to 8 hrs after surgery when hemostasis is established.

Table 35-10 DOSING OF LMWHs FOR VTE PREVENTION AND TREATMENT

	Enoxaparin		Dalteparin	Tinzaparin
Indication	**Standard Dose**	**Dose in Severe Renal Impairment**	**Dose**	**Dose**
VTE prophylaxis				
Hip replacement surgery	30 mg SC q12h (initiated 12–24 hrs after surgery) or 40 mg SC q24h (initiated 10–12 hrs before surgery)	30 mg SC q24h	2500 units SC given 6–8 hrs after surgery, then 5000 units SC q24h or 5000 units SC q24h (initiated the evening before surgery)	75 units/kg SC q24h (initiated the evening before surgery or 12–24 hrs after surgery)* or 4500 units SC q24h (initiated 12 hrs before surgery)*
Knee replacement surgery	30 mg SC q12h	30 mg SC q24h	2500 units SC given 6–8 hrs after surgery, then 5000 units SC q24h*	75 units/kg SC q24h*
Hip fracture surgery	30 mg SC q12h*	30 mg SC q24h*	NA	NA
Abdominal surgery	40 mg SC q24h	30 mg SC q24h	2500 units SC q24h (patients at risk of VTE) or 5000 units SC q24h (patients at high risk of VTE, such as malignancy) or 2500 units SC 1–2 hrs before surgery followed by 2500 units SC 12 hrs later, and then 5000 units SC q24h (patients with malignancy)	3500 units SC q24h*
Acutely ill medical patients	40 mg SC q24h	30 mg SC q24h	5000 units SC q24h	NA
VTE treatment				
DVT +/ PE	1 mg/kg SC q12h or 1.5 mg/kg SC q24h	1 mg/kg SC q24h	100 units/kg SC q12h* or 200 units/kg SC q24h*	175 units/kg SC q24h
Extended VTE treatment in cancer patients	1 mg/kg SC q12h or 1.5 mg/kg SC q24h*	1 mg/kg SC q24h*	200 units/kg SC q24h (first 30 days), then 150 units/kg SC q24h (months 2–6) with a dose cap of 18,000 units per day	175 units/kg SC q24h*

*Non-FDA approved for indication.
DVT, deep venous thrombosis; *NA*, data not available; *PE*, pulmonary embolism; *qh*, every hour; *SC*, subcutaneous; *VTE*, venous thromboembolism.

d. **For treatment** of established VTE, administer a once daily subcutaneous dose as follows:
   (1) Patients with body weight between 50 and 100 kg: 7.5 mg
   (2) Patients with body weight < 50 kg: 5 mg
   (3) Patients with body weight > 100 kg: 10 mg

6. **Cautions**
   a. **Contraindications**
      (1) Severe renal impairment
      (2) Patients weighing < 50 kg when used for prophylaxis
      (3) Patients with active major bleeding

(4) Bacterial endocarditis
(5) Thrombocytopenia associated with positive in vitro test for antiplatelet antibody in the presence of fondaparinux
(6) Known hypersensitivity to fondaparinux

b. Precautions

(1) Conditions or procedures that may enhance the risk of severe bleeding (e.g., trauma, hemophilia, gastrointestinal ulceration, concurrent use of antiplatelet agents, history of cerebrovascular hemorrhage, severe uncontrolled hypertension)
(2) Renal impairment
(3) Heparin-induced thrombocytopenia
(4) Neuraxial anesthesia and indwelling epidural catheter use
(5) Elderly patients
(6) Pregnancy category B and lactating (the drug is excreted into breast milk)
(7) Protamine is **ineffective** as an antidote

E. Oral factor Xa inhibitor

1. Indications

a. Direct factor Xa inhibitor (rivaroxaban [Xarelto])

(1) Thromboprophylaxis against DVT/PE after
(a) elective hip replacement surgery
(b) elective knee replacement surgery
(2) To reduce the risk of stroke and systemic embolism in patients with atrial fibrillation.

2. Chemistry. Direct competitive specific inhibitor of factor Xa

3. Mechanism of action

a. The antithrombotic activity of rivaroxaban is the result of direct specific inhibition of factor Xa.
b. Rivaroxaban potentially inhibits both free and clot-associated factor Xa activity and has no direct effect upon platelet aggregation.

4. Pharmacokinetics

a. After oral administration, the drug is approximately 80% bioavailable and is rapidly absorbed with an onset of action achieved in approximately 2 to 4 hrs after administration of the dose.
b The drug undergoes oxidative metabolism (mainly via CYP3A4) and hydrolysis and is eliminated one-third by renal excretion and two-thirds by hepatic metabolism.
c. The elimination half-life is 5 to 9 hrs, enabling once daily dosing for the orthopedic prophylaxis indication.

5. Administration and dosage

a. For prevention of VTE in adult patients undergoing elective hip or knee replacement surgery, the dosage recommendation is 10 mg orally once daily. For elective hip replacement surgery, the duration of therapy should be 35 days. For elective knee replacement surgery, the duration of therapy should be 12 days minimally.
b. No routine monitoring of INR or aPTT is necessary for this drug.

6. Cautions

a. Contraindications

(1) Hypersensitivity to the active substance or to any of the excipients; clinically significant active bleeding; hepatic disease associated with coagulopathy and clinically relevant bleeding risk, pregnancy, and lactation.

b. Precautions

(1) **Treatment** with rivaroxaban is not recommended in the following patients: concomitantly treated systemically with strong concurrent CYP3A4 inhibitor and plasma glycoprotein (P-gp) inhibitors, i.e., azole antimycotics (such as ketoconazole, itraconazole, voriconazole, and posaconazole) or HIV protease inhibitors (e.g., ritonavir); with severe renal impairment (creatinine clearance [Clcr]<15 mL/min); and, due to lack of data, younger than 18 years of age; undergoing hip fracture surgery.
(2) Strong CYP3A4 inducers (e.g., rifampicin, phenytoin, carbamazepine, phenobarbital, or St. John's Wort) should be used with caution because they may lead to reduced rivaroxaban plasma concentrations and thus may reduce efficacy.
(3) Special care is to be taken when neuraxial anesthesia or spinal/epidural puncture is employed.

F. Oral direct thrombin inhibitor

1. Indications

a. Direct factor IIa (thrombin) inhibitor (dabigatran [Pradaxa])

(1) Reduce the risk of stroke and systemic embolism in patients with nonvalvular atrial fibrillation.

2. Chemistry. The drug binds rapidly and specifically to both free and clot-bound thrombin whose inhibition results in prevention of thrombus.

3. Mechanism of action

a. The antithrombotic activity of dabigatran is the result of directly and selectively inhibiting factor IIa (thrombin).

4. Pharmacokinetics

a. After oral administration, the drug is rapidly absorbed, converted to active drug and eliminated primarily by renal excretion, with an onset of action achieved in approximately 1 hr after administration of the dose.

b. The drug undergoes conjugation (esterase catalyzed hydrolysis in liver or plasma).

c. The elimination half-life is 12 to 17 hrs, requiring twice daily administration for the atrial fibrillation indication.

5. Administration and dosage

a. For reduction of risk of stroke and systemic embolism in patients with nonvalvular atrial fibrillations, the recommendation is 150 mg orally twice daily if renal function is greater than 30 mL/min Clcr. For renal function 15 to 30 mL/min, the recommended dose is 75 mg orally twice daily. For renal function $<$ 15 mL/min, the drug is not recommended. For patients with moderate renal impairment (Clcr 30–50 mL/min) consider reducing the dose of dabigatran to 75 mg orally twice daily if co-administered with dronedarone or systemic ketoconazole.

b. Routine monitoring (INR or aPTT) is not necessary for this drug.

6. Cautions

a. Contraindications

(1) Hypersensitivity to the active substance or to any of the excipients and clinically significant active pathologic bleeding.

b. Precautions

(1) Treatment with dabigatran increases the risk of bleeding and can sometimes cause significant and sometimes fatal bleeding. Risk factors for bleeding include certain medications known, to increase this risk (e.g., antiplatelet agents, heparin, fibrinolytic therapy, chronic use of nonsteroidal anti-inflammatory drugs (NSAIDs), and labor and delivery).

(2) The concomitant use of dabigatran with P-gp inducers (e.g., rifampin) reduces dabigatran exposure and should generally be avoided; P-gp inhibitors (e.g., ketoconazole, verapamil, amiodarone, and clarithromycin) do not require dose adjustment. These results should not be extrapolated to other P-gp inhibitors.

(3) Special care is to be taken when neuraxial anesthesia or spinal/epidural puncture is employed.

Study Questions

Directions for questions 1–4: Each of the questions, statements, or incomplete statements in this section can be correctly answered or completed by **one** of the suggested answers or phrases. Choose the **best** answer.

1. A 67-year-old man who weighs 100 kg (212 lb) and is 60 inches tall presents to his physician after a transatlantic flight complaining of pain and swelling of his right lower extremity. The patient had total knee arthroplasty 2 weeks before his travel. His medical history reveals that he has an ejection fraction of 15%, he is in remission for non-Hodgkin lymphoma, and he had a previous MI. His mother, father, and sister are dead as a result of stroke, pulmonary embolism (PE), and childbirth, respectively. Given this patient's history, he is most likely suffering from which of the following?

(A) ruptured Baker cyst
(B) deep venous thrombosis (DVT) of the lower extremity
(C) torn medial meniscus
(D) septic arthritis

2. Prophylaxis against venous throboembolic disease (VTED) may include

(A) nonpharmacological prophylaxis.
(B) pharmacological prophylaxis.
(C) nonpharmacological and pharmacological prophylaxis.
(D) neither nonpharmacological nor pharmacological prophylaxis.

3. Unfractionated heparin binds to antithrombin III and inactivates clotting factor(s)

(A) Xa
(B) IXa
(C) IIa
(D) All of the above
(E) None of the above

4. Initiation of UFH therapy for the patient described in question 1 would best be achieved with

(A) 5000 U loading dose followed by 1000 U/hr.
(B) 5000 U loading dose followed by 1800 U/hr.
(C) 8000 U loading dose followed by 1800 U/hr.
(D) 1000 U loading dose followed by 1000 U/hr.

Directions for questions 5–11: The questions and incomplete statements in this section can be correctly answered or completed by **one or more** of the suggested answers. Choose the answer, **A–E**.

A if **I only** is correct
B if **III only** is correct
C if **I and II** are correct
D if **II and III** are correct
E if **I, II, and III** are correct

Directions for questions 5–10: Upon confirmation of diagnosis, the attending physician asks you, the pharmacist, to commence low-molecular-weight-heparin (LMWH) therapy for the patient described in question 1 as mentioned earlier. The following questions pertain to your pharmaceutical care for this patient:

5. When choosing an Food and Drug Administration (FDA)-approved LMWH to treat this patient, you would administer

I. enoxaparin 1.0 mg/kg/dose subcutaneously every 12 hrs.
II. enoxaparin 1.5 mg/kg/dose subcutaneously every 24 hrs.
III. tinzaparin 175 IU/kg/dose subcutaneously every 24 hrs.

6. Which of the following tests are used to monitor heparin antithrombotic therapy?

I. international normalized ratio (INR)
II. activated partial thromboplatin time (aPTT)
III. heparin assay

7. A patient to be commenced on oral anticoagulant therapy for DVT would be treated with

I. oral anticoagulant therapy with warfarin for a goal INR of 2.0 to 3.0.
II. oral anticoagulant therapy with warfarin for a goal INR of 2.5 to 3.5.
III. oral anticoagulant therapy with aspirin for a goal INR of 2.0 to 3.0.

8. A patient on oral anticoagulant therapy is commenced on sulfamethoxazole-trimethoprim, double-strength twice daily. One may expect to see the INR

I. increase.
II. decrease.
III. remain unchanged.

9. If a patient has an INR > 20 and active bleeding that is clinically significant (i.e., hematuria), the pharmacist should

I. hold the drug therapy.
II. administer vitamin K.
III. administer fresh frozen plasma.

10. Compared to unfractionated heparin (UFH), LMWHs have

I. preferential binding affinity to factor Xa relative to IIa (thrombin).
II. shorter half-lives.
III. dose-dependent renal clearance.

11. An 87-year-old woman who weighs 49 kg (108 lb) and is 66 inches tall has sustained a hip fracture requiring open reduction with internal fixation (ORIF) surgery. She has a documented serum creatine value recorded in the chart and in the laboratory results as 4.3 mg/dL. The orthopedic surgeon asks you, the pharmacist, about the appropriate fondaparinux dosing for this patient to prevent venous thromboembolism after the surgery. Which of the following are contraindications to the use of fondaparinux in this patient?

I. Patient weighs < 50 kg.
II. Patient has severe renal impairment.
III. Patient is elderly.

36 Infectious Diseases

PAUL F. SOUNEY, ANTHONY E. ZIMMERMANN, LINDA M. SPOONER

I. PRINCIPLES OF ANTI-INFECTIVE THERAPY

A. **Definition.** Anti-infective agents treat infection by suppressing or destroying the causative microorganisms—bacteria, mycobacteria, fungi, protozoa, or viruses. Anti-infective agents derived from natural substances are called **antibiotics**; those produced from synthetic substances are called **antimicrobials**. These two terms are now used interchangeably.

B. **Indications.** Confirm the presence of infection by completing a careful history and physical examination, searching for signs and symptoms of infection as well as predisposing factors. Anti-infective agents should be used only when

1. A significant infection has been diagnosed or is strongly suspected.
2. An established indication for prophylactic therapy exists.

C. **Gram stain**, **microbiological culturing**, and **susceptibility tests** should be performed before anti-infective therapy is initiated. Test materials must be obtained by a method that avoids contamination of the specimen by the patient's own flora.

1. **Gram stain.** Performed on all specimens except blood cultures, the gram stain helps identify the cause of infection immediately. By determining if the causative agent is gram positive or gram negative, the test allows a better choice of drug therapy, particularly when an anti-infective regimen must begin without delay.
   a. **Gram-positive** microorganisms stain **blue** or **purple**.
   b. **Gram-negative** microorganisms stain **red** or **rose-pink**.
   c. **Fungi** may also be identified by gram stain.
2. **Microbiological cultures.** To identify the specific causative agent, specimens of body fluids or infected tissue are collected for analysis.
3. **Susceptibility tests.** Different strains of the same pathogenic species may have widely varying susceptibility to a particular anti-infective agent. Susceptibility tests determine microbial susceptibility to a given drug and thus can be used to predict whether the drug will combat the infection effectively.
   a. **Microdilution method.** The drug is diluted serially in various media containing the test microorganism.
      (1) The lowest drug concentration that prevents microbial growth after 18 to 24 hrs of incubation is called the **minimum inhibitory concentration** (MIC).
      (2) The lowest drug concentration that reduces bacterial density by 99.9% is called the **minimum bactericidal concentration** (MBC).
      (3) **Breakpoint** concentrations of antibiotics are used to characterize antibiotic activity: The interpretive categories are **susceptible**, **moderately susceptible (intermediate)**, and **resistant**. These concentrations are determined by considering pharmacokinetics, serum and tissue concentrations following normal doses, and the **population distribution** of MICs of a group of bacteria for a given drug.
   b. **Kirby–Bauer disk diffusion technique.** This test is less expensive but less reliable than the microdilution method; however, it provides qualitative susceptibility information.
      (1) Filter paper disks impregnated with specific drug quantities are placed on the surface of agar plates streaked with a microorganism culture. After 18 hrs, the size of a clear inhibition zone is determined; drug activity against the test strain is then correlated to zone size.

(2) The Kirby–Bauer technique does not reliably predict therapeutic effectiveness against certain microorganisms (e.g., *Staphylococcus aureus*, *Shigella*).

D. Choice of agent. An anti-infective agent should be chosen on the basis of its pharmacological properties and spectrum of activity as well as on various host (patient) factors (*Figure 36-1*).

1. **Pharmacological properties** include the drug's ability to reach the infection site and to attain a desired level in the target tissue.
2. **Spectrum of activity.** To treat an infectious disease effectively, an anti-infective drug must be active against the causative pathogen. Susceptibility testing or clinical experience in treating a given infection may suggest the effectiveness of a particular drug.

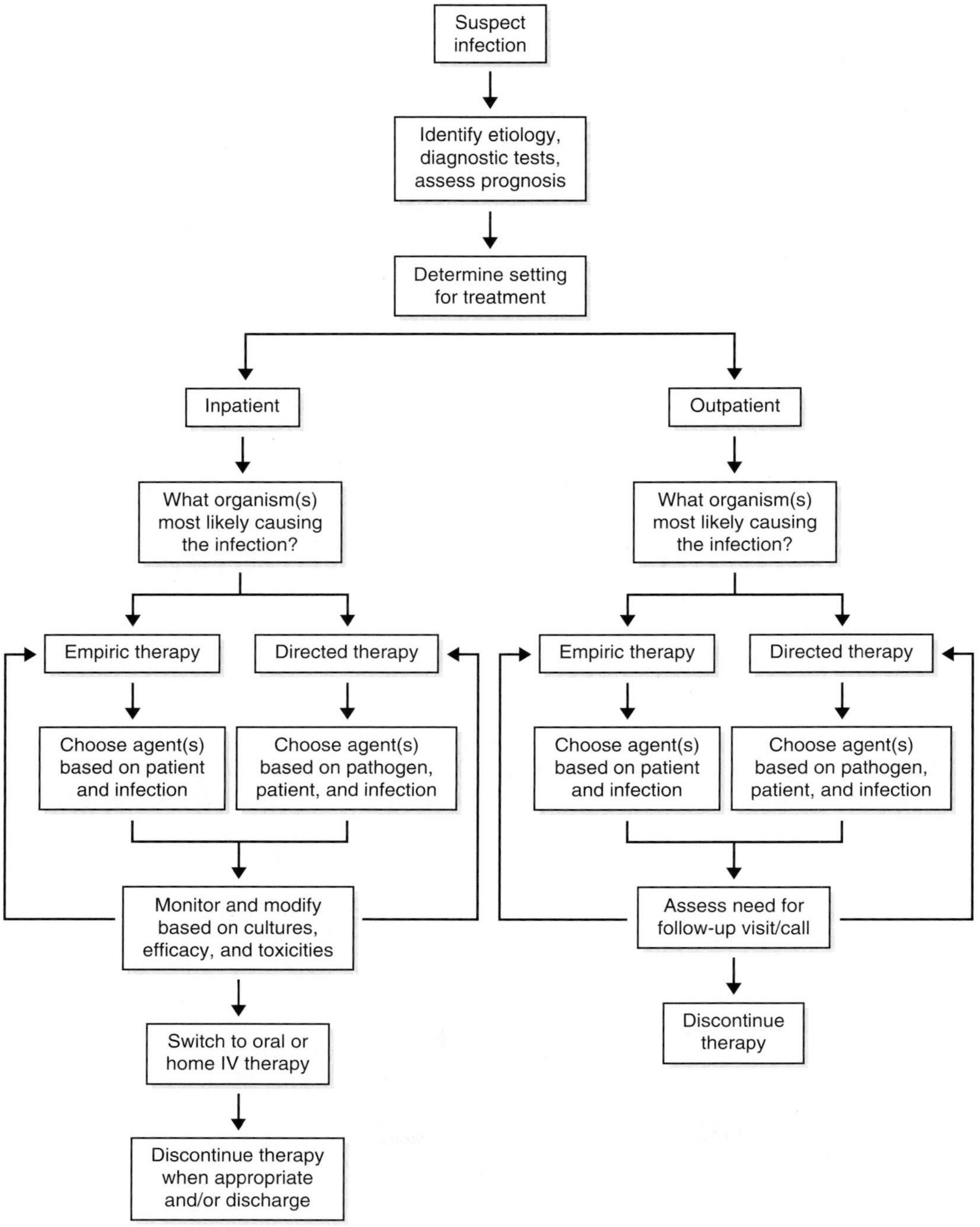

Figure 36-1. Approach to management of infection.

3. **Patient factors.** Selection of an anti-infective drug regimen must take various patient factors into account to determine which type of drug should be administered, the correct drug dosage and administration route, and the potential for adverse drug effects.
   a. **Immunological status.** A patient with impaired immune mechanisms may require a drug that rapidly destroys pathogens (i.e., **bactericidal agent**) rather than one that merely suppresses a pathogen's growth or reproduction (i.e., **bacteriostatic agent**).
   b. **Presence of a foreign body.** The effectiveness of anti-infective therapy is reduced in patients who have prosthetic joints or valves, cardiac pacemakers, and various internal shunts.
   c. **Age.** A drug's pharmacokinetic properties may vary widely in patients of different ages. In very young and very old patients, drug metabolism and excretion commonly decrease. Elderly patients also have an increased risk of suffering ototoxicity when receiving certain antibiotics.
   d. **Underlying disease**
      (1) Preexisting **kidney** or **liver disease** increases the risk of nephrotoxicity or hepatotoxicity during the administration of some antibacterial drugs.
      (2) Patients with **central nervous system (CNS) disorders** may suffer neurotoxicity (motor seizures) during penicillin therapy.
      (3) Patients with **neuromuscular disorders** (e.g., myasthenia gravis) are at increased risk for developing neuromuscular blockade during aminoglycoside or polymyxin B therapy.
   e. **History of drug allergy or adverse drug reactions.** Patients who have had previous allergic or other untoward reactions to a particular antibiotic have a higher risk of experiencing the same reaction during subsequent administration of that drug. Except in life-threatening situations, patients who have had serious allergic reactions to penicillin, for example, should not receive the drug again.
   f. **Pregnancy and lactation.** Because drug therapy during pregnancy and lactation can cause unwanted effects, the mother's need for the antibiotic must be weighed against the drug's potential harm.
      (1) Pregnancy can increase the risk of adverse drug effects for both mother and fetus. Also, plasma drug concentrations tend to decrease in pregnant women, reducing a drug's therapeutic effectiveness.
      (2) Most drugs, including antibiotics, appear in the breast milk of nursing mothers and may cause adverse effects in infants. For example, sulfonamides may lead to toxic bilirubin accumulation in a newborn's brain.
   g. **Genetic traits**
      (1) Sulfonamides may cause hemolytic anemia in patients with glucose-6-phosphate dehydrogenase (G6PD) deficiency.
      (2) Patients who rapidly metabolize drugs (i.e., rapid acetylators) may develop hepatitis when receiving the antitubercular drug isoniazid.

E. **Empiric therapy.** In serious or life-threatening disease, anti-infective therapy must begin before the infecting organism has been identified. In this case, the choice of drug (or drugs) is based on clinical experience, suggesting that a particular agent is effective in a given setting.
   1. A **broad-spectrum antibiotic** usually is the most appropriate choice until the specific organism has been determined.
   2. In all cases, **culture specimens must be obtained** before therapy begins.

F. **Multiple antibiotic therapy.** A combination of drugs should be given only when clinical experience has shown such therapy to be more effective than single-agent therapy in a particular setting. A multiple-agent regimen can increase the risk of toxic drug effects and, in a few cases, may result in drug antagonism and subsequent therapeutic ineffectiveness. Indications for multiple-agent therapy include
   1. **Need for increased antibiotic effectiveness.** The **synergistic** (intensified) effect of two or more agents may allow a dosage reduction or a faster or enhanced drug effect.
   2. **Treatment of an infection caused by multiple pathogens** (e.g., intra-abdominal infection)
   3. **Prevention of proliferation of drug-resistant organisms** (e.g., during treatment of tuberculosis)

G. **Duration of anti-infective therapy.** To achieve the therapeutic goal, anti-infective therapy must continue for a sufficient duration.
   1. **Acute uncomplicated infection.** Treatment generally should continue until the patient has been afebrile and asymptomatic for at least 72 hrs.

2. **Chronic infection** (e.g., endocarditis, osteomyelitis). Treatment may require a longer duration (4 to 6 weeks) with follow-up culture analyses to assess therapeutic effectiveness.

H. **Monitoring therapeutic effectiveness.** To assess the patient's response to anti-infective therapy, appropriate specimens should be cultured and the following parameters monitored.

1. **Fever curve.** An important assessment tool, the fever curve may be a reliable indication of response to therapy. Defervescence usually indicates favorable response.
2. **White blood cell (WBC) count.** In the initial stage of infection, the neutrophil count from a peripheral blood smear may rise above normal (neutrophilia), and immature neutrophil forms ("bands") may appear ("left shift"). In patients who are elderly, debilitated, or suffering overwhelming infection, the WBC count may be normal or subnormal.
3. **Radiographic findings.** Small effusions, abscesses, or cavities that appear on radiographs indicate the focus of infection.
4. **Pain** and **inflammation** (as evidenced by swelling, erythema, and tenderness) may occur when the infection is superficial or within a joint or bone, also indicating a possible focus of infection.
5. **Erythrocyte sedimentation rate (ESR or "sed rate").** Large elevations in ESR are associated with acute or chronic infection, particularly endocarditis, chronic osteomyelitis, and intra-abdominal infections. A normal ESR does not exclude infection; more often, ESR is elevated as a result of noninfectious causes such as collagen vascular disease.
6. **Serum complement concentrations**, particularly the C3 component, are often reduced in serious infections because of consumption during the host defense process.

I. **Lack of therapeutic effectiveness.** When an antibiotic drug regimen fails, other drugs should not be added indiscriminately or the regimen otherwise changed. Instead, the situation should be reassessed and diagnostic efforts intensified. Causes of therapeutic ineffectiveness include the following:

1. **Misdiagnosis.** The isolated organism may have been misidentified by the laboratory or may not be the causative agent for infection (e.g., the patient may have an unsuspected infection).
2. **Improper drug regimen.** The drug dosage, administration route, dosing frequency, or duration of therapy may be inadequate or inappropriate.
3. **Inappropriate choice of antibiotic agent.** As discussed in I.D, patient factors and the pharmacological properties and spectrum of activity of a given drug must be considered when planning anti-infective drug therapy.
4. **Microbial resistance.** By acquiring resistance to a specific antibiotic, microorganisms can survive in the drug's presence. Many gonococcal strains, for instance, now resist penicillin. Drug resistance is particularly common in geographical areas in which a specific drug has been used excessively (and perhaps improperly).
5. **Unrealistic expectations.** Antibiotics are ineffective in certain circumstances.
   a. Patients with conditions that require **surgical drainage** frequently cannot be cured by anti-infective drugs until the drain has been removed. For example, the presence of necrotic tissue or pus in patients with pneumonia, empyema, or renal calculi is a common cause of antibiotic failure.
   b. **Fever** should not be treated with anti-infective drugs unless infection has been identified as the cause. Although fever frequently signifies infection, it sometimes stems from noninfectious conditions (e.g., drug reactions, phlebitis, neoplasms, metabolic disorders, arthritis). These conditions do not respond to antibiotics. One exception to this position is neutropenic cancer patients; such patients with no signs or symptoms of infection other than fever are widely treated with antimicrobial agents.
6. **Infection by two or more types of microorganisms.** If not detected initially, an additional cause of infection may lead to therapeutic failure.

J. **Antimicrobial prophylaxis for surgery**

1. **Definition.** Antibiotic prophylaxis is a short course of antibiotic administered before there is clinical evidence of infection.
2. **General considerations**
   a. **Timing.** The antibiotic should be administered to ensure that appropriate antibiotic levels are available at the site of contamination before the incision. Initiation of prophylaxis is often at induction of anesthesia, within 1 hr or just before the surgical incision. This ensures peak serum and tissue antibiotic levels.

b. **Duration.** Prophylaxis should be maintained for the duration of surgery. Long surgical procedures (e.g., > 3 hrs) may require additional doses. There is little evidence to support continuation of prophylaxis beyond 24 hrs.
c. **Antibiotic spectrum** should be appropriate for the usual pathogens.
(1) In general, **first-generation cephalosporins** (e.g., cefazolin) are the drugs of choice for most procedures and patients. These agents have an appropriate spectrum, a low frequency of side effects, a favorable half-life, and a low cost.
(2) **Vancomycin** is a suitable alternative in penicillin-sensitive patients and in situations in which methicillin-resistant *S. aureus* is a concern.
d. **Route of administration.** Intravenous (IV) or intramuscular (IM) routes are preferred to guarantee good serum and tissue levels at the time of incision.

II. ANTIBACTERIAL AGENTS

A. **Definition and classification.** Used to treat infections caused by **bacteria**, antibacterial agents fall into several major categories: **aminoglycosides**, **carbapenems**, **cephalosporins**, **erythromycins**, **penicillins** (including various subgroups), **sulfonamides**, **tetracyclines**, **fluoroquinolones**, **metronidazole** (see V.C.2.b), **urinary tract antiseptics**, and **miscellaneous anti-infectives** (*Table 36-1*).
B. **Aminoglycosides.** These drugs, containing amino sugars, are used primarily in infections caused by gram-negative enterobacteria and in suspected sepsis. They have little activity against anaerobic and facultative organisms. The toxic potential of these drugs limits their use. Major aminoglycosides include **amikacin (Amikin)**, **gentamicin (Garamycin)**, **kanamycin**, **neomycin**, **netilmicin**, **streptomycin**, and **tobramycin (Nebcin)**.
1. **Mechanism of action.** Aminoglycosides are **bactericidal**; they inhibit bacterial protein synthesis by binding to and impeding the function of the 30S ribosomal subunit. (Some aminoglycosides also bind to the 50S ribosomal subunit.) Their mechanism of action is not fully known.
2. **Spectrum of activity**
a. **Streptomycin** is active against both gram-positive and gram-negative bacteria. However, widespread resistance to this drug has restricted its use to the organisms that cause plague and tularemia, gram-positive streptococci (given in combination with penicillin), and *Mycobacterium tuberculosis* (given in combination with other antitubercular agents as described in VI.C.2).
b. **Amikacin**, **kanamycin**, **gentamicin**, **tobramycin**, **neomycin**, and **netilmicin** are active against many gram-negative bacteria (e.g., *Proteus*, *Serratia*, and *Pseudomonas* organisms).
(1) **Gentamicin** is active against some *Staphylococcus* strains; it is more active than tobramycin against *Serratia* organisms.
(2) **Amikacin** is the broadest spectrum aminoglycoside with activity against most aerobic gram-negative bacilli as well as many anaerobic gram-negative bacterial strains that resist gentamicin and tobramycin. It is also active against *M. tuberculosis* and *Mycobacterium avium-intracellulare* (MAI).
(3) **Tobramycin** may be more active against *Pseudomonas aeruginosa* than gentamicin.
(4) **Netilmicin** may be active against gentamicin-resistant organisms; it appears to be less ototoxic than other aminoglycosides.
(5) **Neomycin**, in addition to its activity against such gram-negative organisms as *Escherichia coli* and *Klebsiella pneumoniae*, is active against several gram-positive organisms (e.g., *S. aureus*). *P. aeruginosa* and most streptococci are now neomycin resistant.
3. **Therapeutic uses**
a. **Streptomycin** is used to treat plague, tularemia, acute brucellosis (given in combination with tetracycline), and tuberculosis (given in combination with other antitubercular agents, as described in VI.C.2).
b. **Gentamicin**, **tobramycin**, **amikacin**, and **netilmicin** are therapeutic for serious gram-negative bacillary infections (e.g., those caused by *Enterobacter*, *Serratia*, *Klebsiella*, and *P. aeruginosa*), bacterial endocarditis caused by *Streptococcus viridans* (given in combination with penicillin), pneumonia (given in combination with a cephalosporin or penicillin), meningitis, complicated urinary tract infections, osteomyelitis, bacteremia, and peritonitis.
c. **Neomycin** is used for preoperative bowel sterilization; hepatic coma (as adjunctive therapy); and, in topical form, for skin and mucous membrane infections (e.g., burns).

Table 36-1 SOME IMPORTANT PARAMETERS OF ANTI-INFECTIVE DRUGS

Agent	Elimination Route	Half-Life	Administration Route	Common Dosage Range (Adults)
Aminoglycosides				
Amikacin	Renal	2–3 hrs	IV, IM	15 mg/kg/day (once daily dose)
Gentamicin	Renal	2 hrs	IV, IM	3 mg/kg/day (standard dose); 6–7 mg/kg/day (once daily dose)
Kanamycin	Renal	2–4 hrs	Oral, IV	15 mg/kg every 8–12 hrs
Neomycin	Renal	2–3 hrs	Oral, topical	50–100 mg/kg/day (oral); 10–15 mg/day (topical)
Netilmicin	Renal	2–7 hrs	IV, IM	3–6 mg/kg/day
Streptomycin	Renal	2–3 hrs	IM	15 mg/kg/day[a]
Tobramycin	Renal	2–5 hrs	IV, IM	3 mg/kg/day (standard dose); 6–7 mg/kg/day (once daily dose)
Carbapenems				
Doripenem	Renal	1 hr	IV	500 mg every 8 hrs
Imipenem	Renal	1 hr	IV	250 mg to 1 g every 6 hrs
Ertapenem	Renal	4 hrs	IV, IM	1 g/day
Meropenem	Renal	1.5 hr	IV, IM	0.5–2 g every 8 hrs
Cephalosporins				
First-generation				
Cefadroxil	Renal	1.5 hr	Oral	1–2 g/day
Cefazolin	Renal	1.4–2.2 hrs	IV	250 mg to 1 g every 8 hrs
Cephalexin	Renal	0.9–1.3 hrs	Oral	250–500 mg every 6 hrs
Cephapirin	Renal (H)	0.6–0.8 hr	IV, IM	500 mg to 2 g every 4–6 hrs
Cephradine	Renal	1.3 hr	Oral, IV	250–500 mg every 6 hrs
Second-generation				
Cefaclor	Renal (H)	0.8 hr	Oral	250–500 mg every 8 hrs
Cefmetazole	Renal	72 mins	IV	2 g every 6–12 hrs
Cefotetan	Renal	2.8–4.6 hrs	IV, IM	1–2 g every 12 hrs
Cefoxitin	Renal	0.8 hr	IV	1–2 g every 6–8 hrs
Cefprozil	Renal	78 mins	Oral	250–500 mg every 12–24 hrs
Cefuroxime	Renal	1.5–2.2 hrs	IV, IM	750 mg to 1.5 g every 8 hrs
Third-generation				
Cefixime	Renal	3–4 hrs	Oral	400 mg/day
Cefdinir	Renal	1.7–1.8 hr	Oral	300 mg every 12 hrs
Cefditoren	Renal	1.6 hr	Oral	400 mg every 12 hrs
Cefoperazone	Hepatic	1.6–2.4 hrs	IV	2–4 g every 12 hrs
Cefotaxime	Renal (H)	1.5 hr	IV	1–2 g every 6–8 hrs
Cefpodoxime	Renal	2.5 hrs	Oral	100–400 mg every 12 hrs
Ceftazidime	Renal	1.8 hr	IV, IM	1–2 g every 8–12 hrs
Ceftibuten	Renal	2.5 hrs	Oral	400 mg/day
Ceftizoxime	Renal	1.7 hr	IV	1–2 g every 8–12 hrs
Ceftriaxone	Renal	8 hrs	IV, IM	1–2 g/day
Fourth-generation				
Cefepime	Renal	2.0–2.3 hrs	IV, IM	1–2 g every 8–12 hrs
Ceftaroline	Renal	2.6 hrs	IV	600 mg every 12 hrs
Erythromycins and other macrolides				
Azithromycin	Hepatic	68 hrs	Oral	250 mg/day
Clarithromycin	Renal	3–7 hrs	Oral	250–500 mg every 12 hrs

(Continued on next page)

Table 36-1 Continued.

Agent	Elimination Route	Half-Life	Administration Route	Common Dosage Range (Adults)
Erythromycins and other macrolides (continued)				
Erythromycin base estolate, ethylsuccinate, and stearate	Hepatic	1.2–2.6 hrs	Oral	250–500 mg every 6 hrs
Erythromycin gluceptate and lactobionate			IV	0.5–2.0 g every 6 hrs
Natural penicillins				
Penicillin G	Renal (H)	0.5 hr	Oral, IV, IM	200,000–500,000 U every 6–8 hrs
Penicillin V	Renal	1 hr	Oral	500 mg to 2 g/day
Penicillin G procaine	Renal	24–60 hrs	IM	300,000–600,000 U/day
Penicillin G benzathine	Renal	24–60 hrs	IM	300,000–600,000 U/day
Penicillinase-resistant penicillins				
Dicloxacillin	Renal (H)	0.5–0.9 hr	Oral	500 mg to 1 g/day
Methicillin	Renal (H)	0.5–1.0 hr	IV, IM	1–2 g every 4–6 hrs
Nafcillin	Hepatic (R)	0.5 hr	Oral, IV, IM	0.25–2.00 g every 6 hrs
Oxacillin	Renal (H)	0.5 hr	Oral, IV, IM	500 mg to 2 g every 4–6 hrs 500–875 mg every 12 hrs
Aminopenicillins				
Amoxicillin	Renal (H)	0.9–2.3 hrs	Oral	250–500 mg every 8 hrs
Amoxicillin/clavulanic acid	Renal	1 hr	Oral	250–500 mg every 8 hrs
Ampicillin	Renal (H)	0.8–1.5 hrs	Oral, IV, IM	250 mg to 2 g every 4–6 hrs
Ampicillin/sulbactam	Renal	1.0–1.8 hr	IV, IM	1.5–3.0 g every 6 hrs
Extended-spectrum penicillins				
Piperacillin	Renal (H)	0.8–1.4 hr	IV, IM	1.0–1.5 mg/kg every 6–12 hrs
Piperacillin/tazobactam	Renal	0.7–1.2 hr	IV	3.375 g every 6 hrs
Ticarcillin/clavulanic acid	Renal	1.0–1.5 hr	IV	3.1 g every 4–6 hrs
Sulfonamides				
Sulfacytine	Renal	4.0–4.5 hrs	Oral	250 mg every 6 hrs
Sulfadiazine	Renal (H)	6 hrs	Oral, IV	2–4 g/day
Sulfamethoxazole	Hepatic (R)	9–11 hrs	Oral	1–3 g/day
Sulfisoxazole	Renal (H)	3–7 hrs	Oral, IV	2–8 g/day
Sulfamethizole	Renal	—	Oral	0.5–1.0 g every 6–8 hrs
Tetracyclines				
Demeclocycline	Renal	10–17 hrs	Oral	300 mg to 1 g/day
Doxycycline	Hepatic	14–25 hrs	Oral, IV	100–200 mg every 12 hrs
Minocycline	Hepatic	12–15 hrs	Oral, IV	100–200 mg every 12 hrs
Oxytetracycline	Renal	6–12 hrs	Oral, IM	250–500 mg every 6 hrs 250–500 mg q.i.d. or 300 mg/day in one or two divided doses
Tetracycline[b]	Renal	6–12 hrs	Oral, IV, IM	1–2 g/day
Fluoroquinolones				
Ciprofloxacin	Renal (H)	5–6 hrs	IV	200–600 mg every 12 hrs
Gemifloxacin	Fecal (R)	4–12 hrs	Oral	320 mg once daily
Levofloxacin	Renal	8 hrs	IV, Oral	250–500 mg every 24 hrs
Moxifloxacin	Hepatic	12 hrs	Oral	400 mg once daily
Ofloxacin	Renal	5.0–7.5 hrs	Oral	100 mg/day–400 mg

Table 36-1 Continued.

Agent	Elimination Route	Half-Life	Administration Route	Common Dosage Range (Adults)
Urinary tract antiseptics				
Cinoxacin	Renal	1.0–1.5 hr	Oral	250 mg every 6 hrs or 500 mg every 12 hrs
Fosfomycin	Renal/fecal	5.7 hrs	Oral	One packet (3 g) in 90–120 mL water × one dose
Methenamine hippurate and mandelate	Renal	1–3 hrs	Oral	0.5–2 g q.i.d.
Nalidixic acid	Renal	8 hrs	Oral	4 g/day
Nitrofurantoin	Renal	0.3–1.0 hr	Oral	5–7 mg/kg/day
Norfloxacin	Hepatic	3–4 hrs	Oral	400 b.i.d.
Miscellaneous anti-infectives				
Atovaquone	Fecal	50–84 hrs	Oral	750 mg b.i.d. 21 days
Aztreonam	Renal	1.7 hr	Oral, IV	50–100 mg/kg/day
Clindamycin	Hepatic	2–4 hrs	Oral, IM, IV	300–900 mg every 6–8 hrs
Clofazimine	Hepatic	70 days	Oral	50–100 mg/day
Dapsone	Hepatic (R)	28 hrs	Oral	50–100 mg/day
Daptomycin	Renal	8 hrs	IV	4 mg/kg/day
Fidaxomicin	Fecal	11.7 hrs	Oral	200 mg b.i.d. × 10 days
Lincomycin	Hepatic (R)	4.4–6.4 hrs	IV, IM	600 mg to 1 g every 8–12 hrs
Linezolid	Renal	4–6 hrs	Oral, IV	600 mg every 12 hrs
Mupirocin	Renal	19–35 mins	Topical	Apply every 8–12 hrs
Quinupristin/dalfopristin	Hepatic	1 hr/0.4–0.5 hr	IV	7.5 mg/kg every 8 hrs
Rifaximin	Fecal	6 hrs	Oral	200 mg t.i.d.
Spectinomycin	Renal	1.2–2.8 hrs	IM	2–4 g (single dose)
Telavancin	Renal	6–8 hrs	IV	10 mg/kg/day
Telithromycin	Hepatic (R)	10 hrs	Oral	800 mg/day
Tigecycline	Biliary (R)	42 hrs	IV	100 mg load, 50 mg every 12 hrs
Trimethoprim	Renal (H)	8–15 hrs	Oral	100–200 mg/day
Vancomycin	Renal	6–8 hrs	Oral, IV	500 mg every 6 hrs
Antifungal agents				
Amphotericin B	Unknown	24 hrs	IV	1.0–1.5 mg/kg/day
Anidulafungin	Fecal (R)	40–50 hrs	IV	Candidemia: 200 mg day 1, then 100 mg/day Esophageal candidiasis: 100 mg day 1, then 50 mg/day
Caspofungin	Hepatic	9–11 hrs	IV	70 mg on day 1, then 50 mg q.d.
Fluconazole	Renal	22–37 hrs	IV, Oral	100–800 mg/day
Flucytosine	Renal	6 hrs	Oral	50–150 mg/kg/day
Griseofulvin	Hepatic (R)	9–24 hrs	Oral	300–375 mg/day
Itraconazole	Hepatic	24–42 hrs	Oral	200–600 mg/day
Ketoconazole	Hepatic/fecal	3.3 hrs	Oral	200–400 mg/day b.i.d.
Micafungin	Hepatic	11–17 hrs	IV	Esophageal candidiasis: 150 mg/day HSCT prophylaxis: 50 mg/day
Miconazole	Hepatic	20–24 hrs	Oral	200–400 mg/day
Nystatin	Fecal	—	Oral	500,000–1,000,000 U t.i.d.
Terbinafine	Hepatic (R)	11–16 hrs	Oral	250 mg/day
Voriconazole	Hepatic	6 hrs	IV, Oral	IV: 6 mg/kg every 12 hrs × two doses, then 4 mg/kg every 12 hrs; oral: 200 mg every 12 hrs for > 40 kg, 100 mg every 12 hrs for < 40 kg

(Continued on next page)

Table 36-1 Continued.

Agent	Elimination Route	Half-Life	Administration Route	Common Dosage Range (Adults)
Antiprotozoal agents				
Atovaquone	Hepatic	67 hrs	Oral	750 mg b.i.d.
Chloroquine	Renal/fecal	72–120 hrs	IM, Oral	Depends on disease
Coartem	Hepatic	3–6 days	Oral	Day 1: four tablets initially and 8 hrs later Day 2 and 3: four tabs b.i.d.
Diloxanide	Renal	—	IM	500 mg t.i.d.
Eflornithine	Renal	3 hrs	IV	100 mg/kg/dose every 6 hrs
Fansidar	Renal	100–231 hrs	Oral	1 tablet every week
Hydroxychloroquine	Renal	72–120 hrs	Oral	310 mg every week
Iodoquinol	Fecal	—	Oral	650 mg t.i.d. for 20 days
Mefloquine	Hepatic	15–33 days	Oral	1250 mg single dose
Metronidazole	Hepatic (R)	6–14 hrs	Oral, IV	250–500 mg every 6–8 hrs
Nitazoxanide	Hepatic	1.0–1.6 hr	Oral	100–200 mg b.i.d. based on age
Paromomycin	Fecal	—	Oral	25–35 mg/kg/day
Pentamidine	Renal	6–9 hrs	IM, IV, inhalation	IV, IM: 3–4 mg/kg every day; inhalation: 300 mg every 4 weeks
Primaquine	Hepatic	3.7–9.6 hrs	Oral	15 mg (base)/day
Pyrimethamine	Renal	111 hrs	Oral	25 mg every week
Quinacrine		5 days	Oral	100 mg/day
Quinine	Renal	12 hrs	Oral	325 mg b.i.d.
Tinidazole	Hepatic (R)	13.2 hrs	Oral	2 g q.d. × 1–3 days
Antitubercular agents				
Aminosalicylic acid	Renal	1 hr	Oral	150 mg/kg daily (maximum acid 12 g/day)
Capreomycin	Renal	4–6 hrs	IM	15 mg/kg/day to 1 g/day maximum
Cycloserine	Renal	10 hrs	Oral	15–20 mg/kg (maximum 1 g/day)
Ethambutol	Hepatic	3.3 hrs	Oral	15–25 mg/kg/day
Ethionamide	Hepatic	3 hrs	Oral	500 mg to 1 g/day
Isoniazid	Hepatic	1–4 hrs	Oral, IV	5–10 mg/kg daily (maximum dose = 300 mg)
Pyrazinamide	Hepatic	9–10 hrs	Oral	15–30 mg/kg daily (maximum 2 g/day)
Rifampin	Hepatic	2–3 hrs	Oral, IV	10 mg/kg (up to 600 mg) q.d.
Rifabutin	Hepatic	45 hrs	Oral	300 mg q.d.
Rifapentine	Hepatic	13.9 hrs (active metabolite /13.4 hrs)	Oral	600 mg every 3 days
Antiviral agents				
Abacavir	Hepatic	1.5 hr	Oral	300 mg b.i.d. or 600 mg every day
Adefovir	Renal	7.5 hrs	Oral	10 mg every day
Acyclovir	Renal	2.2 hrs	Oral, IV, topical	IV: 5–10 mg/kg every 8 hrs; oral: 200–800 mg 3–5 × daily (depending upon indication)
Amantadine	Renal	17 hrs	Oral	100 mg b.i.d. or 200 mg every day
Atazanavir	Hepatic	7 hrs	Oral	400 mg every day or 300 mg plus 100 mg ritonavir every day
Boceprevir	Hepatic	3 hrs	Oral	800 mg every 7–9 hrs
Cidofovir	Renal	6.5 hrs	IV	5 mg/kg/week × 2 (induction); 5 mg/kg every 2 weeks (maintenance)

Table 36-1 Continued.

Agent	Elimination Route	Half-Life	Administration Route	Common Dosage Range (Adults)
Antiviral agents (continued)				
Darunavir	Hepatic	15 hrs	Oral	600 mg plus 100 mg ritonavir b.i.d. or 800 mg plus 100 mg ritonavir every day
Delavirdine	Hepatic	5.8 hrs	Oral	400 mg t.i.d.
Didanosine	Renal	1.5 hrs	Oral	≥ 60 kg: 400 mg every day (EC caps); < 60 kg: 250 mg every day (EC caps)
Emtricitabine	Renal	10 hrs	Oral	200 mg every day (caps)
Enfuvirtide	n/a	3.8 hrs	SC	90 mg b.i.d.
Entecavir	Renal	128–149 hrs	Oral	0.5 mg every day, or 1 mg every day in patients with lamivudine resistance
Efavirenz	Hepatic	40–55 hrs	Oral	600 mg at bedtime
Etravirine	Hepatic	41 hrs	Oral	200 mg b.i.d.
Famciclovir	Renal	2.0–2.3 hrs	Oral	250–500 mg every 8–12 hrs
Fosamprenavir	Hepatic	7.7 hrs	Oral	1400 mg b.i.d. or 1400 mg plus 100–200 mg ritonavir every day or 700 mg plus 100 mg ritonavir every day
Foscarnet	Renal	3–6 hrs	IV	90 mg/kg every 12 hrs × 14–21 days (CMV induction); 90 mg/kg every day (CMV maintenance)
Ganciclovir	Renal	2.9 hrs	IV	5 mg/kg every 12 hrs (induction) × 14–21 days; 5 mg/kg every day (maintenance)
		4.8 hrs	Oral	1000 mg t.i.d. (after induction)
Indinavir	Hepatic	1.5–2.0 hrs	Oral	800 mg every 8 hrs
Lamivudine	Renal	5–7 hrs	Oral	150 mg b.i.d. or 300 mg daily
Lopinavir/ritonavir	Hepatic	5–6 hrs	Oral	200 mg/50 mg per tab (2 tablets b.i.d. or 4 tablets every day)
Maraviroc	Hepatic	14–18 hrs	Oral	150–600 mg b.i.d. (depending upon concomitant medications)
Nelfinavir	Hepatic	3.5–5.0 hrs	Oral	1250 mg b.i.d.
Nevirapine	Hepatic	25–30 hrs	Oral	Immediate-release: 200 mg every day × 14 days, then 200 mg b.i.d. Extended-release: 200 mg every day × 14 days, 400 mg every day
Oseltamivir	Renal	6–10 hrs	Oral	75 mg b.i.d. (treatment); 75 mg every day (prophylaxis)
Raltegravir	Hepatic	9 hrs	Oral	400 mg b.i.d.
Ribavirin	Renal	298 hrs	Oral	800–1200 mg daily, divided into 2 doses
Rilpivirine	Hepatic	50 hrs	Oral	25 mg daily
Rimantadine	Renal	25 hrs	Oral	100 mg b.i.d.
Ritonavir	Hepatic	3–5 hrs	Oral	100–400 mg daily, divided in 1 or 2 doses (as booster agent with other PIs)
Saquinavir	Hepatic	1–2 hrs	Oral	1000 mg (Invirase) plus 100 mg ritonavir b.i.d.
Stavudine	Renal	1 hrs	Oral	≥ 60 kg: 40 mg b.i.d.; < 60 kg: 30 mg b.i.d.
Telaprevir	Hepatic	9–11 hrs	Oral	750 mg every 7–9 hrs

(Continued on next page)

Table 36-1 Continued.

Agent	Elimination Route	Half-Life	Administration Route	Common Dosage Range (Adults)
Antiviral agents (continued)				
Telbivudine	Renal	40–49 hrs	Oral	600 mg every day
Tenofovir	Renal	17 hrs	Oral	300 mg daily
Tipranavir	Hepatic	6 hrs	Oral	500 mg plus 200 mg ritonavir b.i.d.
Valacyclovir	Renal	2.5–3.6 hrs	Oral	0.5–1.0 g every day or b.i.d. or t.i.d.
Valganciclovir	Renal	4 hrs	Oral	900 mg b.i.d. × 21 days (induction), 900 mg every day (maintenance)
Zanamivir	Renal	2.5–5.1 hrs	Inhalation (Diskhaler)	2 inhalations (10 mg) b.i.d. (treatment); 10 mg every day (prophylaxis)
Zidovudine	Renal (H)	1.1 hr	Oral	300 mg b.i.d.
			IV	2 mg/kg over 1 hr, then 1 mg/kg/hr until delivery (intrapartum perinatal prophylaxis for pregnant women)
Anthelmintics				
Albendazole	Hepatic	8–12 hrs	Oral	400–800 mg daily
Diethylcarbamazine	Renal	8 hrs	Oral	25 mg/day for 3 days, then 50 mg/day for 5 days, then 100 mg/day for 3 days, then 150 mg/day for 12 days
Ivermectin	Hepatic	16–35 hrs	Oral	150–200 mcg/kg × 1 dose
Mebendazole	Hepatic	8 hrs	Oral	100 mg b.i.d. × 3 consecutive days
Praziquantel	Hepatic	0.8–3.0 hrs	Oral	60–75 mg/kg in 3 divided doses on the same day
Pyrantel	Hepatic	—	Oral	11 mg/kg (maximum = 1 g) as a single dose

[a]Dosage applies to infections other than tuberculosis; for tuberculosis, dosage is 1 g/day.
[b]Intravenous agent withdrawn from U.S. market.
CMV, cytomegalovirus; *EC cap*, enteric-coated capsule; *H*, additional significant hepatic elimination; *HSCT*, hematopoietic stem cell transplant; *IM*, intramuscular; *IV*, intravenous; *PIs*, protease inhibitors *R*, additional significant renal elimination; *SC*, subcutaneous.

4. **Precautions and monitoring effects.** Aminoglycosides can cause serious adverse effects. To prevent or minimize such problems, blood drug concentrations and blood urea nitrogen (BUN) and serum creatinine levels should be monitored during therapy.
   a. **Ototoxicity.** Aminoglycosides can cause vestibular or auditory damage. The relative ototoxicity is as follows:

      streptomycin = kanamycin > amikacin = gentamicin = tobramycin > netilmicin

      (1) Gentamicin and streptomycin cause primarily **vestibular** damage (manifested by tinnitus, vertigo, and ataxia). Such damage may be bilateral and irreversible.
      (2) Amikacin, kanamycin, and neomycin cause mainly **auditory** damage (hearing loss).
      (3) Tobramycin can result in both vestibular and auditory damage.
   b. **Nephrotoxicity.** Because aminoglycosides accumulate in the proximal tubule, mild renal dysfunction develops in up to 25% of patients receiving these drugs for several days or more. Usually, this adverse effect is reversible. Use of once-daily administration (ODA) has been reported in the literature to be as effective and less nephrotoxic than traditional dosing.
      (1) Neomycin is the most nephrotoxic aminoglycoside; streptomycin is the least nephrotoxic. Gentamicin and tobramycin are nephrotoxic to approximately the same degree.
      (2) **Risk factors** for increased nephrotoxic effects include the following:
         (a) Preexisting renal disease
         (b) Previous or prolonged aminoglycoside therapy
         (c) Concurrent administration of another nephrotoxic drug

(d) Impaired renal flow unrelated to renal disease (e.g., from hypotension, severe hepatic disease)

(3) Trough levels > 2 μg/mL for gentamicin and tobramycin and > 10 μg/mL for amikacin are associated with nephrotoxicity.

c. **Neuromuscular blockade.** This problem may arise in patients receiving high-dose aminoglycoside therapy.

(1) **Risk factors** for neuromuscular blockade include the following:

(a) Concurrent administration of a neuromuscular blocking agent or an anesthetic

(b) Preexisting hypocalcemia or myasthenia gravis

(c) Intraperitoneal or rapid IV drug administration

(2) Apnea and respiratory depression may be reversed with administration of calcium or an anticholinesterase.

d. **Hypersensitivity** and **local reactions** are rare adverse effects of aminoglycosides.

e. **Therapeutic levels**

(1) Gentamicin and tobramycin peak at 6 to 10 μg/mL for traditional dosing; when using the ODA method, the peak is 16 to 20 μg/mL or 8 to 10 times the MIC of targeted bacteria. Their trough level is 0.5 to 1.5 μg/mL for traditional or once-daily regimens.

(2) Amikacin peaks at 25 to 30 μg/mL. The trough level is 5 to 8 μg/mL.

5. **Significant interactions**

a. **IV loop diuretics** can result in increased ototoxicity.

b. **Other aminoglycosides, cisplatin, and amphotericin B** can cause increased nephrotoxicity when given concurrently with streptomycin.

C. **Carbapenems.** These agents are β-lactams that contain a fused β-lactam ring and a five-membered ring system that differs from penicillins in being unsaturated and containing a carbon atom instead of a sulfur atom. The class has a broader spectrum of activity than do most β-lactams. Formerly known as thienamycin, **imipenem (Primaxin)** was the first carbapenem compound introduced in the United States, followed by **meropenem (Merrem)** and, most recently, **ertapenem (Invanz)** and **doripenem (Doribax)**. Because it is inhibited by renal dipeptidases, imipenem must be combined with **cilastatin** sodium, a dipeptidase inhibitor (cilastatin is not required with the others because these are not sensitive to renal dipeptidase).

1. **Mechanism of action.** Carbapenems are **bactericidal**, inhibiting bacterial cell wall synthesis.

2. **Spectrum of activity.** These drugs have the broadest spectrum of all β-lactam antibiotics. The group is active against most gram-positive cocci (including many enterococci), gram-negative rods (including many *P. aeruginosa* strains), and anaerobes. This class has good activity against many bacterial strains that resist other antibiotics. Ertapenem has a narrower spectrum of activity than the other carbapenems. It has little or no activity against *P. aeruginosa* and *Acinetobacter*. These β-lactam antibiotics resist destruction by most β-lactamases.

3. **Therapeutic uses.** Carbapenems are most valued in the treatment of severe infections caused by drug-resistant organisms susceptible to these agents. These agents are effective against urinary tract and lower respiratory infections; intra-abdominal and gynecological infections; and skin, soft tissue, bone, and joint infections.

4. **Precautions and monitoring effects**

a. Carbapenems may cause nausea, vomiting, diarrhea, and pseudomembranous colitis.

b. Seizures, dizziness, and hypotension may develop; seizures appear less frequently with meropenem or ertapenem (1.5% of patients receiving imipenem vs. 0.5% of those receiving meropenem or ertapenem).

c. Patients who are allergic to penicillin or cephalosporins may suffer cross-sensitivity reactions during carbapenem therapy.

D. **Cephalosporins.** These agents are known as **β-lactam antibiotics** because their chemical structure consists of a β-lactam ring adjoined to a thiazolidine ring. Cephalosporins generally are classified in four major groups based mainly on their spectrum of activity (*Table 36-2*).

1. **Mechanism of action.** Cephalosporins are **bactericidal**; they inhibit bacterial cell wall synthesis, reducing cell wall stability and thus causing membrane lysis.

2. **Spectrum of activity**

a. **First-generation** cephalosporins are active against most gram-positive cocci (except enterococci) as well as enteric aerobic gram-negative bacilli (e.g., *E. coli*, *K. pneumoniae*, *Proteus mirabilis*).

Table 36-2 CLASSIFICATION OF CEPHALOSPORINS

First-Generation	Second-Generation	Third-Generation	Fourth-Generation
Cefadroxil* (Duricef, Ultracef)	Cefaclor* (Ceclor)	Cefdinir (Omnicef)*	Cefepime (Maxipime)
Cefazolin (Ancef, Kefzol)	Cefmetazole (Zefazone)	Cefixime (Suprax)*	Ceftaroline (Teflaro)
Cephalexin* (Keflex)	Cefotetan (Cefotan)	Cefoperazone (Cefobid)	
Cephapirin (Cefadyl)	Cefoxitin (Mefoxin)	Cefotaxime (Claforan)	
Cephradine* (Anspor, Velosef)	Cefuroxime (Zinacef)	Cefpodoxime proxetil* (Vantin)	
	Cefuroxime axetil* (Ceftin)	Ceftazidime (Fortaz, Tazicef, Tazidime)	
	Cefprozil* (Cefzil)	Ceftibuten* (Cedax)	
		Ceftizoxime (Cefizox)	
		Ceftriaxone (Rocephin)	
		Cefditoren* (Spectracef)	

*Oral agents.

b. **Second-generation** cephalosporins are active against the organisms covered by first-generation cephalosporins and have extended gram-negative coverage, including β-lactamase–producing strains of *Haemophilus influenzae*.

c. **Third-generation** cephalosporins have wider activity against most gram-negative bacteria, for example, *Enterobacter*, *Citrobacter*, *Serratia*, *Providencia*, *Neisseria*, and *Haemophilus* organisms, including β-lactamase–producing strains. Some members have antipseudomonal activity.

d. **Fourth-generation** cephalosporins include **cefepime (Maxipime) and ceftaroline (Teflaro)**. However, their designation as a fourth-generation cephalosporin is debatable. Cefepime is highly resistant to β-lactamases and has a low propensity for selection of β-lactam–resistant mutant strains. It shows evidence of greater activity versus gram-positive cocci, *Enterobacteriaceae*, and *Pseudomonas* than third-generation cephalosporins. Ceftaroline has extended coverage of gram-positive bacteria including methicillin-resistant *Staphylococcus aureus* (MRSA), multidrug-resistant *Streptococcus pneumonia* (MDRSP), and common gram-negative bacteria. However, it has poor activity against anaerobes; atypical bacteria; and *Stenotrophomonas*, *Acinetobacter*, and *Pseudomonas* species. It is not stable against several β-lactamases.

e. Each generation of cephalosporin has shifted toward increased gram-negative activity but has lost activity toward gram-positive organisms. Fourth-generation agents should have improved activity toward gram-positive organisms (including MRSA) over third-generation agents, as well as greater aerobic and anaerobic gram-negative coverage.

3. **Therapeutic uses**

a. **First-generation** cephalosporins commonly are administered to treat serious *Klebsiella* infections and gram-positive and some gram-negative infections in patients with mild penicillin allergy. These agents also are used widely in perioperative prophylaxis. For most other indications, they are not the preferred drugs.

b. **Second-generation** cephalosporins are valuable in the treatment of urinary tract infections resulting from *E. coli* organisms, acute otitis media, sinusitis, and gonococcal disease caused by organisms that resist other agents.

(1) **Cefaclor (Ceclor)** is useful in otitis media and sinusitis in patients who are allergic to ampicillin and amoxicillin. **Cefprozil (Cefzil)**, a second-generation cephalosporin can be administered twice daily but offers no important spectrum differences.

(2) **Cefoxitin (Mefoxin)** is therapeutic for mixed aerobic–anaerobic infections, such as intra-abdominal infection. The **cefotetan (Cefotan)** spectrum is similar, but this agent can be given twice daily.

(3) **Cefuroxime (Zinacef)** is commonly administered for outpatient community-acquired pneumonia.

c. **Third-generation** cephalosporins penetrate the cerebrospinal fluid (CSF) and thus are valuable in the treatment of meningitis caused by such organisms as meningococci, pneumococci, *H. influenzae*, and enteric gram-negative bacilli.
   (1) These agents also are used to treat sepsis of unknown origin in immunosuppressed patients and to treat fever in neutropenic immunosuppressed patients (given in combination with an aminoglycoside).
   (2) Third-generation cephalosporins are useful in infections caused by many organisms resistant to older cephalosporins.
   (3) These agents are frequently administered as empiric therapy for life-threatening infection in which resistant organisms are the most likely cause.
   (4) Initial therapy of mixed bacterial infections (e.g., sepsis) commonly involves third-generation cephalosporins.

d. The **fourth-generation** agent, cefepime, is approved for treatment of urinary tract infections, uncomplicated skin and skin structure infections, pneumonia, and empiric use in febrile neutropenic patients. Cefepime has a spectrum of activity similar to third-generation agents but is more resistant to some β-lactamases. Ceftaroline is approved only for the treatment of community-acquired bacterial pneumonia and acute bacterial skin and skin structure infections caused by susceptible isolates.

4. **Precautions and monitoring effects**
   a. Because all cephalosporins (except cefoperazone) are eliminated renally, doses must be adjusted for patients with renal impairment.
   b. Cross-sensitivity with penicillin has been reported in up to 10% of patients receiving cephalosporins. More recent information indicates that true cross-reactivity is rare.
   c. Cephalosporins can cause hypersensitivity reactions similar to those resulting from penicillin (see II.F.1.e.[1]). Manifestations include fever, maculopapular rash, anaphylaxis, and hemolytic anemia.
   d. Other adverse effects include nausea, vomiting, diarrhea, superinfection, nephrotoxicity, and *Clostridium difficile*–induced colitis; with cefoperazone, cefmetazole, and cefotetan, bleeding diatheses may occur. Bleeding can be reversed by vitamin K administration.
   e. Cephalosporins may cause false-positive glycosuria results on tests using the copper-reduction method.
   f. Ceftriaxone now contraindicated in newborns receiving concurrent administration of calcium-containing solutions or products due to risk of fatal precipitation in lungs and kidneys. New warning added also stating that ceftriaxone and IV calcium-containing solutions should not be administered within 48 hrs of each other.

5. **Significant interactions**
   a. **Probenecid** may impair the excretion of cephalosporins (except ceftazidime), causing increased cephalosporin levels and possible toxicity.
   b. **Alcohol consumption** may result in a disulfiram-type reaction in patients receiving cefmetazole, cefotetan, and cefoperazone.
   c. Plasma concentrations of cefaclor extended-release tablets, cefdinir, and cefpodoxime may be reduced by coadministration with **antacids**.
   d. **H_2-antagonists** may reduce plasma levels of cefpodoxime and cefuroxime.
   e. **Iron supplements** and **iron-fortified foods** reduce absorption of cefdinir by 80% and 30%, respectively.

E. **Erythromycins.** The chemical structure of these macrolide antibiotics is characterized by a lactone ring to which sugars are attached. Erythromycin base and the estolate, ethylsuccinate, and stearate salts are given orally; erythromycin lactobionate and gluceptate are given parenterally.

1. **Mechanism of action.** Erythromycins may be **bactericidal** or **bacteriostatic**; they bind to the 50S ribosomal subunit, inhibiting bacterial protein synthesis.
2. **Spectrum of activity.** Erythromycins are active against many gram-positive organisms, including streptococci (e.g., *Streptococcus pneumoniae*), and *Corynebacterium* and *Neisseria* species as well as some strains of *Mycoplasma*, *Legionella*, *Treponema*, and *Bordetella*. Some *Staphylococcus aureus* strains that resist penicillin G are susceptible to erythromycins.
3. **Therapeutic uses**
   a. Erythromycins are the preferred drugs for the treatment of *Mycoplasma pneumoniae* and *Campylobacter* infections, Legionnaires disease, chlamydial infections, diphtheria, and pertussis.

b. In patients with penicillin allergy, erythromycins are important alternatives in the treatment of pneumococcal pneumonia, *S. aureus* infections, syphilis, and gonorrhea.
c. Erythromycins may be given prophylactically before dental procedures to prevent bacterial endocarditis.

4. **Precautions and monitoring parameters**
a. Gastrointestinal (GI) distress (e.g., nausea, vomiting, diarrhea, epigastric discomfort) may occur with all erythromycin forms and are the most common adverse effects.
b. Allergic reactions (rare) may present as skin eruptions, fever, and eosinophilia.
c. Cholestatic hepatitis may arise in patients treated for 1 week or longer with erythromycin estolate; symptoms usually disappear within a few days after drug therapy ends. There have been infrequent reports of hepatotoxicity with other salts of erythromycin.
d. IM injections of more than 100 mg produce severe pain persisting for hours.
e. Transient hearing impairment may develop with high-dose erythromycin therapy.

5. **Significant interactions**
a. Erythromycin inhibits the hepatic metabolism of **theophylline**, resulting in toxic accumulation.
b. Erythromycin interferes with the metabolism of **digoxin**, **corticosteroids**, **carbamazepine**, **cyclosporin**, and **lovastatin**, possibly potentiating the effect and toxicity of these drugs.
c. **Clarithromycin (Biaxin)** may potentiate **oral anticoagulants** (monitor prothrombin time), increase **cyclosporine** levels with increased toxicity, and increase **digoxin** and **theophylline** levels.
d. Coadministration of clarithromycin and **cisapride** may increase risk of serious cardiac arrhythmias; coadministration is contraindicated.
e. Sudden deaths have been reported when clarithromycin was added to ongoing **pimozide** therapy; coadministration is contraindicated.

6. **Alternatives to erythromycin**
a. **Clarithromycin and azithromycin (Zithromax)** are semisynthetic macrolide antibiotics. These expensive but well-tolerated alternatives to erythromycin are administered once daily.
(1) **Clarithromycin**
(a) **Spectrum of activity.** Clarithromycin is more active than erythromycin against staphylococci and streptococci. In addition to activity against other organisms covered by erythromycin, it is also active in vitro against MAI, *Toxoplasma gondii*, and *Cryptosporidium* spp.
(b) **Therapeutic uses.** This agent is indicated for the prevention of *Mycobacterium avium* complex (MAC) infection and is useful in otitis media, sinusitis, mycoplasmal pneumonia, and pharyngitis. Clarithromycin is also used with proton pump inhibitors (PPIs) for *Helicobacter pylori* eradication.
(2) **Azithromycin**
(a) **Spectrum of activity.** Azithromycin is less active than erythromycin against gram-positive cocci but more active against *H. influenzae* and other gram-negative organisms. Azithromycin concentrates within cells, and tissue levels are higher than serum levels.
(b) **Therapeutic uses.** This agent is useful in nongonococcal urethritis caused by chlamydia, lower respiratory tract infections, *Mycobacterium avium-intracellulare* (MAC or MAI) infection and prophylaxis, pharyngitis, pelvic inflammatory disease, and Legionnaires disease. Azithromycin is also indicated for pediatric use.

F. **Penicillins**

1. **Natural penicillins.** As with cephalosporins and all other penicillins, natural penicillins are β-lactam antibiotics. Among the most important antibiotics, natural penicillins are the preferred drugs in the treatment of many infectious diseases.
a. **Available agents**
(1) **Penicillin G** sodium and potassium salts can be administered orally, intravenously, or intramuscularly.
(2) **Penicillin V (Pen-Vee K),** a soluble drug form, is administered orally.
(3) **Penicillin G procaine** and **penicillin G benzathine** are repository drug forms. Administered intramuscularly, these insoluble salts allow slow drug absorption from the injection site and thus have a longer duration of action (12 to 24 hrs).
b. **Mechanism of action.** Penicillins are **bactericidal**; they inhibit bacterial cell wall synthesis in a manner similar to that of the cephalosporins.

c. Spectrum of activity

(1) Natural penicillins are highly active against gram-positive cocci and against some gram-negative cocci.

(2) Penicillin G is 5 to 10 times more active than penicillin V against gram-negative organisms and some anaerobic organisms.

(3) Because natural penicillins are readily hydrolyzed by penicillinases (β-lactamases), they are ineffective against *S. aureus* and other organisms that resist penicillin.

d. Therapeutic uses

(1) Penicillin G is the preferred agent for all infections caused by penicillin-susceptible *S. pneumoniae* organisms, including

(a) Pneumonia

(b) Arthritis

(c) Meningitis

(d) Peritonitis

(e) Pericarditis

(f) Osteomyelitis

(g) Mastoiditis

(2) Penicillins G and V are highly effective against other streptococcal infections, such as pharyngitis, otitis media, sinusitis, and bacteremia.

(3) Penicillin G is the preferred agent in gonococcal infections, syphilis, anthrax, actinomycosis, gas gangrene, and *Listeria* infections.

(4) Administered when an oral penicillin is needed, penicillin V is most useful in skin, soft tissue, and mild respiratory infections.

(5) Penicillin G procaine is effective against syphilis and uncomplicated gonorrhea.

(6) Used to treat syphilis infections outside the CNS, penicillin G benzathine also is effective against group A β-hemolytic streptococcal infections.

(7) Penicillins G and V may be used prophylactically to prevent streptococcal infection, rheumatic fever, and neonatal gonorrheal ophthalmia. Patients with valvular heart disease may receive these drugs preoperatively.

(8) There is emerging resistance to penicillin G by *S. pneumoniae* in some areas of the United States. The alternative therapy is vancomycin.

e. Precautions and monitoring effects

(1) Hypersensitivity reactions. These occur in up to 10% of patients receiving penicillin. Manifestations range from mild rash to anaphylaxis.

(a) The rash may be urticarial, vesicular, bullous, scarlatiniform, or maculopapular. Rarely, thrombopenic purpura develops.

(b) Anaphylaxis is a life-threatening reaction that most commonly occurs with parenteral administration. Signs and symptoms include severe hypotension, bronchoconstriction, nausea, vomiting, abdominal pain, and extreme weakness.

(c) Other manifestations of hypersensitivity reactions include fever, eosinophilia, angioedema, and serum sickness.

(d) Before penicillin therapy begins, the patient's history should be evaluated for reactions to penicillin. A positive history places the patient at heightened risk for a subsequent reaction. In most cases, such patients should receive a substitute antibiotic. (However, hypersensitivity reactions may occur even in patients with a negative history.)

(2) Other adverse effects of natural penicillins include GI distress (e.g., nausea, diarrhea), bone marrow suppression (e.g., impaired platelet aggregation, agranulocytosis), and superinfection. With high-dose therapy, seizures may occur, particularly in patients with renal impairment.

f. Significant interactions

(1) Probenecid increases blood levels of natural penicillins and may be given concurrently for this purpose.

(2) Antibiotic antagonism occurs when **erythromycins**, **tetracyclines**, or **chloramphenicol** is given within 1 hr of the administration of penicillin. The clinical significance of such antagonism is not clear.

(3) With penicillin G procaine and benzathine, precaution must be used in patients with a history of hypersensitivity reactions to penicillins because prolonged reactions may occur. Intravascular injection should be avoided. Procaine hypersensitivity is a contraindication to the use of procaine penicillin G.

(4) Parenteral products contain either potassium (1.7 mEq/million units) or sodium (2 mEq/million units).

2. **Penicillinase-resistant penicillins.** These penicillins are not hydrolyzed by staphylococcal penicillinases (β-lactamases). These agents include **methicillin**, **nafcillin**, and the **isoxazolyl penicillins—dicloxacillin (Dynapen)** and **oxacillin**.

a. **Mechanism of action** (see II.F.1.b)

b. **Spectrum of activity.** Because these penicillins resist penicillinases, they are active against staphylococci that produce these enzymes.

c. **Therapeutic uses**

(1) Penicillinase-resistant penicillins are used solely in staphylococcal infections resulting from organisms that resist natural penicillins.

(2) These agents are less potent than natural penicillins against organisms susceptible to natural penicillins and thus make poor substitutes in the treatment of infections caused by these organisms.

(3) **Nafcillin** is excreted by the liver and thus may be useful in treating staphylococcal infections in patients with renal impairment.

(4) **Oxacillin** and **dicloxacillin** are most valuable in long-term therapy of serious staphylococcal infections (e.g., endocarditis, osteomyelitis) and in the treatment of minor staphylococcal infections of the skin and soft tissues.

d. **Precautions and monitoring effects**

(1) As with all penicillins, the penicillinase-resistant group can cause hypersensitivity reactions (see II.F.1.e.[1]).

(2) Methicillin may cause nephrotoxicity and interstitial nephritis.

(3) Oxacillin may be hepatotoxic.

(4) Complete cross-resistance exists among the penicillinase-resistant penicillins.

e. **Significant interactions. Probenecid** increases blood levels of these penicillins and may be given concurrently for that purpose.

3. **Aminopenicillins.** This penicillin group includes the semisynthetic agents **ampicillin** and **amoxicillin (Amoxil)**. Because of their wider antibacterial spectrum, these drugs are also known as **broad-spectrum penicillins**.

a. **Mechanism of action** (see II.F.1.b)

b. **Spectrum of activity.** Aminopenicillins have a spectrum that is similar to but broader than that of the natural and penicillinase-resistant penicillins. Easily destroyed by staphylococcal penicillinases, aminopenicillins are ineffective against most staphylococcal organisms. Against most bacteria sensitive to penicillin G, aminopenicillins are slightly less effective than this agent.

c. **Therapeutic uses.** Aminopenicillins are used to treat gonococcal infections, upper respiratory infections, uncomplicated urinary tract infections, and otitis media caused by susceptible organisms.

(1) For infections resulting from penicillin-resistant organisms, **ampicillin** may be given in combination with sulbactam (**Unasyn**).

(2) **Amoxicillin** is less effective than ampicillin against shigellosis.

(3) **Amoxicillin** is more effective against *S. aureus*, *Klebsiella*, and *Bacteroides fragilis* infections when administered in combination with clavulanic acid—amoxicillin/potassium clavulanate (**Augmentin**) because clavulanic acid inactivates penicillinases.

d. **Precautions and monitoring effects**

(1) Hypersensitivity reactions may occur (see II.F.1.e.[1]).

(2) Diarrhea is most common with ampicillin.

(3) In addition to the urticarial hypersensitivity rash seen with all penicillins, ampicillin and amoxicillin frequently cause a generalized erythematous, maculopapular rash. (This occurs in 5% to 10% of patients receiving ampicillin.)

e. **Significant interactions** (see II.F.2.e)

4. **Extended-spectrum penicillins.** These agents have the widest antibacterial spectrum of all penicillins. Also called **antipseudomonal penicillins**, this group includes the **carboxypenicillin** (e.g., **ticarcillin**) and the **ureidopenicillin** (e.g., **piperacillin**).
   a. **Mechanism of action** (see II.F.1.b)
   b. **Spectrum of activity.** These drugs have a spectrum similar to that of the aminopenicillins but also are effective against *Klebsiella* and *Enterobacter* spp., some *B. fragilis* organisms, and indole-positive *Proteus* and *Pseudomonas* organisms.
      (1) **Ticarcillin** is active against *P. aeruginosa.* Combined with clavulanic acid (**Timentin**), ticarcillin has enhanced activity against organisms that resist ticarcillin alone.
      (2) **Piperacillin** is more active than ticarcillin against *Pseudomonas* organisms.
      (3) **Piperacillin and tazobactam (Zosyn).** Tazobactam is a β-lactamase inhibitor that expands the spectrum of activity to include some organisms not sensitive to piperacillin alone (if resistance is the result of β-lactamase production), including strains of staphylococci, *Haemophilus*, *Bacteroides*, and *Enterobacteriaceae*. Generally, tazobactam does not enhance activity against *Pseudomonas*.
   c. **Therapeutic uses.** Extended-spectrum penicillins are used mainly to treat serious infections caused by gram-negative organisms (e.g., sepsis; pneumonia; infections of the abdomen, bone, and soft tissues). Piperacillin/tazobactam is effective in the treatment of nosocomial pneumonia.
   d. **Precautions and monitoring effects**
      (1) Hypersensitivity reactions may occur (see II.F.1.e.[1]).
      (2) Ticarcillin may cause hypokalemia.
      (3) The high sodium content of ticarcillin may pose a danger to patients with heart failure (HF).
      (4) All inhibit platelet aggregation, which may result in bleeding.
   e. **Significant interactions** (see II.F.2.e)

G. **Sulfonamides.** Derivatives of sulfanilamide, these agents were the first drugs to prevent and cure human bacterial infection successfully. Although their current usefulness is limited by the introduction of more effective antibiotics and the emergence of resistant bacterial strains, sulfonamides remain the drugs of choice for certain infections. The major sulfonamides are **sulfadiazine**, **sulfamethoxazole**, **sulfisoxazole**, and **sulfamethizole**.

1. **Mechanism of action.** Sulfonamides are **bacteriostatic**; they suppress bacterial growth by triggering a mechanism that blocks folic acid synthesis, thereby forcing bacteria to synthesize their own folic acid.
2. **Spectrum of activity.** Sulfonamides are broad-spectrum agents with activity against many gram-positive organisms (e.g., *S. pyogenes*, *S. pneumoniae*) and certain gram-negative organisms (e.g., *H. influenzae*, *E. coli*, *P. mirabilis*). They also are effective against certain strains of *Chlamydia trachomatis*, *Nocardia*, *Actinomyces*, and *Bacillus anthracis*.
3. **Therapeutic uses**
   a. Sulfonamides most often are used to treat urinary tract infections caused by *E. coli*, including acute and chronic cystitis and chronic upper urinary tract infections.
   b. These agents have value in the treatment of nocardiosis, trachoma and inclusion conjunctivitis, and dermatitis herpetiformis.
   c. **Sulfadiazine** may be administered in combination with pyrimethamine to treat toxoplasmosis.
   d. **Sulfamethoxazole** may be given in combination with trimethoprim (**Bactrim**) to treat such infections as *Pneumocystis carinii* pneumonia, *Shigella* enteritis, *Serratia* sepsis, urinary tract infections, respiratory infections, and gonococcal urethritis. It is the drug of choice in the treatment of *Stenotrophomonas maltophilia*.
   e. **Sulfisoxazole** is sometimes used in combination with erythromycin ethylsuccinate to treat acute otitis media caused by *H. influenzae* organisms. For the initial treatment of uncomplicated urinary tract infections, sulfisoxazole may be given in combination with phenazopyridine for relief of symptoms of pain, burning, or urgency.
   f. Prophylactic sulfonamide therapy has been used successfully to prevent streptococcal infections and rheumatic fever recurrences.
4. **Precautions and monitoring effects**
   a. Sulfonamides may cause blood dyscrasias (e.g., hemolytic anemia—particularly in patients with G6PD deficiency, aplastic anemia, thrombocytopenia, agranulocytosis, and eosinophilia).

b. Hypersensitivity reactions to sulfonamides probably result from sensitization and most commonly involve the skin and mucous membranes. Manifestations include various types of skin rash, exfoliative dermatitis, and photosensitivity. Drug fever and serum sickness also may develop.
c. Crystalluria and hematuria may occur, possibly leading to urinary tract obstruction. (Adequate fluid intake and urine alkalinization can prevent or minimize this risk.) Sulfonamides should be used cautiously in patients with renal impairment.
d. Life-threatening hepatitis caused by drug toxicity or sensitization is a rare adverse effect. Signs and symptoms include headache, nausea, vomiting, and jaundice.
e. AIDS patients have increased frequency of cutaneous hypersensitivity reactions to sulfamethoxazole.

5. **Significant interactions.** Sulfonamides may potentiate the effects of **phenytoin**, **oral anticoagulants**, and **sulfonylureas**.

H. **Tetracyclines.** These broad-spectrum agents are effective against certain bacterial strains that resist other antibiotics. Nonetheless, they are the preferred drugs in only a few situations. The major tetracyclines include **demeclocycline (Declomycin)**, **doxycycline (Vibramycin)**, **minocycline (Minocin)**, and **oxytetracycline (Terramycin)**.

1. **Mechanism of action.** Tetracyclines are **bacteriostatic**; they inhibit bacterial protein synthesis by binding to the 30S ribosomal subunit.
2. **Spectrum of activity.** Tetracyclines are active against gram-negative and gram-positive organisms, spirochetes, *Mycoplasma* and *Chlamydia* organisms, rickettsial species, and certain protozoa.
   a. *Pseudomonas* and *Proteus* organisms are now resistant to tetracyclines. Many coliform bacteria, pneumococci, staphylococci, streptococci, and *Shigella* strains are increasingly resistant.
   b. Cross-resistance within the tetracycline group is extensive.
3. **Therapeutic uses**
   a. Tetracyclines are the agents of choice in rickettsial (Rocky Mountain spotted fever), chlamydial, and mycoplasmal infections; amebiasis; and bacillary infections (e.g., cholera, brucellosis, tularemia, some *Salmonella* and *Shigella* infections).
   b. Tetracyclines are useful alternatives to penicillin in the treatment of anthrax, syphilis, gonorrhea, Lyme disease, nocardiosis, and *H. influenzae* respiratory infections.
   c. Oral or topical tetracycline may be administered as a treatment for acne.
   d. **Doxycycline** is highly effective in the prophylaxis of "traveler's diarrhea" (commonly caused by *E. coli*). Because the drug is excreted mainly in the feces, it is the safest tetracycline for the treatment of extrarenal infections in patients with renal impairment.
   e. **Demeclocycline** is used commonly as an adjunctive agent to treat the **syndrome of inappropriate antidiuretic hormone (SIADH)** secretion.
4. **Precautions and monitoring effects**
   a. GI distress (e.g., diarrhea, abdominal discomfort, nausea, anorexia) is a common adverse effect of tetracyclines. This problem can be minimized by administering the drug with food or temporarily decreasing the dosage.
   b. Skin rash, urticaria, and generalized exfoliative dermatitis signify a hypersensitivity reaction. Rarely, angioedema and anaphylaxis occur.
   c. Cross-sensitivity within the tetracycline group is common.
   d. Phototoxic reactions (severe skin lesions) can develop with exposure to sunlight. This reaction is most common with demeclocycline and doxycycline.
   e. Tetracyclines may cause hepatotoxicity, particularly in pregnant women. Manifestations include jaundice, acidosis, and fatty liver infiltration.
   f. Renally impaired patients may experience a significant increase in BUN secondary to catabolic effects of tetracyclines.
   g. Tetracyclines may induce permanent tooth discoloration, tooth enamel defects, and retarded bone growth in infants and children.
   h. Use of outdated and degraded tetracyclines can lead to renal tubular dysfunction, possibly resulting in renal failure.
   i. Minocycline can cause vestibular toxicity (e.g., ataxia, dizziness, nausea, vomiting).
   j. IV tetracyclines are irritating and may cause phlebitis.

5. **Significant interactions**
   a. **Dairy products** and other foods, **iron preparations**, and **antacids** and **laxatives** containing aluminum, calcium, or magnesium can cause reduced tetracycline absorption. Absorption of doxycycline is not inhibited by these factors.
   b. **Methoxyflurane** may exacerbate the tetracyclines' nephrotoxic effects.
   c. **Barbiturates** and **phenytoin** decrease the antibiotic effectiveness of tetracyclines.
   d. Demeclocycline antagonizes the action of **antidiuretic hormone (ADH)** and may be given as a diuretic in patients with SIADH.

I. **Fluoroquinolones** are agents related to nalidixic acid—see II.J.1.c; II.J.2.c; II.J.4.c—and include **ciprofloxacin (Cipro)**, **norfloxacin (Noroxin)**, **ofloxacin (Floxin)**, **moxifloxacin (Avelox)**, **levofloxacin (Levaquin)**, and **gemifloxacin (Factive)**. They are bactericidal for growing bacteria.
   1. **Mechanism of action.** Fluoroquinolones inhibit DNA gyrase.
   2. **Spectrum of activity.** Fluoroquinolones are highly active against enteric gram-negative bacilli, *Salmonella*, *Shigella*, *Campylobacter*, *Haemophilus*, and *Neisseria*.
      a. **Ciprofloxacin** has activity against *P. aeruginosa*, but the fluoroquinolones as a group have variable activity against non–*P. aeruginosa*. Ciprofloxacin is active against some anaerobes; it has moderate activity against *M. tuberculosis*.
      b. Gram-positive organisms are less susceptible than gram-negative organisms but usually are sensitive, except for *Enterococcus faecalis* and methicillin-resistant staphylococci.
      c. **Ofloxacin** has the greatest activity against *Chlamydia*.
   3. **Therapeutic uses** (*Table 36-3*)
      a. Norfloxacin is indicated for the oral treatment of urinary tract infections, uncomplicated gonococcal infections, and prostatitis.
      b. Ciprofloxacin, ofloxacin, and levofloxacin are available orally and intravenously. Ciprofloxacin is approved for use in urinary tract infections; lower respiratory infections; sinusitis; bone, joint, and skin structure infections; empiric use in febrile neutropenic patients; typhoid fever; urethral and cervical gonococcal infections; and infectious diarrhea. Ofloxacin is approved for use in lower respiratory infections, uncomplicated gonococcal and chlamydial cervicitis and urethritis, skin and skin structure infections, prostatitis, and urinary tract infections.
      c. Levofloxacin is approved for the treatment of urinary tract infections. Gemifloxacin, moxifloxacin, and levofloxacin are also used in lower respiratory tract infections. Gemifloxacin is only available orally.
      d. Moxifloxacin is approved for the treatment of complicated intra-abdominal infections but should not be used for urinary tract infections.
   4. **Precautions and monitoring effects**
      a. Occasional adverse effects include nausea, dyspepsia, headache, dizziness, insomnia, cardiac QT prolongation, arthropathy, tendonitis, CNS effects, photosensitivity, and hypoglycemia.

Table 36-3 QUINOLONE AGENTS CLASSIFIED BY GENERATION

	Agent	Spectrum of Coverage	Site of Infection
First-generation	Cinoxacin (Cinoxacin, Cinobac) Nalidixic acid (NegGram) Norfloxacin (Noroxin)	Gram negatives	Urinary tract
Second-generation	Ciprofloxacin (Cipro) Ofloxacin (Floxin)	Gram negatives Gram positives	Systemic, urinary tract
Third-generation	Levofloxacin (Levaquin)	Gram positives Gram negatives Atypicals	Systemic, urinary tract
	Gemifloxacin (Factive) Moxifloxacin (Avelox)	Gram negatives Gram positives Atypicals	Systemic only

b. Infrequent adverse effects include rash, urticaria, leukopenia, and elevated liver enzymes. Crystalluria occurs with high doses at alkaline pH.
c. The FDA has added a black box warning about the increased risk of developing tendinitis and tendon rupture in patients taking this class of medications.

5. **Significant interactions**
a. Ciprofloxacin has been shown to increase **theophylline** levels. Variable effects on theophylline levels have been reported from other members of the group. In patients requiring fluoroquinolones, theophylline levels should be monitored.
b. **Antacids** and **sucralfate** and divalent or trivalent cations such as iron significantly decrease the absorption of fluoroquinolones.
c. Fluoroquinolones may increase prothrombin times in patients receiving **warfarin**.
d. Concurrent use with **nonsteroidal anti-inflammatory drugs** (NSAIDs) may increase the risk of CNS stimulation (seizures).
e. Fluoroquinolones may produce prolonged QT interval when administered with **antiarrhythmic agents**. Some fluoroquinolones (i.e., gemifloxacin, moxifloxacin) should be avoided in patients with known prolongation of the QTC interval, with uncorrected hypocalcemia, or who are receiving class IA or class III antiarrhythmic drugs.
f. Some fluoroquinolones have been reported to enhance the effects of oral anticoagulants.
g. Hyperglycemia and hypoglycemia have been reported in patients receiving quinolones and an antidiabetic agent. Blood glucose monitoring is recommended in such patients.

J. **Urinary tract antiseptics.** Concentrating in the renal tubules and bladder, these agents exert local antibacterial effects; most do not achieve blood levels high enough to treat systemic infections. However, some new quinolone derivatives, such as ciprofloxacin and ofloxacin, are valuable in the treatment of certain infections outside the urinary tract (see II.I.3.b).

1. **Mechanism of action**
a. **Methenamine** is hydrolyzed to ammonia and formaldehyde in acidic urine; formaldehyde is antibacterial against gram-positive and gram-negative organisms. Mandelic and hippuric acids, with which methenamine is combined, provide supplementary antibacterial action.
b. **Nitrofurantoin** is **bacteriostatic**; in high concentrations, it may be **bactericidal**. Presumably, it disrupts bacterial enzyme systems.
c. **Quinolones. Nalidixic acid** and its analogs and derivatives—**oxolinic acid, norfloxacin, cinoxacin, ciprofloxacin,** and others—interfere with DNA gyrase and inhibit DNA synthesis during bacterial replication.
d. **Fosfomycin tromethamine** is bactericidal in the urine at therapeutic doses. The bactericidal action is because of its inactivation of the enzyme enolpyruvyl transferase, thereby blocking the condensation of uridine diphosphate-*N*-acetylglucosamine with p-enolpyruvate, one of the first steps in bacterial cell wall synthesis.

2. **Spectrum of activity**
a. **Methenamine** is active against both gram-positive and gram-negative organisms (e.g., *Enterobacter, Klebsiella, Proteus, P. aeruginosa, S. aureus*).
b. **Nitrofurantoin** is active against many gram-positive and gram-negative organisms, including some strains of *E. coli, S. aureus, Proteus, Enterobacter*, and *Klebsiella*.
c. **Quinolones** (see II.I.2)
(1) **Nalidixic acid** and **oxolinic acid** are active against most gram-negative organisms that cause urinary tract infections, including *P. mirabilis, E. coli, Klebsiella*, and *Enterobacter* organisms. These drugs are not effective against *Pseudomonas* organisms.
(2) **Norfloxacin** is active against *E. coli, Enterobacter, Klebsiella, Proteus, P. aeruginosa, S. aureus, Citrobacter*, and some *Streptococcus* organisms.
(3) **Cinoxacin** is active against *E. coli, Klebsiella, P. mirabilis, Proteus vulgaris, Proteus morganii, Serratia*, and *Citrobacter* organisms.

3. **Therapeutic uses**
a. **Methenamine** and **nitrofurantoin** are used to prevent and treat urinary tract infections.
b. **Quinolones** are administered to treat urinary tract infections; some also are used in such diseases as osteomyelitis and respiratory tract infections.
c. **Fosfomycin** is indicated for treatment of uncomplicated urinary tract infection (acute cystitis) in women caused by susceptible strains of *E. coli* or *E. faecalis*.

4. **Precautions and monitoring effects**
   a. **Methenamine** may cause nausea, vomiting, and diarrhea; in high doses, it may lead to urinary tract irritation (e.g., dysuria, frequency, hematuria, albuminuria). Skin rash also may develop.
   b. **Nitrofurantoin** may cause various adverse effects.
      (1) GI distress (e.g., nausea, vomiting, diarrhea) is relatively common.
      (2) Hypersensitivity reactions to nitrofurantoin may involve the skin, lungs, blood, or liver; manifestations include fever, chills, hepatitis, jaundice, leukopenia, hemolytic anemia, granulocytopenia, and pneumonitis.
      (3) Adverse CNS effects include headache, vertigo, and dizziness. Polyneuropathy may develop with high doses or in patients with renal impairment.
   c. **Quinolones**
      (1) **Nalidixic acid** and **oxolinic acid** may cause nausea; vomiting; abdominal pain; urticaria; pruritus; skin rash; fever; eosinophilia; and CNS effects such as headache, dizziness, confusion, vertigo, drowsiness, and weakness.
      (2) **Cinoxacin** may induce nausea, vomiting, diarrhea, headache, insomnia, skin rash, pruritus, and urticaria.
5. **Significant interactions**
   a. The effects of methenamine are inhibited by **alkalinizing agents** and are antagonized by **acetazolamide**.
   b. Nitrofurantoin absorption is decreased by **magnesium-containing antacids**. Nitrofurantoin blood levels are increased and urine levels decreased by **sulfinpyrazone** and **probenecid**, leading to increased toxicity and reduced therapeutic effectiveness.
   c. **Quinolones**
      (1) Cinoxacin urine levels are decreased by **probenecid**, reducing therapeutic effectiveness.
      (2) Norfloxacin is rendered less effective by **antacids**.

K. **Miscellaneous antibacterial agents**
1. **Aztreonam (Azactam).** This agent was the first commercially available monobactam (monocyclic β-lactam compound). It resembles the aminoglycosides in its efficacy against many gram-negative organisms but does not cause nephrotoxicity or ototoxicity. Other advantages of this drug include its ability to preserve the body's normal gram-positive and anaerobic flora, activity against many gentamicin-resistant organisms, and lack of cross-allergenicity with penicillin.
   a. **Mechanism of action.** Aztreonam is **bactericidal**; it inhibits bacterial cell wall synthesis.
   b. **Spectrum of activity.** This drug is active against many gram-negative organisms, including *Enterobacter* and some strains of *P. aeruginosa*.
   c. **Therapeutic uses.** Aztreonam is therapeutic for urinary tract infections, septicemia, skin infections, lower respiratory tract infections, and intra-abdominal infections resulting from gram-negative organisms. Increased incidence of *P. aeruginosa* resistant to aztreonam has been reported.
   d. **Precautions and monitoring effects**
      (1) Aztreonam sometimes causes nausea, vomiting, and diarrhea.
      (2) Liver enzymes may increase transiently during aztreonam therapy.
      (3) This drug may induce skin rash.
2. **Chloramphenicol.** A nitrobenzene derivative, this drug has broad activity against rickettsia as well as many gram-positive and gram-negative organisms. It also is effective against many ampicillin-resistant strains of *H. influenzae*.
   a. **Mechanism of action.** Chloramphenicol is primarily **bacteriostatic**, although it may be bactericidal against a few bacterial strains.
   b. **Spectrum of activity.** This agent is active against rickettsia and a wide range of bacteria, including *H. influenzae, Salmonella typhi, Neisseria meningitidis, Bordetella pertussis, Clostridium, B. fragilis, S. pyogenes*, and *S. pneumoniae*.
   c. **Therapeutic uses.** Because of its toxic side effects, chloramphenicol is used only to suppress infections that cannot be treated effectively with other antibiotics. Such infections typically include
      (1) Typhoid fever
      (2) Meningococcal infections in cephalosporin-allergic patients
      (3) Serious *H. influenzae* infections, particularly in cephalosporin-allergic patients
      (4) Anaerobic infections (e.g., those originating in the pelvis or intestines)

(5) Anaerobic or mixed infections of the CNS

(6) Rickettsial infections in pregnant patients, tetracycline-allergic patients, and renally impaired patients

d. **Precautions and monitoring effects**

(1) Chloramphenicol can cause bone marrow suppression (dose-related) with resulting pancytopenia; rarely, the drug leads to aplastic anemia (not related to dose).

(2) Hypersensitivity reactions may include skin rash and, in extremely rare cases, angioedema or anaphylaxis.

(3) Chloramphenicol therapy may lead to gray baby syndrome in neonates (especially premature infants). This dangerous reaction, which stems partly from inadequate liver detoxification of the drug, is manifested by vomiting, gray cyanosis, rapid and irregular respirations, vasomotor collapse, and in some cases death.

e. **Significant interactions**

(1) Chloramphenicol inhibits the metabolism of **phenytoin**, **tolbutamide**, **chlorpropamide**, and **dicumarol**, leading to prolonged action and intensified effect of these drugs.

(2) **Phenobarbital** shortens chloramphenicol's half-life, thereby reducing its therapeutic effectiveness.

(3) **Penicillins** can cause antibiotic antagonism.

(4) **Acetaminophen** elevates chloramphenicol levels and may cause toxicity.

3. **Clindamycin (Cleocin).** This agent has essentially replaced lincomycin, the drug from which it is derived. It is used to treat skin, respiratory tract, and soft tissue infections caused by staphylococci, pneumococci, and streptococci.

a. **Mechanism of action.** Clindamycin is **bacteriostatic**; it binds to the 50S ribosomal subunit, thereby suppressing bacterial protein synthesis.

b. **Spectrum of activity.** This agent is active against most gram-positive and many anaerobic organisms, including *B. fragilis.*

c. **Therapeutic uses.** Because of its marked toxicity, clindamycin is used only against infections for which it has proven to be the most effective drug. Typically, such infections include abdominal and female genitourinary tract infections caused by *B. fragilis.*

d. **Precautions and monitoring effects**

(1) Clindamycin may cause rash, nausea, vomiting, diarrhea, and pseudomembranous colitis as evidenced by fever, abdominal pain, and bloody stools.

(2) Blood dyscrasias (e.g., eosinophilia, thrombocytopenia, leukopenia) may occur.

e. **Significant interactions.** Clindamycin may potentiate the effects of **neuromuscular blocking agents**.

4. **Dapsone.** A member of the sulfone class, this drug is the primary agent in the treatment of all forms of leprosy.

a. **Mechanism of action.** Dapsone is **bacteriostatic** for *Mycobacterium leprae*; its mechanism of action probably resembles that of the sulfonamides.

b. **Spectrum of activity.** This drug is active against *M. leprae*; however, drug resistance develops in up to 40% of patients. Dapsone also has some activity against *P. carinii* organisms and the malarial parasite *Plasmodium.*

c. **Therapeutic uses**

(1) Dapsone is the drug of choice for treating leprosy.

(2) This agent may be used to treat dermatitis herpetiformis, a skin disorder.

(3) Maloprim, a dapsone–pyrimethamine product, is valuable in the prophylaxis and treatment of malaria.

(4) Dapsone, with or without trimethoprim, is used for prophylaxis of *P. carinii* pneumonia in patients with AIDS.

d. **Precautions and monitoring effects**

(1) Hemolytic anemia can occur with daily doses $>$ 200 mg. Other adverse hematological effects include methemoglobinemia and leukopenia.

(2) Nausea, vomiting, and anorexia may develop.

(3) Adverse CNS effects include headache, dizziness, nervousness, lethargy, paresthesias, and psychosis.

(4) Dapsone occasionally results in a potentially lethal mononucleosis-like syndrome.
(5) Paradoxically, this drug sometimes exacerbates leprosy.
(6) Other adverse effects include skin rash, peripheral neuropathy, blurred vision, tinnitus, hepatitis, and cholestatic jaundice.

e. **Significant interactions. Probenecid** elevates blood levels of dapsone, possibly resulting in toxicity.

5. **Clofazimine** is phenazine dye with antimycobacterial and anti-inflammatory activity.
   a. **Mechanism of action.** Clofazimine appears to bind preferentially to mycobacterial DNA, inhibiting replication and growth. It is **bactericidal** against *M. leprae*, and it appears to be **bacteriostatic** against MAI.
   b. **Spectrum of activity.** Clofazimine is active against various mycobacteria, including *M. leprae*, *M. tuberculosis*, and MAI.
   c. **Therapeutic uses.** Clofazimine is used to treat leprosy and a variety of atypical *Mycobacterium* infections.
   d. **Precautions and monitoring effects**
      (1) Pigmentation (pink to brownish) occurs in 75% to 100% of patients within a few weeks. This skin discoloration has led to severe depression (and suicide).
      (2) Urine, sweat, and other body fluids may be discolored.
      (3) Other effects include ichthyosis and dryness of skin (8% to 28%), rash and pruritus (1% to 5%), and GI intolerance (e.g., abdominal/epigastric pain, diarrhea, nausea, vomiting) in 40% to 50% of patients. Clofazimine should be taken with food.
6. **Daptomycin (Cubicin)** is a unique lipopeptide antibiotic with clinical activity in the treatment of resistant gram-positive infections.
   a. **Mechanism of action.** Daptomycin is bactericidal; unlike other antibiotics, it binds to the bacterial cell membrane, causing depolarization of the membrane potential leading to inhibition of RNA, DNA, and protein synthesis.
   b. **Spectrum of activity.** This drug is active against vancomycin-susceptible *E. faecium* and *S. aureus* (including methicillin-resistant strains) as well as other aerobic gram-positive bacteria.
   c. **Therapeutic uses.** Daptomycin is indicated for the treatment of complicated skin and skin structure infections and intravascular line and *S. aureus* bacteremia. It is *not* indicated for the treatment of pneumonia.
   d. **Precautions and monitoring effects**
      (1) Reported side effects are generally mild and self-limiting and include constipation, abnormal liver function tests, and renal failure.
      (2) Cases of myalgia and/or muscle weakness, exacerbations of myasthenia gravis, and increases in creatine phosphokinase (CPK) have been reported.
7. **Fidaxomicin (Dificid)** is the first of a new class of antibiotics called macrocycles.
   a. **Mechanism of action.** Fidaxomicin is bactericidal against *C. difficile* in vitro, inhibiting RNA synthesis by RNA polymerases.
   b. **Spectrum of activity.** Fidaxomicin eradicates *C. difficile* selectively with minimal disruption to normal GI flora.
   c. **Therapeutic uses.** To reduce the development of drug-resistant bacteria and maintain the effectiveness of fidaxomicin and other antibacterial drugs, fidaxomicin should be used only to treat infections that are proven or strongly suspected to be caused by *Clostridium difficile*. Fidaxomicin is indicated in adults ($\geq$ 18 years of age) for treatment of *C. difficile*–associated diarrhea (CDAD).
   d. **Precautions and monitoring effects.** Because there is minimal systemic absorption of fidaxomicin, it is not effective for treatment of systemic infections. The most common adverse reactions are nausea (11%), vomiting (7%), abdominal pain (6%), gastrointestinal hemorrhage (4%), anemia (2%), and neutropenia (2%).
8. **Linezolid (Zyvox)** is a synthetic oxazolidinone that has clinical use in the treatment of infections caused by aerobic gram-positive bacteria.
   a. **Mechanism of action.** Linezolid is bacteriostatic against *Enterococci* and *Staphylococci*, and bactericidal against *Streptococci*. Linezolid binds to the 23S ribosomal RNA of the 50S subunit and thus inhibits protein synthesis.

b. **Spectrum of activity.** The drug is active against vancomycin-resistant *Enterococcus faecium* and *S. aureus* (methicillin-susceptible and -resistant strains) as well as other aerobic gram-positive bacteria.
c. **Therapeutic uses.** Linezolid is indicated for treatment of infections caused by vancomycin-resistant *E. faecium*, nosocomial pneumonia caused by methicillin-susceptible and -resistant strains of *S. aureus*, community-acquired pneumonia caused by penicillin-susceptible strains of *S. pneumoniae*, and skin and skin structure infections owing to these organisms.
d. **Precautions and monitoring effects**
   (1) Safety data are limited. Adverse effects generally are minor (e.g., gastrointestinal complaints, headache, rash).
   (2) Thrombocytopenia or a significant reduction in platelet count has been reported (2.4%) and is related to duration of therapy. Monitor platelets in patients with risk of bleeding, preexisting thrombocytopenia, platelet disorders (including those caused by concurrent medications) and in patients receiving linezolid lasting longer than 2 weeks.
   (3) Myelosuppression owing to direct bone marrow suppression has been reported rarely.
e. **Significant interactions.** Patients receiving concomitant therapy with adrenergic or serotonergic agents or consuming more than 100 mg of tyramine a day may experience an enhancement of the drug's effect or serotonin syndrome.

9. **Quinupristin/dalfopristin (Synercid)** is an intravenous streptogramin antibiotic composed of two chemically distinct compounds.
   a. **Mechanism of action.** Quinupristin binds to the 50S subunit, and dalfopristin binds tightly to the 70S ribosomal particle.
   b. **Spectrum of activity.** Synercid has activity against *Staphylococci* spp., including resistant strains. This combination has better activity against *E. faecium* than *Enterococcus faecalis* and is also active against some gram-negative organisms and anaerobes; activity has not been shown against *Enterobacteriaceae*.
   c. **Therapeutic uses.** It is used for treatment of vancomycin-resistant *E. faecium* (VREF) bacteremia and skin and skin structure infections caused by *S. aureus* and *S. pyogenes*.
   d. **Precautions and monitoring effects**
      (1) Reported side effects are generally mild and infusion related: pain, erythema, or itching at the infusion site; increases in pulse and diastolic pressure; headache; nausea or vomiting; and diarrhea. It may increase liver function tests slightly.
      (2) Drug interactions are a result of cytochrome P450 3A4 inhibition. Potential drug interactions include **cyclosporin**, **nifedipine**, and **midazolam**.
      (3) Concomitant use of medications that may prolong QTc interval should be avoided.
      (4) Mild to life-threatening pseudomembranous colitis has been reported.

10. **Rifaximin.** Is a semisynthetic antibiotic that is structurally related to rifamycin.
    a. **Mechanism of action.** It inhibits bacterial RNA synthesis by binding to the β subunit of bacterial DNA-dependent RNA polymerase.
    b. **Spectrum of activity.** This nonsystemically absorbed drug has activity against both enterotoxigenic and enteroaggregative strains of *Escherichia coli*.
    c. **Therapeutic uses.** Rifaximin is used in the treatment of travelers diarrhea with noninvasive strains of *E. coli* and prophylaxis of hepatic encephalopathy. High resistance rates have been reported after 5 days of treatment.
    d. **Precautions and monitoring effects.** Because of its limited systemic absorption, adverse effects are few but include constipation, vomiting, flatulence, and headache.

11. **Spectinomycin.** An aminocyclitol agent related to the aminoglycosides, this antibiotic is useful against penicillin-resistant strains of gonorrhea.
    a. **Mechanism of action.** Spectinomycin is **bacteriostatic**; it selectively inhibits protein synthesis by binding to the 30S ribosomal subunit.
    b. **Spectrum of activity.** This agent is active against various gram-negative organisms.
    c. **Therapeutic uses.** Spectinomycin is used only to treat gonococcal infections in patients with penicillin allergy or when such infection stems from penicillinase-producing gonococci (PPNG).
    d. **Precautions and monitoring effects.** Because spectinomycin is given only as a single-dose IM injection, it causes few adverse effects. Nausea, vomiting, urticaria, chills, dizziness, and insomnia occur rarely.

12. **Telavancin (Vibativ)** is the first of a new class of antimicrobials known as the lipoglycopeptides. It is a semisynthetic derivative of vancomycin.
    a. **Mechanism of action.** Telavancin is bacteriocidal; it inhibits peptidoglycan and cell wall synthesis as well as disrupts membrane potential.
    b. **Spectrum of activity.** This drug is active against gram-positive bacteria, including MRSA and vancomycin-susceptible *Enterococcus faecalis*.
    c. **Therapeutic uses.** Telavancin is indicated for the treatment of complicated skin and skin structure infections caused by susceptible gram-positive bacteria, including MRSA.
    d. **Precautions and monitoring effects**
        (1) Taste disturbance, nausea and vomiting, and foamy urine were the most common side effects.
        (2) Nephrotoxicity and QT prolongation have been reported in patients.
        (3) Use of telavancin should be avoided in pregnant women.
13. **Telithromycin (Ketek)** is the first of a new class of antimicrobials called the ketolides. It is an oral semisynthetic derivative of erythromycin.
    a. **Mechanism of action.** Telithromycin may be bactericidal or bacteriostatic; it inhibits bacterial protein synthesis.
    b. **Spectrum of activity.** This drug is active against many aerobic and anaerobic gram-positive organisms, including multidrug-resistant *S. pneumoniae*, some gram-negative organisms, as well as atypical pathogens.
    c. **Therapeutic uses.** Telithromycin is indicated for the treatment of mild to moderate community-acquired pneumonia only. The FDA removed the previous two approved indications and added a black box warning.
    d. **Precautions and monitoring effects**
        (1) GI effects (including diarrhea, nausea, and vomiting) were the most common side effects followed by dizziness and visual disturbances (such as diplopia and blurred and abnormal vision); serious liver toxicity has been reported.
        (2) Cross-sensitivity with the other macrolides occurs.
        (3) Concomitant use of drugs or conditions that may prolong the QTc interval should be avoided.
        (4) Contraindicated in patients with myasthenia gravis, hepatitis, or jaundice.
    e. **Significant interactions**
        (1) Coadministration of telithromycin with either cisapride or pimozide is contraindicated.
        (2) Concomitant administration of drugs metabolized by cytochrome P450 3A4 in patients with telithromycin should be closely monitored.
        (3) Patients on bepridil, mesoridazine, terfenadine, thioridazine, or ziprasidone should not be prescribed telithromycin owing to the high potential for toxicity.
        (4) **This agent has a high potential to interact with many drugs. Check product information for the most current interaction information.**
14. **Tigecycline (Tygacil).** An intravenous glycylcycline antibiotic developed as a semisynthetic analogue of tetracycline with a broad spectrum of activity.
    a. **Mechanism of action.** Tigecycline is bacteriostatic; it inhibits bacterial protein synthesis by reversibly binding to the 30S ribosome subunit.
    b. **Spectrum of activity.** The drug is active against vancomycin-susceptible *E. faecalis*, methicillin-resistant *S. epidermidis*, and *S. aureus* (methicillin-susceptible and -resistant strains) as well as some gram-negative aerobes and anaerobes.
    c. **Therapeutic uses.** Tigecycline is indicated for the treatment of complicated intra-abdominal infections caused by *E. coli*, vancomycin-susceptible *E. faecalis*, *S. aureus* (methicillin-susceptible strains only) and *B. fragilis*. Also indicated for the treatment of complicated skin and skin structure infections caused by *E. faecalis* (vancomycin-susceptible strains), *S. pyogenes* and *S. aureus* (methicillin-susceptible and -resistant strains).
    d. **Precautions and monitoring effects**
        (1) Safety data are limited. Side effects are generally mild with GI disturbances—for example, nausea (22% to 35%) and vomiting (13% to 19%)—the most commonly reported. The mechanism of these reactions is uncertain.
        (2) May cause permanent discoloration of the teeth similar to the tetracyclines.
        (3) Caution in patients with a history of hypersensitivity reactions to tetracyclines.
        (4) Phototoxic reactions, pancreatitis, and increases in BUN may occur.

e. **Significant interactions.** Closely monitor the prothrombin time or international sensitivity index (INR) in patients on warfarin during concomitant administration of tigecycline.

15. **Trimethoprim.** A substituted pyrimidine, trimethoprim is most commonly combined with sulfamethoxazole (a sulfonamide discussed in II.G) in a preparation called co-trimoxazole. However, it may be used alone for certain urinary tract infections.
    a. **Mechanism of action.** Trimethoprim inhibits dihydrofolate reductase, thus blocking bacterial synthesis of folic acid.
    b. **Spectrum of activity**
        (1) Trimethoprim is active against most gram-negative and gram-positive organisms. However, drug resistance may develop when this drug is used alone.
        (2) Trimethoprim–sulfamethoxazole is active against a variety of organisms, including *Streptococcus pneumoniae*, *N. meningitidis*, and *Corynebacterium diphtheriae*; some strains of *Staphylococcus aureus*, *Staphylococcus epidermidis*, *P. mirabilis*, *Enterobacter*, *Salmonella*, *Shigella*, *Serratia*, and *Klebsiella* spp.; and *Escherichia coli*.
        (3) The trimethoprim–sulfamethoxazole combination is synergistic; many organisms resistant to one component are susceptible to the combination.
    c. **Therapeutic uses**
        (1) Trimethoprim may be used alone or in combination with sulfamethoxazole to treat uncomplicated urinary tract infections caused by *Escherichia coli*, *P. mirabilis*, and *Klebsiella* and *Enterobacter* organisms.
        (2) Trimethoprim–sulfamethoxazole is therapeutic for acute gonococcal urethritis, acute exacerbation of chronic bronchitis, shigellosis, and *Salmonella* infections.
        (3) Trimethoprim–sulfamethoxazole may be given as prophylactic or suppressive therapy in *P. carinii* pneumonia. It is the drug of choice for the treatment of *Stenotrophomonas maltophilia* infections.
    d. **Precautions and monitoring effects**
        (1) Most adverse effects involve the skin (possibly from sensitization). These include rash, pruritus, and exfoliative dermatitis.
        (2) Rarely, trimethoprim–sulfamethoxazole causes blood dyscrasias (e.g., acute hemolytic anemia, leukopenia, thrombocytopenia, methemoglobinemia, agranulocytosis, aplastic anemia).
        (3) Adverse GI effects including nausea, vomiting, and epigastric distress glossitis may occur.
        (4) Neonates may develop kernicterus.
        (5) Patients with AIDS sometimes suffer fever, rash, malaise, and pancytopenia during trimethoprim therapy.

16. **Vancomycin.** This glycopeptide destroys most gram-positive organisms.
    a. **Mechanism of action.** Vancomycin is **bactericidal**; it inhibits bacterial cell wall synthesis.
    b. **Spectrum of activity.** This drug is active against most gram-positive organisms, including methicillin-resistant strains of *S. aureus and Enterococci*.
    c. **Therapeutic uses.** Vancomycin usually is reserved for serious infections, especially those caused by methicillin-resistant staphylococci. It is particularly useful in patients who are allergic to penicillin or cephalosporins. Typical uses include endocarditis, osteomyelitis, and staphylococcal pneumonia.
        (1) Oral vancomycin is valuable in the treatment of antibiotic-induced pseudomembranous colitis caused by *C. difficile* or *S. aureus* enterocolitis. Because vancomycin is not absorbed after oral administration, it is not useful for systemic infections. Because of resistance, the Centers for Disease Control and Prevention (CDC) recommend vancomycin as the second choice to metronidazole for *C. difficile* infections.
        (2) Because 1 g provides adequate blood levels for 7 to 10 days, IV vancomycin is particularly useful in the treatment of anephric patients with gram-positive bacterial infections.
    d. **Precautions and monitoring effects**
        (1) Ototoxicity may arise; nephrotoxicity is rare but can occur with high doses.
        (2) Vancomycin may cause hypersensitivity reactions, manifested by such symptoms as anaphylaxis and skin rash.
        (3) Therapeutic levels peak at 20 to 40 μg/mL. The trough is $<$ 15 μg/mL.

(4) Red man's syndrome may occur. This is facial flushing and hypotension owing to too rapid infusion of the drug. Infusion should be over a minimum of 60 mins for a 1-g dose.

(5) IV solutions are very irritating to the vein.

e. **Vancomycin-resistant enterococci.** A few strains of vancomycin-resistant enterococci are susceptible to teicoplanin (investigational by Hoechst Marion Roussel), linezolid (Zyvox), or quinupristin/dalfopristin (Synercid). These agents may be useful for multiple-drug–resistant *E. faecium*.

III. SYSTEMIC ANTIFUNGAL AGENTS

A. **Definition.** These agents treat systemic and local fungal (mycotic) infections—diseases that resist treatment with antibacterial drugs.

B. **Amphotericin B (Fungizone).** This polyene antifungal antibiotic is therapeutic for various fungal infections that frequently proved fatal before the drug became available. It is used increasingly in the empiric treatment of severely immunocompromised patients in certain clinical situations.

1. **Mechanism of action.** Amphotericin B is both **fungistatic** in clinically obtained concentrations and may be fungicidal in the presence of susceptible organisms. It binds to sterols in the fungal cell membrane, thereby increasing membrane permeability and permitting leakage of intracellular contents. Other mechanisms may be involved as well.

2. **Spectrum of activity.** Amphotericin B is a broad-spectrum antifungal agent with activity against *Aspergillus*, *Blastomyces*, *Candida* spp. (*albicans*, *krusei tropicalis*, and *glabrata*), *Cryptococcus*, *Coccidioides*, *Histoplasma*, *Paracoccidioides*, *Phycomycetes* (*mucor*), and *Sporothrix*. It is also useful against some protozoa such as *Leishmania*, *Naegleria*, and *Acanthamoeba*.

3. **Therapeutic uses.** Amphotericin B is the most effective antifungal agent in the treatment of systemic fungal infections, especially in immunocompromised patients.

   a. It is the treatment of choice for pulmonary *Aspergillus* infections; *Blastomyces* infections, which are life-threatening with AIDS or CNS involvement; deep-organ infections with *Candida*; *Coccidioides* infections with severe pulmonary involvement or with disseminated nonmeningeal immunocompetent or immunocompromised patients; all *Cryptococcus* infections; disseminated *Histoplasma* infections involving CNS or immunosuppressed patients; *Malassezia furfur* fungemia; pulmonary and extrapulmonary *Phycomycetes* (mucormycosis); *Penicillium marneffei*; and extracutaneous *Sporothrix*.

   b. This agent may be used to treat coccidioidal arthritis.

   c. Topical preparations are given to eradicate cutaneous and mucocutaneous candidiasis.

   d. It may be used as empiric therapy in febrile, neutropenic patients.

   e. It is used as secondary prophylaxis of fungal infections in HIV-positive patients, guarding against recurrence of infection.

   f. It may be used prophylactically in neutropenic cancer patients and bone marrow transplant or solid-organ transplant patients to reduce the incidence of *Aspergillus* and *Candida* infections.

4. **Precautions and monitoring effects.** Because amphotericin B can cause many serious adverse effects, it should be administered in a hospital setting—at least during the initial therapeutic stage. The adverse effects are divided into infusion reactions and others.

   a. Infusion reactions occur while the drug is being administered and include fever, shaking chills, hypotension, anorexia, nausea, vomiting, headache, dyspnea, and tachypnea. Premedication with acetaminophen and diphenhydramine has been helpful in prophylaxing against infusion reactions. In addition, hydrocortisone 10 to 50 mg may be added to the infusion as prophylaxis against infusion-related reactions. Meperidine 25 to 50 mg IV is effective treatment of active shaking chills/rigors. Meperidine is also effective in prophylaxis of rigors.

   b. Nephrotoxicity frequently occurs. Dosage adjustment or drug discontinuation or changing to a liposomal amphotericin B product may be necessary as renal impairment progresses.

   c. Electrolyte abnormalities, including hypokalemia, hypomagnesemia, and hypocalcemia, are common. Monitor and replace electrolytes as needed.

   d. Normocytic, normochromic anemia will develop over long-term use (10 weeks). Monitor hematocrit periodically.

   e. Bronchospasm, wheezing, and anaphylaxis or anaphylactoid reactions have occurred. A test dose of 1 mg of amphotericin B is often administered before infusion of large quantities of the drug.

f. Phlebitis or thrombophlebitis is reported with conventional amphotericin B. Heparin (500 to 1000 U) can be added to the infusion to aid in prevention.
g. CNS effects include headache, peripheral neuropathy, malaise, depression, seizure, myasthenia, and hallucinations.
h. Elevated liver transaminases, aspartate aminotransferase (AST), alanine aminotransferase (ALT), alkaline phosphatase, bilirubin, γ-glutamyltransferase (GGT), and lactate dehydrogenase (LDH) may occur.
i. Amphotericin B parenteral use should be mixed only in dextrose 5% in water (D_5W) and should be protected from light.

5. **Significant interactions.** Other nephrotoxic drugs (aminoglycosides, capreomycin, colistin, cisplatin, cyclosporine, methoxyflurane, pentamidine, polymyxin B, and vancomycin) may cause additive nephrotoxicity.
6. Amphotericin B lipid complex (Abelcet), amphotericin B cholesterol sulfate complex (Amphotec), and liposomal amphotericin B (AmBisome) offer alternative formulations of amphotericin B for the treatment of severe fungal infections in patients who are intolerant of or whose disease is refractory to conventional treatment.

C. **Echinocandins.** Three echinocandins are approved in the United States: caspofungin (Cancidas), micafungin (Mycamine), and anidulafungin (Eraxis). These agents have a broad spectrum of activity against *Candida* species with micafungin and anidulafungin having similar MICs that are generally lower than the MIC of caspofungin.

1. **Mechanism of action.** Caspofungin works by causing fungal cell wall lysis. By being a noncompetitive inhibitor of β (1,3) synthase, which is an essential component of fungal cell wall synthesis, it causes osmotic instability within the fungus and fungal cell wall lysis.
2. **Spectrum of activity.** Echinocandins have fungicidal activity against Candida species and fungistatic activity against *Aspergillus* species. All three agents in this class appear to have good activity in vitro for most isolates of Candida species, including those that are either Amphotericin-B or fluconazole and itraconazole-resistant, such as *C. glabrata*.
3. **Therapeutic uses.** All three agents are indicated for the treatment of esophageal candidiasis.
   a. Caspofungin and anidulafungin are also indicated for the treatment of candidemia and other infections caused by *Candida* species, including intra-abdominal abscesses and peritonitis.
   b. Caspofungin may also be used for the treatment of candidal pleural space infections, empiric treatment of presumed fungal infections in neutropenic patients, and treatment of invasive aspergillosis in patients refractory to or intolerant of other antifungals (i.e., amphotericin B, itraconazole).
   c. Micafungin is indicated for the prophylaxis of candidal infections in patients undergoing hematopoietic stem cell transplantation (HSCT).
4. **Precautions and monitoring effects.** Although this class has adverse events associated with its use, the overall toxicity profile is significantly better than that of amphotericin B.
   a. Infusion vein complications (not defined by manufacturer) and thrombophlebitis have been seen on infusion of caspofungin.
   b. Hematological decreases in hemoglobin and hematocrit may occur; however, the incidence does not differ from that of having a fungal disease.
   c. Headache may occur.
   d. Slight decreases in serum potassium may occur, but nowhere near the magnitude of that caused by amphotericin B.
   e. Anorexia, nausea, vomiting, and diarrhea have occurred.
   f. Rare increases in serum creatinine; however, there have been no reported cases of nephrotoxicity.
   g. Possible slight increases in serum aminotransferases
   h. Allergic reactions occur in $< 5\%$ of patients and anaphylaxis in $< 2\%$ of patients.
   i. Pregnancy category C embryotoxic reactions have occurred in animals.
5. **Significant interactions**
   a. When cyclosporine is combined with caspofungin, clinically significant rises in ALT were observed. Serum transaminases should be monitored, and this combination should be avoided in patients with preexisting liver disease.
   b. When used in combination, carbamazepine, nelfinavir, nevirapine, phenytoin, and rifampin increases the clearance of caspofungin. Higher doses of caspofungin (70 mg every day) should be considered when this combination is administered.

c. Tacrolimus clearance will be increased when the combination is used; monitor tacrolimus serum levels closely.

D. **Flucytosine (Ancobon).** This fluorinated pyrimidine usually is given in combination with amphotericin B.

1. **Mechanism of action.** Flucytosine penetrates fungal cells and is converted to fluorouracil, a metabolic antagonist. Incorporated into the RNA of the fungal cell, flucytosine causes defective protein synthesis. It is either **fungistatic** or **fungicidal**, depending on the concentration of the drug.
2. **Spectrum of activity.** This drug is primarily active against *Cryptococcus* and *Candida*. It is most commonly used in conjunction with amphotericin B. Fungal resistance against flucytosine alone has been well documented. Flucytosine may also possess some activity against chromomycosis and some strains of *Aspergillus* (in vitro testing only).
3. **Therapeutic uses.** Flucytosine is adjunctively used with amphotericin B for severe systemic infections (e.g., septicemia, endocarditis, pulmonary and urinary tract infections, meningitis). Use of flucytosine alone is not recommended.
4. **Precautions and monitoring effects**
   a. Frequent adverse effects include GI intolerance with nausea, vomiting, and diarrhea.
   b. Occasional adverse reactions are more severe and include marrow suppression with leukopenia or thrombocytopenia (dose related, especially with renal failure or concurrent amphotericin B use). Confusion, rash, hepatitis, enterocolitis, headache, and photosensitivity reactions can also occur.
   c. Rare reactions include hallucinations, blood dyscrasias with agranulocytosis and pancytopenia, fatal hepatitis, anaphylaxis, and anemia.
   d. Flucytosine may cause a markedly false elevation of serum creatinine if an Ektachem analyzer is used.
5. **Significant interactions.** Beneficial drug interactions occur with flucytosine. Flucytosine has demonstrated synergy with **amphotericin B** and **fluconazole** against *Cryptococcus* and *Candida* spp.

E. **Griseofulvin (Fulvicin).** Produced from *Penicillium griseofulvin Dierckx*, this drug is deposited in the skin, bound to keratin.

1. **Mechanism of action.** This agent is **fungistatic**; it inhibits fungal cell activity by interfering with mitotic spindle structure. Its mechanism of action is similar to colchicine.
2. **Spectrum of activity.** Griseofulvin is active against various strains of *Microsporum*, *Epidermophyton*, and *Trichophyton*.
3. **Therapeutic uses.** Griseofulvin is effective in tinea infections of the skin, hair, and nails (including athlete's foot, jock itch, and ringworm) caused by *Microsporum*, *Epidermophyton*, and *Trichophyton*.
   a. Generally, this agent is given only for infections that do not respond to topical antifungal agents.
   b. Griseofulvin is available only in oral form.
   c. It possesses vasodilatory activity and may be used in Raynaud disease.
   d. It may be used to treat gout.
4. **Precautions and monitoring effects**
   a. Griseofulvin rarely results in serious adverse effects. However, the following problems have been reported.
      (1) *Common*: headache, fatigue, confusion, impaired performance, syncope, and lethargy, which generally resolve with continued use
      (2) *Occasional*: leukopenia, neutropenia, and granulocytopenia
      (3) *Rare*: serum sickness, angioedema, urticaria, erythema, and hepatotoxicity
   b. The dosage depends on the particle size of the product: 250 mg of ultramicrosize (Fulvicin P/G) is equivalent in therapeutic effects to 500 mg of microsize (Fulvicin U/F).
5. **Significant interactions**
   a. Griseofulvin may increase the metabolism of **warfarin**, leading to decreased prothrombin time.
   b. **Barbiturates** may reduce griseofulvin absorption.
   c. **Alcohol consumption** may cause tachycardia and flushing.
   d. **Oral contraceptives** may cause amenorrhea or increased breakthrough bleeding.

F. **Imidazoles.** The substituted imidazole derivatives **ketoconazole (Nizoral)**, **miconazole (Monistat)**, **fluconazole (Diflucan)**, **itraconazole (Sporanox)**, **voriconazole (Vfend)** and **posaconazole (Noxafil)** are valuable in the treatment of a wide range of systemic fungal infections.

1. **Mechanism of action.** Imidazoles inhibit sterol synthesis in fungal cell membranes and increase cell wall permeability; this in turn makes the cell more vulnerable to osmotic pressure. These agents are **fungistatic**.

2. **Spectrum of activity.** These agents are active against many fungi, including yeasts, dermatophytes, actinomycetes, and some *Phycomycetes*.
3. **Therapeutic uses**
   a. **Ketoconazole,** an oral agent, successfully treats many fungal infections that previously yielded only to parenteral agents.
      (1) It is therapeutic for systemic and vaginal candidiasis, mucocandidiasis, candiduria, oral thrush, histoplasmosis, coccidioidomycosis, chromomycosis, dermatophytosis (tinea), and paracoccidioidomycosis.
      (2) Because ketoconazole is slow acting and requires a long duration of therapy (up to 6 months for some chronic infections), it is less effective than other antifungal agents for the treatment of severe and acute systemic infections.
   b. **Miconazole,** primarily administered as a topical agent, the parenteral form has been discontinued in the United States. It was a relatively toxic formulation which has been replaced by other members of this class (e.g., fluconazole).
      (1) Topical miconazole is highly effective in vulvovaginal candidiasis, ringworm, and other skin infections.
   c. **Fluconazole.** Available in oral and parenteral forms, fluconazole can be used against systemic and CNS infections involving *Cryptococcus* and *Candida*. *Candida* oropharyngeal infection and esophagitis may also be treated with fluconazole. *Aspergillus*, *Coccidioides*, and *Histoplasma* have demonstrated in vitro sensitivity.
   d. **Itraconazole** is available as an oral agent with activity against systemic and invasive pulmonary aspergillosis without the hematological toxicity of amphotericin B. Other deep mycotic infections susceptible to itraconazole include blastomycosis, coccidioidomycosis, cryptococcosis, and histoplasmosis.
   e. **Voriconazole.** Voriconazole is available as both an intravenous and an oral agent for the treatment of fungal infections involving invasive aspergillosis, *Scedosporium apiospermum*, and *Fusarium* spp., including those species that are refractory to other therapy.
   f. **Posaconazole.** Available as an oral suspension indicated for the prevention of invasive infections caused by *Aspergillus* and *Candida* species in patients receiving HSCT or with neutropenis. Posaconazole may also be used to treat invasive fungal infections in patients who have previously failed or are intolerant to other antifungals.
4. **Precautions and monitoring effects**
   a. **Ketoconazole** may cause nausea, vomiting, diarrhea, abdominal pain, and constipation. Rarely, it leads to headache, dizziness, gynecomastia, and fatal hepatotoxicity.
   b. **Fluconazole** commonly causes GI disturbances (e.g., nausea, vomiting, epigastric pain, diarrhea). Reversible elevations in serum aminotransferase, exfoliative skin reactions, and headaches have been reported.
   c. **Itraconazole** may cause nausea, vomiting, hypertriglyceridemia, hypokalemia, rash, and elevations in liver enzymes.
   d. **Voriconazole.** Visual disturbances, fever, rash, vomiting, nausea, diarrhea, headache, sepsis, peripheral edema, abdominal pain, and respiratory disorders rarely occurred. Liver function test abnormalities have occurred.
   e. **Posaconazole.** Most common adverse events have been nausea and headache. Rash, dry skin, taste disturbances, abdominal pain, dizziness, hypokalemia, thrombocytopenia, and flushing can occur. Posaconazole can cause abnormalities in liver function and has been associated with prolongation of the QT interval.
5. **Significant interactions**
   a. Both **ketoconazole** and **miconazole** may enhance the anticoagulant effect of **warfarin**.
   b. **Ketoconazole** may antagonize the antibiotic effects of **amphotericin B**.
   c. **Fluconazole** has been shown to elevate serum levels of **phenytoin, cyclosporine, warfarin,** and **sulfonylureas.** Concurrent hepatic enzyme inducers, such as **rifampin**, have resulted in increased elimination of both fluconazole and itraconazole.
   d. Coadministration of **itraconazole** or **ketoconazole** with **astemizole** or **terfenadine** may result in increased astemizole or terfenadine levels, possibly leading to life-threatening dysrhythmias and death.
   e. Both **ketoconazole** and **itraconazole** need the presence of stomach acid for adequate absorption. Use with antacids, H_2-blockers, or proton pump inhibitors is contraindicated.

f. Concomitant use of imidazole antifungal agents with **cisapride** may result in increased concentrations of cisapride, which has been associated with adverse cardiac events such as torsades de pointes leading to sudden death.

g. **Voriconazole.** Cytochrome P450 2C19 is the major enzyme involved in metabolism. Voriconazole inhibits cytochrome P450 2C19, 2C9, and 3A4. Any medication that is metabolized via these routes may be affected, and monitoring of blood levels (if appropriate) or clinical signs and symptoms is necessary when taking concomitant medications.

h. **Posaconazole** serum levels are reduced by concurrent administration with cimetidine, phenytoin or rifabutin; avoid concomitant use if possible. Posaconazole may increase concentrations of cyclosporine, tacrolimus, rifabutin, midazolam, and phenytoin; dosage adjustments may be required.

(1) Food increases the oral bioavailability; take posaconazole with a full meal or liquid nutritional supplement

G. **Nystatin (Mycostatin).** A polyene antibiotic, nystatin has a chemical structure similar to that of amphotericin B.

1. **Mechanism of action.** Nystatin is **fungicidal** and **fungistatic**; binding to sterols in the fungal cell membrane, it increases membrane permeability and permits leakage of intracellular contents.
2. **Spectrum of activity.** Nystatin is active primarily against *Candida* spp.
3. **Therapeutic uses**

a. This drug is used primarily as a topical agent in vaginal and oral *Candida* infections.

b. Oral nystatin is therapeutic for *Candida* infections of the GI tract, especially oral and esophageal infections; because the drug is not readily absorbed, it maintains good local activity.

4. **Precautions and monitoring effects.** Oral nystatin occasionally causes GI distress (e.g., nausea, vomiting, diarrhea). Rarely, hypersensitivity reactions occur.

H. **Terbinafine (Lamisil)** is a synthetic allylamine with structure and activity related to naftifine.

1. **Mechanism of action.** Terbinafine inhibits squalene monooxygenase, leading to an interruption of fungal sterol biosynthesis. Terbinafine may be **fungicidal** or **fungistatic**, depending on drug concentration and species.
2. **Spectrum of activity.** Terbinafine has activity against dermatophytic fungi (*Trichophyton*, *Microsporum*, and *Epidermophyton*), filamentous fungi (*Aspergillus*), and dimorphic fungi (*Blastomyces*). It may also possess some activity against yeasts.
3. **Therapeutic uses**

a. Oral terbinafine is useful against infections of the toenail and fingernail (onychomycosis, tinea unguium). Time to cure is reduced over imidazole antifungals for these indications. It is useful in patients who may not tolerate the adverse effect profile of imidazole antifungals.

b. It is also used in tinea capitis and tinea corporis infections.

4. **Precautions and monitoring effects.** Adverse effects include taste or ocular disturbances, symptomatic hepatobiliary dysfunction, decrease in lymphocyte count and neutropenia, and serious skin reactions.

IV. TOPICAL ANTIFUNGAL AGENTS

A. **Definition.** These agents are for topical use for fungal infections.

B. **Amphotericin B (Fungizone)** is available as a 3% cream or lotion or an oral suspension that is not absorbed through the GI tract.

1. **Mechanism of action.** See III.B.1.
2. **Spectrum of activity.** See III.B.2.
3. **Therapeutic uses.** Amphotericin B is used for oropharyngeal candidiasis, cutaneous and mucocutaneous candidal infections, or as a local irrigant for the bladder and intrapleural or intraperitoneal areas.
4. **Precautions and monitoring effects.** Compared with systemic administration, the topical formulations have relatively low toxicity.

a. Dry skin and local irritation with erythema, pruritus, or burning, along with mild skin discoloration, has occurred with the lotion and cream.

b. Rash and GI effects (e.g., nausea, vomiting, steatorrhea, diarrhea) tend to occur with the suspension. In addition, there have been case reports of urticaria, angioedema, Stevens–Johnson syndrome, and toxic epidermal necrolysis.

C. **Butenafine (Mentax)** is a synthetic benzylamine related to the allylamine antifungal agents (naftifine, terbinafine).

1. **Mechanism of action.** Butenafine alters fungal membrane permeability and growth inhibition, interferes with sterol biosynthesis by allowing squalene to accumulate within the cell, and may be fungicidal in certain concentrations against susceptible organisms such as the dermatophytes.
2. **Spectrum of activity.** Butenafine is active against *Trichophyton rubrum*, *T. mentagrophytes*, *Microsporum canis*, *Sporothrix schenckii*, and yeasts, including *Candida parapsilosis* and *C. albicans*.
3. **Therapeutic uses.** The 1% cream is used in dermatophytoses, including tinea corporis, tinea cruris, and tinea pedis.
4. **Precautions and monitoring effects.** If clinical improvement of fungal infection does not improve after the treatment period, the diagnosis should be reevaluated.

D. **Butoconazole (Mycelex)** is an azole antifungal cream available for vaginal use.

1. **Mechanism of action.** Butoconazole has fungistatic activity against susceptible organisms. The drug interferes with membrane permeability, secondary metabolic effects, and growth inhibition. Butoconazole contains antibacterial effects against some gram-positive organisms.
2. **Spectrum of activity.** Butoconazole is active against dermatophytes (*Trichophyton concentricum*, *T. mentagrophytes*, *T. rubrum*, *T. tonsurans*, *Epidermophyton floccosum*, *M. canis*, *M. gypseum*), yeasts (*C. albicans*, *C. glabrata*), and some gram-positive organisms (*S. aureus*, *E. faecalis*, and *S. pyogenes*).
3. **Therapeutic uses.** A 2% cream is used for vulvovaginal candidiasis and complicated, recurrent vulvovaginal candidiasis.
4. **Precautions and monitoring effects**
   a. Vulvovaginal burning and itching are the most common; however, their incidence is low. Headache; itching of fingers; urinary frequency and burning; and vulvovaginal discharge, irritation, soreness, stinging, odor, and swelling rarely occur.
   b. Butoconazole may damage birth-control devices such as condoms and diaphragms, leading to inadequate protection. Consider alternative methods of birth control.
   c. Tampon use should be avoided with the use of butoconazole.

E. **Ciclopirox (Loprox)** is a synthetic antifungal agent that is chemically unrelated to any other antifungal agent. The ethanolamine contained in ciclopirox appears to enhance epidermal penetration.

1. **Mechanism of action.** Ciclopirox causes intracellular depletion of amino acids and ions necessary for normal cellular function.
2. **Spectrum of activity.** Ciclopirox is active against dermatophytes, yeasts, some gram-positive and gram-negative bacteria, *Mycoplasma*, and *Trichomonas vaginalis*. Specifically, ciclopirox has activity against *T. mentagrophytes*, *T. rubrum*, *E. floccosum*, *M. canis*, *M. furfur*, and *C. albicans*.
3. **Therapeutic uses.** Ciclopirox is used topically for the treatment of tinea pedis, tinea cruris, tinea corporis, tinea versicolor (from *Malassezia*), and cutaneous candidiasis (moniliasis) from *C. albicans*.
4. **Precautions and monitoring effects.** Local irritation manifested by erythema, pruritus, burning, blistering, swelling, and oozing has occurred. If this occurs, ciclopirox should be discontinued.

F. **Clioquinol** (formerly iodochlorhydroxyquin) is a topical antifungal in a 3% ointment that can be used alone or in combination with hydrocortisone.

1. **Mechanism of action.** Unknown
2. **Spectrum of activity.** It is active against dermatophytic fungi.
3. **Therapeutic uses.** It is used topically against the following:
   a. Tinea pedis and tinea cruris (ringworm infections)
   b. Previously used to treat diaper rash; however, it is no longer recommended, and use in children $<$ 2 years of age is contraindicated
4. **Precautions and monitoring effects**
   a. Local irritation, rash, and sensitivity reactions are common.
   b. Systemic absorption after topical application may occur.
   c. High doses of clioquinol over long periods have been associated with oculotoxic/neurotoxic effects, including optic neuritis, optic atrophy, and subacute myelo-optic neuropathy.

G. **Clotrimazole (Lotrimin)** is an azole antifungal agent that is an imidazole derivative. It is related to other azole antifungal agents, such as **butoconazole**, **econazole**, **ketoconazole**, **miconazole**, **oxiconazole**, **sulconazole**, and **tioconazole**.

1. **Mechanism of action.** Clotrimazole alters fungal cell membrane permeability by binding with phospholipids in the membrane.

2. **Spectrum of activity.** It is active against yeasts, dermatophytes (*T. rubrum*, *T. mentagrophytes*, *E. floccosum*, *M. canis*), and some gram-positive bacteria. At higher concentrations, clotrimazole inhibits *M. furfur*, *Aspergillus fumigatus*, *C. albicans*, and some strains of *S. aureus*, *S. pyogenes*, *Proteus vulgaris*, and *Salmonella*. At very high concentrations, clotrimazole has an effect on *Sporothrix*, *Cryptococcus*, *Cephalosporium*, *Fusarium*, and *T. vaginalis*.
3. **Therapeutic uses**
    a. The lozenges, which are administered five times per day, are useful in treating oropharyngeal candidiasis. Lozenges are also used for primary prophylaxis of mucocutaneous candidiasis in HIV-infected infants or children with severe immunosuppression.
    b. The cream, lotion, or solution is used to treat dermatophytoses, superficial mycoses, and cutaneous candidiasis.
    c. Intravaginal dosage forms are useful in treating vulvovaginal candidiasis.
4. **Precautions and monitoring effects**
    a. Cutaneous reactions with topical administration may include blistering, erythema, edema, pruritus, burning, stinging, peeling, skin fissures, and general irritation.
    b. The vaginal tablets are associated with mild burning, skin rash, itching, vulval irritation, lower abdominal cramps, bloating, slight cramping, vaginal soreness during intercourse, and an increase in urinary frequency.
    c. Cross-sensitization occurs with imidazole; however, it is unpredictable.
    d. Abnormal liver function tests (elevated AST) have occurred in patients taking the lozenges.

H. **Econazole (Spectazole)** is an azole antifungal agent that is an imidazole derivative.
1. **Mechanism of action.** Econazole alters cell membranes and increases permeability (like many other azole agents).
2. **Spectrum of activity.** Econazole is active against dermatophytes, yeasts, some gram-positive bacteria, and *T. vaginalis*.
3. **Therapeutic uses**
    a. The 1% topical cream, lotion, or solution is useful in treating dermatophytoses and cutaneous candidiasis (tinea corporis and tinea cruris).
    b. Econazole is also used to treat pityriasis (tinea) versicolor (*M. furfur*).
4. **Precautions and monitoring effects.** In general, there is a low incidence of toxicity. Topically, a patient may experience burning, stinging sensations, pruritus, and erythema (after 2 to 4 days).

I. **Gentian violet** is a dye that possesses the ability to kill fungi, yeasts, and some gram-positive bacteria.
1. **Mechanism of action.** None known
2. **Spectrum of activity.** Gentian violet is active against *Candida*, *Epidermophyton*, *Cryptococcus*, *Trichophyton*, and some *Staphylococcus* spp.
3. **Therapeutic uses.** It is used to treat cutaneous *C. albicans* infections (monilia or thrush).
4. **Precautions and monitoring effects**
    a. Gentian violet may cause irritation or sensitivity reactions or possibly ulceration of the mucous membranes. If the solution is swallowed, esophagitis, laryngitis, or tracheitis may occur.
    b. Skin tattooing may occur if gentian violet is applied to granulation tissue.
    c. Gentian violet should not be used in areas of extensive ulceration.
    d. This drug is a dye and will stain clothing.

J. **Ketoconazole (Nizoral)** is an imidazole-derived antifungal drug that is available topically as a cream and a shampoo.
1. **Mechanism of action.** See III.E.1.
2. **Spectrum of activity.** See III.E.2.
3. **Therapeutic uses**
    a. The 2% topical cream is used in treating tinea corporis, tinea cruris, and tinea pedis caused by the dermatophytes (*E. floccosum*, *T. mentagrophytes*, and *T. rubrum*).
    b. It is used for cutaneous candidiasis.
    c. The 2% topical cream or 2% shampoo may be used in treating tinea versicolor (*M. furfur*). Selenium-based shampoos may also be useful in this area.
    d. The 2% topical cream is useful against seborrheic dermatitis. The 2% shampoo is useful in reducing scaling caused by dandruff.

e. When combined with a steroid, ketoconazole is useful in treating the following: atopic dermatitis, diaper rash, eczema, folliculitis, impetigo, intertrigo, lichenoid dermatitis, and psoriasis.
f. An ophthalmic suspension can be extemporaneously prepared to treat fungal keratitis.

4. **Precautions and monitoring effects**
   a. Reactions from the 2% topical cream include local irritation, pruritus, and stinging. Contact dermatitis is possible and occurs with other imidazole derivatives.
   b. The 2% shampoo may lead to increased hair loss, irritation, abnormal hair texture, scalp pustules, dry skin, pruritus, and oiliness or dryness of hair and scalp. It may in addition straighten otherwise curly hair.

K. **Miconazole (Monistat)** is an imidazole-derived antifungal drug that is available topically as a 2% aerosol, 2% aerosol powder, 2% cream, a kit, 2% powder and 2% tincture, 2% vaginal cream, and 100 mg and 200 mg vaginal suppositories.

1. **Mechanism of action.** See III.E.1.
2. **Spectrum of activity.** See III.E.2.
3. **Therapeutic uses.** Miconazole is advantageous over other agents such as nystatin and tolnaftate in that its activity covers dermatophytes as well as *Candida*.
   a. Topical use is effective against tinea pedis, tinea cruris, and tinea corporis caused by dermatophytes (*T. mentagrophytes*, *T. rubrum*, and *E. floccosum*).
   b. It is also effective against tinea versicolor from *M. furfur*.
   c. Like other imidazole derivatives, it is useful in treating cutaneous fungal infections.
   d. The vaginal cream and vaginal suppositories are effective in treating vulvovaginal candidiasis.
4. **Precautions and monitoring parameters**
   a. Topical creams have caused local irritation and burning.
   b. Vaginal preparations have led to vulvovaginal burning, itching, irritation, pelvic cramps, vaginal burning, headache, hives, and skin rash.
   c. If vulvovaginal candidiasis persists for longer than 3 days, seek further medical attention.
   d. Tampons should be avoided in patients using vaginal suppositories or cream; sanitary pads should be substituted.
   e. Vaginal suppositories are manufactured from a vegetable oil base that may interact with latex products. Avoid using diaphragms or condoms concurrently with suppositories. Seek an alternative form of birth control.

L. **Naftifine (Naftin)** is a synthetic allylamine similar to terbinafine. It is available as a 1% topical cream and a 1% topical gel.

1. **Mechanism of action.** Naftifine is **fungistatic** and interferes with sterol biosynthesis by accumulating squalene in the fungal cell. Naftifine also possesses some local anti-inflammatory activity.
2. **Spectrum of activity**
   a. Naftifine is active against *T. mentagrophytes*, *T. rubrum*, *T. tonsurans*, *Trichophyton verrucosum*, *Trichophyton violaceum*, *E. floccosum*, *Microsporum audouinii*, *M. canis*, and *M. gypseum*.
   b. *C. albicans*, *Candida krusei*, *Candida parapsilosis*, and *Candida tropicalis* are affected by naftifine; however, the concentrations of naftifine vary for *Candida* killing, depending on the species.
   c. In vitro activity has been demonstrated against *Aspergillus flavus* and *Aspergillus fumigatus*. Others include *Sporothrix schenckii*, *Cryptococcus neoformans*, *Petriellidium boydii*, *Blastomyces dermatitidis*, and *Histoplasma capsulatum*.
3. **Therapeutic uses.** Naftifine is active against dermatophytoses and cutaneous candidiasis.
   a. It is also used to treat tinea cruris, tinea pedis, tinea corporis, and tinea manus (*T. mentagrophytes*, *T. rubrum*, *T. verrucosum*, *T. violaceum*, *E. floccosum*, or *M. canis*).
   b. It is also useful in treating tinea unguium (onychomycosis).
4. **Precautions and monitoring effects.** Transient burning and stinging

M. **Nystatin (Mycostatin).** A polyene antibiotic, nystatin has a chemical structure similar to that of amphotericin B. It is available as an oral suspension, tablet, lozenge, topical cream, ointment, topical powder, and vaginal tablet.

1. **Mechanism of action.** Nystatin is **fungicidal** and **fungistatic**; binding to sterols in the fungal cell membrane, it increases membrane permeability and permits leakage of intracellular contents.

2. **Spectrum of activity.** Nystatin is active primarily against *Candida* spp.
3. **Therapeutic uses.** This drug is used primarily as a topical agent in vaginal and oral *Candida* infections.
4. **Precautions and monitoring effects.** Irritation has occurred in extremely rare instances.

N. **Oxiconazole (Oxistat)** is an imidazole-derived antifungal drug that is available as a 1% topical cream or 1% topical lotion.
1. **Mechanism of action.** See III.E.1.
2. **Spectrum of activity.** See III.E.2.
3. **Therapeutic uses**
   a. The 1% cream or lotion is useful in treating tinea cruris, tinea corporis, tinea manus, and tinea pedis from dermatophytes.
   b. Oxiconazole is also effective against tinea versicolor caused by *M. furfur*.
4. **Precautions and monitoring effects**. Adverse effects are rare and are confined to local irritation.

O. **Sulconazole (Exelderm)** is an imidazole-derived antifungal drug that is available as a 1% topical cream and a 1% topical solution.
1. **Mechanism of action** (see III.E.1). The antibacterial effects exerted by sulconazole are thought to be the result of a direct physicochemical effect on the destruction of unsaturated fatty acids present in bacterial cell membranes.
2. **Spectrum of activity**
   a. Sulconazole has activity against dermatophytes, including *E. floccosum*, *M. audouinii*, *M. canis*, *M. gypseum*, *T. mentagrophytes*, *T. rubrum*, *T. tonsurans*, and *T. violaceum*. It also has activity against *M. furfur*.
   b. Sulconazole also has activity against selected gram-positive aerobes (*S. aureus*, *S. epidermidis*, *Staphylococcus saprophyticus*, *E. faecalis*, *Micrococcus luteus*, and *Bacillus subtilis*) and anaerobes (*Clostridium* and *Propionibacterium acnes*, *Clostridium perfringens*, *Clostridium tetani*, and *Clostridium botulinum*).
3. **Therapeutic uses**
   a. The 1% topical cream or 1% topical solution is useful in treating tinea corporis and tinea cruris.
   b. The 1% topical cream has been studied for use against tinea pedis; the solution has not been evaluated for this indication.
   c. The 1% cream is useful against tinea versicolor (*M. furfur*).
   d. There is not an approved indication for cutaneous candidiasis; however, sulconazole 1% is as effective as miconazole 2% or clotrimazole 1% in treating cutaneous candidiasis.
   e. Sulconazole is useful in treating infections caused by bacteria such as impetigo (*S. pyogenes*) and ecthyma (*S. aureus*).
4. **Precautions and monitoring effects.** Adverse reactions include local effects such as burning and irritation, skin edema, dryness, scaling, fissuring, cracking, generalized red papules, and severe eczema.

P. **Terbinafine (Lamisil AT)** is a synthetic allylamine available as a 1% cream with structure and activity related to naftifine.
1. **Mechanism of action.** Terbinafine inhibits squalene monooxygenase, leading to an interruption of fungal sterol biosynthesis. Terbinafine may be **fungicidal** or **fungistatic**, depending on drug concentration and species.
2. **Spectrum of activity.** Terbinafine has activity against dermatophytic fungi (*Trichophyton*, *Microsporum*, and *Epidermophyton*), filamentous fungi (*Aspergillus*), and dimorphic fungi (*Blastomyces*). It may also possess some activity against yeasts.
3. **Therapeutic uses**. It is useful for tinea pedis, tinea corporis, and tinea cruris.
4. **Precautions and monitoring effects.** It can cause local irritation.

Q. **Terconazole (Terazol 7)** is an imidazole-derived antifungal drug that is available as a 0.4% and 0.8% vaginal cream and an 80-mg vaginal suppository.
1. **Mechanism of action.** It is **fungicidal** against *C. albicans*. Like other imidazole agents, terconazole alters cellular membranes, resulting in increased membrane permeability.
2. **Spectrum of activity.** It is active against dermatophytes; yeasts; and, at high concentrations, gram-positive and gram-negative bacteria.
3. **Therapeutic uses** are for complicated and uncomplicated vulvovaginal candidiasis.

4. **Precautions and monitoring effects.** Adverse reactions include burning, pruritus, irritation, headache, body pain, and pain of female genitalia.

R. **Tioconazole (Vagistat-1)** is an imidazole-derived antifungal drug that is available as a 6.5% vaginal ointment.

1. **Mechanism of action.** Tioconazole is **fungicidal** against *C. albicans*. Like other imidazole agents, tioconazole alters cellular membranes, resulting in increased membrane permeability.
2. **Spectrum of activity**
   a. Activity against fungi includes most strains of *Candida* and the dermatophytes. There is also activity against *Aspergillus* and *C. neoformans*.
   b. Tioconazole is active against the following aerobic gram-positive bacteria: *Gardnerella vaginalis*, *Corynebacterium minutissimum*, *E. faecalis*, *S. aureus*, *S. epidermidis*, and some *Streptococci* spp. Gram-negative bacteria: it is active against *H. pylori*, *Haemophilus ducreyi*, *Moraxella catarrhalis*, *Neisseria gonorrhoeae*, and *N. meningitidis*.
   c. Other organisms that tioconazole has activity against are *T. vaginalis*, *Lymphogranuloma venereum*, and *Chlamydia trachomatis*.
3. **Therapeutic uses.** Tioconazole is used for simple and complicated vulvovaginal candidiasis. Other uses have been explored; however, topical creams for use in those scenarios are not available in the United States.
4. **Precautions and monitoring effects.** Local irritation has been manifested as vulvovaginal burning, vaginitis, and pruritus.

S. **Tolnaftate (Tinactin)** is available topically as a 1% aerosol, 1% powder, 1% cream, and 1% solution.

1. **Mechanism of action.** It may distort hyphae and stunt mycelial growth in susceptible fungi.
2. **Spectrum of activity.** Tolnaftate may be either **fungistatic** or **fungicidal** to the following organisms: *M. gypseum*, *M. canis*, *M. audouinii*, *Microsporum japonicum*, *T. rubrum*, *T. mentagrophytes*, *Trichophyton schoenleinii*, *T. tonsurans*, *E. floccosum*, *Aspergillus niger*, *C. albicans*, *C. neoformans*, and *A. fumigatus*.
3. **Therapeutic uses.** Tolnaftate is used for dermatophytoses and tinea versicolor.
4. **Precautions and monitoring effects.** There may be slight local irritation.

V. ANTIPROTOZOAL AGENTS

A. **Classification.** These drugs fall into two main categories: **antimalarial agents**, used to treat malaria infection, and **amebicides** and **trichomonacides**, used to treat amebic and trichomonal infections.

B. **Antimalarial agents.** Still a leading cause of illness and death in tropical and subtropical countries, malaria results from infection by any of four species of the protozoal genus *Plasmodium*. Antimalarial agents are selectively active during different phases of the protozoan life cycle. Major antimalarial drugs include **chloroquine (Aralen)**, **hydroxychloroquine (Plaquenil)**, **primaquine**, **pyrimethamine (Daraprim)**, **quinine**, and **mefloquine (Lariam)**. In addition, three combination brands are available: sulfadoxine plus pyrimethamine (Fansidar), atovaquone plus proguanil (Malarone), and artemether plus lumefantrine (Coartem).

1. **Mechanism of action**
   a. **Chloroquine** and **hydroxychloroquine** bind to and alter the properties of microbial and mammalian DNA.
   b. The mechanism of action of **primaquine**, **quinine**, **Fansidar**, and **mefloquine** is unknown.
   c. **Pyrimethamine** impedes folic acid reduction by inhibiting the enzyme dihydrofolate reductase.
2. **Spectrum of activity**
   a. **Chloroquine** and **hydroxychloroquine** are suppressive blood **schizonticidal** agents and are active against the asexual erythrocyte forms of *Plasmodium vivax* and *Plasmodium falciparum* and gametocytes of *P. vivax*, *Plasmodium malariae*, and *Plasmodium ovale*.
   b. **Primaquine**, a curative agent, is active against liver forms of *P. vivax* and *P. ovale* and the primary exoerythrocytic forms of *P. falciparum*.
   c. **Pyrimethamine** is active against chloroquine-resistant strains of *P. falciparum* and some strains of *P. vivax*.
   d. **Quinine**, a generalized protoplasmic poison, is toxic to a wide range of organisms. In malaria, this drug has both suppressive and curative action against chloroquine-resistant strains.

e. **Fansidar** (sulfadoxine plus pyrimethamine) is a blood **schizonticidal** agent that is active against the erythrocytic forms of susceptible plasmodia. It is also active against *T. gondii*.

f. **Malarone** (atovaquone plus proguanil) is active against the erythrocytic and exoerythrocytic forms of *Plasmodium* spp.

g. **Mefloquine** is a blood **schizonticidal** agent that is active against *P. falciparum* (both chloroquine-susceptible and -resistant strains) and *P. vivax*.

h. Coartem is a fixed dose oral combination of artemether (20 mg), an artemisinin derivative, and lumefantrine (120 mg), two antimalarials. Both components are blood schizontocides **active against *P. falciparum***.

3. **Therapeutic uses**

a. **Chloroquine** is the preferred agent used to suppress malaria symptoms and to terminate acute malaria attacks resulting from *P. falciparum* and *P. malariae* infections.
   (1) It is more potent and less toxic than quinine.
   (2) Except where drug-resistant *P. falciparum* strains are prevalent, chloroquine is the most useful antimalarial agent.

b. **Hydroxychloroquine** is used as an alternative to chloroquine in patients who cannot tolerate chloroquine or when chloroquine is unavailable.

c. **Primaquine** is used to cure relapses of *P. vivax* and *P. ovale* malaria and to prevent malaria in exposed persons returning from regions where malaria is endemic.

d. **Pyrimethamine** is effective in the prevention and treatment of chloroquine-resistant strains of *P. falciparum*. It is now used almost exclusively in combination with a sulfonamide or sulfone.

e. **Quinine**
   (1) Quinine sulfate, an oral form, is therapeutic for acute malaria caused by chloroquine-resistant strains.
   (2) Quinine dihydrochloride, a parenteral form, is used in severe cases of chloroquine-resistant malaria (it is available only from the CDC).
   (3) Quinine is almost always given in combination with another antimalarial agent.

f. **Fansidar**
   (1) Fansidar is used for the suppression or prophylaxis of chloroquine-resistant *P. falciparum* malaria.
   (2) It has been used for the prophylaxis of *P. carinii* infections in AIDS patients unable to tolerate cotrimoxazole (trimethoprim–sulfamethoxazole).

g. **Mefloquine** is indicated for the treatment of acute malaria and the prevention of *P. falciparum* and *P. vivax* infections.

h. Coartem is indicated for treatment of acute, uncomplicated malaria infections due to *Plasmodium falciparum* in patients of 5 kg body weight and above.

i. **Malarone**
   (1) Prophylaxis of *P. falciparum* malaria, including areas where chloroquine resistance has been reported.
   (2) Treatment of acute, uncomplicated *P. falciparum* malaria. This combination has been shown to be effective in regions where the drugs chloroquine, halofantrine, mefloquine, and amodiaquine may have unacceptable failure rates, presumably because of drug resistance.

4. **Precautions and monitoring effects**

a. **Chloroquine and hydroxychloroquine**
   (1) Because these drugs concentrate in the liver, they should be used cautiously in patients with hepatic disease.
   (2) Chloroquine must be administered with extreme caution in patients with neurological, hematological, or severe GI disorders.
   (3) Visual disturbances, headache, skin rash, and GI distress have been reported.

b. **Primaquine**
   (1) This agent is contraindicated in patients with rheumatoid arthritis and lupus erythematosus and in those receiving other potentially hemolytic drugs or bone marrow suppressants.
   (2) Primaquine may cause agranulocytosis, granulocytopenia, and mild anemia. In patients with G6PD deficiency, it may cause hemolytic anemia.
   (3) Abdominal cramps, nausea, vomiting, and epigastric distress sometimes occur.

c. **Pyrimethamine**
   (1) In high doses, this drug may cause agranulocytosis, megaloblastic anemia, aplastic anemia, and thrombocytopenia.
   (2) Erythema multiforme (Stevens–Johnson syndrome), nausea, vomiting, and anorexia may develop during pyrimethamine therapy.

d. **Quinine**
   (1) Quinine is contraindicated in patients with G6PD deficiency, tinnitus, and optic neuritis.
   (2) Quinine overdose or hypersensitivity reactions may be fatal. Manifestations of quinine poisoning include visual and hearing disturbances; GI symptoms (e.g., nausea, vomiting); hot, flushed skin; headache; fever; syncope; confusion; shallow, then depressed, respirations; and cardiovascular collapse.
   (3) Quinine must be used cautiously in patients with atrial fibrillation.
   (4) Renal damage and anuria have been reported.

e. **Fansidar**
   (1) Severe, sometimes fatal, hypersensitivity reactions have occurred. In most cases, death resulted from severe cutaneous reactions, including erythema multiforme, Stevens–Johnson syndrome, and toxic epidermal necrolysis.
   (2) Adverse hematological and hepatic effects as seen with sulfonamides have been reported.

f. **Mefloquine**
   (1) Concomitant use of mefloquine with quinine, quinidine, or β-adrenergic blockade may produce electrocardiographic abnormalities or cardiac arrest.
   (2) Concomitant use of mefloquine and quinine or chloroquine may increase the risk of convulsions.

g. **Coartem**
   (1) Coartem tablets should be taken with food.
   (2) Avoid use in patients with known QT prolongation, those with hypokalemia or hypomagnesemia, and those taking other drugs that prolong the QT interval.
   (3) The most common adverse reactions in adults (> 30%) are headache, anorexia, dizziness, asthenia, arthralgia, and myalgia. The most common adverse reactions in children (> 12%) are pyrexia, cough, vomiting, anorexia, and headache.

h. **Malarone**
   (1) Concomitant administration with tetracycline has been associated with 40% reduction in plasma concentrations of atovaquone. Similarly, concurrent rifampin is known to reduce atovaquone levels by 50%.
   (2) Take malarone with food or milk.

C. **Amebicides and trichomonacides.** These agents are crucial in the treatment of amebiasis, giardiasis, and trichomoniases—the most common protozoal infections in the United States. The major amebicides include **diloxanide, iodoquinol (Yodoxin), metronidazole (Flagyl), nitazoxanide (Alinia), paromomycin (Humatin), quinacrine, and tinidazole (Tindamax)**.

1. **Mechanism of action**
   a. **Diloxanide**, a dichloroacetamide derivative, is **amebicidal**; its mechanism of action is unknown. (Not available commercially but can be compounded by Panorama Compounding Pharmacy, Van Nuys, CA—per Medical Letter 8/04.)
   b. **Metronidazole** is a synthetic compound with direct **amebicidal** and **trichomonacidal** action; it works at both intestinal and extraintestinal sites. Its mechanism of action involves disruption of the helical structure of DNA.
   c. **Nitazoxanide** is designated by the U.S. Food and Drug Administration (FDA) as an orphan drug. Its antiprotozoal activity is believed to be the result of interference with the pyruvate: ferredoxin oxidoreductase (PFOR) enzyme-dependent electron transfer reaction essential for energy metabolism.
   d. **Quinacrine** is an acridine derivative that inhibits DNA metabolism.
   e. **Iodoquinol** is a luminal or contact amebicide that is effective against the trophozoites of *Entamoeba histolytica* located in the lumen of the large intestine.
   f. **Paromomycin** is a poorly absorbed amebicidal aminoglycoside whose mechanism of action parallels other aminoglycosides (i.e., protein synthesis inhibitor). It is also effective against enteric bacteria *Salmonella* and *Shigella*.
   g. **Tinidazole** precise mechanism of action is unknown.

2. **Spectrum of activity and therapeutic uses**
   a. **Diloxanide**
      (1) This drug is used to treat asymptomatic carriers of amebic and *Giardia* cysts.
      (2) Diloxanide is therapeutic for invasive and extraintestinal amebiasis (given in combination with a systemic or mixed amebicide).
      (3) Diloxanide is not effective as single-agent therapy for extraintestinal amebiasis.
   b. **Metronidazole**
      (1) This agent is the preferred drug in amebic dysentery, giardiasis, and trichomoniasis.
      (2) Metronidazole also is active against all anaerobic cocci and gram-negative anaerobic bacilli.
      (3) This agent is the treatment of choice by the CDC for the treatment of *C. difficile* colitis infections owing to the emerging use of broad-spectrum antibiotics. This therapy is cost-effective.
   c. **Quinacrine** is useful in the treatment of giardiasis and tapeworms.
   d. **Iodoquinol** is indicated for treatment of intestinal amebiasis. It is active against the protozoa *E. histolytica*.
   e. **Nitazoxanide** is indicated for treatment of diarrhea caused by *Cryptosporidium parvum* and *Giardia lamblia* in children.
   f. **Paromomycin** is indicated for acute and chronic intestinal amebiasis; it is not useful for extraintestinal amebiasis because it is not absorbed. Paromomycin has been used for *Dientamoeba fragilis*, *Taenia saginata*, *Dipylidium caninum*, and *Hymenolepis nana*.
   g. **Tinidazole** is a second-generation synthetic nitroimidazole active against trichomoniasis, *Giardia duodenalis*/*G. lamblia, and E. histolytica*.
3. **Precautions and monitoring effects**
   a. **Diloxanide** rarely causes serious adverse effects. Vomiting, flatulence, and pruritus have been reported.
   b. **Metronidazole**
      (1) The most common adverse effects of this drug are nausea, epigastric distress, and diarrhea.
      (2) Metronidazole is carcinogenic in mice and should not be used unnecessarily.
      (3) Headache, vomiting, metallic taste, and stomatitis have been reported.
      (4) Occasionally, neurological reactions (e.g., ataxia, peripheral neuropathy, seizures) develop.
      (5) A disulfiram-type reaction may occur with concurrent ethanol use.
   c. **Quinacrine**
      (1) This drug frequently causes dizziness, headache, nausea, and vomiting. Nervousness and seizures also have been reported.
      (2) Quinacrine should not be taken in combination with primaquine because this may increase primaquine toxicity.
      (3) Quinacrine should be administered with extreme caution in patients with psoriasis because it may cause marked exacerbation of this disease.
   d. **Iodoquinol** may produce optic neuritis or atrophy or peripheral neuropathy with high-dose, long-term use. Protein-bound iodine levels may be increased during treatment and may interfere with the results of thyroid tests for 6 months after treatment. Iodoquinol should not be used in patients who are hypersensitive to 8-hydroxy-quinolone (e.g., iodoquinol, iodochlorhydroxyquin) or iodine-containing agents or in patients with hepatic disorders.
   e. **Paromomycin** may cause nausea, cramping, and diarrhea at high doses (> 3 g/day). Inadvertent absorption through ulcerative bowel lesions may result in ototoxicity or renal damage.
   f. **Nitazoxanide** may cause abdominal pain, diarrhea, vomiting, headache, flatulence, fever, eye discoloration, rhinitis, and discolored urine.
   g. **Tinidazole** may produce metallic taste, nausea, anorexia, dyspepsia, vomiting, weakness, dizziness, and headache.

D. **Pentamidine isethionate (Pentam 300)** is an aromatic diamide antiprotozoal agent. It can be administered intramuscularly, intravenously, or by inhalation.
   1. **Mechanism of action** is not fully understood, but in vitro studies indicate interference with nuclear metabolism and inhibition of DNA, RNA, phospholipid, and protein synthesis.

2. **Therapeutic uses**
   a. Pentamidine is indicated for the prevention and treatment of infections caused by *P. carinii.*
   b. Unlabeled uses include treatment of trypanosomiasis, visceral leishmaniasis, and babesiosis.
3. **Precautions and monitoring effects**
   a. Nephrotoxicity, bronchospasm, and cough are the most common effects produced by intravenous or inhaled pentamidine.
   b. Severe hypotension may occur after a parenteral dose of pentamidine. Cardiorespiratory arrest can occur after a single rapid infusion of the drug.
   c. Pain, erythema, and tenderness may occur after an IM administration of the drug. This can be minimized by using the Z-track technique of drug administration. Phlebitis may occur following IV administration.
   d. Hypoglycemia may occur with initial administration of drug via the IV, IM, or inhalational route. After the patient has been on the drug for a period, hyperglycemia will result. The effect of the drug may actually induce a reversible insulin-dependent diabetes mellitus.
   e. Leukopenia and thrombocytopenia, which can be severe, occur occasionally.
   f. Pentamidine may result in elevated liver function tests, AST, and ALT.
   g. GI effects can also occur, including nausea, vomiting, abdominal discomfort, pain, diarrhea, and dysgeusia.
   h. Neurological effects can occur with parenteral administration and may include dizziness, tremors, confusion, anxiety, insomnia, and seizures.
   i. Hypocalcemia and fever have also been reported and may be severe at times.

E. **Atovaquone (Mepron)** is a hydroxynaphthoquinone initially synthesized as an antimalarial drug.
1. **Mechanism of action.** Atovaquone blocks mitochondrial electron transport at complex III of the respiratory chain of protozoa, resulting in inhibition of pyrimidine synthesis.
2. **Spectrum of activity.** It is active against *P. carinii, T. gondii, C. parvum, P. falciparum*, isosporidia, and microsporidia.
3. **Therapeutic uses.** Atovaquone is used for second-line treatment of mild to moderate *P. carinii* pneumonia in patients intolerant of co-trimoxazole or other sulfonamides or who are nonresponsive to co-trimoxazole.
4. **Precautions and monitoring effects**
   a. Oral absorption significantly increases when administered with food (especially a high-fat meal).
   b. Rash, nausea, diarrhea, headache, fever, abdominal pain, dizziness, and elevated liver function tests commonly are reported.
5. **Significant interactions.** Atovaquone is highly bound to plasma protein. It should be used with caution when administered with other highly protein-bound drugs with a narrow therapeutic range.

F. **Eflornithine HCl (Ornidyl).** This is an IV antiprotozoal agent. Its activity has been attributed to the inhibition of the enzyme ornithine decarboxylase.
1. **Mechanism of action.** This is a specific, enzyme-activated, irreversible inhibitor of ornithine decarboxylase.
2. **Spectrum of activity and therapeutic uses.** Eflornithine is active in the treatment of the meningoencephalitic stage of *Trypanosoma brucei gambiense* (sleeping sickness).
3. **Precautions and monitoring effects**
   a. Myelosuppression is the most frequent serious side effect.
   b. Seizures occur in about 8% of treated patients.
   c. Cases of hearing impairment have been reported.

VI. ANTITUBERCULAR AGENTS

A. **Definition and classification.** Drugs used to treat tuberculosis suppress or kill the slow-growing mycobacteria that cause this disease. Antitubercular agents fall into two main categories: first-line and second-line drugs. Because the causative organisms tend to develop resistance to any single drug, combination drug therapy has become standard in the treatment of tuberculosis.
1. The **incidence** of tuberculosis in the United States is increasing owing to shifts in populations considered to be endemic for tuberculosis, the rise in HIV-positive patients, and drug resistance.

2. Agents chosen for **therapy** must eradicate mycobacterium. First-line agents available include isoniazid, ethambutol, pyrazinamide, rifampin, rifabutin, and rifapentine. **Combination chemotherapy** is essential. Agents showing the lowest incidence of resistance (isoniazid, rifampin) are usually used in combination with pyrazinamide or ethambutol.
3. Choice of therapy depends on many patients and disease factors (e.g., duration of therapy needed, likelihood of drug resistance, and HIV status).
4. **Treatment choices based on CDC recommendations** (*Table 36-4*).

B. First-line. These drugs, isoniazid, ethambutol, rifampin, rifabutin, rifapentine, and pyrazinamide, usually offer the greatest effectiveness with the least toxicity; they are successful in most tuberculosis patients. At least three to four drug combinations are recommended. The CDC recommends daily treatment with isoniazid, rifampin, pyrazinamide, and ethambutol for the initial phase of 2 months, followed by a continuation phase of isoniazid and rifampin for 4 to 5 months (*Table 36-4*).

1. **Ethambutol (Myambutol)** is a synthetic water-based compound.
   a. **Mechanism of action.** This drug is **bacteriostatic**. Its precise mechanism of action is unknown; however, it has demonstrated activity only against susceptible bacteria actively undergoing cell division.
   b. **Spectrum of activity and therapeutic uses.** Ethambutol is active against many *M. tuberculosis* strains as well as many other mycobacterial species. However, drug resistance develops fairly rapidly when it is used alone. In most cases, ethambutol is given adjunctively in combination with isoniazid or rifampin for tuberculosis. It is also useful in combination with other agents such as clarithromycin or azithromycin and rifabutin in treating MAC.
   c. **Precautions and monitoring effects.** Rarely, ethambutol causes such adverse effects as reversible dose-related (= 15 mg/kg/day) optic neuritis, drug fever, abdominal pain, headache, dizziness, and confusion. Liver function tests should be periodically monitored. Visual testing and renal function (reduce dose with impairment) should also be monitored.

Table 36-4 TREATMENT FOR ACTIVE TUBERCULOSIS

	Initial Phase		Continuation Phase	
Rank	**Agent**	**Dosage**	**Agent**	**Dosage**
1	INH RIF PZA EMB	7 days a week × 8 weeks *or* 5 days a week × 8 weeks	INH/RIF	7 days a week × 18 weeks *or* 5 days a week × 18 weeks
2	INH RIF PZA EMB	7 days a week × 2 weeks, *then* 2 times a week × 6 weeks *or* 5 days a week × 2 weeks, *then* 2 times a week × 6 weeks	INH/RIF	2 times a week × 18 weeks
3	INH RIF PZA EMB	3 times a week × 8 weeks	INH/RIF	3 times a week × 19 weeks
4	INH RIF EMB	7 days a week × 8 weeks *or* 5 days a week × 8 weeks	INH/RIF	7 days a week × 31 weeks *or* 5 days a week × 31 weeks *or* 2 times a week × 31 weeks

EMB, ethambutol; *INH*, isoniazid; *PZA*, pyrazinamide; *RIF*, rifampin.
Adapted with permission from CDC guidelines for treatment of tuberculosis. *MMWR.* 2003;52 (RR11);1–77.

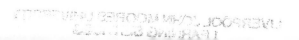

2. **Isoniazid (Nydrazid)** is a hydrazide of isonicotinic acid. The mainstay of antitubercular therapy, this drug should be included (if tolerated) in all therapeutic regimens.
   a. **Mechanism of action.** Isoniazid is **bacteriostatic** for resting bacilli and **bactericidal** for rapidly dividing organisms. Its mechanism of action is not fully known; the drug probably disrupts bacterial cell wall synthesis by inhibiting mycolic acid synthesis.
   b. **Spectrum of activity.** Isoniazid has activity only against organisms in the genus *Mycobacterium*. More specifically, it has demonstrated activity against *M. tuberculosis*, *Mycobacterium bovis*, and select strains of *Mycobacterium kansasii*.
   c. **Therapeutic uses**
      (1) The most widely used antitubercular agent, isoniazid should be given in combination with other antitubercular drugs (such as rifampin, ethambutol, and pyrazinamide) to prevent drug resistance in tuberculosis.
      (2) **Treatment of latent infection** (previously referred to as preventive therapy of chemoprophylaxis). Isoniazid may be administered alone for up to 1 year in adults or children who have a positive tuberculin test result but lack active lesions.
   d. **Precautions and monitoring effects**
      (1) The most common adverse effects of isoniazid are skin rash, fever, jaundice, and peripheral neuritis.
      (2) Hepatitis, an occasional reaction, can be severe and, in some cases, fatal. The risk of hepatitis increases with the patient's age and rises with alcohol abuse. Monitor liver function tests.
      (3) Blood dyscrasias (e.g., agranulocytosis, aplastic or hemolytic anemia, thrombocytopenia) may occur. Monitor complete blood count (CBC) routinely.
      (4) Adverse GI effects include nausea, vomiting, and epigastric distress.
      (5) CNS toxicity may result from pyridoxine deficiency. Signs and symptoms include insomnia, restlessness, hyperreflexia, and convulsions. Pyridoxine 15 to 50 mg/day should be administered to patients taking isoniazid to minimize the peripheral neuropathy associated with its use (especially in patients with diabetes, HIV, uremia, alcoholism, malnutrition, pregnancy, or seizure disorder).
   e. **Significant interactions**
      (1) With concurrent **phenytoin** therapy, blood levels of both phenytoin and isoniazid may increase, possibly causing toxicity.
      (2) **Aluminum-containing antacids** may reduce isoniazid absorption.
      (3) Concurrent **carbamazepine** therapy may increase the risk of hepatitis.
      (4) Use of isoniazid with other antitubercular agents, such as cycloserine or ethionamide, may cause additive nervous system effects.
      (5) There is the potential for the serotonin syndrome to exist when isoniazid is used in combination with selective serotonin reuptake inhibitors or in patients taking meperidine. Isoniazid has been shown to have some monoamine oxidase (MAO)–inhibiting activity.
3. **Rifampin (Rimactane)** is a complex macrocyclic agent.
   a. **Mechanism of action.** This drug is **bactericidal**; it impairs bacterial RNA synthesis by binding to DNA-dependent RNA polymerase.
   b. **Spectrum of activity.** Rifampin has activity against most mycobacterial strains. In addition, rifampin has activity against many other organisms, including *N. meningitidis*, *S. aureus*, *H. influenzae*, *Legionella pneumophila*, and *C. trachomatis*.
   c. **Therapeutic uses**
      (1) In recommended combinations for treatment of active tuberculosis
      (2) Prophylactic rifampin is effective when administered to carriers of *N. meningitidis* disease and chemoprophylaxis of patients with *H. influenzae* type b organisms.
      (3) Rifampin may be used in combination with dapsone for the treatment of leprosy.
   d. **Precautions and monitoring effects**
      (1) Serious hepatotoxicity may result from rifampin therapy. Liver function tests should be routinely conducted.
      (2) In rare cases, this drug induces an influenza-like syndrome.
      (3) Other adverse effects include skin rash, drowsiness, headache, fatigue, confusion, nausea, vomiting, and abdominal pain.
      (4) Rifampin colors urine, sweat, tears, saliva, and feces orange-red.

e. **Significant interactions**
   (1) Rifampin induces hepatic microsomal cytochrome P450 isoenzymes and thus may decrease the therapeutic effectiveness of **corticosteroids, warfarin, oral contraceptives, quinidine, digitoxin, protease inhibitors (PIs), nonnucleoside reverse transcriptase inhibitors, ketoconazole, verapamil, methadone, oral antidiabetic agents, cyclosporine, dapsone, chloramphenicol,** and **barbiturates.**
   (2) **Probenecid** may increase blood levels of rifampin.
   (3) **Aminosalicylic acid** may impair absorption of rifampin secondary to bentonite, an excipient used in preparation of aminosalicylic granules.

f. The newer rifamycins, **rifabutin (Mycobutin)** and **rifapentine (Priftin)** may be substituted for rifampin in special situations, for example, intolerance or serious drug interactions.

4. **Rifabutin (Mycobutin)** is an antimycobacterial agent that is similar to rifampin, with activity against both tubercular and nontubercular mycobacterial, and offers no clear advantage over rifampin.
   a. **Mechanism of action.** In addition to its antimycobacterial activity against tubercular and nontubercular mycobacterial, rifabutin has been reported to inhibit reverse transcriptase and block the in vitro infectivity and replication of HIV.
   b. **Therapeutic uses.** Rifabutin is indicated for the prevention of disseminated MAI complex disease in patients with advanced HIV infections.
   c. **Precautions and monitoring effects.** The use of rifabutin has resulted in mild elevation of liver enzymes and thrombocytopenia.
   d. **Significant interactions**
      (1) Rifabutin antagonizes and potentially negates the immune response mediated by the bacillus Calmette–Guérin (BCG) vaccine.
      (2) Rifabutin may increase the clearance of drugs by inducing hepatic microsomal enzymes, but does so to a lesser extent than rifampin. The concentrations of the following drugs may be reduced while taking rifabutin: **cyclosporine, zidovudine, prednisone, digitoxin, quinidine, ketoconazole, protease inhibitors, propranolol, phenytoin, sulfonylureas,** and **warfarin.** Serum cyclosporine levels should be monitored in patients receiving both agents.

5. **Rifapentine (Priftin)** is a long-acting rifamycin-derivative and has a similar profile of microbiological activity to rifampin. It is usually administered once or twice weekly.
   a. **Mechanism of action.** Rifapentine is bactericidal against intracellular and extracellular *M. tuberculosis* at therapeutic levels.
   b. **Spectrum of activity and therapeutic uses.** Indicated for treatment of primary tuberculosis. Rifapentine should always be used in conjunction with $\geq$ 1 other antituberculosis drug to which the isolate is susceptible.
   c. **Precautions and monitoring effects.** Rifapentine induces cytochrome P450 isoenzymes 3A4 and 2C8/9 responsible for inactivation of certain calcium channel–blocking agents (verapamil, diltiazem, nifedipine), antifungals (ketoconazole, fluconazole, itraconazole), sulfonylurea antidiabetic agents, methadone, corticosteroids, cardiac glycosides, certain antiarrhythmic agents (disopyramide, mexiletine, quinidine, tocainide), quinine, dapsone, chloramphenicol, clarithromycin, doxycycline, fluoroquinolones, transcriptase inhibitor cyclosporin, tacrolimus, and warfarin. Concomitant use of rifapentine with these drugs may decrease plasma concentrations, and dosage adjustments may be required.

6. **Pyrazinamide** is a pyrazine analog of nicotinamide.
   a. **Mechanism of action.** This drug is **bactericidal** and/or **bacteriostatic**, depending on the cell concentration achieved.
   b. **Spectrum of activity and therapeutic uses.** Pyrazinamide is a highly specific agent and has activity only against *M. tuberculosis.* Pyrazinamide is used as a primary agent with isoniazid and rifampin for at least 2 months, followed by isoniazid and rifampin.
   c. **Precautions and monitoring effects.** This agent may result in hepatotoxicity and, rarely, hepatic necrosis resulting in death. Anorexia, nausea, vomiting, malaise, and fever have been reported. Hyperuricemia may result in gouty exacerbations. Both liver function tests and uric acid levels should routinely be monitored.

C. **Second-line agents.** These agents include aminosalicylic acid **(Paser)**, capreomycin **(Capastat)**, cycloserine **(Seromycin)**, ethionamide **(Trecator-SC)**, quinolones (ciprofloxacin, ofloxacin, levofloxacin, sparfloxacin), streptomycin, and kanamycin. Second-line drugs are mainly substituted or added to preferred therapy owing to intolerance or drug resistance. These agents are less effective, more toxic, and are used in combination with primary agents.

1. **Mechanism of action**
   a. **Aminosalicylic acid** is **bacteriostatic**; it probably inhibits the enzymes responsible for folic acid synthesis.
   b. **Cycloserine** can be **bacteriostatic** or **bactericidal**, depending on its concentration at the infection site; it impairs amino acid use, thereby inhibiting bacterial cell wall synthesis.
   c. The mechanism of action of capreomycin (**bacteriostatic**), ethionamide (**bactericidal**), and pyrazinamide (**bactericidal**) is unknown.
2. **Spectrum of activity and therapeutic uses.** Second-line antitubercular agents are active against various microorganisms, including *M. tuberculosis*. These agents generally are reserved for patients with extensive extrapulmonary or drug-resistant disease or for patients who need retreatment. These drugs are almost always administered in combination.
3. **Precautions and monitoring effects**
   a. Adverse effects of **aminosalicylic acid** include leukopenia, agranulocytopenia, thrombocytopenia, hemolytic anemia, mononucleosis-like syndrome, malaise, joint pain, fever, and skin rash.
   b. **Capreomycin** and **streptomycin** are ototoxic and nephrotoxic; they should not be administered together.
   c. **Cycloserine** may cause adverse CNS effects including headache, suicidal and psychotic tendencies, hyperirritability, confusion, paranoia, and nervousness.
   d. **Ethionamide** may induce nausea, vomiting, orthostatic hypotension, metallic taste, epigastric distress, and peripheral neuropathy.
   e. **Streptomycin.** See II.B.3.

D. **Alternative agents**

1. **Rifater.** A combination of rifampin 120 mg, isoniazid 50 mg, and pyrazinamide 300 mg in one tablet is used in patients expected to have low compliance with tuberculosis drug therapy. One **disadvantage** is that many patients are required to take as many as five to six tablets daily, which may reduce compliance.
2. **Quinolones.** Ciprofloxacin and levofloxacin are used in tuberculosis therapy. Levofloxacin is preferred owing to increased serum concentrations. Levofloxacin is usually used in combination with other tuberculosis agents for active treatment. For prophylaxis, levofloxacin is combined with pyrazinamide.
3. **Macrolides.** Clarithromycin and azithromycin have shown limited activity against *M. tuberculosis*.

VII. ANTIVIRAL AGENTS

A. **Definition.** These drugs treat viral infections by affecting viral replication. Because viruses lack independent metabolic activity and can replicate only within living host cells, antiviral agents tend to injure host as well as viral cells. Although most antiviral drugs are active against either DNA or RNA viruses, some (e.g., adefovir, ribavirin) are active against both.

B. **DNA viruses.** Currently approved antiviral therapies against the Herpesviridae family of DNA viruses—herpes simplex virus 1 and 2 (HSV-1, HSV-2), varicella zoster virus (VZV), cytomegalovirus (CMV)—are **virustatic** and arrest DNA synthesis by inhibiting viral DNA polymerase. Many of these agents are prodrugs and require viral and host cellular enzymes (e.g., thymidine, deoxyguanosine kinase) to phosphorylate them into the active triphosphate form before exerting their antiviral activity. Hence, a common mechanism of resistance is a deficiency or structural alteration in viral thymidine kinase (*Table 36-5*). Some of these agents also demonstrate activity against RNA viruses, including hepatitis C and HIV.

1. **Acyclovir (Zovirax)** is a synthetic acyclic analog of guanosine with activity against various herpes viruses.
   a. **Mechanism of action.** Acyclovir monophosphate is phosphorylated to the triphosphate, where it becomes incorporated into viral DNA and inhibits viral replication.
   b. **Spectrum of activity.** This agent is active against herpes viruses, particularly HSV-1, HSV-2, VZV, and chickenpox (varicella).

Table 36-5 ACTIVITY OF VARIOUS ANTI-DNA VIRAL AGENTS

Agent	HSV-1	HSV-2	VZV	CMV	Influenza A	Influenza B
Acyclovir[a]	+	+	+	—	—	—
Amantadine	—	—	—	—	+	—
Cidofovir	—	—	—	+	—	—
Famciclovir	+	+	+	—	—	—
Foscarnet	+	+	+	+	—	—
Ganciclovir[a]	—	—	—	+	—	—
Oseltamivir	—	—	—	—	+	+
Rimantadine	—	—	—	—	+	—
Valacyclovir[a]	+	+	+	—	—	—
Valganciclovir[a]	—	—	—	+	—	—
Zanamivir	—	—	—	—	+	+

[a]Requires activation into triphosphate form.
HSV, herpes simplex virus; *VZV*, varicella zoster virus; *CMV*, cytomegalovirus.

c. **Therapeutic uses**

(1) Acyclovir is used to treat initial and recurrent HSV-1 and HSV-2 infections and for acute treatment of herpes zoster (shingles) and chickenpox. It is also used orally for long-term suppression of genital HSV infections.

(2) This agent is available in topical, oral, and IV forms. Topical acyclovir is applied directly on herpes lesions in recurrent herpes labialis (cold sores). It is not recommended for use on genital herpes lesions due to poor efficacy.

(3) Acyclovir may be administered intravenously in the treatment of initial and recurrent mucocutaneous HSV infection and VZV infection in immunocompromised patients as well as in the treatment of HSV infections that are disseminated or affect the central nervous system.

d. **Precautions and monitoring effects**

(1) Oral acyclovir may induce nausea, vomiting, diarrhea, and headache.

(2) IV administration may cause dose-dependent renal impairment, crystalline nephropathy, neurological effects (e.g., lethargy, confusion, tremors, agitation, seizures, coma, obtundation), hypotension, rash, itching, and phlebitis at the injection site.

(3) Local discomfort and pruritus may result from topical administration.

(4) Acyclovir is removed by hemodialysis. Doses should be adjusted in renal impairment and hemodialysis.

e. **Significant interactions. Probenecid** reduces the renal clearance of acyclovir, resulting in increases in acyclovir half-life and serum concentration. Acyclovir may decrease plasma concentrations of **phenytoin** and **valproic acid**.

2. **Adefovir dipivoxil** (Hepsera) is a phosphonate nucleotide analog with activity against various DNA and RNA viruses.

a. **Mechanism of action.** Adefovir is phosphorylated to the active diphosphate form by cellular kinases. It is then incorporated into viral DNA, resulting in termination of replication.

b. **Spectrum of activity and therapeutic uses**

(1) Adefovir is active against hepatitis B virus (including lamivudine-resistant strains), herpes viruses, and HIV.

(2) However, adefovir is approved for use only for treatment of chronic hepatitis B infection in adults with evidence of active viral replication with persistently elevated liver function tests or histologically active disease.

c. **Precautions and monitoring effects**

(1) Severe acute hepatitis exacerbations have occurred in patients who discontinue therapy (**black box warning**). If therapy is discontinued, liver function tests must be monitored closely.

(2) Nephrotoxicity has been reported with adefovir, especially in patients with underlying renal dysfunction or those taking concomitant nephrotoxins (**black box warning**).
(3) Other adverse effects include rash, GI disturbances, headache, and weakness.
(4) Dose adjustment is required for renal insufficiency.

3. **Amantadine (Symmetrel)** is a synthetic tricyclic amine with a unique chemical structure similar to rimantadine. It demonstrates activity against influenza A viral infection.
   a. **Mechanism of action.** Amantadine inhibits replication of the influenza A virus by interfering with viral attachment and uncoating.
   b. **Spectrum of activity and therapeutic uses**
      (1) Due to increasing rates of resistance, amantadine is no longer recommended for prophylaxis or treatment of influenza A virus.
      (2) This drug may also be used to treat parkinsonism as well as drug-induced extrapyramidal symptoms.
   c. **Precautions and monitoring effects**
      (1) The most pronounced adverse effects of amantadine are ataxia, nightmares, and insomnia. Other CNS effects include depression, confusion, dizziness, fatigue, anxiety, and headache. Elderly patients may be at increased risk of CNS adverse reactions. Patients with a history of seizures or psychiatric disorders should be monitored closely during therapy.
      (2) Anticholinergic reactions (e.g., dry mouth, blurred vision) have been reported.
      (3) Dosage adjustment is needed for patients with impaired renal function.
4. **Cidofovir (Vistide)** is a synthetic acyclic purine nucleoside phosphonate derivative.
   a. **Mechanism of action.** Cidofovir diphosphate suppresses CMV replication by selective inhibition of viral DNA synthesis.
   b. **Spectrum of activity.** In vitro activity has been demonstrated against CMV, VZV, Epstein–Barr virus (EBV), and HSV-1 and HSV-2. Controlled clinical studies are limited to patients with AIDS and CMV retinitis.
   c. **Therapeutic use** includes the treatment, but not the cure, of CMV retinitis in patients with AIDS.
   d. **Precautions and monitoring effects**
      (1) Cases of acute renal failure leading to dialysis or death have occurred (**black box warning**). It is also carcinogenic and teratogenic.
      (2) Avoid using this drug in patients with serum creatinine > 1.5 mg/dL or creatinine clearance (CrCl) < 55 mL/min or in patients who are receiving (or have received in the past 7 days) nephrotoxic agents.
      (3) Cidofovir is contraindicated in patients with a history of severe hypersensitivity to probenecid or sulfa-containing medications.
      (4) The dose-limiting toxicity of cidofovir is **nephrotoxicity**; neutropenia, peripheral neuropathy, and diarrhea are common adverse effects.
      (5) Probenecid must be administered before and after each cidofovir dose. The patient must be hydrated with 1 L of normal saline before infusing. Cidofovir is available only in IV form.
5. **Entecavir (Baraclude)** is a carbocyclic analog of guanosine used for treatment of chronic hepatitis B infection.
   a. **Mechanism of action.** Once phosphorylated to the active triphosphate form, entecavir inhibits hepatitis B viral polymerase and ultimately halts hepatitis B DNA synthesis.
   b. **Spectrum of activity.** Entecavir exhibits activity against hepatitis B virus, including lamivudine-resistant strains. Development of HIV resistance to nucleoside reverse transcriptase inhibitors is possible if entecavir is used without antiretroviral treatment in HIV and hepatitis B virus coinfection.
   c. **Therapeutic uses**
      (1) Entecavir is approved for treatment of chronic hepatitis B infection in adults with evidence of active viral replication and persistent elevations in liver function tests or histologically active disease.
      (2) It is effective for patients who have failed treatment with lamivudine owing to resistance development.
      (3) Entecavir is not recommended for use in patients with hepatitis B virus infection who are coinfected with HIV and are not receiving antiretroviral therapy.

d. Precautions and monitoring effects

(1) Severe acute exacerbations of hepatitis B have been observed in patients who discontinue therapy, necessitating close monitoring (**black box warning**).

(2) Common adverse effects include dizziness, fatigue, headache, and nausea.

(3) Dose adjustment is required for renal insufficiency.

(4) Counsel patients to take entecavir on an empty stomach.

6. **Famciclovir (Famvir)** is a prodrug of the antiviral agent penciclovir.

a. Mechanism of action. Famciclovir is rapidly phosphorylated in virus-infected cells by viral thymidine kinase to penciclovir monophosphate. Penciclovir is a competitive inhibitor of viral DNA polymerase and prevents viral replication by inhibition of herpes virus DNA synthesis.

b. Spectrum of activity and therapeutic uses

(1) Famciclovir has activity against HSV-1, HSV-2, and VZV. The drug is indicated for management of acute herpes zoster (shingles) and oral and genital herpes.

(2) Therapy must be promptly initiated as soon as herpes zoster is diagnosed (within 48 to 72 hrs), at a dose of 500 mg every 8 hrs for 7 days.

c. Precautions and monitoring effects

(1) **Common adverse events** include fatigue, GI complaints (nausea, diarrhea, vomiting, constipation), and anorexia. Headache is also commonly reported.

(2) Dose adjustment is necessary in patients with renal dysfunction. Famciclovir is removed by hemodialysis.

7. **Foscarnet (Foscavir)** is a synthetic pyrophosphate analog that directly inhibits enzymes involved in viral DNA synthesis without incorporation into viral DNA. It is a broad-spectrum antiviral agent and is an option in cases of acyclovir or ganciclovir resistance.

a. Mechanism of action

(1) Viral DNA replication requires the addition of deoxynucleoside triphosphates at the end of the DNA strand by DNA polymerase and the subsequent cleavage of pyrophosphate from the newly attached nucleotide. Foscarnet binds noncompetitively to DNA polymerase to form an inactive complex and prevents pyrophosphate cleavage. Viral DNA chain elongation is thus terminated.

(2) Foscarnet is also active against HIV. It is a noncompetitive, reversible inhibitor of HIV reverse transcriptase, the enzyme responsible for converting viral RNA to viral DNA.

b. Spectrum of activity and therapeutic uses. Foscarnet has in vitro activity against HSV-1 and HSV-2, CMV, VZV, EBV DNA polymerases, influenza polymerase, and HIV reverse transcriptase. Therapeutically, the drug is used to treat CMV disease as well as acyclovir-resistant HSV and VZV infections.

(1) Foscarnet is an alternative to ganciclovir and valganciclovir for treatment of CMV infection in immunocompromised patients. Foscarnet causes less hematologic toxicity than ganciclovir in patients who have received allogeneic stem cell transplants. An initial induction therapy lasts 2 to 3 weeks. Maintenance therapy is needed to prevent relapse.

(2) Foscarnet is indicated for the treatment of acyclovir-resistant mucocutaneous HSV in immunocompromised patients. It is not, however, a cure for HSV infections.

(3) Foscarnet is able to cross the blood–brain barrier.

c. Precautions and monitoring effects

(1) IV foscarnet is highly **nephrotoxic**, causing acute tubular necrosis. The incidence of acute renal failure can be markedly reduced if adequate hydration and daily monitoring of BUN and serum creatinine are maintained throughout therapy.

(2) Other common adverse effects include electrolyte abnormalities (e.g., hypocalcemia, hypomagnesemia, hypophosphatemia and hyperphosphatemia, hypokalemia), anemia, fever, headache, and seizures.

(3) Dose adjustment for renal dysfunction is required. Foscarnet is removed by hemodialysis.

(4) Foscarnet must be administered using an infusion pump over at least 1.5 to 2 hrs. Do not administer the drug as an IV bolus.

d. **Significant interactions**
   (1) Concomitant nephrotoxins (aminoglycosides, amphotericin B, etc.) increase the risk of renal toxicity.
   (2) Foscarnet is exclusively eliminated by glomerular filtration; concurrent nephrotoxic agents should be avoided whenever possible.

8. **Ganciclovir (Cytovene)** is a synthetic purine nucleoside analog that is approved for the treatment and prophylaxis of CMV infections in immunocompromised patients (e.g., HIV-positive patients, transplant recipients).
   a. **Mechanism of action.** After conversion to ganciclovir triphosphate, ganciclovir is incorporated into viral DNA, which inhibits viral DNA polymerase, thereby terminating viral replication.
   b. **Spectrum of activity.** Ganciclovir has in vitro activity against HSV-1 and HSV-2, VZV, EBV, and CMV (owing to its enhanced ability to penetrate host cells).
   c. **Therapeutic uses.** It is indicated for treatment of CMV retinitis in patients with HIV/AIDS. It is also used for prophylaxis of CMV infection in HIV-positive patients (secondary prophylaxis) and transplant recipients at risk for CMV disease.
      (1) Conversion into the triphosphate form is greater in infected host cells, even though drug penetration occurs in both uninfected and infected cells.
      (2) Inhibitory concentrations for the viral DNA polymerase are lower than those for the host cellular polymerase.
      (3) It is available in oral and IV formulations as well as an intraocular implant. Although the oral formulation is approved for prevention and maintenance treatment of CMV, its poor bioavailability has limited its use. Valganciclovir has become the drug of choice for these indications, owing to its markedly improved bioavailability.
   d. **Precautions and monitoring effects**
      (1) Ganciclovir has a **black box warning** concerning increased potential for neutropenia, anemia, and thrombocytopenia. It is also teratogenic, carcinogenic, and mutagenic.
      (2) Adverse effects commonly include fever, rash, and GI disturbances. Phlebitis and pain may occur at the site of infusion.
      (3) Because ganciclovir is cleared by glomerular filtration and tubular secretion, renal function and adequate hydration should be monitored. Doses should be adjusted in cases of renal impairment and hemodialysis.
      (4) Solutions of ganciclovir are extremely alkaline. Avoid direct contact with skin.
   e. **Significant interactions**
      (1) **Probenecid** may increase ganciclovir concentrations and possibly toxicity.
      (2) Use of **zidovudine**, **azathioprine**, or **mycophenolate mofetil** in combination with ganciclovir may result in neutropenia; careful monitoring of neutrophil count is required when these are taken concurrently with ganciclovir.
      (3) **Imipenem–cilastatin** in combination with ganciclovir may increase the potential for seizures.

9. **Oseltamivir (Tamiflu)** is pharmacologically similar to zanamivir but structurally different. Both of these agents are in a class known as the neuraminidase inhibitors and have a unique mechanism of action.
   a. **Mechanism of action.** Oseltamivir is a prodrug that must be hydrolyzed to oseltamivir carboxylate in vivo to exert its antiviral activity. It is a potent selective inhibitor of the influenza virus enzyme, neuraminidase. Inhibition of this enzyme prevents viral replication and spread to other host cells.
   b. **Spectrum of activity.** This agent is active against both influenza A and B viruses. It is one of the preferred agents for use against the 2009 H1N1 strain of influenza.
   c. **Therapeutic uses**
      (1) It is approved for the symptomatic treatment of influenza A and B infections in patients 1 year of age and older who present with symptoms within 48 hrs.
      (2) Oseltamivir has been shown to decrease the duration of symptoms by 1 to 2 days if taken within 48 hrs of onset of viral symptoms.
      (3) It is also approved for the prophylaxis of influenza infections in patients 1 year of age and older. Dosing recommendations are available for prevention and treatment of H1N1 influenza in children younger than 1 year of age. *Note:* The influenza virus vaccine is still the gold standard for prophylaxis.

(4) Oseltamivir demonstrates some activity against strains of avian influenza, making it a possible option for treatment and prophylaxis.

d. Precautions and monitoring effects

(1) The most common adverse effects are nausea and vomiting. There have been postmarketing reports of self-injury and delirium (mostly in Japan) among pediatric patients. Close monitoring for abnormal behavior is recommended.

(2) Dosage adjustments are required for patients with impaired renal function.

(3) Cross-resistance between oseltamivir and zanamivir has been reported.

(4) Dosing errors have resulted when prescribers dosed oseltamivir suspension in mL instead of mg. Be sure to verify and communicate doses in mg only.

10. Ribavirin (Rebetol, Copegus) is a synthetic nucleoside analog.

a. Mechanism of action. Ribavirin may inhibit RNA and DNA synthesis by depleting intracellular nucleotide reserves.

b. Spectrum of activity. This agent is active in vitro against a broad spectrum of DNA and RNA viruses, including influenza A and B, RSV, herpes simplex, and hepatitis C virus.

c. Therapeutic uses. The aerosolized form of ribavirin is no longer recommended for treatment of RSV in infants and children, owing to inconsistent clinical benefits observed in clinical trials. Combination therapy with oral ribavirin and subcutaneous interferon-alpha is effective in treatment of non-genotype1 chronic hepatitis C.

d. Precautions and monitoring effects

(1) Common adverse effects of oral ribavirin include hemolytic anemia (**black box warning**) and GI disturbances. Hemoglobin and hematocrit should be monitored carefully, especially during the first 4 weeks of treatment.

(2) Ribavirin is teratogenic; its use is contraindicated in pregnancy and in the male partners of pregnant women.

(3) Ribavirin should be avoided in patients with a CrCl $<$ 50 mL/min.

(4) Ribavirin should never be used as monotherapy in treatment of chronic hepatitis C.

11. Rimantadine (Flumadine) is a synthetic antiviral agent and an α-methyl derivative of amantadine that blocks the early step in the replication of the influenza A virus.

a. Mechanism of action. Rimantadine inhibits the early viral replication cycle, possibly inhibiting the uncoating of the virus. It has the same mechanism of action and spectrum of activity as amantadine.

b. Spectrum of activity and therapeutic uses

(1) Due to increasing rates of resistance, rimantadine is no longer recommended for prophylaxis or treatment of influenza A virus.

(2) Influenza vaccination is the method of choice for prevention of influenza infection.

c. Precautions and monitoring effects

(1) Rimantadine may increase the incidence of seizure in patients with seizure disorder.

(2) The most frequent adverse reactions include GI disturbance (e.g., nausea, vomiting, anorexia) and CNS toxicity (e.g., insomnia, dizziness, headache), which are less than those observed with amantadine.

(3) Dose reductions are recommended in patients with hepatic or renal dysfunction.

12. Telbivudine (Tyzeka) is a synthetic thymidine nucleoside analog used for treatment of chronic hepatitis B infection.

a. Mechanism of action. Telbivudine is phosphorylated into the active triphosphate form that inhibits hepatitis B viral DNA polymerase, with ultimate termination of the DNA chain and inhibition of viral replication.

b. Spectrum of activity

(1) Telbivudine exhibits activity against hepatitis B virus but not HIV.

(2) There is a high incidence of cross-resistance between lamivudine-resistant hepatitis B virus and telbivudine.

c. Therapeutic uses

(1) Telbivudine is indicated for treatment of chronic hepatitis B infection in adults with active viral replication and persistent elevations in liver function tests or histologically active disease.

(2) When compared with lamivudine, telbivudine produced a greater virologic response in controlled clinical trials.

d. **Precautions and monitoring effects**
   (1) There is a **black box warning** regarding severe exacerbations of hepatitis B in patients discontinuing therapy, requiring close monitoring.
   (2) Common adverse effects include elevations in creatine phosphokinase, headache, fatigue, nausea, and vomiting.
   (3) Dosage adjustment is required in patients with renal insufficiency.
   (4) May be taken without regard to meals.

13. **Valacyclovir (Valtrex)** is the L-valyl ester prodrug of the antiviral agent acyclovir.
   a. **Mechanism of action.** Valacyclovir is rapidly converted to acyclovir. Acyclovir is selective for the thymidine kinase enzyme, beginning the conversion of acyclovir to acyclovir triphosphate, stopping the replication of herpes viral DNA.
   b. **Spectrum of activity and therapeutic uses**
      (1) Valacyclovir is active against HSV-1, HSV-2, and VZV.
      (2) This agent is used for the acute treatment of herpes zoster (shingles), herpes labialis (cold sores), and genital herpes in immunocompetent adults. It is also effective for suppression of recurrent episodes of genital herpes in immunocompetent and HIV-infected people as well as reduction of transmission of genital herpes.
      (3) Advantages over acyclovir include oral dosing of only once to three times daily and attainment of higher plasma concentrations than oral acyclovir. A disadvantage is that there is no IV form available.
   c. **Precautions and monitoring effects**
      (1) Valacyclovir has caused thrombotic thrombocytopenic purpura/hemolytic uremic syndrome in immunocompromised individuals, including those with advanced HIV and transplant recipients.
      (2) Begin therapy within 72 hrs of herpes zoster rash onset.
      (3) Most commonly reported adverse reactions are mild and include nausea, headache, and vomiting. Dosage adjustment is needed in patients with renal dysfunction.

14. **Valganciclovir (Valcyte)** is the L-valyl ester prodrug of the antiviral agent ganciclovir.
   a. **Mechanism of action.** Valganciclovir is converted in vivo to ganciclovir. After conversion to the active form, ganciclovir triphosphate, ganciclovir is incorporated into viral DNA, which inhibits viral DNA polymerase, thereby terminating viral replication.
   b. **Spectrum of activity and therapeutic uses**
      (1) For in vitro activity, see VII.B.8.b.
      (2) Valganciclovir is indicated for the treatment of CMV retinitis in patients with AIDS and for prevention of CMV after transplantation of kidney, heart, and kidney-pancreas. It is not indicated for liver transplant recipients, due to an increased risk of tissue-invasive CMV as compared with ganciclovir.
      (3) The markedly improved bioavailability of valganciclovir over oral ganciclovir has resulted in the widespread use of valganciclovir for treatment and prevention of CMV disease.
   c. **Precautions and monitoring effects**
      (1) Same **black box warnings** as for ganciclovir.
      (2) Doses should be adjusted in cases of renal impairment. Do not use in hemodialysis patients; ganciclovir must be used.
      (3) Only available orally. Do not substitute doses of oral valganciclovir 1:1 for oral ganciclovir; they are not equivalent.
      (4) A potential carcinogen and teratogen; common adverse effects are the same as for ganciclovir.
      (5) If the tablet is broken, avoid contact with skin owing to teratogenic and carcinogenic potential.
      (6) Be aware of the potential for errors as a result of the look-alike and sound-alike names of valganciclovir and valacyclovir.
   d. **Significant interactions.** Same as for ganciclovir; see VII.B.8.e.

15. **Zanamivir (Relenza)** is the first of a class of antiviral agents called neuraminidase inhibitors approved by the FDA for the treatment of influenza A and B infections in adults and children at least 7 years of age. It is also indicated for prevention of influenza in adults and children at least 5 years of age.
   a. **Mechanism of action.** Zanamivir inhibits replication of the influenza A and B viruses by selective inhibition of the influenza virus neuraminidase enzyme.

b. **Spectrum of activity.** This agent is active against both the influenza A and B viruses. It demonstrates activity against avian influenza in animal studies. It is one of the preferred agents for use against the 2009 H1N1 strain of influenza.

c. **Therapeutic uses**

(1) It is approved for the treatment of uncomplicated influenza A and B infection for patients who have been symptomatic for < 48 hrs. It is also indicated for influenza prophylaxis.

(2) Zanamivir is approved for oral inhalation use only, using the Diskhaler device provided by the manufacturer.

(3) Zanamivir may be considered for prevention or treatment of avian and swine (H1N1) influenza.

(4) Shown to decrease duration of symptoms by approximately 1.5 days if taken within 48 hrs of onset of viral symptoms.

d. **Precautions and monitoring effects**

(1) The use of zanamivir is not recommended in patients with a history of asthma or chronic obstructive pulmonary disease, owing to the risk of bronchospasm and acute decline in lung function.

(2) The most common adverse effects were mild and included diarrhea, nausea, and vomiting. The incidence of these was no different than placebo.

(3) Do not puncture the Rotadisk blister until immediately before administering the dose to ensure full dosage. Manual dexterity required for this device.

(4) Do not use in a nebulizer or mechanical ventilator.

C. **HIV (RNA virus)**

1. Currently, six classes of antiretroviral agents are approved. These drugs are active against HIV and include the nucleoside reverse transcriptase inhibitors (NRTIs) **abacavir, didanosine, emtricitabine, lamivudine, stavudine,** and **zidovudine**; the nucleotide reverse transcriptase inhibitor (NtRTI) **tenofovir disoproxil fumarate**; the nonnucleoside reverse transcriptase inhibitors (NNRTIs) **delavirdine, efavirenz, etravirine, nevirapine**, and **rilpivirine** and the protease inhibitors (PIs) **atazanavir, darunavir, fosamprenavir, indinavir, lopinavir/ritonavir, nelfinavir, ritonavir, saquinavir**, and **tipranavir**; the fusion inhibitor **enfuvirtide**; the entry inhibitor **maraviroc**; and the integrase inhibitor **raltegravir**.

2. These agents are virustatic and require lifelong therapy. They are currently approved for use in various combinations known as potent combination antiretroviral therapy.

a. Appropriate combinations include those that have demonstrated efficacy and safety in controlled clinical trials (*Table 36-6*).

b. Monotherapy with any single antiretroviral agent is unacceptable in the treatment of HIV infection owing to rapid development of viral resistance.

c. Before designing a treatment plan, a $CD4^+$ cell count, an HIV RNA level (viral load), genotypic resistance testing, along with baseline lab values (e.g., basic chemistry, complete blood count, etc.) should be obtained to determine if treatment should be initiated. After starting therapy, repeat these measurements in 2 to 8 weeks, followed by every 3 to 6 months once undetectable.

d. A minimum of 0.5 to log_{10} copies/mL decline in HIV RNA levels should be seen after the first 2 to 8 weeks of therapy for clinical response; a subsequent decrease to undetectable levels should be achieved by 12 to 24 weeks.

3. **Reverse transcriptase inhibitors** are classified as either nucleosides or nucleotides. These agents are competitive inhibitors of reverse transcriptase, which leads to chain termination when incorporated into the viral DNA chain. They are inactive until phosphorylated by human cellular kinases into the active triphosphate metabolite. Each agent has a corresponding three-letter acronym as well as a brand name. With the exception of abacavir, each agent in this class of antiretrovirals requires dosage adjustment in patients with renal dysfunction. **All agents in this class have a black box warning concerning the potential for development of lactic acidosis and severe hepatomegaly with steatosis.**

a. **Abacavir (ABC; Ziagen)** is a synthetic carbocyclic nucleoside analog indicated for the treatment of both adult and pediatric patients with HIV.

(1) **Mechanism of action.** See VII.C.3.

Table 36-6 DEPARTMENT OF HEALTH AND HUMAN SERVICES (DHHS) GUIDELINES FOR THE USE OF ANTIVIRAL AGENTS IN HIV-1-INFECTED ADULTS AND ADOLESCENTS

When to begin treatment

Treat all individuals, regardless of $CD4^+$ cell count

Treat individuals who are pregnant, have HIV-associated nephropathy, those co-infected with hepatitis B virus (when treatment for hepatitis B is indicated), and those with a history of an AIDS-defining illness

Treat individuals who are at risk for transmitting HIV to a sexual partner, as effective treatment has been shown to prevent transmission

Regimen selection

Selection of a treatment regimen should be individualized for each patient based on adverse effect profiles, drug interactions, comorbidities, pill burden, etc. Preferred and alternative treatment regimens in previously untreated patients are as follows:

NNRTI-based regimens	
Preferred regimen	efavirenz[a] + tenofovir + emtricitabine[b]
Alternative regimens	efavirenz[a] + abacavir + lamivudine[b]
	rilpivirine[c] + tenofovir + emtricitabine[b]
	rilpivirine[c] + abacavir + lamivudine[b]
PI-based regimens	
Preferred regimen	atazanavir/ritonavir + tenofovir + emtricitabine[b]
	darunavir/ritonavir + tenofovir + emtricitabine[b]
Alternative regimens	atazanavir/ritonavir + abacavir + lamivudine[b]
	darunavir/ritonavir + abacavir + lamivudine[b]
	fosamprenavir/ritonavir + either [abacavir + lamivudine[b]] or [tenofovir + emtricitabine[b]]
	lopinavir/ritonavir + either [abacavir + lamivudine[b]] or [tenofovir + emtricitabine[b]]
Integrase inhibitor-based regimen	
Preferred regimen	raltegravir + tenofovir + emtricitabine[b]
Altertnative regimen	raltegravir + abacavir + lamivudine[b]
Regimen for pregnant patients	
Preferred regimen	lopinavir/ritonavir (twice daily) + zidovudine + lamivudine[b]

Agents or combinations that should not be offered at any time

Monotherapy with NRTI
2-NRTI regimens
Abacavir + zidovudine + lamivudine as a triple NRTI regimen in treatment-naïve patients
Abacavir + zidovudine + lamivudine as a quadruple NRTI regimen in treatment-naïve patients
Zidovudine + stavudine
Didanosine + stavudine
Didanosine + tenofovir
Didanosine + lamivudine or emtricitabine
Lamivudine + emtricitabine
Atazanavir + indinavir
Efavirenz in first trimester of pregnancy or those with significant childbearing potential
Unboosted darunavir, saquinavir, indinavir, or fosamprenavir
Nevirapine in treatment-naive women with $CD4^+$ cell counts $> 250/mm^3$ or men with $CD4^+$ cell counts $> 400/mm^3$
Delavirdine, etravirine, nelfinavir, enfuvirtide in treatment-naïve patients

Table 36-6 Continued.

Monitoring
Before initiating drug therapy, must obtain CD4+ cell count and plasma HIV RNA levels plus complete blood count, chemistry, lipid profile, liver enzymes, and genotypic resistance testing
HIV RNA level should be checked within 2–8 weeks of initiating treatment and repeated every 4–8 weeks until it reaches undetectable levels (<20–75 copies/mL)

[a]Cannot be used in first trimester of pregnancy or in those women not using consistent and effective contraception who may become pregnant.
[b]May substitute lamivudine for emtricitabine or vice versa.
[c]Must be used with caution in patients with pretreatment HIV RNA >100,000 copies/mL.
NNRTI, nonnucleoside reverse transcriptase inhibitor; *NRTI*, nucleoside reverse transcriptase inhibitor; *PI*, protease inhibitor.

(2) **Spectrum of activity and therapeutic uses.** Abacavir is approved for use in adults and children ≥ 3 months of age only in combination with other antiretroviral agents.
   (a) Abacavir is available alone or coformulated as a combination tablet with lamivudine and zidovudine (Trizivir), which is dosed twice daily.
   (b) Abacavir is also available in a combination tablet with lamivudine (Epzicom) which is dosed once daily.

(3) **Precautions and monitoring effects**
   (a) Abacavir has a **black box warning** for a life-threatening hypersensitivity reaction that can lead to death. It occurs in approximately 5% of patients taking this drug, typically within the first 6 weeks of therapy. This reaction involves respiratory symptoms, fever, rash, and GI complaints. Reexposure following these symptoms can mimic anaphylaxis and may result in death. Therefore, rechallenge is contraindicated. A medication guide describing this reaction should be dispensed with each new prescription and refill of abacavir-containing products. The HLA-B*5701 screening test should be used prior to initiating therapy to determine if a patient is at risk for having this reaction.
   (b) There are cohort studies indicating increased risk of myocardial infarction with abacavir; however, this has not been shown in other studies, and this remains a controversial association.

(4) **Significant interactions.** Alcohol increases the area under the curve (AUC) of abacavir by 41%.

b. Didanosine (ddI; Videx), a synthetic purine analog, inhibits HIV replication and has a longer intracellular half-life (> 20 hrs) than zidovudine (7 hrs).

(1) **Mechanism of action.** See VII.C.3.

(2) **Spectrum of activity and therapeutic uses.** Didanosine is approved for the treatment of adults and children only in combination with other antiretroviral agents.

(3) **Precautions and monitoring effects**
   (a) Didanosine can cause reversible peripheral neuropathy and acute, potentially lethal pancreatitis (**black box warning**). Serum triglycerides should be monitored, and didanosine should be withheld when initiating potential pancreatitis-inducing agents (e.g., IV pentamidine, sulfonamides). Transiently elevated serum amylase may not reflect pancreatitis.
   (b) Didanosine has been associated with noncirrhotic portal hypertension, with some patients presenting with esophageal varices.
   (c) Other adverse effects include headache, diarrhea, nausea, and hyperuricemia (because didanosine is catalyzed to uric acid).
   (d) Didanosine is available in an enteric-coated capsule or buffered oral tablet formulation to prevent degradation at acidic pH. It must be taken on an empty stomach.
   (e) Do not use in combination with stavudine because of additive potential for toxicity.
   (f) Do not use the combination regimen of didanosine and tenofovir in treatment-naive patients, owing to high rates of early virologic failure and toxicity.

(4) **Significant interactions.** Pancreatitis-inducing drugs, **alcohol**, and **those known to cause peripheral neuropathy** should not be used with didanosine. Ribavirin should not be coadministered with didanosine.

c. **Emtricitabine (FTC; Emtriva)** is a synthetic nucleoside analog structurally related to lamivudine with activity against HIV infection.

(1) **Mechanism of action.** See VII.C.3.

(2) **Spectrum of activity and therapeutic uses.** Emtricitabine is indicated for use in HIV-infected adults and children in combination with other antiretroviral agents. It is available by itself or as a combination tablet with tenofovir (Truvada), as a combination tablet with tenofovir and efavirenz (Atripla), and as a combination tablet with tenofovir and rilpivirine (Complera). Although it demonstrates activity against hepatitis B virus, it is not approved for use in treatment of this infection. Emtricitabine and tenofovir are approved for daily use in combination to prevent HIV infection in HIV-negative men who have sex with men.

(3) **Precautions and monitoring effects**

(a) Adverse effects most commonly observed in clinical trials were mild-moderate and include headache, rash, diarrhea, and nausea. Hyperpigmentation of the palms or soles may occur.

(b) Serious acute exacerbations of hepatitis B have been documented in HIV/hepatitis B coinfected patients who discontinued therapy with emtricitabine (**black box warning**); therefore, liver function tests should be monitored for several months after discontinuation.

(c) Do not use in combination with lamivudine, due to similar resistance profiles and no additional benefits.

(4) **Significant interactions.** None have been identified.

d. **Lamivudine (3TC; Epivir)** is a synthetic nucleoside analog with activity against HIV and hepatitis B virus.

(1) **Mechanism of action.** See VII.C.3.

(2) **Spectrum of activity and therapeutic uses.** Lamivudine is indicated for use in HIV-positive adults and children > 3 months of age in combination with other antiretroviral agents. It is also used in a lower dosage for the treatment of chronic hepatitis B in patients with active liver inflammation and evidence of hepatitis B viral replication.

(a) Lamivudine is available alone or within a twice daily combination tablet containing lamivudine, zidovudine, and abacavir (Trizivir).

(b) Lamivudine is also available as a combination tablet with abacavir (Epzicom) and zidovudine (Combivir).

(3) **Precautions and monitoring effects**

(a) Reported adverse reactions are minor and include headache, fatigue, and GI reactions such as nausea, vomiting, and diarrhea. CNS toxicity includes neuropathy, dizziness, and insomnia.

(b) Do not use in combination with emtricitabine, due to similar resistance profiles and no additional benefits.

(c) Lamivudine has the same **black box warning** regarding acute exacerbations of hepatitis B as emtricitabine (see VII.C.3.c).

(4) **Significant interactions.** Coadministration with **co-trimoxazole** results in increased lamivudine levels. No dose adjustment is required.

e. **Stavudine (d4T; Zerit)** is a synthetic thymidine nucleoside analog that is active against HIV.

(1) **Mechanism of action.** See VII.C.3.

(2) **Spectrum of activity and therapeutic uses.** Stavudine is indicated for use in combination with other antiretroviral agents in adults and children of all ages.

(3) **Precautions and monitoring effects**

(a) The major toxicity with stavudine is a dose related, but reversible peripheral neuropathy occurring in up to 21% of patients.

(b) Other adverse effects include headache, rash, diarrhea, nausea, and vomiting.

(c) Fatal episodes of pancreatitis have been reported.

(4) **Significant interactions.** Do not use in combination with zidovudine.

f. **Tenofovir disoproxil fumarate (TDF; Viread)** is an acyclic nucleoside phosphonate diester analog (**nucleotide**) with antiviral activity against HIV and hepatitis B virus.

(1) **Mechanism of action.** Tenofovir (a prodrug) is rapidly hydrolyzed by plasma esterases to tenofovir, with subsequent conversion to the active tenofovir diphosphate. *Note:* NtRTIs are active as the diphosphate, unlike the NRTIs, which require conversion to the triphosphate.

(2) **Spectrum of activity and therapeutic uses.** Tenofovir is approved for use in combination with other antiretroviral agents for the treatment of HIV in adults. It is also available as a once daily combination tablet containing tenofovir and emtricitabine (Truvada) as well as tenofovir, emtricitabine, and efavirenz (Atripla) and tenofovir, emtricitabine, and rilpivirine (Complera). Tenofovir and emtricitabine are approved for daily use in combination to prevent HIV infection in HIV-negative men who have sex with men.

(3) **Precautions and monitoring effects**

(a) Minor adverse effects have been reported in clinical trials. These include complaints of diarrhea, nausea, vomiting, headache, and asthenia.

(b) Additional adverse effects observed during postmarketing surveillance include renal insufficiency and decreases in bone mineral density.

(c) Tenofovir has the same **black box warning** that emtricitabine has for patients with concomitant hepatitis B (see VII.C.3.c).

(d) Dose adjustment is required for renal insufficiency.

(4) **Significant interactions**

(a) Tenofovir increases **didanosine** serum concentrations, resulting in increased risk of toxicity. Additionally, there is a high rate of early virologic failure and development of resistance mutations. Thus, this combination is not recommended for use.

(b) Tenofovir decreases serum concentrations of **atazanavir**. When these two agents are used together, ritonavir must be added to the regimen.

g. Zidovudine (AZT; Retrovir) is a synthetic thymidine analog. This agent was the first available drug for the treatment of HIV infection.

(1) **Mechanism of action.** See VII.C.3.

(2) **Spectrum of activity and therapeutic uses**

(a) Zidovudine is indicated in the treatment of adults and children for the treatment of HIV.

(b) It is indicated for the prevention of maternal–fetal HIV transmission.

(c) Zidovudine is available as oral capsules, tablets, and solution as well as an IV solution.

(d) Oral zidovudine is also available as a coformulation with lamivudine (Combivir) and with lamivudine and abacavir (Trizivir).

(3) **Precautions and monitoring effects**

(a) Zidovudine can cause severe bone marrow suppression, including macrocytic anemia and neutropenia after the first few weeks to months of therapy. The risk is increased in patients with preexisting bone marrow suppression or who are taking concomitant medications that cause bone marrow suppression.

(b) Erythropoietin can be considered as an adjunctive therapy in patients with zidovudine-induced anemia, in cases for which it cannot be discontinued.

(c) Other adverse effects include headache, malaise, seizures, anxiety, fever, and rash.

(d) Prolonged use may lead to symptomatic myopathy.

(4) **Significant interactions**

(a) **Co-trimoxazole**, **atovaquone**, **valproic acid**, **methadone**, and **probenecid** may increase zidovudine concentrations, causing increased risk of zidovudine toxicity.

(b) Other **cytotoxic drugs**, such as **ganciclovir**, **dapsone**, **ribavirin**, and **interferon-alpha**, can cause additive bone marrow suppression.

(c) Rifabutin and rifampin may decrease levels of zidovudine.

4. Nonnucleoside reverse transcriptase inhibitors (NNRTIs). The NNRTI class binds directly to and produces a noncompetitive inhibition of the HIV reverse transcriptase, leading to chain termination. These agents are indicated for use in adults and pediatric patients in combination with NRTIs or possibly protease inhibitors (PIs). Efavirenz is the preferred NNRTI for initial treatment, whereas the others are currently recommended as alternatives. NNRTI-based regimens provide potent antiviral activity with less pill burden than many PI-based regimens. All NNRTIs may cause **rash and hepatotoxicity**; patients should be monitored closely for these adverse effects.

a. Delavirdine (Rescriptor)

(1) **Mechanism of action.** See VII.C.3.

(2) **Spectrum of activity and therapeutic uses.** Delavirdine is approved for use in adults in the treatment of HIV in combination with other antiretroviral agents. Its use has fallen out of favor owing to its three times daily dosing schedule.

(3) **Precautions and monitoring effects**
  (a) In clinical trials, 4.3% of patients discontinued delavirdine because of rash. Cases of Stevens–Johnson syndrome have been reported.
  (b) Other adverse effects include headache and nausea.
(4) **Significant interactions**
  (a) The concentrations of the following medications are greatly increased by delavirdine and must be avoided: **alprazolam**, **midazolam**, **triazolam**, **simvastatin**, **lovastatin**, **rifabutin**, and **cisapride**.
  (b) Decreased delavirdine concentrations result when it is administered with **St. John's wort**, **carbamazepine**, **phenobarbital**, **phenytoin**, or **rifampin**. Concomitant use should be avoided.
  (c) Because delavirdine requires an acidic GI tract for optimal absorption, its use should be avoided with **proton pump inhibitors** and **H_2-receptor antagonists**.

b. **Efavirenz (Sustiva)**
(1) **Mechanism of action.** See VII.C.3.
(2) **Spectrum of activity and therapeutic uses.** Efavirenz is approved for use in combination with other antiretroviral agents for the treatment of HIV infection in adults and pediatric patients. One advantage over other NNRTIs is its once-daily dosing. It is available alone or as a combination tablet with tenofovir and emtricitabine (Atripla).
(3) **Precautions and monitoring effects**
  (a) Most common adverse effects are CNS-related (52%), including insomnia, dizziness, drowsiness, nightmares, and hallucinations, necessitating a bedtime dosing to minimize these effects. These effects typically subside after 2 to 4 weeks of treatment.
  (b) Owing to its teratogenic effects, efavirenz should be avoided in the first trimester of pregnancy and in women of childbearing potential who wish to conceive or who are using unreliable contraception.
  (c) Other adverse effects include rash, increased transaminases, and GI disturbances.
  (d) False-positive results may occur with screening tests for cannabinoids and benzodiazepines.
(4) **Significant interactions**
  (a) Efavirenz induces and inhibits the cytochrome P450 3A4 isoenzyme system. It should not be used concomitantly with **cisapride**, **midazolam**, **triazolam**, or **ergot derivatives**.
  (b) **St. John's wort** decreases efavirenz concentrations and should be avoided.
  (c) Efavirenz decreases **methadone** AUC by 52%; patients should be monitored for opiate withdrawal and have their doses titrated accordingly.
  (d) Efavirenz decreases **levonorgestrel** concentrations, resulting in possible decreased effectiveness of emergency postcoital contraception.

c. **Etravirine (Intelence)**
(1) **Mechanism of action.** See VII.C.3.
(2) **Spectrum of activity and therapeutic uses.** Etravirine is indicated for use in combination with at least two additional antiretroviral agents in treatment-experienced adults who demonstrate viral replication and documented resistance to other NNRTIs. It is not for use in treatment-naive patients.
(3) **Precautions and monitoring effects**
  (a) Adverse effects include nausea and rash. Hypersensitivity reactions have occurred, resulting in rash, constitutional symptoms, and possible hepatic failure.
  (b) Because food increases the absorption of etravirine by 50%, it should be taken following a meal.
(4) **Significant interactions**
  (a) Etravirine induces and inhibits a variety of cytochrome P450 isoenzymes. It should not be used concomitantly with **carbamazepine**, **phenobarbital**, **phenytoin**, **unboosted PIs**, **atazanavir/ritonavir**, **fosamprenavir/ritonavir**, **tipranavir/ritonavir**, **ritonavir**, or **other NNRTIs**.

(b) **St. John's wort** and **rifampin** decrease etravirine concentrations and should be avoided.

(c) Etravirine may decrease serum concentrations of **phosphodiesterase Type 5 (PDE 5) inhibitors** used for erectile dysfunction, requiring a dosage increase.

(d) Etravirine may decrease **clopidogrel** activation and should not be used concomitantly.

d. Nevirapine (Viramune) was the first NNRTI approved for use by the FDA for the treatment of HIV infection.

(1) **Mechanism of action.** See VII.C.3.

(2) **Spectrum of activity and therapeutic uses.** Nevirapine is indicated in combination with other antiretrovirals in adult and pediatric HIV patients. An extended-release tablet became available in early 2011.

(3) **Precautions and monitoring effects**

(a) Nevirapine has the highest incidence of Stevens–Johnson syndrome of all NNRTIs.

(b) Symptomatic hepatitis, including fatal hepatic necrosis, has been observed with nevirapine (**black box warning**). The frequency of this adverse effect is increased in women with pre-nevirapine $CD4^+$ counts > 250 cells/mm^3 and men with $CD4^+$ counts > 400 cells/mm^3. Nevirapine should not be initiated in these patients.

(c) Other adverse effects include fever, nausea, and headache.

(d) To decrease the frequency of adverse effects, a 2-week dose escalation is required.

(4) **Significant interactions**

(a) Nevirapine induces cytochrome P450 3A4, resulting in decreased concentrations of **oral contraceptives**, **efavirenz, atazanavir ± ritonavir**, **and ketoconazole**. These combinations should be avoided.

(b) Use of **rifampin** and **St. John's wort** should be avoided, as they decrease the serum concentrations of nevirapine.

(c) **Methadone** concentrations decrease significantly with nevirapine, often necessitating a dose increase.

e. Rilpivirine (Edurant)

(1) **Mechanism of action.** See VII.C.3

(2) **Spectrum of activity and therapeutic uses.** Rilpivirine is approved for use in combination with other antiretroviral agents for the treatment of HIV infection in treatment-naïve adults. It is available alone and as a combination tablet with tenofovir and emtricitabine (Complera).

(3) **Precautions and monitoring effects**

(a) In clinical trials, virologic failure was more likely with rilpivirine in those patients with high viral loads (e.g.: $> 100{,}000$ copies/mL) as compared to those with viral loads $< 100{,}000$ copies/mL. Therefore, it is especially important to consider the patient's baseline viral load prior to initiating therapy with rilpivirine.

(b) In clinical trials, virologic failure with rilpivirine was more likely to result in resistance to other NNRTIs as compared to efavirenz.

(c) In order to improve absorption, rilpivirine should be taken with a meal.

(d) Most common adverse effects are nausea, dizziness, insomnia, headache, and rash. The incidence of rash and CNS adverse effects is lower than efavirenz.

(4) **Significant interactions**

(a) At therapeutic doses, rilpivirine does not inhibit or induce the CYP450 isoenzyme system.

(b) Since rilpivirine is a substrate of CYP450 3A4, concomitant use with inducers of this enzyme system, including **rifampin, carbamazepine, phenobarbital, phenytoin, dexamethasone, and St. John's wort** should be avoided.

(c) Because rilpivirine requires an acidic GI tract for optimal absorption, its use should be avoided with **proton pump inhibitors**. If other acid suppressants are used with rilpivirine, the doses should be separated by as much time as possible (e.g: 12 hours before or 4 hours after rilpivirine dosing).

5. Protease inhibitors (PIs). The PIs competitively inhibit the viral protease enzyme, preventing the enzyme from cleaving the gag and gag-pol polyproteins necessary for virion production. PIs are used in combination with other antiretroviral agents, including other PIs, to suppress HIV replication. All of the PIs are cytochrome P450 inhibitors; ritonavir is the most potent inhibitor. All PIs are contraindicated with numerous drugs, including **simvastatin**, **lovastatin**, **rifampin**, **cisapride**, **pimozide**, **midazolam**, **triazolam**, **ergots**, **alfuzosin**, **salmeterol**, and **St. John's wort**. Concomitant therapy with antiepileptic drugs, erectile dysfunction drugs, colchicine, and azole antifungals must be undertaken with caution. Most PIs interact with warfarin, necessitating close INR monitoring and warfarin dosage adjustment. Owing to the wide array of drug interactions with PIs, always assess medication profiles carefully for drug interactions before initiation. Many PIs require dose adjustment for hepatic insufficiency.

a. **Atazanavir (Reyataz)**
   (1) **Mechanism of action.** See VII.C.5.
   (2) **Spectrum of activity and therapeutic uses.** Atazanavir is a component of preferred and alternative PI-based regimens for HIV. It is dosed once daily.
   (3) **Precautions and monitoring effects**
      (a) Atazanavir may prolong the PR interval and possibly cause first-degree AV block. Caution should be used in patients with underlying conduction defects or in those taking concomitant medications that prolong the PR interval.
      (b) Other adverse effects include fat maldistribution, hyperglycemia, and indirect hyperbilirubinemia. Atazanavir may increase lipids when used with ritonavir booster doses. Rash may occur in up to 20% of patients.
      (c) Dose adjustment is required for hepatic insufficiency.
   (4) **Significant interactions** (see VII.C.5). Atazanavir is the most problematic of all PIs in terms of drug interactions.
      (a) Because atazanavir requires an acidic GI tract for optimal absorption, concomitant use of **proton pump inhibitors** is contraindicated when used without ritonavir booster doses or in PI-experienced patients. In PI-naive patients, atazanavir/ritonavir may be used with proton pump inhibitors in a dosage equivalent to no more than omeprazole 20 mg daily. Dosing of the proton pump inhibitor should be separated by 12 hrs from the atazanavir/ritonavir. If other acid suppressants are used with atazanavir, the doses must be separated by as much time as possible (up to 12 hrs apart).
      (b) Atazanavir substantially increases concentrations of **clarithromycin**, resulting in possible QTc prolongation. The dose of clarithromycin should be decreased by 50%, or alternative therapy considered.
      (c) Concentrations of **buprenorphine** and its active metabolite are substantially increased by atazanavir; concomitant use with unboosted atazanavir must be avoided.

b. **Darunavir (Prezista)**
   (1) **Mechanism of action.** See VII.C.5.
   (2) **Spectrum of activity and therapeutic uses.** Darunavir is the newest PI to receive FDA approval for the treatment of HIV. It is considered a preferred PI for use in treatment-naive patients. Its dosing is dependent on treatment experience and number of resistance mutations present.
   (3) **Precautions and monitoring effects**
      (a) Darunavir must be coadministered with ritonavir.
      (b) Because darunavir contains a sulfonamide moiety, cross-reactivity may occur in sulfa-allergic patients.
      (c) Adverse effects include nausea, increased amylase, hepatotoxicity, hyperlipidemia, hyperglycemia, and rash.
   (4) **Significant interactions.** See VII.C.5.

c. **Fosamprenavir (Lexiva)**
   (1) **Mechanism of action.** See VII.C.5. Fosamprenavir is the prodrug of amprenavir.
   (2) **Spectrum of activity and therapeutic uses.** Fosamprenavir has largely replaced amprenavir because of its improved dosing convenience. It is recommended as one of the alternative components in PI-based regimens for initial treatment of HIV.

(3) **Precautions and monitoring effects**
   (a) Fosamprenavir may be dosed once daily in treatment-naive patients. PI-experienced patients require twice daily dosing. In most cases, fosamprenavir is administered with low-dose ritonavir.
   (b) Adverse effects include hyperlipidemia, hyperglycemia, fat maldistribution, rash, and GI disturbances.
(4) **Significant interactions** see VII.C.3.

d. Indinavir (Crixivan)
(1) **Mechanism of action.** See VII.C.5.
(2) **Spectrum of activity and therapeutic uses.** Indinavir, in combination with ritonavir, is no longer recommended as part of regimen for patients receiving initial treatment for HIV due to a high incidence of nephrolithiasis.
(3) **Precautions and monitoring effects**
   (a) Because indinavir may cause **nephrolithiasis** (kidney stones), patients should be instructed to drink at least 1.5 L of water daily to prevent this adverse effect.
   (b) Indinavir can cause **indirect hyperbilirubinemia.** Combination therapy with atazanavir is not recommended owing to the potential for additive effects.
   (c) Other adverse effects include hyperglycemia, hyperlipidemia, fat maldistribution, headache, and GI intolerance.
   (d) Dose adjustment is required for hepatic insufficiency.
(4) **Significant interactions** (see VII.C.5). Vitamin C in doses > 1 g daily decreases indinavir concentrations. Caution patients not to exceed the recommended daily allowance for vitamin C.

e. Lopinavir/ritonavir (Kaletra)
(1) **Mechanism of action.** See VII.C.5.
(2) **Spectrum of activity and therapeutic uses.** This product is available as a coformulation of lopinavir with a "booster" dose of ritonavir, which inhibits lopinavir metabolism and results in higher serum concentrations. Lopinavir/ritonavir is an alternative PI used in regimens for treatment-naive patients due to its risk of GI adverse effects and hyperlipidemia. It is the preferred PI in pregnancy.
(3) **Precautions and monitoring effects**
   (a) Lopinavir/ritonavir is formulated as a film-coated tablet that does not require refrigeration. It is also available as an oral solution containing 42% alcohol.
   (b) Adverse effects include GI intolerance, hyperlipidemia, hyperglycemia, fat maldistribution, PR interval prolongation, and pancreatitis.
(4) **Significant interactions.** See VII.C.5.
   (a) Lopinavir/ritonavir decreases **methadone** concentrations, possibly necessitating a methadone dose increase to prevent opiate withdrawal.
   (b) Concomitant administration with **voriconazole** is contraindicated because of the risk of decreased voriconazole efficacy.
   (c) Concomitant administration with **efavirenz** or **nevirapine** requires increased doses of lopinavir/ritonavir due to enzyme induction.
   (d) Once daily dosing of lopinavir/ritonavir should not be used in patients receiving **carbamazepine**, **phenytoin**, or **phenobarbital**, due to induction of lopinavir/ritonavir metabolism.

f. Nelfinavir (Viracept)
(1) **Mechanism of action.** See VII.C.5.
(2) **Spectrum of activity and therapeutic uses.** Nelfinavir is not generally recommended for treatment of HIV infection due to inferior virologic efficacy. Unlike the other PIs, it is never used in combination with ritonavir.
(3) **Precautions and monitoring effects**
   (a) Diarrhea is commonly reported with nelfinavir. This can often be managed with antidiarrheals.
   (b) Other adverse effects are similar to those with lopinavir/ritonavir.
   (c) Use caution with look-alike, sound-alike names (nelfinavir and nevirapine).
(4) **Significant interactions** (see VII.C.5). Nelfinavir decreases **methadone** concentrations, necessitating increased monitoring and dose adjustment if indicated.

g. Ritonavir (Norvir)

(1) Mechanism of action. See VII.C.5.

(2) Spectrum of activity and therapeutic uses. Ritonavir is not used as the sole PI in a PI-based regimen owing to its poor tolerability and high pill burden when administered in full doses. Alternatively, it is used in low doses as a pharmacokinetic boosting agent with other PIs. Because it is such a potent cytochrome P450 enzyme inhibitor, ritonavir markedly increases the serum concentrations of other PIs, resulting in higher concentrations with improved viral suppression.

(3) Precautions and monitoring effects

(a) Capsules should be refrigerated before dispensing. Capsules then may be stored at room temperature for up to 30 days. A tablet formulation is also available that does not require refrigeration and should be taken with food.

(b) Oral solution should **not** be refrigerated.

(c) Adverse effects include GI intolerance, circumoral paresthesias, hyperlipidemia, hyperglycemia, fat maldistribution, increased liver function tests, and taste perversion.

(4) Significant interactions (see VII.C.5). Many drug interactions occur with ritonavir because it is such a potent inhibitor of so many cytochrome P450 isoenzymes. Always refer to proper resources to assess for drug interactions.

h. Saquinavir (Invirase)

(1) Mechanism of action. See VII.C.5.

(2) Spectrum of activity and therapeutic uses. Use of saquinavir without booster doses of ritonavir is not recommended because of the poor bioavailability of saquinavir. Because saquinavir/ritonavir has been associated with significant QTc prolongation, its use should be avoided in patients with pretreatment QT intervals $>$ 450 msec, refractory hypokalemia or hypomagnesemia, presence of or at risk for complete heart block, and concomitant medications that prolong QT interval. Thus, its use is greatly limited as compared with other PIs.

(3) Precautions and monitoring effects

(a) Saquinavir/ritonavir prolongs the PR and QT intervals; cases of torsades de pointes have been reported. A baseline electrocardiogram (ECG) should be obtained prior to treatment.

(b) Other adverse effects are similar to lopinavir/ritonavir.

(4) Significant interactions. (See VII.C.5). Saquinavir/ritonavir increases concentrations of **trazodone** and may result in prolonged QT interval. Concomitant use is contraindicated.

i. Tipranavir (Aptivus)

(1) Mechanism of action. See VII.C.5.

(2) Spectrum of activity and therapeutic uses. The use of tipranavir is limited to highly treatment-experienced patients with HIV who are resistant to other PIs as well as to other classes of antiretrovirals.

(3) Precautions and monitoring effects

(a) Owing to the poor bioavailability of tipranavir, it must be coadministered with ritonavir.

(b) Capsules must be refrigerated. Once dispensed, they are stable at room temperature for up to 60 days.

(c) Tipranavir has been associated with clinical hepatitis and fatal hepatic decompensation (**black box warning**). Liver function tests should be monitored closely, especially in patients with underlying liver disease.

(d) Rarely, there have been reports of fatal and nonfatal intracranial hemorrhage with tipranavir (**black box warning**).

(e) Because the structure of tipranavir contains a **sulfonamide** moiety, cross-reactivity may occur in sulfa-allergic patients.

(f) Other adverse effects include rash, hyperlipidemia, hyperglycemia, and fat maldistribution.

(4) Significant interactions. See VII.C.5.

6. **Fusion inhibitors. Enfuvirtide (T-20; Fuzeon)** is the first and only member of this class of antiretrovirals.
   a. **Mechanism of action.** Enfuvirtide inhibits the entry of HIV into $CD4^+$ cells by interfering with the fusion of viral and cellular membranes.
   b. **Spectrum of activity and therapeutic uses.** Enfuvirtide is primarily used in highly treatment-experienced patients with extensive viral resistance. It is not recommended for use as initial therapy in treatment-naive patients, as it has not been studied in this population.
   c. **Precautions and monitoring effects**
      (1) Enfuvirtide is injected subcutaneously twice daily. Local injection site reactions occur in almost all patients, including pain, redness, pruritus, and nodules.
      (2) Other adverse effects include hypersensitivity reactions and increased rate of bacterial pneumonia.
      (3) No dose adjustment is necessary for renal impairment.
   d. **Significant interactions.** There are no significant drug interactions with enfuvirtide.
7. **Entry inhibitor. Maraviroc (Selzentry)** is the first and only member of this class of antiretroviral therapy.
   a. **Mechanism of action.** Maraviroc is a chemokine receptor 5 (CCR5) coreceptor antagonist. It binds to the CCR5 receptor on the CD4 cell membrane, preventing entry of the virus into the cell.
   b. **Spectrum of activity and therapeutic uses.** Maraviroc is used along with other antiretrovirals in adult patients who are infected with HIV that binds to the CCR5 receptor.
   c. **Precautions and monitoring effects**
      (1) **Hepatotoxicity** was observed during clinical trials with maraviroc (**black box warning**). This may be preceded by a systemic allergic reaction. Patients should be evaluated immediately if either occurs.
      (2) Use caution in patients with liver disease or cardiovascular risk factors.
      (3) Adverse effects include cough, rash, fever, musculoskeletal symptoms, dizziness, abdominal pain, and orthostatic hypotension.
      (4) Not recommended for use in patients with severe or end-stage renal disease unless clinically warranted.
   d. **Significant interactions**
      (1) Dosing for maraviroc varies depending upon concomitant medications that interact:
         (a) When used with cytochrome P450 inhibitors, such as **PIs (except tipranavir/ritonavir)**, **delavirdine**, **ketoconazole**, **itraconazole**, and **clarithromycin**, administer maraviroc 150 mg twice daily.
         (b) When used with cytochrome P450 inducers (such as **carbamazepine**, **phenobarbital**, **phenytoin**, **efavirenz**, and **rifampin**) without a strong cytochrome P450 inhibitor, administer maraviroc 600 mg twice daily.
         (c) When used with other medications, including tipranavir/ritonavir, nevirapine, NRTIs, raltegravir, and enfuvirtide, administer maraviroc 300 mg twice daily.
      (2) Concomitant administration with **St. John's wort** or rifapentine is not recommended due to reduction in maraviroc serum concentrations.
8. **Integrase inhibitor. Raltegravir (Isentress)** is the first and only member of this class of antiretroviral therapy.
   a. **Mechanism of action.** Raltegravir inhibits the viral enzyme integrase, thereby preventing the insertion of HIV genetic material into the CD4 cell genome and halting the viral replication process.
   b. **Spectrum of activity and therapeutic uses.** Raltegravir is used along with other antiretrovirals as a preferred agent in treatment-naïve patients with HIV infection.
   c. **Precautions and monitoring effects**
      (1) Because elevations in creatine kinase, along with myopathy and rhabdomyolysis, may occur with raltegravir, use with caution in patients who are receiving concomitant medications that may cause these adverse effects.
      (2) The most common adverse effects include nausea, diarrhea, headache, and fever.

d. **Significant interactions.** Because **rifampin** decreases the serum concentration of raltegravir, the dose of raltegravir should be increased to 800 mg twice daily when used concomitantly.

D. **Hepatitis C virus (RNA virus): Direct-acting antiviral (DAA) agents**

1. Currently, there are two directly acting antiviral agents (DAAs) available for use in combination with interferon alfa and ribavirin for the management of genotype 1 hepatitis C virus (HCV) infection; these include **boceprevir** and **telaprevir**. The addition of either of these agents to standard interferon alfa and ribavirin therapy has resulted in improved sustained virologic response rates and the possibility of a shorter duration of treatment for patients with genotype 1 HCV infection.
2. These agents are inhibitors of the HCV nonstructural 3/4A (NS3/4A) serine protease, an enzyme required for viral replication and virion assembly.
   a. Monotherapy with these agents is unacceptable, as the development of resistance with subsequent virologic failure occurs rapidly.
   b. These agents should only be used for treatment of genotype 1 HCV infection, in combination with interferon alfa and ribavirin.
   c. Limited data exists for use of these agents in patients coinfected with HCV and HIV; caution should be used in this population of patients.
3. Boceprevir (Victrelis)
   a. **Mechanism of action.** See VII.D.2.
   b. **Spectrum of activity and therapeutic uses.** Boceprevir is approved for use in adults with genotype 1 HCV infection who are treatment-naïve or who have failed prior treatment with interferon and ribavirin. It is added to interferon alfa and ribavirin following 4 weeks of t reatment with those two agents. The total treatment duration of this three drug regimen varies from 24-44 weeks, depending upon the patient's previous history of HCV treatment, HCV viral load measurements, and presence of cirrhosis.
   c. **Precautions and monitoring effects.**
      (1) Boceprevir must be administered **every 7-9 hours** with a meal or light snack. Patients should be counseled on how to avoid missing or delaying doses in order to optimize the effectiveness of this agent.
      (2) No dosage adjustments are necessary for renal or hepatic impairment.
      (3) Common adverse effects include headache, nausea, anemia, and taste disturbances.
   d. **Significant interactions**
      (1) Boceprevir is a substrate and strong **inhibitor** of CYP450 3A4/5, resulting in numerous drug-drug interactions. Avoid concomitant use with **alfuzosin, rifampin, phenobarbital, carbamazepine, phenytoin, ergot alkaloids, St. John's wort, simvastatin, lovastatin, drosperinone, triazolam, and oral midazolam.**
      (2) Careful review of concomitant medications is required during treatment with boceprevir, so that appropriate monitoring can be performed.
4. **Telaprevir (Incivek)**
   a. **Mechanism of action.** See VII.D.2.
   b. **Spectrum of activity and therapeutic uses.** Telaprevir is approved for use in adults with genotype 1 HCV infection who are treatment-naïve or who have not responded to prior treatment with interferon-based therapy, including prior null responders, partial responders, and relapsers. It is added to interferon alfa and ribavirin at the start of therapy and continued for the first 12 weeks of treatment, depending upon response. The interferon and ribavirin are then continued for an additional 12 or 36 weeks, depending upon the virologic response observed.
   c. **Precautions and monitoring effects.**
      (1) Telaprevir must be administered **every 7–9 hours** with a meal or snack containing **at least 20 grams of fat**. The product labeling and educational materials provided with this agent include numerous examples of these food combinations.
      (2) No dosage adjustment is necessary for renal impairment.
      (3) Use of telaprevir is not recommended in moderate to severe hepatic impairment, owing to a lack of pharmacokinetic data in this population.

(4) Adverse effects include rash, anemia, nausea, diarrhea, rectal discomfort, dysgeusia, and fatigue.

d. Significant interactions.

(1) Telaprevir is a substrate and strong **inhibitor** of CYP450 3A, resulting in numerous drug-drug interactions. Avoid concomitant use with **alfuzosin, rifampin, ergot alkaloids, St. John's wort, simvastatin, lovastatin, triazolam, and oral midazolam.**

(2) Careful review of concomitant medications is required during treatment with telaprevir, so that appropriate monitoring can be performed.

VIII. ANTHELMINTICS

A. **Definition.** These drugs are used to rid the body of worms (**helminths**). These agents may act locally to rid the GI tract of worms or work systemically to eradicate worms that are invading organs or tissues.

B. **Mebendazole (Vermox)** is a synthetic benzimidazole-derivative anthelmintic. This project was discontinued in early 2012, although it will likely remain on pharmacy shelves until the last lots expire in mid-2014.

1. **Mechanism of action.** Mebendazole interferes with reproduction and survival of helminths by inhibiting the formation of microtubules and irreversibly blocking glucose uptake, thereby depleting glycogen stores in the helminth.
2. **Spectrum of activity.** Mebendazole is active against various nematodes that are pathogenic to humans, including *Ancylostoma duodenale* (common hookworm), *Ascaris lumbricoides* (roundworm), *Capillaria philippinensis* (Philippine threadworm), *Enterobius vermicularis* (pinworm), *Necator americanus* (American hookworm), and *Trichuris trichiura* (whipworm).
3. **Therapeutic uses.** Mebendazole is used for the treatment of single or mixed infections with the helminths listed in VIII.B.2. Immobilization and subsequent death of helminths are slow, with complete GI clearance up to 3 days after therapy.
4. **Precautions and monitoring effects**
   a. In cases of massive infection, abdominal pain, nausea, and diarrhea associated with expulsion of organisms may result.
   b. Myelosuppression (neutropenia and thrombocytopenia) can occur with high doses (40 to 50 mg/kg/day).
   c. If the patient is not cured in 3 weeks, retreatment is necessary.
5. **Significant interactions.** Agents that may reduce the serum concentrations and subsequent efficacy of mebendazole include carbamazepine and phenytoin.

C. **Albendazole (Albenza)** is a synthetic benzimidazole-derivative anthelmintic.

1. **Mechanism of action.** See VIII.B.1.
2. **Spectrum of activity.** Albendazole is active against *Taenia solium* (pork tapeworm) and *Echinococcus granulosus* (dog tapeworm).
3. **Therapeutic uses.** Albendazole is used to treat parenchymal neurocysticercosis in combination with corticosteroids as well as cystic hydatid disease (before and after surgical removal of the disease).
4. **Precautions and monitoring effects**
   a. The drug should be administered with a fatty meal to achieve optimal absorption.
   b. Hepatotoxicity occurs in 16% of patients; liver function tests every 2 weeks are recommended while taking albendazole.
   c. Rarely, leukopenia, thrombocytopenia, granulocytopenia, pancytopenia, and agranulocytosis occur. A CBC should be checked every 2 weeks while taking albendazole.

D. **Diethylcarbamazine citrate (Hetrazan)**

1. **Mechanism of action.** Diethylcarbamazine citrate is a synthetic organic compound highly specific for several common parasites.
2. **Spectrum of activity.** This agent is active against *Wuchereria bancrofti*, *Onchocerca volvulus*, *Brugia malayi*, *Mansonella perstans*, *Mansonella ozzardi*, *Ascaris lumbricoides*, and *Loa loa*.
3. **Therapeutic uses.** Diethylcarbamazine citrate is used for the treatment of Bancroft's filariasis, onchocerciasis, ascariasis, and loiasis. It is available directly from the Centers for Disease Control and Prevention.

4. **Precautions and monitoring effects**
   a. Patients treated for *W. bancrofti* infection often present with headache and general malaise. Severe allergic phenomena in conjunction with a skin rash have been reported.
   b. Patients treated for onchocerciasis present with pruritus, facial edema, and systemic symptoms secondary to the inflammatory response caused by pathogen death (known as a **Mazzotti reaction**). Severe reactions may be noted after a single dose. For this reason, ivermectin is used to treat onchocerciasis.
   c. Children who are undernourished or are suffering from debilitating ascariasis infection may experience giddiness, malaise, nausea, and vomiting after treatment. Other drugs are available to treat *Ascaris* (mebendazole and albendazole).

E. **Pyrantel (Pin-X)** is a pyrimidine-derivative anthelmintic.
1. **Mechanism of action.** Pyrantel is a depolarizing neuromuscular blocking agent that causes a spastic paralysis of the helminth.
2. **Spectrum of activity.** Pyrantel is active against *A. lumbricoides* (roundworm), *E. vermicularis* (pinworm), *A. duodenale* (hookworm), *N. americanus* (hookworm), and *Trichostrongylus orientalis* (hairworm).
3. **Therapeutic uses.** Pyrantel is used for the treatment of roundworm, pinworm, and hookworm infections.
4. **Precautions and monitoring effects**
   a. Most commonly reported reactions include anorexia, nausea, vomiting, diarrhea, headache, and rash.
   b. A single dose may be mixed with food, milk, juice, or taken on an empty stomach.

F. **Ivermectin (Stromectol)**
1. **Mechanism of action.** Ivermectin potentiates the inhibitory effects of γ-aminobutyric acid (GABA) in various nematodes and arthropods, resulting in paralysis and death of the organisms.
2. **Spectrum of activity.** This agent is active against *S. stercoralis* (intestinal forms only) and *O. volvulus* (immature forms only). It is also useful for treatment of infections with *A. lumbricoides*, *E. vermicularis*, *M. ozzardi*, *T. trichiura*, and *W. bancrofti*.
3. **Therapeutic uses**
   a. Ivermectin is useful for treatment of infections with the parasites listed in VIII.G.2.
   b. Two studies demonstrated that ivermectin was more effective than albendazole for treatment of strongyloidiasis.
   c. Ivermectin is often favored over diethylcarbamazine citrate owing to its less severe adverse effect profile.
4. **Precautions and monitoring effects**
   a. May cause a **Mazzotti reaction** (see VIII.D.4.b) that is less severe than with diethylcarbamazine citrate.
   b. Reports of serious and possibly fatal encephalopathy have occurred in patients with concomitant *L. loa* infection.
   c. Other adverse effects include edema, dizziness, headache, rash, and GI disturbances.
   d. Counsel patients to take ivermectin with water.

G. **Praziquantel (Biltricide)**
1. **Mechanism of action.** Praziquantel increases cell membrane permeability in susceptible helminths, with loss of intracellular calcium and paralysis of their musculature. Vacuolization and disintegration of the schistosome tegument results, followed by attachment of phagocytes to the parasite and death.
2. **Spectrum of activity.** Praziquantel is active against trematodes (flukes), including all *Schistosoma* spp. and *Clonorchis sinensis*, *Opisthorchis viverrini*, *Fasciola hepatica* (liver flukes), *Paragonimus uterobilateralis*, *Paragonimus westermani* (lung flukes), *Metagonimus yokogawai*, *Fasciolopsis buski*, and *Heterophyes heterophyes* (intestinal flukes).
3. **Therapeutic uses.** Praziquantel is active in treating all types of schistosomiasis that are pathogenic to humans; clonorchiasis and opisthorchiasis (Chinese and southeast Asian liver flukes); many other types of infections involving intestinal, liver, and lung flukes; and cestodiasis (tapeworm) infections.

4. **Precautions and monitoring effects**
   - **a.** Treatment of ocular cysticercosis is contraindicated because parasite destruction within the eyes may cause irreparable lesions.
   - **b.** In general, adverse effects are generally mild and well tolerated. It is difficult to differentiate between effects caused by the praziquantel versus effects demonstrated by dying parasites.
   - **c.** The most common side effects are transient and may include malaise, headache, dizziness, and abdominal discomfort.
   - **d.** Praziquantel may impair activities that require mental alertness.

Study Questions

Directions for questions 1–12: Each of the questions, statements, or incomplete statements in this section can be correctly answered or completed by **one** of the suggested answers or phrases. Choose the **best** answer.

1. Isoniazid is a primary antitubercular agent that

(A) requires pyridoxine supplementation.
(B) may discolor the tears, saliva, urine, or feces orange-red.
(C) causes ocular complications that are reversible if the drug is discontinued.
(D) may be ototoxic and nephrotoxic.
(E) should never be used because of hepatotoxic potential.

2. All of the following factors may increase the risk of nephrotoxicity from gentamicin therapy *except* which one?

(A) age > 70 years
(B) prolonged courses of gentamicin therapy
(C) concurrent amphotericin B therapy
(D) trough gentamicin levels < 2 mg/mL
(E) concurrent cisplatin therapy

3. In which of the following groups do all four drugs warrant careful monitoring for drug-related seizures in high-risk patients?

(A) penicillin G, imipenem, amphotericin B, metronidazole
(B) penicillin G, chloramphenicol, tetracycline, vancomycin
(C) imipenem, tetracycline, vancomycin, sulfadiazine
(D) cycloserine, metronidazole, vancomycin, sulfadiazine
(E) metronidazole, imipenem, doxycycline, erythromycin

4. AC is a 34-year-old male admitted with a diagnosis of peritonitis. Cultures are positive for *Bacteroides fragilis*, *Enterococcus faecalis*, and *Staphylococcus aureus*. Which of the following would be the best initial therapy to recommend?

(A) telithromycin
(B) quinupristin/dalfopristin
(C) tigecycline
(D) trimethoprim/sulfamethoxazole
(E) kanamycin

5. TJ is a 45-year-old female presenting with an *Enterobacter aerogenes* bacteremia with a low-grade fever (101.6°F). The most appropriate management of her fever would be to

(A) give acetaminophen 1000 mg orally every 6 hrs.
(B) give aspirin 650 mg orally every 4 hrs.
(C) give alternating doses of aspirin and acetaminophen every 4 hrs.
(D) withhold antipyretics and use the fever curve to monitor her response to antibiotic therapy.
(E) use tepid water baths to reduce the fever.

6. BC has an upper respiratory infection. Two years ago, she experienced an episode of bronchospasm after penicillin therapy. Current cultures are positive for a strain of *Streptococcus pneumoniae* that is sensitive to all of the following drugs. Which of these drugs would be the best choice for this patient?

(A) amoxicillin/clavulanate
(B) telithromycin
(C) ampicillin
(D) cefaclor
(E) loracarbef

7. All of the following drugs are appropriate therapies for a lower urinary tract infection owing to *Pseudomonas aeruginosa except*

(A) norfloxacin.
(B) trimethoprim–sulfamethoxazole.
(C) ciprofloxacin.
(D) tobramycin.
(E) methenamine mandelate.

8. BT is a 43-year-old female seen by her primary-care physician for a mild staphylococcal cellulitis on the arm. Which of the following regimens would be appropriate oral therapy?

(A) dicloxacillin 125 mg every 6 hrs
(B) vancomycin 250 mg every 6 hrs
(C) methicillin 500 mg every 6 hrs
(D) cefazolin 1 g every 8 hrs
(E) penicillin V 500 mg every 6 hrs

9. RC is a 33-year-old male with a history of HIV for 10 years who now presents with *Mycobacterium avium-intracellulare* (MAI). Which of the following drugs has demonstrated in vitro activity against MAI?

(A) daptomycin
(B) clarithromycin
(C) erythromycin base
(D) cloxacillin
(E) minocycline

10. All of the following statements regarding pentamidine isethionate are true *except* which one?

(A) It is indicated for treatment or prophylaxis of infection owing to *Pneumocystis carinii.*
(B) It may be administered intramuscularly, intravenously, or by inhalation.
(C) It has no clinically significant effect on serum glucose.
(D) It is effective in the treatment of leishmaniasis.

11. RE is a 23-year-old male with a history of severe asthma. An outbreak of H1N1 influenza has just been reported in his community, and he is exhibiting initial symptoms of the infection. Which agent would be the most useful to treat RE?

(A) cidofovir
(B) famciclovir
(C) oseltamivir
(D) zanamivir
(E) ribavirin

12. Dr. Jones requests your help in selecting a protease inhibitor as part of a regimen for a treatment-naive male patient. Which of the following would you recommend?

(A) darunavir/ritonavir
(B) lopinavir/ritonavir
(C) nelfinavir
(D) saquinavir/ritonavir
(E) tipranavir/ritonavir

Directions for questions 13–14: The questions and incomplete statements in this section can be correctly answered or completed by **one or more** of the suggested answers. Choose the answer, **A–E**.

A if **I only** is correct
B if **III only** is correct
C if **I and II** are correct
D if **II and III** are correct
E if **I, II, and III** are correct

13. Drugs usually active against penicillinase-producing *Staphylococcus aureus* include which of the following?

I. piperacillin–tazobactam
II. amoxicillin–clavulanate
III. nafcillin

14. Antiviral agents that are active against cytomegalovirus (CMV) include which of the following?

I. ganciclovir
II. foscarnet
III. acyclovir

Directions for questions 15–17: Each description listed in this section is most closely associated with **one** of the following drugs. The drugs may be used more than once or not at all. Choose the **best** answer, **A–E**.

A clofazimine
B itraconazole
C levofloxacin
D neomycin

15. It may be administered once per day for the treatment of urinary tract infections.

16. It may cause pink to brownish skin pigmentation within a few weeks of initiation of therapy.

17. Coadministration with astemizole or terfenadine may lead to life-threatening cardiac dysrhythmias.

Answers and Explanations

1. **The answer is A** *[see VI.B.2.d.(5)]*.
Isoniazid increases the excretion of pyridoxine, which can lead to peripheral neuritis, particularly in poorly nourished patients. Pyridoxine (a form of vitamin B_6) deficiency may cause convulsions as well as the neuritis, involving synovial tenderness and swelling. Treatment with the vitamin can reverse the neuritis and prevent or cure the seizures.

2. **The answer is D** *[see II.B.4.b]*.
Trough serum levels < 2 mg/mL are considered appropriate for gentamicin and are recommended to minimize the risk of toxicity from this aminoglycoside. Because aminoglycosides accumulate in the proximal tubule of the kidney, nephrotoxicity can occur.

3. **The answer is A** *[see II.C.4.6; II.F.e.2; V.C.3.b.(4); VI.B.2.d.(5)]*.
Seizures have been attributed to the use of penicillin G, imipenem, amphotericin B, and metronidazole. Seizures are especially likely with high doses in patients with a history of seizures and in patients with impaired drug elimination.

4. **The answer is C** *[see II.K.14]*.
Although active against various gram-positive and negative organisms, tigecycline is only agent approved for the treatment of intra-abdominal infections caused by these organisms.

5. **The answer is D** *[see I.H.1]*.
The fever curve is useful for monitoring a patient's response to antimicrobial therapy. Antipyretics can be used to reduce high fever in patients at risk for complications (e.g., seizures) or, in some cases, to make the patient more comfortable.

6. **The answer is B** *[see II.K.13; II.D.4.6]*.
Amoxicillin and ampicillin are all penicillins and should be avoided in patients with histories of hypersensitivity to other penicillin compounds. Although the risk of cross-reactivity with cephalosporins (e.g., cefaclor, loracarbef) is now considered low, most clinicians avoid the use of these agents in patients with histories of type I hypersensitivity reactions (e.g., anaphylaxis, bronchospasm, giant hives).

7. **The answer is B** *[see II.B.2.b.(3); II.I.2.a; II.J.2.a; II.J.2.c.(1)]*.
Norfloxacin, ciprofloxacin, tobramycin, and methenamine mandelate achieve urine concentrations high enough to treat urinary tract infections caused by *P. aeruginosa*. Trimethoprim–sulfamethoxazole is not useful for treating infection caused by this organism, although the combination is useful for treating certain other urinary tract infections.

8. **The answer is A** *[see II.F.2.c.(4)]*.
Although vancomycin, methicillin, and cefazolin have excellent activity against staphylococci, they are not effective orally for systemic infections. Vancomycin is prescribed orally for infections limited to the gastrointestinal tract, but because it is poorly absorbed orally, it is not effective for systemic infections. Most hospital- and community-acquired staphylococci are currently resistant to penicillin. Thus, of the drugs listed, the most appropriate drug for oral therapy of staphylococcal cellulitis is dicloxacillin.

9. **The answer is B** *[see II.D.6.a–b]*.
Clarithromycin, an alternative to erythromycin, has demonstrated in vitro activity against MAI. Clarithromycin is also used against *Toxoplasma gondii* and *Cryptosporidium* spp., and it is more active than erythromycin against staphylococci and streptococci. Vancomycin and cloxacillin are used to treat staphylococci and streptococci, but has no demonstrated activity versus MAI.

10. **The answer is C** *[see V.D]*.
Pentamidine isethionate is indicated for both treatment and prophylaxis of infection from *P. carinii*. It can be administered intramuscularly, intravenously, or by inhalation. Inhalation may produce bronchospasm. Blood glucose should be carefully monitored because pentamidine may produce either hyperglycemia or hypoglycemia.

11. **The answer is C** *[see VII.B.9]*.
Cidofovir and famciclovir have little or no in vivo activity against H1N1 influenza. Ribavirin has some activity but is not used for influenza and is mainly indicated for treatment of hepatitis C in combination with interferon. Zanamivir and oseltamivir are agents that demonstrate activity against H1N1 influenza and are indicated for the treatment of influenza infections. Zanamivir is an inhaled agent that should be avoided in patients with a history of asthma or chronic obstructive pulmonary disease, due to the risk of bronchospasm and acute decline in lung function. Oseltamivir is an oral agent that is most appropriate in this case.

12. **The answer is A** *[see VII.C.5.a–i]*.
Lopinavir/ritonavir is a PI used in alternative regimens for treatment-naïve patients and is only a preferred PI in pregnant women. Nelfinavir, saquinavir/ritonavir, and tipranavir/ritonavir are not preferred PIs due to inferior virologic potency and/or adverse effects. Darunavir/ritonavir is considered a preferred PI.

13. **The answer is E (I, II, III)** *[see II.E.2–4]*.
Piperacillin and amoxicillin each include a β-lactamase inhibitor. These combinations offer activity against *S. aureus* similar to that of the penicillinase-resistant penicillins, such as nafcillin.

14. **The answer is C (I, II)** *[see VII.B.1; VII.B.7–8]*.
Only ganciclovir and foscarnet are active against CMV infections. These agents are virustatic and arrest DNA synthesis by inhibiting viral DNA polymerase. Foscarnet is a broad-spectrum antiviral agent and is used in patients with ganciclovir resistance. Acyclovir is not clinically useful for the treatment of CMV infections because CMV is relatively resistant to acyclovir in vitro.

15. **The answer is C** *[see II.I.3.c]*.
Levofloxacin is appropriate for treatment of urinary tract infections, and may be dosed once daily.

16. **The answer is A** *[see II.K.5.d.(1)]*.
Because clofazimine contains phenazine dye, it can cause pink to brown skin pigmentation. This change in pigmentation occurs in 75% to 100% of patients taking clofazimine, and it occurs within a few weeks of the initiation of therapy. The discoloration of skin has reportedly led to severe depression and even suicide in some patients. Clofazimine is used in the treatment of leprosy and several atypical *Mycobacterium* infections.

17. **The answer is B** *[see III.F.5.d]*.
Administration of itraconazole or ketoconazole with astemizole or terfenadine may increase the level of astemizole or terfenadine, which can lead to life-threatening dysrhythmias and death. Itraconazole, which is an imidazole, is a fungistatic agent. Specifically, itraconazole can be taken orally to treat aspergillosis infections and other deep fungal infections, such as blastomycosis, coccidioidomycosis, cryptococcosis, and histoplasmosis.

37 Seizure Disorders

AZITA RAZZAGHI

I. INTRODUCTION

A. Definitions

1. **Seizures** are characterized by an excessive, hypersynchronous discharge of cortical neuron activity, which can be measured by the electroencephalogram (EEG). In addition, there may be disturbances in consciousness, sensory motor systems, subjective well-being, and objective behavior; seizures are usually brief, with a beginning and an end, and may produce post-seizure impairment.
2. **Epilepsy** is defined as a chronic seizure disorder or group of disorders characterized by seizures that usually recur unpredictably in the absence of a consistent provoking factor. The term *epilepsy* is derived from the Greek word meaning "to seize upon" or "taking hold of." It was first described by Hughlings Jackson in the 19th century as an intermittent derangement of the nervous system due to a sudden, excessive, disorderly discharge of cerebral neurons.
3. **Convulsions** are violent, involuntary contractions of the voluntary muscles. A patient may have epilepsy or a seizure disorder without convulsions.

B. Classification.

An alternative seizure classification is being developed that is purely symptom based. This consists of four categories: sensorial (auras), consciousness, autonomic, and motor. Also, the international league against epilepsy is establishing a four-level descriptive seizure classification based on symptoms, a pathophysiological seizure, an epileptic syndrome, and functional disability. At present, there are two systems of classification of seizure disorder: one is based on the seizure type and characteristics (*Table 37-1*), and the other is based on the characteristics of the epilepsy (including age at onset, etiological factors, and frequency) and characteristics of the seizure (*Table 37-2*).

1. **Partial seizures** are the most common seizure type, occurring in approximately 80% of patients with epilepsy.
   a. **Clinical and EEG changes** indicate initial activation of a system of neurons limited to part of one cerebral hemisphere that may spread to other or all brain areas. Manifestations of the seizures depend on the site of the epileptogenic focus in the brain.
   b. Partial seizures are subclassified as **simple** (usually unilateral involvement) or **complex** (usually bilateral involvement). Impairment of consciousness is a feature of complex seizures. Consciousness is defined as the degree of awareness and responsiveness of the patient to externally applied stimuli.
      (1) **Simple partial seizures** generally do not cause loss of consciousness. **Signs and symptoms** of simple partial seizures may be primarily motor, sensory, somatosensory, autonomic, or behavioral. These signs and symptoms may help pinpoint the site of the abnormal brain discharge; for example, localized numbness or tingling reflects a dysfunction in the sensory cortex, located in the parietal lobe.
         (a) **Motor signs** include convulsive jerking, chewing motions, and lip smacking.
         (b) **Sensory and somatosensory manifestations** include paresthesias and auras.
         (c) **Autonomic signs** include sweating, flushing, and pupil dilation.
         (d) **Behavioral manifestations**, which are sometimes accompanied by impaired consciousness, include déjà vu experiences, structured hallucinations, and dysphasia.

Table 37-1 INTERNATIONAL CLASSIFICATION OF EPILEPTIC SEIZURES

I. **Partial seizures** (seizures beginning locally)
   A. **Simple partial seizures** (consciousness not impaired)
      1. With motor symptoms
      2. With somatosensory or special sensory symptoms
      3. With autonomic symptoms
      4. With behavioral symptoms
   B. **Complex partial seizures** (with impairment of consciousness)
      1. Beginning as simple partial seizures and progressing to impairment of consciousness
         a. Without automatisms
         b. With automatisms
      2. With impairment of consciousness at onset
         a. With no other features
         b. With features of simple partial seizures
         c. With automatisms
   C. **Partial seizures** (simple or complex), secondarily generalized
II. **Generalized seizures** (bilaterally symmetric, without localized onset)
   A. **Absence seizures**
      1. **True absence seizures (petit mal)**
      2. **Atypical absence seizures**
   B. **Myoclonic seizures**
   C. **Clonic seizures**
   D. **Tonic seizures**
   E. **Tonic–clonic seizures (grand mal)**
   F. **Atonic seizures**
III. **Unclassified seizures**

Reprinted from Commission on Classification and Terminology of the International League against Epilepsy. Proposal for classification of epilepsies and epileptic syndromes. *Epilepsia*. 1985;26:268–278.

(2) **Complex partial seizures** are accompanied by impaired consciousness; however, in some cases, the impairment precedes or follows the seizure. These seizures have variable manifestations.
   (a) Purposeless behavior is common.
   (b) The affected person may have a glassy stare, may wander about aimlessly, and may speak unintelligibly.
   (c) Psychomotor (temporal lobe) epilepsy may lead to aggressive behavior (e.g., outbursts of rage or violence).
   (d) Postictal confusion usually persists for 1 to 2 mins after the seizure ends.
   (e) Automatism (e.g., picking at clothes) is common and may follow visual, auditory, or olfactory hallucinations.

2. **Generalized seizures** are diffuse, affecting both cerebral hemispheres.
   a. **Clinical and EEG changes** indicate initial involvement of both hemispheres.
      (1) Consciousness may be impaired, and this impairment may be the initial manifestation.
      (2) Motor manifestations are bilateral.
      (3) The ictal EEG patterns initially are bilateral and presumably reflect neuronal discharge, which is widespread in both hemispheres.
   b. There are three **types** of generalized seizures.
      (1) **Idiopathic epilepsies** have an age-related onset, typical clinical and EEG characteristics, and a presumed genetic origin.
      (2) **Symptomatic epilepsies** are considered the consequence of a known or suspected underlying disorder of the central nervous system (CNS).
      (3) **Cryptogenic epilepsy** refers to a disorder for which the cause is hidden or occult; it is presumed to be symptomatic, but the causal factors are unknown. It is age related but often does not have well-defined clinical and EEG characteristics.

Table 37-2 CLASSIFICATION OF EPILEPSIES AND EPILEPTIC SYNDROMES

- **I. Localized-related (focal, local, partial) epilepsies and syndromes**
  - **A. Idiopathic** (with age-related onset)
    - **1.** Benign childhood epilepsy with centrotemporal spikes (rolandic epilepsy)
    - **2.** Childhood epilepsy with occipital paroxysms
  - **B. Symptomatic**
    - **1.** Chronic progressive epilepsia partialis continua of childhood
    - **2.** Syndromes characterized by specific modes of precipitation
    - **3.** Temporal lobe epilepsies
    - **4.** Frontal lobe epilepsies
    - **5.** Parietal lobe epilepsies
    - **6.** Occipital lobe epilepsies
  - **C. Cryptogenic**
- **II. Generalized epilepsies and syndromes**
  - **A. Idiopathic** (with age-related onset)
    - **1.** Benign neonatal familial convulsions
    - **2.** Benign neonatal convulsions
    - **3.** Benign myoclonic epilepsy in infancy
    - **4.** Childhood absence epilepsy (pyknolepsy)
    - **5.** Juvenile absence epilepsy
    - **6.** Juvenile myoclonic epilepsy
    - **7.** Epilepsy with generalized tonic–clonic seizures on awakening
    - **8.** Other generalized idiopathic epilepsies not defined above
    - **9.** Epilepsies with seizures precipitated by specific modes of activation
  - **B. Cryptogenic or symptomatic** (in order of age)
    - **1.** West syndrome (infantile spasms)
    - **2.** Lennox–Gastaut syndrome
    - **3.** Epilepsy with myoclonic–astatic seizures
    - **4.** Epilepsy with myoclonic absences
  - **C. Symptomatic**
    - **1. Nonspecific etiology**
      - **a.** Early myoclonic encephalopathy
      - **b.** Early infantile epileptic encephalopathy with suppression burst
      - **c.** Other symptomatic generalized epilepsies not defined above
    - **2. Specific syndromes and generalized seizures complicating other disease states**
- **III. Epilepsies and syndromes undetermined whether focal or generalized**
  - **A. With both focal and generalized seizures**
    - **1.** Neonatal seizures
    - **2.** Severe myoclonic epilepsy in infancy
    - **3.** Epilepsy with continuous spike waves during slow-wave sleep
    - **4.** Acquired epileptic aphasia (Landau–Kleffner syndrome)[a]
    - **5.** Other undetermined epilepsies not defined above
  - **B. Without unequivocal generalized or focal features**
- **IV. Special situations**
  - **A.** Febrile convulsions
  - **B.** Isolated seizures or isolated status epilepticus
  - **C.** Seizures occurring only when there is an acute metabolic or toxic event due to such factors as alcohol, drugs, eclampsia, and nonketotic hyperglycemia

[a]Believed to be a localized-related epilepsy.
Reprinted with permission from Bleck TP. Convulsive disorders: the use of anticonvulsant drugs. *Clin Neuropharmacol.* 1990;1:198–209.

c. **Signs and symptoms** of generalized seizures may be minor or major.

(1) **Absence (petit mal) seizures** present as alterations of consciousness (absences) lasting 10 to 30 secs.

(a) Staring (with occasional eye blinking) and loss or reduction in postural tone are typical. If the seizure takes place during conversation, the individual may break off in midsentence.

(b) Enuresis and other autonomic components may occur during absence seizures.

(c) Some patients experience 100 or more absences daily.

(d) Onset of this seizure type occurs from age 3 to 16 years; in most patients, absence seizures disappear by age 40.

(2) **Myoclonic (bilateral massive epileptic myoclonus) seizures** present as involuntary jerking of the facial, limb, or trunk muscles, possibly in a rhythmic manner.

(3) **Clonic seizures** are characterized by sustained muscle contractions alternating with relaxation.

(4) **Tonic seizures** involve sustained tonic muscle extension (stiffening).

(5) **Generalized (grand mal) tonic–clonic seizures** cause sudden loss of consciousness.

(a) The individual becomes rigid and falls to the ground. Respirations are interrupted. The legs extend, and the back arches; contraction of the diaphragm may induce grunting. This tonic phase lasts for about 1 min.

(b) A clonic phase follows, marked by rapid bilateral muscle jerking, muscle flaccidity, and hyperventilation. Incontinence, tongue biting, tachycardia, and heavy salivation sometimes occur.

(c) During the postictal phase, the individual may experience headache, confusion, disorientation, nausea, drowsiness, and muscle soreness. This phase may last for hours.

(d) Some patients with epilepsy have serial grand mal seizures, regaining consciousness briefly between attacks. In some cases, grand mal seizures occur repeatedly with no recovery of consciousness between attacks (**status epilepticus**); this disorder is discussed in III.A.

(6) **Atonic seizures (drop attacks)** are characterized by a sudden loss of postural tone so that the individual falls to the ground. They occur primarily in children.

C. **Epidemiology**

1. **Most common neurological disorder**
2. Epilepsy has a prevalence of approximately 1% (i.e., 500,000 cases per 50 million persons worldwide).
3. In the United States, the prevalence of epilepsy is 6.42 cases per 1000 people.
4. The onset of seizures is greatest during the first year of life; this probability decreases each decade after the first year until age 60. Approximately 1 of 50 children and 1 of 100 adults are affected.
5. Approximately 70% of people with epilepsy have only one seizure type; the remainder have two or more seizure types.

D. **Cause.** Some seizures arise secondary to other conditions. However, in most cases, the cause of the seizure is unknown.

1. **Primary (idiopathic) seizures** have no identifiable cause.

a. This type of seizure affects about 75% of people with epilepsy.

b. The onset of primary seizures typically occurs before age 20.

c. Birth trauma, hereditary factors, and unexplained metabolic disturbances have been proposed as possible causes.

2. **Secondary seizures (symptomatic or acquired seizures)** occur secondary to an identifiable cause.

a. Disorders that may lead to secondary seizures include

(1) Intracranial neoplasms

(2) Infectious diseases, such as meningitis, influenza, toxoplasmosis, mumps, measles, and syphilis

(3) High fever (in children)

(4) Head trauma

(5) Congenital diseases

(6) Metabolic disorders, such as hypoglycemia and hypocalcemia

Table 37-3 PROBABLE CAUSES OF RECURRENT SEIZURES BY AGE GROUP

Age at Seizure Onset	Probable Cause of Seizure
Birth to 1 month	Birth injury or anoxia, congenital hereditary diseases, and metabolic disorders
1–6 months	As above, plus infantile spasms
6 months to 2 years	Infantile spasms, febrile convulsions, birth injury or anoxia, meningitis, and head trauma
3–10 years	Birth injury or anoxia, meningitis, cerebral vessel thrombosis, and idiopathic epilepsy
10–18 years	Idiopathic epilepsy and head trauma
18–25 years	Idiopathic epilepsy, trauma, neoplasm, and withdrawal from alcohol or drugs
35–60 years	Trauma, neoplasm, vascular disease, and withdrawal from alcohol or drugs
> 60 years	Vascular disease, neoplasm, degenerative disease, and trauma

(7) Alcohol or drug withdrawal

(8) Lipid storage disorders

(9) Developmental abnormalities

b. Age at seizure onset is associated with specific causes (*Table 37-3*).

E. Pathophysiology. Seizures reflect a sudden, abnormal, excessive neuronal discharge in the cerebral cortex. Any abnormal neuronal discharge could precipitate a seizure (*Figure 37-1*).

1. Normal firing of neurons, which usually originate from the gray matter of one or more cortical or subcortical areas, requires the following elements:

a. Voltage-dependent ion channels are involved in action-potential propagation or burst generation.

b. Neurotransmitters control neuronal firing, including excitatory neurotransmitters, acetylcholine, norepinephrine, histamine, corticotropin-releasing factors (CRFs), inhibitory neurotransmitters, γ-aminobutyric acid (GABA), and dopamine; therefore, normal neuronal

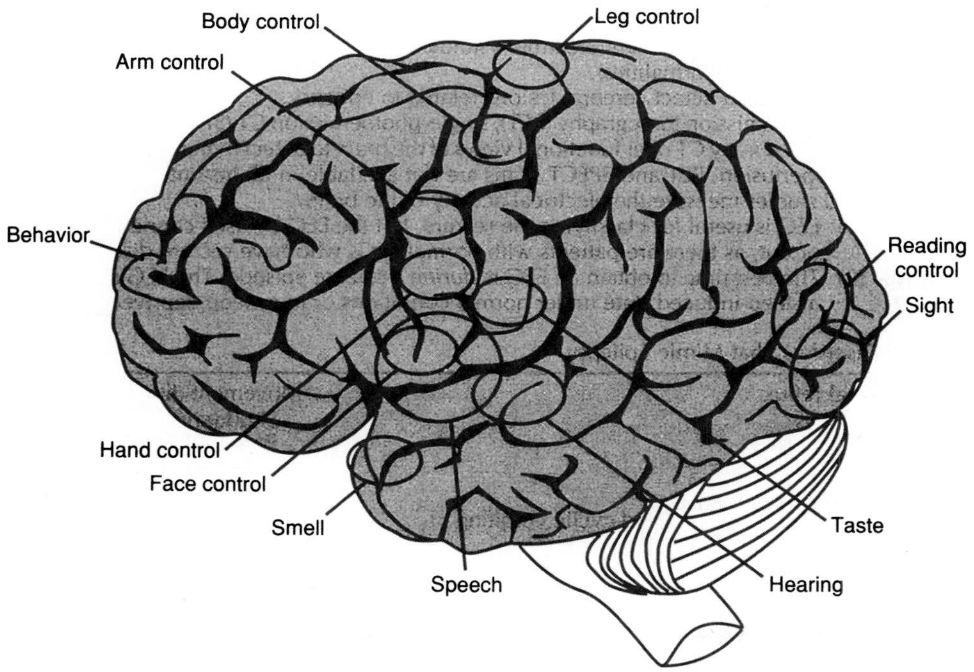

Figure 37-1. Gross anatomy of the brain. Clinical manifestation of seizures depends on the area of the cortex that is affected and its function, the degree of irritability, and the identity of the impulse.

activity requires adequate ions (e.g., sodium, potassium, calcium); excitatory and inhibitory neurotransmitters; and glucose, oxygen, amino acids, and adequate systemic pH.

c. People with epilepsy may be **genetically** predisposed to a **lower seizure threshold**.

d. **A diencephalic nerve group** that normally suppresses excessive brain discharge may be deafferentated, hypersensitive, and vulnerable to activation by various stimuli in individuals with epilepsy.

e. During seizures, there is an increased use of energy, oxygen, and, consequently, an increased production of carbon dioxide. Because of the limited capacity to increase the blood flow to the brain, the blood supply may be **oxygen deficient**. The ratio of supply to demand decreases when the seizure episode is prolonged, leading to increased ischemia and neuronal destruction. Thus, it is crucial to diagnose seizures and treat them as soon as possible.

2. **Abnormal electrical brain activity** occurring during a seizure usually produces **characteristic changes on the EEG**. Each part of the cortical area has its own function, and the clinical presentation of a seizure depends on the site, the degree of irritability of the area, and the intensity of the impulse.

3. Seizure activity may include three major **phases**.

a. **A prodrome** may precede the seizure by hours or days.

(1) Changes in behavior or mood typically occur during the prodrome.

(2) This phase may include an aura—a subjective sensation, such as an unusual smell or flashing light.

b. The **ictal phase** is the seizure itself. In some cases, its onset is heralded by a scream or cry.

c. The **postictal phase** takes place immediately after the seizure.

(1) Extensor plantar reflexes may appear.

(2) The patient typically exhibits lethargy, confusion, and behavioral changes.

F. **Clinical evaluation**

1. **History** includes an evaluation of the seizure, including interviews of the patient's family and eyewitness accounts to establish.

a. The frequency and duration of the episodes

b. Precipitating factors

c. The times at which episodes occur

d. The presence or absence of an aura

e. Ictal activity

f. Postictal state

2. **Physical and neurological examinations** are the tools with which to identify an underlying cause to rule out diseases that manifest as seizures (*Table 37-4*).

3. **Laboratory tests** may also identify an underlying cause.

a. Liver and kidney function tests, complete blood count (CBC), urinalysis, and serum drug levels (e.g., antidepressants and amphetamines may precipitate seizures) are necessary.

Table 37-4 DISORDERS THAT MIMIC EPILEPSY

Gastroesophageal reflux	Movement disorders
Breath-holding spells	Shuddering attacks
Migraine	Paroxysmal choreoathetosis
Confusional	Nonepileptic myoclonus
Basilar	Tics and habit spasms
With recurrent abdominal pain and cyclic vomiting	Psychological disorders
Sleep disorders (especially parasomnias)	Panic disorder
Cardiovascular events	Hyperventilation attacks
Pallid infantile syncope	Pseudoseizures
Vasovagal attacks	Rage attacks
Vasomotor syncope	
Arrhythmias	

b. Lumbar puncture may be required for evidence of cerebrospinal fluid (CSF) infection for patients with a fever who have seizures.

4. Neurological imaging studies, including MRI and/or CT, complement electrophysiological studies and can identify structural brain disorders (anatomical abnormalities).

a. An MRI can detect cerebral lesions related to epilepsy and should be used in all cases, especially in patients with partial seizure, to exclude brain abnormalities.

b. Positron-emission tomography (PET), single-photon emission CT (SPECT), and stable xenon-enhanced x-ray CT offer functional views of the brain to detect hypometabolism or relative hypoperfusion. PET and SPECT scans are not available in all institutions.

c. EEG studies measure the electrical activity of the brain. These studies help identify functional cerebral changes underlying structural abnormalities and are useful with MRI for patients considered for epilepsy surgery.

(1) An EEG is useful for classifying the seizure or as an additional diagnostic tool, but the EEG by itself cannot rule seizures in or out, because some patients with normal interictal EEGs have seizure disorders.

(2) The best time to obtain an EEG is *during* a seizure episode. EEG recordings done while the patient is asleep can often record the abnormal activity; therefore, EEGs performed during a sleep-induced state under normal conditions or in a sleep-deprived state can be more sensitive for making a diagnosis.

G. Treatment objectives

1. To prevent or suppress seizures or reduce their frequency through drug therapy.

2. To control or eliminate the factors that cause or precipitate seizures.

3. To prevent serious consequences of seizures, such as anoxia, airway occlusion, or injury by protecting the tongue and placing a pillow under the victim's head.

4. To encourage a normal lifestyle and prevent the patient from feeling like or being treated as an invalid.

5. Short- and long-term side effects

6. Drug interactions

II. THERAPY

A. Principles of drug therapy

1. Seizure control. Approximately 50% of patients with epilepsy achieve complete seizure control through drug therapy. In another 25%, drugs reduce the frequency of seizures. People with epilepsy generally require continuous drug therapy for at least 2 seizure-free years before the drug discontinuation can be considered.

2. Initial treatment

a. Before anticonvulsive drug treatment is instituted, treatable underlying causes of the seizure activity should be excluded.

b. A single primary drug that is most appropriate for the seizure type must be selected. If there is more than one appropriate primary drug, then age, sex, and compliance of the patient must be considered.

c. For patients with newly diagnosed epilepsy, administer low doses for a few days. Patients may respond to a dosage that is lower than that traditionally prescribed initially by their physicians, and this may have important implications in terms of limiting adverse effects. The incidence of adverse effects increases with increasing drug levels, even when the plasma concentrations are maintained within the so-called therapeutic or optimal range.

d. Between one-fourth and one-third of the maintenance dose of a single medication is used to begin therapy; it is then increased over 3 to 4 weeks. The exceptions are phenytoin and phenobarbital, which can be started with the loading or maintenance dose. The dose should be titrated until seizure control or intolerable side effects occur.

e. With the initiation of therapy, blood concentrations of medications should be measured.

(1) To establish therapeutic ranges and dosage regimens based on symptomatic toxicity or seizure frequency.

(2) To assess the patient's compliance with therapy.

(3) To control the correlation among the dose, blood levels, and clinical therapeutic levels or toxicity.

(a) Phenytoin follows nonlinear kinetics, as drug levels increase dramatically (more than onefold) with only a small increase in the dose. However, before this twofold increase in drug level with a small increase in dose, there is a predictable linear increase with dose increases; for this reason, it is recommended to increase the dose in small increments to be able to predict when the drug follows the nonlinear kinetic. When this happens, that means the maximum rate of hepatic enzyme clearance is reached and the body can no longer clear the drug as it is introduced into the body.

(b) If physical examination reveals a new onset of nystagmus (except with phenytoin, in which nystagmus develops before clinical intoxication), ataxia, and unsteady wide gait, the next dose increase should be minimal.

(c) There is no justification for increasing drug dosage when a patient's seizures are fully controlled, even if the plasma concentration is below the lower limit of the therapeutic range. If the patient continues to have seizures without any evidence of adverse effects at a plasma concentration near the toxic range, there are two approaches:

(i) Some clinicians increase the dosage according to clinical response up to the highest tolerated limit.

(ii) Some clinicians do not increase the dosage because of the likelihood of producing adverse effects.

(d) Carbamazepine has an autoinduction metabolism property, which means that if the dose is increased twofold, blood levels increase less than twofold because of increased metabolism.

(4) To determine the free drug level, which is helpful in patients who are in the therapeutic range but have side effects or no response. The plasma protein binding may be altered in these patients by some other disease state or medication. Because of this alteration, there is more free drug available in the system than the total level shows, especially with phenytoin, valproic acid, and carbamazepine.

3. **Paradoxical intoxication** occurs when a high concentration of a single drug causes an increased frequency of seizures without classical adverse events. This is common with hydantoins and carbamazepine. The proposed reason is that their effect on the cerebellum is blocked at high concentrations. Management usually requires no more than withholding enough doses of the drug to allow the concentration to drift down.

4. When seizures cannot be controlled, there are two options.

a. The initial drug can be substituted with another agent. This is accomplished by gradually discontinuing the initial drug while simultaneously increasing the dosage of the second agent. Then the dosage of the second agent is titrated up to the maintenance level as the initial agent is gradually discontinued. There are three main advantages of gradual substitution.

(1) It allows evaluation of the effects of individual drugs.

(2) It reduces the risk of toxicity.

(3) It reduces the risk of adverse drug interactions.

b. A second drug can be added. Combination therapy is reserved for patients with severe epilepsy to rapidly control the seizures. Rapid control can be important for psychosocial reasons as well as for the possibility of a more favorable prognosis.

5. **Long-term drug treatment.** Most physicians review the patient's condition when the patient has been seizure free for 2 years. This has important implications in children because early termination of treatment has better remission rates compared with adults. It is recommended to gradually decrease the dose, over at least 6 months. The age of onset of epilepsy, the presence of an underlying neurological condition, and any abnormal EEGs should be considered.

6. **Diseases and conditions that alter antiepileptic drug–protein bindings**

a. Liver disease

b. Hypoalbuminemia

c. Burns

d. Pregnancy
e. High protein-binding drugs or antiepileptic agents. (Most important interactions are discussed under individual agents.)

7. **Medications.** Some medications decrease levels of phenytoin, carbamazepine, phenobarbital, and primidone by enhancing their metabolism. These drugs also cause false decreases in thyroid function tests.
   a. Oral contraceptives
   b. Oral hypoglycemics
   c. Glucocorticoids
   d. Tricyclic antidepressants
   e. Azathioprine
   f. Cyclosporine
   g. Quinidine
   h. Theophylline
   i. Warfarin
   j. Doxycycline
   k. Levodopa
8. **Overview of drug therapy in seizure disorder**
   a. Monotherapy. Start the drug therapy as single agent.
   b. Dosage treatment. Use a low dose for a few days. Patients with newly diagnosed epilepsy may respond to dosages that are lower than those prescribed initially by their physicians, and this may have important implications in terms of adverse effects. The incidence of adverse effects increases with increasing drug dosage, even when the plasma concentration is maintained within the so-called therapeutic or optimal range.
   c. Drug monitoring. There is no justification for increasing drug dosage when a patient is fully controlled, even if the plasma concentration is below the lower limit of the therapeutic range. If the patient continues to have seizures without any evidence of adverse effects at a plasma concentration near the toxic range, there are two approaches.
      (1) Some clinicians increase the dosage according to clinical response up to the highest tolerated limit.
      (2) Some clinicians do not increase the dosage because of the likelihood of producing adverse events.
9. **Adverse effects of anticonvulsive drugs**
   a. Alternation in cognition and mentation
      (1) Sedation and depression are the most common symptoms of overdose of anticonvulsive drugs, but they are difficult to assess. For example, barbiturates commonly cause depression, with primidone being the worst offender; diazepam and clorazepate are less likely to cause depression. Barbiturates, clonazepam, and trimethadione commonly cause cognitive impairment, ranging from sensation to confusion.
      (2) Excitation can be a paradoxical effect of barbiturates with younger children and the elderly. For example, felbamate can cause restlessness and hyperactivity.
   b. Deterioration of motor performance and primary coordination includes trembling hands, staggering when rounding corners, and mild limb ataxia. Drugs associated with these effects include hydantoins, methsuximide, carbamazepine, and primidone. These effects are less common with barbiturates and lamotrigine and are rarely seen with gabapentin.
   c. Gastrointestinal symptoms include nausea and vomiting. Two purposed mechanisms include
      (1) A local effect on the stomach, as in the case of valproic acid; divalproex acid, however, has less incidence compared with valproic acid. These symptoms decrease in incidence if the drug is given with meals.
      (2) A brainstem effect, as in the cases of felbamate and carbamazepine. Nausea and vomiting caused by these drugs are associated with brainstem involvement; therefore, drug levels play a role in these symptoms. Administration in smaller, more frequent doses decreases the incidence of these symptoms by lowering the transient peak concentration.

d. **Appetite and body weight.** Few anticonvulsants affect appetite separate from nausea and vomiting, including anorexia or increased appetite.
   (1) **Drugs that cause anorexia** are felbamate, and to a lesser extent, carbamazepine, ethosuximide, and valproic acid.
   (2) **Drugs that cause increased appetite** are valproic acid and to a lesser extent, carbamazepine.
e. **Headache and dizziness**
   (1) **Diffuse headaches** may be caused by ethosuximide and, to a lesser extent, by methsuximide and felbamate.
   (2) **Dizziness** seen in association with anticonvulsants is caused by a combination of ataxia and loss of eye movement coordination, which is part of motor coordination symptoms.
f. **Suicidability:** increased risk in patients who start receiving anticonvulsive as single and combination with other anticonvulsive medications.
g. Some products have REM program.
   Risk Evaluation and Mitigation Strategies (REM)
   - Minimize risk of a specific adverse effect with a drug or drug class
   May contain one or all of the following tools:
   <u>Medication Guide (MedGuide)-Level 1</u>
   - Patient education about risks
   <u>Communication Plan-Level 2</u>
   - **Health care provider** (HCP) letters (Dear Doctor and Dear Pharmacist letters)
   - HCP education (professional societies)
   - Web-based on-demand education materials
   - Medical science liaison presentations
   <u>Elements to Assure Safe Use (ETASU)-Level 3</u>—one or any combination of:
   - Specialized HCP training, education, or certification
   - Certification of pharmacies, HCPs, or health care settings
   - Dispensing only to patients within certain settings (hospital)
   - Evidence or documentation of safe-use conditions
   - Patient monitoring and/or patient registry
   - Implementation system such as registry programs for sponsor
   - Timetable for submission of assessments to regulatory agency by sponsor

B. **Specific antiseizure agents.** *Table 37-5* lists the uses of antiepileptic medications based on seizure type. *Table 37-6* lists classifications of anticonvulsive drugs. *Table 37-7* lists dosage characteristics of antiepileptic medications.
   1. **Carbamazepine (Tegretol)**
      a. **Mechanisms of action.** Carbamazepine is chemically related to tricyclic antidepressants. Its mechanism of action is unknown in the treatment of seizure disorders, but it is thought to act by reducing polysynaptic responses and blocking the posttetanic potentiation.
      b. **Administration and dosage** (*Table 37-7*)
         (1) **Adults and children > 12 years of age** receive an initial oral dose of 200 mg twice daily. This may be increased gradually to 800 to 1200 mg daily (usually given in divided doses).
         (2) **Children < 12** usually receive 10 to 35 mg/kg daily in two or three divided doses.
      c. **Precautions and monitoring effects**
         (1) Carbamazepine should be used with caution in patients with bone marrow depression. A CBC should be obtained and platelets measured to determine baseline levels before therapy, and levels should be monitored during therapy. Aplastic anemia and agranulocytosis have been reported.
         (2) Tricyclic antidepressants should be avoided if there is a history of hypersensitivity to tricyclics. Monoamine oxidase (MAO) inhibitors should be discontinued 2 weeks before carbamazepine therapy.
         (3) Carbamazepine should be used cautiously in patients with glaucoma because of its mild anticholinergic effects that may result in increase of intraocular pressure.
         (4) Carbamazepine is an enzyme inducer; therefore, the half-life ($t_{½}$) decreases over 3 to 4 weeks ($t_{½}$ 18 to 54 hrs; $t_{½}$ 10 to 25 hrs); for maximal enzyme induction, levels should be rechecked to avoid breakthrough seizures.

Table 37-5 USES OF ANTIEPILEPTIC MEDICATIONS BASED ON SEIZURE TYPE

	Drug Therapy			
Seizure Type	**Choice 1**	**Choice 2**	**Choice 3**	**Choice 4**
Simple partial	Carbamazepine (alone or combination)	Phenytoin	Primidone Lamotrigine Oxcarbazepine Lacosamide	Gabapentin, levetiracetam Zonisamide Tiagabine
Complex partial	Carbamazepine Lamotrigine	Phenytoin	Phenobarbital Zonisamide Oxcarbazepine	Valproic acid Primidone Topiramate[a] Tiagabine Vigabatrin[b]
Primary generalized Tonic–clonic	Valproic acid Lamotrigine	Carbamazepine	Phenytoin Valproic acid	Phenobarbital Topiramate Tiagabine
Absence	Lamotrigine,[a] ethosuximide	Zonisamide, valproic acid		
Myoclonic atonic	Valproic acid Valproic acid	Clonazepam Clonazepam	Zonisamide	Felbamate[a] (alone or in combination)
Status epilepticus	Diazepam	Phenytoin	Phenobarbital	
Psychomotor	Phenytoin			
Lennox–Gastaut syndrome	Valproic acid felbamate	Lamotrigine Topiramate Rufinamide		

[a]Also indicated for treatment of Lennox–Gastaut syndrome in children.
[b]Also indicated for treatment infantile spasms.

(5) Carbamazepine is metabolized in the liver to 10,11-epoxid, which also has anticonvulsant activity; carbamazepine may induce its own metabolism.

(6) Potential for drug interaction in elderly patients.

(7) **Adverse effects:**

(a) The physician should be notified if any of the following adverse effects occur: jaundice, abdominal pain, pale stool, darkened urine, unusual bruising and bleeding, fever, sore throat, or an ulcer in the mouth. The most common side effects are dizziness, drowsiness, unsteadiness, nausea, and vomiting.

(b) **CNS effects.** These include dizziness, ataxia, and diplopia. If diplopia and ataxia are common and occur after a dose, the schedule could be adjusted to include more frequent administration or a larger proportion of the dose at night. CNS side effects may decrease with chronic administration.

(c) **Gastrointestinal (GI) effects.** These most commonly include nausea, vomiting, and anorexia.

(d) **Metabolic effects.** Hyponatremia occurs after several weeks to months of therapy, and the incidence increases with age. The antidiuretic hormone (ADH) level may be low. Levels of 125 to 135 mEq/L without symptoms should be monitored. Fluid restriction should be instituted when levels decrease to $<$ 125 mEq/L with or without symptoms. Another agent should be used if fluid dose reduction does not help or the seizures recur.

(e) **Hematopoietic effects.** Aplastic anemia is rare. Thrombocytopenia and anemia have a 5% incidence, and they respond to a cessation of drug therapy. Leukopenia is the most common hematopoietic side effect: 10% of cases are transient, and about 2% of patients have persistent leukopenia but do not seem to have increased infections even with white blood cell (WBC) counts of 3000/mL.

Table 37-6 ANTICONVULSIVE DRUG CLASSIFICATION

Barbiturates	Hydantoins	Succinimides	Sulfonamides	Oxazolidinediones	Benzodiazepine	Miscellaneous
Phenobarbital	Phenytoin	Ethosuximide	Zonisamide	Paramethadione	Clonazepam	Lamotrigine
Primidone	Mephenytoin	Methsuximide	Trimethadione	Diazepam	Felbamate	Gabapentin
Mephobarbital	Ethotoin	Phensuximide		Lorazepam	Clorazepate dipotassium	Pregabalin
	Fosphenytoin				Carbamazepine	Oxcarbazepine
					Valproic acid	Lacosamide
					Topiramate	Rufinamide
					Tiagabine	Vigabatrin
					Levetiracetam	

Table 37-7 DOSAGES CHARACTERISTIC OF ANTIEPILEPTIC MEDICATIONS

Drug	Enzyme Inducer	Enzyme Inhibitor	Loading Dose	Usual Adult Dose (mg/day)	Half-life (hr)	Therapeutic Range of Total Plasma Concentration (μg/mL)	Major Mode of Elimination	Protein-Binding Level (%)
Carbamazepine	+/−	−	No	800–1200	11[a]–22	4–12	Hepatic	75–80
Phenytoin	+/−	−	Yes	300–700	22–72 1–2 (free)	5–20	Hepatic	90
Phenobarbital	+/−	−	Yes	90–300	100	15–40	Hepatic > renal	40–60
Primidone	+/−	−	No	750–3000	15[a,b]	5–12	Hepatic	20–25
Valproic acid	+/−	+	Yes	1000–3000	15–20	50–150	Hepatic	75–90
Ethosuximide	+/−	−	No	750–1000	30–60[c]	40–100	Hepatic > renal	0
Felbamate	+/−	+	No	2400	20–23	30–100	Hepatic > renal	22–25
Gabapentin	−	−	Yes	900–1000	5–7	5–7	Renal	< 3
Lamotrigine	+/−	−	No	200–400	25 12.6[d] 70[e]	2–6	Hepatic > renal	55
Topiramate	+/−	−	No	200–400	15–23	n/a	Renal > hepatic	9–15
Tiagabine	−	−	No	32–56	6–8	n/a	Hepatic	96
Levetiracetam	−	−	Yes	500–3000	7	n/a	Renal	< 10
Zonisamide	−	−	No	100–600	24–50	n/a	Hepatic	40–60
Oxcarbazepine	+/−	+	No	900–1800	4–9	n/a	Hepatic	40–60
Lacosamide	+/−	−	Yes	200–400	13	n/a	Renal	15
Rufinamide	+/−	−	Yes	3200	6–10	n/a	Renal > liver	34
Lacosamide	+/−	−	Yes	200–400 mg	13	n/a	Renal	15

[a]The half-life decreases autometabolism after chronic use.
[b]Metabolized in part to phenobarbital.
[c]Lower range in children and higher range in adults.
[d]Receiving other enzyme-inducing drugs.
[e]Valproic acid slows the metabolism.

(f) **Dermatological effects.** Pruritic and erythematous rashes, the Stevens–Johnson syndrome, and lupus erythematosus have been reported.

(g) **Cardiovascular effect** such as congestive heart failure, hypertension, syncope, AV block, second- and third-degree heart block.

(8) **REM program**

(a) To inform patients regarding serious dermatological reactions (toxic epidermal necrolysis, Stevens–Johnson syndrome), blood dyscrasias, and suicidal thoughts and behavior that could occur during treatment.

(b) **Medication Guide** must be dispensed with this product.

d. **Significant interactions**

(1) **Antiepileptic drugs**, such as **phenytoin**, **primidone**, and **phenobarbital**, decrease the level of carbamazepine (increase metabolism).

(2) **Valproic acid** increases the level of carbamazepine (decreases metabolism).

(3) Other medications such as **erythromycin**, **isoniazid**, **cimetidine**, **propoxyphene**, **diltiazem**, and **verapamil** increase the level of carbamazepine (decrease metabolism).

(4) Carbamazepine decreases levels of **calcium-channel blockers**, increasing its own level.

(5) Carbamazepine decreases the effect of warfarin.

(6) Antibiotics increase the level of carbamazepine.

(7) Carbamazepine decreases tricyclic antidepressant levels.

(8) Carbamazepine an inducer of CYP34A drugs that metabolized within this pathway such as acetaminophen, alprazolam, and levothyroxine would increase plasma concentration of other drugs.

(9) Grapefruit juice will increase concentration of carbamazepine.

2. **Phenytoin (Dilantin)**

a. **Mechanism of action**

(1) Phenytoin inhibits the spread of seizures at the motor cortex and blocks posttetanic potentiation by influencing synaptic transmission. There is an alternation of ion fluxes in depolarization, repolarization, and membrane stability phase and alternating calcium uptake in presynaptic terminals.

(2) Phenytoin is effective for the treatment of generalized tonic–clonic (grand mal) seizures and for partial seizures, both simple and complex. It is not effective for absence seizures.

b. **Administration and dosage** (*Table 37-7*)

(1) The usual daily dose for **adults** is 300 to 700 mg, with adjustments made as needed.

(a) Regular daily doses above 500 mg are poorly tolerated.

(b) A loading dose of 900 mg to 1.5 g may be given intravenously (IV). The infusion rate should not exceed 50 mg/min. (Alternatively, an oral loading dose may be given.)

(2) The usual daily dose for **children** is 4 to 7 mg/kg divided every 12 hrs. An IV loading dose of 15 mg/kg may be given.

(3) Phenytoin sodium is available as capsules and parenteral solution. Phenytoin is available as tablets and oral suspension.

c. **Precautions and monitoring effects**

(1) IV phenytoin should not be used in patients with sinus bradycardia, sinoatrial block, second- and third-degree atrioventricular (AV) block, or Adams–Stokes syndrome.

(2) Phenytoin should be used cautiously in patients with myocardial insufficiency and hypotension.

(3) Elimination of phenytoin converts from first-order elimination (proportional to its concentration) to zero-order elimination (a fixed amount per unit time), usually at high therapeutic levels. The daily dose of phenytoin can be increased 100 mg daily until therapeutic blood levels are attained, after which increases of 30 to 50 mg will avoid twofold to threefold increases in blood levels.

(4) It is necessary to measure free drug levels or correct the total level when aluminum levels are abnormal or the patient has renal failure.

(5) Potential for drug interaction in elderly patients.

(6) Lymphadenopathy (local or generalized), including benign lymph node hyperplasia, Hodgkin disease, and lymphoma, has been associated with use of phenytoin.

(7) Phenytoin have been associated with exacerbation of porphyria (an enzyme deficiency that involves skin and CNS).

(8) **Adverse effects:**

(a) The physician should be notified if any of the following adverse effects occur: swollen or tender gums, skin rash, nausea and vomiting, swollen glands, bleeding, jaundice, fever, or sore throat (i.e., signs of infection or bleeding).

(b) **CNS effects** include ataxia (limiting side effect), dysarthria, and insomnia. Transient hyperkinesia may follow IV phenytoin infusion. Alcoholic beverages should be avoided while on this medication.

(c) **GI effects** most commonly include nausea and vomiting. Phenytoin should be taken with food to enhance absorption and decrease GI upset.

(d) **Dermatological effects** include maculopapular rashes sometimes with fever, Stevens–Johnson syndrome, and lupus erythematosus. Gingival hyperplasia may be reduced by frequent brushing and appropriate oral care.

(e) **Connective tissue disorders** include a coarsening of the facial features.

(f) **Hematopoietic effects** include thrombocytopenia, leukopenia, and granulocytopenia.

(g) **Miscellaneous effects** include hyperglycemia and increased body hair.

d. Significant interactions

(1) **Antiepileptic drugs**, such as **carbamazepine**, **valproic acid**, **clonazepam**, and **phenobarbital**, decrease the level of phenytoin (increase metabolism).

(2) Phenytoin increases the **conversion of primidone to phenobarbital** (increases metabolism).

(3) Other medications such as **disulfiram**, **isoniazid**, **chloramphenicol**, and **propoxyphene** increase the level of phenytoin (decrease metabolism).

(4) Drugs whose efficacy is impaired by phenytoin include **corticosteroids**, **digitoxin**, **doxycycline**, **estrogens**, **furosemide**, **oral contraceptives**, **quinidine**, **rifampin**, **theophylline**, **vitamin D**, and **enteral nutritional therapy**.

(5) **Coumarin** and **warfarin** anticoagulants increase the serum phenytoin levels and prolong the serum half-life of phenytoin by inhibiting its metabolism.

(6) Phenytoin decreases **tricyclic antidepressant** levels.

(7) Phenytoin interacts with **diabetes and arthritis medications**.

3. Fosphenytoin (Cerebyx)

a. Mechanism of action

(1) It is a prodrug of phenytoin.

(2) Water-soluble prodrug of phenytoin. It is converted to phenytoin by the bloodstream phosphatases, with a half-life of about 8 mins in both adults and children.

(3) Fosphenytoin sodium 1.5 mg = 1 mg phenytoin sodium

(4) It is indicated for patients who cannot take oral drugs, and in the acute treatment for status epilepticus.

(5) Administered via IV or intramuscular (IM) injection

(6) A dose conversion table should be used to convert the phenytoin dose to fosphenytoin.

(7) Characteristics similar to phenytoin

(8) Severe cardiovascular reactions such as asystole, ventricular fibrillation, and cardiac arrest. Hypotension could occur with IV administration, which could be controlled by decrease the rate of infusion.

(9) QT prolongation and torsade de pointes when administrated with antiarrhythmic agents such as amiodarone and quinidine

(10) **Advantages**

(a) Fosphenytoin is an aqueous solution, unlike phenytoin, which is an alkaline solution; therefore, there is no need to add propylene glycol and ethanol to the solution.

(b) Fosphenytoin causes less soft tissue injury at the site of injection. When administered by IM injection, it is completely absorbed and has more predictable serum concentration than IM-injected phenytoin.

4. **Valproic acid (Depakote)**
   a. **Mechanism of action**
      (1) Increases levels of GABA
      (2) Potentiates a postsynaptic GABA response by inhibiting the enzymatic response for the catabolism of GABA.
      (3) Affects the potassium channel, creating a direct membrane-stabilizing effect.
   b. **Administration and dosage** (*Table 37-7*)
      (1) For **adults**, valproic acid is administered orally in a usual dose of 1000 to 3000 mg daily in divided doses.
      (2) For **children**, valproic acid is administered orally in a dose of 15 to 60 mg/kg daily, divided into two or three doses.
      (3) Medication should be taken with food to reduce GI upset.
      (4) Tablets or capsules should be swallowed, not chewed, to avoid irritation of the mouth and throat.
   c. **Precautions and monitoring effects.** There are some reports of hepatotoxicity and increased liver function tests, which are mostly reversible. The severity and incidence of hepatotoxicity increase when the patient is younger than 2 years of age.
   d. **Adverse effects.**
      (1) Contact the physician if abdominal pain, nausea, vomiting, or anoxia occurs; these could be symptoms of pancreatitis.
      (2) **CNS effects** include tremor, ataxia, diplopia, lethargy, drowsiness, behavioral changes, and depression.
      (3) **GI effects** include nausea and increased appetite. Enteric-coated divalproex sodium may reduce these side effects.
      (4) **Dermatological effects** include alopecia and petechiae.
      (5) **Hematopoietic effects** include thrombocytopenia, bruising, hematoma, and bleeding.
      (6) **Hepatic effects** include minor elevations of aspartate aminotransferase (AST), alanine aminotransferase (ALT), and lactate dehydrogenase (LDH).
      (7) **Endocrine effects** include decreased levels of prolactin, resulting in irregular menses and secondary amenorrhea.
      (8) **Pancreatic effects** include acute pancreatitis.
      (9) **Metabolic effects** include hyperammonemia owing to renal origin. Discontinuation may be considered if lethargy develops.
   e. **Significant interactions**
      (1) **Antiepileptic drugs**
         (a) **Primidone** decreases valproic acid clearance (increases metabolism).
         (b) **Phenobarbital** and **phenytoin** displace protein binding, resulting in an increased total phenytoin level and an increase or no change of free phenytoin.
         (c) **Clonazepam** increases CNS toxicity in patients on valproic acid.
      (2) **Other medications**
         (a) **Aspirin** increases the level of valproic acid.
         (b) **Warfarin** inhibits the secondary phase of platelet aggregation.
         (c) **Antacids** increase the level of valproic acid.
      (3) **Laboratory tests**
         (a) False-positive urine ketone tests may result in patients taking valproic acid; thus, patients with diabetes must use caution when using urine tests.
         (b) Thyroid function tests may be altered by antiepileptic drugs.
5. **Phenobarbital (Luminal)**
   a. **Mechanism of action.** Phenobarbital increases the seizure threshold by decreasing postsynaptic excitation by stimulating postsynaptic GABA-A receptor inhibitor responses as a CNS depressant.
   b. **Administration and dosage** (*Table 37-7*)
      (1) For **adults**, phenobarbital is administered orally at 90 to 300 mg daily (in three divided doses or as a single dose at bedtime).
      (2) **Children** typically receive 3 to 6 mg/kg daily in two divided doses. Adjustment is made as needed.

c. Precautions and monitoring effects

(1) Phenobarbital produces respiratory depression, especially with parenteral administration.

(2) Phenobarbital should be used with caution in patients with hepatic disease who may need dose adjustments.

(3) Phenobarbital has sedative effects in adults and produces hyperactivity in children.

(4) Abrupt discontinuation of phenobarbital produces withdrawal convulsions. If the drug must be discontinued, another GABA-A agonist (e.g., benzodiazepine, paraldehyde) should be substituted.

(5) Potential for drug interaction in elderly patients.

(6) **Adverse effects.** The physician should be notified if any of the following adverse effects occur: sore throat, mouth sores, easy bruising or bleeding, and any signs of infection.

(a) **CNS effects** include agitation, confusion, lethargy, and drowsiness. Patients should avoid alcohol and other CNS depressants.

(b) **Respiratory effects** include hypoventilation and apnea.

(c) **Cardiovascular effects** include bradycardia and hypotension.

(d) **GI effects** include nausea, diarrhea, and constipation. If GI upset is experienced, phenobarbital should be taken with food.

(e) **Hematological effects** include megaloblastic anemia after chronic use (a rare side effect).

(f) **Miscellaneous effects** include osteomalacia and Stevens–Johnson syndrome, both of which are rare.

d. Significant interactions

(1) **Antiepileptic drugs**, such as **valproic acid** and **phenytoin**, increase the level of phenobarbital (decrease metabolism).

(2) Other drugs such as **acetazolamide**, **chloramphenicol**, **cimetidine**, and **furosemide** increase the level of phenobarbital (decrease metabolism).

(3) **Rifampin**, **pyridoxine**, and **ethanol** decrease the level of phenobarbital (increase metabolism).

6. Primidone (Mysoline)

a. Mechanism of action. Primidone is a metabolite of phenobarbital and phenylethylmalonamide (PEMA), which has some anticonvulsive effects. It has drug characteristics similar to phenobarbital, with some differences in dose and half-life.

b. Administration and dosage (*Table 37-7*)

(1) Primidone has a short half-life of 7 hrs, which may require three times daily dosing.

(2) Primidone is tolerated better if started at 50 mg at night for 3 days until the target daily dose is reached.

7. Ethosuximide (Zarontin)

a. Mechanism of action

(1) Ethosuximide may inhibit the sodium–potassium adenosine triphosphatase (Na^+/K^+ ATPase) system and the reduced form of nicotinamide adenine dinucleotide phosphate (NADPH) linked aldehyde reductase (which is necessary for the formation of γ-hydroxybutyrate, which is associated with the induction of absence seizures).

(2) Ethosuximide reduces or eliminates the EEG abnormality; however, absence seizures are the only seizures in which the normal EEG has clinical value (i.e., when the EEG abnormality is corrected, the seizures are also controlled).

(3) Ethosuximide is a relatively benign anticonvulsant with minimum protein binding.

b. Administration and dosage (*Table 37-7*). Ethosuximide is usually given orally in an initial dose of 500 mg daily in **adults and older children** and 250 mg daily in **children ages 3 to 6 years**. The dose may be raised by 250 mg every week to a maximum of 1.5 g daily in adults.

c. Precautions and monitoring effects

(1) Blood dyscrasias have been reported, making periodic blood counts necessary.

(2) There have been reports of hepatic and renal toxicity; thus periodic renal and liver function monitoring is necessary.

(3) Cases of systemic lupus erythematosus have been reported.

d. **Adverse effects**
   (1) **GI effects** include nausea and vomiting. Small doses may lessen these effects. Ethosuximide should be taken with food if GI upset occurs.
   (2) **Hematopoietic effects** include eosinophilia, granulocytopenia, leukopenia, and lupus.
   (3) **CNS effects** include drowsiness, blurred vision, fatigue, lethargy, hiccups, and headaches. Alcoholic beverages should be avoided with this medication.
   (4) **Psychiatric–psychological** effects include confusion and emotional instability.
   (5) **Dermatological effects include** pruritus, photosensitivity, urticaria, and Stevens–Johnson syndrome.
   (6) **Genitourinary effects include** increased frequency of urination, vaginal bleeding, renal damage, and hematuria.
   (7) **Miscellaneous effects include** periorbital edema and muscle weakness. Patients should also be advised of the risks of exposure to sunlight and ultraviolet light.
   (8) **REM program**
      (a) To inform patients of potential adverse effects, including blood dyscrasias, systemic lupus erythematosus, and suicidal thoughts and behavior, that could occur during treatment.
      (b) **Medication Guide** must be dispensed with this product.

e. **Significant interactions**
   (1) **Antiepileptic drugs**, such as **carbamazepine**, decrease the level of ethosuximide (increases metabolism).
   (2) **Valproic acid** increases the level of ethosuximide (decreases metabolism).

8. **Clonazepam (Klonopin)**

a. **Mechanism of action.** Clonazepam is a potent GABA-A agonist, but its efficacy decreases over several months of treatment.

b. **Administration and dosage**
   (1) For **adults**, clonazepam is an oral agent that may be given in an initial dose of 1.5 mg daily divided two or three times. The dose may be increased to a maximum of 20 mg daily.
   (2) **Children** should receive 0.01 to 0.03 mg daily in two or three doses. The dosage may be increased to a maximum of 0.2 mg/kg daily.

c. **Precautions and monitoring effects**
   (1) Patients with psychoses, acute narrow-angle glaucoma, and significant liver disease should use this medicine cautiously.
   (2) **Adverse effects**
      (a) **CNS effects** include drowsiness, ataxia, and behavior disturbances in children; these may be corrected by dose reduction.
      (b) **Respiratory effects** include hypersalivation and bronchial hypersecretion.
      (c) **Miscellaneous effects** include anemia, leukopenia, thrombocytopenia, respiratory depression, anorexia, and weight loss.
   (3) **REM program**
      (a) To increase awareness of potential risks, including the occurrence of withdrawal symptoms with abrupt discontinuation and suicidal thoughts and behavior, that could occur during treatment.
      (b) **Medication Guide** must be dispensed with this product.

d. **Significant interactions**
   (1) **Antiepileptic drugs**, such as **phenytoin**, increase the level of clonazepam (decrease metabolism).
   (2) **Other drugs.** Clonazepam decreases the efficacy of **levodopa** and increases the serum level of **digoxin**.

9. **Felbamate (Felbatol)**

a. **Mechanism of action.** A proposed mechanism of action is that the drug interacts with glycine modulatory site on *N*-methyl-D-aspartate (NMDA) receptors. Blockade of NMDA may contribute to neuroprotective effects of felbamate. Felbamate is used as monotherapy or adjunctive therapy or without secondary generalization in adults and generalized seizures associated with Lennox–Gastaut syndrome in children. The U.S. Food and Drug

Administration (FDA) recommended that use of felbamate be restricted to only those patients who are refractory to other medications and in whom the risk–benefit relationship warrants its use because of severe hepatotoxicity, aplastic anemia.

b. Administration and dosage (*Table 37-7*)

(1) **Adults and children** > 14 years of age

(2) Monotherapy, initially 1.2 g in three to four doses daily. The dosage may be increased in 600-mg increments every 2 weeks to 2.4 g daily based on clinical response and, thereafter, 3.6 g daily if necessary.

(3) Adjunctive therapy, 1.2 g in three to four doses daily, with reduction of the dosage of other antiepileptic drugs by 20% to 33%. The dosage of felbamate may be increased in increments of 1.2 g at weekly intervals to a maximum of 3.6 g daily.

(4) Conversion to monotherapy initially 1.2 g daily in three to four doses, with reduction of the dosage of other antiepileptic drugs by 33% at week 3. The felbamate dosage may be increased to 3.6 g daily, and other antiepileptic drugs discontinued or dosage further reduced in stepwise fashion.

(5) Children 2 to 14 years of age with Lennox–Gastaut syndrome, as adjunctive therapy, initially 15 mg/kg daily in three to four doses. The dosage of other antiepileptic drugs is reduced by 20%. The amount of felbamate may be increased in increments of 15 mg/kg at weekly intervals to 45 mg/kg daily. Further reduction in the dosage of other antiepileptic drugs may be necessary.

c. Precaution and monitoring effects. There are two very serious toxic effects, aplastic anemia and liver failure, which lead to death for some patients.

(1) For aplastic anemia, the onset range from 5 to 30 weeks of initiation of therapy. Weekly or biweekly CBCs are recommended initially.

(2) For liver, toxicity time between initiation of treatment and diagnosis of these cases ranges from 2 to 3 weeks after initiation of therapy. It is recommended that liver function tests be performed before initiation of therapy to identify patients who have evidence of preexisting liver damage. Liver function tests should also be performed weekly or biweekly. The FDA recommends that this drug be used only in patients who are refractory to other medications and in whom the risk–benefit relationship warrants its use.

(3) **Adverse effects:**

(a) Contact the physician if signs of infection (e.g., bleeding or bruising) occur.

(b) This drug has the potential to cause aplastic anemia (bone marrow).

(c) The patient should be monitored for these toxicities by CBCs and liver function tests weekly or biweekly until discontinuation of any sign of these toxicities occurs.

(d) **CNS effects** are insomnia, headache, anxiety, hyperactivity, and fatigue.

(e) **Cardiovascular effects** are peripheral edema, vasodilation, hypotension, and hypertension.

(f) **Ocular** effects are diplopia and blurred vision.

(g) **GI effects** are anorexia, weight decrease, and nausea.

(h) **Hematological effects** may include lymphadenopathy, leukopenia, and thrombocytopenia.

(i) **Metabolic/nutrition effects** may include hypokalemia and hyponatremia.

(j) **QT prolongation and torsade de pointes**

d. Significant interactions

(1) **Felbamate and phenytoin.** Felbamate causes an increase in phenytoin plasma concentration. Phenytoin doubles felbamate clearance, resulting in 45% decrease in felbamate levels.

(2) **Felbamate and carbamazepine.** Felbamate causes a decrease in carbamazepine levels and an increase in carbamazepine metabolites. In addition, carbamazepine causes a 50% increase in felbamate clearance, resulting in a 40% decrease in steady-state trough levels.

(3) **Felbamate and valproic acid.** Felbamate causes an increase in valproic acid levels, but valproic acid does not affect felbamate levels.

(4) **Adverse effects.** Signs and symptoms associated with increased plasma level and toxicity are anorexia, nausea, vomiting, insomnia, and headache.

10. Gabapentin (Neurontin)

a. **Mechanism of action.** It is an analog of GABA. It increases GABA turnover, but it does not bind to GABA or any other established neurotransmitter receptor. Its mechanism of action is currently unknown, although it binds to a specific receptor in the brain and inhibits voltage-dependent sodium currents. It has been shown to be effective as an add-on drug in patients with partial seizure with or without secondary generalization.

b. **Administration and dosage** (*Table 37-7*)

(1) Patients > **12 years** receive 900 mg to 1.8 g daily, administered as adjunctive therapy in three divided doses. Titrating to an effective dose normally can be achieved within 3 days by initiating therapy with 300 mg and then increasing the dose in 300-mg increments over the next 2 days to establish a dosage of 900 mg daily in three doses. If necessary, the dosage may be increased to 1.8 g daily. To minimize potential side effects, especially somnolence, dizziness, or fatigue, the first dose on day 1 may be administered at bedtime.

(2) Patients 3 to 12 years of age should receive 10 to 15 mg/kg/day in three divided doses up to 25 to 50 mg/kg/day.

(3) The drug is primarily excreted renally; therefore, the dosage should be adjusted for patients who have compromised renal function.

(4) The drug does not bind to plasma protein. There are no significant pharmacokinetic interactions with other commonly used antiepileptic drugs.

(5) If gabapentin is discontinued or an alternate anticonvulsant medication is added, it should be done gradually over a minimum of 1 week.

c. **Precautions and monitoring effects**

(1) Gabapentin is useful in patients who are taking other medications for epilepsy or other chronic diseases. It may be especially useful for elderly patients.

(2) Gabapentin is well absorbed orally; it can be taken with or without food. However, patients who have GI problems might have problems with absorption.

(3) Taper off over at least 1 week; may cause withdrawal symptoms such as anxiety, insomnia, and nausea.

(4) May cause false-positive result with some urinary protein tests

(5) **Adverse effects:**

(a) Common side effects are somnolence, dizziness, ataxia, fatigue, weight gain, and nystagmus.

(b) **CNS effects** are somnolence, dizziness, ataxia, and fatigue.

(c) **GI effects** include dyspepsia, dryness of mouth, constipation, and increased appetite.

(d) **Ocular effects** are diplopia, blurred vision, and nystagmus.

(e) **Cardiovascular**: congestive heart failure, hypertension/hypotension

(f) **Dermatologic**: Dry skin, fungal dermatitis, herpes infection, Steven–Johnson syndrome

(g) **Endocrine:** diabetes melitus

(6) **REM program**

(a) To inform patients of the potential risk of suicidal thoughts and behavior that could occur during treatment.

(b) **Medication Guide** must be dispensed with this product.

d. **Significant interactions**

(1) **Antacids and gabapentin.** Antacids reduce the bioavailability of gabapentin by 20%; gabapentin could be taken 2 hrs after antacid use.

(2) **Cimetidine and gabapentin.** Cimetidine decreases the renal excretion of gabapentin by 14% and consequently increases gabapentin plasma levels (however, this amount is not clinically significant).

(3) **Oral contraceptives and gabapentin.** Oral contraceptives increase the level of norethindrone by 13%; this amount may not be clinically significant.

11. Lamotrigine (Lamictal)

a. **Mechanism of action.** Its antiepileptic effect is similar to that of phenytoin. Its effect may be the result of inhibition of voltage-dependent sodium currents and reduction of sustained repetitive neuronal activity. It is indicated for the treatment of partial seizures and secondary generalized tonic–clonic seizures that are not controlled with other drugs. It is also used to treat Lennox–Gastaut syndrome. Lamotrigine is broad spectrum, as well tolerated as monotherapy, and probably the least teratogenic of the first-line agents. It may aggravate severe myoclonic epilepsy.

b. Administration and dosage (*Table 37-7*)

(1) **Adults** (> 16 years), initially 50 mg/day in two divided doses (patients taking valproic acid should be given 25 mg every other day), up to 100 mg/day (up to 25 mg daily with valproic acid treatment). Monotherapy: 9 (Adults-12 years) 25 mg daily for 14 days, 50 mg for 14 days, up to 500 mg daily.

(2) **Children** 2 to 12 years 0.6 mg/kg/day in two divided doses (0.15 mg/kg/day on valproic acid treatment), up to 1.2 mg/kg/day (up to 0.3 mg/kg/day with valproic acid treatment).

(3) The smallest available chewable dispersible tablet is 5 mg. Then, after 2 weeks, increase by 0.3 mg/kg/day in one to two divided doses, up to 200 mg/day.

(4) Swallow chewable dispersible tablet whole, chewed, or in dispersing water or diluted fruit juice. If chewed, consume a small amount of water or diluted fruit juice to aid in swallowing. To disperse, add the chewable dispersible tablet to a small amount of liquid (1 teaspoon or enough to cover the medication). Approximately 1 min later, when the tablet is completely dispersed, swirl the solution and consume the entire quantity immediately.

(5) For patients taking valproic acid, the initial dose is 50 mg daily for 2 weeks, followed by maintenance doses of 100 to 200 mg daily in two divided doses.

(6) Reduced clearance in the elderly necessitates dosage reduction.

(7) Patients with hepatic impairment may require dosage reduction because of reduction in metabolism.

c. Precautions and monitoring effects

(1) Caution should be used for patients taking this drug. It may adversely affect the patient's metabolism or complicate the elimination of the drug because of renal, hepatic, or cardiac impairment.

(2) Lamotrigine binds to melanin and can accumulate in melanin-rich tissue over time. Periodic ophthalmological monitoring is recommended.

(3) Photosensitization (photoallergy and phototoxicity) patients should take protective measures against exposure to ultraviolet light or sunlight.

(4) Serious rashes requiring hospitalization have been reported. The incidence of rashes, including Stevens–Johnson syndrome, is approximately 1% in patients < 16 years old and 0.3% in adults. Rare cases of toxic epidermal necrolysis or rash-related death have occurred. Most rashes occur within 2 to 8 weeks of initial treatment.

(5) **Adverse effects:**

(a) The most common side effects are dizziness, diplopia, ataxia, blurred vision, nausea, dose-related rash, and vomiting.

(b) **CNS effects** are headache, dizziness, and ataxia tics (in children).

(c) **GI effects** are nausea, vomiting, diarrhea, and dyspepsia.

(d) **Ocular effects** are diplopia, blurred vision, and vision abnormality.

(e) **Dermatological effects** are pruritus, and a rash may form similar to that found when using phenytoin and carbamazepine. In many cases, the rash disappears during continued therapy, but 1% to 2% of patients with the rash represent a more serious allergic reaction. Occasionally, patients have developed the Stevens–Johnson syndrome. Concomitant use with valproic acid may increase the likelihood of serious rash. The occurrences of life-threatening rash that were reported developed within 2 to 8 weeks following therapy; other cases of rash have been reported developing up to 6 months after therapy. The incidence of rash is higher in children than in adults.

(f) Monotherapy during pregnancy found no teratogenic effect.

d. Significant interactions

(1) Carbamazepine decreases lamotrigine concentration by 70% and increases carbamazepine levels.

(2) Phenobarbital or primidone decreases lamotrigine concentration by 40%.

(3) Valproic acid decreases the metabolism of lamotrigine and extends its half-life to 60 hrs, which necessitates a dose reduction.

12. **Topiramate (Topamax)**
    a. **Mechanism of action.** Topiramate is a derivative of fructose. It decreases rapid hippocampal neuronal firing, possibly because of sodium- or calcium-channel inhibition. It is also a weak carbonic anhydrase inhibitor and a sodium-channel blocking agent. Topiramate potentiates the activity of GABA. It has been shown to be effective adjunctive therapy for partial seizure treatment in adults, tonic–clonic seizure, infantile spasms, and Lennox–Gastaut syndrome.
    b. **Administration and dosage** (*Table 37-7*)
        (1) **Adults** 17 years and older, 25 to 50 mg/day, up to 400 mg/day in two divided doses. **Children** 2 to 16 years, 1 to 3 mg/kg/day, up to 5 to 9 mg/kg/day in two divided doses.
        (2) Topiramate is 80% bioavailable, and food does not affect its bioavailability.
        (3) Dose adjustment is necessary for patients with renal or hepatic impairments.
        (4) Enzyme-inducing anticonvulsive drugs can decrease topiramate levels, but topiramate has a significant effect on metabolism of other anticonvulsive drugs.
        (5) Initial treatment is 50 mg daily, followed by titration to an effective dosage. More than 400 mg daily has not been shown to improve response.
    c. **Precaution and monitoring effects**
        (1) Increased incidence of kidney stones (renal calculus) in older patients who received this drug. Patients should be advised to increase intake of fluids while taking topiramate.
        (2) Paresthesia is a common side effect of anhydrase inhibitors.
        (3) Due to effect of topiramate, renal bicarbonate loss and metabolic acidosis could occur.
        (4) Topiramate could cause oligohidrosis and hyperthermia (decrease sweating and increase temperature).
        (5) Acute myopia with secondary angle closure glaucoma could occur, typically occur within 1 month of therapy in which the drug should be discontinued.
        (6) **Adverse effects**
            (a) The physician should be notified if any of the following adverse effects occur:
                (i) Breast pain in females
                (ii) Nausea or tremor, which are dose-related side effects.
                (iii) Back pain, chest pain, dyspepsia, or leg pain
            (b) **CNS effects** mostly seen in 600 mg/day dose include psychomotor slowing, difficulty with concentration and speech, somnolence, fatigue, asthenia, weight loss, cognitive disturbances and difficulties, tremors, dizziness, ataxia, and headache.
            (c) **GI effects** include upset, such as nausea, vomiting, and gastroenteritis.
            (d) **Genitourinary effects** polyuria, oliguria and renal calculi.
            (e) **Cardiovascular effects** include chest pain, palpitation, and vasodilation.
            (f) **Ocular effects** include abnormal vision, eye pain, diplopia, and glaucoma.
            (g) **Hematological effects** include anemia, epistaxis, leukopenia, and aplastic anemia.
            (h) **Other**: metabolic acidosis, hypohidrosis (in children)
        (7) **REM program**
            (a) To inform patients of the potential risk for adverse effects, including suicidal thoughts and behavior and teratogenic effects (i.e., cleft lip, cleft palate), that may occur during treatment.
            (b) **Medication Guide** must be dispensed with this product.
    d. **Significant interactions**
        (1) Phenytoin and carbamazepine will increase clearance.
        (2) Topiramate increases the clearance of other drugs that are cleared by cytochrome P450.
13. **Tiagabine (Gabitril)**
    a. **Mechanism of action.** Tiagabine is designed to act on the inhibitory action of GABA by blocking its uptake, thereby prolonging its action after synaptic release. It is indicated as adjunctive therapy for partial seizures.
    b. **Administration and dosage** (*Table 37-7*)
        (1) Starting dose of 4 mg daily for 2 weeks may be increased 4 to 8 mg weekly thereafter, to a maintenance dose of 32 to 56 mg daily.
        (2) Maximum recommended dosage for **children** is 32 mg daily; maximum recommended dosage for **adults** is 56 mg daily.

(3) A high-fat meal decreases the rate of tiagabine absorption but does not affect the extension of absorption. Tiagabine should be taken with food.

c. **Precautions and monitoring effects**

(1) Moderately severe to severe **generalized weakness** has been reported. It resolves in all cases after reduction in dose or discontinuation of therapy.

(2) **Ophthalmic effects**, as indicated by animal studies, include the possibility for residual binding to retina and melanin binding; this finding, however, has not been confirmed in human studies. Periodic ophthalmological monitoring is necessary.

(3) **Dermatological effects** include the possibility of severe rash to Stevens–Johnson syndrome, as reported in clinical studies.

(4) **Sudden unexpected death** have been reported (as many as 10 cases) among 2531 patients with epilepsy (3831 patient years of exposure).

(5) **EEG abnormalities.** Spike and wave discharges on EEG have been reported to have exacerbations of their EEG abnormalities associated with cognitive/neuropsychiatric events. Patients usually continued tiagabine but required dosage adjustment.

(6) **Adverse effects**

(a) **CNS effects** are confusion, dizziness, and fatigue.

(b) **GI effects** are upset stomach, nausea, mouth ulceration, and anorexia.

(7) **REM program**

(a) To raise awareness of the risk of suicidal thoughts and behavior that could occur during treatment. There have also been case reports of seizures in patients without a history of epilepsy who were receiving **tiagabine** for unapproved indications.

(b) **Medication Guide** must be dispensed with this product.

d. **Significant interactions.** Phenobarbital, phenytoin, and carbamazepine will increase tiagabine clearance.

14. **Zonisamide (Zonegran)**

a. **Mechanism of action.** It is not well known. It may block the sensitive sodium channels and T-type calcium channels. It is indicated for adjunct therapy for partial seizure for adults.

b. **Administration and dosage** (*Table 37-7*)

(1) **Adults and children** > 16 years of age, 100 mg daily; within 2 weeks, increase to 200 mg/daily in 2-week bases, up to 600 mg daily.

(2) Can be taken with or without food.

c. **Precautions and monitoring effects**

(1) **Potentially fatal reactions to sulfonamides.** Fatalities have occurred, although rarely, as a result of severe reactions to sulfonamides (a sulfonamide) including Stevens–Johnson syndrome, toxic epidermal necrolysis, fulminant hepatic necrosis, agranulocytosis, aplastic anemia, and other blood dyscrasias.

(2) **Serious hematologic events.** Very rare cases of aplastic anemia and agranulocytosis were reported.

(3) **Cognitive/neuropsychiatric adverse reactions.** The most significant of these can be classified into three general categories: (1) psychiatric symptoms, including depression and psychosis; (2) psychomotor slowing, difficulty with concentration, and speech or language problems, in particular, word-finding difficulties; and (3) somnolence or fatigue.

(4) **Creatine phosphokinase (CPK) elevation and pancreatitis.** Rare adverse events have been observed (less than 1:1000). Severe muscle pain and/or weakness, either in the presence or absence of a fever, markers of muscle damage should be assessed, including serum CPK and aldolase levels, consideration should be given to tapering and/or discontinuation of zonisamide.

(5) **Kidney stones** have been reported in 4% of patients in clinical trials.

(6) May increase mean concentration of serum creatinine and blood, urea, nitrogen; renal function should be monitored periodically.

(7) **Sudden unexplained death in epilepsy.** Nine sudden unexplained deaths occurred among 991 patients with epilepsy (representing 7.7 deaths per 1000 patient years).

(8) Oligohidrosis and hyperthermia have been reported in pediatric patients.

(9) **Side effects**

(a) **CNS effects** are dizziness, headache, somnolence, ataxia, confusion, tremor, and abnormal thinking.

(b) **Cardiovascular effects** are palpitation, tachycardia, and vascular insufficiency.

(c) **Dermatologic effects** are maculopapular rash, acne, alopecia, and photosensitivity.

(d) **Other effects:** nausea, agitation/irritability

(10) **REM program**

(a) To communicate the increased risk of suicidal thoughts and behavior associated with treatment.

(b) **Medication Guide** must be dispensed with this product.

d. **Significant interactions**

(1) Zonisamide induces **liver enzymes** by increasing metabolism and through clearance of zonisamide and decreases half-life.

(2) **Food** will delay absorption but will not affect the bioavailability of the drug.

15. **Levetiracetam (Keppra)**

a. **Mechanism of action.** It is a pyrrolidone derivative and is chemically unrelated to other antiepileptic drugs. It displays inhibitory properties in the kindling model in rats. It is used as adjunctive therapy in the treatment of partial seizure, myoclonic, and generalized seizure.

b. **Administration and dosage** (*Table 37-7*)

(1) **Adult 16 and older.** Starting dose of 1000 mg/day given in two divided doses may be increased every 2 weeks, to a maximum of 3000 mg/day.

(2) **Children 4 to 16 years of age.** Initiate therapy with 10 mg/kg twice daily; dose may be increased by 20 mg/kg daily every 2 weeks (maximum, 30 mg/kg twice daily).

c. **Precautions and monitoring effects**

(1) **Hematological effects** are minor, but there is a statistically significant decrease compared to placebo in total mean RBC count, mean hemoglobin, and mean hematocrit.

(2) Decrease in WBC count and neutrophil count.

(3) It also causes drowsiness.

(4) **Adverse effects**

(a) Most commonly reported adverse events are somnolence, weakness (asthenia), hostility, infection, and fatigue.

(b) **CNS effects** are somnolence, dizziness, depression, and nervousness.

(c) Dermatologic: pruritis, skin discoloration, rash, and alopecia

(d) **Respiratory effects** are pharyngitis, rhinitis, and increased cough.

d. **Significant interactions.** Levetiracetam does not influence the **plasma concentration** of existing antiepileptic drugs, and other **antiepileptic drugs** do not influence the pharmacokinetic effects of levetiracetam.

16. **Oxcarbazepine (Trileptal)**

a. **Mechanism of action.** This drug produces blockade of voltage-sensitive sodium channels, resulting in stabilization of hyperexcited neural membranes, inhibition of repetitive neuronal firing, and diminution of propagation of synaptic impulses. These actions are thought to be important in the prevention of seizure spread in the intact brain. In addition, increased potassium conductance and modulation of high-voltage activated calcium channels may contribute to the anticonvulsant effects of the drug. Indicated for partial seizures in adults and as monotherapy in the treatment of partial seizures in children 4 years of age and older with epilepsy, and as adjunctive therapy in children 2 years of age and older with epilepsy.

b. **Administration and dosage** (*Table 37-7*)

(1) **Children** 4 to 16 years, 8 to 10 mg/kg/day to 600 mg/day as adjunctive therapy and 8 to 10 mg/kg/day as monotherapy.

(2) **Adults** 600 mg/day as adjunctive therapy and 1200 mg/day as monotherapy. A dosage adjustment is needed for patients with renal failure; no dosage adjustment is needed for patients with mild to moderate hepatic impairment.

(3) Can be taken with or without food.

c. **Precaution and monitoring effects**
   (1) Clinically significant **hyponatremia** (sodium < 125 mmol/L) can develop during therapy.
   (2) **Serious dermatological reactions** including Stevens–Johnson syndrome and toxic epidermal necrolysis have been reported in children and adults.
   (3) **Adverse effects**
      (a) **CNS effects** are dizziness, somnolence, headache, ataxia, fatigue, cognitive symptoms (psychomotor slowing, difficult concentrating) and vertigo.
      (b) **GI effects** are vomiting, nausea, and abdominal pain.
      (c) **Neuromuscular and skeletal effects** are abnormal gait and tremor.
      (d) **Ocular effects** are diplopia, nystagmus, and abnormal vision.
      (e) **Endocrine and metabolic effects** common in elderly include hyponatremia (low level of sodium in the blood).
      (f) **Dermatologic:** rash
d. **Significant interactions**
   (1) Oxcarbazepine inhibits **cytochrome P450 2C19** and induces **cytochrome P450 3A4/5** with potentially important effects on plasma concentrations of other drugs.
   (2) Serum concentrations of **phenytoin** and **phenobarbital** are increased.
   (3) It decreases **oral contraceptive** effects, benzodiazepine, and calcium-channel blockers.
   (4) Cross-sensitivity with **carbamazepine** (25% to 30%).

17. **Lacosamide (Vimpat)**
   a. **Mechanism of action**
      (1) Enhances the slow inactivation of voltage-gated sodium channels and binding collapsing response mediator protein 2
      (2) It is water soluble (20 mg/mL)
      (3) Completely orally bioavailable
   b. **Administration and dosage**
      (1) **Adults.** Initially, 50 mg twice daily (100 mg/day). The dose may be increased, at weekly intervals by 100 mg/day given as two divided doses to a daily dose of 200 to 400 mg/day. The safety and effectiveness in children younger than 17 of age have not been established.
      (2) **Oral-intravenous replacement therapy.** When switching from oral dose, the initial total daily intravenous dosage should be equivalent to the total daily dosage and frequency of oral dose.
   c. **Precaution and monitoring effects**
      (1) **Suicidal behavior and ideation:** observed as early as 1 week after starting treatment.
      (2) **Cardiovascular effects:**
         (a) **PR interval prolongation.** Dose-dependent, asymptomatic AV block was observed in 0.4% of patients who received drug.
         (b) Atrial fibrillation and flutter observed in 0.5% of patients who been treated with lacosamide.
      (3) **Syncope:** observed in 1.2% patients who been treated with lacosamide, mostly in patients who received dosage above 400 mg/day.
      (4) **Side effects:** dizziness, headache, diplopia, nausea and vomiting, ataxia, vertigo, blurred vision, and rash.
      (5) **REM program**
         (a) To inform patients of the potential risk of suicidal thoughts and behavior that could occur during treatment.
         (b) **Medication Guide** must be dispensed with this product.
   d. **Significant interactions**
      (1) Does not effect plasma concentration of concomitant anticonvulsive medications.
      (2) Low potential for drug–drug interaction.

18. **Rufinamide (Banzel).** Does not effect the plasma concentration of other antiseizure drugs.
   a. **Mechanism of action**
      (1) Limits excessive firing of sodium-dependent action potentials, in particular prolongation of the inactive state of the channel.
      (2) Its oral bioavailability increases when administrated with food.

b. **Administration and dosage**
   (1) **Adults.** Initially, 400 to 800 mg every 2 days until the maximum daily dosage of 3200 mg daily (administrated in two equally divided doses).
   (2) **Children.** Four years and older, initially 10 mg/kg increments every other day to a target dosage of 45 mg/kg/day or 3200 mg/day (administrated in two equally divided doses).
c. **Precaution and monitoring effects**
   (1) Suicidal behavior and ideation observed as early as 1 week after starting treatment.
   (2) **Cardiovascular effects.** Shortening of the QT interval (up to 20 msec)
   (3) Multiorgan hypersensitivity reactions such as rash and fever.
   (4) **Adverse effects:** dizziness, nausea, diplopia and ataxia, oligomenorrhea, lymphadenopathy, and hematuria.
   (5) **REM program**
      (a) To inform patients of the potential risk of suicidal thoughts and behavior that could occur during treatment.
      (b) **Medication Guide** must be dispensed with this product.
d. **Significant interactions**
   (1) Does not effect plasma concentration of concomitant anticonvulsive of medications.
   (2) Low potential for drug–drug interaction.

19. **Vigabatrin (Sabril)**
   a. **Mechanism of action**
      (1) Irreversible inhibition of GABA-transaminase responsible for the catabolism of GABA.
   b. **Administration and dosage**
      (1) **Adults and 16 years of age:** Initially, 1000 mg daily (in two divided dosage); total daily dose could be increased in 500-mg increments at weekly intervals depending on response.
      (2) **16 years of age and older:** same as adult dosage administration
   c. **Precaution and monitoring effects**
      (1) Vision loss and peripheral visual field defect observed in 30% of adult population. In some cases, it could damage the central retina and may decrease visual acuity. A baseline vision testing should be conducted not later than 4 weeks after starting vigabatrin and then followed every 3 months. The onset of vision loss and occurrence of it varies and cannot be predicted. The vision loss is irreversible and may get worse after discontinuation of the therapy. If the patient does not show substantial clinical benefit with 2 to 4 weeks of initiation when used in children and in adult as within 3 months, the drug should be discontinued.
      (2) Abnormal magnetic resonance imaging (MRI) signal changes characterized by increased T2 signal and restricted diffusion in a symmetric pattern involving deep gray matter areas of the brain (thalamus, basal ganglia, brainstem, cerebellum) have been reported in some infants receiving vigabatrin for infantile spasms; these abnormalities are generally transient and resolves upon drug discontinuation.
      (3) Adverse effect: are somnolence, fatigue, light-headedness, peripheral neuropathy, and anemia. Depression developed in 12% of patients. There were no significant cognitive adverse effects.
      (4) **REM program**
         (a) To increase awareness and reduce risks of treatment, including vision loss and suicidal thoughts and behavior.
         (b) The FDA-approved REM program includes a medication guide, communication plan, elements to ensure safe use, and implementation system requiring prescriber and pharmacy certification and patient enrollment.
   d. **Significant interactions**
      (1) Does not effect plasma concentration of concomitant anticonvulsive of medications.
      (2) Suppresses ALT and AST enzyme activity in up to 90% of the patient's which may preclude the use of these tests to detect hepatic injury.

20. **Less common drugs** are listed in *Table 37-8.*
21. **Vagus nerve stimulation (VNS)**
   a. It is used as adjunctive therapy for adults and children > 12 years of age whose partial seizures are refractory to antiepileptic medications.

Table 37-8 LESS COMMON DRUGS USED IN PRACTICE

Drug	Labeled Indication	Half-Life (hr)	Total Plasma Concentration (mg/L)	Therapeutic Range of Adult Dose (mg/day)	Usual Mode of Elimination	Major Protein Binding Level
Mephobarbital	• Grand mal • Petit mal • Gets converted to phenobarbital • Indicated when phenobarbital must be decreased because of excessive drowsiness • Hyperexcitability • Mood disturbances	11–67	n/a	400–600	Liver	40–60
Mephenytoin	• Tonic–clonic • Psychomotor • Status epilepticus • Used with phenytoin; together more sedative compared to phenytoin alone	95 (active metabolite)	n/a	200–600	Liver > renal	90
Ethotoin	• Tonic–clonic • Psychomotor • Used as second-line therapy; less toxic and less effective than phenytoin (alone or combined)	3–9[a]	15–50	2000–3000	Liver	n/a
Methsuximide	• Absence • Does not precipitate tonic–clonic (compared to other succinimides)	2–40[b]	n/a	1200	Liver	n/a
Phensuximide	• Absence • Less toxic and less effective compared to other succinimides	8[b]	n/a	1000–3000	Urine, bile	n/a
Paramethadione[c]	• Absence • Useful when other seizures exist with absence seizure • *Note*: Do not use with mephenytoin	n/a	n/a	900–2400	Liver ≥ renal	n/a
Trimethadione[c]	• Absence • Useful when other seizures exist with absence seizure • *Note*: Do not use with mephenytoin	6–13 days	≥ 700	900–2400	Liver	0
Pregabalin	• Simple partial seizure	6	n/a	150–600	Renal	0

[a]At high doses, nonlinear kinetic like phenytoin.
[b]Active metabolite.
[c]Possible fetal malformation if used during pregnancy.

b. A programmable signal generator that is implanted in the patient's left upper chest has a bipolar VNS lead that connects the generator to the left vagus nerve in the neck, a programming wand that uses radio-frequency signals to communicate noninvasively with the generator, and hand-held magnets used by the patient or caregiver to manually turn the stimulator on or off.

c. The implantation procedure usually lasts 1 hr under general anesthesia. Once programmed, the generator will deliver intermittent stimulation at the desired setting until any additional programming is entered.

C. **Surgery.** If seizures do not respond to drug therapy, surgery may be performed to remove the epileptogenic brain region. The most common is cortical excision (lobectomy). Between 70% and 80% of patients who have anterior temporal lobectomy have fewer seizures. Between 30% and 40% patients who have frontal lobectomy have fewer seizures.

1. **Indications** for surgery are intractable or disabling seizures recurring for 6 to 12 months. Should be considered for patients with medically refractory seizures.
2. In **stereotaxic surgery**, the surgeon uses three-dimensional coordinates to guide a needle through a hole drilled in the skull, then destroys abnormal pathways via small intracerebral incisions.
3. **Other surgical approaches** include temporal lobe resection, removal of the temporal lobe tip, and cerebral hemispherectomy.

III. COMPLICATIONS

A. **Convulsive status epilepticus.** This disorder is characterized by rapid repetition of generalized tonic–clonic seizures with no recovery of consciousness between seizures. This life-threatening condition may persist for hours or even days; if it lasts longer than 1 hr, severe permanent brain damage may result.

1. **Causes** of status epilepticus include poor therapeutic compliance, intracranial infection or neoplasm, alcohol withdrawal, drug overdose, and metabolic imbalance.
2. **Management**

a. A patent airway must be maintained.

b. If the cause of the condition is unknown, dextrose 50% in water (25 to 30 mL) is given via IV in case hypoglycemia is the cause.

c. If the seizures persist, **diazepam** (10 mg) is administered via IV at a rate not exceeding 2 mg/min until the seizures stop or 20 mg has been given.

d. **Phenytoin or fosphenytoin** is then administered via IV no faster than 50 mg/min to a maximum dose of 11 to 18 mg/kg. Blood pressure is monitored to detect hypotension.

e. If these measures do not stop the seizures, one of the following drugs is given:

(1) **Diazepam** is given as an IV drip of 50 to 100 mg diluted in 500 mL dextrose 5% in water, infused at 40 mL/hr until the seizures stop.

(2) **Phenobarbital** is given as an IV infusion of 8 to 20 mg/kg no faster than 100 mg/min.

f. If seizures continue despite these measures, one of the following steps is then taken:

(1) **Paraldehyde** is given via IV in a dosage of 0.10 to 0.15 mL/kg diluted to a 4% solution in normal saline solution.

(2) **Lidocaine** is given in an IV loading dose of 50 to 100 mg, followed by an infusion of 1 to 2 mg/min.

(3) **General anesthesia** is induced with ventilatory assistance and neuromuscular junction blockade.

B. **Nonconvulsive status epilepticus.** This condition presents as repeated absence seizures or complex partial seizures. The patient's mental state fluctuates; confusion, impaired responses, and automatisms are prominent. **Initial management** typically involves intravenous diazepam. Complex partial status epilepticus may also necessitate administration of such drugs as phenytoin or phenobarbital.

IV. SEIZURE DISORDER AND PREGNANCY

A. **Epidemiology.** About 0.5% of all pregnancies occur in women with epilepsy.

B. **Preconception counseling.** The risks for mother and fetus should be discussed, including the risks of fetal malformation associated with antiepileptic drugs and other genetic factors.

C. **Drug therapy**

1. If the patient is seizure free for at least 2 years, withdrawal of the drug should be considered. If antiepileptic drug therapy is necessary, a switch to monotherapy should be made if possible.
2. Five antiepileptic medications have been used or studied in pregnant patients: carbamazepine, phenobarbital, phenytoin, primidone, and valproic acid. Monotherapy of lamotrigine during pregnancy found no teratogenic effect. Congenital malformations associated with these drugs include craniofacial abnormalities, cardiac defects, and neuronal tube defects. Most of the studies did not consider paternal genetic factors, environmental factors, drug dosing, or combination therapy.
3. Antiepileptic drugs interfere with folate metabolism. Administration of folic acid, 4 mg daily, and multivitamins decreases the risk of malformation, especially of the neuronal tube.
4. Vitamin K, 10 mg/day for the last 1 to 2 months of gestation, will help prevent neonatal hemorrhage, especially in cases of phenytoin or phenobarbital use.
5. **Seizure disorder and oral contraceptives.** Gabapentin, levetiracetam, ethosuximide, valproate, zonisamide, pregabalin, vigabatrin, and tiagabine do not affect the efficacy of oral contraceptives.
6. **Seizure disorder and the elderly population.** The new generation of antiepileptic drugs such as levetiracetam and gabapentin may be more useful owing to low levels of protein binding and safer side effects. Also, the newer agents have less potential for drug interactions than agents eliminated from the liver.

D. **Monitoring**

1. Free serum antiepileptic drug levels should be monitored monthly, immediately before the next dose, and the dose should be adjusted to the lowest dose providing adequate control.
2. Serum α-fetoprotein levels should be checked, and ultrasonography should be performed at 16 weeks of gestation to evaluate for fetal neuronal tube defects. An alternative to these tests is amniocentesis, especially if the mother is taking valproate or carbamazepine.
3. Comprehensive ultrasonography should be performed at 18 and 22 weeks of gestation for patients taking antiepileptic drugs that cause cardiac anomalies.
4. Intrapartum plans should include IV administration of a short-acting benzodiazepine. If there is concern about fetal or maternal respiratory depression, administering IV phenytoin or IM phenobarbital should be considered. Clotting studies should be performed, and 1 mg vitamin K should be given to the infant. Nurses and physicians should be alerted for possible hemorrhage of the infant and apprised that the infant may experience antiepileptic drug withdrawal.

Study Questions

Directions: Each of the questions, statements, or incomplete statements in this section can be correctly answered or completed by **one** of the suggested answers or phrases. Choose the **best** answer.

1. Phenytoin is effective for the treatment of all of the following types of seizures *except*

   (A) generalized tonic–clonic.
   (B) simple partial.
   (C) complex partial.
   (D) absence.
   (E) grand mal.

2. Which of the following anticonvulsants is contraindicated in patients with a history of hypersensitivity to tricyclic antidepressants?

   (A) phenytoin
   (B) ethosuximide
   (C) acetazolamide
   (D) carbamazepine
   (E) phenobarbital

3. Which anticonvulsive drug requires therapeutic monitoring of phenobarbital serum levels as well as its own serum level?

   (A) phenytoin
   (B) primidone
   (C) clonazepam
   (D) ethotoin
   (E) carbamazepine

4. Which anticonvulsive drug treatment has a higher incidence of kidney stones?
   (A) phenytoin
   (B) carbamazepine
   (C) topiramate
   (D) tiagabine

5. What are the most common adverse effects of anticonvulsive drugs?
   (A) headache and dizziness
   (B) gastrointestinal symptoms
   (C) alternation of cognition and mentation
   (D) adverse effects on appetite and body weight
   (E) all of the above

6. Which antiepileptic drug has the least effect on the efficacy of oral contraceptives?
   (A) phenytoin
   (B) tiagabine
   (C) gabapentin
   (D) lamotrigine
   (E) C and D

7. Which of the following drugs could cause hyponatremia?
   (A) carbamazepine
   (B) phenytoin
   (C) oxcarbazepine
   (D) felbamate
   (E) topiramate
   (F) A, C, and D

Answers and Explanations

1. **The answer is D** *[see II.B.2.a.(2)].*
   Phenytoin (diphenylhydantoin) is the most commonly prescribed hydantoin for seizure disorders. It is one of the preferred drugs for generalized tonic–clonic (grand mal) seizures and for partial seizures, both simple and complex. However, phenytoin is not effective for absence (petit mal) seizures.

2. **The answer is D** *[see II.B.1.c.(2)].*
   Carbamazepine is structurally related to the tricyclic antidepressants (e.g., amitriptyline, desipramine, imipramine, nortriptyline, protriptyline) and should not be administered to patients with hypersensitivity to any of the tricyclic antidepressants.

3. **The answer is B** *[see II.B.5–6].*
   Primidone's antiseizure activity may be partly attributable to phenobarbital. In patients receiving primidone, serum levels of both primidone and phenobarbital should be measured.

4. **The answer is C** *[see II.B.12].*
   There is a higher incidence of kidney stones (renal calculus) with topiramate administration.

5. **The answer is E** *[see I.B.1–9].*
   Alternation in cognition and mentation, gastrointestinal symptoms, appetite and body weight, and headache and dizziness are all common adverse effects of anticonvulsive drugs.

6. **The answer is E** *[see IV.C.5].*
   Gabapentin and lamotrigine do not increase the metabolism of oral contraceptives to a clinically significant level; therefore, they could be used with oral contraceptives.

7. **The answer is F** *[see II.B.1; II.B.9; II.B.16].*
   Carbamazepine, oxcarbazepine, and felbamate all cause hyponatremia.

38 Parkinson Disease

AZITA RAZZAGHI

I. DISEASE STATE AND PATHOLOGY

A. **Definition.** Parkinson disease is a slowly progressive degenerative neurological disease characterized by tremor, rigidity, bradykinesia (sluggish neuromuscular responsiveness), and postural instability. Parkinson disease was first described by Dr. James Parkinson in 1817 as "shaking palsy."

B. **Incidence**

1. It has a prevalence of 1 to 2 per 1000 of the general population and 2 per 100 among people $>$ 65 years.
2. Onset generally occurs between age 50 and 65; it usually occurs in the 60s.

C. **Pathogenesis.** Parkinson disease is a neurodegenerative disease associated with **depigmentation of the substantia nigra** and the **loss of dopaminergic input to the basal ganglia** (extrapyramidal system); it is characterized by distinctive **motor disability**. The basal ganglia are responsible for initiating, sequencing, and modulating motor activity.

1. In healthy individuals, dopamine is produced by neurons that project from the substantia nigra to the neostriatum (which includes caudate and putamen) and globus pallidus. In these areas, dopamine acts as an inhibitory neurotransmitter.
2. Lewy bodies are widespread but occur especially in the basal ganglia, brainstem, spinal cord, and sympathetic ganglia.
3. In Parkinson disease, the loss of dopamine-producing neurons in the substantia nigra results in an imbalance between dopamine, an inhibitory neurotransmitter, and the excitatory neurotransmitter acetylcholine. Alterations in the concentrations of other neurotransmitters, such as norepinephrine, serotonin, and γ-aminobutyric acid (GABA) are also involved in the pathophysiology of Parkinson disease (*Figure 38-1*).

D. **Cause**. Several forms of Parkinson disease have been recognized.

1. **Primary (idiopathic) Parkinson disease**
   a. This is also called classic Parkinson disease or **paralysis agitans**.
   b. The cause is unknown; and although treatment may be palliative, the disease is incurable.
   c. Most patients suffer from this type of parkinsonism.
   d. **Hypotheses of neuronal loss** in idiopathic Parkinson disease are as follows:
      (1) **Absorption of highly potent neurotoxins (environmental)**, such as carbon monoxide, manganese, solvents, and *N*-methyl-4-phenyl-1,2,3,6-tetrahydropyridine (MPTP), which is a product of improper synthesis of a synthetic heroin-like compound. Exposure to these agents, alone or in combination with the neuronal loss of age, may be the cause of Parkinson disease.
      (2) **Exposure to the free radicals**. Normally, dopamine is catabolized by monoamine oxidase (MAO). Hydrogen peroxide and production of free radicals—both toxic to cells—are products of catabolism. Protective mechanisms, enzymes, and free radical scavengers, such as vitamins E and C, protect cells from damage. It is proposed that either a decrease in these protective mechanisms or an increase in the production of dopamine causes a destruction of the neurons by free radicals.
   e. **Genetics factors.** Genes that link to Parkinson disease, such as alpha-synuclein and parkin, are further being studied in treatment and diagnosis of Parkinson disease.

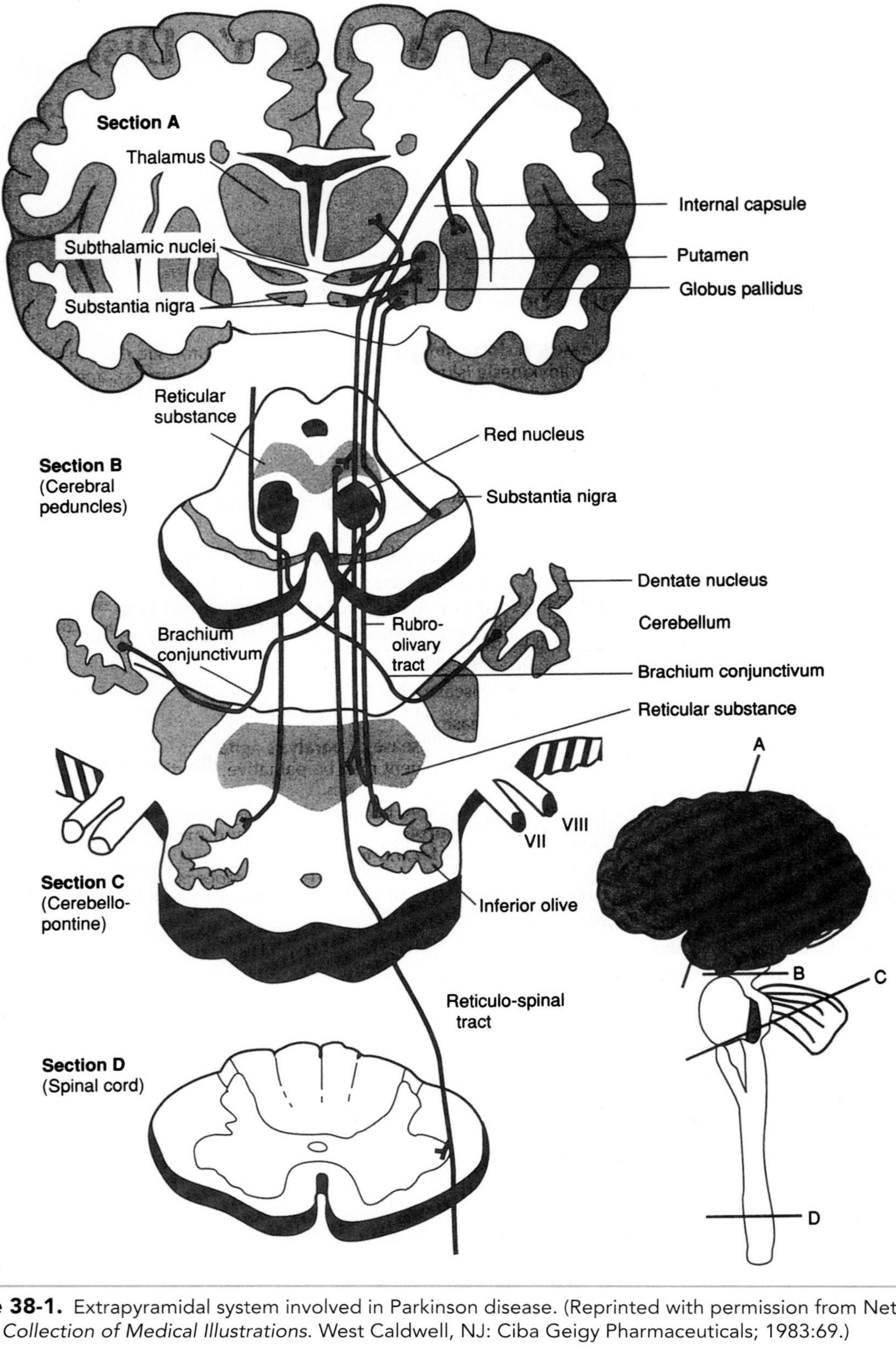

Figure 38-1. Extrapyramidal system involved in Parkinson disease. (Reprinted with permission from Netter F. *Ciba Collection of Medical Illustrations*. West Caldwell, NJ: Ciba Geigy Pharmaceuticals; 1983:69.)

2. **Secondary parkinsonism—from a known cause**
   a. Only a small percentage of cases are secondary, and many of these are curable.
   b. Secondary parkinsonism may be caused by drugs, including dopamine antagonists, such as the following:
      (1) Phenothiazines (e.g., chlorpromazine, perphenazine)
      (2) Butyrophenones (e.g., haloperidol)
      (3) Reserpine
   c. Poisoning by chemicals or toxins may be the cause; these include
      (1) Carbon monoxide poisoning
      (2) Heavy-metal poisoning, such as that by manganese or mercury
      (3) MPTP, a commercial compound used in organic synthesis and found (as a side product) in an illegal meperidine analog
   d. Infectious causes include
      (1) Encephalitis (viral)
      (2) Syphilis
   e. Other causes include
      (1) Arteriosclerosis
      (2) Degenerative diseases of the central nervous system (CNS), such as progressive supranuclear palsy
      (3) Metabolic disorders such as Wilson disease

E. **Signs and symptoms**

1. **Tremor**
   a. Tremor may be the initial complaint in some patients. It is most evident at rest (**resting tremor**) and with low-frequency movement. When the thumb and forefinger are involved, it is known as the **pill-rolling tremor**. Before pills were made by machine, pharmacists made tablets (pills) by hand, hence the name (*Figure 38-2*).
   b. Some patients experience **action tremor** (most evident during activity), which can exist with or before the resting tremor develops.
2. **Limb rigidity** is present in almost all patients. It is detected clinically when the arm responds with a ratchet-like (i.e., cogwheeling) movement when the limb is moved passively. This is owing to a tremor that is superimposed on the rigidity.
3. **Akinesia or bradykinesia.** Akinesia is characterized by difficulty in initiating movements, and bradykinesia is a slowness in performing common voluntary movements, including standing,

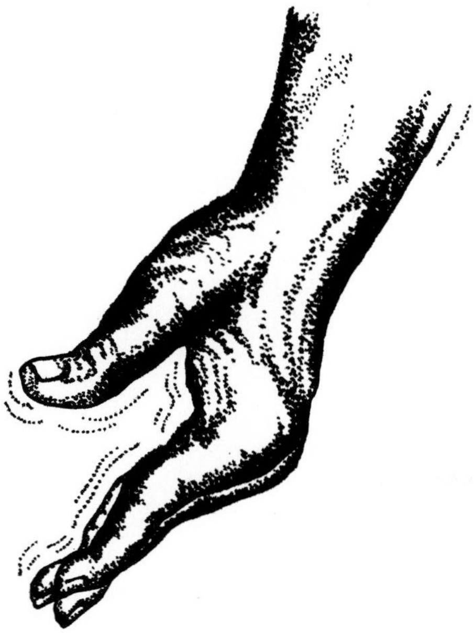

Figure 38-2. Resting (or static) tremors. (Adapted from Bates B. *A Guide to Physical Examination and History Taking*. 5th ed. Philadelphia, PA: Lippincott Williams & Wilkins; 1991:197.)

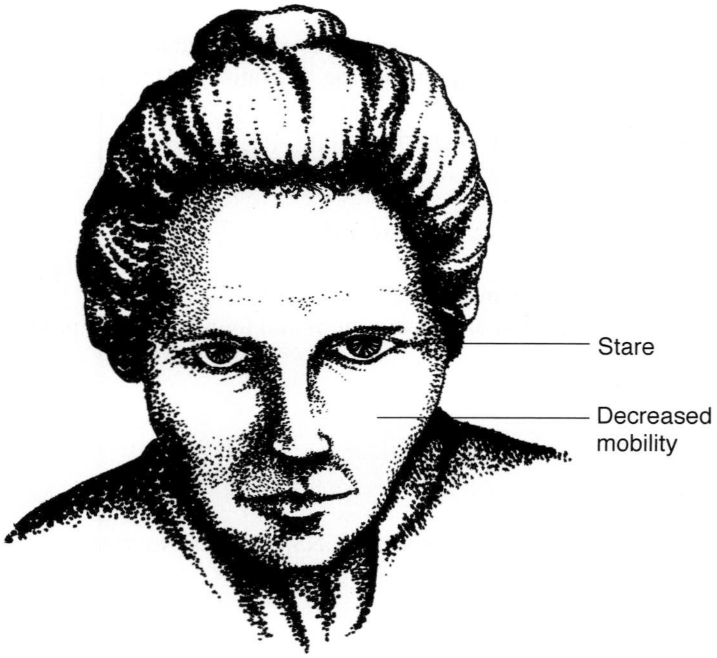

Figure 38-3. Masked face of Parkinson disease. (Adapted from Bates B. *A Guide to Physical Examination and History Taking*. 5th ed. Philadelphia, PA: Lippincott Williams & Wilkins; 1991:197.)

walking, eating, writing, and talking. The lines of the patient's face are smooth, and the expression is fixed (**masked face**) with little evidence of spontaneous emotional responses (*Figure 38-3*).

4. **Gait and postural difficulties.** Characteristically, patients walk with a stooped, flexed posture; a short, shuffling stride; and a diminished arm swing in rhythm with the legs. There may be a tendency to accelerate or festinate (*Figure 38-4*).
5. **Changes in mental status.** Mental status changes, including depression (50%), dementia (25%), and psychosis are associated with the disease and may be precipitated or worsened by drugs.

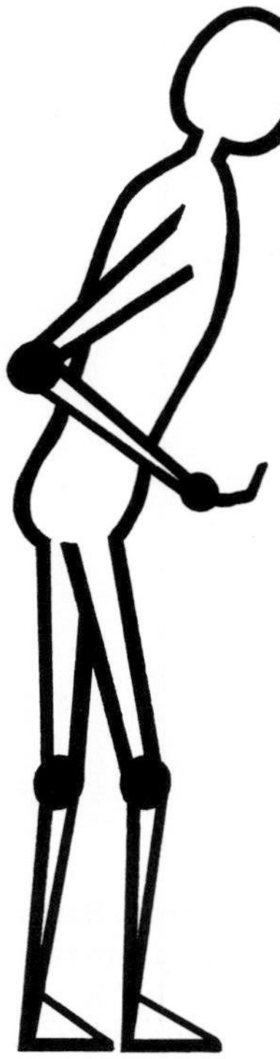

Figure 38-4. Characteristic walk of patients with Parkinson disease. (Adapted from Bates B. *A Guide to Physical Examination and History Taking*. 5th ed. Philadelphia, PA: Lippincott Williams & Wilkins; 1991:553.)

6. **Unified Parkinson disease rating scale (UPDRS)**
   a. **To evaluate the clinical efficacy** of antiparkinson drugs and **to monitor disease progression**, most investigators have used the UPDRS.
      (1) The disadvantages associated with the use of scales for rating the functional and motor disabilities of patients with Parkinson disease include the potential of interrater variability and imprecision because of the semiquantitative scoring.
      (2) The result of testing depends highly on the stage of the disease, whether the patient is being evaluated during an on or off period, and the relative distribution of the improvement across all the items evaluated.
   b. **Part I** of the UPDRS is an **evaluation of mentation**, **behavior**, and **mood**.
   c. **Part II** is a **self-reported evaluation of the activities of daily living (ADLs)** and includes speech, swallowing, handwriting, ability to cut food, dressing, hygiene, falling, salivating, turning in bed, and walking.
   d. **Part III** is a **clinician-scored motor evaluation**.
      (1) Patients are evaluated for speech, rest-tremor facial expression and mobility, action or postural tremor of hands, rigidity, finger taps, hand movements, rapid alternative pronation–supination movement of hands, leg agility, ease of arising from a chair, posture, postural stability, gait, and bradykinesia.
      (2) Each item is evaluated on a scale of 0 to 4.
         (a) **A rating of 0** on the motor performance evaluation scale indicates **normal performance**.
         (b) **A rating of 4** on the motor performance evaluation scale indicates **severely impaired performance**.
   e. **Part IV** is the **Hoehn and Yahr** staging of severity of Parkinson disease (*Table 38-1*).
   f. **Part V** is the **Schwab and England ADL scale**.

F. **Diagnosis**
   1. Diagnosis depends on clinical findings.
   2. Tests (including imaging) are most often used to rule out an origin of secondary Parkinson disease.
   3. New technologies—for example, positron emission tomography (PET) scan—are used to visualize dopamine uptake in the substantia nigra and basal ganglia. The PET scan measures the extent of neuronal loss in these areas.
   4. A specific form of single photon emission computed tomography (SPECT) can be helpful for diagnosis of parkinsonian syndromes and nonparkinsonian syndromes, particularly essential tremor.
   5. Other diseases that are similar to Parkinson disease are multiple system atrophy (striatonigral degeneration, olivopontocerebellar atrophy, Shy-Drager syndrome), corticobasal ganglionic degeneration, and progressive supranuclear palsy.
   6. **Other investigational diagnostic tools.** (1) transcranial ultrasound, (2) examine deficits in olfaction, and (3) detection of oligometric alpha-synuclein in blood of patients with Parkinson disease.

G. **Treatment** (*Figure 38-5*)
   1. **Nondrug treatment**
      a. **Exercise** is an important adjunctive therapy and is most beneficial. Although exercise does not help with the symptoms of Parkinson disease, regular focused exercise, stretching, and strengthening activities can have a positive effect on mobility and mood.

Table 38-1 STAGES OF PARKINSON DISEASE

Stage	Characteristics
0	No clinical signs evident
I	Unilateral involvement, including the major features of tremor, rigidity, or bradykinesia; minimal functional impairment
II	Bilateral involvement but no postural abnormalities
III	Mild to moderate bilateral disease, mild postural imbalance, but still ability to function independently
IV	Bilateral involvement with postural instability; patient requires substantial assistance
V	Severe disease; patient restricted to bed or wheelchair unless aided

Reprinted with permission from Hoehn MM, Yahr MD. Parkinsonism: onset, progression, and mortality. *Neurology*. 1967;17:427.

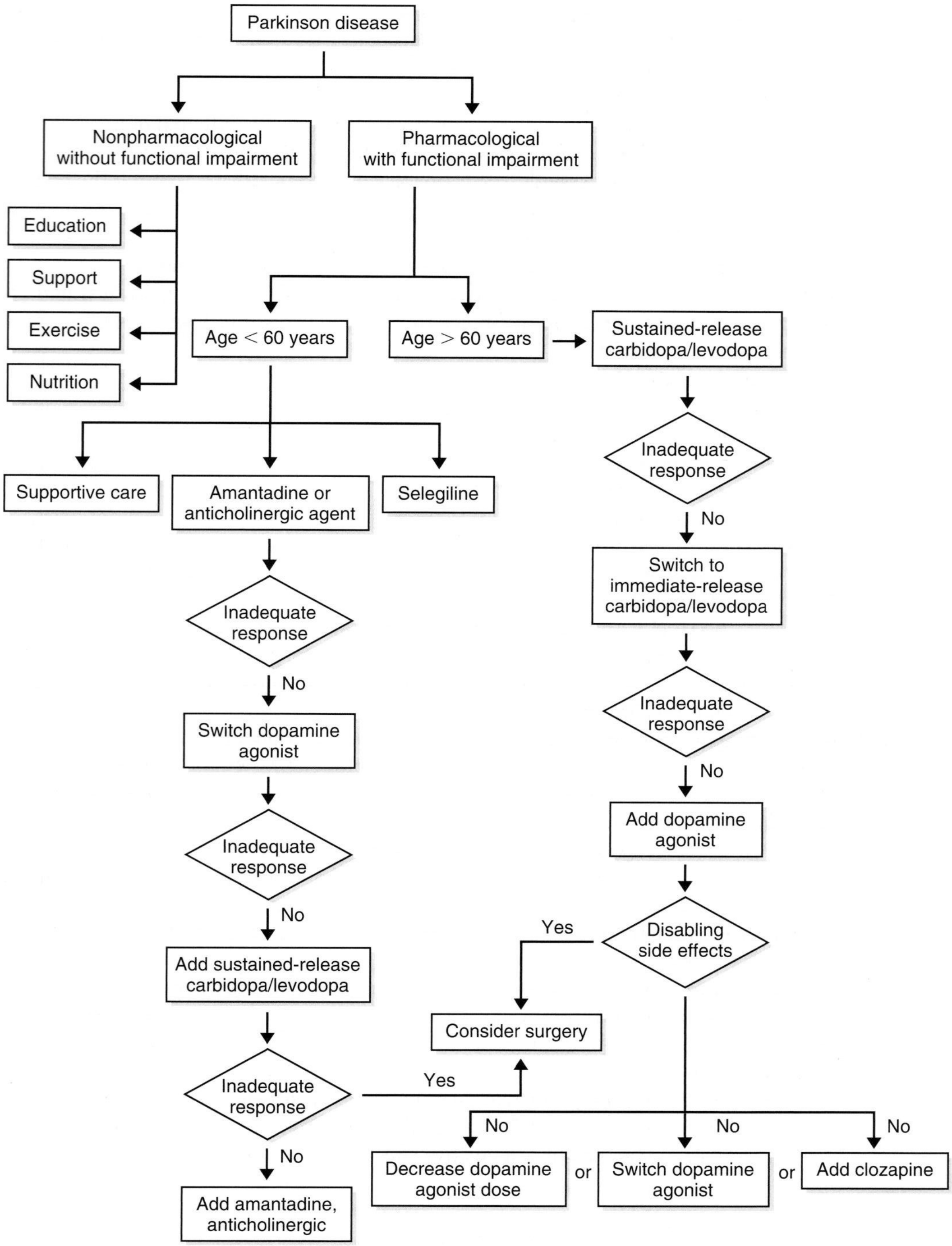

Figure 38-5. Management of Parkinson disease.

b. Nutrition. Patients with Parkinson disease are at increased risk of poor nutrition, weight loss, and reduced muscle mass. Examples of the beneficial effects of proper nutrition in this group of patients include the following:

(1) Sufficient fiber and fluid intake help prevent constipation associated with Parkinson disease and the medications used to treat the disease.

(2) Calcium supplementation helps maintain the existing bone structure.

(3) Excessive dietary protein in the late stages of the disease causes erratic responses to levodopa therapy.

(4) A large body of literature supports the pathophysiological role of antioxidants as a neuroprotective agent and its role in decreasing progression of Parkinson disease. Products such as α-tocopherol or vitamin, creatine, coenzyme Q10 act as scavengers of free radical which are harmful to cells.

2. **Drug therapy for symptomatic relief.** Treatment is divided into two generalized categories: symptomatic therapies and preventive or protective measures. Neuroprotective strategies are used to slow the development and progression of the disorder.

H. Drug treatment: Neuroprotective treatment

1. MAO-Bs, such as selegiline and tocopherol (vitamin E), act as a scavenger of free radicals.
2. Dopamine agonists serve as scavengers of free radicals and decrease dopamine turnover, which reduces oxidative stress. During early development of the disease, there are increases in oxidative stress. Four classes of drugs are available.
   - **a.** Anticholinergics (for resting tremor)
   - **b.** Precursor of dopamine (e.g., carbidopa/levodopa)
   - **c.** Direct-acting dopamine agonists (e.g., bromocriptine)
   - **d.** Indirect-acting dopamine agonists
     - **(1)** Decrease reuptake (e.g., amantadine)
     - **(2)** Decrease metabolism (e.g., selegiline)
3. **Drug therapy for treating associated symptoms**
   - **a. Tricyclic antidepressants** are used to treat **depression**. They exhibit some dopaminergic and anticholinergic effects.
   - **b. β-Blockers**, especially **propranolol** with its high lipophilicity, **benzodiazepines**, and **primidone**, are medications used for **action tremor**. Usually, patients show a clinical response in low doses.
   - **c. Antihistamines**. Diphenhydramine hydrochloride has some mild anticholinergic effects and is used for symptomatic release of mild tremor; because of its adverse reaction in the CNS, it should be used with caution in the elderly.
4. **General principles of drug therapy**
   - **a.** If a patient does not respond to an agent in one class, another class should be tried. Studies show that some patients respond to one agent when they fail to respond to the other.
   - **b.** Therapy should be started with a low dose and titrated up. Response usually is seen within a few days after starting therapy.
   - **c.** If a second agent is added to the drug therapy, the dose of the first medication should be decreased to minimize side effects.
   - **d.** Drug therapy should never be discontinued suddenly because withdrawal may exacerbate the symptoms.
5. **Definitions concerning drug therapy**
   - **a. Dyskinesia/dystonia** typically presents as oral-facial movements, grimacing, or jerky and writhing movements of the trunk and extremities. They are always reversible with antiparkinsonian medications, and they decrease or diminish with dose reduction. Symptoms of Parkinson disease may reappear by reducing the dose, and it is the clinical judgment of the physician or the preference of the patient whether to continue with the drug regimen or tolerate the side effects. There are three types of dyskinesia/dystonia: peak-dose dyskinesia, biphasic dyskinesia, and off-period dystonia. All could benefit from sustained-release preparations.
     - **(1)** Peak-dose dyskinesia
       - **(a)** Could be corrected with sustained-release preparations.
       - **(b)** Decrease L-dopa dose or add catechol-*O*-methyltransferase (COMT) inhibitor.
       - **(c)** Add amantadine.
       - **(d)** Perform surgery.
     - **(2)** Biphasic dyskinesia
       - **(a)** Could be corrected with sustained-release preparations.
       - **(b)** Decrease L-dopa dose and increase dopaminergic dose. If symptoms are still present, a COMT inhibitor should be added.
       - **(c)** Amantadine may be helpful.
     - **(3)** Off-period dystonia
       - **(a)** Decrease L-dopa dose.
       - **(b)** Increase dopaminergic dose.

b. **On–off effect** describes oscillations in response (at the receptor site) and sudden changes in mobility from no symptoms to full parkinsonian symptoms in a matter of minutes. No direct relationship between the on–off effect and drug levels has been found. Usually, a second drug is added to the therapy regimen to correct the effect. Reducing the dose of one drug and adding a second drug may also be useful. Could be managed by adding entacapone, dopamine agonist, amantadine, or selegiline.

c. **End-dose effect**, known also as the **wearing-off effect**, occurs at a latter part of the dosing interval; it happens after a few years of L-dopa therapy. Reduce the single L-dopa dose and spread the total L-dopa dose over a larger number of single doses. Change to a dopamine agonist and use a sustained-release formulation of L-dopa. Could be managed by adding entacapone, dopamine agonist, amantadine, or selegiline.

d. **Drug holiday**. Long-term levodopa use results in down regulation of dopamine receptors. A drug holiday allows striatal nigra dopamine receptors to be resensitized, although controversy exists regarding the consequences and the outcome of this holiday.

6. **Physical rehabilitation** restores patients' physical function and independence through physical and occupational therapy. Such therapy helps patients with managing big and small muscle groups by focusing on maintaining coordination, dexterity, flexibility, and range of motions.

7. **Psychological rehabilitation** provides support for patients and their families. Keep in mind that patients with Parkinson disease have a high incidence of depression and that, in later stages of the disease, they develop dementia (*Table 38-2*).

8. **Secondary effects of Parkinson disease include**
   a. **Cardiovascular effects**, including orthostatic hypotension and arrhythmia.
   b. **Gastrointestinal effects**, including constipation and hypersalivation.
   c. **Genitourinary effects**, including increased urinary frequency and impotence.
   d. **Central nervous system effects**, including hallucinations, depression, and psychosis. Could be treated with reducing or eliminating amantadine, selegiline, anticholinergics, or dopamine agonists.

9. **Late disabilities of Parkinson disease** can be divided into two groups.
   a. **Levodopa-related disabilities**, which include motor fluctuation, dyskinesia, neuropsychiatric toxicity, and reduced response

Table 38-2 OVERVIEW OF PARKINSON DISEASE MANAGEMENT

		Treatment Considerations	
Stage	**Characteristics**	**Physical**	**Psychosocial**
Early	Fully functional May have unilateral tremor, rigidity	Preventive exercise program	Education Information
Early middle	Symptoms bilateral, bradykinesia rigidity Mild speech impairment Axial rigidity, stooped posture, stiffness Gait impairment begins	Corrective exercise program	Counseling Support group Monitor for depression
Late middle	All symptoms worse but independent in ADLs May need minor assistance Balance problems	Compensatory and corrective exercise Speech therapy Occupational therapy	Caregiver issues (medications, mobility) Monitor for dementia
Late	Severely disabled, impaired Dependent with ADLs	Compensatory exercise Dietary concerns Skin care Hygiene Pulmonary function	Dementia Depression

ADLs, activities of daily living.
Reprinted with permission from Custin TM. Overview of Parkinson's disease management. *Phys Ther.*1995;75:363–373.

b. **Non-levodopa–related disabilities**, which include cognitive impairment, instability resulting in more frequent falls, gait disturbance, incontinence, dysphagia, and speech disturbance

c. Late disabilities management therapies include the following:

   (1) **Motor fluctuation**. Altering the levodopa dosage and timing, using alternative means of levodopa administration, delivery, and absorption; using direct-acting dopamine agonists or experimental agonists; altering metabolism of dopamine and levodopa parental agonists; using glutamate antagonists; and performing functional neurosurgery

   (2) **Miscellaneous** late disabilities and management therapies include

      (a) **Urinary urgency**: oxybutynin
      (b) **Urinary retention**: apomorphine
      (c) **Constipation**: fiber, polyethylene glycols
      (d) **Tenesmus**: clonazepam, apomorphine
      (e) **Hypersalivation**: antihistamine, anticholinergic
      (f) **Dysphagia**: liquid levodopa
      (g) **Sweating crises**: β-blockers, anticholinergic agents
      (h) **Daytime sleepiness**: selegiline
      (i) **Nightmares**: amitriptyline, clonazepam
      (j) **Panic attacks and depression**: liquid levodopa, amitriptyline
      (k) **Orthostatic hypotension**: domperidone, desmopressin
      (l) **Dysphonia**: reduce levodopa dosage, speech therapy
      (m) **Pain**: amitriptyline, fluvoxamine

II. INDIVIDUAL DRUGS

A. **Anticholinergic agents** are used for mild symptoms, predominantly tremors.

1. **Mechanism of action**. This class of drugs blocks the excitatory neurotransmitter cholinergic influence in the basal ganglia. These drugs are more effective for tremor and rigidity than for bradykinesia and less effective for postural imbalance.

2. **Administration and dosage** (*Table 38-3*)

3. **Precautions and monitoring effects**

   a. Anticholinergics should be used with caution in patients with obstructed gastrointestinal (GI) or genitourinary (GU) tracts, narrow-angle glaucoma, or severe cardiac disease. Physicians should be notified if a rapid heartbeat or eye pain is experienced. (Frequent ophthalmological visits are recommended.)

   b. The sedative side effects of antihistamines may be beneficial in some patients.

   c. Alcohol and other CNS depressants should be used with caution.

   d. **Adverse effects** of anticholinergic therapy include the following:

      (1) **Peripheral anticholinergic effects** include dry mouth (hard candies may be helpful); decreased sweating, resulting in decreased tolerance to heat; urinary retention; constipation (stool softeners may be helpful); increased intraocular tension; and nausea. Because of patients' decreased tolerance to heat, these agents should be used with caution in hot weather. They should also be taken with food to minimize GI upset.

      (2) **CNS effects** include dizziness, delirium, disorientation, anxiety, agitation, hallucinations, and impaired memory. The incidence of CNS effects increases in elderly individuals.

      (3) **Cardiovascular effects** include hypotension and orthostatic hypotension.

4. **Significant interactions**

   a. Side effects may be potentiated by other drugs with anticholinergic activity, such as **antihistamines, antidepressants**, and **phenothiazines**.

   b. Anticholinergic agents increase **digoxin** levels.

   c. When anticholinergic agents are taken with **haloperidol**, the following occurs:

      (1) Schizophrenic symptoms may increase.
      (2) Haloperidol levels may decrease.
      (3) The severity of (not the risk of) tardive dyskinesia may increase.

   d. When **phenothiazines** are taken with anticholinergic drugs, the effects of the phenothiazines decrease and the anticholinergic symptoms increase.

   e. Patients on high doses of anticholinergics combined with **levodopa** should be watched for decreased levodopa activity because of a delayed gastric emptying time.

Table 38-3 DOSAGE RANGE AND CHARACTERISTICS OF DRUG TREATMENT

Drug	Time to Peak Concentration (hr)	Half-Life (hr)	Daily Dosage Range (mg/day)
Anticholinergic agents			
Benztropine	n/a	n/a	1–6
Biperiden	1.0–1.5	18.4–24.3	2–8
Procyclidine	1.1–2.0	11.5–12.6	6–20
Trihexyphenidyl	1.0–1.3	5.6–10.2	2–15
Ethopropazine	n/a	n/a	50–400
Dopamine agents			
Carbidopa/levodopa	1	1.0–1.75	10/100–200/2000
Carbidopa/levodopa, sustained-release	2	> standard treatment	10/400–25/1000, in 2–3 divided doses
Amantadine	4–8	9.7–14.5	100–400
Bromocriptine	1–3	3–8	2.5–40.0
Selegiline	0.5–2.0	2.0–20.5	5–10
Selegiline Oral Disintegrating table*	1	1–3 hrs	0.5–1.0 mg
Rasagiline	1	1.3–3.0 hrs	0.5–1.0 mg
Non-ergot dopamine agents			
Pramipexole	1–2 (3–4[a])	8–12[b]	1.5–4.5, in 3 divided doses
Ropinirole	1–2(3–4[a])	6	3–24, in 3 divided doses
COMT inhibitor	0.5–4.0	70	0.5–6.0
Tolcapone	2	2–3	300–600
Entacapone	1	2–3	200–1600
Rotigotine	15–27	5–7 hrs	2–6 mg
Apomorphine hydrochloride injection (SC)	1	40 mins	2–6 mg

[a]With food.
[b]Older than 65 years of age.
COMT, catechol-*O*-methyltransferase; *n/a*, not available.
*avoids first-pass effect
SC, subcutaneous injection.

B. Dopamine precursor. Levodopa/carbidopa is the most effective drug for managing Parkinson disease; however, prolonged use decreases its therapeutic effects (there is a decline in efficacy after 3 to 5 years) and increases adverse drug reactions. Dopamine does not cross the blood–brain barrier; therefore, a precursor is used. Peripheral conversion of levodopa to dopamine causes adverse reactions like nausea, vomiting, cardiac arrhythmias, and postural hypotension. To decrease the peripheral conversion and peripheral adverse effects, a peripheral dopa decarboxylase inhibitor (carbidopa) is added to levodopa.

1. Mechanism of action

a. Levodopa is converted to dopamine by the enzyme dopa decarboxylase, which elevates CNS levels of dopamine.

b. The sustained-release formulation is designed to release the drug over 4 to 6 hrs, thereby inhibiting variation in plasma concentration and decreasing motor fluctuation "off" time or improving overall dose response in patients with advanced disease.

2. Administration and dosage (*Table 38-3*)

a. It is necessary to give at least 100 mg daily of carbidopa to decrease the incidence of the peripheral conversion of levodopa and GI side effects (e.g., nausea) and increase the bioavailability of levodopa for the CNS.

b. If carbidopa is given in a separate dosage form, the dose of levodopa can be decreased by 75%.

c. Carbidopa given separately or in addition permits to lower dose of levodopa with decrease in GI side effect and more rapid dosage titration (max dose 200 mg/day).

d. Sustained-release preparations are approximately 30% less bioavailable as compared with levodopa/carbidopa. Because of this lower bioavailability, the daily dosage should be higher. If a patient is receiving a standard preparation and needs to be converted to the sustained-release dose, approximately 10% more levodopa should initially be added to the daily dosage and at least 3 days should pass between increased dosages; then gradually increase the levodopa dose up to 30% of standard preparation.

e. With the sustained-release preparation, the peak plasma concentration is lower and the trough plasma concentration is higher.

f. The sustained-release preparation could be divided in half at the scored point only. The tablet should not be chewed or crushed.

g. When carbidopa is given to patients being treated with levodopa, give the two drugs at the same time, starting with no more than 20% to 25% of the previous daily dosage of levodopa and initiating therapy with carbidopa and levodopa.

h. Long-term treatment could lead to motor fluctuation and dyskinesias, especially at high doses.

3. **Precautions and monitoring effects**

a. Levodopa must be used with caution in patients with narrow-angle glaucoma.

b. Levodopa may activate a malignant melanoma in patients with suspicious undiagnosed skin lesions or a history of melanoma.

c. The efficacy of levodopa declines with long-term therapy by desensitizing the receptors or because of the decreased number of receptors, resulting from the progression of the disease.

d. **Adverse drug reactions**

(1) **GI effects** include anorexia, nausea and vomiting, and abdominal distress. Levodopa should be taken with food to minimize stomach upset.

(2) **Cardiovascular effects** include postural hypotension and tachycardia.

(3) **Musculoskeletal effects** include dystonia or choreiform muscle movement.

(4) **CNS effects** include confusion, memory changes, depression, hallucinations, and psychosis. Physicians should be notified if any of these symptoms occur.

(5) **Hematological effects** include hemolytic anemia, leukopenia, and agranulocytosis (rare).

4. **Significant interactions**

a. **Antacids** cause rapid and complete intestinal levodopa absorption (by decreasing gastric emptying time).

b. **Hydantoin** decreases the effectiveness of levodopa.

c. **Methionine** increases the clinical signs of Parkinson disease.

d. **Metoclopramide** increases the bioavailability of levodopa, which decreases the effects of metoclopramide on gastric emptying and on lower esophageal pressure. As a dopamine blocker, it may also precipitate parkinsonian symptoms.

e. False-positive results are seen with the Coombs test.

f. The uric acid test increases with the calorimetric method but not with the uricase method.

g. Hypertensive reactions may occur if levodopa is administered to patients receiving **MAO inhibitors**. MAO inhibitors must be discontinued 2 weeks before starting levodopa.

h. Administering **papaverine** may decrease the effect of levodopa.

i. **Tricyclic antidepressants** decrease the rate and extent of absorption of levodopa; hypertensive episodes have been reported when levodopa is combined with tricyclic antidepressants.

j. **Food** decreases the rate and extent of absorption and transport to the CNS across the blood–brain barrier. A **protein-restricted diet** may also help minimize the "fluctuations" (i.e., the decreased response to levodopa) at the end of each day or at various times of the day.

k. **Antihypertensive agents increase risk of postural hypotension**.

C. **Direct-acting dopamine agonists** are classified as ergot derivatives (such as bromocriptine) and nonergolines (such as pramipexole and ropinirole).

1. These agents mimic dopamine agonist and reduce motor fluctuations.
2. Drugs in this class have a range of half-lives, and the half-life of any particular drug can vary among patients.
3. These drugs are not metabolized by the oxidative pathway and do not produce free-radical metabolites.
4. Dopamine agonists may have a direct antioxidative effect.
5. They take longer than L-dopa to reach effective doses and require supplementary L-dopa for relief of symptoms after a varying period.

6. Common side effects are nausea and psychiatric side effects similar to L-dopa, such as hallucinations and delusions; dyskinesias are less common.
7. Other adverse effects are headache, nasal congestion, erythromelalgia, pleural and retroperitoneal fibrosis, pulmonary infiltrates, and vasospasm (except with the new, nonergot derivatives such as ropinirole).
8. Annual chest radiographs have been recommended for patients on high-dose therapy with bromocriptine to detect pleuropulmonary changes.
9. New dopaminergic agonists (non-ergot derivatives) cause postural hypotension, sleep disturbances, peripheral edema, constipation, nausea, dyskinesias, and confusion.
10. **Bromocriptine (Parlodel)**
    a. **Mechanism of action**. Bromocriptine is responsible for directly stimulating postsynaptic dopamine receptors; it is most commonly used as an adjunct to levodopa therapy in patients
        (1) with a deteriorating response to levodopa,
        (2) with a limited clinical response to levodopa secondary to an inability to tolerate higher doses, and
        (3) who are experiencing fluctuations in response to levodopa.
    b. **Administration and dosage** (*Table 38-3*)
        (1) Initially, patients are given one-half of a tablet twice daily, which is then increased to one tablet twice daily every 2 to 3 days.
        (2) Patients' responses are extremely variable. Many patients show a dopamine antagonist response at both low and high doses, with the desirable agonist response in the midrange.
        (3) Because postural hypotension may result from the first few doses of bromocriptine, the first dose should be administered with the patient lying down, and sudden changes in posture should be avoided.
    c. **Precautions and monitoring effects**
        (1) Bromocriptine may cause a first-dose phenomenon that can trigger sudden cardiovascular collapse. It should be used with caution in patients with a history of myocardial infarction or arrhythmias.
        (2) Early in therapy, dizziness, drowsiness, and fainting may occur, so patients should be cautious about driving or operating machinery. A physician should be notified if these symptoms appear.
        (3) **Cardiac dysrhythmias**. Patients on bromocriptine were found to have significantly more episodes of atrial premature contractions and sinus tachycardia.
        (4) **Other adverse effects**
            (a) **GI effects**, including anorexia, nausea, vomiting, and abdominal distress, may be decreased by taking bromocriptine with food.
            (b) **Cardiovascular effects** include postural hypotension (to which tolerance develops) and tachycardia. Blood pressure must be monitored, particularly for patients taking antihypertensive medication.
            (c) **Pulmonary effects**, including reversible infiltrations, pleural effusions, and pleural thickening, may develop after long-term treatment, so pulmonary function should be monitored in patients treated longer than 6 months.
            (d) **CNS effects**, including confusion, memory changes, depression, and hallucinations, as well as psychosis, may be exacerbated by bromocriptine; thus, patients with psychiatric illnesses must be monitored.
    d. **Significant interactions**
        (1) A combination of **antihypertensive drugs** and bromocriptine could decrease blood pressure.
        (2) **Dopamine antagonists** increase the effect of bromocriptine.

D. **Indirect-acting dopamine agonists**
1. **Selegiline (Eldepryl)**
    a. **Mechanism of action**
        (1) MAO catabolizes various catecholamines (e.g., dopamine, norepinephrine, epinephrine), serotonin, and various exogenous amines (e.g., tyramines) found in foods (e.g., aged cheese, beer, wine, smoked meat) and drugs. Lack of MAO in the intestinal tract causes absorption of these amines, creating a hypertensive crisis. MAO type A is predominantly found in the

intestinal tract, and MAO type B in the brain. They differ in their substrate specificity and tissue distribution. This specificity decreases with selegiline as the dose increases. Most patients experience side effects at doses of selegiline higher than 30 to 40 mg/day.

(2) Selegiline is a selective inhibitor of MAO-B, which prevents the breakdown of dopamine selectively in the brain at recommended doses.

(3) Selegiline is most commonly used as an adjunct with levodopa/carbidopa when patients experience a "wearing-off" phenomenon; it decreases the amount of off time and decreases the dose needed of levodopa/carbidopa by 10% to 30%.

(4) Results of some studies show that selegiline delays the time before treatment with a more potent dopaminergic drug like levodopa is needed; the proposed mechanism of action is that an oxidation mechanism contributes to the emergence and progression of Parkinson disease.

b. Administration and dosage (*Table 38-3*). Exceeding the recommended dose of 10 mg/day increases the risk of losing MAO selectivity.

(1) **Oral capsule/tablet**: 5 mg (maximum of 10 mg/day)

(2) **Oral disintegrating tablet**: 1.25 mg daily may be increased up to 2.5 mg daily. Disintegrating tablets maximum of 2.5 mg daily.

(3) **Transdermal:** 6 mg/24 hrs apply upper torso, high on the outer surface of the upper arm, avoid exposure of application site to external heat resources. Excessive heat will increase absorption.

c. Precautions and monitoring effects

(1) **Hypertensive crisis.** See II.D.1.a.(1).

(2) Levodopa-associated side effects may be increased because the increased amounts of dopamine react with supersensitive postsynaptic receptors. Reducing the dose of levodopa/carbidopa by 10% to 30% may decrease levodopa side effects.

(3) Patients should be educated about foods and drugs containing tyramine and the signs and symptoms of hypertensive reactions.

(4) **CNS effects** include dizziness, confusion, headache, hallucinations, vivid dreams, dyskinesias, behavioral and mood changes, and depression. Patients who experience insomnia should avoid taking the drug late in the day.

(5) **Cardiovascular effects** include orthostatic hypotension, hypertension, arrhythmia, palpitations, sinus bradycardia, and syncope.

(6) **GI effects** include nausea and abdominal pain and **lead to GI bleeding**, weight loss, poor appetite, and dysphagia.

(7) **GU effects** include slow urination, transient nocturia, and prostatic hypertrophy.

(8) **Dermatological effects** include increased sweating, diaphoresis, and photosensitivity.

(9) **Hepatic effects** include mild and transient elevations in liver function tests.

d. CYP2B6 inhibitors may increase level of selegiline. Also, selegiline has active metabolites (n-desmethylselegeline and amphetamine); examples of such significant interactions are

(1) MAO inhibitors are contraindicated with **meperidine** and other opioids. Administration with opioids should be avoided (serotonin syndrome). **Death has occurred after initiation of selegiline shortly after discontinuation of fluoxetine**. At least 5 weeks should elapse between discontinuation of fluoxetine and initiation of selegiline (serotonin syndrome).

(2) Rasagiline: similar to selegiline. The different is 5- to 10-fold greater potency, higher oral absorption. Unlike selegiline, it is not metabolites to amphetamine derivatives (see *Table 38-3*).

2. Amantadine (Symmetrel)

a. Mechanism of action. Amantadine is an antiviral agent (used to prevent influenza).

(1) Amantadine increases dopamine levels at postsynaptic receptor sites by decreasing presynaptic reuptake and enhancing dopamine synthesis and release.

(2) It may also have some anticholinergic effects. It decreases tremor, rigidity, and bradykinesia.

(3) It can be given in combination with levodopa as Parkinson disease progresses.

(4) Clinical effects of amantadine can be seen within the first few weeks of therapy, unlike the other antiparkinsonian medications (e.g., carbidopa/levodopa), which need weeks to months to show their full clinical effects.

b. **Administration and dosage** (*Table 38-3*)
   (1) Amantadine should be started at 100 mg/day. This may be increased to 200 to 300 mg/day as a maintenance dose.
   (2) Patients experiencing a decline in response may benefit from the following:
      (a) Discontinuing the drug for a few weeks, then restarting it
      (b) Using the drug episodically, only when the patient's condition most needs a therapeutic boost
   (3) Amantadine is also available in liquid form for patients with dysphagia.

c. **Precautions and monitoring effects**
   (1) Amantadine should be used with caution in patients with renal disease, congestive heart failure (CHF), peripheral edema, history of seizures, and mental status changes. It may be necessary to modify dosages in patients with renal failure.
   (2) Tolerance usually develops within 6 to 12 months. If tolerance occurs, another drug from a different class can be added, or the dose may be increased.
   (3) Patients should be informed about the side-effect profile.
      (a) **Peripheral anticholinergic effects** include those mentioned in II.A.3.d.(1).
      (b) **CNS effects** include seizures as well as those mentioned in II.A.3.d.(2).
      (c) **Cardiovascular effects.** Patients may develop CHF. Periodic blood pressure monitoring and electrocardiograms (ECGs) are necessary in patients with myocardial infarction or arrhythmias.
      (d) **Dermatological effects** include **livedo reticularis**, a diffuse rose-color mottling of the skin, which is reversible on discontinuation of the drug.
      (e) **Hematological effects.** Periodic complete blood counts (CBCs) should be done for patients with long-term therapy.
   (4) **Renal function impairment.** Dose adjustment is necessary in patients with renal function impairment.

d. **Significant interactions**
   (1) Amantadine increases the anticholinergic effects of **anticholinergic drugs**, requiring a decrease in the dosage of the anticholinergic drug.
   (2) **Hydrochlorothiazide** plus **triamterene** decreases the urinary excretion of amantadine and increases its plasma concentration.

E. **Non-ergot dopamine agonists**

1. Pramipexole and ropinirole are indicated for both early and advanced stages of Parkinson disease.
2. Both selectively bind to dopamine receptors and activate the D_2-receptor but have little or no affinity to the D_1-receptor. They have greater affinity for the D_3-receptor than for the D_2-receptor. The incidence of adverse events (such as pleuropulmonary fibrosis and retroperitoneal fibrosis, coronary vasoconstriction, erythromelalgia, and Raynaud phenomenon) is low compared to non-selective dopamine agonists.
3. **Non-ergot dopamine agonists** have a low potential for the development of motor fluctuations and dyskinesia.
   a. **Pramipexole (Mirapex)**
      (1) **Mechanism of action**
         (a) **D_2** subfamily of dopamine receptors. Pramipexole fully stimulates the dopamine receptors to which it binds. Its action may be related to its capacity to function as an antioxidant and oxygen free-radical scavenger.
         (b) Pramipexole also has antidepressant activity in moderate depression, which may be related to its preferential binding to the dopamine D_1-receptor subtype.
         (c) Long-acting dopamine agonists appear to have a lower risk of inducing abnormal movements. Their use as initial treatment in early Parkinson disease seems warranted, particularly for those with disease onset at a younger age.
      (2) **Administration and dosage**
         (a) Initial treatment: starting dose of 0.375 mg daily given in three divided doses.
         (b) Do not increase more frequently than every 5 to 7 days.
         (c) Maintenance treatment: 1.5 to 4.5 mg daily in three divided doses with or without levodopa.

(d) When given in combination with levodopa, consider reduction of levodopa dose by an average of 27% from baseline.
(e) Titrate slowly to balance benefits and side effects, such as dyskinesia, hallucinations, somnolence, and dry mouth.
(f) May be taken with food to reduce the occurrence of nausea. Food decreases the rate of absorption but not the extent of absorption.
(g) Dosage adjustment is necessary in patients with renal function impairment.
(h) Weak protein bound 15%
(i) Not extensively metabolized; more than 90% of the dose is excreted unchanged in urine.
(j) Dose needs to be decreased by 25% in the elderly.

(3) **Precautions and monitoring effects**
(a) Dose reduction necessary in patients > 65 years and in patients with renal function impairment or failure
(b) Symptomatic hypotension
(i) Dopaminergic agents appear to impair the systemic regulation of blood pressure, which results in orthostatic hypotension.
(ii) Monitoring and education of the patient is necessary, especially during dose-escalation periods.
(c) Hallucinatory effects are increased in patients > 65 years of age with early or advanced stages of Parkinson disease.
(d) Other effects include nausea, insomnia, constipation, dizziness, somnolence, GI side effects, and visual hallucinations. Sleep attack by falling asleep during activity daily living.
(e) Compulsive behavior related to D_3 activities have been seen without prior history, such as compulsive gambling, hypersexuality, and overreacting.
(f) Falling asleep during activities of daily living

(4) **Significant interactions**
(a) Cimetidine reduces renal clearance of pramipexole.
(b) No interaction with selegiline, probenecid, or domperidone.
(c) When combined with levodopa, the dosage of levodopa must be decreased by 27%.

b. Ropinirole (Requip)

(1) **Mechanism of action** is similar to pramipexole.

(2) **Administration and dosage**
(a) Initial treatment: 0.25 mg three times daily
(b) Titrate weekly increments
(c) After week 4, if necessary, daily dosage may be increased by 1.5 mg/day on a weekly basis up to 9 mg/day, to a total of 24 mg/day.
(d) Discontinue gradually over a 7-day period. Decrease the frequency of administration from three times to two times daily for 4 days and then once daily for the remainder of the week.
(e) When given in combination with levodopa, consider reduction of levodopa dose.
(f) May be taken with food to reduce the occurrence of nausea. Food decreases the rate of absorption but not the extent of absorption.
(g) Metabolized by the liver (cytochrome P450 1A2) and first-pass effect
(h) Smoking induces the liver metabolism.
(i) Between 30% and 40% protein bound

(3) **Precautions and monitoring effects**
(a) **Syncope.** Bradycardia is observed in patients treated with ropinirole. Most cases occur within the first 4 weeks of therapy and are usually associated with a recent increase of dose.
(b) Binds to melanin-containing tissues like the eyes and skin
(c) Symptomatic hypotension
(i) Dopaminergic agents appear to impair the systemic regulation of blood pressure, which results in orthostatic hypotension.
(ii) Monitoring and education of the patient is necessary, especially during dose-escalation periods.

(d) Hallucinatory effects are increased in patients > 65 years of age with early or advanced stages of Parkinson disease.
(e) Other side effects include nausea, dizziness, somnolence, headache, fatigue, and abnormal vision. Sleep attack, by falling asleep during activity daily living.

(4) Significant interactions
(a) Smoking induces the liver metabolism, but the effect of smoking on clearance of ropinirole has not been studied.
(b) There is no interaction between levodopa, theophylline, digoxin, or domperidone.
(c) Estrogens decrease the clearance of ropinirole by approximately 36%.
(d) Ciprofloxacin increases ropinirole area under the curve (AUC) by 84% and maximum plasma concentration by 60%.

c. Apomorphine Hydrochloride Injection SC (Apokyn)

(1) Mechanism of action
(a) Stimulating of postsynaptic dopamine D_2-type receptors within caudate and putamen in brain.
(b) Subcutaneous injection is indicated for acute intermittent treatment if hypomobility "off" episodes (end of dose wearing, unpredictable on/off episodes).

(2) Administration and dosage
(a) Doses more than 6 mg is not recommended.
(b) Dose should be started at 2 mg increase to maximum of 6 mg.
(c) It should be administrated at "off" state and should begin test dose at 2 mg where blood pressure can be monitored. Blood pressure should be monitored predose and at 20, 40, and 60 mins postdose standing up.
(d) If patient developed orthostatic hypotension, patient should not received apomorphine.
(e) Patients who have a significant interruption in therapy (more than a week) should be restarted on a 0.2 mL (2 mg) dose and gradually titrated to effect.

(3) Precautions and monitoring
(a) Profound hypotension and loss of consciousness when given with 5-HT_3-antagonist **class (including ondansetron, granisetron)**
(b) QT prolongation and potential proarrhythmia effect. Patient should be monitored for palpitation syncopy and signs for episode of torsades de pointes.
(c) Sleep attack, falling asleep during daily activities.
(d) Hallucination
(e) **Sulfite sensitivity**: contains a sulfite that may cause allergic-type reactions, including anaphylactic symptoms and life-threatening or less severe asthmatic episodes in certain susceptible people

(4) Drug interactions
(a) 5-HT_3-antagonist such as ondansetron, granisetron, dolasetron, palonosetron results in hypotension.
(b) Antihypertensive medications and vasodilators may result in hypotension.
(c) Contraindicated when used with other drugs that have potential to prolong QT, QTC interval. It increases risk of life-threatening arrhythmias.

4. COMT inhibitors

a. Tolcapone (Tasmar)

(1) Mechanism of action
(a) Tolcapone is a selective and reversible inhibitor of COMT and is used as an adjunct to levodopa/carbidopa therapy.
(b) Tolcapone inhibits COMT both peripheral and centrally.
(c) COMT is the main enzyme responsible for peripheral and central metabolism of catecholamines, including levodopa. Addition of a COMT inhibitor results in the doubling of the elimination half-life of levodopa and in increased oral bioavailability of levodopa by 40% to 50%.
(d) Tolcapone is indicated as an adjunct therapy to carbidopa/levodopa therapy.

(2) Administration and dosage
(a) Starting dose of 100 to 200 mg three times daily
(b) Usual daily dose of 200 mg three times daily

(c) If patient fails to show expected benefit after 3 weeks of treatment, discontinue drug because of associated risk of liver failure. Rapid withdrawal or abrupt reduction dose could lead to hyperpyrexia and confusion symptoms such as high fever and severe rigidity similar to those in neuroleptic malignant syndrome.

(3) Precautions and monitoring

(a) **Liver toxicity.** High risk of fatal liver failure has been reported with tolcapone. Discontinue use if substantial benefit is not seen within 3 weeks of commencement of therapy.

(b) Do not use in patients with liver disease or in patients who have two alanine aminotransferase (ALT) or aspartate aminotransferase (AST) values greater than the upper limit of normal.

(c) Advise patient regarding self-monitoring for liver disease (i.e., clay-colored stool, jaundice, fatigue, appetite loss, or lethargy).

(d) Monitor AST and ALT every 2 weeks for the first year, then every 4 weeks for the next 6 months and every 8 weeks thereafter.

(e) MAO and COMT are two major enzyme systems involved in the metabolism of catecholamines; combination of tolcapone with a nonselective MAO inhibitor will result in inhibition of the pathway responsible for normal catecholamine metabolism.

(f) Tolcapone can be taken concomitantly with a selective MAO-B inhibitor, such as selegiline in recommended dose of less or equal to 10 mg/day.

(g) Fibrolic complications, such as retroperitoneal fibrosis, pulmonary infiltrates or effusion, or pleural thickening.

(4) Other side effects

(a) **Orthostatic hypotension.** Tolcapone enhances levodopa bioavailability and, therefore, may increase the occurrence of orthostatic hypotension.

(b) Diarrhea usually manifests within 6 to 12 weeks after administration of tolcapone but can develop as early as 2 weeks after administration. Diarrhea normally resolves after discontinuation of the drug.

(c) Hallucinations are sometimes accompanied by confusion, insomnia, and excessive dreaming. Hallucinatory effects usually occur after initiation of tolcapone and are usually resolved by decreasing the dose of levodopa.

(d) Tolcapone may potentiate the dopaminergic side effect of levodopa and may cause or exacerbate preexisting dyskinesia. Decreased doses of levodopa may or may not alleviate the symptoms.

(e) Severe cases of rhabdomyolysis have been reported, which present as fever, alternation of consciousness, and muscular rigidity.

(f) **Others.** Dyspepsia, abdominal cramping, mild paresthesia of the legs, and temporary discoloration of urine have also been noted but are not considered clinically important.

(g) **Drug interactions**. Although no drug interaction studies have been conducted, concurrent use of tolcapone and drugs that are metabolized by the COMT system (i.e., methyldopa, dobutamine, apomorphine) should be monitored. Tolcapone also has affinity for the cytochrome P450 2C9 isoenzyme, similar to warfarin. Coagulation parameters should be monitored when tolcapone is administered with warfarin.

b. Entacapone (Comtan)

(1) Mechanism of action

(a) Entacapone is a selective and reversible inhibitor of COMT and permits additional levodopa to reach the brain. It does not have any anti-Parkinson effect of its own.

(b) It acts only peripherally by inhibiting COMT.

(c) It improves the duration of on time and decreases the duration of off time.

(d) It is indicated as an adjunct to those on levodopa/carbidopa therapy who experience the signs and symptoms of end-of-dose wearing-off.

(2) Administration and dosage

(a) Dosage: 200 mg with each dose of L-dopa up to eight times daily with a maximum dose of 1600 mg daily.

(b) Rapid withdrawal could lead to emergency signs and symptoms of Parkinson disease, such as hyperpyrexia and confusion (symptoms resembling neuroleptic malignant syndrome).

(c) Levodopa + carbidopa and entacapone: Available in four strengths, each in a 1:4 ratio of carbidopa to levodopa and combined with entacapone 200 mg in a standard-release formulation, 50, 100, 150, and 200 mg of levodopa.

(3) **Precautions and monitoring effects**

(a) **MAO.** COMT and MAO are two major enzymes in the metabolism of catecholamines. Do not use together.

(b) **Drugs metabolized by COMT.** Drugs that are metabolized by this pathway, such as isoproterenol, epinephrine, norepinephrine, dopamine, and dobutamine, as well as methyldopa, may interact and may result in increased heart rate, arrhythmias, and an excessive increase in blood pressure.

(c) **Hepatic function impairment.** The majority of the drug is metabolized by the liver; therefore, use caution in patients who have liver function abnormalities.

(d) **Fibrotic complication.** Cases of retroperitoneal fibrosis, pulmonary infiltrates, pleural effusion, and pleural thickening have been reported. These complications may resolve when the drug is discontinued, but complete resolution may not always occur.

(e) **Biliary excretion.** Entacapone is excreted by bile; therefore, use caution with drugs known to interfere with biliary excretion, such as probenecid, erythromycin, and ampicillin.

(f) **Patients may be at increased risk for cardiovascular events such as myocardial infarction, stroke, and cardiovascular death.**

(g) **Patients may be at increased risk of developing prostate cancer**.

(4) **Other side effects.** Dyskinesia/hyperkinesia, nausea, urine discoloration (brownish orange), diarrhea, and abdominal pain

(5) **Drug interactions**

(a) May interact with drugs that are metabolized by the liver cytochrome P450.

(b) Iron salts and digoxin reduces bioavailability of carbidopa/levodopa/entacapone.

(c) After ingestion of carbidopa/levodopa/entacapone, the saliva, sweat, or urine may appear dark (red, brown, or black). This is clinically insignificant, garments may become discolored.

III. SURGICAL TREATMENT.

All surgeries require needle insertion into the brain, which in turn increases the risk of hemorrhage.

A. Globus pallidus internus (Gpi) pallidotomy

1. **Definition.** A pallidotomy entails the surgical resection of parts of the globus pallidus.
2. **Advantages.** Improves contralateral dyskinesia.
3. **Disadvantages.** Increased risk of damage to other parts of the brain, including optic nerve and internal capsule, and risk of emotional, behavioral, and cognitive deficits.

B. Deep-brain stimulation

1. **Definition.** High-frequency stimulation that induces functional inhibition of target regions of the brain by implanting an electrode into a target site and connecting the lead to a subcutaneously placed pacemaker.
2. **Advantages.** No destructive lesion is formed. Stimulation parameters can be readjusted at any time to improve efficacy or decrease adverse events.
3. **Disadvantages.** Side effects associated with equipment (such as lead breaks, infection, skin erosion, mechanical malfunction, and need for battery replacement). Other side effects include paresthesia, limb dystonia, ataxia, intracerebral hemorrhage, seizure, and confusion.

C. Fetal nigral transplantation

1. **Definition.** Implantation of embryonic dopaminergic cells into the denervated striatum to replace degenerated neuronal cells.
2. **Advantages.** Implanted cells all survive, and innervation of the striatum is accomplished in an organotypic manner. Does not necessitate making a destructive lesion.

3. **Disadvantages.** Optimal transplant variables and target site not defined. Also, clinical studies showed development atypical dyskinesias during off period.

D. Use of genetically engineered viruses (adeno-associated virus, AAV) to carry levodopa-dopamine converting enzyme aromatic L-amino decarboxylase (AADC) to increase effectiveness of levodopa; as a result, decrease doses of levodopa and subsequently decrease dyskinesia and other side effects associated with levodopa.

E. Neuronal regeneration: delivering either growth factors or stem cells to produce dopamine-producing neurons.

Study Questions

Directions: Each of the questions, statements, or incomplete statements in this section can be correctly answered or completed by **one** of the suggested answers or phrases. Choose the **best** answer.

1. Which of the following drugs is a catechol-*O*-methyltransferase (COMT) inhibitor and has reports of fatal liver toxicity with it?
   (A) tolcapone
   (B) entacapone
   (C) rasagiline
   (D) selegiline

2. Levodopa is associated with which of the following problems?
   (A) Gastrointestinal side effects
   (B) Involuntary movements
   (C) Decline in efficacy after 3 to 5 years
   (D) All of the above

3. Amantadine has which of the following advantages over levodopa?
   (A) More rapid relief of symptoms
   (B) Higher success rate
   (C) Better long-term effects

4. Which drug is a non-ergot dopamine agonist and has a side-effect profile different from the rest of the dopaminergic agents?
   (A) entacapone
   (B) levodopa/carbidopa
   (C) ropinirole
   (D) selegiline

5. Which of the following medications is indicated as an adjunct to carbidopa/levodopa therapy?
   (A) pramipexole
   (B) bromocriptine
   (C) amantadine
   (D) tolcapone

Answers and Explanations

1. **The answer is A** *[see II.E.4.a.(3).(a)–(c)]*.
   High risk of fatal liver failure use with caution with patients with liver abscess. Patients should be monitored and instructed to look for signs of liver disease such as clay-colored stool, jaundice, fatigue, loss of appetite, and lethargy.

2. **The answer is D** *[see II.B.3.c–d]*.
   Levodopa can cause GI side effects such as nausea and vomiting, particularly when starting treatment. Bowel irregularity and gastrointestinal bleeding can also occur. With long-term levodopa therapy, involuntary choreiform movements can develop, and the efficacy of the drug declines. Other unwanted effects of levodopa include tachycardia and cardiac arrhythmias, postural hypotension, and psychiatric disturbances such as confusion or depression.

3. **The answer is A** *[see II.D.2.a.(4); II.D.2.c–d]*.
   Amantadine is most efficacious within the first few weeks, whereas benefits from levodopa may not be seen for weeks to months. Amantadine is more beneficial than the anticholinergics but is less effective than levodopa. Unfortunately, the efficacy of amantadine declines after 6 to 12 months of therapy. The efficacy of levodopa declines after 3 to 5 years of therapy.

4. **The answer is C** *[see II.E.3.a–b]*.
Non-ergot dopamine agonists such as ropinirole are indicated for both early and advanced stages of Parkinson disease. These drugs selectively bind to dopamine receptors and activate the D_2-receptor but have little or no affinity for the D_1-receptor. They have a greater affinity for the D_3-receptor than for the D_2-receptor. The incidence of adverse events (e.g., pleuropulmonary fibrosis and retroperitoneal fibrosis, coronary vasoconstriction, erythromelalgia, and Raynaud phenomenon) is low compared to nonselective dopamine agonists. Non-ergot dopamine agonists have a low potential for the devolvement of motor fluctuations and dyskinesia.

5. **The answer is D** *[see II.E.4.a.(1).(d)]*.
Tolcapone is an inhibitor of COMT enzyme used to metabolize catecholamines, including levodopa. It is indicated as an adjunct therapy to carbidopa/levodopa therapy.

Schizophrenia

REBEKAH R. ARTHUR GRUBE, ANDREW J. MUZYK

39

I. INTRODUCTION

A. **Schizophrenia** is a major psychiatric disorder affecting approximately 1% to 2% of the world population. This complex condition was first described in the late 1800s and exists as a constellation of symptoms that includes hallucinations, delusions, decreased affect, disorganized behavior, and impaired functioning.

II. DIAGNOSIS AND CLINICAL FEATURES

A. Schizophrenia is **diagnosed** based on *Diagnostic and Statistical Manual of Mental Disorders*, 4th ed. (*DSM-IV-TR*) criteria.
  1. A patient must have at least two of the following symptoms: delusions, hallucinations, disorganized speech, disorganized or catatonic behavior, and negative symptoms.
  2. The symptoms should be present for at least 1 month, with at least 6 months of continuous prodromal or residual symptoms.
  3. At least one area of the patient's social or occupational functioning should be significantly affected.
  4. Other conditions causing similar symptoms such as schizoaffective disorder, mood disorders, substance abuse, and general medical conditions should be ruled out.

B. Five **types** of schizophrenia exist (*Table 39-1*).

C. The clinical features of schizophrenia are categorized as **positive**, **negative**, or **disorganized** symptoms (*Table 39-2*). The most common symptoms are **hallucinations** and **delusions**.
  1. A **hallucination** is a perception disturbance in sensory experiences of the environment. Hallucinations can be auditory, visual, olfactory, or tactile. Auditory hallucinations are most common.

Table 39-1 TYPES OF SCHIZOPHRENIA

Type	Presentation
Catatonic	Motor symptoms are most notable. The patient may either demonstrate rigid immobility or excessive purposeless movement. The patient may be silent and withdrawn or may become loud and shout. Bizarre voluntary movements such as posturing may also occur. The patient may fluctuate between the two extremes.
Disorganized	The patient tends to have disorganized speech and behavior with a flat affect. Hallucinations and delusions are not well formed and fragmented. The patient may also have bizarre mannerisms and grimacing.
Paranoid	The most common type of schizophrenia. Patients are usually preoccupied with paranoid delusions or auditory hallucinations. Cognitive function is usually preserved; if thought disorder is present, it does not prevent description of delusions or hallucinations.
Residual	The patient does not have acute psychosis, but some symptoms of schizophrenia remain. Largely negative symptoms are seen, such as flat affect, social withdrawal, and loose associations. Prominent delusions or hallucinations are not present.
Undifferentiated	The patient meets the criteria for a diagnosis of schizophrenia but does not meet the criteria for a specific type, or the patient may meet the criteria for multiple types of schizophrenia. No one type appears to be dominant.

Table 39-2 SYMPTOMS OF SCHIZOPHRENIA

Positive Symptoms	Negative Symptoms	Disorganized Symptoms
Delusions	Affective flattening	Disorganized speech
Hallucinations	Alogia	Thought disorder
Combativeness	Anhedonia	Disorganized behavior
Insomnia	Amotivation	Poor attention
	Apathy	
	Asocial behavior	

2. A **delusion** is an incorrect or false belief. Delusions can be religious, paranoid/persecutory, grandiose, somatic, influential, or sexual. Persecutory or paranoid delusions are the most common.

III. TREATMENT GOALS AND OBJECTIVES.

There is currently no known cure for schizophrenia. Treatment options include **psychotherapy** as well as **pharmacotherapy**. The goals and objectives of treatment are as follows:

A. Minimize symptoms of schizophrenia
B. Improve quality of life and social/occupational functioning
C. Prevent relapse and hospitalization
D. Minimize adverse effects of medications
E. Prevent suicide attempts or self-harm

IV. PHARMACOTHERAPY: ANTIPSYCHOTIC MEDICATIONS

A. Two generations of antipsychotic medications are available for treatment: **first-generation (typical antipsychotics)** and **second-generation (atypical antipsychotics)**.
   1. The choice of an appropriate antipsychotic agent depends on the patient's previous experiences with antipsychotic medications, adverse effects, the patient's concomitant medical conditions, medication interactions, and the patient's preference.
   2. Current American Psychiatric Association (APA) guidelines recommend using an atypical antipsychotic first, owing to less risk for extrapyramidal symptoms (EPS). Patients who prefer or have a history of response to typical antipsychotics may first use typical antipsychotics.
   3. Response to medications is not immediate, and maximal treatment response may take 6 months or longer to be seen.
   4. After a treatment response is seen, patients should be maintained on the current therapy for a minimum of 6 months. Most patients will require chronic therapy, because 80% of first-episode patients who do not receive antipsychotic treatment will relapse within 5 years.

B. **Typical antipsychotic medications** (*Table 39-3*)
   1. **Mechanism of action.** The antipsychotic effect of these medications is primarily mediated through the blockade of dopamine type 2 (D2) receptors. Agents within this medication class vary in their activity at histamine, muscarinic, and α-receptors, although these receptors are not responsible for desired therapeutic activity.
   2. **Potency.** Typical antipsychotic agents are classified by their potency for the dopamine receptor into high-, moderate-, and low-potency antipsychotics. High-potency agents have a higher affinity for the dopamine receptor and are associated with higher risk for the development of EPS. Low-potency agents have less affinity for dopamine receptors; and although they have less risk for causing EPS, they are associated with more adverse effects from their activity at histamine, muscarinic, and α-receptors.
   3. **Efficacy.** When dosed in equivalent doses, the various typical antipsychotics have similar efficacy. Equivalent doses are described using **chlorpromazine (CPZ) equivalents** (*Table 39-3*). Typical antipsychotics are thought to be as effective as atypical antipsychotics for positive symptoms but are less effective for negative symptoms.
   4. **Adverse effects.** Typical antipsychotics are associated with several adverse effects (*Tables 39-3 and 39-4*).

Table 39-3 PROPERTIES OF TYPICAL ANTIPSYCHOTICS

Agent	CPZ[a] Equivalent	Dose Range[a] (mg/day)	Sedation	EPS	Anticholinergic Side Effects	Orthostatic Hypotension
Chlorpromazine (Thorazine)	100	300–1000	+++	++	++	+++
Trifluoperazine (Stelazine)	5	5–15	+	+++	+	+
Thioridazine (Mellaril)	100	300–800	+++	+	+++	+++
Perphenazine (Trilafon)	10	16–64	++	++	+	+
Fluphenazine (Prolixin)	2	5–20	+	+++	+	+
Thiothixene (Navane)	5	15–50	+	+++	+	++
Haloperidol (Haldol)	2	5–20	+	+++	+	+
Molindone (Moban)	10	30–100	++	++	+	+
Loxapine (Loxitane)	10	30–100	+	++	+	+

[a]Data from Lehman AF, Lieberman JA, Dixon LB, et al. Practice guideline for treatment of patients with schizophrenia. 2nd ed. *Am J Psych.* 2004;161:1–56.
CPZ, chlorpromazine; *EPS*, extrapyramidal symptoms; + + +, high; + +, moderate; +, low.

Table 39-4 GENERAL ADVERSE EFFECTS OF ANTIPSYCHOTICS

Typical Antipsychotics	Atypical Antipsychotics
Sedation	Sedation
Anticholinergic effects	Anticholinergic effects (clozapine, olanzapine)
Blurred vision	Orthostatic hypotension
Constipation	Moderate to severe weight gain
Dry mouth	Diabetes mellitus
Urinary retention	Hypercholesterolemia
Extrapyramidal symptoms	Hyperprolactinemia (risperidone)
Lowered seizure threshold	Lowered seizure threshold
Orthostatic hypotension	QT prolongation
Hyperprolactinemia	Neuroleptic malignant syndrome
Moderate weight gain	Extrapyramidal symptoms
QT prolongation	Sexual dysfunction
Photosensitivity	
Temperature dysregulation	
Neuroleptic malignant syndrome	
Sexual dysfunction	
Elevated liver enzymes	

Table 39-5 ADVERSE EFFECTS BY RECEPTOR AFFINITIES

Receptor Antagonized	Adverse Effects
Histamine	Sedation Weight gain
Dopamine	Extrapyramidal symptoms Hyperprolactinemia
Muscarinic	Anticholinergic adverse effects Cognitive impairment Tachycardia
Alpha	Orthostatic hypotension Reflex tachycardia
Serotonin	Weight gain

a. The activity of the various typical antipsychotics at the dopamine, α-, muscarinic, and histamine receptors is responsible for many of the adverse effects of these medications (*Table 39-5*).

b. **Extrapyramidal side effects** can occur with all the typical antipsychotics, especially with high-potency typical antipsychotics. Four types of extrapyramidal side effects have been described: acute dystonia, akathisia, pseudoparkinsonism, and tardive dyskinesia.

(1) **Acute dystonia** describes sudden muscle spasms that primarily occur in the eye, neck, face, and throat muscles. An acute dystonic reaction can be a medical emergency; therefore, use of an intravenous or intramuscular treatment may be warranted for quick symptom resolution.

(a) Acute dystonias can occur within hours of initiating the medication or increasing the dose. This is most common in young men and in patients using high doses of high-potency typical antipsychotics.

(b) Management includes the use of anticholinergic agents like benztropine and diphenhydramine; if ineffective, benzodiazepines can also be used. Prevention of future reactions may be achieved by decreasing the dose of antipsychotic, using oral anticholinergics, or changing therapy to an atypical antipsychotic.

(2) **Akathisia** is described as inner restlessness associated with feelings of having to move.

(a) Patients with akathisia may pace or be unable to sit still. This may occur within days to a few months after the initiation of therapy or increase in dose.

(b) Treatment of akathisia includes dose reduction of the antipsychotic, lipophilic β-blockers or benzodiazepines. Therapy may also be changed to an atypical antipsychotic. Anticholinergic agents may not be useful in the treatment of akathisia.

(3) **Pseudoparkinsonism** clinically appears similar to idiopathic Parkinson disease and includes symptoms like shuffling gait, masklike face, cogwheel rigidity, and resting or pill-rolling tremor.

(a) This can occur within 1 to 3 months after starting therapy or increasing the dose of the antipsychotic agent.

(b) This is treated by changing to an atypical antipsychotic, decreasing the dose, and/or adding an anticholinergic agent.

(4) **Tardive dyskinesia (TD)** usually does not occur until the patient has been taking antipsychotics for a year or more. It is a movement disorder that can occur in various locations of the body, including the face, tongue, hips, and extremities.

(a) Movements can be dystonic (fixed) or choreoathetoid (rhythmic). Common movement disorders include tongue chewing, lip smacking, and rhythmic movements of the trunk.

(b) TD may be irreversible, so patients taking antipsychotics should be monitored closely for the appearance of any movement disorders.

(c) A tool such as the Abnormal Involuntary Movement Scale (AIMS) is available to assist in monitoring TD.

(d) Vigilant monitoring for signs of TD is the best way to prevent it from occurring. Stopping the causative agent (if possible) and switching to an atypical antipsychotic may be the best treatment for preventing irreversible TD. Multiple treatments have been used to attempt to treat TD, although none have been definitively proven to be effective. These include vitamin E, benzodiazepines, baclofen, and reserpine.

c. **Neuroleptic malignant syndrome (NMS)** is an uncommon but potentially fatal adverse effect of antipsychotics. Signs and symptoms include fever, severe rigidity, altered mental status, unstable blood pressure, tachycardia, incontinence, elevated creatine kinase, and increased white blood count.

(1) NMS has a sudden onset, and should prompt immediate discontinuation of all antipsychotics. Antipsychotics are recommended not to be restarted for at least 2 weeks following the resolution of NMS. It is also recommended to restart antipsychotic therapy with a different medication.

(2) Treatment includes supportive care and the use of bromocriptine and/or dantrolene.

C. **Atypical antipsychotic medications** (*Table 39-6*)

1. Ten atypical antipsychotics are currently on the U.S. market: clozapine (Clozaril), risperidone (Risperdal), olanzapine (Zyprexa), quetiapine (Seroquel), ziprasidone (Geodon), aripiprazole (Abilify), paliperidone (Invega), asenapine (Saphris), iloperidone (Fanapt), and lurasidone (Latuda).

2. The **mechanism of action** for atypical antipsychotics is different from that of the typical antipsychotics. With the exception of aripiprazole, the atypical antipsychotics are dopamine antagonists but also potently block 5-HT_{2A}-receptors. They block 5-HT to a greater extent than dopamine. Aripiprazole is a partial dopamine and 5-HT_{1A}-agonist and a 5-HT_{2A}-antagonist. Asenapine has a high affinity for 5-HT, dopamine, alpha, and histaminergic receptors with low affinity for muscarinic receptors. Iloperidone acts at numerous 5-HT and dopamine receptors and has high affinity for alpha-1 receptors. Lurasidone is a partial agonist 5-HT_{1A}-receptor with no affinity for muscarinic or histaminergic receptors.

3. **Receptor affinity** differs for the various atypical antipsychotics. All atypical antipsychotics have activity at the 5-HT_{2A}-receptor and dopamine receptor. Different agents have different activity for histamine, α-, and muscarinic receptors (*Table 39-6*).

4. Atypical antipsychotics may have increased efficacy for negative symptoms compared to typical antipsychotics. Clozapine has demonstrated efficacy for treatment-refractory schizophrenia.

5. **Adverse effects.** Atypical antipsychotics differ from typical antipsychotics in their adverse effect profile (*Table 39-4*). Owing to their higher affinity for 5-HT_2-receptors compared to dopamine receptors, they are associated with less EPS and hyperprolactinemia than typical antipsychotics. However, they have problematic adverse effects, which limit their use (*Table 39-6*).

   a. Atypical antipsychotics have been linked with weight gain, hyperlipidemia, and hyperglycemia. The risk for the development of these metabolic adverse effects differs among agents.

6. Clozapine was the first atypical antipsychotic to be marketed in the United States, is the only antipsychotic with no risk of EPS or TD and is the only antipsychotic with proven efficacy for treatment-refractory schizophrenia. Clozapine has also been shown to reduce suicidal behavior. However, clozapine is indicated only in patients who have failed at least two previous antipsychotics (including typical and atypical antipsychotics) because of its risk of agranulocytosis. Complete blood count (CBC) must be monitored at baseline, every week for the first 6 months of therapy, every other week for the next 6 months, and then every month thereafter. Clozapine may also lower seizure threshold in patients, especially with higher doses. Clozapine should be used with caution in patients at risk for seizures or with a history of a seizure disorder. Clozapine can cause numerous other side effects, especially early in therapy, therefore additional reading is required for a better understanding of its benefits and risks.

Table 39-6 PROPERTIES OF ATYPICAL ANTIPSYCHOTICS

Medication	Dose Range[a] (mg/day)	Receptor Affinity[a]	Sedation	EPS	Anticholinergic Effects	Orthostatic Hypotension	Weight Gain
Clozapine	150–600	D, 5-HT, M, H_1, α	+++	0	+++	+++	+++
Risperidone	2–8	D, 5-HT, H_1, α	+	+ to ++	0	+	++
Olanzapine	10–30	D, 5-HT, M, H_1, α	++	+	++	+	+++
Quetiapine	300–800	D, 5-HT, H_1, α	++	+	0	++	++
Ziprasidone	120–200	D, 5-HT, H_1, α	0	+	0	0	0
Aripiprazole	10–30	D, 5-HT, H_1, α	+	+	0	0	0
Paliperidone[b]	3–12	D, 5-HT, H_1, α	+	+ to ++	0	+	unknown

[a]Data from Lehman AF, Lieberman JA, Dixon LB, et al. Practice guideline for treatment of patients with schizophrenia. 2nd ed. *Am J Psych.* 2004;161:1–56.
[b]Data from Invega package insert, 2007. Titusville, NJ: Janssen, L.P.
5-HT, 5-hydroxytryptamine (serotonin); α, alpha; *D*, dopamine; *EPS*, extrapyramidal symptoms; *H_1*, histamine; *M*, muscarinic; +++, high; ++, moderate; +, low.

7. Unique formulations of atypical antipsychotics are available for patients.
   a. **Orally disintegrating tablets.** Risperidone, olanzapine, aripiprazole, and asenapine are available as orally disintegrating tablets. Asenapine must be given sublingually to increase its absorption. If the tablet is swallowed, its bioavailability significantly decreases from 35% to less than 2%.
   b. **Intramuscular formulations.** Ziprasidone, olanzapine, and aripiprazole are available in intramuscular formulations for use in acutely agitated patients with schizophrenia.
      (1) Ziprasidone may be given as 10 or 20 mg. The 10 mg dose may be repeated in 2 hrs, and the 20 mg dose may be repeated in 4 hrs. The maximum daily dose is 40 mg.
      (2) Olanzapine may be given as 10 mg. The 10 mg dose may be repeated every 2 hrs up to a maximum of 30 mg daily.
      (3) **Aripiprazole may be given as 9.75 mg. The 9.75 mg dose may be repeated every 2 hrs up to a maximum of 30 mg daily.**

D. **Noncompliant patients.** Those patients with a history of noncompliance or who have frequent hospitalizations secondary to noncompliance may be candidates for a long-acting intramuscular formulation of antipsychotic. Currently five options exist: haloperidol decanoate, fluphenazine decanoate, long-acting risperidone (Risperdal Consta), paliperidone palmitate (Invega Sustenna), and olanzapine pamoate (Zyprexa Relprevv).
   1. **Haloperidol decanoate** is given intramuscularly every 3 to 4 weeks. The starting dose should be 10 to 15 times the total daily dose of oral haloperidol. Oral overlap should continue for 1 month. Loading a patient with 20 times the total daily dose of oral haloperidol is another strategy and it does not require oral overlap. Doses should be administered as 100 or 200 mg subsequent doses every 3 to 7 days until the full dose is given. Follow-up intramuscular doses are then decreased by 25% after this initial loading dose has been given.
   2. **Fluphenazine decanoate** is administered intramuscularly every 2 to 3 weeks. The starting dose is 1.2 to 1.6 times the total daily dose of oral fluphenazine. Oral overlap is recommended for 1 week. The maximum dose of fluphenazine decanoate is 100 mg at any one time. The lowest effective dose of this formulation should be used.
   3. **Long-acting risperidone** is administered intramuscularly every 2 weeks. An effective dose of oral risperidone should first be identified before changing to the long-acting formulation. Patients should be started at 25 mg every 2 weeks and covered with oral medications for 3 weeks after initiation. Doses may be increased to a maximum of 50 mg every 2 weeks.
   4. Paliperidone palmitate is administered intramuscularly in the deltoid or gluteal muscle. Therapy is initiated with a loading dose of 234 mg followed by a second injection of 156 mg 1 week later. Subsequent doses are given every 4 weeks and range from 39 to 234 mg.
   5. Olanzapine pamoate is administered intramuscularly at a dose of 210 mg or 300 mg every 2 weeks or 405 mg every 4 weeks during the first 8 weeks of therapy. After 8 weeks, doses can range from 150 mg to 300 mg every 2 weeks or 300 mg to 405 mg every 8 weeks. Olanzapine pamoate can only be administered at a registered health care facility and patients must be monitored for at least 3 hours following injection. This monitoring is required due to delirium/sedation syndrome.

E. **Antipsychotic agents** may be switched for several reasons, such as lack of efficacy and adverse effects. When switching antipsychotic agents, the original agent should be titrated down while the new agent is titrated up. If changing from a typical antipsychotic to an atypical antipsychotic secondary to EPS, anticholinergic agents may be continued until the typical agent is completely discontinued.

F. **Adjunctive therapy.** In patients with partial or no response to therapy after an adequate trial, approximately 4 weeks, of an antipsychotic, a second antipsychotic should be tried. After the failure of two to three antipsychotics, the patient meets the criteria for clozapine, and its use should be considered. Augmentation is an option for those patients unable to take clozapine or with partial/no response. Clozapine has been studied in combination with typical and atypical antipsychotics. Other options for augmentation include mood stabilizers, such as lithium, valproic acid, and carbamazepine. Antidepressants have also been used in patients suffering from depressive symptoms. Electroconvulsive therapy (ECT) has also been used as an adjunctive therapy in patients with partial or no response to antipsychotics.

Study Questions

Directions: Each of the questions, statements, or incomplete statements in this section can be correctly answered or completed by one of the suggested answers or phrases. Choose the best answer.

For questions 1–5: DG is a 23-year-old female committed to the inpatient psychiatric ward by her parents. They state that she has recently been under a large amount of stress from college, and they have noticed over the past year that she has become more withdrawn from her friends and social activities. They also state that she angers more easily than she used to as a child, and this morning they found her with a knife trying to slit her wrists. DG states that the voices keep telling her she is bad and that she should kill herself. She does not admit to any visual hallucinations but describes multiple voices (male and female) talking to her continuously telling her that she should harm herself or that people are out to get her. She keeps telling you that her parents are trying to get rid of her, and she wants to leave. She appears to be a healthy young woman although noticeably agitated. Her medical history is significant only for smoking one pack/day since age 16. DG is diagnosed with schizophrenia.

1. Which type of schizophrenia is DG likely experiencing based upon her presenting signs and symptoms?

(A) catatonic
(B) disorganized
(C) paranoid
(D) residual

2. Which of the following of DG's symptoms is best described as a negative symptom of schizophrenia?

(A) social withdrawal
(B) auditory hallucinations
(C) delusions
(D) agitation

3. The medical team decides to initiate treatment for DG. Which of the following antipsychotic medications is the best initial treatment for this patient?

(A) haloperidol
(B) risperidone
(C) thioridazine
(D) clozapine

4. Which of the following is *not* a potential adverse effect of the medication selected for DG in question 3?

(A) weight gain
(B) pseudoparkinsonism
(C) sedation
(D) urinary retention

5. DG is stabilized on the medication prescribed and is discharged home. DG is readmitted into the psychiatric ward 1 year later for auditory and visual hallucinations secondary to noncompliance on her current treatment regimen. Which of the following treatment options is most appropriate for DG at this time?

(A) haloperidol decanoate
(B) long-acting risperidone
(C) clozapine monotherapy
(D) adjunctive clozapine with haloperidol

For questions 6–8: TW is a 52-year-old female with a history of schizophrenia and diabetes mellitus type 2. She has been treated for many years with haloperidol with good response; however, she has recently developed lip smacking and tongue chewing.

6. What type of adverse effect is TW experiencing?

(A) akathisia
(B) acute dystonia
(C) pseudoparkinsonism
(D) tardive dyskinesia

7. Which of the following medications has been used to treat the adverse effect described in question 6?

(A) vitamin E
(B) propranolol
(C) diphenhydramine
(D) amantadine

8. Now that TW is experiencing this reaction, her health care providers want to change her therapy to a different antipsychotic. Which of the following antipsychotics is the best treatment option for her?

(A) olanzapine
(B) risperidone
(C) quetiapine
(D) fluphenazine

9. Which of the following atypical antipsychotics would be the least likely to cause weight gain?
   (A) risperidone
   (B) olanzapine
   (C) quetiapine
   (D) aripiprazole

10. Which of the following statements does not describe a way in which atypical antipsychotics differ from typical antipsychotics?
   (A) Atypical antipsychotics have a higher affinity for serotonin receptors than dopamine receptors.
   (B) Atypical antipsychotics are more efficacious for positive symptoms than typical antipsychotics.
   (C) Atypical antipsychotics are more likely to cause weight gain and hyperlipidemia than typical antipsychotics.
   (D) Atypical antipsychotics are less likely to cause extrapyramidal symptoms (EPS) than typical antipsychotics.

11. Which of the following long-acting injectable antipsychotics requires a 3-week overlap with oral antipsychotic medication following the first injection?
   (A) paliperidone
   (B) olanzapine
   (C) haloperidol
   (D) risperidone

12. Which of the following antipsychotics is the only agent shown to produce benefit in WELL-DEFINED treatment-resistant schizophrenia?
   (A) risperidone
   (B) clozapine
   (C) olanzapine
   (D) chlorpromazine

13. Which of the following antipsychotics is most likely to cause anticholinergic side effects?
   (A) aripiprazole
   (B) olanzapine
   (C) paliperidone
   (D) risperidone

14. XY is currently being treated for schizophrenia and was recently started on haloperidol (Haldol) 20 mg daily 1 week ago. You notice that he is pacing the unit floors; and upon talking to him, he confesses being unable to sit still. He says he feels like he has a motor running inside him that is relieved only by walking. Your team thinks he is agitated from his hallucinations and wants to increase the haloperidol to 30 mg. You recommend which of the following?
   (A) Disagree with the team, he is experiencing a manic episode and needs to have valproic acid added to his treatment regimen.
   (B) Disagree with the team, he is experiencing a dystonic reaction related to the haloperidol dose. Recommend decreasing the dose and starting an IV anticholinergic medication
   (C) Disagree with the team, he is experiencing akathisia related to the haloperidol dose. Recommend decreasing the dose and starting a benzodiazepine.
   (D) Disagree with the team, he is experiencing tardive dyskinesia related to the haloperidol dose. Recommend decreasing the dose and stating an anticholinergic medication

15. Which of the following antipsychotics acts as a partial agonist at 5-HT_{1A} receptors?
   (A) aripiprazole
   (B) olanzapine
   (C) haloperidol
   (D) risperidone

Answers and Explanations

1. **The answer is C** *[see Table 39-1].*
   DG's prominent symptoms include well-formed hallucinations and delusions. These hallucinations and delusions are characteristics of paranoid schizophrenia. DG also does not meet the criteria for any other type of schizophrenia.

2. **The answer is A** *[see Table 39-2].*
   Social withdrawal or asocial behavior is a negative symptom of schizophrenia. Hallucinations, delusions, and agitation are all positive symptoms of schizophrenia.

3. **The answer is B** *[see IV.A.2; IV.C.1; IV.C.6].*
   The American Psychiatric Association currently recommends using atypical antipsychotics first over typical antipsychotics, unless the patient has a preference. Haloperidol and thioridazine are typical antipsychotics. Clozapine should be used only for treatment refractory patients because of its adverse effect profile.

4. **The answer is D** *[see Table 39-4; Table 39-6].*
   Risperidone has been associated with moderate weight gain, low to moderate risk of EPS, and low risk of sedation. It has not been associated with anticholinergic effects such as urinary retention.

5. **The answer is B** *[see IV.D.3].*
DG has a history of response with risperidone; however, she is experiencing a relapse of symptoms owing to noncompliance. A long-acting formulation is indicated to assist with medication compliance. As she has not failed multiple antipsychotics, DG is not a candidate for clozapine or adjunctive clozapine. Long-acting risperidone is preferred in this patient over haloperidol decanoate owing to the patient's response history and its preferable adverse effect profile.

6. **The answer is D** *[see IV.B.4.b.(1)–(4)].*
TW is experiencing lip smacking and tongue chewing of a late onset, which is best described as tardive dyskinesia.

7. **The answer is A** *[see IV.B.4.b.(4).(d)].*
Vitamin E, benzodiazepines, baclofen, and reserpine have all been used in the treatment of tardive dyskinesia, although none has been definitively proven to be effective.

8. **The answer is C** *[see Table 39-3; Table 39-6].*
Because TW is experiencing tardive dyskinesia, her therapy should be changed to an atypical antipsychotic. Her medical history is significant for type 2 diabetes mellitus. Olanzapine is associated with a high risk of causing weight gain, and other metabolic symptoms and should not be used in this patient. Risperidone has a low to moderate risk of EPS. Other atypical antipsychotics, such as quetiapine, that carry a lower risk of EPS would be preferable.

9. **The answer is D** *[see Table 39-6].*
Olanzapine has a high risk of causing weight gain. Risperidone and quetiapine have a moderate risk of causing weight gain. Aripiprazole is associated with a low risk of weight gain.

10. **The answer is B** *[see IV.C.2–5.a; Table 39-4].*
Atypical antipsychotics have a higher affinity for serotonin receptors than dopamine receptors, whereas typical antipsychotics have no activity at serotonin receptors. Atypical and typical antipsychotics have similar efficacy for positive symptoms of schizophrenia; however, atypical antipsychotics have increased efficacy against negative symptoms. Atypical antipsychotics are more likely to cause significant weight gain and hyperlipidemia and less likely to cause EPS than typical antipsychotics.

11. **The answer is D** *[see IV.D.3].*
Risperdal Consta is the only injectable that requires a 3-week overlap with oral risperidone following the first injection. The other injectables either do not require an oral overlap or it is less/greater than 3 weeks.

12. **The answer is B** *[see IV.C.6].*
Clozapine is the only antipsychotic to be effective in treatment-resistant schizophrenics.

13. **The answer is B** *[see Table 39-6].*
Olanzapine is the only antipsychotic listed that is a strong antagonist of cholinergic receptors. The other three agents have no to minimal blockage of the cholinergic receptors.

14. **The answer is C** *[see IV.B.4.b.(2)].*
The patient is experiencing akathisia from too high of a haloperidol dose. The haloperidol dose should be decreased and a benzodiazepine should be started. Akathisia is described as an inner restlessness coupled with an inability to sit still or a need to move.

15. **The answer is A** *[see IV.C.2].*
Aripiprazole is the only antipsychotic listed that in addition its blocking of 5-HT and dopamine receptors, it also acts as an agonist at 5-HT1A receptors.

40

Mood Disorders, Anxiety Spectrum Disorders, Attention-Deficit Hyperactivity Disorder (ADHD), and Insomnia

REBEKAH R. ARTHUR GRUBE, ANDREW J. MUZYK

I. TREATMENT OF MAJOR DEPRESSIVE DISORDER.

Major depressive disorder is defined as a mood disorder in which the patient has one or more episodes of major depression but has no history of mania, mixed, or hypomania episodes. Major depressive episodes are described in II.D.

A. Diagnosis and clinical features

1. Major depressive episodes are diagnosed using the *Diagnostic and Statistical Manual of Mental Disorders*, 4th ed. (*DSM-IV-TR*) criteria. To meet the criteria for a major depressive episode, patients should experience at least five or more persistent symptoms for at least 2 weeks. These symptoms include depressed mood, loss of interest or pleasure in activities, change in appetite, unintentional weight gain or loss, insomnia or excess sedation, psychomotor agitation or retardation, decreased energy or fatigue, feelings of worthlessness or inappropriate guilt, decreased ability to concentrate, and recurrent thoughts of suicide, death, or suicide attempt.[1]
2. Symptoms should impair social or occupational functioning and should not be related to a general medical condition or substance abuse.

B. Treatment options. Three treatment options exist for the treatment of depression: **pharmacotherapy**, **psychotherapy**, and **electroconvulsive therapy (ECT)**. Complementary or alternative treatments used in major depression include St. John's wort, S-adenosyl methionine, omega-3 fatty acids, and folate.

1. **Pharmacotherapy options (antidepressants).** Pharmacotherapy can be used for mild to severe major depression and produces a response in 50% to 75% of patients. Some evidence suggests antidepressants are more effective in patients with moderate to severe depression. Antidepressants have similar efficacy; however, they differ in adverse effects, mechanism of action, drug–drug interactions, and cost. Therefore, selection of an antidepressant should take these factors into consideration. Patients with a history of response to a particular agent may restart that agent if desired.
   a. **Monoamine oxidase inhibitors (MAOIs)** (*Table 40-1*)
      (1) **Indications.** MOAIs have numerous adverse effects and medication interactions and are indicated only in patients refractory to other antidepressants. These agents also have

Table 40-1 MONOAMINE OXIDASE INHIBITORS

Agent	Starting Dose (mg/day)	Usual Dose[a] (mg/day)	Anticholinergic Effects	Sedation	Weight Gain
Phenelzine (Nardil)	15	45–90	++	++	+++
Isocarboxazid (Marplan)	10–20	30–60	++	++	++
Tranylcypromine (Parnate)	10	30–60	++	+	++
Selegiline (Emsam) patch	6	6–12	++	0	+

[a]For normal adults. Doses may need to be adjusted for elderly patients or those with impaired renal or hepatic function.
+++, high; ++, moderate; +, slight.

a role in patients presenting with atypical depression. Recently, the FDA approved a transdermal patch formulation of selegiline (Emsam), which may be useful in patients unable to take oral antidepressants.

(2) **Mechanism of action.** MAOIs inhibit monoamine oxidase, which is responsible for the breakdown of neurotransmitters such as dopamine (DA), serotonin (5-HT), and norepinephrine (NE).

(3) **Adverse effects** include hypertensive crises, serotonin syndrome, orthostatic hypotension, peripheral edema, weight gain, and sexual dysfunction.

(a) **Hypertensive crises** can occur when increased levels of sympathetic amines, such as NE, build up in the body, which can be the result of ingestion of tyramine-containing foods like wine and cheese or the administration of sympathomimetic agents (e.g., decongestants). Patients should be counseled regarding the risk for drug and food interactions when taking MAOIs. A tyramine-restricted diet is not required with the 6 mg/day selegiline patch, however at doses of 9 mg/day or greater it is recommended.

(b) **Serotonin syndrome.** MAOIs in combination with selective serotonin reuptake inhibitors, tricyclic amines, serotonin and norepinephrine reuptake inhibitors, and any other agent with serotonergic activity can lead to serotonin syndrome. The clinical manifestations of serotonin syndrome are given in *Table 40-2*.

(c) Other common side effects include orthostatic hypotension, sexual dysfunction (anorgasmia, decreased libido, and erectile/ejaculatory dysfunction), and insomnia.

(4) **Medication interactions**

(a) MAOIs are substrates of various cytochrome P450 (CYP450) enzymes and levels can be affected by enzyme inhibitors and inducers.

b. Many tricyclic amines (TCAs) can be classified as tertiary and secondary (*Table 40-3*). Tertiary and secondary amines have pharmacological differences, although this mainly influences their adverse effect profile.

(1) **Indications.** Owing to their numerous adverse effects, TCAs are not usually indicated first line for the treatment of depression.

Table 40-2 SIGNS AND SYMPTOMS OF SEROTONIN SYNDROME

Cognitive-Behavioral Dysfunction	Autonomic Nervous System Dysfunction	Neuromuscular Dysfunction
Confusion	Diarrhea	Myoclonus
Hypomania	Shivering	Hyperreflexia
Agitation	Fever	Tremor
	Diaphoresis	Seizure
	Change in blood pressure	Death
	Nausea and vomiting	

Table 40-3 TRICYCLIC AMINES

Agent	Usual Dose[a] (mg/day)	Anticholinergic Effects	Sedation	Orthostatic Hypotension	Cardiac Effects	Weight Gain
Tertiary amine						
Amitriptyline (Elavil)	100–300	++++	++++	++++	+++	++++
Doxepin (Sinequan)	100–300	+++	++++	++	++	++++
Imipramine (Tofranil)	100–300	+++	+++	++++	+++	++++
Trimipramine (Surmontil)	75–300	++++	++++	+++	+++	++++
Secondary amine						
Nortriptyline (Pamelor)	50–200	++	++	+	++	+
Desipramine (Norpramin)	100–300	+	++	++	++	+
Protriptyline (Vivactil)	20–60	++	+	++	+++	+

[a]For normal adults. Doses may need to be adjusted for elderly patients or those with impaired renal or hepatic function.
++++, very high; +++, high; ++, moderate; +, slight.

(a) TCAs may be considered for patients with a history of response to TCAs, patients refractory to other medications, or patients with comorbidities that might benefit from TCAs, such as neuropathic pain and migraines.

(b) TCAs can be lethal in overdose and should not be used in patients with suicidal ideations. Additionally, TCAs should be avoided or used with caution in patients with cardiovascular conditions, closed-angle glaucoma, urinary retention, or severe prostate hypertrophy.

(2) Mechanism of action. TCAs produce their antidepressant effect by inhibiting the reuptake of 5-HT and NE. TCAs also have effect at α-adrenergic, histamine, and cholinergic receptors. Tertiary and secondary amines have equal potency in blocking NE reuptake. Tertiary amines possess greater potency for blocking 5-HT reuptake and greater affinity for these other receptors.

(3) Adverse effects. Several adverse effects exist for TCAs and may differ between agents, depending on their affinity for α-adrenergic, cholinergic, and histamine receptors (*Table 40-3*).

(a) Tertiary amine TCAs have been associated with a higher risk of causing anticholinergic adverse effects (blurred vision, constipation, urinary retention, dry mouth), sedation, weight gain, and orthostatic hypotension than secondary amine TCAs. Elderly patients may experience memory impairment and confusion due to anticholinergic effects of this medication class. Anticholinergic-induced delirium may be seen in overdose.

(b) Additional adverse effects include tachycardia, orthostatic hypotension, arrhythmias (especially in overdose), cardiac conduction abnormalities, decreased seizure threshold, sedation, falls, and sexual dysfunction. Nortriptyline may be the least likely to cause orthostatic blood pressure changes.

(c) Owing to their activity on serotonin, TCAs have the potential for causing serotonin syndrome when used in combination with other serotonergic agents.

(4) Medication interactions. TCAs are substrates of various cytochrome P450 (CYP450) enzymes, and levels can be affected by enzyme inhibitors and inducers. Drug–drug interactions occurring at CYP3A4 and CYP2D6 are most common with TCAs.

Table 40-4 SELECTIVE SEROTONIN REUPTAKE INHIBITORS AND SEROTONIN AND NOREPINEPHRINE REUPTAKE INHIBITORS

Agent	Starting Dose (mg/day)	Usual Dose (mg/day)	Half-Life	CYP450 Isoenzyme Inhibition
Fluoxetine (Prozac)	10–20	20–60; 80 mg weekly[a]	7–9 days[b]	2D6, 2C9/19 (potent); 3A4 (mild)
Paroxetine (Paxil)	10–20	20–60	21 hrs	2D6 (potent)
Sertraline (Zoloft)	25–50	50–200	24 hrs	2D6 (mild)
Citalopram (Celexa)	10–20	20–60	35 hrs	2D6 (mild)
Escitalopram (Lexapro)	5–10	10–20	27–32 hrs	2D6 (mild)
Venlafaxine (Effexor)	75	75–375	11 hrs	2D6 (mild)
Desvenlafaxine (Pristiq)	50	50	10 hrs	34A (mild)
Duloxetine (Cymbalta)	40	60–120	9–19 hrs	2D6 (moderate)

[a]Fluoxetine can be given in a once-weekly formulation in patients stabilized on fluoxetine 20 mg daily; should be started 1 week after the last dose of fluoxetine.
[b]Norfluoxetine is an active metabolite of fluoxetine and has a half-life of 7–9 days. The half-life of fluoxetine alone is 2–3 days.
CYP450, cytochrome P450.

c. Selective serotonin reuptake inhibitors (SSRIs). Five SSRIs are currently available in the United States for the treatment of depression (*Table 40-4*). SSRIs are considered to be first-line antidepressants for the treatment of depression and many are also indicated for other comorbid psychiatric disorders.

(1) Mechanism of action. SSRIs exert their antidepressant effect by blocking the reuptake of serotonin. SSRIs due differ in the pharmacological actions (such as fluoxetine blocking NE reuptake and paroxetine blocking cholinergic receptors).

(2) Adverse effects

(a) SSRIs have been associated with nausea, vomiting, insomnia, sedation, sexual dysfunction, headache, falls, osteopenia, akathisia, agitation, and tremor.

(b) Paroxetine has also been associated with anticholinergic adverse effects.

(c) These agents have been associated with serotonin syndrome when used in combination with other serotonergic agents.

(d) Abrupt discontinuation of SSRIs can cause withdrawal symptoms, such as nightmares, vivid dreams, tremor, anxiety, and nausea. Fluoxetine is the least likely to cause withdrawal, while paroxetine causes the greatest discontinuation syndrome. SSRIs should be slowly tapered when discontinued to prevent this syndrome.

(3) Medication interactions

(a) SSRIs are metabolized by the liver mainly by CYP3A4 and CYP2D6 enzymes. Fluoxetine and paroxetine are strong inhibitors of CYP2D6.

(b) SSRIs alone and in combination with NSAIDs have been associated with gastrointestinal bleeding.

d. Serotonin and norepinephrine reuptake inhibitors (SNRIs) (*Table 40-4*). Three SNRIs are currently available for the treatment of depression: venlafaxine (Effexor), desvenlafaxine (Pristiq), and duloxetine (Cymbalta). Data have shown these medications to have efficacy for the treatment not only of depression but also for peripheral neuropathies. Duloxetine carries an FDA-approved indication for the treatment of pain in diabetic neuropathy and fibromyalgia.

(1) Mechanism of action. SNRIs inhibit the reuptake of 5-HT and NE, thereby increasing their levels. These medications differ from TCAs in that they have little activity for α-adrenergic, cholinergic, or histamine receptors. Duloxetine is a potent inhibitor of 5-HT and NE at clinical doses, whereas venlafaxine requires higher doses (> 150 mg/day) to affect both 5-HT and NE.

Table 40-5 MISCELLANEOUS ANTIDEPRESSANTS

Agent	Starting Dose (mg/day)	Usual Dose (mg/day)	Cytochrome P450 Isoenzyme Inhibition
Bupropion (Wellbutrin)	75–150	300–450	2D6
Mirtazapine (Remeron)	15	15–45	Does not inhibit
Trazodone (Desyrel)	50–100	150–600	Does not inhibit

(2) **Adverse effects.** SNRIs have an adverse effect profile similar to that of the SSRIs. Venlafaxine has been associated with elevations of diastolic blood pressure, particularly with the immediate release formulation and at higher doses. Abrupt discontinuation of SNRIs can lead to withdrawal symptoms, particularly with immediate-release venlafaxine.

(3) **Medication interactions.** Venlafaxine and duloxetine are both mainly substrates for the CYP2D6 liver enzymes. Duloxetine is a moderate inhibitor of CYP2D6 (*Table 40-4*). SNRIs should not be used with MAOIs or other serotonergic agents owing to risk of serotonin syndrome.

e. **Bupropion (Wellbutrin)** (*Table 40-5*). In addition to its indication for major depression, bupropion is also FDA approved for smoking cessation.

(1) The mechanism of action for bupropion is not completely understood. Bupropion is known to inhibit the reuptake of NE and dopamine.

(2) Common adverse effects associated with the use of bupropion include nausea, vomiting, headaches, activation, agitation, hypertension, and insomnia.

(a) Bupropion has been associated with less sexual dysfunction than other antidepressant medications.

(b) Bupropion has been associated with an increased risk for seizures and is contraindicated in patients at risk for seizures. This includes patients with the following medical disorders: seizure disorder, history of anorexia or bulimia, or using or withdrawing from medications such as alcohol or benzodiazepines. Doses $>$ 450 mg should not be used, and dose increases should be gradual.

(3) **Medication interactions.** Bupropion is a substrate of CYP2B6 liver enzymes and is a strong inhibitor of CYP2D6.

f. **Mirtazapine (Remeron)** (*Table 40-5*)

(1) Mirtazapine antagonizes α-adrenergic and 5-HT_2- and 5-HT_3-receptors, causing an increase in NE and 5-HT. In addition, mirtazapine has activity at histamine (H) receptors.

(2) Adverse effects for mirtazapine include sedation, weight gain, constipation, dry mouth, and increased appetite. Sedation, increased appetite, and weight gain can be problematic, particularly at lower doses. Mirtazapine has a lower risk for causing sexual dysfunction compared to SSRIs.

(3) **Medication interactions.** Mirtazapine is a substrate of CYP3A4 and CYP2D6 liver enzymes. Mirtazapine is a weak inhibitor of CYP1A2 and CYP3A4 enzymes.

g. **Trazodone (Desyrel)** (*Table 40-5*). Trazodone is indicated for the treatment of depression. It is more frequently used in low doses as adjunctive treatment for insomnia in depressed patients.

(1) The mechanism of action for trazodone is not completely understood, but is mainly thought to block 5-HT reuptake, increase in 5-HT neurotransmission, and block 5-HT_2-postsynaptic receptors.

(2) The most common adverse effects of trazodone include sedation, nausea, sexual dysfunction, and orthostatic hypotension. Trazodone has rarely been associated with priapism and QT prolongation.

(3) **Medication interactions.** Trazodone is metabolized mainly by CYP3A4, whereas active metabolite *m*-chlorophenylpiperazine (mCCP) is metabolized by CYP2D6.

h. Nefazodone (Serzone). Nefazodone is a medication structurally similar to trazodone. It was considered to be first line for treatment of depression; however, recent reports of hepatotoxicity have limited its use and led to a black box warning for possible liver failure leading to death.

- **(1) Mechanism of action.** Nefazodone has a mechanism of action similar to trazodone.
- **(2) Adverse effects.** Common adverse effects for nefazodone include dry mouth, nausea, constipation, visual alterations, orthostatic hypotension, and sedation. The most severe adverse effect associated with nefazodone is hepatic failure.
  - **(a)** Reported rates by the FDA estimate one case of liver failure resulting in death or transplant per 250,000 to 350,000 patient-years. Liver function enzymes should be monitored routinely.
  - **(b)** The generic product is still available, although brand name nefazodone was withdrawn from the U.S. market in 2004.
- **(3) Medication interactions.** Nefazodone is highly protein bound and is an inhibitor of CYP3A4.

i. Atypical antipsychotics have recently been the subject of multiple studies in the treatment of major depression. For information regarding dosing, adverse effects, and mechanism of action see Chapter 39. Olanzapine is available in a formulation with fluoxetine (Symbyax) and is FDA approved for treatment-resistant depression. Quetiapine and aripiprazole are FDA approved for adjunct therapy to antidepressants.

- **(1) Duration of treatment.** Treatment is divided into three phases: acute phase, continuation phase, and maintenance phase.
  - **(a)** The acute phase begins with the initiation of therapy until remission is reached, typically lasting between 6 and 12 weeks.
  - **(b)** The continuation phase begins after remission is reached and typically lasts between 4 and 9 months. Medication from the acute phase is continued during this phase to prevent relapse of depression.
  - **(c)** A maintenance phase is used in patients with a high risk of recurrence of depression, such as those with a history of multiple episodes of depression, history of suicidal thoughts, and severe depression. These patients should receive maintenance treatment for 2 to 3 years, and many may receive lifelong therapy.
- **(2) Administration and dosage**
  - **(a)** Antidepressants are usually started at low doses and slowly titrated up to reach target doses over a period of a few weeks to prevent adverse reactions. Clinical response determines if the dose should be further titrated. Although full effects may not be seen for 4 to 6 weeks, often some signs and symptoms of depression such as insomnia may resolve within 1 to 2 weeks of starting an antidepressant. Patients must receive maximum tolerated doses for 4 to 8 weeks without response to be classified as ineffective.
  - **(b)** If patients receive only a partial or no response, other antidepressants may be considered. When changing to another antidepressant agent, caution should be used to prevent serotonin syndrome.
- **(3) Augmentation of therapy.** When patients fail to fully or partially respond to two or more medications, augmentation of antidepressant therapy with another agent may be considered.
  - **(a)** Lithium and thyroid hormone have been used for augmentation of antidepressant medications.
  - **(b)** Dual antidepressant augmentation has also been used. Agents that have been used include bupropion, TCAs, and mirtazapine.
- **(4) Suicide risk.** The FDA has now issued a black box warning for all antidepressants that an increase in suicidal thoughts and actions may occur with therapy and that adolescents and children receiving this therapy should be closely monitored.
- **(5) Treatment options in pregnancy**
  - **(a)** Benefit needs to be weighed against risk of teratogenicity.
  - **(b)** SSRIs and ECT are recommended treatment options.
  - **(c)** Paroxetine is pregnancy category D due to cardiac malformations.

(d) Bupropion is pregnancy category B.
(e) Antidepressants are considered compatible with breastfeeding, but mothers should be warned of possible risks to their newborn.

II. TREATMENT OF BIPOLAR DISORDER

A. **Definition.** Bipolar disorder is a syndrome in which patients suffer from episodes of mania and depression.

B. **Diagnosis.** Bipolar disorder is diagnosed using *DSM-IV-TR* criteria. The symptoms should impair social or occupational functioning and should not be related to a general medical condition or use of a substance.

1. Mania is described as at least a 1-week period of a continuously elevated or irritable mood, although shorter durations of symptoms are acceptable if the patient is hospitalized. In addition to elevated mood, the patient should experience at least three of the following symptoms: elevated self-esteem or grandiose ideations, reduced need for sleep, pressured speech, racing thoughts or flight of ideas, easily distracted, psychomotor agitation, and excessive involvement in high-risk activities.
2. Major depressive episode is diagnosed using the same diagnostic criteria in patients presenting with unipolar depression (see previous section titled Major Depressive Disorder). Depressive episodes are more frequent, last longer, and occur more in bipolar II disorder.
3. Hypomania has similar symptoms to that of mania; however, symptoms are not as severe. Hypomania is diagnosed by an elevated mood present for at least 4 days, with at least three of the same symptoms as described for mania. These symptoms should not interfere with social or occupational functioning and should not cause hospitalization.
4. A mixed disorder is diagnosed when the criteria for both mania and a major depressive episode are met every day for nearly 1 week, affects social and occupational functioning, and is not caused by a general medical condition or substance.
5. Bipolar disorder may be classified into bipolar I disorder, bipolar II disorder, cyclothymia, and rapid cycling.
   a. **Bipolar I disorder.** Patients are classified with bipolar I disorder with a history of at least one mixed or manic episode and at least one major depressive episode.
   b. **Bipolar II disorder.** Patients are classified with bipolar II disorder with a history of at least one episode of hypomania and one major depressive episode but have never experienced mania or a mixed episode.
   c. **Cyclothymic disorder.** Patients are classified with cyclothymic disorder with at least a 2-year history of multiple episodes of hypomania and depressive symptoms. These patients have never met full criteria for a major depressive or manic episode.
   d. **Rapid cycling.** Patients that experience at least four depressive, manic, hypomanic, or mixed episodes within a 12-month period are described as rapid cycling.

C. **Clinical course.** The course of bipolar disorder is lifelong, episodic, and patient specific.

1. Patients usually experience episodes of depression initially. Men are more likely to initially present with mania, but both men and women are more likely to have a first episode of depression. Approximately 95% of bipolar patients will experience a depressive episode during their lifetime.
2. Episodes vary in length and severity; however, they may last from days to months if untreated.
3. The duration of time between episodes varies. Commonly, 4 years or more may separate the first and second episode but subsequent episodes are more frequent.
4. The management of this disorder can be complicated by mixed episodes, rapid cycling, and substance abuse. It is imperative to screen patients for substance use disorders, medical illnesses, medications, and risk-taking behavior as possible causes for acute mood changes. Substance abuse occurs in approximately 45% of patients.
5. Suicide rates are high in bipolar disorder. Approximately 50% of bipolar patients attempt suicide with completed suicide rates of 10% to 15%. Suicide is more likely to be attempted in patients experiencing a depressive or mixed episode.

D. **Treatment options**

1. **Pharmacotherapeutic options.** Mood stabilizers have historically been the mainstays of therapy for bipolar disorder. Agents include lithium, valproic acid and its derivatives (divalproex sodium), and carbamazepine. Recent literature has supported the use of atypical antipsychotics as

Table 40-6 ALGORITHMS FOR TREATMENT OF BIPOLAR I DISORDER

Type of Episode	Monotherapy Options First-Line	Monotherapy Options Second-Line
Acute mania	Lithium, VPA, aripiprazole, quetiapine, risperidone, ziprasidone	Olanzapine, CBZ
Acute mixed	VPA, aripiprazole, quetiapine, risperidone, ziprasidone	Olanzapine, CBZ
Acute depressive	Lamotrigine or lamotrigine plus antimanic	Quetiapine, olanzapinefluoxetine
Maintenance mania or mixed	Lithium, VPA, or lamotrigine	Olanzapine
Depression	Lamotrigine plus antimanic or lamotrigine	

CBZ, carbamazepine; *VPA*, valproic acid.
Adapted from Suppes T, Dennehy EB, Hirschfeld RM, et al. The Texas implementation of medication algorithms: update to the algorithm for treatment of bipolar I disorder. *J Clin Psychiatry.* 2005;66:870–886.

monotherapy or adjunctive treatments in bipolar mania. Agents for the treatment of depressive episodes in patients with bipolar remains more limited, with data supporting the use of lithium, lamotrigine, quetiapine, and olanzapine-fluoxetine. The 2005 Texas Implementation of Medication Algorithms update for the treatment of bipolar I disorder is summarized in *Table 40-6.*

a. Lithium is indicated for the acute and chronic treatment of mania. Lithium may also be effective in the treatment of mixed episodes and depressive episodes.

(1) Lithium carbonate is available as immediate-release (Eskalith), controlled-release (Eskalith CR), or extended-release (Lithobid) tablets, and lithium citrate (Lithonate) is available as syrup.

(2) Pharmacokinetics

(a) Between 60% and 100% of lithium is absorbed from the gastrointestinal tract. The extent of absorption is not affected by food. The rate of absorption varies depending on the formulation.

(b) Lithium is not highly protein bound.

(c) Lithium is eliminated primarily through the kidneys. Changes in renal function can significantly affect the clearance of lithium.

(3) The mechanism of action for lithium is currently unknown, although several theories exist.

(a) Lithium is thought to help correct desynchronized biological rhythms in patients with bipolar disorder.

(b) Lithium may affect membrane stabilization.

(c) Lithium may augment homeostasis by enhancing the function of secondary messenger systems, especially cyclic adenosine monophosphate (cAMP), cyclic guanosine monophosphate (cGMP), and phosphatidylinositol.

(d) Lithium can inhibit NE release and accelerate its metabolism.

(e) Lithium may decrease receptor sensitivity and increase presynaptic reuptake of NE and 5-HT.

(4) Lithium has a narrow therapeutic index, with a therapeutic range of 0.5 to 1.0 mEq/L. Toxicity is associated with levels $>$ 1.5 mEq/L. Patients presenting with acute mania generally require levels in the higher end of the therapeutic range than those on maintenance therapy. Patients treated for bipolar depression require a level $\geq$ 0.8 mEq/L. Maintenance lithium levels can be as low as 0.6 mEq/L if patients are clinically stable.

(a) Patients are generally started on 300 mg two to three times daily of lithium and titrated up by 300 mg increments as needed to achieve therapeutic effects and minimize toxicity. Patients can be switch to a long-acting formulation once a patient is stabilized on treatment.

(b) Patient-specific factors such as age, weight, and renal function should be considered.

Table 40-7 ADVERSE EFFECTS OF LITHIUM

Early Onset	Long-Term Use	Toxicity
Gastrointestinal upset	Morphological kidney changes	Severe drowsiness
Nausea	EKG changes	Coarse hand tremor
Polydipsia	Bradycardia	Muscle twitching
Nocturia	Weight gain	Seizures
Dry mouth	Decreased libido	Choreoathetosis
Hand tremor	Hypothyroidism	Vomiting
Leukocytosis	Rash	Confusion
Polyuria	Acne	Vertigo

(c) Serum concentrations may be monitored 5 days after initiation therapy or changing doses. A level can be checked after 3 days of treatment in patients with suspected toxicity or decreased renal function. Levels should be obtained 12 hrs after the dose, usually in the morning before the first dose of the day. Patients' prescribed extended-release lithium may have a 12-hr trough level that is 12% to 33% higher than regular release lithium.

(d) Once a patient is stabilized, follow-up lithium levels can occur less frequently (every 6 to 12 months) and can be dictated by the clinical status of a patient.

(e) Prior to starting lithium, baseline monitoring should include a medical history, medication history, physical examination, basic metabolic panel, renal function panel, pregnancy test, thyroid panel, complete blood count, and ECG (if risk factors merit ECG).

(f) Follow-up labs should include renal function panel, basic metabolic panel, complete blood count, and a thyroid function panel. These labs can occur less frequently (every 6 to 12 months) in stabilized patients.

(5) Clinical response. Clinical response may be seen within 1 to 2 weeks after lithium initiation for the treatment of acute mania. When used in depression, responses may not occur for 6 to 8 weeks. Lithium has been shown to produce an 8- to 10-fold decrease in suicide rates.

(6) Precautions and adverse effects

(a) Lithium has an absolute contraindication in patients experiencing acute renal failure or women in their first trimester of pregnancy.

(b) Lithium has the following relative contraindications: renal impairment, cardiovascular disease, dehydration, pregnancy, seizure disorder, and thyroid disease.

(c) Lithium has numerous adverse effects (*Table 40-7*). Adverse effects (especially those seen early in therapy) can be related to too high peak levels. Doses should be decreased to minimize these peak-related adverse effects. Certain adverse effects indicate toxicity. If toxicity occurs, lithium should be immediately discontinued, the patient should be properly hydrated, stomach contents should be emptied with gastric lavage, and if severe toxicity occurs (level $\geq$ 3 mEq/L), hemodialysis may be indicated.

(7) Many medications and disease states may affect lithium levels in the body (*Table 40-8*).

(a) Use of lithium with antipsychotics or benzodiazepines may increase the risk for CNS toxicity.

(b) Use of lithium with medications that can increase 5-HT may cause serotonin syndrome.

b. Valproic acid (VPA) is indicated in the acute and chronic treatment of mania. VPA may also be effective in the treatment of hypomania, mixed disorders, and rapid cycling (*Table 40-6*).

(1) Mechanism of action. The mechanism of action for VPA is not entirely known. Efficacy for VPA is thought to be related to its ability to increase levels of GABA.

Table 40-8 FACTORS THAT CHANGE LITHIUM CONCENTRATIONS[a]

Increase Lithium Levels	Decrease Lithium Levels
Angiotensin-converting enzyme inhibitors	Acetazolamide
Angiotensin II receptor blockers	Methylxanthines (e.g., theophylline, caffeine)
Nonsteroidal anti-inflammatory drugs	Osmotic diuretics
Thiazides	Pregnancy (third trimester)
Dehydration	Sodium supplements
Renal dysfunction	Urine alkalinizers (ex. sodium bicarbonate)
Sodium loss	
Fluoxetine	

[a]Not an all-inclusive list.

(2) Many formulations exist for VPA. VPA is formulated as valproic acid (Depakene) in capsules and syrup, as divalproex sodium in delayed-release tablets (Depakote) and extended-release tablets (Depakote ER), and as valproate in intravenous solution (Depacon).

(3) VPA is generally initiated at doses of 20 to 30 mg/kg/day given in divided doses for inpatients and 250 mg three times daily for outpatients. The current therapeutic range (50 to 125 μg/mL) was originally described for the treatment of seizure disorders and has not been established for efficacy in bipolar disorder. The extended-release formulation has a 15% to 25% decreased bioavailability there requiring a 25% dose increase when switching from an immediate-release formulation.

(a) Levels may be first obtained after 3 to 5 days of therapy. These values should be trough values and obtained 12 hrs following a dose. The monitoring of VPA levels can occur less frequently (every 6 to 12 months) in clinical stable patients.

(b) Patients that are treated for 4 to 6 weeks with VPA concentrations of 80 to 120 μg/mL without clinical response may be classified as failures of VPA therapy.

(4) **Adverse effects.** Common adverse effects of VPA include nausea, vomiting, dyspepsia, sedation, elevated liver enzymes, hair loss, and tremor. Less frequent adverse effects include thrombocytopenia, leukopenia, pancreatitis, weight gain, and liver failure. VPA has also been associated with polycystic ovarian syndrome in women of child-bearing age.

(a) Gastrointestinal adverse effects may be minimized by lowering the dose or by using divalproex formulations instead of valproic acid or sodium valproate.

(b) Liver function tests and complete blood counts should be monitored at baseline, every month for the first 2 months of therapy, and then every 6 to 12 months thereafter.

(c) VPA has a wide therapeutic index making a lethal overdose less likely to occur.

(5) **Medication interactions.** VPA has the potential for multiple drug interactions. VPA is highly protein bound in the body; thus, levels can increase in the presence of another medication that is highly protein bound. VPA is also a substrate and inhibitor of the cytochrome P450 isoenzyme 2C9 and can potentially elevate levels of other medications that are metabolized via this isoenzyme.

c. Carbamazepine (CBZ) is indicated in the acute treatment of mania, but is considered to be a second-line agent owing to its numerous adverse effects and medication interactions (*Table 40-6*).

(1) The mechanism of action for CBZ is not completely known; however, its efficacy in bipolar disorder is thought to be the result of its effects on GABA and G protein-linked second messenger systems, such as cAMP.

(2) CBZ should be initiated at doses of 200 to 600 mg/day given in divided doses and increased by 200 mg/day to usual doses of 800 to 1000 mg/day.

(a) A therapeutic range of 4 to 12 μg/mL has been described for seizure disorders. Although correlation between this range and efficacy has not been fully established for bipolar disorder, it is used to minimize adverse effects.

(b) Levels may be obtained 5 to 7 days after initiating therapy. Levels should continued to be obtained in the following few weeks because CBZ concentrations will decrease in the body once autoinduction occurs.

(c) Patients who are treated for 4 to 6 weeks with CBZ concentrations of 6 to 12 μg/mL without clinical response may be classified as failures of CBZ therapy.

(3) **Adverse effects.** CBZ is associated with numerous adverse effects, many of which are dose related.

(a) Frequent adverse effects include dizziness, drowsiness, ataxia, fatigue, blurred vision, diplopia, nystagmus, confusion, headache, nausea, vomiting, diarrhea, and dyspepsia. The gastrointestinal adverse effects of CBZ are often dose related.

(b) Additional adverse effects include rash, leukopenia, thrombocytopenia, hyponatremia, elevation in liver enzymes, and weight gain.

(c) Severe idiosyncratic reactions may also occur, including agranulocytosis, aplastic anemia, severe thrombocytopenia, liver failure, Stevens–Johnson syndrome, and pancreatitis.

(d) Complete blood counts, liver function tests, thyroid tests, and electrolytes should be monitored at baseline and every 3 to 6 months.

(e) Carbamazepine can be lethal with ingestions over ≥ 6 g.

(4) **Medication interactions.** CBZ is an inducer of many hepatic enzymes responsible for metabolism of medications and, therefore, has numerous medication interactions. Oral contraceptive levels in the body can be decreased in patients taking CBZ. Alternative forms of contraception should be used in patients taking CBZ. CBZ can also induce its own metabolism (autoinduction). Decreases in CBZ levels in the body may be seen after 3 to 30 days of therapy. CBZ levels should be monitored and adjusted accordingly.

d. Lamotrigine is indicated in the maintenance treatment of bipolar disorder with benefit in preventing depressive episode relapse. Lamotrigine may be effective in rapid cycling bipolar patients (*Table 40-6*). Lamotrigine has mixed evidence regarding its use in acute depressive episodes.

(1) The mechanism of action for lamotrigine is not completely understood. It is currently thought to be related to its ability to decrease release of glutamate and aspartate by blocking sodium channels.

(2) Owing to the risk of rash, lamotrigine should be initiated at low doses (25 mg/day) and slowly increased by 25 mg every 1 to 2 weeks. Lamotrigine should be administered twice daily in doses > 50 mg. Usual dose range is 50 to 300 mg/d. Patients who are taking lamotrigine with VPA should decrease the dose by half owing to a significant medication interaction. Patients taking lamotrigine with carbamazepine should start at 50 mg/d, because carbamazepine increases the clearance of lamotrigine from the body.

(3) Common adverse effects include dizziness, diplopia, nausea, vomiting, rash, photosensitivity, ataxia, headache, and blurred vision. Rashes may be severe and life-threatening such as Stevens–Johnson rash, and patients should immediately discontinue the medication if a rash appears.

e. Atypical antipsychotics have recently been the subject of multiple studies in the treatment of bipolar disorder. All atypical antipsychotics except clozapine, iloperidone, and lurasidone are approved for the treatment of bipolar disorder (*Table 40-6*). For information regarding dosing, adverse effects, and mechanism of action, see Chapter 39. Olanzapine and quetiapine are approved for maintenance treatment in bipolar. Olanzapine is available in a formulation with fluoxetine (Symbyax), and quetiapine is approved for depressive episodes. Olanzapine and aripiprazole are available in intramuscular injections approved for treatment of agitation associated with bipolar mania.

f. Additional anticonvulsants

(1) Oxcarbazepine is a medication structurally similar to carbamazepine but with fewer adverse effects. It is postulated to have similar therapeutic effects in bipolar disorder to carbamazepine; however, studies demonstrating its efficacy are limited. It currently is recommended only in combination with other mood stabilizers.

g. Antidepressants should be used cautiously in patients with bipolar disorder because of the risk of inducing mania. When possible, patients should be receiving mood stabilizers at goal doses before initiating antidepressants and should be cautiously monitored. Bupropion and paroxetine have been associated with less risk of inducing mania than other antidepressants and may be preferable.

h. Benzodiazepines may be useful adjuncts to a primary treatment in reducing agitation, anxiety, and insomnia. Benzodiazepines should be discontinued once the primary treatment is stabilized because benzodiazepines are ineffective in treating bipolar disorder. Lorazepam is available in an intramuscular formulation, which may be useful in acute agitation.

2. Treatment duration/phases. The treatment of bipolar disorder is structured similarly to that of depression with acute, continuation, and maintenance phases. Maintenance treatment is strongly recommended for all patients with bipolar disorder, especially those with a family history.

3. Treatment augmentation

a. Patients with no or partial response to monotherapy may receive combination therapy with two agents. Agents that can be combined include lithium, VPA, and the atypical antipsychotics. Atypical antipsychotics, if used, should be combined with either VPA or lithium and not combined with another atypical antipsychotic.

b. For depressive episodes, lamotrigine may be combined with another mood stabilizer as first-line therapy, and the olanzapine–fluoxetine combination product is a second-line option.

4. Treatment options in pregnancy

a. Multiple agents used in the treatment of bipolar disorder have been associated with birth defects.

(1) Lithium, VPA, and CBZ are pregnancy category D medications.

(2) Lithium has been associated with birth defects, primarily in the first trimester.

(3) VPA and CBZ should be used during pregnancy only if the benefits outweigh the risks. If the decision is made to use these medications during pregnancy, folic acid should be given to minimize the risk of defects.

(4) Lamotrigine and oxcarbazepine are pregnancy category C medications.

III. TREATMENT OF ANXIETY SPECTRUM DISORDERS. Generalized anxiety disorder, panic disorder, and social anxiety disorder

A. Introduction. Anxiety is a natural response to a real or perceived danger; however, when it causes significant distress or impairment in an individual's life, then it becomes an anxiety disorder. Anxiety disorders are the most commonly encountered psychiatric disorders in health care.

B. Diagnosis/clinical presentation

1. Generalized anxiety disorder (GAD) is diagnosed when an individual experiences unrealistic or excessive anxiety and worry for a period of at least 6 months. Additionally, the individual must have difficult in controlling that anxiety or worry. Accompanying the anxiety or worry more days than not over the 6 month period are 3 or more of following symptoms: feeling tense or restless, easily fatigued or worn-out, difficulty concentrating, irritability, and difficulty with sleep. Lastly, GAD must cause significant distress or impairment and not be accounted for by another medical, psychiatric, or substance use disorder.

2. A patient is diagnosed with a panic disorder when that individual experiences repeated unexpected panic attacks and these attacks are followed by a 1-month period of one or more: persistent concern over future attacks, worry about the consequences of future attacks, and a significant change in behavior related to the attacks. Lastly, panic disorder must cause significant distress or impairment and not be accounted for by another medical, psychiatric, or substance use disorder.

a. A panic attack usually peaks in 10 mins and lasts no longer than 30 mins. Common symptoms experienced during an attack include sweating, chest pain, dizziness, tachycardia, palpitations, and abdominal distress. During an attack an individual will often feel like they are losing control or dying.

3. Social anxiety disorder (SAD) is diagnosed when a person has an intense persistent fear of social situations where an individual may be exposed to unfamiliar people or to scrutiny by others. Exposure to the situation produces anxiety that the individual recognizes is unreasonable or excessive. Usually feared situations are avoided or endured with distress. Lastly, SAD symptoms must cause significant distress or impairment and not be accounted for by another medical, psychiatric, or substance use disorder.

a. Feared situations include public speaking, talking with strangers, and eating or writing in front of others. Common physical symptoms include blushing (cardinal symptom), diarrhea, sweating, and tachycardia.

C. Treatment

1. The mainstay of treatment for GAD, panic disorder, and SAD is the antidepressants. There is emerging evidence with other classes of medications, such as the atypical antipsychotics; however, treatment with antidepressants is still considered first-line treatment. Of the antidepressants, SSRIs and venlafaxine are the first-line treatment options. Nonpharmacological treatments focus on cognitive behavioral therapies (CBT) and are recommended for mild symptoms of these disorders or in combination with pharmacological treatment. The effect of CBT may take weeks to months.
2. The goals of treatment should be a reduction in the frequency and severity of symptoms and relief of a patient's distress and impairment. Full symptom remission should be a realistic goal with treatment.

D. Treatment options

1. **Antidepressants**

 a. **GAD**

 (1) Of the antidepressants, paroxetine, escitalopram, venlafaxine XR, and duloxetine are FDA approved for GAD. The anti-anxiety effect from antidepressants occurs in 2 to 4 weeks. Imipramine (Tofranil), a TCA antidepressant, may be a useful second-line treatment.

 b. **Panic**

 (1) SSRIs are the first-line treatment of panic disorder. Sertraline, paroxetine, and venlafaxine XR are FDA approved. Imipramine has also been shown to be highly effective; however, its use is limited to its adverse effect profile. Treatment effect usually takes at least 4 weeks; however, patients may not respond until 8 to 12 weeks. Initial antidepressant dosing in panic disorder is usually half the initial starting dose used in the treatment of depression.

 c. **SAD**

 (1) Antidepressants are first-line treatment of SAD. Paroxetine, sertraline, venlafaxine XR, and fluvoxamine XR (Luvox XR) are FDA approved. Mirtazapine (Remeron) and phenelzine may be good second-line antidepressants. TCAs are not effective in SAD. Onset of effect may take 4 to 6 weeks with some patients not achieving maximal benefit until 12 weeks. Initial antidepressant dosing in SAD is usually half the initial starting dose used in the treatment of depression.

2. **Other treatment options**

 a. **GAD**

 (1) Benzodiazepines are effective medications due to their anxiolytic properties and may provide rapid symptom relief. All benzodiazepines are considered equally effective and as a class may be most beneficial for somatic and autonomic symptoms. Benzodiazepines may be most useful when used early in treatment in combination with an antidepressant.

 (2) Buspirone (Buspar) is a nonbenzodiazepine anxiolytic useful in the treatment of GAD. Buspirone is a second-line treatment option and may be most useful in patients unable to take benzodiazepines. The anxiolytic properties of buspirone may be due to partial agonism of 5-HT_{1A}-receptors. The effectiveness of buspirone may take up to 4 weeks. Side effects are mild and include dizziness, nausea, and headaches.

 (3) Other treatment options include hydroxyzine (Vistaril), pregabalin, and atypical antipsychotics.

 b. **Panic**

 (1) Benzodiazepines—alprazolam (Xanax) and clonazepam (Klonopin) are FDA approved. Diazepam (Valium) and lorazepam (Ativan) may also be effective. Benzodiazepines provide rapid symptom relief and may be most useful when used early in treatment in combination with an antidepressant.

 (2) Phenelzine (Nardil), an MAOI, may be an alternative treatment option for treatment-resistant patients.

 c. **SAD**

 (1) Benzodiazepines, gabapentin (Neurontin), buspirone (Buspar), pregabalin (Lyrica), and atypical antipsychotics may be useful in SAD.

E. Evaluation of treatment

1. **GAD**
   - **a.** Treatment response should occur within 4 weeks of starting an antidepressant and much more quickly with benzodiazepines.
   - **b.** Treatment should continue for a 1-year period following treatment response.
   - **c.** Treatment should be slowly tapered over several months regardless of the medication chosen. Benzodiazepines require a slow gradual dose reduction due to concerns of withdrawal such as seizures and rebound symptoms.
2. **Panic**
   - **a.** Treatment response should occur within 6 to 8 weeks following antidepressant initiation. Patients receiving antidepressants may need up to 12 weeks of treatment before receiving a full response. Adequate treatment with a benzodiazepine is considered 4 weeks.
   - **b.** Treatment should continue for a period of 12 to 24 months following treatment response.
   - **c.** Treatment should be slowly tapered over several months regardless of the medication chosen.
3. **SAD**
   - **a.** An adequate antidepressant trial is 8 to 12 weeks.
   - **b.** Treatment should continue for a period of 12 to 24 months following treatment response.
   - **c.** Treatment should be slowly tapered over several months regardless of the medication chosen.

IV. OBSESSIVE COMPULSIVE DISORDER (OCD)

A. Introduction. OCD is a psychiatric disorder characterized by intrusive obsessive thoughts and ritualistic behaviors performed to reduce anxiety.

B. Diagnosis

1. *DSM-IV* diagnostic criteria for OCD diagnosis include the following: recurrent obsession or compulsions which are severe enough to be time consuming (> 1 hr/day) or cause marked distress or significant impairment; realizations that obsessions/compulsions are excessive or unreasonable; condition is not the direct result of a psychiatric, medical, or substance abuse disorder.
   - **a.** An obsession is a recurrent, persistent idea, thought, impulse, or image that is experienced as intrusive and inappropriate and causes anxiety or distress.
     - **(1)** Obsessions can have many themes including aggressive impulses, contamination, order, religion, doubts, and sexual imagery.
   - **b.** A compulsion is a repetitive act or mental ritual designed to counteract the anxiety caused by obsessions.
     - **(1)** Common compulsions include hand washing, checking, ordering, need to confess, counting, and repeating.

C. Clinical presentation

1. Patients with OCD will most often present to a nonpsychiatric doctor with physical complaints such as chapped hands from repeated washings or gum bruising from repeated tooth brushing. Irritable bowel syndrome is also commonly seen in patients with OCD.

D. Treatment

1. The mainstay of OCD treatment is the SSRIs. There is emerging evidence with other classes of medications, such as the atypical antipsychotics; however, the SSRIs are still considered first-line treatment. Nonpharmacological treatments focus on cognitive behavioral therapies (CBT) and are recommended for mild symptoms of OCD or in combination with pharmacological treatment. The effect of CBT may take weeks to months.
2. The goal of treatment should be a reduction in the frequency and severity of symptoms. Even a partial resolution of symptoms may provide a remarkable relief to a patient's distress and impairment.
3. **Treatment options**
   - **a. Serotonergic antidepressants**
     - **(1)** All SSRIs are used in the treatment of OCD; however, only four are FDA approved for this indication; fluoxetine (Prozac), fluvoxamine (Luvox), paroxetine (Paxil), and sertraline (Zoloft). Fluoxetine (Prozac), fluvoxamine (Luvox), and sertraline (Zoloft) are FDA approved for children with OCD.

(2) Clomipramine (Anafranil) is a tricyclic antidepressant with strong serotonergic properties. Clomipramine has been shown to be as equal efficacious as SSRIs; however, its use is limited by side effects. Clomipramine is FDA approved for OCD in both children and adults.

(3) Clomipramine is started at 25 mg/day and increased to a maximum dose of 250 mg/day.

b. Other antidepressants

(1) Mixed evidence exists for venlafaxine (Effexor), mirtazapine (Remeron), and phenelzine (Nardil).

c. Atypical antipsychotics

(1) Augmentation with an atypical antipsychotic has been shown to produce a response rate around 50%. Olanzapine (Zyprexa), quetiapine (Seroquel), and risperidone (Risperdal) have the most evidence supporting their use. See Chapter 39 for specific information on atypical antipsychotics.

(2) Augmentation with an atypical antipsychotic is recommended only after a 3-month trial of a maximal dosed antidepressant.

(3) Atypical antipsychotics may be particularly useful for the treatment of tics.

4. Evaluation of treatment

a. Full symptom remission is rare and an unrealistic expectation. Approximately 70% of patients will have some degree of symptom improvement following antidepressant treatment.

b. An adequate trial of an antidepressant is 8 to 12 weeks. Antidepressant medications should be dosed to their maximum tolerated dose for a period of at least 4 to 6 weeks.

c. Treatment should be continued for a period of 1 to 2 years with a slow gradual taper over the course of months to a year.

d. A patient should fail two to three trials with different SSRIs before moving to clomipramine (Anafranil).

e. Combination treatment, SSRI + clomipramine or augmentation of an antidepressant with an atypical antipsychotic, can be tried in patients with treatment-resistant OCD.

f. Lifelong treatment is for patients with two to four severe relapses or three to four mild relapses.

V. POSTTRAUMATIC STRESS DISORDER

A. Introduction. PTSD is a psychiatric disorder with severely debilitating symptoms. Largely recognized as a combat-related phenomenon, PTSD is now widely recognized in civilians as well.

B. Diagnosis/clinical presentation

1. Exposure to a traumatic event is required for a patient to have PTSD. The traumatic event must cause anxiety or impairment that interferes with an individual's ability to function. Lastly, the symptoms cannot be caused by another psychiatric, medical, or substance abuse disorder.

2. Three symptoms domains of PTSD are re-experiencing, avoidance, and increased arousal. For diagnosis, at least one symptom from the re-experiencing domain is required, three symptoms from the avoidance domain are required, and two symptoms from the increased arousal are required.

3. These symptoms must be present for greater than a 1-month period and must cause significant impairment in an individual's life.

4. Common symptoms include: Re-experiencing domain: recurring bad memories, distressing nightmares, flashbacks, and intense fear/anxiety with remembering event; Avoidance domain: Avoidance of people, places, activities, thoughts, feelings associated with traumatic event, restricted affect, sense of doom, and diminished pleasure. Increased arousal domain: insomnia, irritability, anger, and hypervigilance.

5. Subsets of PTSD

a. Acute stress disorder occurs within 2 days of experiencing a traumatic event, but symptoms resolve within 1 month after the event.

b. Acute PTSD is defined as PTSD lasting less than 3 months.

c. Chronic PTSD is defined as PTSD lasting 3 months or more.

C. Treatment

1. The mainstay of treatment is the SSRIs. There is emerging evidence with other classes of medications, such as other antidepressants, atypical antipsychotics, and alpha-1 antagonists; however, the SSRIs are still considered first-line treatment. Nonpharmacological treatments focus on cognitive behavioral therapies (CBT), eye movement desensitization and reprocessing, and stress management. These nonpharmacological treatments are recommended for mild symptoms of OCD or in combination with pharmacological treatment. The effect of CBT may be most useful if initiated within days to weeks following the traumatic event.

2. The goal of treatment should be a reduction in the frequency and severity of symptoms in the three symptom domains. With symptom remission, patients should also have improvement in impairments and quality of life.
3. **Treatment options**
   a. **Antidepressants**
      (1) All antidepressant medications are used in the treatment of PTSD. However, only the SSRIs and venlafaxine (Effexor) are considered first-line treatment options for PTSD. Older TCAs and MAOIs are effective but limited in their use due to their side effect burden. TCAs may be a good second-line treatment option. Mirtazapine (Remeron) may also be a good second-line treatment option due to studies showing benefit in global symptom reduction. MAOIs should be reserved as a third-line treatment option.
      (2) Paroxetine (Paxil) and sertraline (Zoloft) are FDA approved for acute treatment. Sertraline is also FDA approved for long-term treatment.
      (3) Antidepressants may work best on the symptom domains of avoidance and increased arousal. Benefit may also be seen in re-experiencing. Phenelzine (Nardil) may be useful in reducing nightmares, flashbacks, and insomnia.
   b. **Alternative treatment options**
      (1) Atypical antipsychotics, alpha-1 antagonists, anticonvulsants, and β-blockers may be useful augmenting agents.
      (2) Atypical antipsychotics and anticonvulsants may help reduce irritability, impulsivity, and violent behaviors. Atypical antipsychotics have been shown to effectively reduce the core symptoms as well. See Chapter 39 for specific information on atypical antipsychotics.
      (3) The alpha-1 antagonist prazosin (Minipress) dosed between 1 mg and 4 mg may reduce nightmares and insomnia.
      (4) Benzodiazepines have not been shown to be effective. Their use is discouraged use due to their potential for abuse and to cause dissociation.
4. **Evaluation of treatment**
   a. Full symptom remission should be the goal of treatment.
      (1) Full remission is defined as a 70% or greater reduction in symptoms.
      (2) Fifty percent symptom reduction is considered an adequate response.
      (3) Twenty-five percent to 50% symptom reduction is a partial treatment response.
   b. An adequate trial of an antidepressant is 6 to 12 weeks. Antidepressant medications should be dosed to their maximum tolerated dose for a period of at least 4 to 6 weeks.
   c. Treatment should be continued for a period of at least 1 year with a slow gradual taper over the course of months to a year.

VI. TREATMENT OF ATTENTION-DEFICIT HYPERACTIVITY DISORDER (ADHD)

A. **Introduction.** ADHD is a condition characterized by the inability to maintain and sustain attention and control behavior and impulses. ADHD was the first psychiatric disorder to be diagnosed and treated in children rather than in adults. There is increasing recognition that symptoms and impairments of ADHD may persist beyond childhood and into adulthood.

B. **Diagnosis**
1. Symptoms must be present before the age of 7 years old and be present in two or more settings. Symptoms must not result from another psychiatric, developmental, or medical disorder.
2. Six or more symptoms (symptom list in the following text) must be present for a period of at least 6 months. Diagnosis requires evidence of inattention or hyperactivity and impulsivity or both. Evidence of symptoms comes from reports from the child, parents, and teachers. Symptoms include:
   a. **Inattention**
      (1) Often fails to give close attention to details and makes careless mistakes, has difficult sustaining attention, does not seem to listen, does not seem to follow through, has difficulty

organizing tasks, avoids tasks that require sustained attention, loses things necessary for activities, is easily distracted, is forgetful.

b. **Hyperactivity and impulsivity**
   (1) Often fidgets, leaves seat, runs about or climbs excessively, has difficulty with quiet leisure activities, is "on the go" or "driven by motor," talks excessively, blurts out answers, has difficulty awaiting turn, interrupts, or intrudes.

3. These diagnostic criteria are the same for both children and adults. The use of these criteria for adults may present problems since most adults may not remember being diagnosed before the age of 7, some symptoms may not be age appropriate, and the minimal requirement of six criteria may result in underdiagnosis.

C. **Clinical presentation**

1. Eighty percent of children will present with a combination of symptoms of inattention plus hyperactivity/impulsivity. Ten percent to 15% will have only with symptoms inattention, while 5% will only demonstrate symptoms of hyperactivity/impulsivity.
2. Approximately two-thirds of children with ADHD will have impairing levels of symptoms persisting into adulthood.
3. Children with ADHD may also have a comorbid condition; however, children with ADHD have a lower prevalence of comorbid conditions compared to adults.
   a. Most common comorbid conditions in children include: learning and language disorder, oppositional defiant disorder, mood and anxiety disorders, tic, and posttraumatic stress disorder.
4. Adults seek treatment mainly due to the negative impact of ADHD on their own lives, family, and work.
   a. Medical and psychiatric comorbidities are more prevalent in adults and should be included in the differential diagnosis for ADHD symptoms and taken into consideration when patients are being treated with stimulants or nonstimulants.
      (1) Medical conditions include thyroid disorders, head trauma, poisoning, substance intoxication, and seizure disorders.
      (2) Psychiatric conditions include mood disorders, anxiety, substance use, and borderline and antisocial personality disorders.

D. **Treatment**

1. The mainstay of ADHD treatment is pharmacological treatment. Both stimulant and nonstimulant medications are effective in ADHD. Stimulant medications are recommended as first-line treatment because approximately 70% to 90% of patients will have a symptom response. Stimulants have a larger effect size and a lower number needed to treat compared to nonstimulants. Nonstimulants, such as atomoxetine and extended-release guanfacine, are second-line treatment options. Nonpharmacological treatment, mainly behavioral modification, may have the best benefit when used in combination with medication.
2. Stimulant medications (for doses, durations of effect, adverse effects, and contraindications see *Table 40-9*)
   a. This medication class consists of both methylphenidate and amphetamine containing agents. All stimulants mainly work by blocking the reuptake of both dopamine and norepinephrine. The effect of stimulants on ADHD symptoms should occur within days to 1 week. There has little evidence to support any major differences in efficacy, adverse effects, or response rates between stimulants.
   b. Treatment with stimulants is started at the lowest possible dose and titrated slowly up to the maximal tolerated dose. Initiation of therapy usually starts with an immediate-release stimulant and then changes to an extended-release agent to minimize the number of doses per day. Extended-release formulations may improve compliance, decrease the potential for abuse, and remove the stigma associated with taking medication during the school/work day.
   c. If a patient does not have a response to one stimulant, another stimulant should be tried before changing to a nonstimulant medication. It is recommended that a patient try both a methylphenidate and amphetamine containing agent because there are slight differences between these agents that may affect patient response.

Table 40-9 STIMULANT MEDICATIONS USED IN THE TREATMENT OF ADHD

	Usual Dosage (mg)	Duration of Effect (hr)	Adverse Effects	Contraindications
Methylphenidate-based			Growth/appetite suppression, headaches, insomnia, irritability, jitteriness, mild increase in blood pressure and heart rate	Seizures, tics, marked tension, anxiety, aggression glaucoma, MAOIs
Short-acting				
Ritalin, Methylin	10–20	3–5		
Intermediate-acting				
Ritalin SR	20–40	3–8		
Metadate ER	10–20	3–8		
Methylin ER	10–20	3–8		
Long-acting				
Ritalin LA	20–40	6–8		
Concerta	27–54	10–12		
Metadate CD	10–20	4–8		
Daytrana patch	10–30	9–12		
Dexmethylphenidate				
Focalin	5–10	3–5		
Focalin XR	5–20	8–12		
Amphetamine-based			Growth/appetite suppression, headaches, insomnia, irritability, jitteriness, mild increase in blood pressure and heart rate	Cardiovascular disease, hypertension, hyperthyroidism glaucoma, MAOIs
Adderall	5–30	4–6		
Adderall XR	10–30	8–12		
Dextrostat	5–20	3–5		
Dexedrine spansule	5–15	5–8		
Vyvanse	20–70	8–12		

MAOIs, monoamine oxidase inhibitors.

d. Methylphenidate patch (Daytrana) is the only transdermal formulation of a stimulant medication. It is to be worn for a maximum of 9 hrs. The patch should be placed on the hip; alternating placement sites with each use.

e. Pemoline has been withdrawn from the market due to concerns of hepatotoxicity.

f. Special consideration of adverse effects and precautions should be taken before starting an adult on a stimulant medication.

3. Nonstimulant medications (for doses, durations of effect, adverse effects, and contraindications, see *Table 40-10*)

a. Atomoxetine and extended-release guanfacine are the only FDA approved nonstimulant medications for ADHD and are recommended as second-line treatment options. Atomoxetine is also FDA approved for adult ADHD. Nonstimulant medications may be useful in patients unable to tolerate stimulants or their adverse effects, if a contraindication exists for stimulant use, as an adjunctive treatment to stimulants for ADHD symptoms, as treatment of adverse effects from stimulants, or in patients with a comorbid substance use disorder or psychiatric illness (such as a mood disorder or anxiety).

b. Atomoxetine is a selective norepinephrine reuptake inhibitor and its effect on ADHD symptoms may take several weeks. Atomoxetine has no abuse potential and may have less effect on growth and sleep compared to stimulants. Atomoxetine's labeling contains a bolded warning about the potential for severe liver injury and patients should be monitored for signs and symptoms of hepatotoxicity.

Table 40-10 COMMON NONSTIMULANT MEDICATIONS USED IN THE TREATMENT OF ADHD

	Usual Dosage (mg)	Duration of Effect (hr)	Adverse Effects	Contraindications
Atomoxetine (Strattera)	18–60	24	Nausea, vomiting, mild increases in blood pressure and heart rate, suicidality, liver injury	Clinical/laboratory evidence of liver injury, MAOIs, glaucoma
Guanfacine ER (Intuniv)	1–4	24	Mild sedation, dizziness, constipation, hypotension	Hypersensitivity to guanfacine
Bupropion (Wellbutrin SR, XL)	50–300	24	Weight loss, insomnia, agitation, seizure at high doses	Seizure, eating disorders MAOIs, BZ or alcohol use abuse (withdrawal)

MAOIs, monoamine oxidase inhibitors; *BZ*, benzodiasepine.

c. Extended-release guanfacine works by inhibiting central release of norepinephrine and by increasing blood flow to the prefrontal cortex. Benefit in disruptive behavior, aggression, and sleep may also be experienced with this medication.

d. Bupropion is an antidepressant that is a weak dopamine and norepinephrine reuptake inhibitor. Overall, bupropion has shown modest efficacy. In small sample size studies in children, bupropion has demonstrated greater benefit compared to placebo and equal efficacy compared to methylphenidate. Bupropion may cause less appetite suppression compared to methylphenidate.

e. Other nonstimulant agents include clonidine, modafinil, tricyclic antidepressants, anticonvulsants, and antipsychotics. Clonidine may be a useful adjunct to stimulants for symptoms of hyperactivity, impulsivity, aggression, or insomnia. Anticonvulsants and antipsychotics may be most useful in patients with comorbid bipolar disorder, conduct disorder, or aggression.

4. Evaluation of treatment

a. Stimulants are first-line treatment

(1) Stimulants produce an effect on symptoms within days to 1 week.

(2) An adequate trial of a stimulant is considered weeks to 1 month.

(3) A trial of two stimulants (one methylphenidate and one amphetamine) is recommended as a first-line treatment.

b. Nonstimulants are second-line treatment options

(1) Atomoxetine and extended-release guanfacine are FDA-approved treatments. Atomoxetine is FDA approved in adults.

(2) An adequate trial of atomoxetine is 6 weeks; an adequate trial of extended-release guanfacine is 1 to 2 months.

c. Patients prescribed either medication class should be assessed periodically to ensure medication benefit and to monitor for adverse effects.

(1) Height, weight, and eating and sleeping patterns should be assessed at baseline and every 3 months for children prescribed stimulants.

(2) Adults should be appropriately monitored for any changes in their health, for any changes in their comorbid conditions, and for any adverse effects from ADHD medications.

5. Pregnancy and lactation

a. All stimulants and nonstimulants (except bupropion) are pregnancy category C. Bupropion is pregnancy category B.

b. The American Academy of Pediatrics does not recommend the use of methylphenidate and amphetamine in breastfeeding mothers. The effects of nonstimulants in breastfeeding are unknown.

VII. TREATMENT OF INSOMNIA

A. Introduction. Insomnia can refer to a disorder or to a symptom. Insomnia commonly occurs as a symptom experienced in many medical and psychiatric conditions and, as such, is defined as difficulty falling and/or staying asleep or poor quality of sleep. As a disorder, insomnia in addition to these symptoms causes a significant amount of impairment and distress in a person's life.

B. Diagnosis

1. Using the criteria listed by the International Classification of Sleep Disorder, 2nd edition, general criteria for insomnia are the following:
   - **a.** Difficult initiating or maintaining sleep, waking up too early, or sleep that is chronically nonrestorative or poor in quality.
   - **b.** Insomnia occurs despite adequate opportunity and circumstances for sleep.
   - **c.** At least one of the following daytime impairments related to sleep difficulty:
     - **(1)** Fatigue or malaise
     - **(2)** Impairment in attention, memory, or concentration
     - **(3)** Social, work, school performance impairment
     - **(4)** Mood disturbance or irritability
     - **(5)** Daytime sleepiness
     - **(6)** Motivation or energy reduction
     - **(7)** Proneness for errors or accidents
     - **(8)** Tension, headaches, or GI symptoms related to sleep loss
     - **(9)** Concerns or worries about sleep

C. Treatment

1. Treatment of insomnia includes both nonpharmacological and pharmacological treatment options. Nonpharmacological treatment may be a good first-line treatment option or can be useful in combination with medication. Pharmacological treatment options include prescription, OTC medications, and natural remedies. Benzodiazepines and benzodiazepine-receptor agonists are the mainstay of treatment although two new agents, ramelteon (Rozerem) and doxepin (Silenor), have been recently FDA approved. These two agents act through pathways different from the benzodiazepines.
2. **Nonpharmacological treatment**
   - **a.** A number of cognitive behavioral therapies exist including sleep hygiene education, stimulus-control therapy, relaxation therapy, and sleep-restriction therapy.
   - **b.** Sleep hygiene includes maintaining a regular sleep schedule; avoiding vigorous activity, alcohol, and nicotine before bedtime; creating a comfortable bedroom environment; and minimizing negative thoughts or focus on sleep.
   - **c.** Stimulus-control and relaxation therapies are meant to minimize hyperarousal before bedtime and to promote a calm environment used for only for sleep.
   - **d.** Studies have demonstrated the effectiveness of nonpharmacological treatment especially in reducing time to sleep onset, total sleep time, and the number and duration of night awakenings.
3. **Pharmacological treatment**
   - **a.** Prescription medication for insomnia centers on the benzodiazepines and benzodiazepine-receptor agonists. Other medications used for insomnia include ramelton, doxepin, sedating antidepressants and antipsychotics, and miscellaneous medications including barbiturates, chloral hydrate, and ethchlorvynol. The use of barbiturates, chloral hydrate, and ethchlorvynol has largely fallen out favor due to concern over adverse effects. Avoid giving these medications with food as it delays their onset of effect. See *Table 40-11* for doses, onset, half-lives, adverse effects, and contraindications for selected medications.
   - **b.** Benzodiazepines and benzodiazepine-receptor agonists—although all benzodiazepines are used in the treatment of insomnia, only nine agents are FDA approved for this indication.
     - **(1)** Benzodiazepines work by binding nonselectively to benzodiazepine receptors linked to the $GABA_A$ receptor. Nonselective benzodiazepines bind to three different types of benzodiazepine receptors; however, only the benzodiazepine type 1 (BZ type 1) receptor confers sedation.
     - **(2)** Benzodiazepine-receptor agonists only selectively bind to the BZ type 1 receptor and therefore cause sedation without producing an anticonvulsant effect or skeletal muscle relaxation.

Table 40-11 COMMON MEDICATIONS USED IN THE TREATMENT OF INSOMNIA

	Usual Dosage (mg)	Onset (min)	Maximal Half-lives (hr)	Adverse Effects	Contraindications
Benzodiazepines				Drowsiness, dizziness, ataxia, anterograde amnesia, rebound insomnia	None Avoid triazolam with drugs that induce CYP3A4.
Quazepam (Doral)	7.5–15.0	20–45	84		
Temazepam (Restoril)	7.5–30.0	30–60	15		
Triazolam (Halcion)	0.125–0.250	15–30	5		
Estazolam (Prosom)	0.5–2.0	60	24		
Flurazepam (Dalmane)	15–30	15–30	100		
Benzodiazepine-receptor agonists				Same as above. Eszopiclone has an unpleasant taste.	None Avoid with drugs that induce CYP3A4.
Eszopiclone (Lunesta)	1–3	30	7		
Zaleplon (Sonata)	5–20	20	1		
Zolpidem (Ambien)	5–10	30	3		
Extended-release Zolpidem (Ambien XR)	6.25–12.5	30	5.5		
Other medications					
Ramelteon (Rozerem)	8	30–60	5	Drowsiness, dizziness, increased prolactin	Hepatic failure Avoid with drugs that induce CYP1A2.
Doxepin (Silenor)	3–6	30	30	Anticholinergic, dizziness, hypotension, somnolence	MAOIs, glaucoma, severe urinary retention

(3) These medications have been shown to improve sleep latency, total sleep time, number of awakenings, and sleep quality.

(a) Shorter acting agents may have a better effect on reducing time to sleep.

(b) Longer acting agents may have a better effect on total sleep time.

(4) Benzodiazepine-receptor agonists may have less rebound insomnia, potential for abuse and dependence, hangover effect, and rebound insomnia upon drug discontinuation compared to nonselective benzodiazepines. Zolpidem has been associated with parasomnias including sleepwalking, eating, and driving.

(5) Eszopiclone and extended-release zolpidem are not limited to short-term use.

(6) All of these agents should be slowly titrated over the course of weeks to a month.

(7) All of these agents are schedule IV medications.

c. Ramelteon

(1) Ramelteon is a melatonin-receptor agonist selectively targeting the melatonin receptors MT1 and MT2 located in the hypothalamus. Stimulating these receptors is thought to affect the sleep–wake cycle and promote sleep. This is the first and only agent in this medication class.

(2) This medication does not bind to GABA receptors.

(3) Ramelteon has been shown to reduce time to sleep onset and improve total sleep time.

(4) Ramelteon is not limited to short-term use.

(5) Ramelteon is a noncontrolled medication. It is metabolized by CYP1A2 hepatic enzymes. Do not take with a high-fat meal or use in a patient with severe hepatic impairment.

d. Sedating antidepressants and antipsychotics

(1) Doxepin is FDA approved for the treatment of insomnia. Doxepin is a tricyclic antidepressant that produces its effects through histamine blockade.

(2) Tricyclic antidepressants have limited data supporting their use. This medication class may be most effective in patients with insomnia who have a comorbid depression or substance use disorder or in patients who have a contraindication or a poor response to benzodiazepine agents. See Chapter 38 for side effects of this medication class.

(3) The use of antipsychotics may best most effective in insomnia patients with a comorbid psychiatric disorder. See Chapter 37 for side effects of this medication class.

e. OTC medications and natural remedies

(1) Antihistamines such as diphenhydramine and doxylamine are found in nonprescription sleeping aids. There is a paucity of data supporting their use.

(a) Adverse effects include a hangover effect, dizziness, dry mouth, and constipation. Tolerance to these agents develops quickly.

(2) **Natural remedies**

(a) Melatonin and valerian are two commonly used natural remedies. There is minimal data to support the use of these two products for insomnia. The FDA does not strictly regulate nutritional supplements and herbal products therefore ingredients are not standardized.

D. Evaluation of treatment

1. Choice of a sleep agent should be based on a number of patient-specific factors including age, length of treatment, sleep complaint, substance use history, and cost. Pharmacological treatment may be most appropriate for patients with significant impairment and distress.
2. Treatment should focus on both quantitative and qualitative aspects of patient's sleep and daytime function.
3. Short half-life agents may work best in reducing sleep latency, whereas long-acting agents work may work best in improving total sleep time.
4. Ramelteon and doxepin may be best for patients with insomnia and a comorbid substance use disorder.
5. Sedating antidepressants and antipsychotics may work best for patients with insomnia and a comorbid psychiatric disorder.
6. Antihistamines may work best for patients with infrequent symptoms.

E. Pregnancy

1. Benzodiazepines FDA approved for insomnia are all pregnancy category X.
2. Benzodiazepine-receptor agonists are all pregnancy category C.
3. Ramelteon and doxepin are both pregnancy category C.
4. See Chapters 37 and 38 for the pregnancy category ratings for sedating antidepressants and antipsychotics.

Study Questions

Directions: Each of the questions, statements, or incomplete statements in this section can be correctly answered or completed by **one** of the suggested answers or phrases. Choose the **best** answer.

1. Which of the following is correct regarding the *DSM-IV* diagnosis of major depressive disorder?

(A) Patients must have 10 or more symptoms.
(B) Symptoms must be present for at least 2 weeks.
(C) Symptoms do not cause significant social or occupational impairment.
(D) Diagnosis requires a history of mania.

2. A patient with major depression should receive antidepressant therapy for at least

(A) 2 weeks.
(B) 6 weeks.
(C) 2 months.
(D) 6 months.

For questions 3–4: A 36-year-old woman presents with a 2-month history of depressed mood, anhedonia, increased appetite, weight gain, hypersomnolence, and suicidal ideation. This is the patient's first episode of major depression.

3. Which of the following antidepressants would be most appropriate in the treatment of this patient?

(A) amitriptyline
(B) sertraline
(C) phenelzine
(D) mirtazapine

4. Which of the following is *not* a potential adverse effect of the medication selected for the patient in question 3?

(A) sexual dysfunction
(B) nausea
(C) urinary retention
(D) insomnia

5. Which of the following medications would most likely exacerbate a preexisting seizure disorder?

(A) venlafaxine
(B) trazodone
(C) bupropion
(D) paroxetine

6. A patient who has received citalopram 40 mg/day for 2 weeks for the treatment of major depression complains that the medication is not working and would like to be switched to another agent. What is the appropriate recommendation?

(A) Provide the patient with some information on monoamine oxidase inhibitors (MAOIs) and call the physician to recommend switching the patient to phenelzine.
(B) Encourage the patient to continue with the current regimen and inform him or her that it may take 4 to 6 weeks before the full response is evident.
(C) Recommend adding lithium to augment the current regimen.
(D) Recommend switching to mirtazapine because of therapeutic failure with citalopram.

7. A patient diagnosed with depression was unsuccessfully treated with fluoxetine. Fluoxetine was discontinued, and 14 days later, the patient started therapy with phenelzine. Then, 3 days after phenelzine was started, the patient presented with hyperreflexia, fever, elevated blood pressure, confusion, and diarrhea. What is the most likely cause of this clinical presentation?

(A) serotonin syndrome
(B) serotonin withdrawal syndrome
(C) hypertensive crisis
(D) neuroleptic malignant syndrome

8. A patient presents with pressured speech, inability to sleep for 72 hrs, bizarre dress, inappropriate makeup, and grandiose delusions that interfere with social functioning. Which of the following is the most likely diagnosis?

(A) depression
(B) euthymia
(C) hypomania
(D) mania

9. Which of the following medications would be considered first-line monotherapy for an acute episode of mania?

(A) gabapentin
(B) lithium
(C) lamotrigine
(D) haloperidol

10. Which of the following is the appropriate therapeutic range for lithium in the treatment of mania?

(A) 0.4 to 0.6 mEq/L
(B) 0.6 to 1.5 mEq/L
(C) 1.0 to 2.0 mEq/L
(D) 0.5 to 1.2 mEq/L

11. Which of the following mood stabilizers would be most appropriate in a patient with liver disease?

(A) lithium
(B) valproic acid
(C) carbamazepine
(D) none of the above

12. A 32-year-old, 70-kg man diagnosed with bipolar I disorder is being treated with valproic acid (VPA). Which of the following is a reasonable loading dose for VPA in this patient?

(A) 250 mg twice a day
(B) 500 mg twice a day
(C) 250 mg three times a day
(D) 500 mg three times a day

13. Which of the following factors may increase lithium concentration?

(A) caffeine
(B) osmotic diuretics
(C) increased fluid intake
(D) nonsteroidal anti-inflammatory drugs

14. Which of the following is a late adverse effect of lithium?

(A) nausea
(B) hand tremor
(C) seizures
(D) hypothyroidism

15. Which of the following antidepressants is a potent inhibitor of CYP2D6 liver enzyme?

(A) citalopram (Celexa)
(B) paroxetine (Paxil)
(C) trazodone (Desyrel)
(D) venlafaxine (Effexor)

16. The dosage range for selegiline (Emsam) patch is which of the following?

(A) 6 to 12 mg
(B) 12 to 15 mg
(C) 3 to 6 mg
(D) 20 to 40 mg

17. Which of the following tricyclic amine antidepressants (TCAs) causes the most anticholinergic side effects?

(A) nortriptyline (Pamelor)
(B) desipramine (Norpramin)
(C) amitriptyline (Elavil)
(D) protriptyline (Vivactil)

18. Which of the following medications for bipolar disorder is recommended as maintenance treatment?

(A) aripiprazole (Abilify)
(B) carbamazepine (Tegretol)
(C) lamotrigine (Lamictal)
(D) iloperidone (Fanapt)

19. Which of the following medications would have the quickest onset of symptom relief in a patient presenting with generalized anxiety disorder (GAD)?

(A) fluoxetine (Prozac)
(B) buspirone (Buspar)
(C) lorazepam (Ativan)
(D) venlafaxine XR (Effexor XR)

20. Buspirone (Buspar) mechanism of action can best be described as which of the following?

(A) Norepinephrine reuptake inhibitor
(B) 5-HT_2-receptor antagonist
(C) D_2-receptor antagonist
(D) Partial agonist at 5-HT_{1A}-receptors

21. Duration of treatment for panic disorder should be continued for a period of how long after symptom remission?

(A) 3 months
(B) 6 months
(C) 12 months
(D) 12 to 24 months

22. Which of the following medication classes is considered a first-line treatment option for social anxiety disorder?

(A) Atypical antipsychotics
(B) Anticonvulsants
(C) Selective serotonin reuptake inhibitors (SSRIs)
(D) Tricyclic antidepressants

23. Which benzodiazepine is FDA approved for the treatment of panic disorder?

(A) diazepam (Valium)
(B) clonazepam (Klonopin)
(C) lorazepam (Ativan)
(D) chlordiazepoxide (Librium)

Answers and Explanations

1. The answer is D *[see I.A.1]*.
The *DSM-IV-TR* criteria provide the diagnostic guidelines for MDD require a patient have five or more symptoms present for a period of at least 2 weeks. These symptoms must cause significant social and occupational impairment. If a patient had a history of mania as part of his or her symptoms presentation, this patient would be diagnosed as bipolar rather than as unipolar MDD.

2. The answer is D *[see I.B.1]*.
Patients should receive antidepressant therapy through the continuation phase, which is generally 6 to 9 months.

3. The answer is B *[see I.B.1.c]*.
Sertraline, an SSRI, is a good first-line agent, particularly in patients who would benefit from the stimulatory side effects. Amitriptyline and mirtazapine would not be good alternatives because of this patient's hypersomnolence and weight gain. In addition, a TCA (amitriptyline) is not recommended in patients at risk for suicide. Although some aspects of this patient's depression may be considered atypical, an MAOI would not be selected as first-line therapy, given that it is the patient's first episode of depression.

4. **The answer is C** *[see I.B.1.c]*.
Sertraline has been associated with nausea, sexual dysfunction, and insomnia. Sertraline does not express anticholinergic activity and would, therefore, not cause urinary retention. Of the SSRIs, only paroxetine has been associated with causing anticholinergic adverse effects.

5. **The answer is C** *[see I.B.1.e]*.
Although all antidepressants can lower the seizure threshold, bupropion is contraindicated in patients with seizure disorder. Bupropion is specifically contraindicated in patients with a seizure disorder. Paroxetine was associated with a 0.1% incidence of seizures during clinical trials. Seizure associated with venlafaxine occurs infrequently (1/100 to 1/1000 patients). The overdosage of trazodone may be associated with seizures; but at normal doses, trazodone is not thought to alter the seizure threshold.

6. **The answer is B** *[see I.B.1.i]*.
An antidepressant must be given at the maximum tolerated dose for 4 to 6 weeks before it is considered a therapeutic failure; therefore, the best recommendation is to continue with the current regimen for at least 2 more weeks. MAOIs are reserved for refractory depressed patients and are not indicated in this patient scenario. Lithium is an appropriate augmentative agent but is not indicated until the patient has failed two or three different antidepressant trials.

7. **The answer is A** *[see Table 40-2]*.
Serotonin syndrome may result when starting an MAOI immediately after another agent that increases serotonin levels. Generally, a 2-week washout period is recommended; however, fluoxetine requires a 5-week washout period because of norfluoxetine (active metabolite).

8. **The answer is D** *[see II.B.1]*.
The clinical presentation described is consistent with mania. Hypomania generally does not impair functioning. Euthymia implies normal mood, whereas depression typically involves more neurovegetative symptoms.

9. **The answer is B** *[see Table 40-6]*.
Lithium is considered to be first-line monotherapy for euphoric mania. Gabapentin has demonstrated utility as a mood stabilizer but is considered only an adjunctive therapy. Lamotrigine is an anticonvulsant that currently has data supporting its use in depressive episodes of bipolar disorder but not as first-line monotherapy for mania. Haloperidol is a traditional antipsychotic that may be used parenterally to manage acute agitation but is not appropriate as first-line monotherapy.

10. **The answer is D** *[see II.D.1.a.(4)]*.
The therapeutic range of lithium is 0.5 to 1.2 mEq/L. When using lithium in the treatment of acute mania, the upper end of the therapeutic range is typically used.

11. **The answer is A** *[see II.D.1.a.(2)]*.
Lithium is not known to cause hepatic dysfunction, nor is it metabolized via the liver. However, both valproic acid and carbamazepine can impair liver function.

12. **The answer is D** *[see II.D.3]*.
The appropriate loading dose for VPA in acute mania is 20 mg/kg/day; therefore, in this patient, the appropriate loading dose is 1400 mg/day. This equation approximates the need for the patient, and it is appropriate to round up to available dosage forms.

13. **The answer is D** *[see Table 40-8]*.
Caffeine, osmotic diuretics, and increased fluid intake all decrease lithium concentrations. Nonsteroidal anti-inflammatory drugs decrease renal blood flow and decrease lithium clearance, resulting in increased lithium concentrations.

14. **The answer is D** *[see Table 40-7]*.
Hypothyroidism is a late side effect of lithium therapy usually occurring after 18 months of treatment. Thyroid function panel should be checked at baseline and on follow-up to monitor for this adverse effect.

15. **The answer is B** *[see Table 40-4]*.
Paroxetine is a potent inhibitor of CYP2D6. The other antidepressants listed are only mildly potent inhibitors of CYP2D6.

16. **The answer is A** *[see Table 40-1]*.
The recommended dosage range for selegiline patch is 6 to 12 mg/day. Patients should be started on 6 mg and slowly titrated up in dose to a maximum dose of 12 mg/day.

17. **The answer is C** *[see Table 40-3]*.
Tertiary amine TCAs cause more anticholinergic adverse effects than secondary amine TCAs. Of the antidepressants listed, only amitriptyline is a tertiary amine TCA.

18. **The answer is C** *[see Table 40-6]*.
Lamotrigine has been shown to be an effective agent in the preventing relapse into both mania and depression. Therefore, lamotrigine is FDA approved for maintenance treatment of bipolar disorder.

19. **The answer is C** *[see III.E.1]*.
Lorazepam is a benzodiazepine and these agents produce symptom relief in GAD within days to 1 week of treatment. All other medications listed require a period of at least up to 2 weeks or longer for GAD symptom relief.

20. **The answer is D** *[see III.D.2.a]*.
Buspirone main mechanism of action is through partial agonism of 5-HT_{1A}-receptors. Buspirone does not act at all by the other mechanisms of action listed.

21. **The answer is D** *[see III.E.2]*.
Treatment of panic disorder should be continued for a period of 12 to 24 months in order to ensure patients do not have a relapse of symptoms.

22. **The answer is C** *[see III.D.1.c]*.
SSRIs are the first-line treatment option for SAD. These other treatments listed may be used as possible second-line treatments.

23. **The answer is B** *[see III.D.2.b]*.
Clonazepam and alprazolam XR (Xanax XR) are the only benzodiazepines FDA approved for the treatment of panic disorder.

41

Asthma and Chronic Obstructive Pulmonary Disease

ROY A. PLEASANTS II

I. ASTHMA

A. **Definition.** Asthma is a chronic inflammatory disorder of the airways. It involves complex interactions between many cells (e.g., eosinophils, mast cells, macrophages) and inflammatory mediators (e.g., interleukins, leukotrienes) that result in inflammation, obstruction (partially or completely reversible after treatment or resolves spontaneously), increased airway responsiveness (i.e., hyperresponsiveness), and episodic asthma symptoms (see I.G.1). Neutrophils may play an important role in some asthma exacerbations.

B. **Classification.** Asthma severity classifications according to the 2007 expert panel report of the National Heart, Lung, and Blood Institute (NHLBI) include **mild intermittent asthma** in addition to **mild, moderate,** and **severe persistent asthma** (*Table 41-1*). The asthma guidelines highlight that disease severity is used to initiate therapy and asthma control should be used to monitor therapy. The 2007 guidelines have also been modified to incorporate domains of both disease risk and impairment to determine disease severity. The guidelines define impairment as the frequency and intensity of symptoms and functional limitations the patient is currently experiencing or has recently experienced. Risk is defined as the likelihood of asthma exacerbations, progressive decline in lung function (or for children lung growth), or adverse effects from medications. A patient's severity classification plays an important role in determining the most appropriate pharmacotherapeutic approach and is determined by

1. symptoms (short-acting β-agonist use, nocturnal symptoms),
2. interference with normal daily activity,
3. lung function (spirometry to determine FEV_1 and FVC), and
4. frequency of exacerbations.

C. **Incidence.** In 2002, according to CDC data, approximately 31 million Americans had ever been told they had asthma during their lifetime. In 2002, 20 million people in the United States had asthma (~7% of population).

1. It has been estimated that 8.3 million children age 18 years and younger have asthma.
2. Asthma improves in many children as they age; 50% appear to have "outgrown" asthma by their midteens. However, it is incorrect to consider that these individuals no longer have asthma because many eventually have a return of symptoms.
3. Sixty percent of asthmatics have at least one asthma flare each year.
4. Although death from asthma remains uncommon, death rates had been increasing in recent years but appear to have reached a plateau. In 2007, there were 3447 deaths attributed to asthma; this represents a significant decline since 2000. The most common cause of death is believed to be inadequate assessment of the severity of airway obstruction by either practitioner or patient, leading to suboptimal therapy.
5. The cost to society of asthma is substantial. In 2000 alone, it is estimated that direct costs related to asthma exceeded \$8.1 billion. These costs include \$2.4 billion for medications and \$3.5 billion for

Table 41-1 CLASSIFICATION OF ASTHMA SEVERITY

Components of Severity		Classification of Asthma Severity ≥ 12 Years of Age			
			Persistent		
		Intermittent	**Mild**	**Moderate**	**Severe**
Impairment **Normal FEV_1/FVC:** **8–19 yrs 85%** **20–39 yrs 80%** **40–59 yrs 75%** **60–80 yrs 70%**	Symptoms	≤ 2 days/week	> 2 days/week but not daily	Daily	Throughout the day
	Nighttime awakenings	≤ 2×/month	3–4×/month	≥ 1×/week but not nightly	Often 7×/week
	Short-acting β_2-agonist use for symptom control (not prevention of EIB)	≤ 2 days/week	> 2 days/week but not daily, and not more than 1× on any day	Daily	Several times per day
	Interference with normal activity	None	Minor limitation	Some limitation	Extremely limited
	Lung function	• Normal FEV_1 between exacerbations • FEV_1 > 80% predicted • FEV_1/FVC normal	• FEV_1 > 80% predicted • FEV_1/FVC normal	• FEV_1 > 60% but < 80% predicted • FEV_1/FVC reduced 5%	• FEV_1 < 60% predicted • FEV_1/FVC reduced > 5%
Risk	Exacerbations requiring oral systemic corticosteroids	0–1/year (see note)	≥ 2/year (see note) →		
		← Consider severity and interval since last exacerbation. → Frequency and severity may fluctuate over time for patients in any severity category. Relative annual risk of exacerbations may be related to FEV_1.			
Recommended Step for Initiating Treatment		**Step 1**	**Step 2**	**Step 3**	**Step 4 or 5**
				and consider short course of oral systemic corticosteroids	
		In 2–6 weeks, evaluate level of asthma control that is achieved and adjust therapy accordingly.			

EIB, exercise-induced bronchospasm; *FEV_1*, forced expiratory volume 1 sec; *FVC*, forced vital capacity.
Adapted from Expert Panel Report 3: guidelines for the diagnosis and management of asthma. Available online at http://www.nblbi.nih.gov/guidelines/asthma/epr3/index.htm; last accessed April 10, 2008.

hospitalizations. Indirect costs of asthma are estimated at $4.6 billion. Acute care visits (e.g., hospitalizations) account for the majority of health care costs for asthma.

D. Cause. Precipitating factors of an acute asthma exacerbation may include the following:

1. Allergens (e.g., pollen, house dust mite, animal dander, mold, cockroaches, food)
   - **a.** Concurrent predisposition to allergy is highly prevalent in patients with asthma, especially children.
   - **b.** For example, allergic rhinitis is reported in 45% of patients with asthma compared to 20% of the general population.
2. Occupational exposures (e.g., chemical irritants, flour, wood, textile dusts)
3. Viral respiratory tract infections
4. Exercise
5. Emotions (e.g., anxiety, stress, hard laughter, crying)

6. Exposure to irritants (e.g., strong odors, chemicals, fumes)
7. Environmental exposures (e.g., weather changes, cold air, sulfur dioxide, cigarette smoke)
8. Drugs
   a. Reactions to drugs may occur as a result of hypersensitivity or as an extension of the pharmacological effect.
   b. Problematic drugs include
      (1) aspirin and other nonsteroidal anti-inflammatory drugs such as ibuprofen (note: cyclooxygenase 2 inhibitors are not recommended for use in aspirin-sensitive asthma patients)
      (2) antiadrenergic and cholinergic drugs (e.g., β-adrenergic blockers, bethanechol)
      (3) medications (or foods) that contain tartrazine, sulfites, benzalkonium chloride, and other preservatives
      (4) excipients in inhaled drugs that are derivatives of legumes (soybeans) in peanut allergic patients (e.g., oleic acid).

E. **Pathology.** On postmortem examination of patients with asthma, the following characteristics have been identified:
1. Hypertrophy of smooth muscle
2. Airways containing plugs consisting of inflammatory cells and their debris, proteins, and mucus
3. Inflammatory cellular infiltrate with vasodilation, denuded airway epithelium, and microvascular leakage
4. Vasodilation of the vasculature
5. Denuded airway epithelium
6. Microvascular leakage
7. Collagen deposition in basement membranes

F. **Pathophysiology** (*Figure 41-1*)
1. **Major contributing processes**
   a. **Inflammatory cells** (i.e., mast cells, eosinophils, activated T cells, macrophages, and epithelial cells) secrete mediators and influence the airways directly or via neural mechanisms.

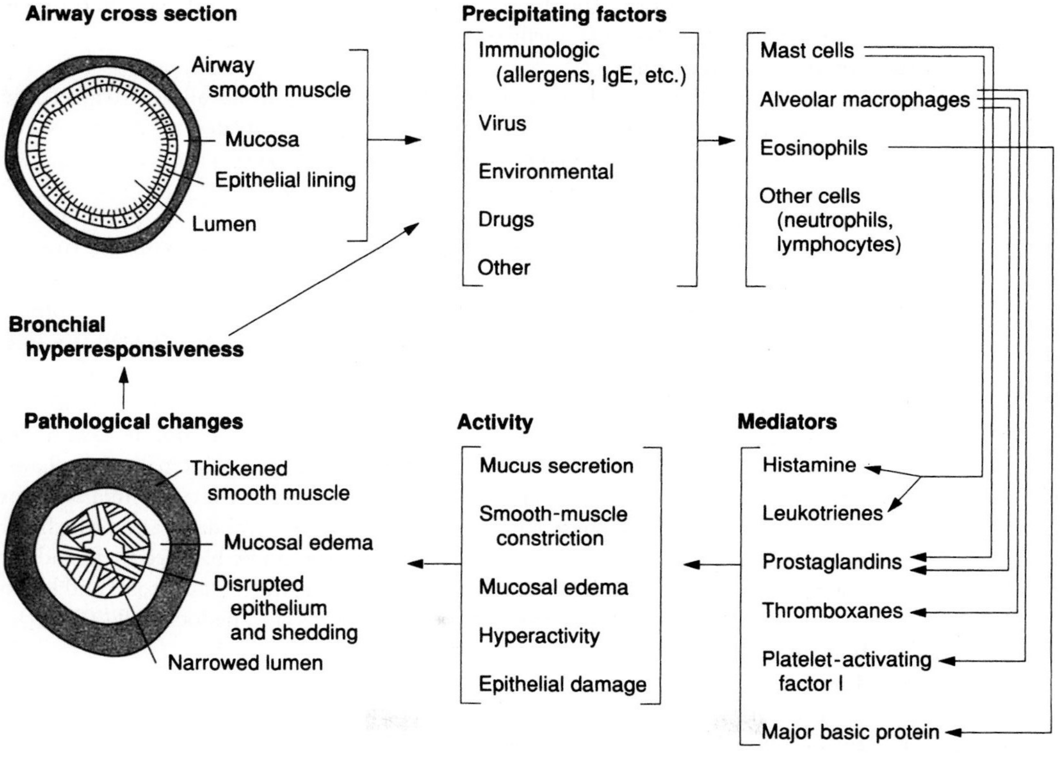

Figure 41-1. The pathophysiology of asthma.

b. **Airway obstruction** is responsible for many of the clinical manifestations of asthma.
   (1) Severity of obstruction is variable and believed to be a result of bronchoconstriction, airway wall edema, mucus plug formation, airway remodeling, smooth muscle hypertrophy, and hyperplasia.
   (2) Airway obstruction reduces ventilation to some lung regions, which causes a ventilation/perfusion (V/Q) imbalance that leads to hypoxemia. This is reflected by a reduction in the partial pressure of arterial oxygen (Pao_2) observed in moderate-to-severe exacerbations.

c. **Hyperresponsiveness**, an exaggerated response to certain stimuli, is an important feature of asthma and appears to correlate with clinical severity and medication requirements. Increased levels of inflammatory mediators and infiltration by inflammatory cells are thought to be the primary mechanisms responsible for airway hyperresponsiveness.

d. **Airway inflammation** is crucial to development of asthma and contributes to airway hyperresponsiveness, airflow obstruction, respiratory symptoms, and disease chronicity. Inflammatory cells and their mediators are responsible for altered mucociliary function, epithelial disruption ranging from minor ciliary loss to severely denuded epithelium, increased airway permeability (to inhaled allergens, irritants, and inflammatory mediators), and reduced clearance of inflammatory mediators.
   (1) Acute inflammation is associated with early recruitment of cells to the airway.
   (2) Subacute inflammation is associated with recruited and resident cell activation, resulting in more persistent inflammation.
   (3) Chronic inflammation is associated with persistent cell damage and ongoing repair, resulting in airway abnormalities that may become permanent.

e. Alteration in **autonomic neural control** also contributes to obstruction.
   (1) Elevated parasympathetic tone and reflex bronchoconstriction may occur as a result of increased cholinergic sensitivity or a change in muscarinic receptor function.
   (2) Increased smooth muscle responsiveness may be the result of smooth muscle hypertrophy. Exposure of the nerve endings, caused by inflammation, may also contribute.

f. **Airway remodeling** can result from persistent inflammation to chronic asthma. The resulting damage can yield permanent airway abnormalities because of subbasement membrane collagen deposition and fibrosis. Hypertrophy of the airway smooth muscle is another form of tissue remodeling in asthma. These events may occur even in the face of mild disease, but airway remodeling does not necessarily occur in all asthma patients.

2. **Sequencing of events in asthma**
   a. **Triggering. In an allergic asthma patient**, after exposure to an allergic trigger, the antigen binds to immunoglobulin E (IgE), which is attached to activated mast cells. Nonallergic factors (e.g., aspirin, viral infections) may also function as triggers. Viral infections serve as an important cause of worsened asthma.
   b. **Early and late responses**
      (1) The **early asthmatic response** begins within 30 mins of trigger exposure (usually only several minutes after exposure) and resolves within 2 hrs. This results in constriction of the airway smooth muscles, bronchospasm, and subsequently asthma symptoms. This response can be blocked by the administration of short-acting β-agonists (albuterol [Proair, Ventolin, Proventil], pirbuterol [Maxair], or levalbuterol [Xopenex]).
      (2) The **late asthmatic response** involves a second decline in lung function, typically 4 to 8 hrs after the initial trigger exposure. The early asthma response does not necessarily progress into the late asthmatic response. The late asthmatic response, principally an inflammatory response, is characterized by persistent airflow obstruction, airway inflammation, and bronchial hyperresponsiveness. The response may last several days, and bronchial hyperreactivity may persist for several weeks. This response can be blocked by the administration of corticosteroids—inhaled steroids such as budesonide (Pulmicort) and leukotriene modifiers such as montelukast (Singulair) or cromones (i.e., nedocromil [Tilade]).

G. **Clinical evaluation**
1. **Physical findings**
   a. In asymptomatic patients, physical findings of asthma are often not present.
   b. Physical findings depend on the severity of the underlying disease and the severity of the exacerbation. Regardless of the underlying disease severity, patients can have mild, moderate, or severe exacerbations (*Table 41-2*).

Table 41-2 STAGES OF SEVERITY OF AN ACUTE ASTHMATIC ATTACK

Stage	Symptoms	FEV_1 or FVC	Arterial pH	$Pa{O_2}$	$Pa{CO_2}$
I Mild	Breathlesness while walking, speaks in sentences, moderate wheezing	> 70% of normal	Normal or ↑	Normal or ↓	Normal or ↓
II Moderate	Dyspnea while at rest, in phrases, loud wheezing throughout expiration	40%–69% of normal	↑	> 60 mm Hg	< 42 mm Hg
III Severe	Breathlessness while at rest, speaks in words loud wheezing, coughing difficulty speaking, accessory chest muscle use, and chest hyperinflation	< 40% of normal	Normal or ↓	< 60 mm Hg	> 42 mm Hg
IV Respiratory failure	Severe respiratory distress, confusion lethargy, cyanosis disappearance of breath sounds, and pulsus paradoxus > 12 mm Hg	< 25% of normal	↓↓	↓	↑↑

FEV_1, forced expiratory volume in 1 sec; *FVC*, forced vital capacity; *$Pa{O_2}$*; partial pressure of arterial oxygen; *$Pa{CO_2}$*; partial pressure of arterial carbon dioxide; ↑, increased; ↓, decreased; ↑↑, markedly increased; ↓↓, markedly decreased.

c. Patients with **chronic**, **poorly controlled**, **severe asthma** may have evidence of chronic hyperinflation, including barrel chest and decreased diaphragmatic excursion, similar to chronic obstructive pulmonary disease.

d. **Acute exacerbations** may have a sudden or gradual onset. Symptoms are frequently nocturnal or occur in the early morning hours.

(1) Common findings in an acute exacerbation include

(a) Shortness of breath

(b) Wheezing (usually occurs at the end of exhalation but may be heard throughout inspiration and exhalation in more severe asthma)

(c) Chest tightness

(d) Cough

(e) Tachypnea and tachycardia (moderate-to-severe exacerbations)

(f) Pulsus paradoxus (severe exacerbations)

(2) Between acute asthma exacerbations, the patient may be asymptomatic.

2. Diagnostic test results

a. Pulmonary function tests determine the degree of airway obstruction and may be normal between exacerbations. The 2007 NHLBI asthma guidelines recommend spirometry in all asthma patients > 5 years old to determine that airway obstruction is at least partially reversible. Breathing tests include spirometry and peak flow meter testing.

(1) **Forced expiratory volume in 1 second (FEV_1)** and forced vital capacity (FVC) both decrease during an acute exacerbation. The spirometer is used to generate the FEV_1 and FVC.

(2) Residual volume (RV) and total lung capacity (TLC) may increase in asthma because of **air trapping** and subsequent **lung hyperinflation**.

(3) **Peak expiratory flow rate (PEFR)**, obtained through the patient forcefully breathing out into a **peak flow meter**, correlates well with FEV_1. However, PEFR measurement is not used in making the diagnosis of asthma. PEFR measurement can be used to monitor control of asthma.

(a) Uses of PEFR monitoring at home include assessment of therapy, trigger identification, and assessment of the need for referral to emergency care.

(b) PEFR monitoring at home is recommended for patients who have had severe exacerbations, who are poor perceivers of asthma symptoms, and who have moderate-to-severe disease.

(c) PEFR is best measured in early morning, before medication administration. More frequent monitoring over a few weeks may also be indicated to identify specific patterns and to identify a patient's personal best PEFR measurement. In this case, measurements are taken before medications are taken in the morning (i.e., on awakening).

(4) **Provocation testing** with **histamine or methacholine challenge** may be performed to assess hyperresponsiveness and to rule out asthma in a patient who has had normal pulmonary function test results but in whom asthma is still suspected.

b. Blood analysis, although not typically undertaken in asthma, typically shows a slightly increased white blood cell (WBC) count during an acute exacerbation; eosinophilia also may be present. Leukocytosis may be present because of WBC demargination that occurs when patients receive systemic corticosteroids.

c. Pulse oximetry is a noninvasive means of assessing the degree of hypoxemia during an acute exacerbation. The oximeter measures oxygen saturation in arterial blood (Sao_2) and pulse.

d. Arterial blood gas measurements may be required to help gauge the severity of the asthma exacerbation (*Table 41-2*).

(1) In the early stages of an asthma exacerbation, **hyperventilation** results in a decrease in the partial pressure of arterial carbon dioxide ($Paco_2$). If the exacerbation progresses and the airways remain narrowed, respiratory muscles may fatigue and the $Paco_2$ level increases.

(2) **Respiratory acidosis** is a poor prognostic sign. It develops if hypoxemia worsens and the patient's respiratory rate is not maintained owing to respiratory fatigue. This results in a rising $Paco_2$ level.

e. An **electrocardiogram (ECG)** may show sinus tachycardia. An ECG may be particularly useful in an older patient.

f. A **chest radiograph** may be normal or could detect accompanying pneumothorax, atelectasis, or pneumonia. Evidence of hyperinflation may be present in acute asthma and in chronic, poorly controlled asthma. A chest radiograph may also be needed to exclude other causes of the patient's symptoms.

3. Signs of respiratory distress include

a. use of accessory muscles,
b. inability to speak in sentences or ambulate owing to dyspnea,
c. declining mental status,
d. PEFR $<$ 50% of predicted (or personal best),
e. cyanosis,
f. suprasternal retractions,
g. absence of respiratory sounds,
h. increasing $Paco_2$, and
i. unable to sleep for extended time because of shortness of breath.

4. Patients with **potentially fatal asthma** should be quickly identified and aggressively managed. These patients have the following characteristics:

a. History of severe exacerbations, particularly exacerbations that develop suddenly
b. Poor self-perception of asthma symptoms and severity
c. History of intubation or intensive care unit (ICU) admission for asthma
d. Two or more hospitalizations, or three or more visits to the emergency department for asthma within 1 year
e. Hospitalization or treatment in the emergency department for asthma within the last month
f. Frequent β-agonist use (i.e., more than two canisters per month), current systemic steroid treatment, or recent systemic steroid withdrawal
g. Concurrent conditions (e.g., cardiovascular or psychiatric disease, substance abuse, low socioeconomic status, particularly in urban areas)

H. Therapy

1. Treatment objectives

a. The goal of therapy is to provide symptomatic control with normalization of lifestyle and to return pulmonary function as close to normal as possible.

b. The treatment goals listed in the 2007 NHLBI's expert panel update report include the following:
   (1) **Reduce impairment**
      (a) Prevent chronic and troublesome symptoms day or night.
      (b) Maintain normal pulmonary function.
      (c) Maintain normal activity levels, including exercise and attendance at work or school.
      (d) Minimal use of short-acting inhaled β_2-agonist (less than two times per week) for quick relief of symptoms (not including use prior to exercise).
      (e) Meet patient and family expectations.
   (2) **Reduce risk**
      (a) Prevent recurrent exacerbations and minimize need for ED visits or hospitalizations.
      (b) Prevent loss of lung function.
      (c) Provide optimal pharmacotherapy and with minimal or no adverse effects from medications.

2. **Management of acute asthma exacerbations**
   a. **Home-based** treatment of an acute asthma exacerbation (*Figure 41-2*)
   b. Treatment of an acute asthma exacerbation in the **hospital or emergency department** (*Figure 41-3*)
3. **Management of persistent asthma**
   a. A stepwise approach to pharmacological therapy is recommended to gain and maintain control of asthma in both the impairment and risk domains (*Table 41-3*). The type, amount, and scheduling of medication is dictated by asthma severity for initiating therapy and the level of asthma control for adjusting therapy.
   b. At each step, patients should control their environment to avoid or control factors, when possible, that make their asthma worse (e.g., allergens, irritants). This requires specific diagnosis and education.
   c. Inhaled steroids are considered to be first-line anti-inflammatory agents in asthma.
   d. Combination products for asthma are formoterol/budesonide (Symbicort), fluticasone/salmeterol (Advair), and mometasone/formoterol (Dulera). These products are indicated for moderate or severe persistent asthma. The 2007 NHLBI asthma guidelines give equal weight to increasing the dose of the inhaled steroid compared to adding a long-acting β_2-agonist to the inhaled steroid in uncontrolled chronic asthma. In the United States, Advair is available as metered dose inhalers (MDIs) and dry-powder inhalers (DPIs) (Diskus); Symbicort is available as an MDI.
   e. Inhaled β-agonists such as albuterol and levalbuterol are used as needed for acute symptoms for all levels of severity.
      (1) Daily or increasing use of a short-acting inhaled β_2-agonist suggests the need for additional long-term controller (i.e., anti-inflammatory) therapy.
      (2) Pretreatment with either an inhaled β-agonist, montelukast, or nedocromil may be used before exercise or allergen exposure.
   f. A rescue course of systemic corticosteroid (e.g., prednisone) may be needed at any time and at any step.
4. **Prevention and treatment of exercise-induced bronchospasm (EIB)**
   a. Steps to prevent EIB should be implemented in all patients with asthma.
   b. Patients should be advised that a warm-up period might be helpful in preventing EIB.
   c. EIB can usually be prevented with one of the following options:
      (1) Short-acting β-agonists (e.g., albuterol) should be administered 15 mins before exercise. These are considered the drug of choice for EIB.
      (2) Long-acting β-agonists—salmeterol (Serevent) and formoterol (Foradil)—should be administered 30 to 60 mins before exercise. When salmeterol is used chronically for EIB, some patients may lose protection toward the end of the 12-hr dosing interval. Because of its rapid onset, formoterol may be dosed 15 mins before exercise. Generally, short-acting agents are preferred over long-acting β-agonists.
      (3) Nedocromil may be used to prevent EIB and exacerbations related to exposure to other asthma triggers. Nedocromil should be administered no more than 1 hr before exercise or exposure.
      (4) Leukotriene modifiers given daily help with EIB but should not be used on an as-needed basis just before exercise.

Table 41-4 Continued.

Agent	Severe Acute: Pediatric	Severe Acute: Adult	Chronic: Pediatric	Chronic: Adult	Site of Action	Duration of Action	Comments
Pirbuterol							
MDI: 0.2 mg/puff	ET: 4–8 puffs q20 mins × 3 doses, then q1–4 hrs with spacer QR: 2 puffs t.i.d. q.i.d. p.r.n. PT: 1–2 puffs 5 mins before exercise	ET: 4–8 puffs q20 mins up to 4 hrs, then q1–4 hrs p.r.n. QR: 2 puffs t.i.d. q.i.d. p.r.n. PT: 2 puffs 5 mins before exercise	Not currently recommended	Not currently recommended	β_1-receptors + β_2-receptors ++++	5 hrs	Thought to be about half as potent as albuterol on a milligram basis.
Salmeterol							
MDI: 0.025 mg/puff	Not currently recommended	Not currently recommended	> 4 yrs: 1–2 puffs q12 hrs	2 puffs q12 hrs	β_1-receptors +	10–12 hrs	Not indicated for acute exacerbations.
DPI: 0.05 mg/inhalation	Not currently recommended	Not currently recommended	> 4 yrs: 1 inhalation q12 hrs	1 inhalation q12 hrs	β_2-receptors ++++		Take 30–60 mins before exercise for EIB prophylaxis.
Terbutaline							
MDI: 0.2 mg/puff	QR: 2 puffs t.i.d. q.i.d. p.r.n. PT: 1–2 puffs 5 mins before exercise	QR: 2 puffs t.i.d. q.i.d. p.r.n. PT: 2 puffs 5 mins before exercise	Not currently recommended	Not currently recommended	β_1-receptors + β_2-receptors ++++	3–6 hrs inhalation 1.5–4 hrs parenteral 4–8 hrs oral	Parenteral solution not FDA approved for nebulization.
SC: 0.1 % (1 μg/mL)	ET: 0.01 mg/kg q20 mins×3 doses, then q2–6 hrs p.r.n.	ET: 0.25 mg q20 mins × 3 doses	Not currently recommended	Not currently recommended			

DPI, dry-power inhaler; *EIB*, exercise-induced bronchospasm; *ET*, emergency treatment; *FDA*, U.S. Food and Drug Administration; *MDI*, metered dose inhaler; *NEB*, solution for nebulizer; *QR*, quick response; *PT*, prophylactic treatment; *SC*, subcutaneous.

Adapted from National Institutes of Health, National Heart, Lung, and Blood Institute, National Asthma Education and Prevention Program expert panel report 2: Guidelines for the diagnosis and management of asthma [NIH Publication 97-4051] July 1997:91, Figure 3–5d (NIH ERR-2, Fig. 35d).

(4) **Hypokalemia** may occur in some patients, particularly those receiving concurrent medications that cause hypokalemia (e.g., diuretics, amphotericin) and high doses, including inhaled agents.

(5) **Paradoxical bronchoconstriction** found with β-agonists may be the result of a "cold freon effect" or the use of additives such as benzalkonium chloride in the formulation.

(6) Unlike albuterol, which is a racemic mixture of albuterol's R- and S-isomers, levalbuterol HCl (Xopenex) is composed of the active *R*-enantiomer.

(7) Systemic adverse reactions when the recommended starting dose of levalbuterol is used appear to be similar to or *slightly less frequent* than the effects of albuterol. When the dose of levalbuterol is increased to 1.25 mg, however, the incidence of adverse reactions is similar to the corresponding dose of albuterol.

(8) It is important to be aware of **significant drug–drug interactions.**

(a) Concomitant use of systemic β-agonists with **monoamine oxidase inhibitors, tricyclic antidepressants**, or **methyldopa** may infrequently lead to severe hypertension. The risk with aerosolized agents may be smaller.

(b) **β-Adrenergic blockers** (especially nonselective agents as propranolol and carvedilol [Coreg]) precipitate bronchospasm and increase the dose of β-agonist necessary to achieve bronchodilation. The risk of bronchospasm should be weighed against the potential benefits of β-blockers. β_1-Selective agents such as metoprolol (Toprol XL) may be used carefully (e.g., in the hospital) in asthma patients when the risk–benefit ratio indicates such, as in an acute myocardial infarction.

(c) **β-Agonists** should not be combined with other sympathomimetic agents because of additive cardiovascular effects. Vasoconstrictor and vasopressor effects of epinephrine are antagonized by **β-adrenergic blocking agents** (e.g., phentolamine).

(9) The effects of β-agonists should be closely monitored in the elderly and in patients with a history of hyperthyroidism, diabetes, seizures, arrhythmias, and coronary artery disease.

2. **Corticosteroids**

a. **Therapeutic effects.** Corticosteroids suppress the inflammatory response and decrease airway hyperresponsiveness.

b. **Mechanism of action.** Corticosteroids bind to glucocorticoid receptors on the cytoplasm of cells. The activated receptor **regulates transcription** of target genes.

(1) Corticosteroids reduce inflammation via

(a) inhibition of transcription and release of inflammatory genes

(b) increased transcription of anti-inflammatory genes that produce proteins that participate in or suppress the inflammatory process

(2) Clinical effects include

(a) reduced production of inflammatory mediators

(b) enhanced β-adrenergic receptor expression (thus making the β_2-agonist work better)

(c) decreased mucus production

(d) prevention of endothelial and vascular leakage

(e) partial reversal of tissue-remodeling

c. **Administration and dosage**

(1) There is no significant difference in the clinical efficacy of the corticosteroid agents currently available. The **route of administration** is determined by the condition of the patient.

(2) **Systemic corticosteroids** are used for rapid response during an exacerbation. Improvement in pulmonary function may begin within 1 to 3 hrs; however, the maximum effect is not achieved until 6 to 9 hrs or longer after administration. Supplemental doses should be administered to patients who are already taking systemic corticosteroids when they experience an exacerbation, even if the exacerbation is mild.

(3) **Intravenous corticosteroids** (e.g., methylprednisolone [Solu-Medrol]) are administered to patients who are unable to take oral medications in severe exacerbations. Large doses (e.g., methylprednisolone 60 mg or 125 mg intravenously [IV]) can be quickly administered; however, patients can usually be switched to oral therapy as soon as they show clinical improvement and can tolerate oral medication.

(4) **Oral corticosteroids** are acceptable as emergency treatment if the patient can tolerate the oral route and is not believed to be in imminent danger of respiratory arrest. **Prednisone** and **prednisolone (Prelone)** are the most frequently used oral corticosteroids.
  (a) Prednisone and prednisolone are frequently administered in short "bursts" over 3 to 10 days [see I.I.2.c.(4).(b)] to treat acute exacerbations in the outpatient setting and in the emergency department. This type of regimen may also be used to rapidly achieve asthma control.
  (b) During burst therapy, these agents may be administered for 3 to 10 days in one or two daily doses and then discontinued. When used in this fashion, tapering is not usually necessary but is often done by physicians. However, if a patient's condition appears to worsen after the last dose has been administered, it is reasonable to reinstitute the corticosteroid and then begin a tapering regimen.

(5) Because **inhaled corticosteroids** are least likely to produce adverse reactions, the inhaled route should be used whenever possible for chronic treatment.
  (a) Inhaled corticosteroids should not be used alone to treat serious acute exacerbations.
  (b) **Inhaled steroids are the preferred anti-inflammatory therapy for chronic asthma.**
  (c) In milder outpatient flares, doses of the inhaled steroids may be increased temporarily (although this is controversial and should not be done if in a combination inhaler of ICS/LABA).
  (d) The number of corticosteroids available for inhalation therapy is increasing. The most recent additions are mometasone (Asmanex) and ciclesonide (Alvesco).
  (e) Dosages of inhaled corticosteroids are provided in *Table 41-5*. When asthma control is achieved, attempts should be made to use the lowest effective dose to maintain

Table 41-5 ESTIMATED COMPARATIVE DAILY DOSAGES FOR INHALED CORTICOSTEROIDS[a]

	Low Daily Dose		Medium Daily Dose		High Daily Dose	
Drug	**Adult**	**Child**	**Adult**	**Child**	**Adult**	**Child**
Beclomethasone						
CFC: 42 or 84 μg/puff	168–504 μg	84–336 μg	504–840 μg	336–672 μg	> 840 μg	> 672 μg
HFA: 40 or 80 μg/puff	80–240 μg	80–160 μg	240–480 μg	160–320 μg	> 480 μg	> 320 μg
Budesonide						
DPI: 200 μg/inhalation	200–600 μg	200–400 μg	600–1200 μg	400–800 μg	> 1200 μg	> 800 μg
Inhalation suspension for nebulization (child dose)		0.5 mg		1.0 mg		2.0 mg
Flunisolide						
250 μg/puff	500–1000 μg	500–750 μg	1000–2000 μg	1000–1250 μg	> 2000 μg	> 1250 μg
Fluticasone						
MDI:[b] 44, 110, or 220 μg/puff	88–264 μg	88–176 μg	264–660 μg	176–440 μg	> 660 μg	> 440 μg
DPI: 50, 100, or 250 μg/inhalation	100–300 μg	100–200 μg	300–600 μg	200–400 μg	> 7600 μg	> 400 μg
Mometasone						
DPI: 200 μg/inhalation (not approved for persons < 12 yrs old)	200 μg	n/a	400 μg	n/a	> 400 μg	n/a
Triamcinolone						
100 μg/puff	400–1000 μg	400–800 μg	1000–2000 μg	800–1200 μg	> 2000 μg	> 1200 μg

[a]In all cases, the lowest dose to maintain control should be used. Some doses are outside package labeling.
[b]MDI doses are actuator doses (i.e., amount leaving actuator).
CFC, chlorofluorocarbons; *DPI*, dry-powder inhaler; *HFA*, hydrofluoroalkanes; *MDI*, metered dose inhaler.
Modified from National Asthma Education and Prevention Program expert panel report guidelines for the diagnosis and management of asthma—NHLBI Asthma Guidelines 2007. August 2007.

control (step-down therapy). Side effects of inhaled steroids (and systemic steroids) are dose-dependent.

(f) Inhaled corticosteroids are considered first-line anti-inflammatory therapy for mild-to-severe persistent asthma in both adults and children.

(6) Treatment of asthma exacerbation in adults

(a) For treatment of a severe exacerbation, prednisone may be given at a dose of 2 mg/kg (maximum of 60 mg/day). For intravenous treatment, methylprednisolone is given at a dosage of 120 to 180 mg/day in three or four divided doses for 48 hrs or until the patient can tolerate oral medications. The dosage is then reduced to 60 to 80 mg/day until PEFR reaches 70% predicted (or personal best).

(b) For outpatient burst therapy, the dosage of prednisone is 1 to 2 mg/kg/day (maximum of 60 mg/day) in one or two divided doses for 3 to 10 days.

(7) Treatment of asthma exacerbation in children

(a) For inpatient treatment of a severe exacerbation, prednisone, methylprednisolone, or prednisolone is given at a dosage of 1 mg/kg every 6 hrs for 48 hrs. The dosage is then reduced to 1 to 2 mg/kg/day (maximum of 60 mg/day) in two divided doses until PEFR is 70% predicted (or personal best).

(b) For outpatient burst therapy, the dosage of prednisone is 1 to 2 mg/kg/day (maximum of 60 mg/day) in one or two divided doses for 3 to 10 days.

d. Precautions and monitoring effects

(1) Systemic corticosteroids

(a) Careful monitoring is necessary in patients with diabetes (steroids commonly increase blood sugar), hypertension, adrenal suppression, congestive heart failure (fluid retention owing to mineralocorticoid effects), peptic ulcer disease, candidiasis, immunosuppression, osteoporosis, chronic infections, cataracts, glaucoma, myasthenia gravis, and psychiatric diseases (e.g., depression, psychosis). Some of these side effects begin shortly after beginning systemic steroids (e.g., hyperglycemia), whereas others (e.g., osteoporosis) only occur with long-term use.

(b) If a prolonged course of systemic therapy is necessary to maintain asthma control, interference with the hypothalamic-pituitary-adrenal axis is lessened by a single morning dose (i.e., 6 to 8 A.M.) or alternate-day therapy. For alternate-day therapy, the dose is twice that of the single morning dose.

(c) Patients on regular systemic therapy should be closely monitored and should receive regular ophthalmological evaluations and osteoporosis screening, and preventative therapy (e.g., calcium, vitamin D, bisphosphonates) if indicated.

(2) Inhaled corticosteroids

(a) Local effects associated with inhaled corticosteroids include hoarseness (dysphonia) and fungal infection (candidiasis) of the mouth and throat. Local side effects can be lessened through mouth rinsing, use of a spacer, and use of certain inhaled steroid products.

(b) The U.S. Food and Drug Administration (FDA) includes warning labels on inhaled corticosteroid products to include dose related slowing of growth velocity in children (approximately one-third in. per year). Shortly after the labeling was revised, two major publications demonstrated short-term growth suppression of approximately 1 cm in the first year of budesonide treatment but without long-term effects on final adult height. However, children should be treated with the lowest effective dose and should be reminded that poorly controlled asthma also slows growth.

(c) Large doses of inhaled corticosteroids may result in systemic effects, such as reduced bone density, changes in adrenal function, skin changes, adrenal suppression, and cataract formation. Further study is needed to fully understand these effects and to determine their clinical significance. However, patients receiving high doses of inhaled corticosteroids should be closely monitored and should receive regular ophthalmological evaluations and osteoporosis screening and treatment (e.g., calcium, vitamin D) if indicated.

(d) Spacers (e.g., AeroChamber) are generally prescribed for patients who receive moderate-to-high doses of inhaled corticosteroids via MDIs. Patients should also gargle, rinse their mouth and throat, and expectorate after administration. Both of these interventions minimize oropharyngeal drug deposition, local adverse reactions, and gastrointestinal absorption.

(i) Steroids in dry-powder inhalers (Pulmicort Flexhaler) generally have a lower incidence of local side effects due to smaller particle size and less oropharyngeal deposition.

(ii) A new form of beclomethasone (Qvar) MDI also has a low incidence of local side effects due to relatively low oropharyngeal deposition.

(3) Significant interactions

(a) Concurrent use of **hepatic microsomal enzyme inducers** (e.g., rifampin, barbiturates, hydantoins) causes enhanced corticosteroid metabolism, reducing therapeutic efficacy.

(b) Concurrent use of **estrogens**, **oral contraceptives**, **itraconazole (Sporanox)**, or **macrolide antibiotics** (e.g., erythromycin, clarithromycin [Biaxin]) may decrease corticosteroid clearance.

(c) **Cyclosporine** may increase the plasma concentration of corticosteroids.

(d) Administration of **potassium-depleting diuretics** (e.g., thiazides, furosemide) or other potassium-depleting drugs (e.g., amphotericin) with corticosteroids causes enhanced hypokalemia. Serum potassium should be closely monitored, especially in patients on **digitalis glycosides**.

3. Leukotriene modifiers are the newest agents with anti-inflammatory properties to be approved for use in asthma. Leukotrienes are important participants in asthma pathophysiology. Cellular effects of leukotrienes include enhanced migration of eosinophils and neutrophils, increased adhesion of leukocytes, and increased monocyte and neutrophil aggregation. Leukotrienes also increase capillary permeability and cause smooth muscle contraction.

a. Leukotriene modifiers currently available in the United States include montelukast, zafirlukast (Accolate), and zileuton (Zyflo).

(1) Therapeutic effects

(a) Leukotriene modifiers have anti-inflammatory and bronchodilator activity. They may allow reduction in corticosteroid doses in some patients.

(b) Because they may be less effective anti-inflammatory agents than inhaled corticosteroids, they are considered second-line agents.

(c) In children, for whom administration of inhaled drugs is challenging, oral leukotriene receptor antagonists may be particularly useful.

(d) They may be useful in patients with concurrent allergic rhinitis and asthma.

(2) Mechanism of action. The leukotriene receptor antagonists are selective cysteinyl leukotriene 1 (cys-LT-1) receptor antagonists; therefore, they prevent leukotrienes from interacting with their receptors. Zileuton, a leukotriene modifier, blocks the effects of 5-lipo-oxygenase and ultimately blocks leukotriene production.

(3) Administration and dosage

(a) The dosage of **zafirlukast** in children $>$ 12 years and adults is 20 mg twice daily. Food reduces bioavailability, so zafirlukast should be taken at least 1 hr before or 2 hrs after meals. Children 5 to 11 years of age should receive 10 mg twice daily.

(b) The dosage of **montelukast** in adolescents 15 years of age or older and adults is one 10-mg tablet once every evening. The dosage for children 6 to 14 years of age is one 5-mg chewable tablet once every evening. Children ages 2 to 5 should receive one 4-mg chewable tablet once every evening. Food does not appear to change bioavailability.

(4) Precautions and monitoring effects

(a) Adverse reactions to montelukast are uncommon and include headache, dizziness, and dyspepsia.

(b) Adverse reactions associated with zafirlukast include headache, dizziness, nausea, and diarrhea.

(c) **Churg–Strauss syndrome**, a form of eosinophilic vasculitis, has rarely been associated with zafirlukast, montelukast, and pranlukast (available in Japan). It has usually, but not always, occurred in patients whose chronic steroid regimens were tapered and discontinued. At-risk patients should be monitored for vasculitic rash; eosinophilia; and increasing pulmonary, cardiac, and neuropathic symptoms.

(d) **Significant drug–drug interactions may occur.**
  (i) **Aspirin** increases zafirlukast levels.
  (ii) **Erythromycin, theophylline**, and **terfenadine** decrease zafirlukast concentrations.
  (iii) Zafirlukast may increase the anticoagulant effect of **warfarin** and levels of dofetilide.
  (iv) Drug interactions appear to be less significant with montelukast. Patients who are receiving montelukast with **hepatic enzyme inducers** (e.g., rifampin, phenobarbital) should be monitored closely.
  (v) The chewable forms of montelukast (4- and 5-mg tablets) contain aspartame and should be avoided in patients with **phenylketonuria**.

b. The only **lipoxygenase inhibitor** approved by the FDA is **zileuton (Zyflo)**. Zileuton may allow reduction in corticosteroid doses in some patients.
(1) **Therapeutic effects.** Lipoxygenase inhibitors have anti-inflammatory and bronchodilator activity.
(2) **Mechanism of action.** Lipoxygenase inhibitors prevent the formation of leukotrienes. Zileuton blocks 5-lipoxygenase, the enzyme responsible for leukotriene formation.
(3) **Administration and dosage.** In adults and children 12 years of age and older, the dosage of zileuton is 600 mg four times daily. It may be taken without regard to meals. A new formulation, Zileuton CR, may be dosed twice daily.
(4) **Precautions and monitoring effects**
  (a) Zileuton is contraindicated in patients with hepatic function impairment and should be monitored closely in patients who drink large quantities of alcohol.
  (b) Adverse effects include headache, abdominal pain, asthenia, nausea, dyspepsia, and myalgia. Drug therapy was discontinued in almost 10% of patients owing to side effects, although this was similar to placebo.
  (c) **Significant drug–drug interactions** may occur.
    (i) Zileuton increases concentrations of **propranolol, terfenadine**, and **theophylline.**
    (ii) The anticoagulant effect of **warfarin** is increased by zileuton.
  (d) Hepatic enzymes (e.g., alanine aminotransferase [ALT]) may become elevated during therapy, with most occurrences during the first several months of therapy. Symptomatic hepatitis has been reported. Therefore, the manufacturer recommends that serum ALT be checked before initiation of treatment, monthly for 3 months, and every 2 to 3 months for the rest of the first year. ALT should be checked periodically thereafter.
    (i) Patients should be monitored closely for signs or symptoms of liver dysfunction (e.g., right upper quadrant abdominal pain, flu-like symptoms, fatigue, nausea, lethargy, itching, jaundice).
    (ii) If ALT increases to more than five times the upper limit of normal, therapy should be discontinued and the patient should be monitored until enzymes normalize.

4. Cromolyn

a. Therapeutic effects. Cromolyn is currently only available as a nebulized solution for the treatment of asthma. Nedocromil and cromolyn MDIs have been removed from the market. Cromolyn is less effective in its anti-inflammatory properties than the inhaled steroids, however, because of its excellent safety profile is sometimes still used in children.
(1) When used prophylactically, cromolyn prevents the early and late response of asthma.
(2) When used as maintenance therapy for asthma, this medication suppresses nonspecific airway reactivity.

b. Mechanism of action. Cromolyn is believed to act locally by stabilizing mast cells and thereby inhibiting mast cell degranulation.

c. Administration and dosage
(1) **Cromolyn** is available as a nebulized solution in 2 ml ampules containing 20 mg and is administered as often as four times a day.
(2) When used as prophylaxis of EIB, it should be used 30 minutes prior to exercise.
(3) After administration, initial improvement is seen within 1 to 2 weeks; however, the maximum effect may take longer.

d. Precautions and monitoring effects

(1) Cromolyn is **not effective during an acute asthma exacerbation.** It should be used only for maintenance therapy of persistent asthma or for prevention of EIB.

(2) It is well tolerated, although paradoxical bronchospasm, wheezing, coughing, nasal congestion, and irritation or dryness of the throat may occur.

5. Theophylline compounds (methylxanthines)

a. Indications

(1) Theophylline compounds may be considered if β-agonists and corticosteroids fail to control an acute asthma exacerbation.

(2) Theophylline is an alternative to long-acting β-agonists in the treatment of persistent asthma.

(3) Theophylline is most beneficial as an adjuvant to inhaled corticosteroids in patients with nocturnal or early morning symptoms.

b. Therapeutic effects

(1) Theophylline compounds produce bronchodilation to a lesser extent than β-agonists.

(2) Nonbronchodilator effects include reduced mucus secretion, enhanced mucociliary transport, improved diaphragmatic contractility, and possibly reduced fatigability.

(3) There may also be notable degree of anti-inflammatory activity.

c. Mechanism of action. Theophylline-induced phosphodiesterase inhibition results in increased levels of cAMP.

d. Administration and dosage

(1) **Oral therapy** (e.g., sustained-release theophyllines) allows for a longer dosing interval and improves compliance. Compliance to oral theophylline also may be better than that of inhaled bronchodilators and corticosteroids.

(a) Because theophylline does not distribute well into fatty tissue, dosages should be calculated using lean body weight.

(b) The initial dose of theophylline for adults and children > age 1 is 10 mg/kg/day (maximum of 300 mg/day) given in divided doses. Usual dosage should be adjusted to achieve serum theophylline concentration of 5 to 15 μg/mL (5 to 10 μg/mL acceptable).

(c) The dosage can be titrated slowly upward and the serum level monitored until a therapeutic level is obtained.

(d) The usual maximal daily dose in adults is 800 mg/day.

(e) The maximum recommended dosage in children < age 1 is 0.2 × (age in weeks) + 5 = mg/kg/day and in children ≥ 1 year is 16 mg/kg/day, given in divided doses.

(f) **Ultra-sustained release theophylline formulations (Theo-24 and Uniphyl) may be dosed once daily.**

(g) In addition to theophylline, other methylxanthine compounds are available (e.g., oxtriphylline, dyphylline) but infrequently used. Dosing of these compounds is based on theophylline content (*Table 41-6*).

(2) **Intravenous therapy.** Although frequently used in the past, IV administration is now uncommon. IV administration is generally used only in hospitalized patients for whom oral therapy is not possible (e.g., vomiting, nothing by mouth).

(a) The usual **loading dose** for adults and children not previously receiving a methylxanthine is 5 mg/kg of theophylline administered over 20 to 30 mins at a rate not exceeding 25 mg/min.

Table 41-6 THEOPHYLLINE CONTENT OF THEOPHYLLINE-CONTAINING PRODUCTS

Preparation	Theophylline Content (%)	Equivalent Dose (mg)
Theophylline anhydrous (most oral solids)	100	100
Theophylline monohydrate (oral solutions)	91	110
Aminophylline anhydrous	86	116
Aminophylline hydrous	79	127
Oxtriphylline	64	156

Table 41-7 FACTORS THAT ALTER THEOPHYLLINE CLEARANCE

Factors that increase theophylline clearance (decrease levels)
- Age 1–9 yrs
- Drugs
  - Carbamazepine
  - Phenobarbital
  - Phenytoin
  - Rifampin
- Fever
- Food (may delay or reduce absorption of some sustained-release products)
- High-protein diet
- Smoking (marijuana and tobacco)

Factors that decrease theophylline clearance (increase levels)
- Age
  - Elderly
  - Premature neonates
  - Term infants < 6 months
- Cor pulmonale
- Congestive heart failure, decompensated
- Drugs
  - Allopurinol
  - β-Blockers (nonselective)
  - Calcium-channel blockers
  - Cimetidine
  - Fluoroquinolones (ciprofloxacin)
  - Influenza virus vaccine
  - Macrolides (clarithromycin, erythromycin)
  - Oral contraceptives
  - Ticlopidine
  - Zafirlukast
- Fever/viral illness
- Fatty foods (may increase rate of absorption of some products)
- High-carbohydrate diet
- Liver dysfunction (e.g., cirrhosis)

(b) The usual **maintenance infusion** rate of theophylline in healthy nonsmoking adults on no interacting drugs is 0.4 mg/kg/hr. This rate should be adjusted for factors that affect theophylline metabolism and serum levels (see *Table 41-7*).

e. **Precautions and monitoring effects**

(1) Theophyllines are contraindicated in patients with hypersensitivity to xanthine compounds and should be used cautiously in patients with a history of peptic ulcer or untreated seizure disorder.

(2) Adverse effects include nausea, vomiting, diarrhea, anorexia, palpitations, dizziness, restlessness, nervousness, insomnia, seizures, reduced lower esophageal sphincter tone, and reduced control of gastroesophageal reflux disease. Patients who experience adverse gastrointestinal effects should be evaluated to rule out theophylline toxicity versus local gastrointestinal effect.

(3) Theophylline clearance can be altered by several factors and drug interactions (*Table 41-7*). Close drug-level monitoring is required for patients with factors that alter theophylline clearance.

(4) Careful monitoring is required in patients with hepatic disease, hypoxemia, hypertension, congestive heart failure, alcoholism, and in the elderly. Because of developmental

changes in the neonate and child, dosing must be carefully established and monitored in these populations as well.

(5) **Therapeutic drug monitoring** of serum levels, adverse reactions, and concomitant drug use is essential for long-term therapy owing to theophylline's age- and condition-specific clearance.

(a) Therapeutic effect is achieved and toxicity minimized by keeping drug concentrations at 5 to 15 μg/mL.

(b) Drug levels should be assessed at steady state (typical half-life 8 hrs, up to 24 hrs in severe heart and liver failure).

(c) During oral therapy, trough drug levels should be obtained at steady state.

(d) Dyphylline serum levels should be monitored during therapy because serum theophylline levels will not measure dyphylline. The minimal effective therapeutic concentration of dyphylline is 12 μg/mL.

6. **Anticholinergics.** Bronchodilation occurs when these drugs block postganglionic muscarinic receptors in the airway. Response to anticholinergics is most pronounced in patients with fixed airway obstruction (e.g., COPD) but may have a role in combination with β-agonists.

a. **Ipratropium bromide** (**Atrovent**) is a quaternary ammonium compound.

(1) **Indications**

(a) Ipratropium bromide is recommended for use in combination with β-agonists for the treatment of an acute asthma exacerbation in the emergency department or hospital settings. However, benefits in the chronic management of asthma have not been established.

(b) Ipratropium bromide may be particularly useful in older patients and patients with coexisting COPD.

(c) Ipratropium should not be used alone to treat an asthma exacerbation.

(d) Ipratropium bromide is an alternative bronchodilator in some patients who cannot tolerate β-agonists and in patients who present with bronchospasm induced by a β-blocker.

(2) **Administration and dosage**

(a) Closed-mouth MDI technique or the use of a spacer is recommended for patients receiving anticholinergic therapy via MDI.

(b) The starting dose of the MDI is two inhalations four times a day. When administered via nebulizer, the dose is 500 μg (2.5 mL) four times a day.

(3) **Precautions and monitoring effects**

(a) If the anticholinergic spray contacts the eye, intraocular pressure may increase.

(b) The onset of action (approximately 15 mins) and peak effect (1 to 2 hrs) are more delayed than for β-agonists.

b. Aerosolized **atropine** is used rarely now that ipratropium bromide nebulization solution is available owing to atropine's high incidence of systemic adverse effects.

7. **Antihistamines** are useful for patients with coexisting allergic rhinitis; however, their role in the treatment of asthma remains unclear. Antihistamines compete with histamine for H_1-receptor sites on effector cells and thus help prevent the histamine-mediated responses that influence asthma.

8. **Antibiotics** are generally not used for the treatment of asthma, unless other signs of infection are present.

9. **Magnesium sulfate**, administered intravenously, may be useful in some patients because of its modest ability to cause bronchodilation. When administered intravenously, it also improves respiratory muscle strength in hypomagnesemic patients. Research has suggested that magnesium may reduce admission rate and improve FEV_1 in severe, acute asthma exacerbations and in stable, chronic asthma.

10. **Immunotherapy** (allergy shots) improves asthma control in some patients and is ineffective in others. A recent meta-analysis demonstrated that immunotherapy may improve lung function, reduce symptoms, and decrease medication requirements in a significant number of patients.

11. **Mucus** may contribute to airway obstruction in asthma. However, because some inhaled mucolytics such as acetylcysteine may precipitate bronchospasm, they should not be used for the treatment of patients with asthma.

12. **Omalizumab** (**Xolair**) is an anti-IgE compound used for severe asthma and concurrent allergies. It is usually administered twice monthly as an injection in a specialty physician's office. Life-threatening anaphylaxis has rarely been reported with this medication.

J. **Drug delivery options**

1. **MDIs**
   a. When administered with good technique and a spacer, the efficacy of MDIs is similar to that of nebulizers, despite the lower doses administered with an MDI and spacer. The only MDI that comes with a built-in spacer is the Azmacort (triamcinolone) inhaler.
   b. For small children to be able to use an MDI, a spacer with a face mask must be used.
   c. MDIs can be difficult to use. Steps for properly using an MDI are outlined in *Table 41-8.*
   d. MDIs can be administered to patients on mechanical ventilation with the use of an attachment device designed for the mechanical ventilator circuit. Higher doses of the β_2-agonist are often used in this setting.
   e. Breath-actuated MDIs (e.g., Maxair Autohaler) require the patient to use a closed-mouth technique. When inhalation has begun, the medication is released automatically. This type of inhaler is useful for a patient who is having problems coordinating actuation and inhalation.
2. **Spacers and holding chambers** (e.g., AeroChamber, AeroVent, Ellipse, InspirEase, OptiChamber)
   a. Spacers and holding chambers reduce the amount of drug deposited in the oral cavity.
   b. The use of spacers and holding chambers may minimize local and systemic adverse reactions.
   c. Addition of a spacer in a patient with poor MDI technique may improve pulmonary delivery of the agent.
   d. Spacers should be considered in all patients who are receiving medium-to-high doses of inhaled corticosteroids.
   e. They are especially beneficial for patients with poor hand–lung coordination, such as very young and old.
   f. Devices vary in construction and efficacy. The presence of a one-way mouthpiece valve, inhalation rate whistle, size, and durability are all factors that should be considered when selecting a particular spacer for a patient. Some new spacers have antistatic interiors to minimize adherence of aerosol particles to the interior of the spacer.
3. **Nebulizers**
   a. Compared to MDI and spacer administration, nebulizers require less patient coordination during administration of multiple inhalations.
   b. Disadvantages of nebulizers include cost, preparation and administration time, size of the device, and drug delivery inconsistencies among devices.
   c. Despite the disadvantages, nebulization is recommended for delivery of high-dose β-agonists and anticholinergics in severe exacerbations.
4. **Dry-powder inhalers**
   a. Dry-powder inhalers (DPIs) are coming to the market as a result of the international move to avoid the use of chlorofluorocarbon (CFC) propellants. They are also being used more frequently because many patients find them easier to use than an MDI.

Table 41-8 PROCEDURE FOR THE PROPER USE OF METERED DOSE INHALERS (MDIs)

Assemble MDI, if necessary.
Remove cap and inspect mouthpiece for foreign objects.
Attach MDI to spacer (if applicable).
Shake MDI (with spacer).
Tilt head back slightly and exhale fully.
Position inhaler:
Wrap lips around spacer mouthpiece.
Position inhaler 1–2 in. from open mouth.
Wrap lips around inhaler mouthpiece.
Just as you begin to inhale, depress canister once to release medication.
Continue inhaling slowly (over 3–5 secs) until lungs are full.
Hold breath for 5–10 secs.
Wait 1 min before repeating steps to deliver additional puffs.
Rinse mouth out after use of inhaled steroids.

b. Dry-powder inhalers require the user to
   (1) first load the dose into the delivery chamber
   (2) exhale fully
   (3) inhale rapidly or slowly, depending on the device (versus only slow inhalation required for MDI administration)
   (4) use the closed-mouth technique
   (5) avoid exhaling into the mouthpiece before inhalation
c. Spacers are not used with DPIs.
d. Patients should be advised to keep these devices away from moisture.

K. **Nonpharmacological treatment**
1. **Humidified oxygen** is administered to all patients with severe, acute asthma to reverse hypoxemia. Although the fraction of inspired oxygen (FIO_2) administered is based on the patient's arterial blood gas status, 1 to 3 L/min is generally given via face mask or nasal cannula. The goal is to keep the $SaO_2 > 90\%$ ($> 95\%$ if the patient is pregnant or has heart disease).
2. **Heliox** is a mixture of helium and oxygen that has a lower density than air. Because of its decreased airflow resistance, heliox may increase ventilation during acute asthma exacerbations. Because conflicting information has been published in studies using heliox, its role in asthma is unclear.
3. **Intravenous fluids** and electrolytes may be required if the patient is volume depleted.
4. **Environmental control** and allergen avoidance are important in the management of a patient with asthma.
   a. Available data suggest that avoidance of known allergens can improve asthma control.
   b. Some measures include use of allergen-resistant mattress and pillow encasements, use of high-filtration vacuum cleaners, removal of carpets and draperies, and avoidance of furry pets.
5. **Vaccines** (e.g., influenza virus, polyvalent pneumococcals) are recommended to prevent infection, which may precipitate an exacerbation.

II. CHRONIC OBSTRUCTIVE PULMONARY DISEASE

A. **Definitions.** The National Heart, Lung, and Blood Institute/World Health Organization (NHLBI/WHO) Global Initiative for Chronic Obstructive Lung Disease (GOLD) definition of COPD is "a disease state characterized by airflow limitation that is not fully reversible. The airflow limitation is usually both progressive and associated with an abnormal inflammatory response of the lungs to noxious particles or gases." The American Thoracic Society definition is similar: A disease state characterized by the presence of airflow limitation owing to chronic bronchitis or emphysema; the airflow obstruction is generally progressive, may be accompanied by airway hyperreactivity, and may be partially reversible. The two major forms of COPD—**chronic bronchitis** and **emphysema**—frequently coexist. COPD also coexists with asthma. These guidelines have been updated annually.
1. **Chronic bronchitis** is characterized by excessive mucus production by the tracheobronchial tree, which results in airway obstruction as a result of edema and bronchial inflammation. Bronchitis is considered chronic when the patient has a cough producing more than 30 mL of sputum in 24 hrs for at least 3 months of the year for 2 consecutive years and other causes of chronic cough have been excluded.
2. **Emphysema** is marked by permanent alveolar enlargement distal to the terminal bronchioles and destructive changes of the alveolar walls. There is a lack of uniformity in airspace enlargement, resulting in loss of alveolar surface area. The collapse of these small airways results in airflow limitation that is independent of exertion.

B. **Incidence.** Approximately 17 million Americans have COPD. COPD is the third leading cause of death in the United States and the leading cause of hospitalization in the older population. It is most commonly diagnosed in older men; however, the incidence is increasing in women owing to an increasing population of women smokers. Women may be more likely to have more rapidly progressive COPD than men. Asthma is a common comorbidity.

C. **Cause.** Various factors have been implicated in the development of COPD, including the following:
1. **Cigarette smoking** is the primary causal factor for the development of COPD, present in $> 90\%$ of patients.
   a. One mechanism suggests that pulmonary hyperreactivity secondary to smoking results in persistent airway obstruction.

b. There is also an increased risk of COPD in people who have α_1-antitrypsin (AAT) deficiency. One in three people with genetic AAT deficiency develop emphysema, usually as young adults.
   (1) AAT is a serine protease inhibitor, and it is also an acute-phase reactive protein. The major physiological function of AAT is inhibition of neutrophil elastase.
   (2) AAT deficiency should be suspected when emphysema develops early in the absence of a significant smoking history.

2. Exposure to irritants such as sulfur dioxide (as in polluted air), noxious gases, and organic or inorganic dusts or combustible fuels in the home.
3. A history of respiratory infections or bronchial hyperreactivity
4. Social, economic, and hereditary factors

D. Pathophysiology

1. Chronic bronchitis

a. **Respiratory tissue inflammation** results in vasodilation, congestion, mucosal edema, and goblet cell hypertrophy. These events trigger goblet cells to produce excessive amounts of mucus.
b. **Changes in tissue** include increased smooth muscle, cartilage atrophy, infiltration of neutrophils and other cells, and impairment of cilia.
c. Airways become blocked by thick, tenacious mucous secretions, which trigger a productive cough.
d. Normally, sterile airways can become colonized with *Streptococcus pneumoniae*, *Haemophilus influenzae*, *Moraxella catarrhalis*, *Staphylococcus aureus*, and *Pseudomonas aeruginosa* species. Recurrent lung infections (viral and bacterial) reduce ciliary and phagocytic activity, increase mucus accumulation, weaken the body's defenses, and further destroy small bronchioles.
e. As the **airways degenerate**, overall gas exchange is impaired, causing **exertional dyspnea**.
f. Hypoxemia results from a V/Q imbalance and is reflected in an increasing arterial carbon dioxide tension (i.e., increasing $Paco_2$).
g. Sustained hypercapnia (increased $Paco_2$) desensitizes the brain's respiratory control center and central chemoreceptors. As a result, compensatory action to correct hypoxemia and hypercapnia (i.e., a respiratory rate or depth increase) does not occur. Instead, hypoxemia serves as the stimulus for breathing. Use of narcotics or benzodiazepines, especially in combination, should be done cautiously in these patients to avoid respiratory failure.

2. Emphysema

a. **Anatomical changes** are the result of loss of tissue elasticity.
   (1) **Inflammation** and **excessive mucus secretion** (as from long-standing chronic bronchitis) cause air trapping in the alveoli. This contributes to breakdown of the bronchioles, alveolar walls, and connective tissue.
   (2) As clusters of alveoli merge, the number of alveoli diminishes, leading to increased space available for air trapping.
   (3) Destruction of alveolar walls causes collapse of small airways on exhalation and disruption of the pulmonary capillary beds.
   (4) These changes result in V/Q abnormalities; blood is shunted away from destroyed areas to maintain a constant V/Q ratio, unlike the case in chronic bronchitis.
   (5) Hypercapnia and respiratory acidosis are uncommon in emphysema because V/Q imbalance is compensated for by an increased respiratory rate.
b. There are **specific regions of the lung** in which characteristic anatomical changes of emphysema occur.
   (1) In **centrilobular** (centriacinar) emphysema associated with cigarette smoking, destruction is central, selectively involving respiratory bronchioles. Typically, bronchioles and alveolar ducts become dilated and merge.
   (2) In **panlobular** (panacinar) emphysema, all lung segments are involved. The alveoli enlarge and atrophy, and the pulmonary vascular bed is destroyed. This form of emphysema is associated with AAT deficiency.
   (3) In **paraseptal** emphysema, the lung periphery adjacent to fibrotic regions is the site of alveolar distention and alveolar wall destruction. This is associated with spontaneous pneumothorax.

E. Clinical evaluation

1. Physical findings

a. **Predominant chronic bronchitis** typically has an insidious onset after age 45.

(1) A **chronic productive cough** is the hallmark of chronic bronchitis. It occurs first in winter, then progresses to year-round. It is usually worse in the morning. Smoking cessation can help lessen the productive cough.

(2) **Exertional dyspnea**, the most common presenting symptom, is progressive. However, the severity of this symptom may not reflect the severity of the disease.

(3) Other common findings include obesity, rhonchi and wheezes on auscultation, prolonged expiration, and a normal respiratory rate. As the disease progresses, right ventricular failure is common, which presents as jugular venous distention, peripheral edema, hepatomegaly, and cardiomegaly. Because patients tend to develop cyanosis, the term *blue bloater* is sometimes used to describe patients with chronic bronchitis.

b. **Predominant emphysema** has an insidious onset, and symptoms occur after age 55.

(1) The **cough** is chronic but less productive than in chronic bronchitis.

(2) **Exertional dyspnea** is progressive, constant, severe, more characteristic of emphysema than chronic bronchitis.

(3) Other common findings include weight loss, tachypnea, pursed-lip breathing, prolonged expiration, accessory chest muscle use, hyperresonance on percussion, diaphragmatic excursion, and diminished breath sounds. Because patients are able to maintain reasonably good oxygenation because of their tachypnea, the term *pink puffer* is sometimes used to describe patients with emphysema. Note however, that the pink puffer and blue bloater presentations are not specific for the respective diseases.

c. Patients may have elements and physical findings from each of these diseases simultaneously. Comorbidities such as CHF, CAD, stroke, DM, and depression are common in COPD patients.

2. Diagnostic test results

a. **COPD** patients with characteristic symptoms of cough, dyspnea, sputum production, and/or exposure to known risk factors (e.g., smoking) should be evaluated for a COPD diagnosis. If the patient has $FEV_1/FVC < 70\%$ and a postbronchodilator $FEV_1 < 80\%$ predicted, he or she has airflow limitation that is not fully reversible. Patients with a smoking history (e.g., > 20 pack/year history and > 45 years old) should be considered for the diagnosis. Spirometry can be used to help make the diagnosis.

b. **Chronic bronchitis**

(1) Blood analysis may reveal polycythemia as a result of to erythropoiesis secondary to hypoxemia. With bacterial infection, the WBC count may be increased.

(2) Sputum inspection reveals thick purulent or mucopurulent sputum tinged yellow, white, green, or gray; an acute change in color and/or quantity suggests infection.

(3) Arterial blood gas studies may show a markedly decreased Pao_2 level (45 to 60 mm Hg), reflecting hypoxemia, and a $Paco_2$ level that is normal or elevated (50 to 60 mm Hg), reflecting hypercapnia.

(4) Pulmonary function tests may be normal in the early disease stages. Later, they show a reduced FEV_1/FVC ratio, increased residual lung volume, a decreased vital capacity, and a decreased FEV_1. Unlike emphysema, chronic bronchitis patients tend to have normal diffusing capacity, normal static lung compliance, and normal TLC.

(5) Chest radiograph typically identifies lung hyperinflation, a barrel chest, and increased bronchovascular markings.

(6) An ECG may reveal right ventricular hypertrophy and changes consistent with cor pulmonale.

c. **Emphysema**

(1) Sputum inspection reveals scanty sputum that is clear or mucoid. Infections are less frequent than in chronic bronchitis.

(2) Arterial blood gas studies typically indicate a reduced or normal Pao_2 level (65 to 75 mm Hg) and, in late disease stages, an increased $Paco_2$ level (50 to 60 mm Hg).

(3) Pulmonary function tests show a reduced FEV_1/FVC ratio, normal or increased static lung compliance, reduced FEV_1 and diffusing capacity, and increased TLC and RV.

(4) Chest radiograph usually reveals bullae, blebs, a flattened diaphragm, lung hyperinflation, vertical heart, enlarged anteroposterior chest diameter, decreased vascular markings in the lung periphery, and a large retrosternal air space.

F. **Treatment objectives** endorsed by GOLD include the following:

1. Prevent disease progression (smoking cessation)
2. Relieve symptoms and improve exercise tolerance (enable the patient to perform normal daily activities)
3. Improve health status
4. Prevent and treat exacerbations
5. Prevent and treat complications
6. Reduce mortality

G. **Therapy**

1. **Pharmacological treatment.** Therapy is based on disease staging, which is determined by spirometry (*Table 41-9*).

a. Short-acting anticholinergics and β-agonists, alone or in combination, are the most commonly used initial agents. Long-acting bronchodilators, such as salmeterol, formoterol, tiotropium (Spiriva), and theophylline are added to the short-acting agents. Methylxanthines are usually added when the response to other agents is inadequate. In addition to bronchodilation, these agents can decrease dyspnea, improve exercise capacity, improve quality of life, and decrease the frequency and severity of exacerbations, especially tiotropium. A new agent was recently approved, roflumilast (Daliresp), in the United States. It is a selective PDE4 inhibitor that is indicated to decrease COPD exacerbations in certain patients.

b. Bronchodilators are the most important therapy for symptoms in COPD. *Figure 41-4* indicates a strategy of use.

c. Inhaled corticosteroids, such as fluticasone and budesonide, have shown small benefits in FEV_1; the majority of their benefit occurs in reducing the severity of exacerbations, not the number of exacerbations.

d. **Anticholinergics** (e.g., ipratropium bromide, tiotropium bromide, atropine)

(1) **Indications.** Anticholinergics may be used as first-line bronchodilators or in conjunction with β-agonists in the treatment of COPD because these agents are the most potent bronchodilators for the condition.

(2) **Mechanism of action.** Ipratropium bromide, tiotropium bromide, and atropine produce bronchodilation by competitively inhibiting cholinergic responses. Ipratropium bromide and tiotropium bromide also reduce sputum volume without altering viscosity. Some studies have shown an increased response to these agents in COPD when they are combined with β-agonists. Tiotropium has greater affinity for cholinergic receptors than ipratropium.

(3) **Administration and dosage**

(a) Ipratropium bromide is three to five times more potent and has significantly fewer side effects than atropine, which is rarely used today since the development of nebulized ipratropium.

(b) Initial MDI dosing of ipratropium bromide is two inhalations (40 μg) four times daily, but dosing can be increased to six inhalations four times daily without significant risk. These higher doses are often required to achieve therapeutic benefit. Administration should be via MDI with spacer or MDI alone using a closed-mouth technique.

(c) Dosing of ipratropium bromide solution is 500 μg/2.5 mL (1 unit dose vial) or more via nebulizer four times daily.

(d) Tiotropium bromide capsules contain 22.5 μg tiotropium bromide monohydrate, equivalent to 18 μg tiotropium.

(i) Tiotropium is an inhalation powder contained in a hard capsule. It should be administered once daily only via a HandiHaler device, which delivers 10 μg tiotropium.

(ii) Patients should generally not be placed on both ipratropium and tiotropium because of the increased risk of anticholinergic side effects, and no additional bronchodilation is likely achieved by adding ipratropium. For example, if a COPD patient is currently on ipratropium/albuterol (Combivent, DuoNeb), and tiotropium is started, the albuterol should be continued as the short-acting bronchodilator and ipratropium discontinued.

Table 41-9 THERAPY AT EACH STAGE OF COPD

Old	**0: At Risk**	**I: Mild**	**II: Moderate IIA**	**IIB**	**III: Severe**
New	**0: At Risk**	**I: Mild**	**II: Moderate**	**II: Severe**	**IV: Very Severe**
Characteristics	Chronic symptoms Exposure to risk factors Normal spirometry	$FEV_1/FVC < 70\%$ $FEV_1 \geq 80\%$ With or without symptoms	$FEV_1/FVC < 70\%$ $50\% \leq FEV_1 < 50\%$ With or without symptoms	$FEV_1/FVC < 70\%$ $30\% \leq FEV_1 < 50\%$ With or without symptoms	$FEV_1/FVC < 70\%$ $FEV_1 < 30\%$ or $FEV_1 < 50\%$ predicted plus chronic respiratory failure
	Avoidance of risk factor(s); influenza vaccination				
		Add short-acting bronchodilator when needed			
			Add regular treatment with one or more long-acting bronchodilators		
			Add rehabilitation		
				Add inhaled glucocorticosteroids if repeated exacerbations	
					Add long-term oxygen if chronic respiratory failure
					Consider surgical treatments

FEV_1, forced expiratory volume in 1 sec; *FEV*, forced vital capacity.
Reprinted with permission from Global Initiative for Chronic Obstructive Lung Disease (GOLD). Global Strategy for the Diagnosis, Management, and Prevention of Chronic Obstructive Pulmonary Disease. Updated 2006. http://www.goldcopd.org.

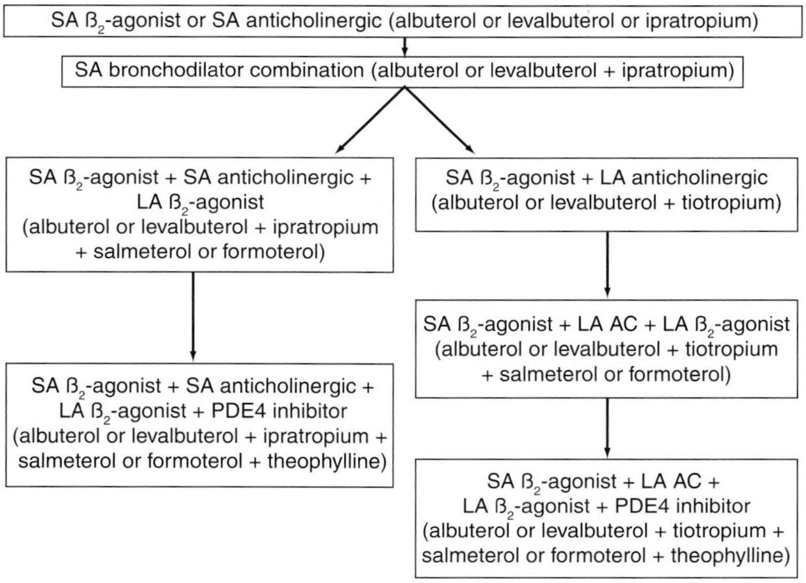

Figure 41-4. Stepped care approach to bronchodilators in COPD. *AC*, anticholinergic; *LA*, long acting; *PDE*, phosphodiesterase; *SA*, short acting.

e. **β-Agonists** (see I.I.1; *Table 41-4*)

(1) **Indications.** β_2-Agonists may be used as first-line bronchodilators or in conjunction with anticholinergic agents in the maintenance treatment of COPD. Short-acting agents are used regularly or on an as-needed basis for symptoms. Some patients may respond clinically to the prolonged treatment with β_2-agonists even after demonstrating lack of acute reversibility (spirometry testing showing $< 12\%$ or < 200-mL increase in FEV_1) to short-acting agents.

(2) **Mechanism of action.** β_2-Agonists relieve dyspnea caused by airway obstruction, although the response is usually not as significant as in patients with asthma. These agents may also increase mucociliary clearance by stimulating ciliary activity (helps patients expectorate sputum).

(3) **Administration and dosage**

(a) β_2-Agonists are administered via inhalation (e.g., DPI, nebulizer, MDI with or without a spacer), unless the patient cannot use the drug properly; then an oral agent is used cautiously.

(b) β_2-Agonists of the same duration should not be used in combination because an adequate dose of a single agent provides peak bronchodilation. However, it is reasonable to administer a long-acting product (e.g., salmeterol, formoterol) on a regular basis with a short-acting agent reserved for as-needed or rescue therapy.

(c) Salmeterol, formoterol, arformoterol (long-acting β-agonist) are administered twice daily. Indacterol (Arcapta®) is a recently marketed long-acting β-agonist that is administered once daily as a dry powder inhaler. They may also be used in combination with ipratropium bromide or tiotropium. Neither agent is used on an as-needed basis for rescue therapy, although formoterol does have a rapid onset of action.

(d) Inhaler devices that require a rapid inspiratory rate may result in suboptimal lung deposition in the COPD patient with limited inspiratory capacity. An MDI or nebulizer may be more optimal in this type of patient.

f. **Theophylline** (see I.I.5)

(1) **Indications.** Theophylline compounds typically are added to the drug regimen after an unsuccessful trial of ipratropium bromide and β-adrenergics. Theophylline appears to have a greater clinical role in COPD than in asthma. Other similar agents (phosphodiesterase inhibitors) are in development.

(2) **Mechanism of action.** In COPD, theophylline compounds are used because they increase mucociliary clearance, stimulate the respiratory drive, enhance diaphragmatic contractility, improve the ventricular ejection fraction, and stimulate renal diuresis. Their bronchodilator properties are modest, at best. Theophylline may be used in lieu of other long-acting bronchodilators or in combination.

(3) **Administration and dosage.** A trial of 1 to 2 months with the serum drug level maintained at 5 to 12 μg/mL and maximized.

- **(a)** Because of the nonbronchodilator effects of methylxanthines, they may be continued in the face of a clinical response, even in the absence of improved FEV_1.
- **(b)** If no change occurs in the patient's clinical condition and/or FEV_1, theophylline therapy should be discontinued owing to the potential for side effects.

(4) **Precautions and monitoring effects.** Serum drug levels should be closely monitored in all patients, especially those with signs of toxicity (tachycardia, nausea, vomiting) as well as with liver impairment, congestive heart failure and/or cor pulmonale as a result of reduced theophylline metabolism. Potential drug interactions (e.g., with ciprofloxacin) may warrant blood testing.

g. Roflumilast (Daliresp)

(1) **Indication.** Roflumilast is indicated as a treatment to reduce the risk of COPD exacerbations in patients with severe COPD associated with chronic bronchitis.

(2) **Mechanism of action.** Roflumilast is a long-acting selective PDE4 inhibitor that provides anti-inflammatory effects and mild bronchodilator effects.

(3) **Administration and dosage.** The dose of roflumilast is 500 mcg once daily, with or without food.

(4) **Precautions and monitoring.** The primary side effects of roflumilast are GI intolerance (diarrhea, nausea). Weight loss, averaging 5 lb, was seen in clinical trials. The PI warns that suicidality was reported in a small number of patients; the relationship with roflumilast is unclear. Drug interactions through CYP450 may occur, analogous to those seen with theophylline.

h. Corticosteroids (see I.I.2; *Table 41-5*)

(1) **Indications**

- **(a)** **Systemic corticosteroids** (preferably oral) are indicated in the treatment of acute COPD exacerbations and chronically in some severe patients.
- **(b)** **Inhaled corticosteroids** play a less prominent role in COPD than in asthma.
- **(c)** Candidates for prolonged use of inhaled corticosteroid therapy should
  - **(i)** be symptomatic and have a documented spirometric response (i.e., an increase in FEV_1 of at least 15% and 200 mL after 6 weeks to 3 months of use).
  - **(ii)** have an $FEV_1 < 50\%$ predicted, with a history of repeated exacerbations requiring systemic corticosteroids or antibiotics.
- **(d)** Long-term use of systemic steroids should be avoided if possible. Osteoporosis of the spine and ribs is especially common in COPD patients receiving frequent or maintenance systemic steroids. It has been recently recognized that inhaled steroids increase the risk of bacterial pneumonia in COPD patients.

(2) **Administration and dosage**

- **(a)** For oral use in outpatient management of acute exacerbations, prednisone or prednisolone is administered at a dosage of 40 mg/day for 10 days.
- **(b)** The dose of oral (e.g., prednisolone) or intravenous corticosteroids (e.g., methylprednisolone) for hospital management of acute COPD exacerbations is not established. However, doses and duration of therapy should be limited (e.g., 30 to 40 mg/day of prednisolone for 10 to 14 days) to avoid significant adverse effects.
- **(c)** In COPD, inhaled steroids are not as efficacious as in asthma patients.
- **(d)** In appropriate patients, corticosteroids may be administered via DPI or MDI with spacer.
- **(e)** Response to oral corticosteroids does not predict response to inhaled corticosteroids.
- **(f)** Medium doses of inhaled corticosteroids are recommended for COPD (e.g., Flovent 110 μg two puffs twice a day or the combination of Advair 250 μg one puff twice a day).
- **(g)** Inhaler devices that require a rapid inspiratory rate (e.g., Pulmicort Flexhaler) are generally not desirable in COPD patients.

i. **Antibiotics**
   (1) **Indications**
      (a) Antibiotics are used to treat exacerbations with suspected infection as evidenced by an increase in volume or change in color or viscosity of the sputum, along with dyspnea.
      (b) Prevention of infection with chronic antibiotic therapy is controversial and should be considered only in patients with multiple exacerbations annually (i.e., more than two per year).
   (2) **Antibiotic therapy**
      (a) Ambulatory antibiotic treatment of exacerbations in patients with COPD is recommended when there is evidence of worsening dyspnea and cough with purulent sputum and increased sputum volume.
         (i) Hospital or laboratory antibiograms should be reviewed when selecting an appropriate agent for *S. pneumoniae*, *M. catarrhalis*, and *H. influenzae*.
         (ii) Agents may include either a second-generation cephalosporin (e.g., cefuroxime, cefaclor), trimethoprim-sulfamethoxazole, a β-lactam with or without a β-lactamase inhibitor (e.g., amoxicillin, amoxicillin-clavulanate), macrolides (azithromycin [Zithromax]), or an oral fluoroquinolone (ciprofloxacin [Cipro], levofloxacin [Levaquin]). (Note that recent evidence indicates chronic macrolides may have a role to decrease COPD exacerbations).
         (iii) If infection with *M. pneumoniae* or *Legionella pneumophila* is a concern, although uncommon in COPD flares, a macrolide or fluoroquinolone may be added.
      (b) Antibiotic treatment of pneumonia in hospitalized patients with COPD includes either a second- or third-generation cephalosporin (e.g., cefuroxime, ceftriaxone, cefotaxime) or a β-lactam with or without a β-lactamase inhibitor (e.g., amoxicillin-clavulanate [Augmentin], piperacillin-tazobactam [Zosyn]), a macrolide, or fluoroquinolone.
      (c) COPD exacerbations are treated for 3 to 10 days, depending on the agent used (e.g., moxifloxacin 400 mg for 5 days) and the patient.

j. **Mucolytics** (e.g., oral *N*-acetylcysteine) may improve sputum clearance and disrupt mucus plugs.

k. **Expectorants** (e.g., guaifenesin) may be used. Potassium iodide should be avoided because of side effects associated with iodine therapy.

l. **Antioxidants** (e.g., oral *N*-acetylcysteine) may reduce exacerbation frequency.

m. **Influenza virus vaccine** is recommended because of its ability to reduce death and serious illness by almost 50%.

2. **Nonpharmacological therapy**

a. **Vaccinations**
   (1) Influenza vaccination administered each fall/winter. **Polyvalent pneumococcal** vaccine is recommended by the American Thoracic Society.

b. **Oxygen therapy**
   (1) Recommended for hypoxemia chronically or during exacerbations. Currently recommended to administer oxygen at least 15 hr/day.
   (2) Reverses hypoxemia (particularly at night and during exercise).
   (3) Indications for home oxygen treatment include
      (a) $Pao_2 < 55$ mm Hg or $Sao_2 < 88\%$
      (b) Pao_2 of 55 to 60 mm Hg or $Sao_2 < 89\%$ with evidence of cor pulmonale, pulmonary hypertension, or polycythemia (hematocrit > 55%).
   (4) Patients hospitalized for COPD exacerbations should receive controlled oxygen to keep $Pao_2 > 60$ mm Hg or $Sao_2 > 90\%$. Arterial blood gas (ABG) tests may be performed 30 mins after placing the patient on oxygen to identify and minimize CO_2 retention.

c. **Chest physiotherapy** loosens secretions, helps reexpand the lungs, and increases the efficacy of respiratory muscle use. Techniques include postural drainage, chest percussion and vibration, coughing, and deep breathing. These efforts may help patients with lobar atelectasis or who produce large quantities (i.e., > 25 mL/day) of sputum.

d. **Physical rehabilitation** improves the patient's exercise tolerance and quality of life. A pulmonary rehabilitation program usually includes physical conditioning and social, psychological, and nutritional interventions. This can be an effective intervention.

e. **Smoking cessation** and avoidance of other irritants has been shown to slow the rate of decline in FEV_1 in COPD patients. It is obviously one of the most important interventions. Nicotine gum, patches, inhalers, lozenges, bupropion, varenicline (Chantix), and clonidine may be useful in smoking cessation. Behavior intervention significantly enhances the effectiveness of pharmacological therapy in smoking cessation.

f. **Surgery.** There is a growing body of evidence that lung volume reduction surgery may be beneficial to patients with severe emphysema. Clinical trials have now delineated proper patient selection for this type of surgery. Lung transplantation is also performed in selected patients.

H. Complications of COPD

1. **Pulmonary hypertension.** With decreased pulmonary vascular bed space (owing to lung congestion), pulmonary arterial pressure increases. In some cases, pressure increases enough to cause **cor pulmonale** (right ventricular hypertrophy) with consequent heart failure.
2. **Acute respiratory failure.** In advanced stages of COPD, the brain's respiratory center may become seriously compromised, leading to poor cerebral oxygenation and an increased $Paco_2$ level. Hypoxia and respiratory acidosis may ensue. If the condition progresses, respiratory failure occurs.
3. **Infection.** In chronic bronchitis, trapping of excessive mucus, air, and bacteria in the tracheobronchial tree sets the stage for infection. In addition, impairment of coughing and deep breathing, which normally cleanses the lungs, leads to destruction of respiratory cilia. Once an infection sets in, reinfection can easily occur.
4. **Polycythemia.** An increase in red blood cells infrequently can lead to hypercoagulable states, embolism, and stroke. This happens uncommonly today due to the widespread use of supplemental oxygen in COPD patients.

Study Questions

Directions for questions 1–7: Each of the questions, statements, or incomplete statements in this section can be correctly answered or completed by **one** of the suggested answers or phrases. Choose the **best** answer.

1. The symptoms of allergen-mediated asthma result from which of the following?

(A) Increased release of mediators from mast cells
(B) Increased adrenergic responsiveness of the airways
(C) Increased vascular permeability of bronchial tissue
(D) Decreased calcium influx into the mast cells
(E) Decreased prostaglandin production

2. Acute exacerbations of asthma can be triggered by all of the following *except*

(A) bacterial or viral pneumonia.
(B) hypersensitivity reaction to penicillin.
(C) discontinuation of asthma medication.
(D) hot, dry weather.
(E) stressful emotional events.

3. A 45-year-old male with a history of asthma has a peak expiratory flow rate (PEFR) of 65%, nocturnal wheezing once a month, and daytime wheezing usually less than twice a week. According to the National Institutes of Health (NIH) guidelines for the treatment of asthma, he has which type?

(A) Mild intermittent
(B) Mild persistent
(C) Moderate persistent
(D) Severe persistent

4. The patient in question 3 should be treated with which *two* agents?

(A) Inhaled steroid and ipratropium
(B) Inhaled steroid and albuterol MDI (as needed)
(C) Inhaled steroid and aspirin

5. A 15-year-old female is brought to the emergency department. She is breathing 30 times per minute, is unable to speak in full sentences, and has a peak expiratory flow rate (PEFR) $< 50\%$ predicted. The preferred first-line therapy for her asthma exacerbation is
   - (A) theophylline.
   - (B) β-agonist.
   - (C) corticosteroid.
   - (D) cromolyn sodium.
   - (E) A and B
   - (F) B and C

6. The primary goals of asthma therapy in an adult patient include all of the following *except*
   - (A) maintain normal activity levels.
   - (B) maintain control of symptoms.
   - (C) avoid adverse effects of asthma medications.
   - (D) prevent acute exacerbations and chronic symptoms.
   - (E) prevent destruction of lung tissue.

7. Which of the following tests is used at home to assess therapy and determine if a patient with asthma should seek emergency care?
   - (A) Forced expiratory volume in 1 sec (FEV_1)
   - (B) Forced vital capacity (FVC)
   - (C) Total lung capacity (TLC)
   - (D) Peak expiratory flow rate (PEFR)
   - (E) Residual volume (RV)

Directions for question 8: The incomplete statement in this section can be correctly answered or completed by **one or more** of the suggested answers. Choose the answer, **A–E.**

- (A) if **I only** is correct
- (B) if **III only** is correct
- (C) if **I and II** are correct
- (D) if **II and III** are correct
- (E) if **I, II, and III** are correct

8. The disease process of chronic bronchitis is characterized by
   - I. the destruction of central and peripheral portions of the acinus.
   - II. an increased number of mucous glands and goblet cells.
   - III. edema and inflammation of the bronchioles.

Directions for questions 9–11: Each description in this section is most closely associated with **one** of the following agents. The agents may be used more than once or not at all. Choose the **best** answer, **A–E.**

- (A) cimetidine
- (B) albuterol
- (C) ipratropium bromide
- (D) epinephrine
- (E) atropine

9. Decreases theophylline clearance

10. Has anticholinergic activity with few side effects

11. Has high β_2-adrenergic selectivity

Answers and Explanations

1. **The answer is A** *[see I.F; Figure 41-1].*
In asthma, airborne antigen binds to the mast cell, activating the IgE-mediated process. Mediators (e.g., histamine, leukotrienes, prostaglandins) are then released, causing bronchoconstriction and tissue edema.

2. **The answer is D** *[see I.D; Figure 41-1].*
Exacerbations of asthma can be triggered by allergens, respiratory infections, occupational stimuli (e.g., fumes from gasoline or paint), emotions, and environmental factors. Studies have shown that cold air can cause release of mast cell mediators by an undetermined mechanism. Hot, dry air does not cause this release.

3. **The answer is C** *[see Table 41-3].*
The patient has moderate persistent asthma. All three parameters are consistent with mild persistent asthma. If any one of the three parameters indicated moderate persistent asthma, then the patient would be classified as moderate asthma (PEFR = 65%).

4. **The answer is B** *[see Figure 41-3].*
Inhaled steroids are the anti-inflammatory drug of choice owing to proven efficacy. All patients should be prescribed a short-acting β_2-agonist to use as rescue therapy for worsening symptoms. If chronic symptoms worsen, a long-acting β_2-agonist can be added (e.g., Advair). Remember that increasing the dose of the inhaled steroid may not improve symptoms, a long-acting bronchodilator is more likely to do so.

5. **The answer is F** *[see Figure 41-3].*
Patient is obviously in respiratory distress. Aggressive treatment with oxygen, systemic steroids, and short-acting bronchodilators is indicated. Ipratropium could also be added to the albuterol in the acute setting.

6. **The answer is E** *[see I.F; I.H.1; II.D].*
Asthma is characterized by reversible airway obstruction in response to specific stimuli. Mast cells release mediators, which trigger bronchoconstriction. After an acute attack, in most cases symptoms are minimal and pathological changes are not permanent. Unlike asthma, COPD does cause progressive airway destruction, chronic bronchitis by excessive mucus production and other changes, and emphysema by destruction of the acinus.

7. **The answer is D** *[see I.G.2.a.(3)].*
For home monitoring, PEFR is the best test for assessment of therapy, trigger identification, and the need for referral to emergency care. It is recommended for patients who have had severe exacerbations of asthma, who are poor perceivers of asthma symptoms, and those with moderate-to-severe disease.

8. **The answer is D (II, III)** *[see II.D.1–2].*
Chronic bronchitis is characterized by an increase in the number of mucous and goblet cells owing to bronchial irritation. This results in increased mucus production. Other changes include edema and inflammation of the bronchioles and changes in smooth muscle and cartilage. Emphysema is a permanent destruction of the central and peripheral portions of the acinus distal to the bronchioles. In this disease, adequate oxygen reaches the alveolar duct, owing to increased rate of breathing, but perfusion is abnormal.

9. **The answer is A** *[see Table 41-8].*

10. **The answer is C** *[see II.G.1.a].*

11. **The answer is B** *[see Table 41-4].*
Cimetidine, an H_2-receptor antagonist, decreases theophylline clearance by inhibiting hepatic microsomal mixed-function oxidase metabolism, thus increasing serum theophylline concentrations. Theophylline clearance can be decreased by 40% during the first 24 hrs of concurrent therapy. Anticholinergic agents such as atropine and ipratropium bromide produce bronchodilation by competitively inhibiting cholinergic receptors. The disadvantages of atropine include dry mouth, tachycardia, and urinary retention. Ipratropium bromide is three to five times more potent than atropine and does not have these side effects. Albuterol is one of the most β_2-selective adrenergic agents available. Other such agents include terbutaline, bitolterol, and pirbuterol. Agents with β_2-selectivity dilate bronchioles without causing side effects related to β_1-stimulation (e.g., increased heart rate).

42

Osteoarthritis and Rheumatoid Arthritis

TINA HARRISON THORNHILL

I. DEFINITION AND CAUSE

A. **Osteoarthritis (OA)** is a common chronic condition of articular cartilage degeneration. Secondary changes can occur in the bone, leading to pain, decreased functioning, and even disability. OA affects nearly 21 million middle-aged and elderly Americans. It is the most common form of arthritis. Although not always symptomatic, most people older than the age of 55 years have radiological evidence of the disease. Until age 55 years, OA affects men more frequently than women, but after age 55, women are more likely to have the disease.

B. **Rheumatoid arthritis (RA)** is a chronic, systemic autoimmune disease that involves inflammation in the membrane lining of the joints and often affects internal organs. Most patients exhibit a chronic fluctuating course of disease that can result in progressive joint destruction, deformity, and disability. RA affects between 1 and 2 million Americans. It occurs three times more often in women, and peaks at age 35 to 50 years.

II. NORMAL JOINT ANATOMY AND PHYSIOLOGY

A. The **synovial joint** consists of two bone ends covered by articular cartilage. The roles of articular cartilage include
   1. Enabling frictionless movement of the joint.
   2. Distributing the load across the joint (shock absorber), to prevent damage.
   3. Promoting stability during use.

B. **Cartilage** is avascular and aneural. It is metabolically active and undergoes continual internal remodeling. It is composed primarily of water but is also made from chondrocytes and extracellular matrix.

C. **Chondrocytes** control the synthesis and degradation of the matrix. They produce proteoglycans and collagen in the extracellular matrix to maintain the integrity of the matrix in healthy cartilage.

D. The **joint capsule** is a fibrous outer layer that encapsulates the joint. The joint capsule is lined by **synovium**, a membrane that produces a viscous fluid that lubricates the joint.

E. The **synovial fluid** is composed, in part, of hyaluronic acid. Glucosamine is a component of hyaluronic acid. The role of hyaluronic acid is to maintain functional and structural characteristics of the extracellular matrix.

F. **Bursae** are small sacs that are lined with synovial membrane and filled with fluid to provide cushioning and lubrication for the movement of the joint.

III. OSTEOARTHRITIS

A. **Pathophysiology.** Many age-related changes contribute to the development of OA.
   1. The strength of tendons, ligaments, and muscles declines with advancing age and may contribute to the development of the disease.
   2. The number of chondrocytes declines owing to apoptosis (cell death), decreased proliferation, or both.

3. The synthesis of normal proteoglycans is reduced.
4. Chondrocytes lose the ability to promote healing and cartilage remodeling, resulting in cartilage matrix degradation. Proteoglycans are depleted.
5. Matrix metalloproteinases (MMPs) and proinflammatory cytokines promote cartilage degradation.
6. Interleukin 1 (IL-1) has several roles in the development of OA
   a. Induction of chondrocytes and synovial cells to synthesize MMPs
   b. Inhibits the synthesis of type II collagen and proteoglycans, preventing collagen from repairing itself
   c. Enhances nitric oxide production and induces chondrocyte apoptosis
7. Pain occurs as a result of
   a. Osteophytes (spurs of cartilage and bone at the joint)
   b. Synovitis
   c. Bursitis
   d. Tendonitis

B. **Risk factors** for OA include advanced age, female gender, muscle weakness, obesity, joint trauma, heredity, congenital or developmental anatomical defects, and repetitive stress.

C. **Clinical presentation.** OA is characterized by a deep, localized ache in a joint. Pain and stiffness usually occurs with rest or immobility and lasts < 30 mins. Inflammation, if present, is mild. Patients will often complain of crepitus, a popping or cracking noise heard in the joint upon moving. OA most commonly affects the hips, knees, spine, feet, and hands.

D. **Diagnosis**
1. **Physical examination.** Joint tenderness, diminished range of motion, crepitus, and misshaped joints.
2. **Laboratory tests.** No specific lab tests are diagnostic for OA; however, if arthrocentesis is performed, synovial fluid will reveal mild leukocytosis with predominance of mononuclear lymphocytes.
3. **Radiography.** Narrowing of joint space (owing to loss of cartilage), subchondral sclerosis, and osteophytes are seen.
4. The American College of Rheumatology (ACR) has defined **criteria for OA of the hip, knee, and hand**:
   a. OA of the hip is characterized by hip pain and at least two of the following:
      (1) Erythrocyte sedimentation rate (ESR) < 20 mm/hr
      (2) Radiographic evidence of femoral or acetabular osteophytes
      (3) Radiographic evidence of joint space narrowing
   b. OA of the knee is characterized by knee pain, radiographic evidence of osteophytes, and at least one of the following:
      (1) Age > 50 years
      (2) Morning stiffness that lasts < 30 mins
      (3) Articular crepitus on motion
   c. OA of the hand is characterized by hand pain, aching, or stiffness and at least three of the following:
      (1) Hard tissue enlargement of ≥ 2 distal interphalangeal (DIP) joints.
      (2) Hard tissue enlargement of ≥ 2 selected joints (second and third DIP and/or proximal interphalangeal [PIP], and the first carpometacarpal joints of both hands).
      (3) Fewer than three swollen metacarpophalangeal (MCP) joints.
      (4) Deformity of at least one of ten selected joints.

E. **Treatment**
1. **Goals**
   a. Control pain and other symptoms
   b. Maintain or improve joint mobility
   c. Correct or minimize functional limitations and disability
2. **Nonpharmacological treatments.** The mainstay of OA therapy should focus on these nondrug therapies.
   a. **Patient education** may include tips on joint protection and exercise programs.
   b. **Weight loss** (if overweight) can decrease pain and OA symptoms.

c. **Aerobic exercise programs** to increase muscle strength.
d. **Physical therapy** for range-of-motion exercises and strengthening.
e. **Assistive devices** (e.g., canes, walkers) may help decrease joint load.
f. **Acupuncture** leads to improvements in pain and function after 26 weeks, compared to placebo or arthritis education in patients with mild knee OA.
g. **Wedge insoles** can help reduce mechanical stress in persons with medial knee OA.
h. **Thermal therapy** (e.g., hot shower or tub, ice pack) may be of benefit for some patients with OA.

3. **Pharmacological treatment**
a. **Acetaminophen** (APAP) is considered first-line therapy by the ACR for OA. It has excellent analgesic and antipyretic activity, but no anti-inflammatory effects.
(1) A dose of $\leq$ 4 g/day is recommended to avoid toxicity. Concomitant use of other medications with acetaminophen should be evaluated closely to avoid overdose.
(2) Hepatotoxicity can occur in patients taking $>$ 4 g APAP a day. Symptoms can include nausea, vomiting, abdominal pain, malaise, and diaphoresis.
(3) Because there is little, if any, inflammation in the OA joint, APAP has been shown to be equally efficacious as ibuprofen and naproxen in patients with mild to moderate OA pain.
(4) Studies have shown either APAP immediate-release or extended-release is effective in treating mild to moderately severe OA pain.
b. **Nonsteroidal anti-inflammatory drugs (NSAIDs)** and **cyclooxygenase 2 (COX-2) specific inhibitors** are indicated in OA treatment when the response to APAP is inadequate (*Table 42-1*).
(1) **Mechanism of action.** NSAIDs are nonselective inhibitors of COX-1 and COX-2 as well as thromboxane synthetase.
(2) **Analgesia** is seen with short treatment duration and at lower doses (e.g., ibuprofen $\leq$ 1200 mg/day).
(3) **Anti-inflammatory** response is seen with higher doses and usually requires several days of therapy to achieve anti-inflammatory effect.
(4) **Adverse effects.** The FDA mandates that a published NSAID Medication Guide be issued with all NSAID prescriptions informing patients about the potential adverse effects.
(a) **Gastrointestinal** (GI) toxicity is caused by direct mucosal injury and inhibition of prostaglandins. Symptoms include dyspepsia, ulceration, and bleeding.
(i) COX-2 inhibitors may be an option for patients with a history of peptic ulcer disease; however, the GI safety of these agents has not been demonstrated long term.
(ii) People at risk for GI toxicity include the elderly and those with a history of peptic ulcer disease, chronic alcohol use, high-dose or multiple NSAID use, and concomitant corticosteroid use.

Table 42-1 SELECTED ANTI-INFLAMMATORY DRUGS

Generic (Brand)	Initial Daily Dose	Maximum Daily Dose
Nonacetylated salicylates		
Salsalate (Disalcid)	1000 mg twice a day	3000 mg
Nonsteroidal anti-inflammatory drugs		
Aspirin (various)	650 mg every 4 hrs	4000 mg
Diclofenac (Voltaren)	75 mg twice a day	200 mg
Ibuprofen (Motrin, Advil)	400 mg three times a day	3200 mg
Naproxen (Naprosyn, Aleve)	500 mg twice a day	1100 mg
Nabumetone (Relafen)	1000 mg once a day	2000 mg
Sulindac (Clinoril)	150 mg twice a day	400 mg
Tolmetin (Tolectin)	400 mg three times a day	1800 mg
Cyclooxygenase 2 inhibitor		
Celecoxib (Celebrex)	100 mg twice a day	400 mg

(b) **Renal** toxicity results from the inhibition of prostaglandins. Although the risks are low (~5%), it does not appear to be dose dependent and is usually reversible.
(i) Effects can include hyperkalemia, hyponatremia, increased serum creatinine, sodium and water retention, and acute renal failure.
(ii) People at risk for renal toxicity include the elderly and those with preexisting renal disease, hypertension, diabetes mellitus, congestive heart failure, cirrhosis, and volume depletion (e.g., hemorrhage, sepsis, diuretics, and diarrhea).

(c) **Hematological** effects are the result of decreased platelet aggregation.

(d) **Hepatic** toxicity, although not common, can include elevated liver enzymes. Patients at risk include those with a history of hepatitis, alcoholism, and heart failure.

(e) **Central nervous system** effects can include sedation, confusion, and mental status changes and are primarily seen in the elderly.

(f) **Allergic reactions**, such as asthma, urticaria, and photosensitivity, may be seen. Cross-sensitivity has been seen in patients allergic to aspirin.

(g) **Cardiovascular (CV)** effects (e.g., myocardial infarction, stroke, hypertension, and heart failure) have been reported. Studies of celecoxib have shown a dose-related increase in CV events in patients with a history of colorectal neoplasia who were at risk of recurrent adenomatous polyps. The U.S. Food and Drug Administration (FDA) recommends using celecoxib at the lowest possible dose for the least time possible.

c. **Other oral analgesics**

(1) **Tramadol (Ultram).** Considered a good choice when the patient's pain is unrelieved by NSAIDs, when the patient cannot take NSAIDs, or when the patient experiences breakthrough pain while taking NSAIDs.

(a) **Mechanism of action.** Centrally acting analgesic that inhibits the reuptake of norepinephrine and serotonin and mildly binds to the μ-receptor.

(b) **Dose.** 50 to 100 mg every 4 to 6 hrs, not to exceed 400 mg/day; and 300 mg/day in the elderly. In patients with impaired renal function (creatinine clearance [CrCl] < 30 mL/min), the dosage interval should be every 12 hrs, with a maximum dose of 200 mg. The extended-release formulation is dosed 100 mg daily with a maximum dose of 300 mg/day.

(c) **Adverse effects.** Although it is not an opioid analgesic, its side effects are similar: nausea, constipation, rash, dizziness, somnolence, and orthostatic hypotension.

(d) **Drug interactions.** Concomitant use with selective serotonin reuptake inhibitors (SSRIs; e.g., citalopram, sertraline, fluoxetine) may cause serotonin syndrome. Tramadol is metabolized by CYP3A4.

(2) **Opiate analgesics** (e.g., codeine, oxycodone) are usually reserved for patients who fail single- or multiple-analgesic therapy. They may also be useful for acute exacerbations of pain. Side effects can include constipation, sedation, nausea, confusion, and respiratory depression.

(3) **Topical analgesics** are effective in relieving OA pain in some patients. Topical therapy can be used as monotherapy or in conjunction with oral therapy.

(a) **Capsaicin** (e.g., Zostrix) is derived from hot chili peppers and with chronic use (> 2 weeks) works by depleting stores of substance P. Patients should be counseled to wash hands thoroughly after application to avoid contact with other skin to avoid burning and stinging.

(b) **Diclofenac** (e.g., Voltaren Gel) is a topical NSAID approved for OA of the knee (4 gm QID) and hands (2 gm QID). The max daily dose is 32 gm/day. The same adverse effects as oral NSAIDs are possible, but studies show that they are rare.

(4) **Intra-articular injections**

(a) **Corticosteroids** may be useful in knee OA when inflammation is present, but are not routinely recommended in hip OA owing to administration difficulties. Duration of action is up to 4 weeks. Because of adverse effects on the bone, injections should be limited to three or four per year. Long-term benefits and safety have not been established definitively.

(b) **Hyaluronic acid derivatives** are intended to improve elasticity and viscosity of synovial fluid. They are indicated for the treatment of knee OA when treatment failure to other therapies occurs. **Sodium hyaluronate (Hyalgan**; 20 mg weekly for 5 weeks) and **hylan polymers** (**Synvisc**; 16 mg weekly for 3 weeks) are two agents currently available. Most benefits are seen after the last dose; effects are superior to placebo. These agents should be used with caution in patients with allergies to avian proteins, feathers, and egg products.

(5) **Adjunctive treatments.** These agents are widely used by patients; however, efficacy has not been consistently demonstrated in controlled trials.

(a) **Glucosamine** acts as a substrate for and promotes the synthesis of the glycosaminoglycans.

(i) The dose is 500 mg three times a day.

(ii) **Side effects** may include GI discomfort, fatigue, and skin rash.

(b) **Chondroitin** helps protect against the breakdown of collagen and proteoglycans. It is usually found in combination with glucosamine, but the added benefits are not clear.

(i) The dose is 1200 mg/day.

(ii) **Side effects** can include prolonged bleeding time and nausea.

(6) **Surgical interventions** (e.g., arthroscopy, joint replacement) are considered when pain is severe and not responding to medical treatment or when disability interferes with daily activities.

IV. RHEUMATOID ARTHRITIS

A. **Etiology and pathogenesis.** The cause of RA is not fully understood but appears to be multifactorial. It is considered an autoimmune disease in which the body loses its ability to distinguish between synovial and foreign tissue. Other factors involved in RA are as follows:

1. **Environmental influences**, such as infections or trauma, are thought to trigger the development of RA.
2. **Genetic markers**, such as human leukocyte antigen DR4 (HLA-DR4), have been associated with triggering the inflammatory process in RA. Such markers, however, are not considered diagnostic because ~30% of people with HLA-DR4 never develop RA.
3. Antigen-dependent activation of **T lymphocytes** leads to proliferation of the synovial lining, activation of proinflammatory cells from the bone marrow, cytokine and protease secretion, and autoantibody production.
4. **Anticitrullinated proteins** and peptides are high specific for RA.
5. **Tumor necrosis factor** α (TNF-α), **IL-1**, **IL-6**, **IL-8**, and **growth factors** propagate the inflammatory process, and agents found to alter these cytokines show promise in reducing pain and deformity.
6. **Inflamed synovium** is a hallmark of the pathophysiology of RA. Synovium proliferates abnormally, growing into the joint space and into the bone, forming a pannus. The pannus migrates to the articular cartilage and into the subchondral bone leading to destruction of cartilage, bone, tendons, and blood vessels.

B. **Clinical manifestations**

1. The onset of RA is insidious. In early disease, symptoms include malaise and anorexia, accompanied by symmetrically tender and swollen joints. Pain in the joints is common and aggravated by movement.
2. Most commonly, the joints first affected by RA include the MCP and PIP joints of the hands, the metatarsophalangeal (MTP) joints, and the wrists. Other areas affected by RA include the spine, shoulder, ankle, and hip.

C. **Clinical course.** The severity of the disease is variable.

1. Within 4 months of diagnosis, irreversible joint damage is detectable on radiographic images. The rate at which joint damage occurs is greatest during the first year.
2. Extra-articular manifestations can include rheumatoid nodules, anemia, peripheral neuropathy, kidney disease, CV effects, and pulmonary disease.
3. Causes of mortality in RA are cardiovascular disease, infection, respiratory disease, and malignancy.

D. **Laboratory assessment**

1. **Rheumatoid factor (RF)** is found in > 60% of patients with RA; however, as many as 5% of healthy individuals will have elevated titers of RF. If initially negative, the test can be repeated in 6 to 12 months. RF is not an accurate measure of disease progression.

2. **Erythrocyte sedimentation rate (ESR) and C-reactive protein (CRP)** are markers of inflammation and are usually elevated in patients with RA. They can also help indicate the activity of the disease, but they do not indicate disease severity.
3. **Anticyclic citrullinated peptide antibodies** (ACPA) are found in most patients with RA and are useful in predicting erosive disease.

E. **Diagnosis and clinical evaluation.** In 2010, the ACR and EULAR (European League Against Rheumatism) established a score-based algorithm criteria aimed at diagnoses before joint damage occurs. Providing the patient has at least one joint with active synovitis (swelling) than cannot be explained by another diagnosis. Definitive RA is defined as a score ≥ 6/10 based on four domains:
1. **Joint involvement** (e.g., number and location of involved joints)
2. **Serology** (e.g., RF, ACPA)
3. **Acute phase reactants** (e.g., CRP, ESR)
4. **Duration of symptoms**

F. **Radiographic examination** can reveal the extent of bone erosion and cartilage loss. An MRI can detect proliferative pannus.

G. **Treatment objectives.** The goals in the management of RA are
1. To prevent or control joint damage
2. To prevent loss of function
3. To decrease pain
4. To maintain the patient's quality of life
5. To avoid or minimize adverse effects of treatment

H. **Prognosis.** Poor prognostic factors include active disease with multiple tender and swollen joints, evidence of erosions seen on radiographs, elevated RF and/or ACPA, and elevated ESR and/or CRP. Additionally, worse outcomes, including disability and morbidity, are associated with female gender, advancing age, cigarette smoking, and genotype.

I. **Therapy.** The ACR published updated treatment recommendations in 2008 on nonbiological and biological disease modifying drugs. Nonpharmacological therapy (e.g., exercise, joint protection, physical therapy) and NSAIDs (*Table 42-1*) were not included in the report as these do nothing to alter the course of the disease or prevent joint destruction. Consideration, however, may be made to include these as adjuvant therapy for mild to moderate pain relief.
1. **Corticosteroids.** Low-dose systemic corticosteroids (e.g., prednisone, methylprednisolone) have excellent anti-inflammatory activity and are immunosuppressant. The lowest effective dose should be used because of adverse effects (e.g., hyperglycemia, GI toxicity, osteoporosis). These agents have shown to slow joint damage; however, they are often used as "bridge" therapy as patients start on disease-modifying antirheumatic drugs (DMARDs) or during an acute RA flare.
2. **Nonbiological disease-modifying antirheumatic drugs (NBDMARDs)** (*Table 42-2*) are used to reduce or prevent joint damage and preserve joint function and should be considered within 3 months of diagnosis. NOTE—the 2008 recommendations only assessed the use of methotrexate (MTX), leflunomide, sulfasalazine, hydroxychloroquine, and minocycline. Other NBDMARDs were not mentioned because of lack of clinical efficacy, side effects, or both.
   a. **Methotrexate (MTX; Rheumatrex)** works by inhibiting dihydrofolate reductase and is considered standard therapy for RA. MTX is recommended for all patients with RA (as monotherapy or with other DMARDs) regardless of disease duration, disease burden, or prognostic factors. Concomitant use with folic acid may reduce side effects.
   b. **Leflunomide (Arava)** inhibits pyrimidine synthesis and is recommended for all patients with RA (as monotherapy or with other DMARDs) regardless of disease duration, disease burden, or prognostic factors. Because of its long elimination half-life, cholestyramine is recommended as a binding agent if serious toxicities occur or if the patient wishes to become pregnant.
   c. **Sulfasalazine** is cleaved by bacteria in the colon into sulfapyridine and 5-aminosalicylic acid. It is recommended for all disease durations and degrees of illness without poor prognosis.
   d. **Hydroxychloroquine's** mechanism of action for RA is unknown. It is recommended for those without poor prognosis and low disease activity of ≤ 2 years.
3. **Biological DMARDs (BDMARDs)** (*Table 42-2*) can reduce or prevent joint damage, preserve joint integrity and function in patient with moderate to severe RA. They are used primarily in those failing an adequate trial of one or more NBDMARDs or in patients with high disease

Table 42-2 DISEASE-MODIFYING ANTIRHEUMATIC DRUGS (DMARDs)

Agent (Brand)	Time to Effect (months)	Starting Dose	Adverse Effects	Monitoring Parameters	Some Drug Interactions
Traditional DMARDs					
Methotrexate (Rheumatrex)	0.5–6.0	7.5–15.0 mg PO weekly	Nausea, diarrhea, mouth ulcers, hepatotoxicity, pulmonary toxicity, myelosuppression	LFTs, SrCr, CBC, chest x-ray Hepatitis B and C serology	Penicillin, cyclosporine, NSAIDs
Sulfasalazine (Azulfidine)	1–3	500 mg PO b.i.d.; gradually increase to 2–3 g/day in 2–4 divided doses	Nausea, diarrhea, rash, photosensitivity	CBC, LFTs, SrCr	Iron, digoxin, warfarin
Hydroxychloroquine (Plaquenil)	2–6	200–300 mg PO b.i.d.	Ocular toxicity, rash, nausea, myopathy	Eye exam, SrCr, CBC, LFTs	Cimetidine
Minocycline (Dynacin)	n/d	100 mg PO b.i.d.	GI, rash	CBC, LFTs	Calcium, magnesium, aluminum, iron
Biologicals					
Leflunomide (Arava)	1–4	100 mg/day PO × 3 days (load), then 10–20 mg/day	Diarrhea, nausea, infection, rash, HTN, alopecia, liver toxicity	LFTs, CBC, SrCr, PPD, hepatitis B and C serology	MTX, rifampin, warfarin
Etanercept (Enbrel)	0.25–3.00	50 mg SC weekly	Abdominal pain, HA, injection site reactions, infections	PPD, CBC, LFTs, SrCr	Cyclophosphamide
Infliximab (Remicade)	0.5	3 mg/kg IV over 2 hrs at weeks 0, 2, and 6; then every 8 weeks	Nausea, HA, abdominal pain, dizziness, hepatic, hematologic, infections	PPD, CBC, LFTs, SrCr	None known
Adalimumab (Humira)	0.25–1.00	40 mg SC every 2 wks	Injection site reactions, infection, rash, HA	PPD, CBC, LFTs, SrCr	None known

(Continued on next page)

Table 42-2 Continued

Agent (Brand)	Time to Effect (months)	Starting Dose	Adverse Effects	Monitoring Parameters	Some Drug Interactions
Anakinra (Kineret)	0.25–1.00	100 mg/day SQ	HA, injection site reactions, infection	CBC with neutrophil counts, LFTs, SrCr	Entanercept, thalidomide
Abatacept (Orencia)	n/d	10 mg/kg IV at day 0; then 2 weeks, 4 weeks, and continuing every 4 weeks	Injection site reactions, infections, HA, nausea, HTN, nasopharyngitis	PPD, CBC, LFTs, SrCr	Anakinra, TNF-antagonists
Rituximab (Rituxan)	n/d	1000 mg IV at days 0 and 14	Injection site reactions, HTN, infections, nausea, arthralgia	Hepatitis B serology, CBC, LFTs, SrCr	Cisplatin
Less Frequently Used DMARDs					
Gold Salts (Aurolate)	3–6	25–50 mg IM every 2–4 weeks	Itching, rash, stomatitis, proteinuria, conjunctivitis	CBC with differential, SrCr, urinalysis	Penicillamine
D-penicillamine (Cuprimine)	3–6	125–250 mg PO daily; increase gradually to 250 mg t.i.d.	Nausea, rash, photosensitivity, myelosuppression	CBC, SrCr	Gold, iron, zinc, antacids, digoxin, antimalarials
Azathioprine (Imuran)	2–3	50–150 mg/day	Chills, fever, N/V, diarrhea, leucopenia	CBC, LFTs	Allopurinol
Cyclosporine (Neoral)	2–4	3–10 mg/kg/day	HTN, HA, nausea, paresthesia, leukopenia	BP, SrCr, LTFs, serum drug levels	CYP450 3A/4 inhibitors, MTX, digoxin, allopurinol, glucocorticoids

BP, blood pressure; *CBC*, complete blood count; *HA*, headache; *HTN*, hypertension; *IM*, intramuscularly; *IV*, intravenously; *LFTs*, liver function tests; *MTX*, methotrexate; *n/d*, no data available; *N/V*, nausea and vomiting, *NSAIDs*, nonsteroidal anti-inflammatory drugs; *PO*, by mouth; *PPD*, tuberculosis skin test; *SC*, subcutaneously; *SrCr*, serum creatinine; *TNF*, tumor necrosis factor; including 2008 recommendations by the ACR.

activity and poor prognosis. *Note*: the only BDMARDs included in the 2008 guidelines are abatacept, adalimumab, etanercept, infliximab, and rituximab. The remaining BDMARDs were not included either because they were not FDA approved at the time of the publication or because of very infrequent use, high incidence of side effects, or both.

a. **TNF-α blockers** (e.g., etanercept [Enbrel], infliximab [Remicade], adalimumab [Humira], golimumab [Simponi], and certolizumab pegol [Cimzia]) inhibit the inflammatory response mediated in immune cells. Etanercept, adalimumab, and certolizumab can be used as monotherapy or in conjunction with MTX. Infliximab and golimumab is only FDA approved for use with MTX in RA. These drugs are recommended if high disease activity is present early in the course of the illness (< 3 months) with poor prognosis. These drugs are usually considered when patients do not achieve an acceptable response to MTX or other NBDMARDs.
b. **Abatacept (Orencia)** is the first T-cell costimulation blocker. It is used as monotherapy or NBDMARDs. Abatacept is recommended with MTX + NBDMARD does not work in the presence of moderate disease with poor prognosis.
c. **Rituximab (Rituxan)** is an anti-CD20 monoclonal antibody. Depletion of the CD20+ B cells appears to affect the autoimmune response and helps with the chronic synovitis associated with RA. It is used when the patient fails MTX and/or multiple DMARDs and has high disease burden and poor prognosis. Severe, even fatal, infusion reactions have been reported.
d. **Anakinra (Kineret)** is an IL-1 receptor antagonist. It is used as monotherapy or in conjunction with any DMARD except a TNF-blocker.
e. **Tocilizumab (Actemra)** is an IL-6 receptor monoclonal antibody. It is indicated for moderate-to-severe RA in adults who have not achieved response with one or more TNF-antagonists. It can be used as monotherapy or with MTX or other NBDMARDs.

4. **Combination therapy.** Concurrent use of several NBDMARDs has been studied. The 2008 guidelines support the following combinations: MTX + HCQ, MTX + sulfasalazine, MTX + leflunomide, and sulfasalazine + HCQ + MTX. Some patients currently receiving DMARD therapy with new or worsening symptoms have benefited from combination therapy. Combination therapy with multiple biological DMARDs were not recommended in the 2008 guidelines because of increased side effects and/or lack of efficacy.
5. **Treatment recommendations** are published by the ACR and are available at http://www.rheumatology.org.
6. **Surgical treatment** (e.g., carpal tunnel release, total joint arthroplasty, joint fusion) may be considered when pain is severe, range of motion is lost, or joint function is poor.

Study Questions

1. Which of the following statements best characterizes osteoarthritis (OA)?
   (A) OA is a common disorder characterized by diffuse inflammation leading to increased disability.
   (B) OA is a systemic disorder characterized by degenerative changes in the joint(s) and typically exhibits extra-articular involvement.
   (C) OA is a common disorder that affects the normal synthesis and degradation of cartilage.
   (D) OA is a common disorder that adversely affects bone density and leads to falls and fractures.
   (E) OA is a systemic disorder frequently associated with localized inflammation and pannus formation.

2. Which of the following agents is recommended as first-line drug therapy by the American College of Rheumatology for patients with mild to moderate osteoarthritis?
   (A) Ibuprofen (Motrin)
   (B) Celecoxib (Celebrex)
   (C) Diclofenac gel (Voltaren Gel)
   (D) Tramadol (Ultram)
   (E) Acetaminophen (Tylenol)

3. When consideration is given to diagnosing osteoarthritis, which of the following statements is FALSE?

(A) Joint tenderness, diminished range of motion, and/or articular crepitus can be assessed
(B) Radiographical evidence will show joint space narrowing
(C) Common patient complaints include a deep, localized ache in a joint
(D) Laboratory evidence reveals a high sedimentation rate, positive rheumatoid factor, and anti-cyclic citrullinated peptide antibody
(E) Morning stiffness lasts < 30 mins

4. Which of the following disease modifying anti-rheumatic drugs are recommended by the American College of Rheumatology for all patients with rheumatoid arthritis regardless of disease duration and degrees of disease activity?

(A) Methotrexate and sulfasalazine
(B) Methotrexate and hydroxychloroquine
(C) Methotrexate and etanercept
(D) Methotrexate and leflunomide
(E) Methotrexate and minocycline

5. In order to reduce toxicity with methotrexate, concomitant administration with what vitamin is recommended?

(A) Folic acid
(B) Thiamine
(C) Ascorbic acid
(D) Pyridoxine
(E) Riboflavin

6. All of the following statements are true about the use of hyaluronic acid derivatives in osteoarthritis (OA) *except*:

(A) Should be considered in those not responding to simple analgesics
(B) Should be considered for the treatment of knee OA
(C) Should be considered as disease-modifying agents
(D) Should be considered if no allergies exist to feathers or egg products
(E) Should be considered to improve elasticity of synovial fluid

7. Which of the following agents used for osteoarthritis or rheumatoid arthritis require dosage adjustment in patients with renal impairment?

(A) Prednisone
(B) Acetaminophen
(C) Oxycodone
(D) Glucosamine
(E) Tramadol

8. Which of the following disease modifying antirheumatic drugs can be administered orally?

(A) Certolizumab (Cimzia)
(B) Anakinra (Kineret)
(C) Abatacept (Orencia)
(D) Leflunomide (Arava)
(E) Etanercept (Enbrel)

9. What is the recommended starting dose of methotrexate when used for rheumatoid arthritis?

(A) 2.5 mg PO daily
(B) 2.5 mg PO weekly
(C) 7.5 mg PO daily
(D) 7.5 mg PO weekly
(E) 25 mg PO weekly

10. Ocular toxicity is associated with

(A) leflunomide (Arava)
(B) methotrexate (Rheumatrex)
(C) hydroxychloroquine (Plaquenil)
(D) infliximab (Remicade)
(E) adalimumab (Humira)

11. A baseline PPD is recommended to rule-out latent tuberculosis before initiating:

(A) leflunomide, etanercept, infliximab
(B) methotrexate, sulfasalazine, hydroxychloroquine
(C) leflunomide, methotrexate, etanercept
(D) methotrexate, infliximab, anakinra
(E) abatacept, leflunomide, sulfasalazine

12. Before initiating therapy with a nonsteroidal anti-inflammatory drug, it is important to evaluate:

(A) hematocrit, sodium, triglycerides
(B) serum creatinine, hematocrit, blood pressure
(C) blood pressure, serum folate, potassium
(D) liver function tests, serum creatinine, and serum folate
(E) sodium, hematocrit, respiration

13. All of the following statements are true about disease modifying antirheumatic drugs *except*:

(A) Should be started within 3 to 4 months of diagnosis of RA
(B) Can reduce or prevent joint damage
(C) Shown to work within 1 to 2 days of starting therapy
(D) Classified as nonbiological or biological
(E) Can preserve joint function

Answers and Explanations

1. **The answer is C** *[see III.C]*.
Inflammation is generally not present in osteoarthritis. It is a localized (not systemic) disorder that affects the cartilage and can eventually affect the underlying bone causing severe pain and disability.

2. **The answer is E** *[see III.E.3.a]*.
The ACR recommends acetaminophen (≤ 4 gm/day) as the first drug treatment option in patients with mild to moderate OA pain.

3. **The answer is D** *[see III.D.2]*.
No specific lab tests are diagnostic for OA.

4. **The answer is D** *[see IV.I.2.a & b]*.
Based on the ACR's 2008 RA Treatment Guidelines, both MTX and leflunomide are recommended for all patients with RA regardless of disease duration, disease burden, or prognostic factors.

5. **The answer is A** *[see IV.I.2.a]*.
MTX inhibits dihydrofolate reductase. Research has shown supplemental doses of folic acid (e.g., 1 mg/day) can reduce side effects.

6. **The answer is C** *[see III.E.3.c.(4)(b)]*.
To date, no drug treatment (including hyaluronic acid derivatives) has demonstrated

7. **The answer is E** *[see III.E.3]*.
Tramadol's maximum daily dose is 200 mg and should be given every 12 hrs if creatinine clearance is ≤ 30 mL/min.

8. **The answer is D** *[see Table 42-2]*.
Leflunomide is available for oral administration. The other agents must be given SC or IV.

9. **The answer is D** *[see Table 42-2]*.
The initial starting dose of MTX when treating RA is 7.5 mg PO weekly.

10. **The answer is C** *[see Table 42-2]*.
An ophthalmic exam is recommended when patients are receiving hydroxychloroquine.

11. **The answer is A** *[see Table 42-2]*.
Some biological DMARDs have been linked with reactivating latent TB; therefore, before starting therapy with leflunomide, etanercept, or infliximab, patients should have a PPD placed.

12. **The answer is B** *[see III.E.3.b.(4)]*.
Common side effects of NSAIDs include GI toxicity (e.g., bleeding), acute renal failure, and fluid retention (leading to hypertension).

13. **The answer is C** *[see IV.I.3; Table 42-2]*.
The main disadvantage to DMARD therapy is the time it takes for the medication to work. In general, nonbiological agents can take 3 to 4 months for affect; whereas biological agents can take 1 to 2 months (or more).

43 Hyperuricemia and Gout

LARRY N. SWANSON

I. INTRODUCTION

A. Definitions

1. **Hyperuricemia** refers to a serum uric acid level that is elevated more than two standard deviations above the population mean. In most laboratories, the upper limit of normal is 7 mg/dL (uricase method). However, the level varies with the laboratory method used; the upper limit of normal is about 1 mg/dL lower for women than for men.
2. **Gout** is a disease that is characterized by recurrent **painful acute attacks** of urate crystal-induced arthritis. It may include **tophi**—deposits of monosodium urate—in and around the joints and cartilage and in the kidneys, as well as uric acid nephrolithiasis.

B. General information

1. The prevalence of gout is believed to be between 3 and 5 million individuals in the United States.
2. Most gout victims are men (7 to 9 times more often than women); most women with the disease are postmenopausal.
3. The mean age at disease onset is 47 years.
4. The risk of developing gout increases as the serum uric acid level rises. Virtually all gout patients have a serum uric acid level > 7 mg/dL.
5. Research shows that among patients with a serum uric acid level above 9 mg/dL, the cumulative incidence of gout reached 22% after 5 years.
6. Gout has a familial tendency; 10% to 60% of cases occur in family members of patients with the disease.
7. Obesity, hypertension, hyperlipidemia, atherosclerosis, diabetes, and alcohol abuse are often associated with hyperuricemia and gout. Certain nutritional approaches (i.e., achieving ideal body weight or limitation of alcohol intake) can treat both the hyperuricemia and the associated conditions.

C. Uric acid production and excretion

1. Uric acid, an end product of **purine metabolism**, is produced from both dietary and endogenous sources. Its formation results from the conversion of adenine and guanine moieties of nucleoproteins and nucleotides (*Figure 43-1*).
2. **Xanthine oxidase** catalyzes the reaction that occurs as the final step in the degradation of purines to uric acid.
3. The body ultimately excretes uric acid via the kidneys (300–600 mg/day; two-thirds of total uric acid) and via the gastrointestinal (GI) tract (100–300 mg/day; one-third of the total uric acid).
4. Uric acid has no known biological function.
5. The body has a total uric acid content of 1.0 to 1.2 g; the daily turnover rate is 600 to 800 mg.
6. At a pH of 4.0 to 5.0 (i.e., in urine), uric acid exists as a poorly soluble free acid; at physiological pH, it exists primarily as **monosodium urate salt**.
7. Uric acid filtration, reabsorption, and secretion sites are shown in *Figure 43-2*.

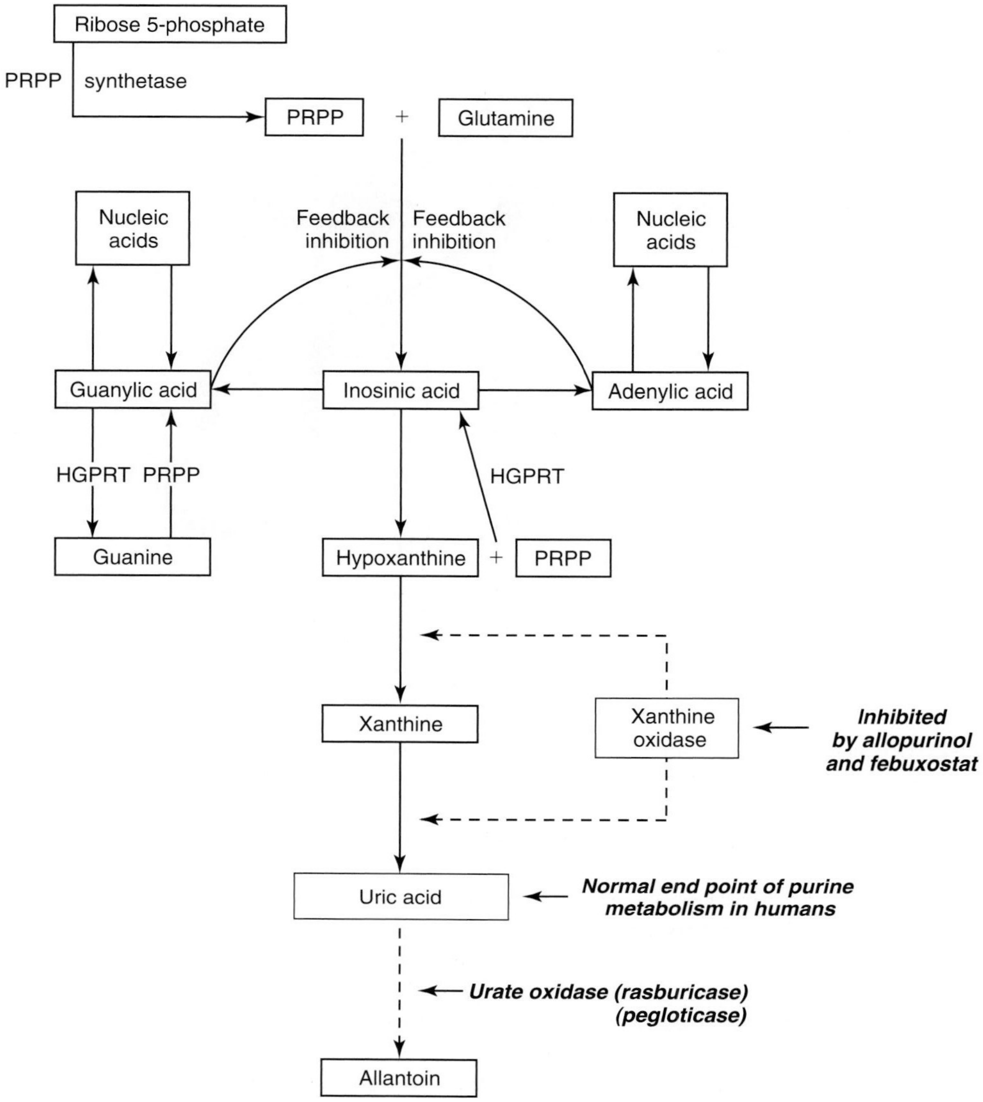

Figure 43-1. Uric acid formation. *HGPRT*, hypoxanthine–guanine phosphoribosyltransferase; *PRPP*, phosphoribosyl-1-pyrophosphate. (Adapted with permission from DiPiro J, Talbert R, Yee G, et al. *Pharmacotherapy—A Pathophysiologic Approach*. 8th ed. New York, NY: McGraw-Hill; 2011:1622.)

D. Cause. Hyperuricemia and gout may be primary or secondary.

1. **Primary hyperuricemia** and **gout** apparently result from an innate **defect in purine metabolism** or **uric acid excretion**. The exact cause of the defect usually is unknown.
   a. Hyperuricemia may result from **uric acid overproduction**, **impaired renal clearance of uric acid**, or a **combination** of these.
   b. Some patients with primary hyperuricemia and gout have a known enzymatic defect, such as hypoxanthine–guanine phosphoribosyltransferase (HGPRT) deficiency or phosphoribosyl-1-pyrophosphate (PRPP) synthetase excess (*Figure 43-1*).
   c. Principally for therapeutic purposes, patients with primary hyperuricemia and gout can be classified as **overproducers** or **underexcretors** of uric acid.
      (1) **Overproducers** (about 10% of patients) synthesize abnormally large amounts of uric acid and excrete excessive amounts: > 800 to 1000 mg daily on an unrestricted diet or > 600 mg daily on a purine-restricted diet. These individuals generally have a markedly increased miscible urate pool (> 2.5 g).

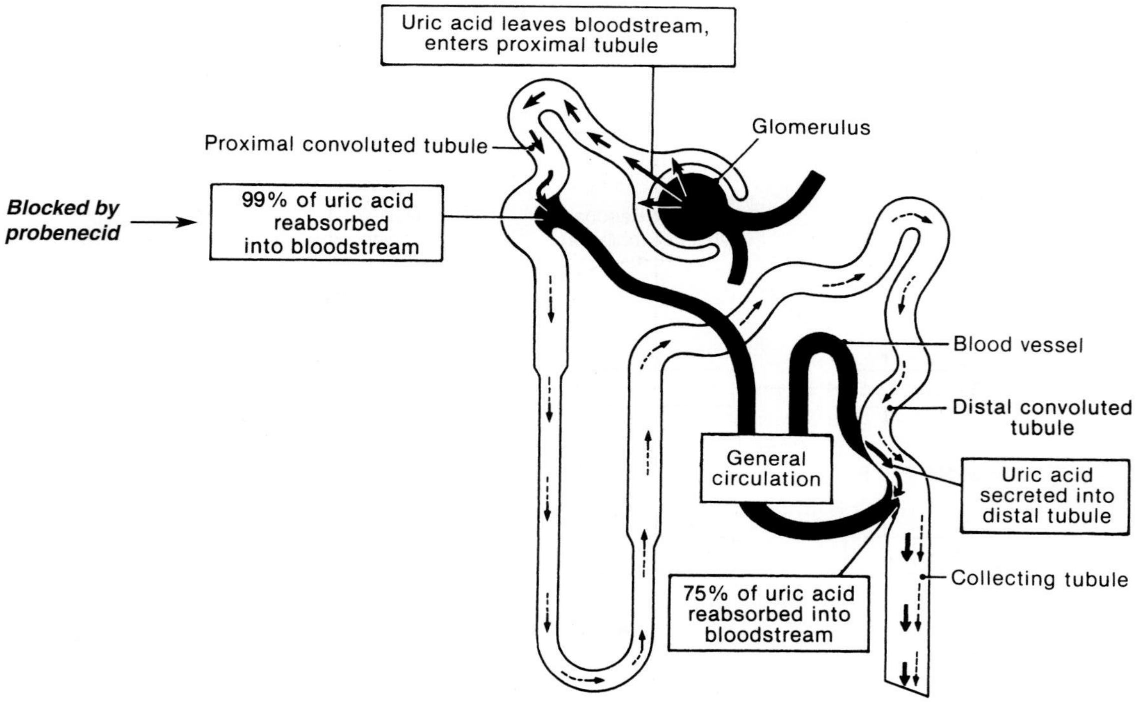

Figure 43-2. Uric acid filtration, reabsorption, and secretion sites. At the glomerulus, uric acid is filtered and enters the proximal tubule. There, approximately 99% of uric acid is reabsorbed into the bloodstream. At the distal tubule, uric acid is secreted; subsequently, about 75% of the amount secreted is reabsorbed. Therefore, almost all urinary uric acid is excreted at the distal tubule.

(2) **Underexcretors** (about 90% of patients) generally produce normal or nearly normal amounts of uric acid but excrete < 600 mg daily on a purine-restricted diet. They generally have only a slightly increased miscible urate pool. Some underexcretors are also overproducers.

2. **Secondary hyperuricemia** and **gout** develop during the course of another disease or as a result of drug therapy.
   a. **Hematological causes** of hyperuricemia and gout (associated with increased nucleic acid turnover and breakdown to uric acid)
      (1) Lymphoproliferative disorders
      (2) Myeloproliferative disorders
      (3) Certain hemolytic anemias and hemoglobinopathies
   b. **Chronic renal failure.** In this condition, reduced renal clearance of uric acid can lead to hyperuricemia.
   c. **Drug-induced disease**
      (1) **Aspirin** and **other salicylates** inhibit tubular secretion of uric acid when given in low doses (e.g., < 2 g/day of aspirin). At high doses, these agents frequently cause uricosuria.
      (2) **Cytotoxic drugs** increase uric acid concentrations by enhancing nucleic acid turnover and excretion.
      (3) **Diuretics** (except spironolactone) may cause hyperuricemia; most likely, this occurs either via volume depletion, which, in turn, increases proximal tubular reabsorption, or via impaired tubular secretion of uric acid.
      (4) **Ethambutol** and **nicotinic acid** increase uric acid concentrations by competing with urate for tubular secretion sites, thereby decreasing uric acid excretion.
      (5) **Cyclosporine** decreases renal urate clearance, as do **pyrazinamide** and **levodopa**.
      (6) **Ethanol** alters uric acid metabolism both by **increasing uric acid production** through an increase in adenine nucleotide catabolism and by **suppressing renal uric acid excretion** as a result of lactate inhibition of renal tubular uric acid secretion.

d. **Miscellaneous disorders.** Diabetic ketoacidosis, psoriasis, and chronic lead poisoning are examples of conditions that may cause hyperuricemia.

E. **Pathophysiology**

1. Gouty arthritis develops when **monosodium urate crystals** are deposited in the synovium of involved joints.
2. An **inflammatory response** to monosodium urate crystals leads to an attack of acute gouty arthritis; painful joint swelling is characterized by **redness, warmth, and tenderness**. A systemic reaction may accompany joint symptoms.
3. If gout progresses untreated, **tophi**, or **tophaceous deposits** (deposits of monosodium urate crystals) may be noted (**nodules on ears, fingers, elbow, etc., which usually are not painful**) and can eventually lead to joint deformity and disability; kidney involvement may lead to renal impairment. However, these developments are uncommon in the general gout population and represent late complications of hyperuricemia.
4. **Renal complications** of hyperuricemia and gout may have serious consequences.
   a. **Acute tubular obstruction**
      (1) This complication may develop secondary to uric acid precipitation in the collecting tubules and ureters, with subsequent blockage and renal failure. It is most common in patients with gout secondary to myeloproliferative or lymphoproliferative disorders, particularly after chemotherapy when allopurinol is omitted.
      (2) Another agent, **urate oxidase** (rasburicase), may be used in the prophylaxis and treatment of hyperuricemia in pediatric patients with leukemia, lymphoma, and solid-tumor malignancies who are receiving anticancer therapy. This agent works by converting uric acid into allantoin, which is five times more soluble in urine than uric acid.
   b. **Urolithiasis.** This condition is characterized by formation of uric acid stones in the urinary tract. Low urine pH seems to be a contributing factor. The risk of urolithiasis rises as serum and urinary uric acid levels increase. This condition is seen more often in patients who produce significant amount of urinary uric acid ($>$ 1100 mg/day).
   c. **Chronic urate nephropathy.** In this complication, urate deposits arise in the renal interstitium. It is generally agreed, however, that chronic hyperuricemia rarely, if ever, leads to clinically significant nephropathy. The presence of additional disease (e.g., diabetes mellitus, hypertension) may explain the finding of nephropathy in gout patients.

F. **Clinical presentation.** Clinical evaluation and the need for intervention depend on the clinical presentation.

1. **Asymptomatic hyperuricemia**
2. **Acute gouty arthritis**
3. **Intercritical gout**
4. **Chronic tophaceous gout**

II. ASYMPTOMATIC HYPERURICEMIA is characterized by an elevated serum uric acid level but has no signs or symptoms of urate deposition disease (arthritis, tophi, or urolithiasis).

A. **Clinical presentation.** Hyperuricemia in and of itself is not believed to be a disease. There also has to be evidence of deposition of urate in the joints, soft tissues, or kidney to routinely warrant drug therapy intervention. Certainly, the risk of symptom development and complications increases as the serum uric acid level rises. However, as many as two-thirds of patients with elevated serum uric acid levels will continue to remain symptom-free. It is difficult to predict which patients who have asymptomatic hyperuricemia will eventually develop hyperuricemia-related issues. Although hyperuricemia often occurs concurrently in patients with cardiovascular disease, diabetes, and hypertension, it has not been proven to be a causal factor for any of these conditions. Serum urate levels of up to 13 mg/dL in men and 10 mg/L in women have not been shown to cause deterioration in renal function.

B. **Therapy.** Therefore, urate lowering **drug treatment for most patients is not required**, **General interventions** such as encouraging maintenance of good urine output (to prevent uric acid stone formation), avoidance of high purine meats and fish, and regular medical exams to get serum urate levels and to check for clinical evidence of gout related signs.

III. ACUTE GOUTY ARTHRITIS.

This clinical presentation of gout is characterized by **painful arthritic attacks** of sudden onset.

A. **Pathogenesis.** Monosodium urate crystals form in articular tissues; this process sets off an inflammatory reaction. **Trauma, exposure to cold, dietary overindulgence, or another triggering event** may be involved in the development of the acute attack.

B. **Signs and symptoms**

1. The **initial attack** is abrupt, usually **occurring at night** or in the early morning as synovial fluid is reabsorbed. This severe arthritic pain progressively worsens and generally involves only one or a few joints.
    a. The **affected joints** typically become hot, swollen, and extremely tender. Seventeenth-century British physician Thomas Sydenham described his personal experience with gout this way: "Now it is a violent stretching and tearing of the ligaments—now, it is a gnawing pain and now a pressure and tightening. So exquisite and lively . . . is the feeling of the part affected, that it cannot bear the weight of bedclothes nor the jar of a person walking in the room."
    b. The **most common site** of the initial attack is the **first metatarsophalangeal joint**; an attack there is known as **podagra**. Other sites that may be affected include the instep, ankle, heel, knee, wrist, elbow, and fingers.
2. The first few untreated attacks typically last 3 to 14 days. The **joint pain and inflammation completely resolves**, even when not treated and is a hallmark of the condition. Later attacks may affect more joints and take several weeks to resolve.
3. During recovery, as edema subsides, local desquamation and pruritus may occur.
4. **Systemic symptoms** during an acute attack may include fever, chills, and malaise.

C. **Diagnostic criteria**

1. **Definitive diagnosis** of gouty arthritis can be made by demonstration of **monosodium urate crystals** in the synovial fluid of affected joints. These needle-shaped crystals are termed **negatively birefringent** when viewed through a polarized light microscope.
2. **Serum analysis** usually reveals an above-normal uric acid level: however, this finding is not specific for acute gout. Other common serum findings include **leukocytosis** and a moderately **elevated erythrocyte sedimentation rate**.
3. A **dramatic therapeutic response to colchicine** may be helpful in establishing the diagnosis, but this is not absolute because other causes of acute arthritis may respond as well.
4. When fluid cannot be aspirated from the affected joint, a **diagnosis of gout is supported by**:
    a. A prior **history of acute monoarticular arthritis** (especially of the **big toe**) followed by a **symptom-free period**
    b. The presence of **hyperuricemia**
    c. Rapid **resolution of symptoms after colchicine** therapy
5. **Other conditions** that may **mimic** gout include pseudogout (calcium pyrophosphate dihydrate crystal disease) or septic arthritis.

D. **Treatment goals**

1. To relieve pain and inflammation
2. To terminate the acute attack
3. To restore normal function to the affected joints

E. **Therapy**

1. **General therapeutic principles**
    a. The affected joint (or joints) should be immobilized.
    b. **Anti-inflammatory drug therapy** should begin **immediately**. For maximal therapeutic effectiveness, these drugs should be kept on hand so that the patient may begin therapy as soon as a subsequent attack begins.
    c. **Urate-lowering drugs should <u>not</u> be given until the acute attack is controlled**, as these drugs **may prolong the attack** by causing a change in uric acid equilibrium. Urate-lowering agents can begin within 1 to 2 weeks after the resolution of the attack.
2. **Specific drugs.** Any of the following agents may be used:
    a. **Nonsteroidal anti-inflammatory drugs (NSAIDs)**
        (1) **Indications.** Most physicians consider these drugs the agents of choice, especially the newer NSAIDs. These drugs may be preferred when treatment is delayed significantly after

symptom onset or when the patient cannot tolerate the adverse GI effects of colchicine. Begin with high doses for 2 to 3 days, then taper the dose rapidly over the next several days.

(a) **Indomethacin** (Indocin) is usually given in a dose of **50 mg three times daily** initially then the dose is tapered. Significant pain relief is achieved within a few hours. Tenderness and warmth usually decreases over the next day and a half with swelling disappearing within a few days.

(b) **Specific NSAIDs**—such as **naproxen** (Naprosyn) 750 mg followed by 250 mg every 8 hrs until the attack subsides or **sulindac** (Clinoril) 200 mg twice a day to start, reducing the dose with satisfactory response (7 days of therapy are usually adequate)—are specifically approved for this indication, but many other NSAIDs have been used successfully. There is no evidence that any particular NSAID is more effective than others in the treatment of an acute gouty attack. Some have also used selective cyclooxygenase 2 (COX-2) inhibitors for these attacks.

(2) **Precautions and monitoring effects**

(a) **Adverse effects of indomethacin** are usually dose related. These effects occur in 10% to 60% of patients and may require that the drug be stopped. They primarily include GI complaints of nausea and abdominal discomfort and central nervous system (CNS) effects of headaches and dizziness. Because of these CNS effects, it should be avoided in the elderly. Indomethacin should be taken with food or milk to minimize gastric mucosal irritation.

(b) **Precautions.** NSAIDs, in general, require cautious use in patients with a history of hypertension, congestive heart failure (CHF), peptic ulcer disease, or mild to moderate renal failure.

b. Colchicine. The traditional drug for relieving pain and inflammation and ending the acute attack, colchicine is most effective when started within 24 hrs after symptoms begin (the period of maximal leukocyte migration). Some would use this agent only if the patient is intolerant to NSAIDs or for those patients who have used colchicine successfully in the past. Colchicine has been available on the market for many years as non-FDA approved medication. The "standard" dosage regimen had not been carefully studied for effectiveness and safety. In August 2009, Colcrys (brand of colchicine) was approved for the treatment of gout in a new, lower dosage regimen.

(1) **Mechanism of action.** Colchicine apparently **impairs leukocyte migration** to inflamed areas and disrupts urate deposition and the subsequent inflammatory response. **It has no effect on serum urate levels**.

(2) **Dosage and administration**

(a) **Oral regimen**

(i) The **new dosing regimen** approved for Colcrys is as follows: **1.2 mg at the first sign of an acute attack; then give 0.6 mg 1 hr later (maximum of 1.8 mg within 1 hr)**. In the AGREE trial, this dose (1.8 mg total) had similar efficacy to high dose (4.8 mg total), but with less gastrointestinal adverse events (23% vs. 77%).

(ii) Previous older dosing regimens were as follows: 0.6 mg to 1.2 mg initially, followed by 0.6 mg every 1 to 2 hrs until pain relief occurred or abdominal discomfort or diarrhea developed or a total dose of 6 mg had been administered. The effective dose of colchicine in patients with acute gout was considered to be very close to which caused adverse GI symptoms.

(b) **Intravenous (IV) regimen.** In February 2008, the FDA asked that IV preparations of this agent should no longer be manufactured or shipped in the United States because of significant toxicity and fatalities.

(3) **Precautions and monitoring effects**

(a) **GI distress** (e.g., nausea, vomiting, abdominal cramps, diarrhea) has occurred in 50% to 80% of patients receiving oral colchicine in a dose-dependent manner. With the new dosage regimen, these side effects should be lower. Oral colchicine should be avoided in patients with peptic ulcer disease and other GI disorders.

(b) In the process that led to the approval of the marketing of Colcrys, fatal colchicine toxicity was noted in patients on standard therapeutic doses of colchicine taken with certain other drugs such as **clarithromycin. Important drug interactions** can occur in patients taking colchicine with **P-glycoprotein** (P-gp) (amiodarone, cyclosporine, tacrolimus, quinidine, erythromycin) and **cytochrome P450** (**CYP3A4**) inhibitors (azole antifungals, macrolide antibiotics, protease inhibitors).

(c) **Chronic colchicine therapy** (see IV.C.2) may result in **neuromyopathy** (patient notes numbness, paresthesias, and/or weakness), which is more likely in patients with decreased kidney function. It is best to limit colchicine therapy to 6 months duration (after goal serum uric acid is achieved.)

c. **Corticosteroids**

(1) **Corticosteroid intra-articular injections** are particularly effective in patients with acute single-joint gout. The actual act of **aspiration of the joint fluid alone can sometimes greatly reduce the extent of the pain of gout**. Specific doses of these agents corticosteroids is related to joint size. An intra-articular dose of **triamcinolone** 8 mg in smaller joints (10 mg in the knee), **methylprednisolone acetate** (5 to 25 mg per joint), or **betamethasone** 3 to 6 mg can be used.

(2) **Systemic corticosteroid therapy** is another option, especially when either NSAIDs or colchicine cannot be given or have not been effective. As an example, **oral prednisone** (20 to 60 mg/day initially, with the dose tapered during a period of 5 to 7 days) can be useful without producing a rebound effect. **IM betamethasone** (7 mg) or **IV methylprednisolone** 125 mg are examples of other potential agents. **IM ACTH** 40 units (reduces inflammation by stimulating corticosteroid production by the patient's adrenal gland plus it activates melanocortin type 3 receptors) may also be used. This agent may not be preferred because of the short duration of action.

IV. INTERCRITICAL GOUT

is the symptom-free period after the first attack. This phase may be interrupted by the recurrence of acute attacks.

A. **Onset of subsequent attacks varies.** In most untreated patients, the second attack occurs within 2 years of the first, but in some it may be delayed for 5 to 10 years. A small percentage of patients never experience a second attack. If hyperuricemia is insufficiently treated, subsequent attacks may become progressively longer and more severe and may involve more than one joint.

B. **Treatment goals**

1. To reduce the frequency and severity of recurrent attacks
2. To minimize urate deposition in body tissues, thereby preventing progression to chronic tophaceous gout.

C. **Therapy**

1. **Nondrug urate-reducing measures.** The following reversible factors can raise the serum uric acid level and should be addressed: avoid selected **high-purine content foods** (e.g., **primarily meats [including organ-rich foods like liver, sweetbreads, etc.] and seafood**), treat obesity, avoid alcohol consumption, or alter drug therapy that may increase the serum uric acid (i.e., change from a thiazide diuretic to a drug like Losartan). [See IV.C.3.b.(5)]. The purine content of the diet does not usually contribute more than 1.0 mg/dL to the serum urate concentration. Weight reduction sometimes reduces the serum uric acid level slightly; however, crash diets should be avoided. Drinking two or more beers increased the risk of gout by 2.5-fold in one study versus a 1.6-fold increase for other alcohol spirits. Wine intake was *not* associated with an increased risk of gout. High purine content vegetables don't appear to increase the risk of gouty attacks. Increasing low fat dairy products in the diet, however, may lower serum urate.

2. **Prophylaxis** against a future gout flare after resolution of an acute gouty attack may consist of **low-dose colchicine**, 0.6 mg once or twice daily in the patient with normal renal function.

a. **Adverse effects** from colchicine at these doses are usually uncommon. In patients, particularly the elderly, who develop loose or diarrheal stools, 0.6 mg every other day might work.

b. **Low-dose NSAIDs** may also be used alternatively (naproxen 250 mg twice daily or indomethacin 25 mg twice daily).

c. Generally, begin prophylactic drug treatment 2 to 3 weeks before urate lowering drug therapy is begun and administer until the desired serum uric acid level is achieved. Prolonged use of these agents may prevent recurrent episodes of gouty arthritis, but they do not prevent the development of silent bony erosions and tophi deposits.

d. If the patient develops signs and symptoms of an impending gouty arthritis attack, he can increase the dose to 1.2 mg followed by an additional dose of 0.6 mg 1 hr later.

3. Urate-reducing drug therapy. The goal for gouty attack prevention is to reduce the serum urate concentrations to values < 6.0 mg/dL. A reduction to < 5.0 mg/dL may be required for the resorption of tophi. **The decision to begin drug therapy should be carefully considered, as urate-lowering drug treatment should be lifelong**. Urate-reducing drugs include the xanthine oxidase inhibitors, **allopurinol** (Zyloprim) and **febuxostat** (Uloric), which reduce uric acid production and the **uricosuric** agent **probenecid** (Benemid), which increases renal uric acid excretion. Uric acid lowering therapy **should *not* be initiated during an acute gout attack as this action may prolong the attack** by changing the equilibrium of body urate. During the first 6 to 12 months of therapy, these drugs may increase the frequency, severity, and duration of acute attacks. Therefore, some clinicians administer prophylactic colchicine concomitantly during the early months of uricosuric therapy (see IV.C.2.).

a. Indications for therapy with a drug that lowers serum urate concentrations should be considered when **all** of the following criteria are met:

(1) The cause of the hyperuricemia cannot be corrected or, if corrected, does not lower the serum urate concentration to < 7.0 mg/dL.

(2) The patient has had two or three definite attacks of gout or has tophi.

(3) The patient is convinced of the need to take medication regularly and permanently.

b. Specific agents

(1) Allopurinol (Zyloprim)

(a) Mechanism of action. Allopurinol and its long-acting metabolite, **oxypurinol**, **block the final steps in uric acid synthesis by inhibiting xanthine oxidase, an enzyme that converts xanthine to uric acid** (*Figure 43-1*). Thus, the drug reduces the serum uric acid level although increasing the renal excretion of the more soluble oxypurine precursors; this decreases the risk of uric acid stones and nephropathy.

(b) Indications. Allopurinol is considered by many to be **the drug of choice for lowering uric acid levels** because of its effectiveness in both underexcretors and overproducers, but it is specifically the preferred urate-reducing agent for patients in the following categories:

(i) Patients who are clearly overproducers (overexcretors) of uric acid

(ii) Patients with recurrent tophaceous deposits or uric acid stones

(iii) Patients with renal impairment (but dose needs to be decreased)

(c) Dosage and administration. It is recommended by the experts that allopurinol be given initially in a daily dose of 100 mg, then increased by 100 mg/day once every 1 to 4 weeks, if needed. Typically, the uric acid level starts to fall after 2 days with maximal effect for a given dose in about 1 to 2 weeks. **300 mg once daily is the most commonly prescribed dose, but this may be an inadequate dose**. A dose of **up to 800 mg/day** (in two to three divided doses) may be needed to achieve the desired 6 mg/dL serum uric acid level. The drug should be given daily without interruption. The dose should be decreased in patients with impaired renal function: 200 mg/day maximum for the patient with a creatinine clearance (CrCl) of 10−20 mL/min, to 100 mg/day for a patient with a CrCl of less than 10 mL/min, and the dosage interval lengthened if less than 3 mL/min.

(d) Precautions and monitoring effects. Allopurinol is generally well tolerated.

(i) Side effects occurring in 3% to 5% of patients include rash, diarrhea, drug fever, leukopenia or thrombocytopenia. About 2% of patients will develop a **rash**; **some** are **mild** and can be treated by stopping the agent, **others** are more **severe** (**Steven Johnsons or toxic epidermal necrolysis** [**TEN**]). Approximately 20% of patients given both allopurinol and ampicillin together develop a rash.

(ii) The most serious side effect of allopurinol, which occurs in about 0.1% of patients, is the **allopurinol hypersensitivity syndrome** (**AHS**) with exfoliative dermatitis, often with vasculitis, fever, liver dysfunction, eosinophilia, and acute interstitial nephritis. It is **more likely to occur** in patients with **renal disease** who receive "regular" doses along with **diuretic therapy** and may be fatal (~25% of patients).

- **(iii)** Allopurinol may induce more frequent acute gout attacks. This risk can be minimized by administration of low doses and concurrent colchicine therapy.
- **(iv)** Allopurinol can result in enhanced effects of azathioprine and 6-mercaptopurine when taken together.

(2) Febuxostat (Uloric) is a selective **xanthine oxidase inhibitor** and is the first new drug to be approved (2009) for gout in over 40 years.

- **(a)** Unlike allopurinol, it is a thiazolecarboxylic acid derivative and not a purine-like core structure. Thus, it does not share the same severe hypersensitivity reactions with allopurinol.
- **(b)** The usual dose is **40 mg/day** (**comparable efficacy to 300 mg allopurinol**). The dose can be increased to 80 mg/day after 2 weeks if the serum uric acid remains above 6 mg/dL.
- **(c)** No dosage adjustments are needed in patients with mild or moderate renal/hepatic impairment.
- **(d)** It is **much more expensive than allopurinol** and generally should be considered an alternative therapy to allopurinol (allopurinol treatment failure, hypersensitivity or other major side effects).
- **(e)** This agent can increase liver function tests. Baseline liver function tests (LFTs) should be taken upon initiation of therapy and repeated at 2 and 4 months.
- **(f)** A slightly higher incidence of thromboembolic events has been reported with febuxostat compared with allopurinol. Patients should be monitored for signs and symptoms of myocardial infarction or stroke.

(3) Probenecid (Benemid) is now the only available **uricosuric drug** on the U.S. market. This drug is preferred for underexcretors.

- **(a) Mechanism of action.** Probenecid **blocks uric acid reabsorption at the proximal convoluted tubule**, thereby increasing the rate of uric acid excretion (*Figure 43-2*).
- **(b) Indications.** Uricosurics generally are used to reduce hyperuricemia in patients who excrete < 600 mg of uric acid per day.
- **(c) Dosage and administration**
  - **(i) Probenecid** is given initially in two daily oral doses of 250 mg for 1 week, then increased to 500 mg twice daily every 1 to 2 weeks until the serum uric acid level drops below 6 mg/dL. Most patients respond to a dose of 1.5 g/day or less (maximum of 3 g/day).
- **(d) Precautions and monitoring effects**
  - **(i)** Patients should maintain a **high fluid intake** (at least 2 L/day) and a high urine output during uricosuric therapy to decrease renal urate precipitation. This action will minimize the formation of **uric acid crystals** in the urine and deposition of **uric acid** in the **renal tubules**, **pelvis**, or **ureter**, which may cause a reduction in renal function. Alkalinization of the urine is usually not necessary (but can be achieved with 1 g of sodium bicarbonate taken three to four times daily; plus a high fluid intake of at least 2 L/day).
  - **(ii)** Uricosurics are **contraindicated** in patients with urinary tract stones.
  - **(iii)** These drugs generally are ineffective in patients with creatinine clearances below 50 to 60 mL/min.
  - **(iv) Aspirin** and **other salicylates** antagonize the action of uricosurics. **Daily low dose aspirin** for antiplatelet function **probably does not have this effect to any extent.**
  - **(v) Probenecid** is well tolerated by most patients, but it occasionally causes **adverse effects**—for example, GI distress (8%) and hypersensitivity reactions (5%).

(4) Pegloticase (Krystexxa) was also approved in 2009 and is a form of **uricase** (urate oxidase), which catalyzes the oxidation of uric acid to **allantoin**, which is water soluble and easily excreted.

- **(a)** It is **indicated for** the relatively small number of gout patients (~50,000 Americans) who cannot be treated with other urate lowering drugs (**refractory patients**).

(b) It **needs to be given by IV infusion** every 2 to 4 weeks.
(c) Patients need to be closely monitored for anaphylaxis and infusion reactions. Pretreatment with antihistamines and corticosteroids is needed.
(d) A large percentage of patients develop pegloticase antibodies, which results in decreased effectiveness.
(e) Prophylaxis with colchicine or nonsteroidal agents is also appropriate.
(f) It is **much more expensive than other urate lowering drug therapies**.

(5) **Other drugs that increase uric acid excretion**
(a) **Losartan** (Cozaar), an angiotensin II receptor blocker (ARB), might be a useful antihypertensive agent in the patient who has **both hyperuricemia and hypertension** because this agent can lower serum uric acid levels by inhibiting the uptake of uric acid by the urate anion exchange transporter in the proximal tubule. This effect is minimal or not seen in other ARBs.
(b) **Fenofibrate** (TriCor) is a fibric acid agent used to treat elevated cholesterol and triglyceride levels. It has been shown to decrease serum uric levels by increasing renal uric acid clearance and would be a useful agent in the patient with **both hyperlipidemia and hyperuricemia**.
(c) **Vitamin C** may lower the serum uric acid level. One study noted a 0.5 mg/dL decrease when 500 mg was given daily.

V. CHRONIC TOPHACEOUS GOUT.

This **rare** clinical presentation may develop if hyperuricemia and gout remain untreated for many years.

A. **Pathogenesis.** Persistent hyperuricemia leads to the development of tophi in the synovia, olecranon bursae, and various periarticular locations. Eventually, articular cartilage may be destroyed, resulting in joint deformities, bone erosions, deposition of tophi within tissues, and renal disease.

B. **Clinical evaluation**
1. Patients may develop large subcutaneous tophi in the pinna of the external ear (the classic site) as well as in other locations.
2. Typically, the urate pool is many times the normal size.

C. **Therapy.** Allopurinol and probenecid may be given in combination to treat severe cases.

Study Questions

Directions for questions 1–3: Each of the questions, statements, or incomplete statements in this section can be correctly answered or completed by **one** of the suggested answers or phrases. Choose the **best** answer.

1. All of the following statements concerning an acute gouty arthritis attack are correct *except* which one?
   (A) The diagnosis of gout is ensured by a good therapeutic response to colchicine because no other form of arthritis responds to this drug.
   (B) To be ensured of the diagnosis, monosodium urate crystals must be identified in the synovial fluid of the affected joint.
   (C) Attacks frequently occur in the middle of the night.
   (D) An untreated attack may last up to 2 weeks.
   (E) The first attack usually involves only one joint, most frequently the big toe (first metatarsophalangeal joint).

2. A 42-year-old obese man has been diagnosed with gout. He has had three acute attacks this year, and his uric acid level is presently 11.5 mg/dL (upper limit of normal is 7.0 mg/dL). He has no other diseases. Rational treatment of this patient during the interval period between gouty attacks might include any of the following *except*
   (A) acetaminophen or aspirin 650 mg as needed for joint pain.
   (B) probenecid.
   (C) colchicine.
   (D) allopurinol.
   (E) a decrease in caloric intake.

3. A 45-year-old man is admitted to the hospital with the diagnosis of an acute attack of gout. His serum uric acid is 10.5 mg/dL (normal is 3 to 7 mg/dL). Which of the following would be the most effective initial treatment plan?
   - **(A)** Before treating this patient, immobilize the affected joint and obtain a 24-hr urinary uric acid level to determine which drug, either allopurinol or probenecid, would be the best agent to initiate therapy.
   - **(B)** Begin oral colchicine 1.2 mg initially, followed by 0.6 mg every 2 hrs until relief is obtained, gastrointestinal distress occurs, or a maximum of 8 mg has been taken; also, begin probenecid 250 mg twice a day concurrently.
   - **(C)** Administer oral indomethacin 50 mg three times a day for 2 days; then gradually taper the dose over the next few days.
   - **(D)** Administer oral naproxen 750 mg, followed by 250 mg every 8 hrs for 3 weeks.
   - **(E)** Give colchicine 0.5 mg intramuscularly followed by 1.0 mg intravenous piggyback every 12 hrs for 2 weeks.

Directions for question 4: The question in this section can be correctly answered or completed by **one or more** of the suggested answers. Choose the answer, **A–E**.

- **(A)** if **I only** is correct
- **(B)** if **III only** is correct
- **(C)** if **I and II** are correct
- **(D)** if **II and III** are correct
- **(E)** if **I, II, and III** are correct

4. Allopurinol is recommended instead of probenecid in the treatment of hyperuricemia in which of the following situations?
   - **(I)** When the patient has several large tophi on the elbows and knees
   - **(II)** When the patient has an estimated creatinine clearance of 15 mL/min
   - **(III)** When the patient has leukemia and there is concern regarding renal precipitation of urate

Directions for question 5: The incomplete statement in this section can be correctly answered or completed by **one** of the suggested answers or phrases. Choose the **best** answer.

5. In a patient who has had documented gouty arthritis and hyperuricemia and who also has hypertension, a preferred antihypertensive agent would be
   - **(A)** hydrochlorothiazide
   - **(B)** losartan
   - **(C)** clonidine
   - **(D)** lisinopril
   - **(E)** irbesartan

6. Which of the following ***best describes*** a current important point about the use of allopurinol in the treatment of intercritical gout?
   - **(A)** It is best dosed in a "2 months on and 2 months off" pattern
   - **(B)** It needs to be dosed twice daily because of its short half-life.
   - **(C)** It is the only currently available FDA-approved xanthine oxidase inhibitor on the market.
   - **(D)** It should be used in reduced doses if the patient has significant renal impairment.
   - **(E)** It can only be used in patients who are overproducers of uric acid.

Answers and Explanations

1. **The answer is A** *[see III.B.1–2; III.C.1; III.C.3]*.
   Other forms of acute arthritis may respond to colchicine, so that the diagnosis of gout cannot be established unequivocally by a good response to this agent. A definitive diagnosis requires the presence of urate crystals in the affected joint, although the presence of other symptoms or laboratory findings may suggest a probable diagnosis of gout.

2. **The answer is A** *[see I.D.2.c.(1); IV.C]*.
   Aspirin in doses < 2 g/day can inhibit uric acid secretion. Weight reduction, allopurinol or probenecid to lower the serum uric acid levels, and prophylactic colchicine are all appropriate interventions in the interval phase to reduce the incidence of acute gouty attacks.

3. **The answer is C** *[see III.E.1.c; III.E.2.a; III.E.2.b; IV.C]*.
   Of the selections, the most effective initial plan in treating an acute attack of gout is to administer indomethacin orally, giving 50 mg three times a day for 2 to 3 days, then gradually tapering the dosage over the next few days. Although joint immobilization is an appropriate initial step, drugs for pain relief should be administered as soon as possible. Uric acid modification therapy (allopurinol or probenecid) should not be initiated until the acute attack is under control. Initiating therapy with probenecid at this point may prolong the resolution of an acute attack of gouty arthritis, which can usually be accomplished within 7 days of NSAID therapy. Colchicine should never be given intramuscularly because it causes tissue irritation. The IV form of this drug has been removed from the market.

4. **The answer is E (I, II, III)** *[see IV.C]*.
In the treatment of hyperuricemia, allopurinol is indicated rather than probenecid when large tophi are present, when the creatinine clearance is < 50 to 60 mL/min (probenecid would be ineffective, but the allopurinol dosage would have to be decreased), when the patient is an overproducer of uric acid, and when there is a need to prevent the formation of large amounts of uric acid (e.g., when conditions such as leukemia are present).

5. **The answer is B** *[see IV.C.3.b.(5).(a)]*.
Losartan, an angiotensin II receptor blocker has been shown to increase urinary uric acid secretion and can, therefore, lower serum uric acid levels. Hydrochlorothiazide actually decreases urinary uric acid excretion and must be used cautiously in gout patients, if at all. The other antihypertensive agents mentioned have minimal or no effects on the serum uric acid.

6. **The answer is D** *[IV.C.3.b.(1)]*.
Allopurinol must be given daily without interruption, its principal metabolite (oxypurinol) has a long half-life so once a day dosing is appropriate, febuxostat is another xanthine oxidase inhibitor on the market, it can be used for both overproducers and hypoexcreters of uric acid. D. is correct because doses do need to be reduced if the patient has renal impairment.

44 Peptic Ulcer Disease and Related Acid-Associated Disorders

PAUL F. SOUNEY, ANTHONY E. ZIMMERMANN

I. INTRODUCTION

A. **Definition**

1. **Peptic ulcer disease** (PUD) refers to a group of disorders characterized by circumscribed lesions of the mucosa of the upper gastrointestinal (GI) tract (particularly the stomach and duodenum). The lesions occur in regions exposed to gastric juices.
2. **Gastroesophageal reflux disease (GERD)** refers to the retrograde movement of gastric contents from the stomach into the esophagus. Reflux may occur without consequences, and thus be considered a normal physiological process, or it may lead to profound symptomatic or histological conditions (e.g., GERD). When reflux leads to inflammation (with or without erosions or ulcerations) of the esophagus, it is called **reflux (erosive) esophagitis**. Most patients (50% to 70%) report typical symptoms but lack evidence of esophageal mucosal injury **(nonerosive reflux disease; NERD)**.
3. **Dyspepsia** is defined as persistent or recurrent abdominal pain or abdominal discomfort centered in the upper abdomen.

B. **Manifestations**

1. **Duodenal ulcers** almost always develop in the duodenal bulb (the first few centimeters of the duodenum). A few, however, arise between the bulb and the ampulla.
2. **Gastric ulcers** form most commonly in the antrum or at the antral–fundal junction.
3. **Less common forms of peptic ulcer disease**
   a. **Stress ulcers** result from serious trauma or illness, major burns, coagulopathy not related to anticoagulant therapy, need for mechanical ventilation > 48 hrs, or ongoing sepsis. The **most common site** of stress ulcer formation is the proximal portion of the stomach.
   b. **Zollinger–Ellison syndrome** is a severe form of peptic ulcer disease in which intractable ulcers are accompanied by extreme gastric hyperacidity and at least one gastrinoma (a non–β-islet cell tumor of the pancreas or another site).
   c. **Stomal ulcers** (also called marginal ulcers) may arise at the anastomosis or immediately distal to it in the small intestine in patients who have undergone ulcer surgery and have experienced subsequent ulcer recurrence after a symptom-free period.
   d. **Drug-associated ulcers** occur in patients who chronically ingest substances that damage the gastric mucosa, such as nonsteroidal anti-inflammatory drugs (NSAIDs).
4. **Reflux esophagitis** is most often recognized by the presence of recurrent symptoms (e.g., heartburn) or altered epithelial morphology visualized radiologically, endoscopically, or histologically.
   a. Heartburn is substernal burning or regurgitation that may radiate to the neck. Other symptoms include belching, water brash, chest pain, asthma, chronic cough, hoarseness, and laryngitis.
   b. Endoscopic evaluation detected **Barrett esophagus (BE)** in 6% of patients with frequent heartburn. Barrett's esophagus is a premalignant condition that may lead to adenocarcinoma of the esophagus or esophagogastric junction.

C. **Epidemiology**
  1. **Incidence.** Peptic ulcer disease is the most common disorder of the upper GI tract.
    a. **Duodenal ulcers** affect 4% to 10% of the United States population; **gastric ulcers** occur in 0.03% to 0.05% of the population.
    b. Nearly 80% of peptic ulcers are duodenal; the others are gastric ulcers.
    c. Most duodenal ulcers appear in people between age 20 and 50; onset of gastric ulcers usually occurs between age 45 and 55.
    d. The 1-year point prevalence of active gastric or duodenal ulcer in the United States in men and women is about 1.8%; the lifetime prevalence of peptic ulcer ranges from 11% to 14% for men and 8% to 11% for women.
    e. Approximately 10% to 20% of gastric ulcer patients also have a concurrent duodenal ulcer.
    f. In the United States, 44% of the adult population experience **heartburn** at least once a month; 14% take some type of "indigestion" medication at least twice a week. Of patients with GERD symptoms who have undergone endoscopy, 50% to 65% have apparent esophagitis.
    g. The annual prevalence of dyspepsia in Western countries is approximately 25%; 2% to 5% of primary care consultations are for dyspepsia.
  2. **Hospitalization**
    a. Hospitalization rates in the United States for peptic ulcers have been declining; these rates dropped from 25.2 per 10,000 in 1965 to 16.5 per 10,000 in 1981. This reflects a decrease in hospitalization for uncomplicated cases owing to increased outpatient diagnosis and treatment. There has been little change in hospitalization rates since then.
    b. There has been little or no decrease in duodenal ulcer perforations and only a slight decrease in hemorrhages.
  3. **Mortality**
    a. The mortality rate for gastric ulcers declined between 1962 and 1979 from 3.5 per 100,000 to 1.1 per 100,000.
    b. For duodenal ulcer, the mortality rate declined from 3.1 per 100,000 to 0.9 per 100,000.
    c. Although death from GERD is uncommon, morbidity is not, because of the prevalence of the well-recognized complications such as esophageal ulceration (5%), stricture formation (4% to 20%), and the development of Barrett columnar-lined esophagus (8% to 20%).

D. **Description**
  1. **Ulcer size.** The average duodenal ulcer typically has a diameter < 1 cm; most gastric ulcers are somewhat larger (1.0 to 2.5 cm in diameter).
  2. Most ulcers are sharply demarcated and have a round, oval, or elliptical shape.
  3. The mucosa surrounding the ulcer typically is inflamed and edematous.
  4. Ulcers penetrate the **muscularis propria** and, in some cases, extend into the serosa or even into the pancreas.
  5. Fibrous tissue, granulation tissue, and necrotic debris form the ulcer base. During ulcer healing, a scar forms as epithelium from the edges covers the ulcer surface.
  6. Nearly all duodenal ulcers are benign; up to 10% of gastric ulcers are malignant.

E. **Cause.** The two major observations regarding PUD are the causal relationship among NSAID intake; gastroduodenal mucosal injury; the pathogenesis of gastric ulcer and, to a lesser extent, duodenal ulcer; and the association of ***Helicobacter pylori*** infection in the pathogenesis of duodenal ulcer (and to a lesser extent, gastric ulcer).
  1. ***H. pylori*** (formerly *Campylobacter pylori*) is a gram-negative microaerophilic, spiral bacterium with multiple flagella that lives and infects the gastric mucosa. This bacterium is able to survive in the acidic gastric environment by its ability to produce urease, which hydrolyzes urea into ammonia. Ammonia neutralizes gastric hydrochloric acid (HCl), creating a neutral cloud surrounding the organism.
    a. In the United States, the **prevalence** of *H. pylori* increases with age from approximately 10% at 20 years of age to approximately 50% at 60 years of age; approximately 17% of *H. pylori*–positive individuals will develop a duodenal ulcer. Prevalence is higher in developing countries.
    b. *H. pylori* is associated with several common GI disorders.
      (1) Always present in the setting of active chronic gastritis.
      (2) Present in the vast majority of duodenal ($> 90\%$) and gastric (60% to 90%) ulcers. Recent studies indicate a decline in the prevalence of *H. pylori* in duodenal ulcer patients.

(3) Sometimes present with nonulcer dyspepsia (probably in 50% of cases); eradication of *H. pylori*, when present, leads to symptom improvement in only about one-half of treated patients.

(4) In gastric cancer, 85% to 95% (Although the association is strong, no causal relationship has yet been proven in gastric cancer. The World Health Organization has classified *H. pylori* as a group 1 carcinogen.)

c. *H. pylori* **eradication** can cure peptic ulcers and reduce ulcer recurrence; it can eliminate the need for maintenance therapy in many ulcer patients.

2. **Genetic factors**
   a. The lifetime prevalence of developing an ulcer in **first-degree relatives** of ulcer patients is about threefold greater than in the general population. This may be secondary to clustering of *H. pylori* within families.
   b. People with **blood type O** have an above-normal incidence of duodenal ulcers.
3. **Smoking.** Smokers have an increased risk of developing peptic ulcer disease. In addition, cigarette smoking delays ulcer healing and increases the risk and rapidity of relapse after the ulcer heals. Nicotine decreases biliary and pancreatic bicarbonate secretion. Smoking also accelerates the emptying of stomach acid into the duodenum.
4. **NSAIDs.** When ingested chronically, aspirin, indomethacin, and other NSAIDs promote gastric ulcer formation.
   a. These drugs may injure the gastric mucosa by allowing back-diffusion of hydrogen ions into the mucosa.
   b. NSAIDs also inhibit the synthesis of prostaglandins, which are substances with a cytoprotective effect on the mucosa.
   c. Selective cyclooxygenase 2 (COX-2) inhibitors, celecoxib or rofecoxib, are associated with fewer ulcers than nonselective NSAIDs, with rates comparable to placebo at 3 months. Questions regarding long-term safety of COX-2 inhibitors remain. With the recent documentation of increasing COX-2 expression with the progression of BE to cancer, trials have been initiated using COX-2 selective inhibitors in BE patients to prevent development of cancer.
5. **Alcohol.** A known mucosal irritant, alcohol causes marked irritation of the gastric mucosa if ingested in large quantities at concentrations of 20% or greater. The only association between ethanol intake and ulcer disease exists in patients with portal cirrhosis.
6. **Coffee.** Both regular and decaffeinated coffee contain peptides that stimulate release of gastrin, a hormone that triggers the flow of gastric juice. However, a direct link between coffee and peptic ulcer disease has not been proven.
7. **Corticosteroids.** Controversy over whether systemic corticosteroid therapy is associated with increased risk for the development of peptic ulcer disease has, for the most part, been resolved. Evidence for this direct association has always been weak in previous retrospective reviews/trials and reflected the concurrent use of an NSAID. Current data support no link between steroids and peptic ulcer disease in the absence of concurrent NSAID use.
8. **Associated disorders.** Peptic ulcer disease is more common in patients with hyperparathyroidism, emphysema, rheumatoid arthritis, and alcoholic cirrhosis.
9. **Advanced age.** Degeneration of the pylorus permits bile reflux into the stomach, creating an environment that favors ulcer formation.
10. **Psychological factors.** Once assigned key roles in the pathogenesis of PUD, stress and personality type now are viewed as relatively minor influences.

F. **Pathophysiology.** Ulcers develop when an imbalance exists between factors that protect gastric mucosa and factors that promote mucosal corrosion. Approximately 90% of patients with duodenal ulcer and 70% of patients with gastric ulcer have *H. pylori* infection.

1. **Protective factors**
   a. Normally, the mucosa secretes a thick mucus that serves as a barrier between luminal acid and epithelial cells. This barrier slows the inward movement of hydrogen ions, and allows their neutralization by bicarbonate ions in fluids secreted by the stomach and duodenum.
   b. Alkaline and neutral pancreatic biliary juices also help buffer acid entering the duodenum from the stomach.
   c. An **intact mucosal barrier** prevents back-diffusion of gastric acids into mucosal cells. It also has the capacity to stimulate local blood flow, which brings nutrients and other substances to

the area and removes toxic substances (e.g., hydrogen ions). Mucosal integrity also promotes cell growth and repair after local trauma.

2. **Corrosive factors.** Peptic ulcer disease reflects the inability of the gastric mucosa to resist corrosion by irritants, such as pepsin, HCl, and other gastric secretions.
   a. **Exposure to gastric acid** and **pepsin** is necessary for ulcer development.
   b. **Disrupted mucosal barrier integrity** allows gastric acids to diffuse from the lumen back into mucosal cells, where they cause injury.
3. **Physiological defects associated with peptic ulcer disease.** Researchers have identified various physiological defects in patients with duodenal and gastric ulcers.
   a. **Duodenal ulcer patients** may have the following defects:
      (1) Increased capacity for gastric acid secretion
         (a) Some duodenal ulcer patients have up to twice the normal number of parietal cells (which produce HCl).
         (b) Nearly 70% of duodenal ulcer patients have elevated serum levels of **pepsinogen I**, and a corresponding increase in pepsin-secreting capacity.
      (2) Increased parietal cell responsiveness to gastrin
      (3) Above-normal postprandial gastrin secretion
      (4) Defective inhibition of gastrin release at low pH, possibly leading to failure to suppress postprandial acid secretion
      (5) Above-normal rate of gastric emptying, resulting in delivery of a greater acid load to the duodenum
   b. **Gastric ulcer patients** typically exhibit the following characteristics:
         (a) Deficient gastric mucosal resistance, direct mucosal injury, or both
         (b) Elevated serum gastrin levels (in acid hyposecretors)
         (c) Decreased pyloric pressure at rest and in response to acid or fat in the duodenum
         (d) Delayed gastric emptying
         (e) Increased reflux of bile and other duodenal contents
         (f) Subnormal mucosal levels of prostaglandins (these levels normalize once the ulcer heals)
4. **GERD** requires both initiation and perpetuation of the reflux of gastric contents. Esophagitis develops when noxious substances in the refluxate (i.e., acid, pepsin) are in contact with the esophageal mucosa long enough to cause irritation and inflammation.
   a. In patients with GERD, 65% of reflux events occur via transient lower esophageal sphincter relaxation (TLESR). The main difference between normal individuals and those with GERD is the frequency of TLESR. GERD patients have more frequent and prolonged TLESR. TLESR represents a decrease in lower esophageal sphincter (LES) pressure that is not associated with swallowing or peristalsis.
   b. Other mechanisms of LES incompetence are increased abdominal pressure and spontaneous reflux during periods of very low LES pressure.
   c. Such motility problems are permissive—that is, they allow reflux of acid and other noxious substances.
5. Many diseases cause dyspeptic symptoms, including PUD, GERD, gastric cancer, and biliary tract disease. However, in many cases, no clear pathological reason for a patient's symptoms can be determined. Dyspepsia in the absence of an identifiable organic cause is frequently described as "functional" or "nonulcer" dyspepsia.

G. Clinical presentation. Signs and symptoms of PUD vary with the patient's age and the location of the lesion. Only about 50% of patients experience classic ulcer symptoms. The remainder are asymptomatic or report vague or atypical symptoms.

1. **Pain.** Patients typically describe heartburn or a gnawing, burning, aching, or cramp-like pain. Some patients report abdominal soreness or hunger sensations. It is unclear whether peptic ulcer pain results from chemical stimulation or from spasm.
   a. **Duodenal ulcer pain** usually is restricted to a small, midepigastric area near the xiphoid. Pain may radiate below the costal margins into the back or the right shoulder. Pain from a duodenal ulcer frequently awakens the patient between midnight and 2 A.M.; it is almost never present before breakfast.

b. **Gastric ulcer pain** is less localized. It may be referred to the left subcostal region. Gastric ulcer rarely produces nocturnal pain.

c. **GERD** patients most commonly present with heartburn, belching, regurgitation, or water brash; **atypical presentations** include chest pain, hoarseness/laryngitis, loss of dental enamel, asthma, chronic cough, or dyspepsia. Complications of GERD include esophageal ulceration, strictures, BE, and adenocarcinoma of the esophagus or esophagogastric junction.

d. **Dyspepsia** applies broadly to a range of symptoms, including abdominal or retrosternal pain and discomfort, heartburn, nausea, vomiting, and other symptoms referable to the proximal GI tract.

e. **Food** usually relieves duodenal ulcer pain but may cause gastric ulcer pain. This finding may explain why duodenal ulcer patients tend to gain weight, whereas gastric ulcer patients may lose weight. Pain characteristically occurs 90 mins to 3 hrs after meals in duodenal ulcer patients, whereas pain in gastric ulcer patients is usually present 45 to 60 mins after a meal. Food aggravates reflux disease.

2. **Nausea** and **vomiting** may occur with either ulcer type.

3. **Disease course.** Both duodenal and gastric ulcers tend to be chronic, with spontaneous remissions and exacerbations. Within a year of the initial symptoms, most patients experience a relapse.

a. In many cases, relapse is seasonal, occurring more often in the spring and autumn.

b. All patients with a confirmed duodenal or gastric ulcer should be tested for *H. pylori* infection. If the patient is *H. pylori*–positive, eradication therapy will reduce the recurrence rate significantly and preclude the need for maintenance medication.

c. GERD is also a chronic disease; most patients with reflux esophagitis who are healed with antisecretory drug therapy will experience a recurrence within 6 months of discontinuation of the healing regimen. Maintenance therapy reduces the recurrence of esophagitis.

H. Clinical evaluation

1. **Physical findings.** Patients with peptic ulcer disease may exhibit superficial and deep epigastric tenderness and voluntary muscle guarding. With duodenal ulcer, patients also may show unilateral spasm over the duodenal bulb. Gastric ulcer patients may have weight loss.

2. **Diagnostic test results**

a. **Blood tests** may show hypochromic anemia.

b. **Stool tests** may detect occult blood if the ulcer is chronic.

c. **Gastric secretion tests** may reveal hypersecretion of HCl in duodenal ulcer patients and normal or subnormal HCl secretion in gastric ulcer patients.

d. **Upper GI series** (barium x-ray) reveals the ulcer crater in up to 80% of cases. Duodenal bulb deformity suggests a duodenal ulcer.

e. **Upper GI endoscopy**, the most specific test, may be done if barium x-ray yields inconclusive results. This procedure confirms an ulcer in at least 95% of cases and may detect ulcers not demonstrable by radiography.

f. **Biopsy** might be necessary to determine whether a gastric ulcer is malignant.

g. *H. pylori* status is determined by noninvasive tests (not requiring endoscopy) or invasive methods (requiring endoscopy).

(1) **Noninvasive.** Serology, the test of choice when endoscopy is not indicated, is inexpensive. Several office tests are available. Breath tests can also be used to detect the organism, and are uniquely suited as noninvasive means of confirming eradication of *H. pylori* after therapy. False-negative breath tests may occur in patients receiving proton pump inhibitors, antibiotics, or bismuth compounds.

(2) **Invasive.** These methods include histological visualization of *H. pylori* or measurement of urease activity, which require biopsy.

I. Treatment objectives

1. Relieve pain and other symptoms and promote healing
2. Prevent complications
3. Minimize recurrence (eradicate *H. pylori* in PUD)
4. Maintain adequate nutrition
5. Teach the patient about the disease to improve therapeutic compliance
6. Maintain the patient symptom-free

II. THERAPY

A. Drug therapy. Peptic ulcer patients usually are treated with antacids, histamine 2(H_2)-receptor antagonists, or proton pump inhibitors; other drugs are added as necessary. Drug regimens that suppress nocturnal acid secretion are found to result in the highest duodenal ulcer healing rates. Drug therapy typically provides prompt symptomatic relief and promotes ulcer healing within 4 to 6 weeks (*Figure 44-1*). GERD management requires more aggressive acid suppression regimens; the pharmacodynamic end point is to maintain the pH in the esophagus at four or more (*Figure 44-2*).

1. **Antacids.** These compounds, which neutralize gastric acid, are used to treat ulcer pain and heal the ulcer. Studies show antacids and H_2-receptor antagonists to be equally effective. Antacids are available as **magnesium**, **aluminum**, or **calcium**. The most widely used antacids are mixtures of aluminum hydroxide and magnesium hydroxide (*Table 44-1*). Duodenal ulcers rarely occur in the absence of acid or when the hourly maximum acid output is < 10 mEq. Peptic activity decreases

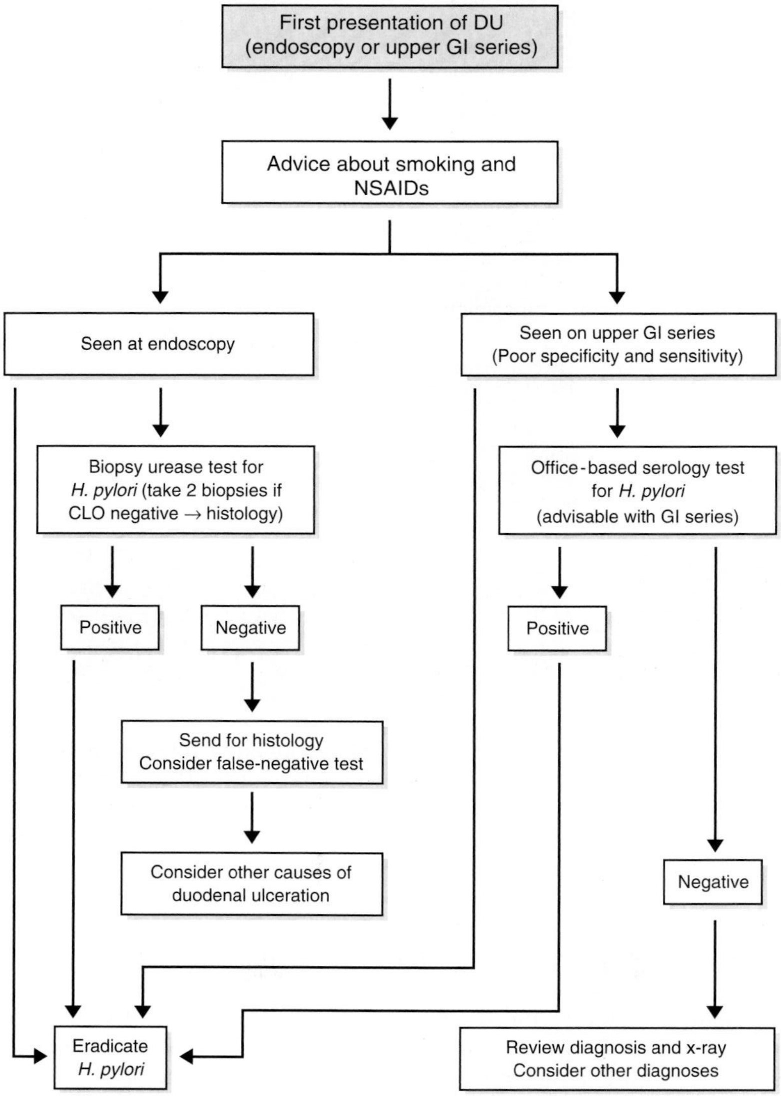

Figure 44-1. Treatment strategy for management of duodenal ulcer. *CLO*, *Campylobacter*-like organism; *DU*, duodenal ulcer; *GI*, gastrointestinal; *NSAIDs*, nonsteroidal anti-inflammatory drugs.

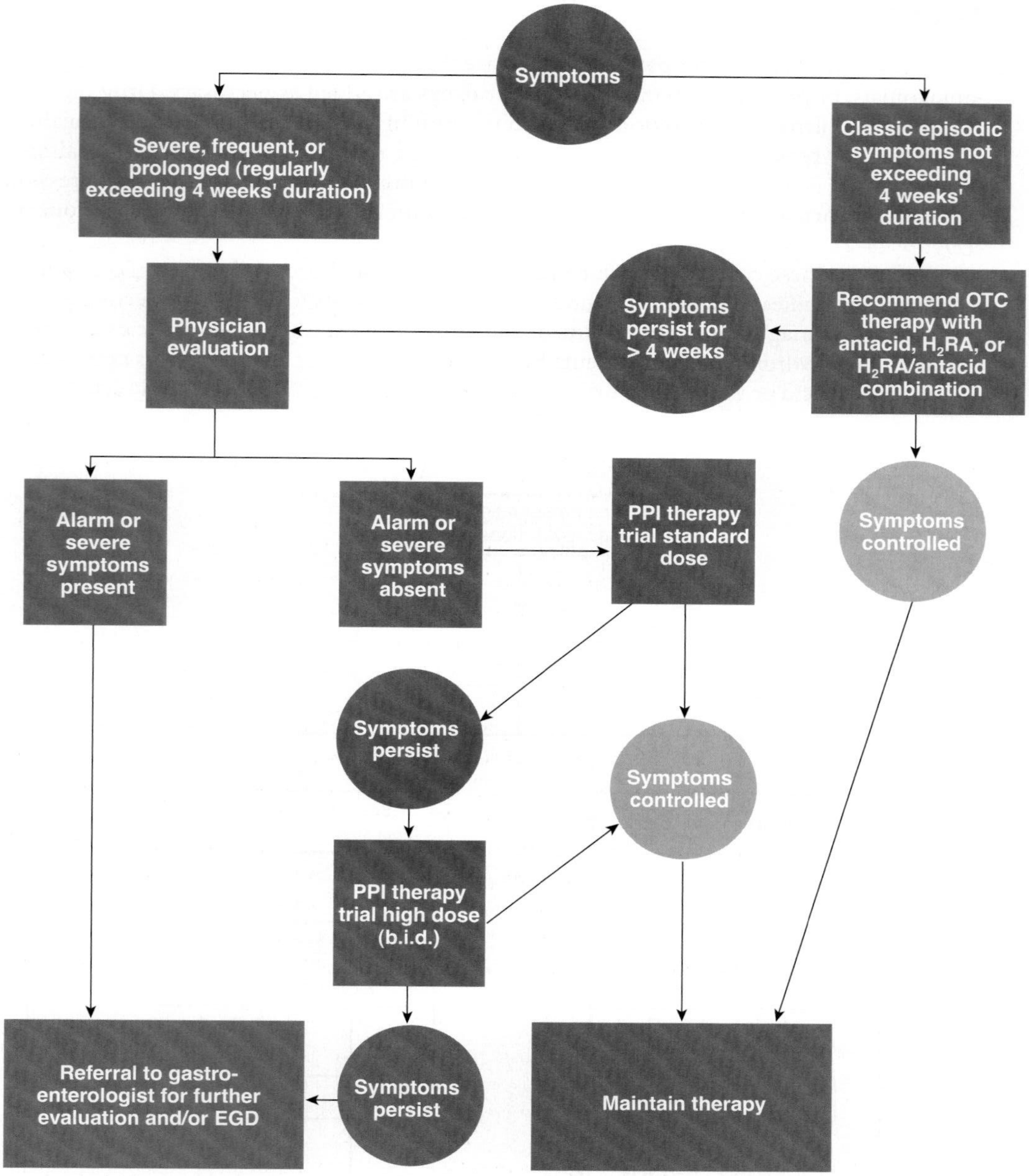

Figure 44-2. Treatment strategy for management of gastroesophageal reflux disease. *EGD*, esophagogastroduodenoscopy; *H_2RA*, histamine 2-receptor antagonist; *OTC*, over the counter; *PPI*, proton pump inhibitor. Adapted with permission from Peterson WL. GERD evidence-based therapeutic strategies (AGA Consensus Development Panel), 2002. Available at http://www.gastro.org/user-assets/documents/GERDmonograph.pdf.

as acidity decreases; experimental ulcer formation is inhibited by antacids; and acid-reducing operations cure ulcers.

a. **Mechanism of action and therapeutic effects.** Antacids reduce the concentration and total load of acid in the gastric contents. By increasing gastric pH, antacids also inhibit pepsin activity. In addition, they strengthen the gastric mucosal barrier.

b. **Choice of agent**

   (1) **Nonsystemic antacids** (e.g., magnesium or aluminum substances) are preferred to systemic antacids (e.g., sodium bicarbonate) for intensive ulcer therapy because they avoid the risk of alkalosis.

Table 44-1 COMPARISON OF COMMON ANTACIDS

Brand Name	Acid-Neutralizing Capacity (mEq/mL or tab)	Therapeutic Amount (140 mEq) (mL or no. of tablets)	Sodium Content (mg/5 mL or tablet)
Regular Liquids			
Aluminum hydroxide, magnesium hydroxide, simethicone			
Gelusil	2.4	58	0.09
Maalox Max	5.2	27	0.00
Mylanta	2.5	56	0.03
Mylanta Max Strength	5.0	28	0.00
Aluminum hydroxide			
Alternagel	4.0	35	0.20
Tablets			
Calcium carbonate			
Maalox Advanced Max Strength	5.0	6.0	0.00
Tums	10.0	14.0	0.00
Tums E-X	15.0	9.3	0.11
Titralac	7.5	18.7	0.00
Calcium carbonate and magnesium hydroxide			
Rolaids	8.5	16.5	0.04
Mylanta Ultra	12.8	8.4	0.00
Aluminum hydroxide and magnesium carbonate			
Gaviscon Extra Strength	8.0	16.0	29.00

(2) **Liquid antacid forms** have a greater buffering capacity than tablets. However, tablets are more convenient to carry. With either dosage form, the size and frequency of doses may limit patient compliance.

(3) **Antacid mixtures** (e.g., aluminum hydroxide with magnesium hydroxide) provide more even, sustained action than single-agent antacids, and permit a lower dosage of each compound. In addition, compounds in a mixture may interact so as to negate each other's untoward effects. For instance, the constipating effect of aluminum hydroxide may counter the diarrhea that magnesium hydroxide frequently produces.

(4) **Calcium carbonate** usually is avoided because it causes acid rebound, may delay pain relief and ulcer healing, and induces constipation. Another potential adverse effect of this compound is hypercalcemia; the risk is increased if calcium carbonate is taken with milk or another alkaline substance. The milk-alkali syndrome (i.e., hypercalcemia, alkalosis, azotemia, nephrocalcinosis) can also occur.

c. **Administration and dosage**

(1) Antacids differ greatly in acid-neutralizing capacity (ANC), defined as the number of milliequivalents (mEq) of a 1 N solution of HCl that can be brought to a pH of 3.5 in 15 mins. For most duodenal ulcer patients, approximately 50 mEq/hr of available antacid is needed for ongoing neutralization of gastric contents. Therefore, the required dosage depends on the ANC of the specific antacid.

(2) In the fasting state, antacids have only a transient intragastric buffering effect (15 to 20 mins). When ingested 1 hr after a meal, they have a much more prolonged effect, about 3 to 4 hrs; therefore, they should optimally be taken 1 and 3 hrs after meals and before sleep. Consequently, the typical antacid regimen calls for doses 1 and 3 hrs after meals and at bedtime.

(3) **Dosage**

(a) Because the ANC of antacid products varies widely, no standard dosage can be given in terms of milliliters of suspension or number of tablets. However, patients with duodenal ulcers generally require individual dosages of 80 to 160 mEq of ANC (equivalent to 30 to 60 mL of Mylanta or Maalox). Thus the total daily dosage may be as much as 420 mL of Mylanta or Maalox if the standard seven-times–daily dosing regimen is used. Because of the large doses required, increase in adverse effects, need for frequent administration, and poor patient compliance, their role in the management of PUD is limited.

(b) Antacid therapy usually continues for 6 to 8 weeks.

d. **Precautions and monitoring effects**

(1) Calcium carbonate- and magnesium-containing antacids should be used cautiously in patients with severe renal disease.

(2) Sodium bicarbonate is contraindicated in patients with hypertension, congestive heart failure (CHF), severe renal disease, and edema. It should not be used for ulcer therapy.

(3) All antacids should be used cautiously in elderly patients (particularly those with decreased GI motility) and renally impaired patients.

(4) Aluminum-containing antacids should be used cautiously in patients who suffer from dehydration or intestinal obstruction.

(5) The combination of calcium carbonate with an alkaline substance (e.g., sodium bicarbonate) and milk may cause the milk-alkali syndrome.

(6) Always check brand name extension products for major ingredient changes (i.e., Maalox Total Stomach Relief contains bismuth subsalicylate).

(7) Chronic administration of calcium carbonate-containing antacids should be avoided because of hypercalcemia and calcium ion stimulation of acid secretion.

(8) Aluminum or magnesium toxicity is unlikely in patients with normal renal function. The encephalopathy of tissue deposition of aluminum occurs only in dialysis patients receiving aluminum hydroxide for control of hyperphosphatemia. Chronic use of magnesium-containing antacids is not advisable in patients with renal insufficiency.

(9) Constipation can occur in patients using calcium carbonate- and aluminum-containing antacids.

(10) Diarrhea is a common adverse effect of magnesium-containing antacids. If diarrhea occurs, the patient may alternate the antacid mixture with aluminum hydroxide.

(11) Hypophosphatemia and osteomalacia can occur with long-term use of aluminum hydroxide, but these conditions can also occur with short-term use in severely malnourished patients, such as alcoholics.

e. **Significant interactions.** Because antacids alter gastric pH and affect absorption of ingested substances, they have a high potential for drug interactions. To ensure consistent absorption and therapeutic efficacy, orally administered drugs should be given 30 to 60 mins before antacids.

(1) Antacids bind with **tetracycline and fluoroquinolones**, inhibiting the absorption and reducing therapeutic efficacy.

(2) Antacids may destroy the coating of **enteric-coated drugs**, leading to premature drug dissolution in the stomach.

(3) Antacids may interfere with the absorption of many drugs, including **cimetidine**, **ranitidine**, **digoxin**, **isoniazid**, **anticholinergics**, **iron products**, and **phenothiazines** (see II.A.2.e.[3]).

(4) Antacids may reduce the therapeutic effects of **sucralfate** (see II.A.3.d).

2. **H_2-receptor antagonists.** These drugs may be preferred to other antiulcer agents because of their convenience and lack of effect on GI motility. Although reasonably effective in treating mild to moderate GERD symptoms, H_2-receptor antagonists are less reliable for healing erosive esophagitis. All current choices require multiple, divided doses for GERD management.

a. **Mechanism of action and therapeutic effects.** H_2-receptor antagonists competitively inhibit the action of histamine at parietal cell receptor sites, reducing the volume and hydrogen ion concentration of gastric acid secretions (*Figure 44-3* and *Table 44-2*). These agonists accelerate the healing of most ulcers.

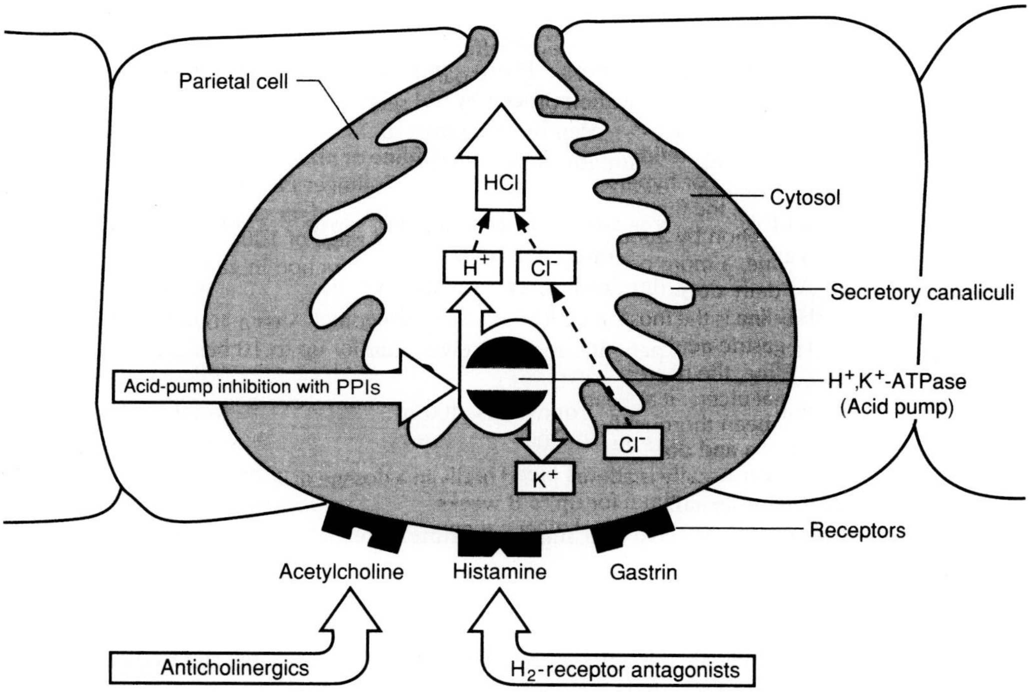

Figure 44-3. Sites of drug action in a parietal cell. *HCl,* hydrochloric acid; *PPIs,* proton pump inhibitors.

b. **Choice of agent. Cimetidine (Tagamet)**, **ranitidine (Zantac)**, **famotidine (Pepcid)**, or **nizatidine (Axid)** may be administered to treat peptic ulcers or hypersecretory states (e.g., Zollinger–Ellison syndrome).

(1) **Cimetidine**, the first H_2-receptor antagonist approved for clinical use, reduces gastric acid secretion by approximately 50% (at a total daily dosage of 1000 mg).

Table 44-2 H_2-RECEPTOR ANTAGONISTS

Characteristic	Cimetidine (Tagamet)	Ranitidine (Zantac)	Famotidine (Pepcid)	Nizatidine (Axid)
Ring structure	Imidazole	Furan	Thiazole	Thiazole
Relative potency	1	4–10	4–10	20–50
Evening dose (mg)				
Active ulcer	800	300	40	300
Maintenance	400	150	20	150
Bioavailability (F) (%)	60–70	50–60	40–45	90–100
Peak time (t_{max}) (hr)	1–3	1–3	1.0–3.5	0.5–3.0
Volume of distribution (L/kg)	1	1.4	1.1–1.4	0.8–1.6
Protein binding (%)	20	15	15–22	32–35
Renal elimination (%)	60–75	30 oral; 70 intravenous	65–70	65–75
Half-life (hr)				
Normal	2	2–3	2.5–4.0	1.6
Anuric	4–5	4–10	20+	6.0–8.5
Clearance (L/hr)	30–48	46	19–29	40–60

Reprinted with permission from Hurwitz A. Clinical pharmacology of agents for the treatment of acid-related disorders. In: Zakim D, Dannenberg AJ, eds. *Peptic Ulcer Disease and Other Acid-Related Disorders.* New York, NY: Academic Research Associates; 1991:343.

(2) **Ranitidine**, a more potent drug, causes a 70% reduction in gastric acid secretion (at a total daily dosage of 300 mg).

(3) **Famotidine** is the most potent H_2-receptor antagonist. After a 40-mg dose, mean nocturnal gastric acid secretion is reduced by 94% for up to 10 hrs.

(4) **Nizatidine**, the last H_2-receptor antagonist marketed, causes a 90% reduction in nocturnal gastric acid secretion for up to 10 hrs.

c. Administration and dosage

(1) **Cimetidine** usually is administered orally in a dosage of 300 mg four times daily (with meals and at bedtime) for up to 8 weeks.

(a) Alternatively, duodenal ulcer patients may receive 400 mg twice daily or 800 mg at bedtime. An 800-mg bedtime dose is also effective in treating gastric ulcers.

(b) Hospitalized patients may receive parenteral doses of 300 mg intravenously every 6 hrs.

(c) For duodenal ulcer prophylaxis, 400 mg may be given orally at bedtime. However, the ulcer recurs in 20–40% of patients. Cimetidine is also FDA approved for the prevention of Upper GI bleeding at a dose of 50 mg/hr continuous infusion.

(2) **Ranitidine** usually is given orally in a dosage of 150 mg twice daily. Duodenal ulcer patients may receive 300 mg at bedtime, alternatively. Therapy continues for up to 8 weeks.

(a) Hospitalized patients may receive ranitidine by the intravenous or intramuscular route (50 mg every 6 to 8 hrs).

(b) Prophylactic therapy may be administered to reduce the risk of ulcer recurrence. The approved prophylactic dosage is 150 mg at bedtime.

(c) Ranitidine 150 mg twice daily can be administered to maintain healing of erosive esophagitis; for this purpose, it is better than placebo but less effective than the proton pump inhibitors.

(d) Ranitidine bismuth citrate, combined with antibiotics such as clarithromycin, is indicated for eradication of *H. pylori* in patients with duodenal ulcer.

(3) **Famotidine**, administered to duodenal ulcer patients, is given in an oral dosage of 40 mg at bedtime for acute therapy for a maximum of 8 weeks. For prophylactic therapy, the dosage is 20 mg at bedtime.

(a) Hospitalized patients may receive an intravenous injection of 20 mg every 12 hrs.

(b) As with cimetidine and ranitidine, the ulcer may recur after drug discontinuation.

(4) **Nizatidine**, for the treatment of duodenal ulcers, is given orally in a dosage of 300 mg once daily at bedtime or 150 mg twice daily for up to 8 weeks. For prophylactic therapy, the dosage is 150 mg at bedtime.

d. Precautions and monitoring effects

(1) Ranitidine must be used cautiously in patients with hepatic impairment. Hepatotoxicity is unusual and occurs most often during intravenous administration. Cimetidine has also been associated with hepatotoxicity.

(2) Cimetidine may cause such hematological disorders as thrombocytopenia, agranulocytosis, and aplastic anemia.

(3) All of these agents may cause headache and dizziness. Cimetidine additionally may lead to confusion, particularly if patients are more than 60 years of age or if the dosage is not adjusted for patients with decreased kidney or liver function. All agents require dosage reductions in patients with impaired renal function.

(4) Cimetidine has a weak androgenic effect, possibly resulting in male gynecomastia and impotence.

(5) Cimetidine and ranitidine rarely can cause bradycardia, which is reversible on discontinuation of therapy.

(6) Evaluate *H. pylori* status in any patient with confirmed ulcer disease; eradication of *H. pylori* reduces the need for maintenance therapy in patients with duodenal or gastric ulcers. Patients with complicated ulcer disease should continue maintenance therapy until the eradication of *H. pylori*.

(7) Tolerance develops frequently to H_2-receptor antagonists (H_2RAs) and may explain diminished responses to these agents over time.

e. **Significant interactions**
   (1) Cimetidine binds the cytochrome P450 system of the liver, and thus may interfere with the metabolism of such drugs as **phenytoin**, **theophylline**, **phenobarbital**, **lidocaine**, **warfarin**, **imipramine**, **diazepam**, and **propranolol**.
   (2) Cimetidine decreases hepatic blood flow, possibly resulting in reduced clearance of **propranolol** and **lidocaine**.
   (3) **Antacids** impair absorption of cimetidine and ranitidine, and should be given 1 hr apart from these drugs.
   (4) **Concomitant use of an H_2RA and an azole drug has resulted in decreased efficacy.**

3. **Sucralfate (Carafate).** This mucosal protectant is a nonabsorbable disaccharide containing sucrose and aluminum.
   a. **Mechanism of action and therapeutic effects.** Sucralfate adheres to the base of the ulcer crater, forming a protective barrier against gastric acids and bile salts.
      (1) Sucralfate's ulcer-healing efficacy compares favorably to that of the H_2RAs.
      (2) Duodenal ulcers respond better than gastric ulcers to sucralfate therapy.
   b. **Administration and dosage**
      (1) An oral agent, sucralfate usually is given in a dosage of 1 g four times daily (1 hr before meals) and at bedtime. Unless radiography or endoscopy documents earlier ulcer healing, therapy continues for 4 to 8 weeks.
      (2) Continued sucralfate therapy after remission postpones ulcer relapse more effectively than cimetidine therapy does.
      (3) There is no evidence that combining sucralfate with H_2RAs improves healing or reduces recurrence rates.
   c. **Precautions and monitoring effects.** Constipation is the most common adverse effect of sucralfate.
   d. **Significant interactions**
      (1) **Antacids** may reduce mucosal binding of sucralfate, decreasing its therapeutic efficacy, and thus should be given 30 to 60 mins apart from sucralfate if used in combination ulcer therapy.
      (2) Sucralfate may interfere with the absorption of orally administered **digoxin**, **tetracycline**, **phenytoin**, **iron**, **ciprofloxacin and other fluoroquinolones**, and **cimetidine** if doses are given simultaneously.

4. **GI anticholinergics** (e.g., belladonna leaf, atropine, propantheline) sometimes are used as adjunctive agents for relief of refractory duodenal ulcer pain. However, these agents have no proven value in ulcer healing.
   a. **Mechanism of action.** Anticholinergics decrease basal and stimulated gastric acid and pepsin secretion.
      (1) Given in combination with antacids, anticholinergics delay gastric emptying, thereby prolonging antacid retention. They are most effective when taken at night and in large doses.
      (2) Anticholinergics occasionally are used in patients who do not respond to H_2RAs alone.
   b. **Administration and dosage**
      (1) Taken 30 mins before food, anticholinergics inhibit meal-stimulated acid secretion by 30% to 50% for a duration of 4 to 5 hrs.
      (2) The optimal effective dose varies from patient to patient.
   c. **Precautions and monitoring effects**
      (1) All anticholinergics have side effects to varying degrees, such as dry mouth, blurred vision, tachycardia, urinary retention, and constipation.
      (2) These drugs are contraindicated in patients with gastric ulcers because they prolong gastric emptying. They also are contraindicated in patients with narrow-angle glaucoma and urinary retention.

5. **Prostaglandins.** These agents suppress gastric acid secretion and may guard the gastric mucosa against damage from NSAIDs. **Misoprostol (Cytotec)** has been approved for use in the prevention of gastric ulcers caused by NSAIDs.
   a. **Mechanism of action.** Misoprostol has both antisecretory (inhibiting gastric acid secretion) and mucosal protective properties. NSAIDs inhibit prostaglandin synthesis, and a deficiency of prostaglandin within the gastric mucosa may lead to diminishing bicarbonate

and mucus secretion, contributing to the mucosal damage caused by NSAIDs. Misoprostol increases bicarbonate and mucus production at doses of 200 mcg and above—doses that can also be antisecretory. Misoprostol also maintains mucosal blood flow.

b. Administration and dosage

(1) Misoprostol is indicated for the prevention of NSAID-induced gastric ulcers in patients at high risk for complications from gastric ulcers (e.g., patients more than 60 years of age, patients with concomitant debilitating disease, patients with a history of ulcers).

(2) Misoprostol has not been shown to prevent duodenal ulcers in patients taking NSAIDs.

(3) The recommended adult dosage is 200 mcg four times daily with food; it must be taken for the duration of NSAID therapy. If this dose cannot be tolerated, 100 mcg four times daily can be used.

(4) Adjustment of dosage in renally impaired patients is not routinely needed.

c. Precautions and monitoring effects

(1) Misoprostol is contraindicated in pregnant women because of its abortifacient property. Patients must be advised of the abortifacient property, and warned not to give the drug to others.

(2) Misoprostol should not be used in women with childbearing potential unless the patient requires NSAID therapy, and is at high risk of complications from gastric ulcers associated with use of the NSAIDs or is at high risk of developing gastric ulceration. In such a patient, misoprostol may be prescribed if the patient:

(a) Is capable of complying with effective contraceptive measures

(b) Has received both oral and written warnings of the hazards of misoprostol, the risk of possible contraception failure, and the danger to other women of childbearing potential should the drug be taken by mistake

(c) Had a negative serum pregnancy test within 2 weeks before beginning therapy

(d) Will begin misoprostol only on the second or third day of the next normal menstrual period

(3) The most frequent adverse effects are diarrhea (14% to 40%) and abdominal pain (13% to 20%). Diarrhea is dose related, usually develops early in the course (> 2 weeks), and is often self-limiting. Discontinuation of misoprostol is necessary in about 2% of patients. Administration with food minimizes the diarrhea.

d. Significant interactions. None has been reported.

6. **Proton pump inhibitors (PPIs). Omeprazole (Prilosec)** was the first PPI available in the United States, followed by **lansoprazole (Prevacid), rabeprazole (AcipHex), pantoprazole (Protonix), esomeprazole (Nexium), and dexlansoprazole (Kapidex)** (*Table 44-3*). The intravenous forms

Table 44-3 PROTON PUMP INHIBITORS

Pharmacokinetics of PPIs

Characteristic	Omeprazole (Prilosec)	Lansoprazole (Prevacid)	Rabeprazole (Aciphex)	Pantoprazole (Protonix)	Esomeprazole (Nexium)	Dexlansoprazole (Kapidex)
Bioavailability (%)	30–40	80–85	52	77	64–89	n/a
Time to peak plasma concentration (hours)	0.5–3.5	1.7	2.0–5.0	1.1–3.1	1.56	First peak 1–2, Second peak 4–5
Plasma elimination half-life (hours)	0.5–1.0	1.3–1.7	1.0–2.0	1.0–1.9	0.85–1.25	1.0–2.0
Protein binding (%)	95	97	96	98	97	98
Urinary excretion of oral dose (%)	77	14–23	30–35	71–80	80	51

PPIs, proton pump inhibitors.

of esomeprazole, lansoprazole, and pantoprazole have been approved by the U.S. Food and Drug Administration (FDA).

a. **Mechanism of action and therapeutic effects.** The gastric proton pump H^+/K^+-ATPase has a sulfhydryl group near the potassium-binding site on the luminal side of the canalicular membrane. Omeprazole sulfonamide (the active form) forms a stable disulfide bond with this specific sulfhydryl, thereby inactivating the ATPase and shutting off acid secretion. All other PPIs exhibit a similar irreversible mechanism of action.
   (1) Because of the potency and marked reduction in gastric acidity, the PPIs are more rapidly effective than other approved agents in treating peptic ulcer disease (i.e., PPIs tend to control symptoms and heal ulcers more rapidly than other antiulcer drugs). PPIs provide effective healing of duodenal ulcers; healing rates at 4 weeks are similar to those reported for H_2-receptor antagonist therapy at 8 weeks.
   (2) All PPIs are effective in healing erosive esophagitis, provide more rapid symptom relief and more consistent healing than H_2-receptor antagonists, and are also effective in maintenance of healing of erosive esophagitis.
   (3) All PPIs except dexlansoprazole and pantoprazole have been approved in various combinations of antibiotics for the eradication of *H. pylori* (*Table 44-4*).
   (4) PPIs have resulted in significant improvement in patients with pathological hypersecretory conditions (e.g., Zollinger–Ellison syndrome) and GERD compared to H_2-receptor antagonists.
   (5) Esomeprazole and lansoprazole have been approved by the FDA for healing and risk reduction of NSAID-induced gastric ulcers.
   (6) **Esomeprazole**, omeprazole and lansoprazole have been approved by the FDA for use in infants and children for the short-term treatment of GERD and erosive esophagitis. Omeprazole is approved for use in children ages 1 to 16 years, and both esomeprazole and lansoprazole are approved for use in children 1 to 11 years old.

Table 44-4 U.S. FOOD AND DRUG ADMINISTRATION (FDA) APPROVED ORAL REGIMENS USED TO ERADICATE *HELICOBACTER PYLORI* AND REDUCE THE RISK OF DUODENAL ULCER RECURRENCE

Drug Combination	Dose and Frequency	Duration
Omeprazole	20 mg b.i.d.	Days 1–10
	20 mg q.d.	Days 11–28[a]
Clarithromycin	500 mg b.i.d.	Days 1–10
Amoxicillin	1 g b.i.d.	Days 1–10
Lansoprazole	30 mg b.i.d.	10 days
Amoxicillin	1 g b.i.d.	10 days
Clarithromycin	500 mg b.i.d.	10 days
Esomeprazole	40 mg q.d.	q.d. 10 days
Amoxicillin	1 g b.i.d.	10 days
Clarithromycin	500 mg b.i.d.	10 days
Rabeprazole	20 mg b.i.d.	7 days
Amoxicillin	1 g b.i.d.	7 days
Clarithromycin	500 m.g b.i.d.	7 days
Bismuth subsalicylate	525 mg q.i.d	Days 1–14
Metronidazole	250 mg q.i.d	Days 1–14
Tetracycline HCl	500 mg q.i.d	Days 1–14
H_2RA of choice	Ulcer healing regimen	Days 1–28

[a]In patients with an ulcer present at the time of initiation of therapy, additional omeprazole treatment is recommended for ulcer healing and relief of symptoms.
b.i.d., twice a day; *H_2RA*, histamine H_2-receptor antagonist; *q.d.*, every day; *q.i.d.*, four times a day.

b. Administration and dosage

(1) PPIs are more potent than H_2-blockers. In the usual dosage (omeprazole 20 mg daily), these agents inhibit > 90% of 24-hr acid secretion in most patients, rarely producing achlorhydria. Esomeprazole 40 mg daily provided significantly higher intragastric pH values above 4 during 24-hr monitoring compared to lansoprazole 30 mg, rabeprazole 20 mg, omeprazole 20 mg, and pantoprazole 40 mg.

(2) PPIs should optimally be taken in the morning 30 to 60 mins before eating; food activates parietal cells, maximizing the effect of the PPI. Optimal binding to proton pumps occurs when the pumps are actively secreting.

(3) Recommended adult dosages

(a) Erosive esophagitis initially is healed with 20 mg omeprazole or equivalent doses of other PPIs for 8 to 12 weeks; only omeprazole has a demonstrated dose response in GERD patients (patients failing omeprazole 20 mg daily may benefit from higher doses; this has not been demonstrated with esomeprazole, lansoprazole, rabeprazole, or pantoprazole). In addition, esomeprazole 40 mg every day has been shown to produce significantly higher healing rates than omeprazole 20 mg or lansoprazole 30 mg across all grades of erosive esophagitis.

(b) **Dexlansoprazole 30 mg**, esomeprazole 20 to 40 mg, lansoprazole 30 mg, omeprazole 20 mg, rabeprazole 20 mg, and pantoprazole 40 mg may be used to manage GERD symptoms in patients who have failed previous therapy with H_2-receptor antagonist therapy.

(c) The recommended dosage to maintain healing of erosive esophagitis is dexlansoprazole 30 mg, esomeprazole 20 mg, omeprazole 20 mg, lansoprazole 15 mg, pantoprazole 40 mg, or rabeprazole 20 mg daily for as long as medically necessary.

(d) Duodenal ulcer healing requires omeprazole 20 mg, lansoprazole 15 mg, or rabeprazole 20 mg once daily. Most patients heal within 4 weeks.

(4) Esomeprazole, lansoprazole, and omeprazole are delayed-release capsules, and should be taken before eating, can be used concomitantly with antacids, and should not be chewed or crushed. Capsule contents can be sprinkled on foods (i.e., applesauce) or mixed with acidic juices. Suspensions of omeprazole or lansoprazole in sodium bicarbonate have been used for administration to patients with nasogastric and jejunostomy tubes.

(5) Rabeprazole and pantoprazole are available as enteric-coated tablets that should not be crushed or chewed.

(6) Lansoprazole is available as the first orally disintegrating tablet formulation. It is placed on the tongue, with or without water, until dissolved. However, it needs to be swallowed to be absorbed.

(7) Dexlansoprazole is the first and only PPI available as a dual delayed-release capsule formulation.

(8) Omeprazole in sodium bicarbonate powder for suspension (Zegerid) is the first PPI approved by the FDA for reduction in the risk of upper GI bleeding in critically ill patients. It has a peach/mint flavor that is tolerable. It is dosed at 40 mg every 6 hrs times two doses (as a loading dose), then 40 mg daily.

(9) Omeprazole (20 mg daily) and lansoprazole (15 mg daily) are approved for the over-the-counter use of heartburn.

(10) No dosing adjustments are necessary in patients with impaired renal or hepatic function or in the elderly.

(11) Intravenous pantoprazole is indicated for management of erosive esophagitis and treatment of Zollinger–Ellison syndrome. Esomeprazole, lansoprazole, and pantoprazole are currently being widely used for the treatment of acute bleeding gastric ulcers, though not FDA approved.

(12) Intravenous esomeprazole (20 to 40 mg daily), lansoprazole (30 mg daily), and pantoprazole (40 mg daily) are FDA approved for the short-term use in patients with GERD with a history of erosive esophagus unable to take oral medications.

(13) In patients with nocturnal signs and symptoms of GERD, twice daily PPIs have been effective when taken appropriately. The addition of an H_2RA to the twice-daily PPI has shown little added benefit and is not recommended.

c. **Precautions and monitoring effects**
   (1) Headache, diarrhea, abdominal pain, nausea and vomiting, and flatulence have been reported in > 1% of patients.
   (2) Fever, fatigue, malaise, elevated liver enzymes, dizziness, vertigo, skin rash, and itching have been reported in < 1% of patients.

d. **Significant interactions**
   (1) Omeprazole interferes with the hepatic microsomal enzyme metabolism (cytochrome P450) of **diazepam**, **warfarin**, and **phenytoin**, **although clinically significant interactions are infrequent**.
   (2) **PPIs may decrease the antiplatelet activity of clopidogrel but the exact clinical significance is still unclear**.
   (3) Because gastric pH plays a role in the bioavailability of **ketoconazole**, **ampicillin esters**, and **iron salts**, prolonged gastric acid inhibition with PPIs may decrease the absorption of these agents.
   (4) Antacids may be used concomitantly with all PPIs.
   (5) Food may reduce the bioavailability of esomeprazole and lansoprazole by 50%; food does not reduce the bioavailability of omeprazole or rabeprazole.

7. **Bismuth compounds.** In the United States, bismuth subsalicylate (Pepto-Bismol) is the only available bismuth product.
   a. **Mechanism of action.** Bismuth prevents adhesion of *H. pylori* to gastric mucosa, decreases resistance when used with other anti–*H. pylori* agents, inhibits release of proteolytic enzymes, and suppresses *H. pylori* growth.
   b. **Administration and dosage**
      (1) Bismuth subsalicylate is highly effective when combined with PPIs and/or antibiotics. Eradication rates with these combinations are > 80% (*Table 44-4*).
      (2) Preferred regimen with bismuth: bismuth subsalicylate 525 mg four times a day, metronidazole 250 mg four times a day, tetracycline 500 mg four times a day plus PPI (omeprazole 20 mg every day or lansoprazole 30 mg every day) for 2 weeks total. This regimen provides consistently high eradication rates (> 90%), and may be useful for patients who have failed previous therapy. This regimen is not currently FDA approved.
   c. **Precautions and monitoring effects**
      (1) CNS toxicity with higher doses, including neurotoxicity
      (2) Tinnitus, hyperpyrexia, tachycardia, and confusion (salicylism) from high doses of bismuth subsalicylate
   d. **Reversible proton pump inhibitors** are currently under development by a number of pharmaceutical companies (AstraZeneca and Altana). When compared with the currently available irreversible proton pump inhibitors, these agents are expected to offer more rapid symptom resolution, control pH more quickly, achieve higher pH levels, and sustain these more aggressive pH levels consistently over a 24-hr period.

8. **Sedatives** are useful adjuncts in promoting rest for highly anxious ulcer patients.

B. **Other therapeutic measures**
   1. **Modification of diet and social habits**
      a. Previously emphasized in ulcer therapy, strict dietary limitations now are considered largely unnecessary.
         (1) Bland or milk-based diets formerly were recommended; however, research indicates that these diets do not speed ulcer healing. In fact, most experts now advise ulcer patients to **avoid milk** because recent studies show that milk increases gastric acid secretion. Also, because milk leaves the stomach quickly, it lacks an extended buffering action.
         (2) Small, frequent meals, also previously recommended, can worsen ulcer pain by causing acid rebound 2 to 4 hrs after eating.
      b. **Current dietary guidelines** emphasize avoiding foods and beverages known to exacerbate gastric discomfort or promote acid secretion. This category typically includes coffee, caffeinated beverages, and alcohol.
      c. **Smoking.** Patients who smoke should be encouraged to quit because smoking markedly slows ulcer healing, even during optimal ulcer therapy.
      d. **NSAIDs** should be avoided by ulcer patients.

2. **Surgery.** An ulcer patient who develops complications may require surgery—sometimes on an emergency basis (see III). Incapacitating recurrent ulcers also may warrant surgery.
   a. **Types of surgical procedures** for ulcer disease include antrectomy and truncal vagotomy (Billroth I procedure), partial gastrectomy and truncal vagotomy (Billroth II procedure), highly selective (proximal gastric) vagotomy, and total gastrectomy (the treatment of choice for Zollinger–Ellison syndrome that is unresponsive to medical management).
      (1) A **vagotomy** severs a branch of the vagus nerve, thereby decreasing HCl secretion.
      (2) An **antrectomy**, by removing the antrum, eliminates some acid-secreting mucosa as well as the major source of gastrin.
   b. The general indications for antireflux surgery are failure of medical therapy to heal or prevent relapse of erosive esophagitis, inability of medical therapy to prevent recurrence of stricture, or a patient whose lifestyle is adversely affected by the need for medical therapy. **Laparoscopic fundoplication** is currently the gold standard for GERD, and successfully relieves symptoms and heals lesions in approximately 85% of patients. However, recent studies have demonstrated that most patients require continued medical therapy after fundoplication.
3. **Emerging endoscopic therapies.** Three endoscopic techniques to treat GERD have recently been introduced.
   a. Augmentation of LES pressure may be achieved by delivery of radio frequency energy to the muscle of the gastroesophageal junction (Stretta procedure). The radio frequency is delivered by means of a flexible catheter made up of a bougie tip, a balloon-basket combination, and four-needle delivery sheaths.
   b. Another endoscopic procedure, the EndoCinch, augments the LES by suturing of the mucosa.
   c. The third endoscopic/endoluminal treatment is by use of Enteryx injection.
   d. Early studies have demonstrated good feasibility in performing these procedures, and an overall satisfactory safety profile. Further studies are necessary to assess long-term failure rate, early versus late complications, and success rate in the different GERD groups.

III. COMPLICATIONS

of peptic ulcer disease cause approximately 7000 deaths in the United States annually.

A. **Hemorrhage.** This life-threatening condition develops from widespread gastric mucosal irritation or ulceration with acute bleeding.
   1. **Clinical features.** The patient may vomit fresh blood or a coffee grounds–like substance. Other signs include passage of bloody or tarry stools, diaphoresis, and syncope. With major blood loss, manifestations of **hypovolemic shock** may appear: The pulse rate may exceed 110, or systolic blood pressure may drop below 100.
   2. **Management**
      a. Patient stabilization, bleeding cessation, and measures to prevent further bleeding are crucial.
         (1) Airway, breathing, and circulation must be ensured.
         (2) Intravenous crystalloids and colloids (e.g., hetastarch) should be infused as needed.
         (3) The patient's electrolyte status must be monitored, and any imbalances should be corrected promptly.
      b. **Gastric lavage** may be performed via a nasogastric or orogastric tube; iced saline solution is instilled until the aspirate returns free of blood.
      c. Vasoconstrictors or continuous infusion proton pump inhibitors have been administered with good response.
         (1) Decrease rebleeding rates were found when the continuous infusion PPI maintained the gastric pH to 6 or above. The doses required were much higher than normal doses (e.g., pantoprazole 80 mg bolus plus 8 mg/hr or lansoprazole 90 mg bolus plus 9 mg/hr). However, none of the intravenous PPIs are currently FDA approved for this indication.
         (2) **Vasopressin**, an agent that causes contraction of the GI smooth muscle, may be given to constrict vessels and control bleeding but only in patients with hemorrhagic gastritis.
      d. **Emergency surgery** usually is indicated if the patient does not respond to medical management.

B. Perforation. Penetration of a peptic ulcer through the gastric or duodenal wall results in this acute emergency. Perforation most commonly occurs with ulcers located in the anterior duodenal wall.

1. **Clinical features.** Sudden acute upper abdominal pain, rigidity, guarding, rebound tenderness, and absent or diminished bowel sounds are typical manifestations. Several hours after onset, symptoms may abate somewhat; this apparent remission is dangerously misleading because peritonitis and shock may ensue.
2. **Management.** Emergency surgery is almost always necessary.

C. Obstruction. Inflammatory edema, spasm, and scarring may lead to obstruction of the duodenal or gastric outlet. The pylorus and proximal duodenum are the most common obstruction sites.

1. **Clinical features.** Typical patient complaints include postprandial vomiting or bloating, appetite and weight loss, and abdominal distention. Tympany and a succussion splash may be audible on physical examination. Gastric aspiration after an overnight fast typically yields more than 200 mL of food residue or clear fluid contents. (Gastric cancer must be ruled out as the cause of obstruction.)
2. **Management**
   a. **Conservative measures** (as in routine ulcer therapy) are indicated in most cases of obstruction.
   b. Patients with marked obstruction may require **continuous gastric suction** with careful monitoring of fluid and electrolyte status. A **saline load test** may be performed after 72 hrs of continuous suction to test the degree of residual obstruction.
   c. If $<$ 200 mL of gastric contents are aspirated, liquid feedings can begin. **Aspiration** is performed at least daily for the next few days to monitor for retention and to guide dietary modifications as the patient progresses to a full regular diet.
   d. **Surgery** is indicated if medical management fails.

D. Postsurgical complications

1. **Dumping syndrome.** Affecting about 10% of patients who have undergone partial gastrectomy, this disorder is characterized by rapid gastric emptying.
   a. **Causes.** The mechanism underlying dumping syndrome is poorly defined. However, intestinal exposure to hypertonic chyme may play a key role by triggering rapid shifts of fluid from the plasma to the intestinal lumen.
   b. **Clinical features.** The patient may experience weakness, dizziness, anxiety, tachycardia, flushing, sweating, abdominal cramps, nausea, vomiting, and diarrhea.
      (1) Manifestations may develop 15 to 30 mins after a meal (early dumping syndrome) or 90 to 120 mins after a meal (late dumping syndrome).
      (2) Reactive hypoglycemia may partly account for some cases of late dumping syndrome.
   c. **Management.** The patient usually is advised to eat six small meals of high protein and fat content and low carbohydrate content. Fluids should be ingested 1 hrs before or after a meal but never with a meal. **Anticholinergics** may be given to slow food passage into the intestine.
2. **Other postsurgical complications** include reflux gastritis, afferent/blind loop syndrome, stomal ulceration, diarrhea, malabsorption, early satiety, and iron-deficiency anemia.

E. Refractory ulcers. Ulcers that fail to heal on a prolonged course of drug treatment should not be confused with ulcers that recur after therapy is stopped. It is difficult to predict which patients will have a refractory ulcer.

1. **Differential diagnosis.** Any compliant patient who continues to have dyspeptic symptoms after 8 weeks of therapy should have gastroscopy and biopsy to exclude rare causes of ulceration in the duodenum, such as Crohn disease, tuberculosis, lymphoma, pulmonary or secondary carcinoma, and cytomegalovirus (CMV) infection in immunodeficient patients. Fasting plasma gastrin concentration should be measured to exclude Zollinger–Ellison syndrome.
2. **Treatment**
   a. Available data indicate that only maximum acid inhibition, with a regimen such as omeprazole (20 mg twice a day) or lansoprazole (30 mg twice a day), offers advantages over continued therapy with standard antiulcer regimens.
   b. Eradication of *H. pylori* infection, when present, is likely to facilitate healing and alter the natural history of refractory ulcers.

c. Every effort should be made to discover and reduce or eliminate NSAID use.
d. Perform surgery.

F. Maintenance regimens

1. Despite healing after withdrawal of therapy, 70% of ulcers recur in 1 year, and 90% in 2 years. Similarly, erosive esophagitis will recur in more than 80% of individuals within 1 year after discontinuation of antisecretory therapy.
2. Candidates for long-term maintenance therapy include patients with serious concomitant diseases; four relapses per year; or a combination of risk factors, producing a more severe natural history of peptic disease (e.g., old age, male sex, a long history of aspirin or NSAID use, heavy alcohol intake, cigarette smoking, a history of peptic ulcer disease in an immediate relative, high maximal acid output, and a history of ulcer complications).
3. Patients with confirmed ulcer disease should be evaluated for presence of *H. pylori*. Eradication of *H. pylori* minimizes the recurrence of ulcer disease. Patients with a history of complicated ulcer disease should have *H. pylori* eradication confirmed.

Study Questions

Directions for questions 1–6: Each of the questions, statements, or incomplete statements in this section can be correctly answered or completed by **one** of the suggested answers or phrases. Choose the **best** answer.

1. ZZ is a 43-year-old female with a chief complaint of hematemesis and abdominal pain. Serology is positive for *H. pylori*. Which of the following would be the best regimens to treat ZZ?
   (A) Omeprazole 20 mg daily plus clarithromycin 500 mg b.i.d. × 14 days
   (B) Lansoprazole 30 mg b.i.d. plus tetracycline 500 mg q.i.d. × 14 days
   (C) Rabeprazole 20 mg b.i.d. plus amoxicillin 1 g b.i.d. plus clarithromycin 500 mg b.i.d. × 7 days
   (D) Esomeprazole 40 mg b.i.d. plus amoxicillin 500 mg b.i.d. plus clarithromycin 500 mg b.i.d. × 7 days
   (E) Pantoprazole 40 mg b.i.d. plus amoxicillin 1 g b.i.d. plus clarithromycin 500 mg t.i.d. × 10 days

2. All of the following statements concerning antacid therapy used in the treatment of duodenal or gastric ulcers are correct *except* which one?
   (A) Antacids may be used to heal the ulcer but are ineffective in controlling ulcer pain.
   (B) Antacids neutralize acid and decrease the activity of pepsin.
   (C) If used alone for ulcer therapy, antacids should be administered 1 hr and 3 hrs after meals and before bedtime.
   (D) If diarrhea occurs, the patient may alternate the antacid product with aluminum hydroxide.
   (E) Calcium carbonate should be avoided because it causes acid rebound and induces constipation.

3. As part of a comprehensive management strategy to treat peptic ulcer disease, patients should be encouraged to do all of the following *except*
   (A) decrease caffeine ingestion.
   (B) eat only bland foods.
   (C) stop smoking.
   (D) avoid alcohol.
   (E) avoid the use of milk as a treatment modality.

4. A gastric ulcer patient requires close follow-up to document complete ulcer healing because
   (A) perforation into the intestine is common.
   (B) spontaneous healing of the ulcer may occur in 30% to 50% of cases.
   (C) there is the risk of the ulcer being cancerous.
   (D) symptoms tend to be chronic and recur.
   (E) weight loss may be severe in gastric ulcer patients.

5. IT is a 58-year-old male admitted to the intensive care unit with acute respiratory failure and thrombocytopenia. He is at high risk for an upper gastrointestinal bleed. Which of the following agents are approved by the U.S. Food and Drug Administration (FDA) for the prevention of this type of bleed?
   (A) Sucralfate
   (B) Famotidine
   (C) Esomeprazole
   (D) Lansoprazole
   (E) Omeprazole

6. All of the following provide acid suppression similar to omeprazole 20 mg every day *except*
   (A) dexlansoprazole 30 mg every day.
   (B) pantoprazole 40 mg every day.
   (C) rabeprazole 20 mg every day.
   (D) ranitidine 150 mg twice a day.
   (E) all provide equivalent acid suppression.

Directions for questions 7–8: The questions and incomplete statements in this section can be correctly answered or completed by **one or more** of the suggested answers. Choose the answer, **A–E**.

A if **I only** is correct
B if **III only** is correct
C if **I and II** are correct
D if **II and III** are correct
E if **I, II, and III** are correct

7. Correct statements concerning cigarette smoking and ulcer disease include which of the following?
   (I) Smoking delays healing of gastric and duodenal ulcers.
   (II) Nicotine decreases biliary and pancreatic bicarbonate secretion.
   (III) Smoking accelerates the emptying of stomach acid into the duodenum.

8. When administered at the same time, antacids can decrease the therapeutic efficacy of which of the following drugs?
   (I) sucralfate
   (II) ranitidine
   (III) cimetidine

Directions for questions 9–13: Each description in this section is most closely associated with **one** of the following agents. Each agent is used only **once**. Choose the **best** answer, **A–E**.

A Sodium bicarbonate
B Aluminum hydroxide
C Calcium carbonate
D Magnesium hydroxide
E Propantheline

9. May cause diarrhea

10. Cannot be used by patients with heart failure

11. If used with milk and an alkaline substance can cause milk-alkali syndrome

12. May cause dry mouth

13. Can be alternated with an antacid mixture to control diarrhea.

Answers and Explanations

1. **The answer is C** *[see Table 44-4]*.
   Though all agents are useful in the treatment of *Helicobacter pylori*, only the combination of rabeprazole with amoxicillin and clarithromycin for 7 days is correct. The other doses and duration of therapy are incorrect.

2. **The answer is A** *[see II.A.1]*.
   Antacids have been shown to heal peptic ulcers, and their main use in modern therapy is to control ulcer pain. Antacids should be taken 1 hr and 3 hrs after meals because the meal prolongs the acid-buffering effect of the antacid. If diarrhea becomes a problem with antacid use, an aluminum hydroxide product can be alternated with the antacid mixture; this takes advantage of the constipating property of aluminum. Because calcium carbonate causes acid rebound and constipation, its use should be avoided.

3. **The answer is B** *[see II.B.1.a.(1)]*.
   Bland food diets are no longer recommended in the treatment of ulcer disease because research indicates that bland or milk-based diets do not accelerate ulcer healing. Studies show that patients can eat almost anything; however, they should avoid foods that aggravate their ulcer symptoms.

4. **The answer is C** *[see I.D.6]*.
   Between 5% and 10% of gastric ulcers may be the result of cancer. The ulcer may respond to therapy; however, failure of the ulcer to decrease satisfactorily in size and to heal with therapy may suggest cancer. Close follow-up is necessary to document complete ulcer healing.

5. **The answer is E** *[see II.6.B]*.
   Though all of these agents have been used with success in the prevention of GI bleeds in critically ill patients, only omeprazole (as a powder for oral suspension) has been FDA approved for this indication.

6. **The answer is D** *[see II.A.6.b.(1)]*.
   Doses of omeprazole 20 mg, dexlansoprazole 30 mg, pantoprazole 40 mg, and rabeprazole 20 mg administered once daily provide similar levels of acid suppression. All provide significantly better acid inhibition than ranitidine, even at doses of 150 mg twice a day or more.

7. **The answer is E** *(I, II, III) [see I.E.3; II.B.1.c]*.
Clinical studies have shown that smoking increases susceptibility to ulcer disease, impairs spontaneous and drug-induced healing, and increases the risk and rapidity of recurrence of the ulcer. These findings may result in part from nicotine's ability to decrease biliary and pancreatic bicarbonate secretion, thus decreasing the body's ability to neutralize acid in the duodenum. Also, the accelerated emptying of stomach acid into the duodenum may predispose to duodenal ulcer and may decrease healing rates.

8. **The answer is E** *(I, II, III) [see II.A.1.e.(3); II.A.3.d]*.
The mean peak blood concentration of cimetidine and the area under the 4-hr cimetidine blood concentration curve were both reduced significantly when cimetidine was administered at the same time as an antacid. The absorption of ranitidine is also reduced when it is taken concurrently with an aluminum-magnesium hydroxide antacid mixture. To avoid this interaction, the antacid should be administered 1 hr before or 2 hrs after the administration of cimetidine or ranitidine. Antacids may reduce mucosal binding of sucralfate, decreasing its therapeutic efficacy. Antacids should, therefore, be given 30 to 60 mins before or after sucralfate.

9. **The answer is D** *[see II.A.1.b.(3)]*.

10. **The answer is A** *[see II.A.1.d.(2)]*.

11. **The answer is C** *[see II.A.1.d.(5)]*.

12. **The answer is E** *[see II.A.4.c.(1)]*.

13. **The answer is B** *[see II.A.1.b.(3)]*.
Magnesium-containing products tend to cause diarrhea, possibly because of magnesium's ability to stimulate the secretion of bile acids by the gallbladder. Because of its sodium content, sodium bicarbonate is contraindicated in patients with CHF, hypertension, severe renal disease, and edema. Sodium bicarbonate is no longer used in peptic ulcer therapy. In addition to causing acid rebound, calcium carbonate, if taken with milk and an alkaline substance for long periods, may cause milk-alkali syndrome. It also may cause adverse effects such as hypercalcemia, alkalosis, azotemia, and nephrocalcinosis. Propantheline, like other anticholinergic agents, may cause dry mouth, blurred vision, urinary retention, and constipation. These agents sometimes are used as adjuncts to relieve duodenal ulcer pain. They are contraindicated in gastric ulcer because they delay gastric emptying. Aluminum hydroxide is constipating and can be alternated with the patient's current antacid when that antacid product is causing diarrhea.

45

Diseases of the Bowel: Inflammatory Bowel Disease and Irritable Bowel Syndrome

DEAN S. COLLIER

I. INTRODUCTION

A. Definition

1. **Inflammatory Bowel Disease** (**IBD**) is a designation commonly used to **describe** two idiopathic diseases of the gastrointestinal tract with closely related clinical presentations. These diseases are **ulcerative colitis** (**UC**) and **Crohn disease** (**CD**).
   - **a.** UC is a chronic inflammatory condition of the gastrointestinal tract mucosa and is primarily found in the rectum and colon.
   - **b.** CD is chronic transmural inflammation of the gastrointestinal mucosa and can be found throughout the gastrointestinal tract from the mouth to the anus. CD most commonly affects the small bowel and colon.
2. **Irritable bowel syndrome** (**IBS**) is a disorder that interferes with the normal motility functions of the gastrointestinal tract. The disorder is characterized by a principle symptom of abdominal pain. Abdominal bloating is another common symptom. These symptoms are associated with various changes in bowel habits, predominantly diarrhea or constipation, though some cases experience both or alternate between the two. Importantly, there is an absence of certain "Alarm signs or symptoms" including unintentional weight loss, anemia, bloody stools, new onset at ≥ 50 years of age and family history of colon cancer, IBD, or celiac disease. Presence of any of these red flags may indicate a disease other than IBS such as colon cancer or IBD.

B. Manifestations

1. **IBD**
   - **a. UC** onset is frequently insidious with increasing stool urgency and frequency. In addition to urgency, bloody stool, and mucus in the stool can also gradually increase. The typical course of UC can be generalized as bouts of varied disease intensity interspersed with asymptomatic periods.
   - **b. CD** onset is typically insidious but can present as severe or fulminate disease. Further, there may be patterns of symptoms, which relate to disease location as well as type (inflammatory, fibrostenotic, or fistulizing for example), which can be useful in determining therapy decisions.
2. **IBS**
   - **a.** IBS can be characterized by pain relieved by defecation, alternating bowel habits, abdominal distention, mucus in the stool, and a sensation of incomplete defecation. IBS usually occurs as either constipation predominant IBS or diarrhea-predominant IBS.

- **b. Constipation predominant (IBS-C)** tends to present with pain and periodic constipation alternating with normal periods of bowel function. Pain has been described as colicky, periodic, and/or as a continuous dull ache. Defecation may relieve the pain and eating can commonly trigger symptoms. Other common symptoms are bloating, nausea, dyspepsia, flatulence, and heartburn.
- **c. Diarrhea predominant (IBS-D)** is commonly characterized by precipitous diarrhea occurring immediately on rising or during meals or immediately postprandially. Nocturnal episodes are rare. Other common presenting complaints are pain, bloating, rectal urgency, and incontinence.
- **d.** Mixed pattern (IBS-M) is used to describe cases where predominant symptoms include both diarrhea and constipation.
- **e.** Alternating pattern (IBS-A) is used to describe cases where predominant symptoms alternate from constipation to diarrhea over a period.

C. Epidemiology of IBD. It has been estimated that more than 1 million Americans have IBD and that roughly half have UC and half have CD.

1. **UC incidence and prevalence rates** have remained relatively constant in North America and northern Europe and appear to be increasing in southern Europe and East Asia. UC historically has been more common than CD.
   - **a.** UC incidence rates in North America range between 9 and 12 cases per 100,000 patients. Recent prevalence rates for UC in North America are reported to be 205 to 240 per 100,000 patients. Rates are comparable in northern European countries.
   - **b.** UC incidence and prevalence rates are lower in southern Europe, Asia, and Central/South America.
2. **CD incidence and prevalence rates** have seen a marked rise since the early 1950s. There is a great variance in published incidence rates of CD. Areas of higher CD incidence are generally similar to those of higher UC incidence. CD has become more common than UC in some areas recently.
   - **a.** Reported CD incidence rate for North America ranges between 6 and 8 cases per 100,000 patients. CD prevalence rates in North America are estimated to be 100 to 200 cases per 100,000 patients. CD rates for northern Europe are comparable to those in North America.
   - **b.** Rates for southern Europe, Asia and Central/South America have been reported to be lower than those seen in North America and northern Europe.
3. **Geographic related components**
   - **a.** Northern regions have historically reported higher rates of IBD than southern regions. Rates in southern Europe have recently seen increasing incidence rates compared to historical rates.
   - **b.** CD rates have been reported to be higher in urban areas.
   - **c.** UC rates have been reported to be higher in rural areas.
   - **d.** IBD rates have historically been higher in developed countries compared to underdeveloped countries. This difference has been shown to decrease as underdeveloped areas are developed and a more western diet is adopted.
4. **Ethnic, racial, and socioeconomic components**
   - **a.** IBD, CD in particular, development risk is higher in Jews of European decent than non-Jews. While IBD prevalence is reported to be higher in Jews compared to non-Jews, there is considerable variation within Jewish populations from different geographic locations.
   - **b.** Non-Jewish Whites historically have been considered to be at higher risk for IBD compared to African Americans but that difference has been questioned in recent published reports. Blacks in Africa tend to be at less risk for IBD than either North American Caucasians or African Americans.
   - **c.** Asians appear to be at lower risk for developing IBD than Caucasians but migrant Asians to the United Kingdom interestingly have been shown to be at higher risk for UC and nearly equal risk of developing CD compared to UK-born Caucasians.
   - **d.** Incidence rates of IBD have historically been reported to be higher in higher socioeconomic classes.
5. **Age and sex related components**
   - **a.** IBD is more common in young adult patients than older patients with peak age of onset between 15 and 30 years.
   - **b.** Men and women are at similar risk to develop IBD, with women having a slightly higher risk to develop CD and men a slightly higher risk of developing UC.

6. **Other contributing factors**
   a. Smoking has been associated with a decrease in UC rates (roughly 60% of rates seen in nonsmokers), but the risk factors to general health do not warrant forgoing counseling patients on the benefits of smoking cessation.
   b. Former smokers are at increased risk of developing UC.
   c. Smoking has been shown to be risk factor for developing CD (more than 1.75 times the rates seen in nonsmokers). CD patients who actively smoke also have increased morbidity compared to CD patients who stop smoking.
   d. Appendectomy has been shown to be protective with regard to development of UC.
   e. Use of oral contraceptives has been associated with increased risk of developing IBD.
7. **Genetic** predisposition to IBD is another area of recent research advances. Genetic predisposition to IBD is suggested by, among other factors, epidemiologic studies, studies of twins, family aggregation studies, and ethnic differences in disease patterns. The CARD15 (NOD2) genetic mutation, for example, is seen more often in CD than in the general population. The mutation has been associated with altered immune response to bacteria. There are limitations to CARD15 usefulness in clinical practice, but the identification of this mutation and others has opened the door for more work around genetic predisposition and possible disease mechanism. These may lead to new modes of therapy.

D. **Epidemiology of IBS**
1. IBS is reported to be more common in women than men.
2. IBS usually presents between the ages of 30 and 50 with significant decreases at ages greater than 50.
3. Prevalence seems to be equal in Caucasians and Blacks and less in Hispanics. Overall prevalence rates are estimated at 7% to 15% of the U.S. population.
4. IBS appears to be as common in Asian, South American, and India as in western countries.

E. **Description**
1. UC is chronic recurring mucosal inflammation of the colon.
   a. **Proctitis**: Inflammation of the rectum.
   b. **Proctosigmoiditis**: Colitis affecting the rectum and sigmoid colon.
   c. **Left-sided colitis**: Disease starting at the rectum and extending retrograde to the splenic flexure of the colon.
   d. **Pancolitis**: Disease affecting the entire colon.
   e. **Backwash ileitis**: Inflammation of the terminal ileum due to retrograde flow of colonic contents in pancolitis patients
2. CD is chronic recurring transmural inflammation of the gastrointestinal tract.
   a. **Ileocolitis**: The most common form of CD, affecting the ileum and colon.
   b. **Ileitis**: CD affecting the ileum.
   c. **Gastroduodenal Crohn disease**: CD affecting the stomach and duodenum.
   d. **Jejunoileitis**: CD producing inflammation of the jejunum and ileum.
   e. **Crohn (granulomatous) colitis**: CD affecting only the colon.
3. **IBS**
   a. IBS is recognized as being part of **functional bowel disease**.
   b. IBS is characterized by symptoms of abdominal pain or discomfort that is associated with disturbed defecation patterns. IBS is typically of a constipation predominant (IBS-C) or diarrhea predominant (IBS-D) type with a minority of patients alternating between the two (IBS-A) or of a mixed presentation (IBS-M).

F. **Etiology**
1. **IBD** is thought to be caused by a poorly understood compilation of environmental, genetic factors, and possibly infectious agents. IBD is likely a result of multiple environmental factors eliciting an abnormal immune response in genetically susceptible individuals. There is significant overlap between the clinical presentation of UC and CD, the two main idiopathic inflammatory disease states, which make up IBD, and as such clear differential diagnosis between UC and CD is not always possible.
   a. There is clear evidence of immune system activation with subsequent infiltration of the tissue by lymphocytes, macrophages, and other cells. The exact trigger of this apparent poorly regulated immune response has yet to be defined.

b. Possible mechanisms postulated for IBD disease initiation include virus or bacterial infection, dietary antigens or inappropriate immune response to normally nonantigenic microbes, and the possibility of an inappropriate immune response to intestinal autoantigens expressed on the intestinal epithelium.
c. Regardless of cause there appears to be failure of normal suppressor mechanisms with a resultant overly vigorous and abnormally long immune response to a disease trigger.
d. IBD occurs 30 to 100 times more frequently in first-degree relatives of IBD patients compared to the general population.
e. **Infectious colitis** can mimic IBD. Differential diagnosis includes bacterial, protozoal, and viral pathogens (notably *Clostridium difficile*, fungal, protozoal, viral, and helminthic pathogens).
f. **Ischemic colitis** and **neoplastic** diseases such as cecal adenocarcinoma, lymphoma, and metastatic cancers may also present like IBD.
g. **Microscopic colitis** and other inflammatory diseases such as **celiac sprue** and **eosinophilic colitis** can present in much the same manner as IBD.
h. **Drug-induced enterocolitis** can induce IBD-like symptoms. The most commonly implicated classes of drugs are nonsteroidal anti-inflammatory drugs (NSAIDs), gold compounds, oral contraceptives, enteric potassium supplements, pancreatic enzymes, phospho soda bowel preps, and thermal injury secondary to colostomy irrigation.
i. Other possibly confounding diseases include **endometriosis** and **diverticular disease**.

2. IBS

a. The exact cause of IBS is unknown and no anatomic cause has yet to be elucidated.
b. Possible comorbid factors such as viral or bacterial gastroenteritis, emotional health, diet, environmental, concurrent drug therapy, and hormones have been implicated in GI dysmotility.
c. Anxiety disorders, particularly panic disorder; major depressive disorder; and somatization disorder, have also been implicated as possible initiating factors for IBS.
d. Learned aberrant illness behavior where patients may tend to express emotional conflict as a GI complaint, usually abdominal pain, may also be a contributing disease state. The clinician evaluating patients with IBS, particularly those with refractory symptoms, should investigate for unresolved psychological issues, including the possibility of sexual or physical abuse.

G. Pathophysiology

1. IBD

a. **UC.** Physiologic changes in UC begin with edema followed by loss of fine vascular pattern and increased mucosal friability. Ulceration, exudates and pseudopolyps may also be present. With longer disease history, the colon may begin to become featureless and tubular in nature. UC tends to occur in a **contiguous** manner.
b. **CD.** Inflammation and subsequent injury of tissue known as cryptitis leads to crypt abscess and subsequently focal aphthoid ulceration. The inflammatory process can progress with influx and proliferation of macrophages and other inflammatory cells. Transmural inflammation may lead to lymphedema and bowel wall thickening. This thickening can lead to fibrosis. Affected areas are usually sharply demarcated from normal adjacent tissue and give rise to the **skip lesion** appearance of CD.

2. IBS

a. Abnormalities in intestinal motility in IBS appear to be related to underlying muscle dysfunction as well as hyperactive response to initiating factors such as food or parasympathomimetic drugs.
b. Abnormal increases in frequency and amplitude of contractions can lead to functional constipation while diminished motor function of the underlying musculature can lead to diarrhea.
c. Hypersensitivity to normal amounts of intraluminal distention exists, as does a heightened perception of pain in the presence of normal quantity and quality of intestinal gas.
d. The pain of IBS may be caused by abnormally strong contraction of the intestinal smooth muscle or by increased sensitivity of the intestine to distention.

e. Hypersensitivity to the hormones gastrin and cholecystokinin may also be present. However, hormonal fluctuations have not correlated with clinical symptoms.
f. The caloric density of food intake may increase the magnitude and frequency of myoelectrical activity and gastric motility. Fat ingestion may cause a delayed peak of motor activity, which can be exaggerated in IBS.
g. The first few days of menstruation can lead to transiently elevated prostaglandin E_2, resulting in increased pain and diarrhea.

H. Clinical presentation

1. **UC.** Most patients will present with symptoms related to altered stool frequency, bowel sensation, and abdominal pain.
   a. Most UC cases begin as mild disease and worsens as the disease course progresses.
   b. UC usually follows a chronic intermittent course.
   c. Quiescent periods tend to be long with acute attacks interspersed.
   d. Attacks or flares can last weeks to months.
   e. Some patients suffer from continuous disease.
   f. Severe UC can result in **toxic megacolon**, a life-threatening condition.
   g. Elderly patients can rarely present with constipation secondary to rectal spasm.
   h. **Typical presenting symptoms of UC are as follows:**
      (1) Increased stool frequency
      (2) Hematochezia
      (3) Tenesmus
      (4) Lower left quadrant pain
      (5) Nausea, vomiting, and weight loss (usually only in severe disease)
   i. **Extraintestinal manifestations of UC**
      (1) Arthralgias
      (2) Ankylosing spondylitis
      (3) Pyoderma gangrenosum, erythema nodosum
      (4) Aphthous ulcers
      (5) Iritis and uveitis
2. **CD.** Many patients present with acute symptoms mimicking appendicitis or intestinal obstruction. CD can be exacerbated by infections, smoking, and NSAID use. While not well correlated in controlled trials, stress is often implicated by patients and family members as a contributing factor.
   a. A significant number of patients have a history of perianal disease, especially fissures and fistulas, which are sometimes the most prominent or even initial complaint.
   b. Extraintestinal manifestations can be more prominent than GI symptoms in pediatric patients.
   c. **Typical presenting symptoms of CD are as follows:**
      (1) Abdominal pain
      (2) Diarrhea
      (3) Weight loss
      (4) Fever
   d. **Extraintestinal manifestations of CD**
      (1) Arthralgias
      (2) Acute peripheral arthritis
      (3) Ankylosing spondylitis, peripheral arthritis
      (4) Erythema nodosum, pyoderma gangrenosum, Sweet syndrome
      (5) Iridocyclitis, uveitis, and episcleritis
3. **IBS**
   a. IBS symptoms are frequent in patients with active disease.
   b. Symptoms may be classified with either the new **Rome III criteria** or may still be classified with the **Rome II criteria**, which center around bowel movement and abdominal pain. The clinical symptoms are the same regardless of how they are classified.
      (1) Abdominal pain has been characterized as crampy, localized to the lower left abdomen with variable intensity. Patient presentation is highly variable with regard to intensity, location, and duration of pain. Some women will have exacerbations coinciding with menstrual periods.

(2) Alteration of bowel habits is the second major identifying symptom of IBS. They include diarrhea, constipation, mixed, and alternating diarrhea and constipation.

(3) IBS can also present with bloating, gas, belching, heartburn, reflux disease, achalasia, early feeling of fullness on eating and nausea, painful menstruation, sexual dysfunction, and frequent or urgent urination.

c. IBS tends to wax and wane over the long term with patients having acute bouts of disease interspersed with periods of no disease. While total prevalence numbers remain relatively constant, studies of defined patient populations at various periods show the same number of active patients, but the individual patients may be different.

I. Clinical evaluation

1. **IBD** differences in typical clinical presentation between UC and CD are summarized in *Table 45-1*.

a. **UC**

(1) Patient symptoms are usually the first signs of disease. Diarrhea, bleeding, tenesmus, mucus in the stool, and pain are the most common.

(2) The severity of symptoms correlates with disease severity.

(3) Acute disease can be associated with increased C-reactive protein, platelet count, erythrocyte sedimentation rate (ESR), and a decrease in hemoglobin.

(4) Serum albumin can fall quickly in severe disease.

(5) Sigmoidoscopy can be useful for assessing disease severity and extent before therapy. Care must be used in severe disease as risk of perforation is increased.

b. **UC disease classification** according to extent (distal versus extensive) and severity is of use in determining therapy.

(1) **Mild** UC has been defined as less than four stools per day with or without blood, normal ESR.

(2) **Moderate** UC has been defined as more than four stools per day but minimal signs of toxicity (fever, tachycardia, anemia, or elevated ESR).

(3) **Severe** UC has been defined as more than six bloody stools per day, evidence of toxicity as demonstrated by fever, tachycardia, anemia, or elevated ESR (elevated ESR is not always present, even in the most severe UC).

Table 45-1 DIFFERENCES OF UC AND CD

	UC	CD
Abdominal pain	Infrequent	Frequent
Bloody diarrhea	Frequent	Occasional
Perianal involvement	Rare	Frequent
Perianal fistula	Rare	Frequent
Rectovaginal fistula	Rare	Common
Fever	Occasional	Frequent
Weight loss	Occasional	Frequent
Palpable mass	Rare	Common
Intra-abdominal abscess	Rare	Common
Bowel obstruction	Rare	Common
Antibiotic response	Rare	Frequent
Skip lesions	Rare	Frequent
Contiguous disease	Frequent	Infrequent
Effect of smoking	Often improves UC	Often worsens CD
Serologic markers		
ASCA+	15%	65%
p-ANCA+	70%	20%

ASCA, anti-*Saccharomyces cerevisiae* antibody; *p-ANCA*, perinuclear antineutrophil cytoplasmic antibody; *UC*, ulcerative colitis; *CD*, Crohn disease.

(4) **Fulminate** UC has been defined as more than 10 bowel movements, continuous bleeding, toxicity, abdominal tenderness and distension, need for blood transfusion, and colonic dilation (toxic megacolon).

(5) In addition to classifying UC as mild to fulminate, it is useful to ascertain the impact the disease is having on patient activity with a global assessment approach including extraintestinal manifestations, (ocular, oral, joint, skin, moods), general health (laboratory evaluation for anemia, liver function tests), quality of life (impairment at work or school, interpersonal relationships).

c. CD

(1) CD patients may present with elevated ESR; C-reactive protein; and, in more severe disease with hypoalbuminemia, anemia, and leukocytosis.

(2) CD can occur throughout the bowel and site of disease affects disease course and treatment choices.

(3) **Ileocolitis** is the most common form of CD. It has been characterized by right lower quadrant pain, diarrhea, and can mimic acute appendicitis. Pain can be colicky and usually precedes defecation and is relieved by defecation.

(4) **Jejunoileitis.** Extensive inflammation can lead to loss of absorptive surfaces with resultant malabsorption and steatorrhea. This malabsorptive state can lead to dietary deficiency, hypoalbuminemia, electrolyte imbalances, coagulopathy, and increased risk of bone fractures.

(5) **Colitis** patients tend to present with low grade fever, diarrhea, vomiting, and epigastric pain.

(6) **Perianal CD** patients may present with incontinence, stricture, anorectal fistula, and perirectal abscess.

d. CD classification based on severity and location is useful for determining therapy.

(1) **Mild-to-moderate disease** has been used to define CD in patients who are ambulatory, able to take food orally, no symptoms of dehydration, no signs of toxicity (high fever, rigors, prostration), no abdominal tenderness or painful mass, no obstruction, or weight loss $>$ 10%.

(2) **Moderate-to-severe disease** describes patients who have failed to respond to therapy for mild to moderate disease or patients with more prominent symptoms of fever, significant weight loss, abdominal pain or tenderness, intermittent nausea or vomiting (without obstruction), or anemia.

(3) **Severe to fulminant disease** describes patients with persisting symptoms despite therapy with steroids as outpatients, or patients with high fever, persistent vomiting, obstruction, rebound tenderness, cachexia, or evidence of abscess.

(4) **Remission** refers to patients who have responded to acute medical therapy or who are postsurgical intervention without gross evidence of residual CD. Patients who require steroids to maintain control of CD are considered **steroid dependant** and are not considered to be in remission.

(5) **CD disease location** is often classified as being ileocolic, small bowel, colonic, or anorectal. The **Vienna classification** of disease location and type of CD is also often used. CD type is recognized to change with regard to type and location during disease course.

(a) **Terminal ileum** disease is CD in less than one-third of small bowel with or without spillover into the cecum.

(b) **Colon** CD is colonic involvement anywhere from the cecum to the rectum without small bowel or upper gastrointestinal disease.

(c) **Ileocolon** is CD of the terminal ileum and any location between the ascending colon and rectum.

(d) **Upper GI** CD is disease in any location proximal to the terminal ileum, with or without involvement distal to the terminal ileum.

(e) Type of disease is described as **inflammatory**, **stricturing**, **or penetrating**.

(6) The **Crohn Disease Activity Index**, or **CDAI**, is a validated measurement tool used to assess clinical improvement. The CDAI is a complete scoring system of subjective aspects

and objective observations. It is not normally used in clinical practice but is extensively used in clinical research. Crohn disease severity, as defined by the CDAI, breaks down into the following stratifications:

(a) A score of 150 or less is considered clinical remission.
(b) A score of more than 150 up to 450 is considered mild to moderate disease.
(c) A score of over 450 is considered severe disease.

2. IBS

a. Diagnosis of IBS commonly includes identifying positive symptoms by medical history. This can be guided by older **Rome II criteria** or the recently published **Rome III criteria**. Physical exam is also done to exclude non-IBS disease (abdominal mass, palpable liver, etc.) as the majority of IBS patients do not have these physical abnormalities. Both patient history and physical exam are also needed to exclude IBD and microscopic and eosinophilic colitis, which can present in similarly to IBS.

b. Rome II diagnostic criteria for IBS

(1) At least 12 weeks, which need not be consecutive, in the preceding 12 months of abdominal discomfort or pain that has two of three features:
(a) Pain relieved by defecation; and/or
(b) pain onset associated with a change in frequency of stool; and/or
(c) pain onset associated with a change in form (appearance) of stool.

(2) Symptoms that cumulatively support the diagnosis of IBS:
(a) Abnormal stool frequency (for research purposes, "abnormal" may be defined as greater than three bowel movements per day and less than three bowel movements per week);
(b) abnormal stool form (lumpy/hard or loose/watery stool);
(c) abnormal stool passage (straining, urgency, or feeling of incomplete evacuation);
(d) passage of mucus; and
(e) bloating or feeling of abdominal distension. The diagnosis of a functional bowel disorder (IBS) always presumes the absence of a structural or biochemical explanation for the symptoms.

c. Rome III diagnostic criteria for IBS

(1) Recurrent abdominal pain or discomfort at least 3 days per month in the last 3 months associated with two or more of the following:
(a) Improvement with defecation
(b) Onset associated with a change in a frequency of stool
(c) Onset associated with a change in form (appearance) of stool

(2) Criteria fulfilled for the last 3 months with symptoms onset at least 6 months prior to diagnosis.

(3) Discomfort means an uncomfortable sensation not described as pain.

(4) In pathophysiology, research, and clinical trials, a pain/discomfort frequency of at least 2 days a week during screening evaluation for subject eligibility

d. Routine blood testing is normal in most suspected IBS patients and helps rule out other possible diagnoses.

e. Sigmoidoscopy and colonoscopy are done to visualize the bowel when clinically appropriate to exclude other possible diagnoses.

J. Treatment objectives

1. IBD

a. Induce remission with control of acute inflammatory flare.
b. Maintain remission as long as possible.
d. Normalize bowel function when possible.
e. Maintain nutritional status.
b. Improve quality of life (QOL).

2. IBS

a. Alleviate discomfort.
b. Normalize bowel habits.
c. Minimize negative impact on patient QOL.

II. THERAPY

A. Overview of **agents used in IBD**

1. **Aminosalicylates** are generally considered to be effective therapy of UC, but are of little to no benefit for CD. The commercially available agents all deliver the active mesalamine or 5-aminosalicyclic acid (5-ASA) moiety. The oldest agent sulfasalazine (Azulfidine®) contains a 5-ASA molecule bound to sulfapyridine. This bond is cleaved by intestinal flora to release the active compound 5-ASA. Newer agents (enteric-coated mesalamine, olsalazine, balsalazide) have been developed to allow dosing without the sulfapyridine moiety, which has been implicated in many of the common adverse events and intolerances to sulfasalazine. Sulfasalazine is considered by many to be the first choice due to longer history of use, more convincing clinical trial data, and lower cost. Disadvantages of sulfasalazine are increased incidence of adverse events. Topical 5-ASA has been added to oral 5-ASA with improved response and time to response.

   a. **Mechanism of action.** The effectiveness of 5-ASA can be attributed to its anti-inflammatory properties. Through varied mechanisms including blockade of the inflammatory mediators interleukin-1 and tumor necrosis factor-alpha (TNF-α) as well as modulation of peroxisome proliferator activated receptor-γ (PPAR-γ) colonic inflammation is reduced. Though 5-ASA differs from salicylic acid by the addition of an amino group, 5-ASA drugs retain some variable effects on prostaglandin and prostacyclin synthesis that may be beneficial in IBD as well.

   b. **Administration and dosage.** There are currently several 5-ASA derivatives available (*Table 45-2*). Dosages in UC are based on disease location, severity, and overall patient condition. Enteric-coated or sustained-release products should not be crushed or chewed.

Table 45-2 AMINOSALICYLATES

Drug	Trade	Strength	Dosing (max)	Formulation	Delivery Site
Oral					
Sulfasalazine	Azulfidine®	500 mg tab	1000 mg t.i.d. (6 g/day)	Prodrug Sulfapyridine: **5-ASA**	Colon
	Azulfidine EN-tabs®	500 mg tab	1000 mg t.i.d. (6 g/day)	Prodrug Sulfapyridine: **5-ASA** enteric coated	Colon
Balsalazide	Colazal®	750 mg cap	2250 mg t.i.d. (6.75 m/day)	Prodrug 4-aminobenzoyl-β-alanine: **5-ASA**	Colon
Olsalazine	Dipentum®	250 mg cap	500 mg b.i.d. (3 gm/day)	Prodrug **5-ASA: 5-ASA**	Colon
Delayed-release					
Mesalamine	Asacol® Asacol HD®	400 mg tab 800 mg tab	800 mg t.i.d. (4.8 g/day)	Eudragit S pH-sensitive coating	Distal ileum, colon
Mesalamine	Apriso®	375 mg cap	1500 mg q.d.	Enteric coat, polymer matrix	Colon
Mesalamine	Lialda®	1200 mg tab	2400 mg q.d. (4.8 g/day)	Multimatrix system	Colon
Sustained-release					
Mesalamine	Pentasa®	250 mg cap 500 mg cap	1000 mg q.i.d.	Ethylcellulose granules	Stomach, colon
Topical					
Mesalamine	Rowasa®	4 gm/60 mL susp		Suspension for rectal administration	Rectum, splenic flexure
Mesalamine	Canasa®	500 mg sup 1000 mg sup		Suppository	Rectum

5-ASA, 5-aminosalicylic acid.

c. **Precautions and adverse effects**

(1) **Sulfasalazine:** The most common adverse events are fever, dizziness, headache, itching, rash, photosensitivity, GI upset, nausea, vomiting, diarrhea, reversible oligospermia and less commonly, Stevens–Johnson syndrome, Lyell syndrome, granulocytopenia, leucopenia, thrombocytopenia, aplastic anemia, hemolytic anemia, and hepatitis. Intolerance of the sulfapyridine moiety of sulfasalazine is common and is implicated in many adverse events associated with sulfasalazine. Sulfasalazine can interfere with the absorption of folic acid, thus it is advisable for such patients to take folic acid supplements.

(2) **Mesalamine, olsalazine, balsalazide:** The most common adverse events are diarrhea, headache, abdominal pain, cramps, flatulence, and less commonly skin rash. Rarely more serious side effects such as hepatotoxicity or acute or chronic renal injury have been reported.

d. **Significant interactions.** The aminosalicylates may increase risk of toxicity and leukopenia when given in combination with mercaptopurine by decreasing mercaptopurine clearance. 5-ASA drugs have also been associated rarely with exacerbation of IBD. Concomitant use of antacids or acid lowering agents may affect release characteristics of some of the formulations.

2. **Steroids.** Steroids are useful for patients refractory to 5-ASA or patients with severe symptoms requiring rapid control.

a. **Systemic corticosteroids** are effective treatment for acute UC and CD. Use as maintenance therapy for IBD is normally avoided as the risk of systemic adverse effects outweighs limited benefit. **Steroid dependency**, when a patient is unable to be tapered completely off of steroids, does occur and should not be confused with maintenance.

b. **Topical and nonsystemic steroids** in the form of enemas, suppositories, and ileal release formulations have been effective in treating IBD. The rectally delivered topical formulations of steroids are of particular use in left-sided disease. Budesonide (Entocort®) is an oral steroid delivered in a controlled release formulation which acts in a topical manner owing to very high first-pass metabolism by the liver. Budesonide has been shown to be effective in acute IBD when the targeted release formulation is able to reach the site of disease.

c. **Mechanism of action.** The glucocorticoid and mineralocorticoid effects of the steroids used in IBD are wide ranging. The anti-inflammatory effects are likely due to glucocorticoid suppression of proinflammatory cytokines.

d. **Precautions and adverse effects.** Therapy with oral and intravenous (IV) corticosteroids produce systemic effects, can impact multiple organ systems, and should be closely monitored for adverse events.

(1) Adverse effects of steroids in IBD therapy are related to dose and length of dosing and are the typical glucocorticoid and mineralocorticoid effects seen with exogenous steroid therapy.

(2) Systemic steroids are more prone to inducing adverse effects. Topical delivery and targeted delivery of low bioavailability steroids have been developed to reduce the risk of adverse effects.

(3) Minimizing duration of therapy as well as tapering patients off of systemic steroids are also methods of minimizing adverse effects as much as possible.

3. **Azathioprine (Imuran®) and 6-mercaptopurine (6-MP; Purinthol®)** are effective at inducing and maintaining remission in IBD. Response is slow and may take months to be fully effective. 6-MP or azathioprine are effective for patients who do not respond to oral steroids but are not so acutely ill so as to require IV therapy.

a. **Mechanism of action.** Azathioprine and 6-MP are purine antimetabolite drugs, which interfere with DNA synthesis, with disruption of the inflammatory response seen in IBD.

b. **Dosing and administration.** There is known metabolic differences with regard to **thiopurine methyltransferase (TPMT)** activity, which can lead to toxicity in patients with low or absent TPMT activity. Testing for TPMT phenotype can be useful in initial dosing. Consensus on the value of monitoring of metabolite levels during therapy has not been reached. Monitoring complete blood counts 4 weeks after starting therapy and then monthly during therapy should be done to monitor for toxicity. Azathioprine is 50% 6-MP by molecular weight and equivalent doses are twice that of 6-MP.

c. **Precautions and adverse effects.** Bone marrow suppression. Both azathioprine and 6-MP have been implicated in increased risk for Epstein Barr related non-Hodgkin lymphoma. This risk appears to be small but is serious.

4. **Methotrexate (Rheumatrex®)** given parenterally is an effective treatment for inducing remission, maintaining remission, and steroid sparing in CD. Parenteral methotrexate is also effective for maintaining remission in CD. Methotrexate appears to be of little use in UC.
   a. **Mechanism of action.** Methotrexate is a folate analog and inhibits dihydrofolate reductase with multiple modes of anti-inflammatory effects.
   b. **Dosing and administration.** A 25 mg intramuscular (IM) weekly has been shown to be effective for inducing remission of active CD, 15 mg IM weekly has been shown to be effective at maintaining remission and as steroid sparing therapy. Oral methotrexate 12.5 to 25.0 mg per week does not appear to be as effective as parenteral dosing.
   c. **Precautions and adverse effects.** Methotrexate is a known teratogen and should be avoided or used with extreme caution in patients of child-bearing age (female and male) and only when all other therapies have been ineffective and the patients understand the risks involved. The doses used in CD are lower than those used in oncology and the adverse events seen are generally less severe. The most common risks are rash, nausea, pneumonitis or *Mycoplasma* pneumonia, and elevated serum transaminases. CD patients treated with methotrexate appear to be at low risk for hepatic toxicity. It is important to avoid alcohol consumption as it can increase the risk of hepatic toxicity in CD patients on methotrexate.

5. **Cyclosporine (Neoral®) and tacrolimus (Prograf®)** are potent immunosuppressive agents that have been shown to be effective in IBD. They are typically used for severe acute IBD as there is little data to support efficacy in mild disease to offset the potential toxicities of these agents.
   a. **Mechanism of action.** Both cyclosporine and tacrolimus are calcineurin inhibitors and are potent inhibitors of T-lymphocyte activation.
   b. **Dosing and administration.** Before therapy is initiated, patients should be screened for potential drug interactions, normal renal function, cholesterol levels, blood pressure, and electrolyte status to help avoid toxicity.
      (1) Cyclosporine is started IV at 2 to 4 mg/kg/day and titrated to levels of 250 to 350 ng/mL.
      (2) Tacrolimus is initiated at 0.1 to 0.15 mg/kg/day by month and titrated to trough concentrations of 10 to 15 ng/mL.
      (3) Patients who respond are discharged on oral drug. Oral cyclosporine is dosed at twice the IV dose divided b.i.d.
      (4) Azathioprine or 6-MP is added as soon as possible and oral systemic steroids are often given concomitantly also for 3 to 4 months.
      (5) Cyclosporine and tacrolimus are normally stopped at 3 to 4 months. A steroid taper is also started at 3 to 4 months and should be done over 4 to 8 weeks.
   c. **Precautions and adverse events.** Cyclosporine and tacrolimus both have short- and long-term adverse events that can be serious. The most commonly seen in IBD patients are paresthesias, hypertension, hypertrichosis, renal insufficiency, infection, gingival hyperplasia and seizure. Patients should be closely monitored for effects on blood pressure, electrolytes, renal function, and cholesterol. Hypocholesterolemia and hypomagnesemia increase the risk of seizure.
   d. **Significant interactions.** Cyclosporine and tacrolimus are substrates of cytochrome P450-3A4 and P-glycoprotein enzymes. Significant and harmful alterations in cyclosporine and tacrolimus blood concentrations have been described as a result of concomitant administration of drugs that are also substrates or modifiers of these enzymes. Care must be used in concomitant dosing of these agents with other drugs that can adversely affect renal function such as NSAID. Cyclosporine has been noted to increase methotrexate and methotrexate metabolite concentrations.

6. **Biologics.** Infliximab (Remicade®), adalimumab (Humira®), and certolizumab pegol (Cimzia®) are currently the main biologic therapies used in IBD (*Table 45-3*). These agents are **anti-tumor necrosis factor-alpha (anti-TNF-α)** antibodies. All three agents are indicated for inducing and

Table 45-3 BIOLOGIC THERAPIES OF NOTE IN IBD

Drug	Trade	Mechanism	Efficacy in IBD
Adalimumab	Humira®	Fully human IgG_1 monoclonal antibody to TNF	Effective in CD
Infliximab	Remicade®	Chimeric (mouse/human) IgG_1 monoclonal antibody to TNF	Effective therapy in CD and UC. Primary biologic therapy used in IBD.
Certolizumab pegol	Cimzia®	Humanized pegylated Fab fragment TNF antibody	Approved for CD in April 2008. Effective in CD.
Natalizumab	Tysabri®	Humanized IgG_4 monoclonal antibody to α4-integrin that selectively inhibits leukocyte adhesion	Removed from U.S. market in 2005 secondary to association with progressive multifocal leukoencephalopathy (PML). Natalizumab was made available again in 2006 via a restrictive company administered access program. Place in therapy is yet to be fully elucidated and the benefit must clearly outweigh the risks.
Etanercept	Enbrel®	is a p75-soluble TNF receptor FC fusion protein that binds TNF	Not of benefit.

CD, Crohn's disease; *IgG*, immunoglobulin G; *TNF*, tumor necrosis factor; *UC*, ulcerative colitis; *FC*, (please spellout); *IBD*, inflammatory bowel disease.

maintaining clinical remission of CD. Infliximab is also indicated in treating enterocutaneous and enterovaginal fistulae and maintaining remission of fistulizing CD. Infliximab is also effective in acute and quiescent UC. A fourth biologic agent, natalizumab (Tysabri®), is a humanized monoclonal antibody directed at α4-integrin on the surface of white blood cells. It is approved for use in CD as well as multiple sclerosis.

a. **Anti-TNF-α therapy mechanism of action.** Tumor necrosis factor-alpha (TNF-α) is a cytokine involved in multiple proinflammatory and proliferative pathways in IBD. These agents bind TNF-α preventing its binding to cell surface receptors and subsequently decreases inflammatory cytokines and increasing apoptosis of activated T lymphocytes and monocytes. Infliximab is a chimeric mouse–human monoclonal anti-TNF-α antibody. It is made up of human IgG_1 constant regions, human κ light chains, and monoclonal murine regions that recognize TNF-α. Adalimumab is a recombinant human IgG_1 monoclonal antibody with human heavy and light chain variable regions and human IgG_1:k constant regions. Certolizumab pegol is a humanized Fab fragment of an anti-TNF-α monoclonal antibody that has been pegylated to increase half-life of the antibody.

b. **Dosing and administration**

(1) Infliximab initial dosing is 5 mg/kg in a three-dose induction regimen of day 0, 2, and 6 weeks. Duration of therapeutic effect appears to be 8 to 10 weeks and dosing every 8 weeks has been advocated following a response to initial dosing. Formation of antibodies to infliximab (ATI) during infliximab use has been described. The presence of ATI may increase infusion-related adverse reactions, delayed-type hypersensitivity reactions, and may decrease the effectiveness of infliximab therapy. Strategies to reduce ATI formation include a regularly scheduled maintenance regimen of infliximab (versus episodic treatment) and the use of concomitant administration of azathioprine, 6-MP, or methotrexate. These immunosuppressant drugs have not been shown to improve clinical disease control when given concomitantly with infliximab.

(2) Adalimumab is initially dosed 160 mg on day 1 as four 40 mg injections on the first day or two 40 mg injections per day for 2 days, followed by 80 mg 2 weeks later or at day 15. Two weeks later (day 29) maintenance therapy is begun at 40 mg every other week. Formation of anti-adalimumab antibodies has been reported in 3% of patients.

(3) Certolizumab pegol is given as a 400 mg injection on day 0 and weeks 2 and 4. If response occurs, dosing may continue with 400 mg every 4 weeks. Formation of anti-certolizumab antibodies has been reported in 8% of certolizumab treated patients.

c. **Precautions and adverse effects.** Anti-TNF-α therapies share similar precautions and adverse effect profiles.
   (1) Acute infusion or injection-related reactions can occur. Risk of such a reaction is greater (22%) with infliximab use than with adalimumab (1%) or certolizumab (rare). Severe anaphylactic reactions are rare.
   (2) Delayed hypersensitivity reactions including myalgias, rash, fever, arthralgias, pruritus, edema, urticaria, sore throat, and dysphagia occur 3 to 12 days after infliximab infusion and are much less common at approximately 2% of patients receiving maintenance infliximab therapy.
   (3) All anti-TNF-α antibodies carry **black box warnings** for increased risk of opportunistic infections (e.g., tuberculosis, invasive fungal infections such as histoplasmosis, blastomycosis, or pneumocystis, viral infections such as hepatitis B). Use of concomitant immunosuppressive agents may increase risk of infection. Patients should be tested for tuberculosis prior to use of these agents and their use should be avoided or discontinued in the case of active infections.
   (4) All anti-TNF-α antibodies carry **black box warnings** for increased risk of lymphomas and other malignancies. Use of concomitant immunosuppressive agents may increase this risk.

d. Anti-α4 integrin antibody mechanism of action. Binding of the α4-integrin protein by natalizumab effectively interrupts normal leukocyte trafficking across endothelial layers to areas of inflammation.

e. Anti-α4 integrin antibody dosing. Natalizumab is given as an intravenous infusion of 300 mg every month. Availability of natalizumab is restricted. It is available only through entities registered with the TOUCH prescribing program.

f. Anti-α4 integrin antibody adverse effects. Common adverse effects include headache, arthralgia, and fatigue. More serious adverse effects include increased risk of opportunistic infections and acute hypersensitivity reactions. Prescribing information for natalizumab also carries a **black box warning** for increased risk of progressive multifocal leukoencephalopathy or PML. There is no treatment for PML. Patients are to be monitored closely for symptoms so that natalizumab may be discontinued. Typical symptoms associated with PML include progressive weakness on one side of the body or clumsiness of limbs, and changes in vision, thinking, memory, and orientation. These lead to confusion and personality changes. PML symptoms progress over days to weeks. Concomitant use of other immunosuppressive agents such as azathioprine, 6-MP, methotrexate, and so forth is not advised due to increased risk of serious adverse effects.

7. **Antibiotics.** No specific infectious agent has been identified as the single causative factor in either UC or CD.
   a. Use of broad-spectrum antibiotics in IBD is limited to empiric treatment of fulminant disease or in patients with toxic megacolon where short-term use of these antibiotics can be justified due to the increased risk of perforation or bacteremia.
   b. Use of select antibiotics such as metronidazole (Flagyl®), ciprofloxacin (Cipro®), clofazimine (Lamprene®), or rifaximin (Xifaxan®) with the specific goal of remission of acute IBD is controversial. While few clinical trials and a recent meta-analysis indicate potential benefit, design limitations temper the strength of those findings.
   c. Metronidazole and ciprofloxacin are used widely by convention as maintenance therapy in CD but controlled trial results do not conclusively support this use.
   d. Metronidazole has been useful in patients suffering from **pouchitis** postbowel resection surgery that involves formation of a pouch.
   e. Metronidazole and ciprofloxacin both would appear to be of some benefit in treating patients with fistulous IBD.

8. **Probiotic and prebiotic therapy.** Probiotic involves using exogenously administered bacteria such as *Lactobacillus GG*, *Saccharomyces boulardii* and nonpathogenic *Escherichia coli* among others in an attempt to normalize the intestinal environment flora and thus decrease inflammatory triggers. Controlled trials of probiotic therapy in IBD have yet to clearly define clinical utility. There is little evidence to support their use in acute IBD. However, recent meta-analyses suggest potential benefit of probiotics, when combined with conventional therapies, for mainte-

nance of UC but not CD. Remission maintenance of pouchitis with VSL #3, a probiotic preparation of four lactobacilli strains and three *Bifidobacterium* and one strain of *Streptococcus* was shown to be of benefit. Prebiotics are orally administered substances like nondigested carbohydrates with the goal of facilitating growth of commensal gut flora to displace possible antigenic microorganisms. There is little data to support prebiotics at this time.

9. **Antispasmodics and antidiarrheals.** Cramping and abdominal IBS-like symptoms are often noted in IBD patients. Use of symptomatic therapies is not well defined in the published IBD literature as most research is aimed at the inflammatory process. Once active inflammation is controlled or ruled out, anticholinergic antispasmodics are frequently used judiciously to treat cramping or discomfort in IBD inflammation, as are antidiarrheals in mild or quiescent disease. All of these agents should be avoided in serious disease as they may further impair intestinal motility and increase risk of toxic megacolon.
10. **Antidepressants and anxiolytics** have been used when specific patient symptoms warrant their use as adjuvant therapy. Universal use of such therapies is not supported by available evidence.
11. **Analgesics.** There is rarely a need for pain control in UC as the disease is limited to the mucosa of the colon with limited involvement of tissue containing pain receptors. Narcotics are to be avoided in UC therapy outside of perioperative situations as they increase the risk of toxic megacolon and can mask signs of perforation. NSAID medications should be avoided as they have been implicated in inducing IBD flares.
12. **Surgery.** Surgical resection of the colon is considered curative in UC. Surgical resection of bowel in CD is not curative as the disease will often recur at the resection site as well as other sites.
    - **a.** Surgery in UC is most commonly indicated for disease refractory to medical therapy, inability to wean the patient off of high corticosteroid dosages, serious drug side effects or intolerance, and occurrence of premalignant or malignant changes in the colon.
    - **b.** Approximately one-third of UC patients eventually undergo colectomy. Patients with extensive disease (pancolitis) undergo colectomy more than patients with less extensive (distal) disease and also usually require colectomy sooner than patients with less extensive disease.
    - **c.** **UC surgery** can be divided into two types, those that preserve continence and those which do not and subsequently require appliances to collect the fecal material.
        - (1) **Proctocolectomy with permanent ileostomy** is the oldest procedure and involves formation of an abdominal stoma connected to the ileum. An external appliance is used to collect fecal material.
        - (2) **Proctocolectomy with continent ileostomy** involves creation of a pouch inside the abdomen using the terminal ileum. A small leakproof opening is created in the abdomen wall, and the pouch is periodically drained.
        - (3) **Colectomy with ileorectal anastomosis** involves removing diseased large bowel and reattaching the remaining small intestine to a preserved rectum. While bowel movements via the rectum are preserved patients are at risk of relapse as the rectum is often involved in UC.
        - (4) **Ileal pouch anal anastomosis (IPAA)** is the most common surgical procedures done for IBD. The large bowel and rectum are removed, with preservation of the anal sphincter. A tubular pouch is formed from the small intestine and attached to the preserved sphincters, which allows bowel movements without external bags or appliances. A temporary ileostomy is often used during healing.
    - **d.** **CD surgery** while not curative, is required in a very high percentage of patients. Surgical intervention can be limited to specific areas of diseased bowel or total ileostomy or colectomy. Surgery is most commonly indicated in CD refractory to medical therapy, medication side effects, or steroid dependency.
        - (1) Small bowel resection is preferred in most patients with ileal or ileocolic CD. Primary anastomosis versus ileostomy (permanent or temporary) choice is based on patient status and CD severity.
        - (2) Large bowel CD may require varying degrees of resection secondary to the typical CD disease course involving "skip lesions." Primary anastomosis of preserved bowel may be preferred for patient QOL reasons but has been linked to earlier reoccurrence of CD.
        - (3) Colectomy with ileorectal anastomosis, while increasing risk of earlier CD recurrence, is useful in young patients where ileostomy may adversely affect QOL.

(4) Proctocolectomy and ileostomy is preferred in patients with extensive perianal disease or pancolitis CD.

(5) Strictureplasty can also be useful in stricturing CD.

e. **Pouchitis** is the most common complication of continent ileostomy and IPAA. It has been characterized as a syndrome including acute nonspecific inflammation of the reservoir pouch formed during surgery with unknown etiology.

(1) Idiopathic pouchitis must be differentiated from inflammation of the pouch due to anastomotic stricture and infection due to known pathogens.

(2) Broad-spectrum antibiotics have been the main medical therapy used for pouchitis. Metronidazole and ciprofloxacin have both been effective for acute pouchitis and have also been used as maintenance therapy.

(3) Probiotic therapy with VSL#3 has been of benefit also.

(4) Pharmacologic therapy used in IBD has been shown to be of mixed efficacy in pouchitis. Surgical revision may be required in chronic pouchitis unresponsive to medical therapy.

13. **Other therapy**

a. **Nutritional** issues are important to consider in IBD. While conclusive evidence does not exist showing particular foods cause IBD, special attention to diet in patients with IBD can be beneficial.

(1) Nutritional and hydration deficiencies can occur secondary to a poorly functioning GI tract and the chronic nature of IBD.

(2) Foods that are known to exacerbate an individual patient's IBD should be avoided and a well-balanced diet should be encouraged to maintain nutritional status. Restrictive diets are not normally required. Simply limiting offending foods while encouraging a balanced diet is usually sufficient to maintain nutritional status.

(3) Parenteral feeding is seldom used long term in IBD but can be useful to improve or maintain nutritional status in severely ill patients.

b. **Emotional factors.** Due to the chronic nature of IBD, many sufferers have need for emotional support during the course of their disease. While IBD does not appear to be directly affected by emotional state, the QOL experienced by these sufferers can be noticeably affected in a negative manner. Many will benefit greatly by support groups, continued open dialogue with their health care providers, and in less common cases, formal counseling or pharmacologic therapy may be needed.

B. **Drug therapy of UC**

1. Classifying UC based on anatomic disease extent is useful for determining medical therapy. Distal disease (below the splenic flexure) can be treated effectively with topical therapy. Extensive disease (extending proximal to the splenic flexure) normally requires systemic therapy. Severity of acute UC is also useful in determining medical therapy. Severity is generally defined as mild, moderate, severe, or fulminate.

2. **Management of acute mild–moderate UC distal disease.** Patients with mild to moderate distal UC respond well to oral or topical 5-ASA or topical steroids for inducing remission (control of inflammation).

a. Topical 5-ASA is superior to topical steroids or oral 5-ASA agents.

b. Topical 5-ASA plus oral 5-ASA is superior to either alone.

c. Topical 5-ASA may be effective in patients refractory to oral 5-ASA or topical steroids.

d. Oral plus topical therapy consisting of oral mesalamine 2.4 g/day in divided doses plus mesalamine 4 g/day enema may induce remission of UC more quickly.

e. Infrequently oral corticosteroids may be needed in patient's refractory to topical/oral 5-ASA agents and topical steroids in maximal doses (see oral corticosteroids under "Mild to moderate extensive or relapsing disease").

f. Therapy is largely determined by patient preference to therapy modality.

g. Oral 5-ASA doses for inducing remission in mild to moderate distal disease

(1) Sulfasalazine 3 to 6 g/day in three divided doses

(2) Mesalamine 2.4 to 4.8 g/day in divided doses where interval varies by product from one to four doses per day (see *Table 45-2*)

(3) Balsalazide 6.75 g/day in three divided doses

(4) Olsalazine 1.0 to 3 g/day in two divided doses

h. The oral 5-ASA drugs tend to work in 2 to 4 weeks and are effective in a high percentage of patients.

i. Clinical efficacy of the different oral agents is very similar. Choice is then influenced by adverse effect profile and cost.

j. Recent evidence suggests there is minimal benefit of 5-ASA oral doses greater than 2.4 g/day.

k. **Oral nonsystemic corticosteroids.** Budesonide is an oral corticosteroid that offers lower systemic exposure compared to prednisone secondary to high first-pass metabolism. Budesonide has been effective in UC treatment but is limited to UC when the ileal release formulation can reach the location of disease.

l. Topical therapy generally induces remission more quickly than oral therapy. Suppositories reach disease approximately 10 cm proximally. Foam products reach disease approximately 15 to 20 cm proximally. Enemas reach disease approximately to the splenic flexure (52 to 56 cm).

m. Topical 5-ASA for inducing and maintaining remission of UC
   (1) Mesalamine suppositories 1 gm/day in one or two divided doses (proctitis)
   (2) Mesalamine enemas 4 g/day (distal colitis proximally to the splenic flexure)

n. **Topical corticosteroids for inducing remission of UC**
   (1) Hydrocortisone enema 100 mg/day
   (2) Hydrocortisone foam, 10% one application (80 mg) q.d. to b.i.d.

3. **Maintenance of distal disease**
   a. **5-ASA** preparation dosages for maintaining remission of distal disease.
      (1) Balsalazide 3 to 6 g/day
      (2) Mesalamine 2.4 g/day
      (3) Mesalamine suppository 500 mg q.d. or b.i.d.
      (4) Mesalamine enema 2 to 4 g daily, every other day or every third day
      (5) Olsalazine 1 g/day
      (6) Sulfasalazine 2 g/day
      (7) Mesalamine 1.6 g orally per day plus 4 g enemas twice weekly is also effective.
   b. Dose reduction from amounts used during induction of remission of acute disease may be explored. Data suggest total daily doses of 5-ASA < 2 g are less effective than total daily doses ≥ 2 g.
   c. Corticosteroids, topical or oral, are not effective in maintaining UC remission and should not be used.

4. Acute **mild to moderate extensive or relapsing disease**
   a. **Oral 5-ASA**
      (1) Sulfasalazine 4 to 6 g/day in four divided doses. Doses less than 2 g/day appear to offer little benefit.
      (2) Newer 5-ASA preparations are generally considered to be equal to sulfasalazine with regard to efficacy, likely superior with regard to adverse events and tolerance but are more expensive. The dosages used are a minimum of 2.4 g/day of active 5-ASA moiety titrated up to a maximum of 4.8 g/day.
   b. **Oral steroids**
      (1) Prednisone 40 to 60 mg/day (modest efficacy gain with 60 mg compared to 40 mg) until significant clinical effect is seen followed by a dose taper of 5 to 10 mg weekly until a daily dose of 20 mg is reached. Tapering generally continues from here at 2.5 mg per week until the patient is weaned from oral steroids.
      (2) Higher doses for longer periods increase risk of corticosteroid-associated complications.
      (3) IBD patients receiving corticosteroids for greater than 3 months should be carefully monitored for presence of corticosteroid-associated complications such as hypertension, dyslipidemia, loss of bone mineral density, etc.
      (4) For patients on long-term corticosteroid, calcium supplementation at 1 to 1.5 g/day and vitamin D supplementation at 800 mg/day should also be considered.

5. **Maintenance of mild to moderate extensive or relapsing disease.** Sulfasalazine is as effective as equivalent doses of newer 5-ASA agents and is less costly in long-term therapy. Systemic corticosteroids as a rule are not accepted as long-term therapy options secondary to adverse events and

questionable therapeutic effect. 6-MP or azathioprine has been useful as steroid sparing agents and as long-term options to wean patients off of corticosteroids.

a. **Oral 5-ASA therapy**
   (1) Balsalazide 3 to 6 g/day
   (2) Mesalamine 2.4 to 4.8 g/day
   (3) Olsalazine 1 g/day
   (4) Sulfasalazine 2 to 4 g/day
b. **Immune modulators**
   (1) 6-MP 0.5 to 1.5 mg/kg once daily
   (2) Azathioprine 0.5 to 2.5 mg/kg once daily
   Doses are titrated to keep white blood cell count > 4000 cells/mm^3. Patients with thiopurine methyltransferase (TPMT) deficiency are at excess risk of bone marrow suppression given usual doses of 6-MP or azathioprine. Allopurinol inhibits metabolism of 6-MP and azathioprine. 6-MP and azathioprine doses should be reduced with concomitant use of allopurinol.

6. **Acute moderate-to-severe disease.** UC patients with moderate-to-severe disease may or may not require hospitalization. Infection with enteric pathogens should be ruled out. 5-ASA should be stopped in the acute setting to avoid intolerance issues and the rare instances of 5-ASA exacerbating colitis.
   a. **Corticosteroids.** Intensive IV steroid therapy is indicated for patients with severe disease who are hospitalized. Doses with prednisolone 40 to 60 mg, hydrocortisone 300 mg, or methylprednisolone 32 to 48 mg/day in divided doses or as continuous infusion have been shown to be effective. Higher doses are of limited benefit and increase risk of steroid toxicity. Patients with moderate-to-severe disease but not requiring hospitalization may be treated with oral doses on an outpatient basis.
   b. **Biologics**
      (1) Infliximab was more effective compared to placebo (reduced need for colectomy) for ambulatory patients refractory to or intolerant of systemic steroids.
      (2) Infliximab 5 mg/kg at 0, 2, and 6 weeks
         (a) ATI formation may be limited with concomitant dosing of azathioprine or 6-MP.
      (3) Other marketed anti-TNF-α antibodies may be effective in this role, however, studies are lacking.
   c. **Immune suppressants.** Failure to demonstrate significant improvement within 7 to 10 days is an indication for surgical resection or alternate IV therapy such as with cyclosporine.
      (1) IV cyclosporine at 2 to 4 mg/kg/day and titrated to blood levels between 200 and 400 ng/mL has been effective in a high percentage of patients who do not respond to maximal parenteral steroids.
         (a) Oral cyclosporine at twice the daily IV dose is given in divided doses (b.i.d.) with oral steroids once clinical remission is reached with IV cyclosporine. However, cyclosporine is not generally recommended for long-term maintenance due to significant adverse effects.
         (b) Sulfamethoxazole/trimethoprim (Bactrim®) should be added as prophylaxis against *Pneumocystis* pneumonia for patients on cyclosporine.
         (c) Relapse on 5-ASA therapy alone after remission induced with cyclosporine is frequent, and azathioprine or 6-MP can be beneficial when added for maintenance.
   d. Topical steroids may provide benefit in patients with rectal urgency or tenesmus.
   e. Empiric broad-spectrum antibiotics are of little use for the treatment of moderate-to-severe UC; however, their use is justified in the case of proven bacterial infection.
   f. When possible patients should be maintained on oral feedings with modified diet to reduce abdominal discomfort, diarrhea and bowel frequency. Total parenteral nutrition is used when oral feeds are not tolerated and can be especially useful in patients with severe nutritional depletion.
   g. In patients with signs of toxicity narcotics, antidiarrheals, and anticholinergics should be avoided as they can increase the risk of worsening colonic dilation and perforation.
7. **Maintenance moderate-to-severe disease**
   a. Oral 5-ASA agents–as with mild to moderate disease, these agents have been shown effective in preventing disease relapse.

b. Immune suppressants

(1) Azathioprine or 6-MP–are modestly effective for patients who have failed or are intolerant of 5-ASA agents. Because of the delay in onset of effect, optimal results are seen when these agents are started during induction of remission and continued into maintenance the phase.

c. Biologics

(1) Infliximab–in early studies, continued injections of infliximab at 5 mg/kg/dose at 8-week intervals have been shown effective in remission maintenance compared to placebo for patients intolerant of 5-ASA, corticosteroids, or azathioprine or 6-MP. Use of infliximab and other anti-TNF-α antibodies in this capacity continues to be investigated.

8. **Fulminant disease.** Patients with fulminant colitis or toxic megacolon are treated as severe and generally kept on bowel rest. Broad-spectrum antibiotics are often used empirically due to high risk of perforation. Any worsening of disease as evidenced by radiologic, clinical, or laboratory changes while on medical therapy is an indication for immediate colectomy.

C. **Drug therapy of CD** is dependant upon disease location, disease severity and complications if present. Patient's response to initial therapy should be evident within weeks. Once control of acute disease occurs, consideration of maintenance therapy is warranted. Failure of continued symptomatic improvement or worsening of symptoms by 3 to 4 months necessitates reconsideration of chosen therapy.

1. Mild to moderate acute CD

a. Budesonide orally

(1) Targeted delivery to ileum, works well in ileal or proximal colonic disease.

(2) 9 mg/day for 8 to 16 weeks

(3) Tapered 3 mg per week over 2 to 4 weeks

b. Oral broad-spectrum antibiotics have been used with limited controlled clinical data to support such use.

(1) Possibly more beneficial in patients with primary colonic involvement.

(2) Metronidazole 750 to 1500 mg/day

(3) Ciprofloxacin 1000 mg/day

c. If these therapies fail, the presentation can be considered refractory and treated as moderate to severe.

d. Historically, 5-ASA products have been used to induce and/or maintain remission of mild to moderate CD. More recent analyses question the benefit of 5-ASA for these patients.

2. Moderate-to-severe acute CD

a. Systemic steroids

(1) Oral prednisone 40 to 60 mg/day until symptom improvement (weeks) then initiate a tapering regimen.

(2) Hospitalization for IV corticosteroids may also be considered.

b. Methotrexate

(1) Methotrexate 25 mg/week IM, taper to 15 mg/week IM after 16 weeks

(2) Methotrexate use trended toward improvement in remission of disease. Best results seen when given with corticosteroids

(3) Methotrexate is an antimetabolite drug and will take considerable time to reach full effect, up to 3 to 4 months may be required.

(4) Concomitant use of oral 5-ASA or antibiotics with immunosuppressant therapy has not been shown to be of benefit in controlled trials.

c. Anti-TNF-α therapy

(1) For patients refractory to or do not tolerate systemic steroids and immunosuppressant therapy.

(2) In perianal fistulizing CD, infliximab is effective therapy.

(3) Infliximab 5 mg/kg at 0, 2, and 6 weeks

(a) Relapse at 1 year is high if infliximab stopped.

(b) ATI formation is common in noncontinuous therapy and may decrease efficacy of future courses of therapy. ATI formation may be limited with concomitant dosing of azathioprine, 6-MP, or methotrexate.

(c) Concomitant therapy with 5-ASA, steroids, or antibiotics is of little added benefit.

(4) Adalimumab 160 mg day 1 and 80 mg day 15 followed by 40 mg every other week starting on day 29.

(5) Certolizumab pegol is given as a 400 mg injection on day 0 and weeks 2 and 4.

d. **Other biologics**
   (1) Natalizumab has been shown successful in inducing remission of CD. Due to the risk of PML, its use is limited to cases failing all other therapies.

3. **Severe or fulminant acute CD** includes active disease of a severe nature, toxic enteritis or colitis, megacolon, small bowel obstruction, and abdominal abscess. The patients often require hospitalization secondary to severity of disease and risk of complications.
   a. Typical therapy may include
      (1) IV fluids and bowel rest (parenteral nutrition);
      (2) IV antibiotics with metronidazole, aminoglycosides, and broad-spectrum penicillin or third-generation cephalosporins empirically for possible abscess or infections; and
      (3) IV corticosteroids.
   b. Anti-TNF-α therapy with infliximab may be useful for patients who do not respond to IV corticosteroids.
   c. Natalizumab may be useful for patients not responding to anti-TNF-α therapy.
   d. Surgical intervention may be required in patients who do not respond to IV corticosteroids and infliximab.

4. **Maintenance of CD remission** strategies have been of questionable efficacy. Historically, long-term treatment with 5-ASA agents and broad-spectrum antibiotics has been advocated with a lack of convincing controlled clinical data to support these measures. Newer evidence-based approaches may change therapy strategies.
   a. **Immunosuppressants**
      (1) Azathioprine, 6-MP, or methotrexate have been used in maintenance but adverse events must be weighed carefully, especially in patients with mild disease.
      (2) Azathioprine, 6-MP, and methotrexate may be useful in patients unable to wean off systemic steroids.
   b. **Biologics.** Anti-TNF-α therapy is effective at inducing and maintaining clinical remission in Crohn disease.
      (1) **Infliximab 5 mg/kg infused every 8 weeks**
      (2) **Adalimumab 40 mg injection every 2 weeks**
      (3) **Certolizumab pegol 400 mg injection monthly**
      (4) Concomitant azathioprine, 6-MP, or methotrexate can also reduce ATI formation with infliximab injections and may increase efficacy.
      (5) Skillful monitoring is essential to successful use of these agents. All anti-TNF-α antibodies have black box warnings regarding infection and malignancies.
      (6) Efficacy of natalizumab for maintenance of CD remission appears to be similar to anti-TNF-α antibodies, however, due to risk of PML, its use is limited to those who have failed treatment with the former.
   c. Systemic steroids are normally avoided in long-term therapy secondary to systemic toxicity and lack of convincing data to support their use.
   d. Antibiotics have not been shown in controlled clinical trials to be effective in maintaining medically induced remission.

D. **IBS**

1. The treatment of IBS is based on the nature and severity of symptoms, correlation of symptoms to food intake and/or defecation, degree of functional impairment, and the presence of psychosocial or psychiatric disorders. Treatment is highly personalized, symptom based, and can be generalized as follows.

2. **Mild IBS** is the most common disease presentation and is normally associated with few psychosocial problems.
   a. Education about disease and support can be of great benefit.
   b. Diet and lifestyle changes
      (1) Specific foods are usually not as important as the size of meals with smaller meals being preferable. Care should be used and restrictive diets should be avoided.
      (2) Decrease fatty foods, gas-producing foods
      (3) Decrease alcohol
      (4) Decrease caffeine
      (5) Avoid dairy in lactose intolerant patients

(6) Excess fiber can also increase IBS symptoms
(7) Prepare strategies to handle stress

3. **Moderate IBS** symptoms, which are normally intermittent but can be disabling at times. These patients suffer from more symptom-related distress. Patient symptoms historically are also associated with more gut reactivity (worse with eating and better with defecation). Consider management strategies described earlier with drug therapy targeted predominant symptoms.

a. **Pain.** Consider use of anticholinergics or antispasmodics. These agents have shown benefit in relief of IBS-related abdominal pain. Caution of anticholinergic adverse effects (dry mouth, dizziness, visual changes, etc.) is advised with their use.
(1) Dicyclomine (Bentyl®) 10 to 20 mg PO 2 to 4 times daily
(2) Hyoscyamine (Anaspaz®, Levsin®) 0.125 to 0.25 mg PO q.i.d. (max 1.5 mg/day)
(3) Clidinium + chlordiazepoxide 2.5/5.0 mg (Librax®) 1 to 2 tabs PO a.c. & h.s.
(4) Hyoscyamine + scopalamine, atropine, phenobarbital (Donnatal®) 1 to 2 tabs q6 to 8 hrs
(5) Low dose tricyclic antidepressants (TCAs) can be effective for pain control. The dosages typically used are below effective doses used for clinical depression. TCA also may slow GI transit time and be useful in diarrhea predominate patient cases.
(a) Amitriptyline initially 10 mg at bedtime.
(b) Desipramine initially 10 mg at bedtime.

b. **Diarrhea.** Consider use of conventional antidiarrheals prior to trial of other agents.
(1) Diphenoxylate + atropine (Lomotil®) 0.025/2.5 mg two tabs PO q.i.d., maximum of eight tabs per day
(2) Loperamide (Imodium®) 4 mg followed by 2 mg after each unformed bowel movement up to a maximum of 16 mg/day
(3) Alosetron (Lotronex®) is a 5-HT_3-antagonist and is available in the United States through a manufacturer-sponsored access program and is only to be used for diarrhea-predominant IBS in women.
(a) Access to prescribe is restricted in the United States to a manufacturer administered program.
(b) Severe IBS dose in **women only** is 0.5 to 1.0 mg PO b.i.d.
(4) Rifaximin (Xifaxan®) is a nonabsorbable antibiotic indicated for traveler's diarrhea and hepatic encephalopathy. Rifaximin has been shown in phase III trials to be more effective than placebo in relieving symptoms in non–IBS-C patients.
(a) Rifaximin 550 mg t.i.d. for 2 weeks

c. **Constipation**
(1) **Fiber and bulking agents.** This class is often recommended as the first line for treating IBS-C. Various agents have shown some minimal benefit. Fiber supplementation can worsen bloating symptoms, so low-starting doses with upward titration are recommended.
(a) Psyllium 2.5 to 30.0 gm daily in divided doses.
(b) Methylcellulose 0.5 to 3.0 gm daily in divided doses
(c) Calcium polycarbophil 1.25 to 5.0 gm daily in divided doses
(2) **Laxatives.** Laxatives are an alternative first-line therapy for IBS-C. Their efficacy is less well-studied than bulking agents. Concerns with their use include worsening bloating or cramps and electrolyte loss. Osmotic laxatives are favored over stimulant laxatives.
(a) Polyethylene glycol (PEG, Miralax® and others) is an osmotic laxative solution that increases the amount of water in the intestinal tract to stimulate bowel movements. Potassium, sodium, and other minerals are also included to replace electrolytes that are passed from the body in the stool. Polyethylene glycol is available by prescription or OTC and is generally considered to be very safe for constipation and may be of benefit to IBS-C patients. Caution should be used in severely constipated patients or patients who may have an obstruction.
(b) Senna alkaloids or bisacodyl may be tried to relieve constipation where PEG was unsuccessful.
(3) **Chloride channel activators.** Activation causes for movement of chloride, sodium, and water into the lumen of the intestine.
(a) Lubiprostone (Amitiza) is a chloride channel activator indicated for idiopathic constipation. It is approved for use in women with IBS-C at a dose of 8 mcg twice daily.

4. **Severe IBS** is a very small proportion of the entire IBS population. GI complaints can be refractory and of continuous nature. Psychosocial and psychiatric comorbidities are common.
   a. Antidepressants, including the selective serotonin reuptake inhibitors, are often useful in severe IBS patients due to the increase in psychosocial components to patient presentation.
   b. Anxiolytic drugs, including diazepam, are occasionally used for IBS when patients are experiencing acute anxiety that is worsening their symptoms. In light of the risk of dependency, these drugs should only be taken for short periods.
   c. **5-HT$_4$-receptor agonist**
   Tegaserod (Zelnorm®) is a 5-HT$_4$-agonist for constipation predominant IBS in women and is only available in the United States for emergency situations via petition of the FDA. Use of this drug is so restricted due to its cardiovascular risk profile.
      (1) IBS-C dosing (**women only**) is 6 mg PO b.i.d. before meals.

III. COMPLICATIONS

A. **IBD**
   1. **UC and CD** have many similar presenting features as well as commonalities in complications. The majority of UC patients will have a chronic relapsing disease course. Length of disease is related to risk of colectomy and colorectal cancer. Mortality is similar to rates in non-UC populations. CD may impose a slight increase in mortality with long-standing disease.
   2. **Musculoskeletal** manifestations of IBD are the most common extraintestinal manifestations of the disease. Arthralgias in the absence of arthritis signs are the most common complaint. Five percent to 20% of IBD patients experience peripheral arthritis pain that is self-limiting and coincides with IBD disease flares and resolves with successful treatment of IBD. Occurrence is nearly equal between males and females. Ankylosing spondylitis in IBD is less common at approximately 5% and is equal in UC and CD. Males are affected more than females and course is usually not related to the course of IBD.
   3. **CD fistulas and abscess.** Long-standing inflammation may progress into penetrating disease, abscess formation, and fistula formation. These penetrating communications can be from diseased organ to neighboring organ, peritoneum, and to the skin. Fistula types include perianal fistula, enteroenteric, enterocutaneous, enterovesical, and rectovaginal.
   4. **Hemorrhage** in the colon is relatively rare in UC but is serious. Acute hemorrhage accounts for a significant percentage of urgent colectomies in UC. Severe bleeding tends to occur early in the course of disease. Hemorrhage in CD is extremely rare.
   5. **Strictures** or narrowing of the colon or rectum occurs in a small percentage of the UC population. Importantly nearly one-third of strictures may be related to malignancy and as such strictures should be carefully evaluated.
   6. **Toxic megacolon** is a serious complication mainly seen in UC but occasionally in CD as well. It occurs when the inflammatory process causes the colon to dilate with subsequent bowel wall thinning. This results in the bowel becoming more fragile. The major risk is bowel perforation. Bowel dilation that does not respond to therapy within 72 hrs is considered an indication for surgical resection.
   7. **Cancer.** Overall UC patients are at higher risk of developing **colorectal cancer** compared to patients without IBD. The risk to individuals is variable and is related to duration and extent of UC as well as patient specific history risk factors. Risk is greatest in patients with pancolitis of long-standing duration. Colorectal cancer is also a risk in CD patients, especially if it is CD involving the colon. Risk of cancer of the small intestine has been noted in CD also.
   8. **Primary sclerosing cholangitis** (PSC) is the most common hepatobiliary complication of IBD. PSC affects men more than woman. PSC is more common in UC than CD.
   9. **Osteoporosis** as evidenced by increased fractures and diminished bone density has been shown in CD patients.
   10. **Quality of life impact.** While most IBD patients are able to lead nearly normal lives, many do suffer significantly during active flares of disease. The chronic nature of disease also has a negative impact on patient QOL.

B. **IBS.** Although IBS has been shown to produce substantial physical discomfort and emotional distress, most patients with IBS do not develop serious or long-term health complications. Most patients also learn to control their individual symptoms with diet and lifestyle modification or medical therapy as needed.

Study Questions

For questions 1–2: A 35-year-old male presents to his physician with a primary complaint of abdominal pain and frequent bowel movements over the past few weeks. Upon examination and routine laboratory testing, he is found to have a low-grade fever and an elevated erythrocyte sedimentation rate. Further questioning reveals he is having four to five loose bowel movements each day. The patient is a past smoker. Stool antigen tests are negative for known GI pathogens. Physical examination and colonoscopy reveal contiguous inflammation of the rectum and most of the descending colon. The physician diagnosis is mild to moderate ulcerative colitis.

1. Which therapy would be the most effective for inducing remission?

(A) Topical corticosteroids
(B) Topical 5-ASA
(C) Oral budesonide
(D) Topical 5-ASA plus oral 5-ASA

2. Once remission is achieved, which therapy is most appropriate for maintenance?

(A) Sulfasalazine 2 g/day
(B) Balsalazide 2 g/day
(C) Olsalazine 4 g/day
(D) Topical corticosteroids

For questions 3–4: An 18-year-old female with newly diagnosed mild Crohn's disease within the ileum returns to her physician for her first follow-up since starting treatment. Three weeks ago she started oral sulfasalazine 4 g/day and azathioprine 25 mg/day. Since starting these meds, her symptoms have not improved. If anything, they are slightly worse. She is ambulatory with no signs of toxicity (blood per rectum, pain, anemia, etc.) or weight loss.

3. What would be a logical next step in therapy?

(A) Stop azathioprine and begin IV corticosteroids
(B) Stop sulfasalazine and begin oral budesonide 9 mg/day
(C) Stop azathioprine and begin prednisone 40 mg orally per day
(D) Stop sulfasalazine and begin Lialda® 4.8 gm/day

4. Remission of her first episode was successful. Unfortunately, fulldose azathioprine alone has been unable to maintain effective control of her CD. Over the past 18 months she has had numerous flare-ups. They resolve with each burst of acute therapy but return with azathioprine alone. Her symptoms are increasing (moderate disease) and her schooling is beginning to suffer. What would be a logical next step in therapy?

(A) Change azathioprine to 6-MP at 1.5 mg/kg/day
(B) Add metronidazole 750 mg/day
(C) Surgical resection with ostomy
(D) Add infliximab 5 mg/kg every 8 weeks

For question 5: A man with diarrhea-predominant IBS is experiencing interruption of his work as a truck driver secondary to frequent bouts of diarrhea. He states his symptoms are worse after eating, especially fried foods. His physician discusses the possible benefit of avoiding fat in his diet. The patient agrees to try but also asks for something to uses in emergencies.

5. What would be the most appropriate therapy to use?

(A) Alosetron 0.5 mg b.i.d.
(B) Hyoscyamine 0.15 mg PO p.r.n.
(C) Loperamide 4 mg then 2 mg p.r.n. up to 16 mg/day
(D) Fluoxetine 40 mg q.d.

6. Which of the following is the most appropriate initial therapy for a woman with severe constipation-predominant IBS?

(A) A restrictive bland diet
(B) Tegaserod 6 mg PO b.i.d.
(C) Alosetron 1 mg PO b.i.d.
(D) Psyllium 2.5 g in divided doses

7. Ulcerative colitis and Crohn's disease present in very similar ways. There are several clinical differences between the diseases that can help differentiate them. Which of the following clinical features is more common in Crohn's disease than in ulcerative colitis?
   (A) abnormal bowel movements
   (B) slow onset of disease
   (C) joint pain
   (D) fistula formation

8. Patient prescribed anti-TNF-α agents such as adalimumab should be monitored carefully for which of the following adverse events according to black box warnings included in prescribing information?
   (A) Increased risk of severe loss of bone density
   (B) Increased risk of critically high potassium levels
   (C) Increased risk of toxic megacolon
   (D) Increased risk of pneumonia

Answers and Explanations

1. **The answer is D** *[see II.B.2]*.
   Topical 5-ASA therapy plus oral 5-ASA therapy has been shown to be superior to either alone or topical steroids at inducing remission in mild to moderate UC. Budesonide ileal release will not likely reach the site of disease in this patient as he has left-sided disease.

2. **The correct answer is A** *[see II.B.3]*.
   The correct doses for balsalazide would be 3 to 6 g/day and for olsalazine would be 1 g/day. Topical steroids have no place in maintenance of UC.

3. **The correct answer is B** *[see II.C.1]*.
   This patient has not responded to 5-ASA therapy for inducing remission of her mild disease. Additionally, recent evidence indicates there are more effective treatments than 5-ASA for acute CD. As such, Lialda would not be an effective treatment either. The patient is not showing signs of severe disease or toxicity and as such neither IV or oral therapy with systemic corticosteroids is warranted at this time. Azathioprine is an appropriate agent for CD maintenance but not acute CD as it may take several months to induce remission. Continuing azathioprine is a reasonable approach to transition the patient to maintenance therapy. Budesonide is an ileal release therapy and her disease is mainly confined to the ileum. Budesonide has been shown to be effective in acute mild and moderate CD. Budesonide will help control the acute disease and then it can be withdrawn as she transitions to the maintenance phase.

4. **The correct answer is D** *[see II.C.4]*.
   Azathioprine is a first-line therapy for maintenance of CD but in this case is not working. Switching to 6-MP will not be effective as the two agents are mechanistically similar. Broad-spectrum antibiotics such as metronidazole are unlikely to be of any benefit in this patient and should not be used. In addition, long-term adverse effects associated with metronidazole may not be tolerable. While likely to be beneficial, surgery with a permanent ostomy would also be severely limiting to a young patient due to social and QOL concerns. Infliximab has been shown to be effective for refractory CD and maintenance of CD.

5. **The correct answer is C** *[see II.D.3]*.
   This patient is male and as such alosetron is not an appropriate option for him. Hyoscyamine is an effective antispasmodic but will likely do little for his diarrhea. The patient makes no complaint of serious impact on his life and does not show signs of severe disease. Full dose antidepressant fluoxetine dosing is not warranted. Loperamide can be of use in managing mild to moderate symptoms of IBS.

6. **The correct answer is B** *[see II.D.4]*.
   Tegaserod has been withdrawn from the market and is available only for emergency use upon appeal to the FDA. Alosetron is effective in women with diarrhea-predominant IBS. Restrictive diets are not normally of benefit. Increasing dietary fiber is a reasonable choice prior to prescription therapy. Dietary fiber may increase bloating symptoms with IBS-C, these can be lessened by starting with smaller doses and titrating to effect. If fiber fails, laxative or lubiprostone (Amitiza) could be tested.

7. **The correct answer is D** *[see Table 45.1]*.
   While the overlap of clinical presentation of these two diseases is substantial, fistula formation is extremely rare in ulcerative colitis.

8. **The correct answer is D** *[see II.A.6.c]*.
   Black box warnings for all of the anti-TNF-α therapies include increased risk of serious infections such as pneumonia or reactivation of tuberculosis or hepatitis and increased risk of malignancies such as lymphoma. Changes in potassium or bone density are not adverse effects commonly associated with anti-TNF-α therapies and are not included in black box warnings. Toxic megacolon is a complication usually associated with UC and also is not included in black box warnings with anti-TNF-α use.

46 Diabetes Mellitus

JENNIFER D. SMITH

I. INTRODUCTION

A. **Definition.** The American Diabetes Association (ADA) defines diabetes mellitus as a group of metabolic diseases characterized by inappropriate hyperglycemia resulting from defects in insulin secretion, insulin action, or both. Symptoms of acute hyperglycemia include polyuria, polydipsia, polyphagia, weight loss, blurred vision, fatigue, headache, and poor wound healing. Chronic hyperglycemia can lead to damage and potentially failure of various organs, including the eyes, heart, kidneys, blood vessels, and nerves.

B. **Classification.** There are four clinical classes of diabetes: type 1, type 2, gestational, and other specific types.

1. **Type 1.** Type 1 diabetes mellitus (T1DM) is typically characterized by an absolute insulin deficiency attributed to an autoimmune destruction of the β-cells of the islets of Langerhans. Affected individuals will have autoantibodies to glutamic acid decarboxylase, pancreatic islet β cells, and/or insulin. T1DM may be diagnosed at any age, but is most likely to be diagnosed prior to the age of 30 years.
2. **Type 2.** Type 2 diabetes mellitus (T2DM) is the most common form of DM and is typically identified in individuals over the age of 30 years; however, it has become a more prominent diagnosis in adolescents of certain ethnic origins (e.g., Hispanic, African American). Those diagnosed with T2DM are typically overweight or obese, have a positive family history of diabetes, and/or exhibit signs of insulin resistance (e.g., truncal obesity, high triglycerides, low high-density lipoprotein cholesterol [HDL-C], acanthosis nigricans); autoantibodies found in T1DM are absent in T2DM.
3. **Gestational diabetes mellitus.** Gestational diabetes mellitus (GDM) is a condition in which women first exhibit levels of elevated plasma glucose during pregnancy. Women previously diagnosed with diabetes prior to pregnancy are excluded from this classification. After pregnancy, the diagnostic classification of GDM may be changed based on postpartum testing (*see III.B.2.b*).
4. **Other specific types.** Secondary diabetes occurs when the diagnosis of diabetes is a result of other disorders (e.g., Cushing syndrome, acromegaly, cystic fibrosis, Down syndrome, pancreatic disorders) or treatments (e.g., glucocorticoids, antipsychotics). **Monogenic DM** (formerly maturity-onset diabetes of the young) should be considered in children with an atypical presentation or response to therapy. Adults may present with **Latent Autoimmune Diabetes of the Adult (LADA)**, which is a slow destruction of the pancreatic β-cells similar to T2DM, but autoantibodies are present as in T1DM.
5. **Categories of increased risk for diabetes (prediabetes):** Individuals who have elevated blood glucose levels that do not meet diagnostic criteria for diabetes, but that are too high to be considered normal, are classified as having prediabetes. Prediabetes is a high-risk category for the future development of T2DM.

C. **Diabetes demographics and statistics**

1. In the United States, an estimated 8.3% of the population has DM and 35% of adults (age 20 years and older) have prediabetes.
2. Disparities exist in the diagnosis of diabetes across ethnic groups and minority populations, with Native Americans and Alaska Natives having the highest rates of diagnosed diabetes (16.1%), followed by blacks (12.6%) and Hispanics (11.8%).
3. T2DM accounts for more than 90% of the cases of diabetes.

II. PATHOPHYSIOLOGY OF THE DIABETIC STATE

A. **Normal glucose regulation** involves many factors including insulin, counterregulatory hormones, incretin hormones, and amylin. Changes to any of these factors may result in an imbalance in glucose levels.

1. **Insulin** regulates the metabolism of carbohydrate, protein, and fat as follows:
   a. Promotes the cellular uptake of plasma glucose
   b. Stimulates conversion of glucose into energy storage molecules (e.g., glycogen, fat) in the liver, muscles, and adipose cells
   c. Facilitates cellular uptake of amino acids and their incorporation into proteins
   d. Inhibits production of glucose from liver, muscle glycogen, or amino acids
   e. Decreases the breakdown of fatty acids to ketone bodies
2. **Counterregulatory hormones** in diabetes are hormones that work against insulin. Thus, where insulin lowers blood glucose, counterregulatory hormones **increase blood glucose**. The counterregulatory hormones include:
   a. Glucagon
   b. Growth hormone
   c. Catecholamines (epinephrine and norepinephrine)
   d. Cortisol
3. **Incretin hormones:** Ingested glucose promotes a more rapid release of insulin from the pancreas than when glucose is given by intravenous injection. This occurs because the incretin hormones, gastric inhibitory peptide (**GIP**) and glucagon-like peptide-1 (**GLP-1**) are secreted by the intestines in response to glucose ingestion, before the glucose is absorbed. Postprandial secretion of GLP-1 is diminished in DM, whereas GIP secretion is normal or increased. Actions of GLP-1 include:
   a. Increases glucose-dependent insulin secretion
   b. Inhibits inappropriate glucagon secretion
   c. Increases β-cell growth/replication
   d. Slows gastric emptying
   e. Suppresses appetite
4. **Amylin** is a hormone that is **cosecreted with insulin** from the pancreatic β-cells. Thus, in individuals with T1DM, little to no amylin is produced, whereas in T2DM, amylin is produced, but in an insufficient quantity. Amylin lowers postprandial blood glucose levels by the following actions:
   a. Prolongs gastric emptying time
   b. Decreases postprandial glucagon secretion
   c. Suppresses appetite

B. **Development of diabetes**

1. **T1DM.** Genetic predisposition, environmental factors, and autoimmunity have been proposed as causes that lead to progressive β-cell dysfunction and eventually, overt diabetes mellitus. T1DM is the result of immune-mediated destruction of the β-cells and is characterized by the abrupt onset of clinical signs and symptoms.
   a. **Genetics.** Human leukocyte antigens (HLAs) DQA and DQB appear to code for either disease susceptibility (DR3, DR4, HLA-DQA1*0301, and HLA-DQA1*0302) or resistance (DRB1*04008-DQB1*0302, DRB1*0411-DQB1*0302). Greater than 90% of Caucasians diagnosed with T1DM have HLA-DR3 and/or HLA-DR4 present, but 95% of these individuals have HLA-DQA1*0301 and HLA-DQA1*0302 present. However, in studies of identical twins, there is a 50% discordance rate, suggesting that other factors such as the environment (e.g., infectious agents, chemical agents, dietary agents) may be contributing factors to disease development. The risk of developing T1DM is increased in the offspring of individuals diagnosed with diabetes.
   b. **Environment.** Environmental triggers such as viral (e.g., rubella, Coxsackie B), chemical, or dietary (e.g., cow's milk) have been suspected in the development of T1DM.
   c. **Autoimmunity.** An autoimmune component, possibly triggered by an environmental factor, is involved in the development of T1DM. Anti-insulin or anti-β-cell antibodies are present in the blood of most individuals at the time of diagnosis of T1DM. Antibodies to glutamic acid decarboxylase (GAD) are found in the blood of approximately 70% of individuals diagnosed with T1DM. Thus, the presence of these antibodies may serve as an immunologic predictor of the future development of the disease.

2. **T2DM.** Genetic factors, a β-cell defect, and peripheral site defects have been implicated.
   a. **Genetics.** There is greater than a 90% concordance rate in identical twins if one has T2DM, suggesting that the development of T2DM is predominately dependent on genetics. The risk of offspring development of T2DM is at least 15%.
   b. A primary β-**cell dysfunction** has been postulated in the development of T2DM because at diagnosis, typically only about 50% of β-cells are functioning. The number of functioning β-cells continues to decline with duration of the disease.
   c. A **peripheral site defect** may also contribute to the expression of T2DM. Defects in postreceptor binding or a decreased number of insulin receptors can lead to hyperglycemia.
3. **Secondary diabetes** may arise from other disorders (e.g., Cushing syndrome, acromegaly, cystic fibrosis, Down syndrome, pancreatic disorders) or treatments (e.g., glucocorticoids, antipsychotics).

III. CLINICAL EVALUATION

A. **Physical findings** include the "polys" (e.g., polyuria, polydipsia, and polyphagia), weight loss, blurred vision, fatigue, headache, frequent vaginal infections, and poor wound healing. Because hyperglycemia typically exists for extended periods prior to the diagnosis of T2DM, these persons may also present with signs and symptoms of chronic complications from diabetes (*see section X*).

B. **Diagnostic testing** should be performed from **venipuncture** testing. Home blood glucose monitors and point-of-care (POC) A1c monitors are not sufficiently accurate for diagnostic purposes. A1c tests reflect the average blood glucose level over the preceding 2 to 3 months and correlate with an estimated average glucose (eAG = 28.7 × A1C − 46.7). **A1c testing for diagnostic purposes should not be done in individuals with abnormal red cell turnover** (e.g., pregnancy, recent blood loss or transfusion, some anemias). These individuals should only be diagnosed with glucose criteria. **Repeat testing**, preferably with the same method, must be performed **to confirm diagnosis**, unless there is unequivocal hyperglycemia (e.g., random blood glucose sample > 200 in a symptomatic individual, hyperglycemia crisis). Fasting is defined as no caloric intake for at least 8 hrs.

1. **Diabetes in nonpregnant adults and children**
   a. **Fasting** blood glucose **≥ 126 mg/dL**
   b. **Random** (casual) blood glucose and symptoms of hyperglycemia: **≥ 200 mg/dL**
   c. **Oral glucose tolerance test** (OGTT) using oral glucose load equivalent to 75 g anhydrous glycerin dissolved in water: **> 200 mg/dL**
   d. **A1c ≥ 6.5%**
2. **Gestational diabetes mellitus (GDM)** screening should occur **between weeks 24 to 28 gestation** if not previously diagnosed with overt diabetes. A fasting 75-g oral glucose tolerance test (OGTT) should be performed in the morning. Venipuncture should be measured at fasting and 1- and 2-hr post-oral glucose solution ingestion.
   a. Diagnosis of GDM based on OGTT: Fasting ≥ 92 mg/dL; 1 hr ≥ 180 mg/dL; 2 hrs ≥ 153 mg/dL.
   b. If diagnosed with GDM, screening for persistent diabetes should occur between 6 to 12 weeks postpartum and, if negative, at least every 3 years thereafter.
3. **Prediabetes:** relatively high risk for the future development of diabetes
   a. **Impaired fasting glucose (IFG):** fasting blood glucose **100 to 125 mg/dL**
   b. **Impaired glucose tolerance (IGT):** OGTT results of **140 to 199 mg/dL**
   c. **A1c 5.7 to 6.4%**
4. **Testing in asymptomatic individuals:**
   a. Adults who are overweight (BMI ≥ 25 kg/m^2) or who have one or more risk factors for diabetes should be tested immediately and at least every 3 years thereafter if tests are negative. Risk factors for diabetes include:
      (1) Physical inactivity
      (2) First degree relative with diabetes
      (3) High-risk ethnicity (e.g., African American, Latino, Native American, Asian American, Pacific Islander)
      (4) Women who delivered a baby weighing ≥ 9 lb or were diagnosed with GDM
      (5) Hypertension (≥ 140/90 mm Hg or on therapy for hypertension)
      (6) HDL cholesterol level < 35 mg/dL and/or a triglyceride level > 250 mg/dL
      (7) Women with polycystic ovarian syndrome (PCOS)

(8) Previous testing indicative of prediabetes
(9) Clinical conditions associated with insulin resistance (e.g., severe obesity, acanthosis nigricans)
(10) History of CVD

b. Asymptomatic adults without risk factors should have screenings beginning at the age of 45 years.

c. Testing for T2DM in the asymptomatic **pediatric population** should occur at the **age of 10 years or the onset of puberty** (whichever comes first) in children who are **overweight** (BMI > 85th percentile for age and sex; weight for height > 85th percentile; weight > 120% for height) and have **at least two risk factors** (e.g., family history of diabetes in first or second degree relative, race/ethnicity of African, Asian, or Native American or Latino, signs of insulin resistance, or maternal history of GDM during child's gestation). If negative, repeat testing should occur every 3 years.

IV. GLYCEMIC TREATMENT GOALS.

The two available techniques for monitoring glycemic control are patient self-monitoring blood glucose (SMBG) and A1c. Important measurements for SMBG include fasting plasma glucose (FPG) and 2-hr postprandial glucose (PPG). Guideline recommendations for the use of these two techniques are provided by the American Diabetes Association (ADA) and the American Association of Clinical Endocrinologists (AACE). The guideline recommendations differ slightly, with those of AACE being more stringent (*Table 46-1*). All glucose targets should be individualized, taking into account other disease states, age of person, duration of disease, and risk for hypoglycemia.

A. Outpatient glucose targets for nonpregnant adults:
   1. ADA: A1c < 7.0%; FPG 70 to 130 mg/dL; 1- to 2-hr PPG < 180 mg/dL
   2. AACE: A1c ≤ 6.5%; FPG < 110 mg/dL; 2-hr PPG < 140 mg/dL

B. Inpatient glucose targets for nonpregnant adults is specified by ADA and AACE as a glucose range of 140 to 180 mg/dL

C. Outpatient glucose targets for pregnant adults are the same for ADA and AACE guidelines. These goals should be implemented, only if they can be achieved safely.
   1. GDM: Preprandial ≤ 95 mg/dL; 1-hr PPG ≤ 140 mg/dL; 2-hr PPG ≤ 120 mg/dL
   2. Preexisting T1DM or T2DM: A1c ≤ 6.0%; pre-meal, bedtime, and overnight values between 60 to 99 mg/dL; peak PPG of 100 to 129 mg/dL; A1c < 6%

V. PHARMACOLOGIC TREATMENT OF DIABETES MELLITUS

A. **Insulin and insulin analog** (*Table 46-2*)
   1. **Types of insulin**
      a. **Rapid-acting** insulin. Lispro (Humalog), aspart (NovoLog), and glulisine (Apidra) insulins
      b. **Short-acting** insulin. Regular insulin (Humulin regular, Novolin regular)
      c. **Intermediate-acting** insulin. Isophane insulin suspension (neutral protamine Hagedorn; NPH) insulin
      d. **Long-acting** insulins. Glargine (Lantus) and detemir (Levemir) insulins.

Table 46-1 GUIDELINE RECOMMENDATIONS FOR OUTPATIENT GLYCEMIC GOALS IN NONPREGNANT ADULTS[1,2]

	American Diabetes Association (ADA)	American Association of Clinical Endocrinologists (AACE)
A1c goal	< 7.0%	≤ 6.5%
Fasting plasma glucose goal	70–130 mg/dL	< 110 mg/dL
Postprandial glucose goal	< 180 mg/dL	< 140 mg/dL

[1]American Diabetes Association. Standards of medical care in diabetes—2012. *Diabetes Care* 2012;35:s11–63.
[2]AACE Diabetes Care Plan Guidelines. *Endocrine Practice* 2011;17(Suppl 2):1–53.

Table 46-2 TYPES OF INSULIN—ONSET, PEAK, AND DURATION OF ACTION[a]

Agent	Onset (hr)	Peak (hr)	Effective Duration (hr)	Variability in Absorption and Duration
Rapid acting				
Lispro (Humalog)	< 0.5	0.5–1.5	3–4	Minimal
Aspart (NovoLog)	< 0.5	0.7–1.0	3–5	Minimal
Glulisine (Apidra)	< 0.5	0.5–1.5	3–5	Minimal
Short-acting				
Regular	0.5–1.0	2–4	5–8	Moderate
Intermediate-acting				
NPH	2–4	6–10	10–16	High
Long-acting				
Glargine (Lantus)	5	n/a	20–24	Minimal-to-moderate
Detemir (Levemir)	3–4	6–12	12–24	Minimal

[a]Approximate time action in nonpregnant adult, with normal renal function.
n/a, not applicable; *NPH*, neutral protamine Hagedorn.

e. **Premixed insulin products.** Each mixture gives rapid- or short-acting insulin as a premeal bolus plus an intermediate-acting insulin to control later hyperglycemia or the subsequent meal.
   (1) 50/50 insulin: 50% protamine lispro insulin with 50% lispro insulin
   (2) 70/30 insulin: 70% insulin aspart protamine with 30% aspart insulin or 70% NPH with 30% regular insulin
   (3) 75/25 insulin: 75% protamine lispro insulin with 25% lispro insulin

f. **Extemporaneous mixtures.** Two insulins mixed in one syringe, before administration.
   (1) Glargine and detemir should never be mixed in the same syringe with another insulin.
   (2) When rapid-acting insulins (e.g., lispro, aspart, glulisine) are mixed with another insulin, the preparation should be used immediately.
   (3) Extemporaneous mixtures which include regular-acting and intermediate-acting insulin are stable for 14 days refrigerated or 7 days at room temperature.

2. **Chemical sources** of commercial insulin available in the United States
   a. **Biosynthetic human, also called human insulin.** Produced by recombinant DNA techniques
   b. **Insulin analog.** Produced by chemical alteration of human insulin
3. **Concentration** of insulin products available in the United States
   a. U-100: a concentration of 100 units/mL
   b. U-500: a concentration of 500 units/mL
      (1) Recommended for individuals with marked insulin resistance, requiring greater than 200 units of U-100 insulin daily.
      (2) U-500, a highly concentrated insulin, is available by prescription only.
      (3) Currently U-500 syringes are not available in the United States. Patients should be taught to use the mL markings on a tuberculin or U-100 syringe to prevent dosing errors in units.
4. **Indications.** Insulin is required for glycemic management in individuals with T1DM and may be used in combination with oral agents (e.g., metformin) or amylin agonists (e.g., pramlintide) as necessary. Insulin may be an initial or adjunctive agent for individuals with T2DM and may be used in combination with oral agents, GLP-1 agonists (e.g., exenatide), or amylin agonists to achieve glycemic control.
5. **Mechanism of action.** Insulin exerts its effects in several ways, including the following:
   (1) Stimulates hepatic glycogen synthesis
   (2) Increased protein synthesis
   (3) Facilitates triglyceride synthesis and storage by adipocytes; inhibits lipolysis
   (4) Stimulates peripheral uptake of glucose
6. **Initial dosage of insulin**
   a. **T1DM, without concomitant infection or physiologic stress condition.** Insulin should be dosed based on weight and requires a calculation of the total daily dose (TDD). The total daily

dose for an adult with T1DM is estimated as 0.6 units/kg/day, which can then be applied to determine an initial starting dose of insulin.

(1) **50/50 rule:** 50% of the TDD is given as a basal (e.g., NPH, glargine, detemir) dose and the remaining 50% is given as the bolus (e.g., regular, lispro, aspart, glulisine) dose, divided between the meals. For example, if a person who weighs 120 lb is to start insulin, the estimated TDD would be approximately 32 units. Half of the TDD (16 units) would be initiated as the basal insulin and the remaining 16 units would be divided into an approximate bolus dose as follows:

(a) Glargine or detemir as a basal with short- or rapid-acting insulin as bolus: 16 units once daily of basal insulin; 5 units t.i.d. of bolus insulin with meals.

(b) NPH as a basal requires twice daily dosing in persons with T1DM. Also, when using NPH, the total bolus dose should be decreased by 20% and given twice daily to prevent hypoglycemia. Thus, the regimen for this example would be 8 units of NPH and 6 units of bolus, each given b.i.d.

(2) **Premixed insulin** should be initiated as two-third of the TDD in the morning and the remaining one-third of the TDD in the evening, prior to meals. This means for the same example used earlier with a TDD of 32 units, the insulin regimen would be 21 units in the morning prior to breakfast and 11 units in the evening prior to the evening meal. It should be noted that this type of dosing is not preferred for the individual with T1DM because it cannot be easily adjusted for changes in diet, exercise, or health (e.g., sick days), nor does it allow the titration of one insulin type to target the specific phase of insulin release that is primarily contributing to the impaired glycemic control.

b. **Type 2 DM**

(1) Basal insulin alone may be initiated as 10 units once daily in the average-sized individual or 0.1 to 0.2 units/kg/day in the overweight or obese individual. If administered in the evenings, the dose of insulin should be titrated as necessary to achieve fasting blood glucose levels in the target range. Bolus insulin can be added as needed based on pre- and post-meal blood glucose monitoring.

(2) Premixed insulin should be initiated based on TDD of 0.2 units/kg/day, with two-thirds of the TDD given in the morning prior to breakfast and one-third of the TDD given in the evening prior to the last meal.

7. **Insulin adjustment algorithms** allow for the correction of an elevated blood glucose level or dosing for carbohydrate intake. Though useful for optimizing glycemic control, adjustment algorithms are not for everyone.

a. **Adjustment based on blood glucose level:** Several variations exist in the dosing of correction insulin for elevated blood glucose. The rule of 1500 is typically used for dosing short-acting (e.g., Regular) insulin, while the rule of 1800 is used for dosing rapid-acting insulin. However, there are a myriad of algorithms used between 1500 and 2200. The higher the "rule" used, the lower the risk of inducing hypoglycemia.

(1) The **rule of 1800** is used to determine the correction factor (i.e., how many mg/dL the blood glucose will decrease with the injection of 1 unit of insulin). The calculation is: 1800/TDD = **correction factor (CF)**. For example, for the individual with a TDD of 32, one unit of insulin should change the blood glucose level by approximately 56 mg/dL (1800/32 = 56).

(2) The correction factor can then be used as a point-of-care calculation to determine how much insulin to inject. The calculation is: [Current blood glucose—target blood glucose]/CF. For the individual previously mentioned, if the blood glucose level is 230 mg/dL, to achieve a target of 120 mg/dL with the above calculated CF of 56 mg/dL, the individual would need to inject 2 units of rapid-acting insulin to bring the blood glucose back into the target range. The target blood glucose is typically set by practice site protocol. The CF should be rechecked at least once per year or when there is a significant change in weight, as this is a weight-based calculation.

b. **Adjustment based on carbohydrate intake** uses the "**rule of 500.**" The "rule of 500" is as follows: 500/TDD = (x) grams of carbohydrate. This equation estimates how many grams of carbohydrates will be covered by 1 unit of insulin. Use of this rule requires the ability of the individual with diabetes or the caretaker to count carbohydrates.

8. **Insulin adjustments for repeated, time-sequenced events of hypoglycemia or hyperglycemia:** When individuals experience repeated hypoglycemia or hyperglycemia at particular periods, several factors should be taken into consideration (e.g., appropriateness of insulin dose(s), eating habits, changes in exercise routine). Adjustments to insulin dosing should be made based on clinical evaluation of the blood glucose levels and on the knowledge of insulin onset, peak, and duration of action (*Table 46-2*). For example, if an individual who is taking 16 units of NPH insulin and 6 units of regular insulin twice daily (6 A.M. and 6 P.M.) has in-target pre-lunch blood glucose levels, but is having hypoglycemia pre-supper, a downward adjustment to the morning NPH dose would be most appropriate based on its longer duration of action. Adjusting the morning dose of Regular insulin would be inappropriate because the main effect of Regular insulin in this instance would be on the pre-lunch blood glucose value. Changes in insulin doses may also be necessary for the following causes of hyperglycemia:
   a. **Dawn phenomenon** produces **fasting hyperglycemia** due to the release of counterregulatory hormones, which typically occurs during the early morning hours (2:00 A.M. to 4:00 A.M.). Evening basal insulin doses should be increased or moved to bedtime dosing to correct for hyperglycemia attributed to dawn phenomenon.
   b. **Somogyi effect** is considered **rebound hyperglycemia**. This can occur at any time (day or night) and is when the blood glucose goes too low and counterregulatory hormones are released to increase the blood glucose. When the somogyi effect produces fasting hyperglycemia, the evening basal doses of insulin should be decreased to prevent hypoglycemia.
9. **Routes of insulin administration**
   a. **Subcutaneous (SQ) injection** is the method used most often for self-administration of insulin. Vials of insulin with syringes have been the traditional method to deliver a SQ injection; however, the insulin pens are rapidly becoming popular due to the convenience and portability the devices offer (*see section XII*).
      (1) **Site selection:** Insulin may be injected into the subcutaneous tissue of the **abdomen, buttocks, upper arm, and thigh** (upper and outer only). The rate of absorption may differ depending on the anatomical site used. The abdomen is typically the fastest site for insulin absorption, followed by the arm, buttocks, and thigh.
      (2) **Injection site rotation:** Within an anatomical region, the **injection site should be rotated** to avoid lipohypertrophy and fibrosis.
   b. **Continuous intravenous (insulin drip):** The IV route is used to administer regular U-100 insulin, typically in a hospital setting, for the treatment of acute hyperglycemia, hyperglycemic emergency (e.g., DKA or HHS), or during surgical procedures. The following applies to transitioning from IV to SQ insulin:
      (1) Short or rapid-acting insulin should be administered 1 to 2 hrs prior to IV insulin discontinuation.
      (2) Intermediate or long-acting insulin should be administered 2 to 3 hrs prior IV insulin discontinuation.
   c. **Continuous subcutaneous infusion (insulin pump therapy)** is a method to provide tighter glycemic control by continuously infusing rapid-acting insulin into the body. Users must be able to understand the complexity of the pump, check blood glucose levels, and determine bolus insulin doses for dietary intake.

B. **Insulin secretagogues** (oral hypoglycemic agents)
   1. **Agents**
      a. **Sulfonylureas** generally target fasting blood glucose levels and are classified as first- or second-generation agents.
         (1) First-generation agents are typically not prescribed with the evolution of the second-generation agents, which are associated with fewer adverse events. First-generation sulfonylureas have been associated with thrombocytopenia, agranulocytosis, hemolytic anemia, hyponatremia, SIADH, and disulfiram-like reactions. The three agents in this class include tolbutamide (Orinase), tolazamide (Tolinase), and chlorpropamide (Diabinese).
         (2) **Second generation:**
            (a) Glyburide (DiaBeta, Glynase)
            (b) Glipizide (Glucotrol)
            (c) Glimepiride (Amaryl)

b. **Meglitinides:** Repaglinide (Prandin)
c. **Phenylalanine derivatives:** Nateglinide (Starlix)

2. **Indication:** The secretagogues are indicated for the management of T2DM only. The focus of sulfonylureas is overall glycemic control, whereas the meglitinide and phenylalanine derivative target postprandial control. Sulfonylureas have traditionally been seen as a first-line agent for the management of T2DM; however, this class has lost some favor with the evolution of agents that are multifactorial in the management of blood glucose.
3. **Contraindications:** Individuals with severe renal or hepatic dysfunction should avoid the use of secretagogues. Caution should be used in the elderly due to the increased risk of falls with hypoglycemic events. It should be noted that neither repaglinide nor nateglinide are effective in patients who have failed sulfonylurea therapy.
4. **Mechanisms of action: stimulates enhanced secretion of insulin** from pancreatic β-cells, reduces hepatic glucose output
5. **Administration and dosage** (*Table 46-3*)
6. **Patient education and other concerns:**
   a. **Hypoglycemia** is an adverse effect of insulin secretagogues that warrants significant counseling. Sulfonylureas are more likely to cause hypoglycemia, but repaglinide and nateglinide are likely to induce hypoglycemia as well, if taken without food. Education should include signs and symptoms of hypoglycemia and appropriate treatment (*see IX.B and IX.D*).
   b. **Weight gain**, secondary to increased insulin secretion, can occur.

C. **Biguanides**

1. **Agents:** The only available biguanide is **metformin** (Glucophage, Glucophage XR, Fortamet, Glumetza, Riomet).
2. **Indication:** Metformin may be used for the glycemic management of **T1DM or T2DM** and is **recommended to be initiated at diagnosis of T2DM** unless there is an existing contraindication. Metformin primarily targets fasting blood glucose levels.
3. **Contraindications**
   a. **Renal disease:** Metformin is contraindicated in renal disease due to the potential for lactic acidosis. Metformin should be discontinued when the **Scr is ≥ 1.4 mg/dL for females or ≥ 1.5 mg/dL for males**. It should be understood that metformin does not cause renal dysfunction, but rather accumulation of the drug can contribute to toxicity (lactic acidosis) in the individual with renal dysfunction.
   b. **Hepatic impairment** or those with alcoholism or binge drinking
   c. Heart failure: Metformin may be initiated or continued in those with stable heart failure; however, in **unstable or acute heart failure**, the risk of lactic acidosis can be increased secondary to hypoperfusion.
   d. Intravascular **iodinated contrast media:** Metformin should be withheld, if possible, at least 24 hrs prior to the procedure and may be reinitiated 48 hrs after, or when normal renal function returns. However, metformin can be withdrawn as few as 6 hrs prior to the procedure with adequate hydration.
4. **Mechanisms of action:** The primary role of metformin is to **inhibit hepatic glucose output**, thus exerting beneficial effects on fasting blood glucose levels. The secondary role of metformin is to promote glucose uptake by fat and muscles, thereby improving insulin sensitivity. Thirdly, metformin has a minor role in decreasing intestinal absorption of glucose.
5. **Administration and dosage** (*Table 46-3*)
6. **Patient education and other concerns**
   a. **Up to 30% of individuals using metformin are affected by GI effects** (e.g., abdominal bloating, nausea, cramping, feeling of fullness, loss of appetite, or diarrhea). GI effects are self-limiting over 7 to 14 days. Effects can be minimized by taking the medication with food, starting with a low dose, and slow upward titration of dosage.
   b. Minimal weight loss can be seen initially with this agent, but is not a continued effect.
   c. Metformin use has been associated with a reduction in vitamin B_{12} levels. Monitoring of vitamin B_{12} levels should be considered.
   d. Miscellaneous effects include sweating and a metallic taste.

Table 46-3 ORAL AND NONINSULIN INJECTABLE AGENTS[a]

Agent	Initial Dose (Maximum Dose)	Comments
	α-Glucosidase Inhibitors	
Acarbose (Precose)	25 mg t.i.d. with the first bite of each main meal (< 60 kg: 50 mg t.i.d.; > 60 kg: 100 mg t.i.d.)	Adverse effects include diarrhea and abdominal stress, which is dose dependent and subsides with continued use; adverse effects typically limit the favorability of these agents Glucose or lactose should be used to treat hypoglycemia that occurs within 2 hrs of taking medication Dose should be increased slowly as tolerated
Miglitol (Glyset)	25 mg t.i.d. with first bite of each main meal (100 mg t.i.d.)	
	Biguanide	
Metformin (Glucophage, Glucophage XR, Glumetza, Fortamet, Riomet)	500 mg once or twice daily with meals (Short-acting: 2550 mg/day; long-acting: 2000 mg/day)	Adverse effects: transient nausea and abdominal cramping (typically lasts up to 2 weeks); lactic acidosis (rare, but fatal) Contraindicated in persons with renal or hepatic disease, unstable heart failure, or alcoholism
	Thiazolidinediones (TZDs)	
Pioglitazone (Actos)	15–30 mg once daily without regard to meals (45 mg/day)	Adverse effects include weight gain and peripheral edema Contraindicated in hepatic disease and heart failure (class III or IV) Rosiglitazone has restricted access Therapy may take 6–12 weeks for maximum effectiveness
Rosiglitazone (Avandia)	4 mg once daily without regard to meals (8 mg/day)	
	Sulfonylureas	
Glipizide (Glucotrol, Glucotrol XL)	5 mg once daily (Immediate release: 40 mg/day; extended release: 20 mg/day) IR given 30 mins before a meal and > 15 mg/day is given in divided doses	Adverse effects: hypoglycemia, weight gain Micronized tablet (Glynase) formulation is **NOT** bioequivalent to regular glyburide Contraindications: Glyburide is not recommended if CrCl < 50 mL/min; however, glimepiride and glipizide may be used to a lower CrCl
Glyburide (DiaBeta, Glynase PresTab)	DiaBeta: 2.5–5.0 mg/day with a meal (20 mg/day) Glynase 1.5–3.0 mg/day with a meal (12 mg/day)	
Glimepiride (Amaryl)	1–2 mg once daily with a meal (8 mg/day)	
	Meglitinides	
Repaglinide (Prandin)	Not previously treated for DM or A1c < 8%: 0.5 mg before each meal Previously treated for DM or A1c > 8%: 1–2 mg before each meal (16 mg/day)	Primary adverse effect: hypoglycemia Targets postprandial blood glucose values
	Phenylalanine Derivatives	
Nateglinide (Starlix)	120 mg t.i.d., up to 30 mins prior to each meal (180 mg/day) If near goal A1c may initiate 60 mg t.i.d.	Adverse effects: hypoglycemia; increased uric acid levels Targets postprandial blood glucose values

Table 46-3 Continued.

Agent	Initial Dose (Maximum Dose)	Comments
	DPP-IV Inhibitors	
Sitagliptin (Januvia) Saxagliptin (Onglyza) Linagliptin (Tradjenta)	100 mg once daily regardless of a meal (100 mg/day) 2.5–5.0 mg once daily regardless of a meal (5 mg/day) 5 mg once daily regardless of a meal (5 mg/day)	Adverse effects: upper respiratory tract infection, nasopharyngitis, angioedema, urticaria Sitagliptin and saxagliptin require dosage adjustments for CrCl < 50 mL/min All three may be used in mild-to-moderate hepatic impairment Avoid use in persons with pancreatitis Drug–drug interactions: Saxagliptin levels may be increased by strong CYP3A4 inhibitors and the risk of edema is more than doubled when combined with a TZD; saxagliptin dose should be 2.5 mg when initiated with a TZD or strong CYP3A4 inhibitor
	Bile Acid Sequestrants	
Colesevelam (Welchol)	1.875 g (3 tablets) b.i.d. or 3.75 g (6 tablets) once daily	Adjunctive treatment only Take other oral medications 1 hr before or 4 hrs after colesevelam Avoid in persons with obstructive bowel disease or triglyceride levels > 500 mg/dL
	Dopamine Agonists	
Bromocriptine (Cycloset)	0.8 mg once daily (4.8 mg/day) with a meal within 2 hrs of wakening	Adjunctive treatment only Adverse effects: gastrointestinal symptoms Contraindications: use with caution in persons with cardiovascular disease, peptic ulcer disease, psychosis, or dementia
	GLP-1 Agonists	
Exenatide (Byetta) Liraglutide (Victoza)	5 mcg b.i.d. within 60 mins of a meal (10 mcg b.i.d.) 0.6 mg once daily regardless of a meal (1.8 mg/day)	Available in pen devices for subcutaneous injection Adverse effects: Dose-related nausea and/or vomiting that may decrease with continued use, weight loss unrelated to GI symptoms, possible pancreatitis, injection site reaction Contraindications: Liraglutide is contraindicated in persons with or a family history of medullary thyroid cancer or in persons with multiple endocrine neoplasia syndrome type 2 (MEN2). Both liraglutide and exenatide are contraindicated in persons with pancreatitis or a history of pancreatitis, T1DM, and gastroparesis Slow titrations will minimize GI effects: Liraglutide dose of 0.6 mg should be used for 1 week prior to increasing to 1.2 mg/day; exenatide 5 mcg b.i.d. should be used for 30 days prior to increasing to 10 mcg b.i.d. Targets postprandial blood glucose

(Continued on next page)

Table 46-3 Continued.

Agent	Initial Dose (Maximum Dose)	Comments
	Amylin Agonists	
Pramlintide (Symlin)	T1DM: 15 mcg immediately prior to meals (60 mcg t.i.d.) T2DM: 60 mcg immediately prior to meals (120 mcg t.i.d.)	Adverse effects: nausea/vomiting, increased risk of severe hypoglycemia in persons with T1DM within 3 hrs of dosing Indicated for adjunctive therapy to basal and bolus insulin: reduce prandial (bolus) insulin by 50% when initiating pramlintide to avoid hypoglycemia Do not mix together with insulin or inject into the same site as insulin Drug–drug interactions: oral medications needing rapid onset (e.g., analgesics) should be administered 1 hr before or 2 hrs after pramlintide Targets postprandial blood glucose

[a]Consult package insert for detailed prescribing information. Dosage should be reduced if frequent hypoglycemia occurs without apparent cause (e.g., medication error, changes in diet, exercise, timing of regimen).
BID, twice a day; *CrCl*, çcreatinine clearance; *DM*, diabetes mellitus; *DPP*, dipeptidyl peptidase; *GI*, gastrointestinal; *GLP*, glucagon-like peptide; *IR*, immediate release; *TID*, three times a day; *T1DM*, type 1 diabetes mellitus; *T2DM*, type 2 diabetes mellitus.

D. Thiazolidinediones (TZDs)

1. **Agents**
   a. Pioglitazone (Actos)
   b. Rosiglitazone (Avandia)
2. **Indication:** TZDs are indicated for glycemic control in T2DM and primarily affect the fasting blood glucose levels.
3. **Contraindications**
   a. TZDs should be used with caution in patients with **hepatic dysfunction**. Several linked cases of liver toxicity are owed to troglitazone (Rezulin) which was removed from the market in 1999. Manufacturers of Avandia and Actos have taken caution, but have made great strides in overcoming the stigma associated with the class. For instance, when the agents first became available, LFTs had to be monitored every 2 months during the first year. In 2004, manufacturers of the two available TZDs achieved FDA approval for LFTs to be monitored at baseline, at 6 months, and periodically thereafter.
   b. **Class III/IV heart failure:** TZDs may cause **fluid retention**, which can exacerbate or lead to heart failure. Patients should be observed for signs and/or symptoms of heart failure. In 2007, FDA mandated manufacturers of TZDs to add CHF as a black box warning.
   c. Anemia: TZDs may cause plasma volume expansion. This may result in a small **decrease in hemoglobin and hematocrit**. Use cautiously in persons with anemia.
   d. **Fracture risk:** TZDs have been associated with **fractures**, typically in the distal upper or lower limbs of females.
   e. **Rosiglitazone** has been associated with increased risk of **cardiovascular events** (e.g., myocardial infarction, angina) and thus its **use has been restricted** by the Food and Drug Administration (FDA). Rosiglitazone is available only from certain mail order pharmacies for certain individuals under the Avandia-Rosiglitazone Medicines Access Program.
   f. **Pioglitazone** is under an ongoing safety review for the potential increased risk of **bladder cancer**. At this time, the FDA has not concluded an overall associated risk.
4. **Mechanism of action:** promote glucose uptake by fat and muscles and inhibit hepatic glucose output by the stimulation of peroxisome-proliferator-activated receptor-gamma (PPAR-γ).
5. **Administration and dosage** (*Table 46-3*)

6. **Patient education and other concerns**
   a. TZDs as a class cause significant **weight gain** that is likely associated with fluid retention and fat accumulation. **Report unusual weight gain, shortness of breath, or swelling of the lower extremities.**
   b. Benefits may not be seen prior to 2 to 4 weeks of use, with **maximum effectiveness not seen until 6 to 12 weeks of use.**

E. **α-Glucosidase inhibitors**
1. **Agents**
   a. Acarbose (Precose)
   b. Miglitol (Glyset)
2. **Indication:** α-glucosidase inhibitors are for management of **postprandial blood glucose**
3. **Contraindications**
   a. Inflammatory bowel disease, colonic ulceration, or obstructive bowel disorders
   b. Acarbose is not recommended in patients with serum creatinine > 2.0 mg/dL and neither agent is recommended in patients with creatinine clearance of < 25 mL/min.
   c. Acarbose is contraindicated in patients with hepatic impairment; dose-dependent elevation in serum transaminases can be seen.
4. **Mechanism of action:** Competitive **inhibition of alpha-glucosidases** in the intestinal brush border, which leads to a **slower absorption of complex carbohydrates**.
5. **Administration and dosage** (*Table 46-3*)
6. **Patient education and other concerns**
   a. α-glucosidase inhibitors **cause increased gas formation in the colon**, which can result in **flatulence**.
   b. The dose should be **taken with the first bite of the meal** for effectiveness.
   c. If **hypoglycemia** occurs within 2 hrs of dosing, patient should be treated with oral **glucose** if the patient is conscious or intravenous glucose or glucagon if the patient is unconscious. **Lactose** is also an acceptable alternative in the conscious patient.
   d. GI side effects will lessen over time, but timing is variable for each patient.

F. **Dipeptidyl peptidase-IV (DPP-IV) inhibitors**
1. Agents
   a. Sitagliptin (Januvia)
   b. Saxagliptin (Onglyza)
   c. Linagliptin (Tradjenta)
2. Indication: DPP-IV inhibitors are appropriate for use in individuals with T2DM with normal or impaired hepatic and renal function.
3. Contraindications
   a. **Pancreatitis:** use cautiously in an individual with a past medical history of pancreatitis and discontinue use if an individual develops pancreatitis while on a DPP-IV inhibitor.
   b. T1DM: DPP-IV inhibitors provide a glucose-dependent insulin secretion and thus are not appropriate for individuals with T1DM.
4. Mechanisms of action: Prevents the inactivation of incretin hormones (e.g., GLP-1) by the enzyme DPP-IV. GLP-1 works to stimulate insulin secretion and decrease glucagon secretion from the pancreas during hyperglycemia; thus inhibiting the breakdown of GLP-1 would allow for increased insulin secretion and decreased hepatic glucose production.
5. **Administration and dosage** (*Table 46-3*)
6. Patient education and other concerns
   a. Notify prescriber if develop signs/symptoms of pancreatitis (e.g., persistent abdominal pain, nausea, or vomiting).
   b. Hypersensitivity reactions may include angioedema, severe skin rash, or difficulty breathing.

G. **Bile acid sequestrant**
1. Agent: Colesevelam (Welchol)
2. Indication: adjunctive therapy for the management of T2DM
3. Contraindications
   a. Persons with a history of bowel obstruction, hypertriglyceridemia-induced pancreatitis, or serum triglyceride concentration > 500 mg/dL.
   b. Persons with gastroparesis or other severe GI motility disorders due to constipating effects

4. Mechanism of action for improved glycemic control is unknown.
5. **Administration and dosage** (*Table 46-3*)
6. Patient education and other concerns
   a. Oral medications should be taken 1 hr before or 4 hrs after colesevelam.
   b. Constipation is the most common adverse effect.

H. Dopamine agonist

1. Agent: Bromocriptine (Cycloset)
2. Indication: adjunctive therapy for the management of T2DM
3. Contraindications: Use with caution in persons with cardiovascular disease (e.g., myocardial infarction, arrhythmias), dementia, psychosis, or peptic ulcer disease.
4. Mechanism of action for improvement in glycemic control is unknown; however, it is postulated that bromocriptine may affect circadian rhythms, which may play a role in obesity and insulin resistance.
5. **Administration and dosage** (*Table 46-3*)
6. Patient education and other concerns
   a. May cause dizziness and fatigue. Use caution when performing tasks that require mental alertness.
   b. May cause **gastrointestinal discomfort**, nausea, or vomiting. **Take with food** to lessen gastrointestinal discomfort.
   c. **Take within 2 hrs after waking in the morning.** Dose will be increased weekly until the maximum tolerated dose is achieved.

I. Available oral combination products

1. Metformin/glyburide (Glucovance)
2. Metformin/glipizide (Metaglip)
3. Metformin/rosiglitazone (Avandamet): restricted access medication
4. Metformin/pioglitazone (Actoplus Met, Actoplus Met XR)
5. Metformin/repaglinide (PrandiMet)
6. Metformin/saxagliptin (Kombiglyze)
7. Metformin/sitagliptin (Janumet, Janumet XR)
8. Rosiglitazone/glimepiride (Avandaryl): restricted access medication
9. Pioglitazone/glimepiride (Duetact)

J. Incretin mimetics (GLP-1 agonists)

1. **Agents**
   a. Exenatide (Byetta)
   b. Liraglutide (Victoza)
2. **Indication:** management of T2DM
3. **Contraindications**
   a. Individuals with severe GI motility disease (e.g., gastroparesis)
   b. Pancreatitis or a history of pancreatitis
   c. Severe renal impairment or hepatic impairment
   d. Liraglutide is contraindicated in individuals with a history or family history of medullary thyroid carcinoma (MTC) and individuals with multiple endocrine neoplasia syndrome type 2 (MEN2). It may be used in individuals with other thyroid disorders, including hypothyroidism or hyperthyroidism.
4. **Mechanisms of action.** Increases glucose dependent insulin secretion, decreases hepatic glucose output, increases β-cell growth and replication, slows gastric emptying, and enhances satiety.
5. **Administration and dosage** (*Table 46-3*)
6. **Patient education and other concerns**
   a. Exenatide should be administered within 60 mins of a meal twice daily. Liraglutide may be dosed independent of meals once daily.
   b. Administration sites include the upper arm, thigh, or abdomen.
   c. Nausea and vomiting may occur with initiation and dose changes, but is typically a transient effect. Weight loss is a sustained effect unrelated to gastrointestinal effects.
   d. Report unusual lump or swelling of the neck, difficulty swallowing, or unusual hoarseness with the use of liraglutide.

K. Amylin receptor agonist

1. **Agent: Pramlintide** (Symlin)
2. **Indication:** enhanced postprandial control in individuals with **T1DM or T2DM**

3. **Contraindication:** Use should be avoided in individuals with gastric motility disorders, such as **gastroparesis**
4. **Mechanisms of action.** Slows gastric emptying; decreases postprandial glucagon secretion; suppresses appetite
5. **Administration and dosage** (*Table 46-3*)
6. **Patient education and other concerns**
   a. When concomitantly given with insulin, may produce severe hypoglycemia within 3 hrs of administration.
   b. Pre- and post-blood glucose monitoring should be used to determine efficacy of agent.
   c. Administration is into abdomen or thigh; injection into upper arm should be avoided due to variable absorption.
   d. Oral medications needing rapid onset of action (e.g., antibiotics, analgesics) should be administered 1 hr before, or 2 hrs after pramlintide.
   e. Do not mix in same syringe as insulin. Inject at least 2 inches away from insulin injection.

L. **Emerging treatment options**
1. **Once weekly exenatide** (Bydureon)*: Dosed once weekly as a 2 mg subcutaneous injection, this agent targets over-all blood glucose control rather than postprandial as seen with other GLP-1 agonists; because it takes 6 weeks for this agent to hit steady state, there is no dose titration necessary and less pronounced gastrointestinal effects. Onset of action is approximately 2 weeks.
2. **Sodium glucose transporter 2 (SGLT2) inhibitors:** SGLT2 is a transporter in the kidneys that is responsible for approximately 90% of renal glucose reabsorption. The SGLT2 inhibitors are proposed to inhibit this transporter, thus increasing the urinary excretion of glucose and lowering blood glucose levels. These agents are unique in that they provide an insulin-independent mechanism of action with near absence of hypoglycemia. Agents currently in clinical trials include dapagliflozin, sergliflozin, and remogliflozin.

VI. GLYCEMIC MANAGEMENT OF T2DM

A. **Initiation of therapy.** Unless contraindications exist, metformin is the preferred initial agent for the management of T2DM. However, therapy should be individualized, taking into account the significance of the hyperglycemia and the desired target of therapy.
1. **Treatment based on current A1c level:**
   a. **6.5% to 7.5%:** Metformin is the preferred initial agent, but a DPP-IV inhibitor, GLP-1 agonist, or α-glucosidase inhibitor may be considered when the postprandial blood glucose is of most concern. A TZD may also be initial therapy when metabolic syndrome and/or nonalcoholic fatty liver disease (NAFLD) is present. Monotherapy should be tried for 2 to 3 months with the initiating agent prior to adding other agents to the regimen.
   b. **7.6% to 9.0%:** Dual therapy should be initiated with metformin providing the backbone of therapy, unless contraindicated. A GLP-1, DPP-IV inhibitor, TZD, sulfonylurea, or meglitinide may be used in combination with the metformin. The chosen therapy should be continued for 2 to 3 months before consideration of an additional agent for glycemic control.
   c. **> 9.0%**
      (1) Symptomatic: Insulin with or without additional oral agents
      (2) Asymptomatic: Dual or triple oral therapy with metformin as the backbone.
2. **Targeted blood glucose control**
   a. **Fasting blood glucose target:** consider metformin, sulfonylurea, TZD, or long-acting basal insulin
   b. **Postprandial blood glucose target:** consider GLP-1 agonist, meglitinide, rapid-acting insulin, or α-glucosidase inhibitor

B. **Management.** Maintaining glycemic control should also be individualized. Consideration should be given to initiating insulin if more than three oral agents are needed to maintain glycemic control or if the A1c remains > 8.5% with dual oral therapy.

---

*In January 2012, Bydureon (long-acting exenatide) was FDA-approved for once weekly injection as adjunct therapy in the management of type 2 diabetes. Mixing of the agent is required immediately prior to injection.

VII. PHARMACOLOGIC THERAPY OF PREDIABETES.

Therapy with data to delay or prevent the disease progression include metformin, pioglitazone, orlistat, and alpha-glucosidase inhibitors (e.g., miglitol, acarbose).

VIII. HYPERGLYCEMIC EMERGENCIES.

The two most common hyperglycemic emergencies are **diabetic ketoacidosis (DKA)** and **hyperosmolar hyperglycemic state (HHS)**. DKA and HHS **differ in the presence of ketoacidosis and the degree of hyperglycemia** (*Table 46-4*).

A. **DKA**, which is caused by profound insulin deficiency, typically occurs in persons with T1DM, but can also occur in those with T2DM. It is characterized by hyperglycemia, ketosis, dehydration, and electrolyte imbalance.
   1. **Pathophysiology**
      a. **Insulin deficiency** leads to the following actions:
         (1) impairs glucose uptake in the peripheral tissues, resulting in hyperglycemia
         (2) impairs protein synthesis and promotes breakdown of protein, thus leading to a loss of lean body mass
         (3) increases hydrolysis of triglycerides, which leads to increased hepatic glucose production (further hyperglycemia) and formation of ketone bodies
      b. **Hyperglycemia** causes **osmotic diuresis**, which leads to hypotonic fluid losses, dehydration, and electrolyte depletion.
   2. **Precipitating factors:** illness or infection, inadequate dosing of insulin or discontinuation of insulin
   3. **Signs and symptoms** often include those typical of hyperglycemia (e.g., polyuria, polydipsia, weight loss, blurred vision), **Kussmaul respirations** (deep, rapid breathing), dehydration, and mental status changes. Persons may appear **lethargic**, have a fruity odor to the breath, or have **gastrointestinal symptoms** (e.g., nausea, vomiting, abdominal pain).
   4. **Laboratory findings** typically include plasma glucose level > 250 mg/dL, but < 600 mg/dL; positive urine and serum ketones; arterial pH < 7.3; sodium bicarbonate < 15 mEq/L
   5. **Treatment** is focused on correction of dehydration, hyperglycemia, and electrolyte imbalance. Treatment may include any of the following as necessary: IV fluids, insulin, potassium, and/or sodium bicarbonate.

B. **HHS** predominantly **affects elderly** individuals and is an extreme manifestation of impaired glucose regulation. HHS is associated with a **higher mortality** than DKA, likely due to severe metabolic changes, delay in diagnosis, or other medical complications that can affect the elderly individual.
   1. **Pathophysiology:** The pathogenesis of HHS is not as clear as DKA. However, HHS does differ from DKA in that insulin deficiency is not as profound, thus increased lipolysis does not occur.

Table 46-4 RECOGNITION OF DKA AND HHS[3]

	DKA	HHS
Onset	Sudden	Gradual
Affected individuals	T1DM (occasionally T2DM)	Elderly
Plasma glucose	Between 250 mg/dL and 600 mg/dL	> 600 mg/dL
Gastrointestinal symptoms (e.g., nausea, vomiting, abdominal pain)	Present	Negative
Serum or urine ketones (nitroprusside reaction)	Positive	Minimal to none
Kussmaul respirations	Positive	Negative
Arterial pH	< 7.3	> 7.3
Serum osmolality 2[(*sodium* + *glucose*)/18]	Variable	> 320 mOsm/kg
Sodium bicarbonate	< 15 mEq	> 15 mEq

DKA, diabetic ketoacidosis; *HHS*, hyperosmolar hyperglycemic state; *T1DM*, type 1 diabetes mellitus; *T2DM*, type 2 diabetes mellitus.
[3]American Diabetes Association. Position statement: Hyperglycemic crises in patients with diabetes. Diabetes Care 2003;26:s109–117.

Individuals with HHS do have osmotic diuresis that produces dehydration, electrolyte depletion, and hypotonic fluid loss to a greater extent than seen in DKA.

2. **Precipitating factors:** illness or infections, hypertonic feedings, excessive fluid loss secondary to hyperglycemia, severe burns, severe diarrhea, dialysis, or the use of diuretics
3. **Signs and symptoms** may include hyperglycemic symptoms (e.g., polyuria, polydipsia, polyphagia, blurred vision, decreased wound healing), **decreased mentation** (e.g., lethargy and mild confusion), or **focal neurological signs** that mimic a cerebrovascular accident.
4. **Laboratory findings** typically include **plasma glucose levels > 600 mg/dL**, normal sodium bicarbonate level, **minimal to no ketones**, **normal arterial pH**, and **high serum osmolality** (measure of dehydration).
5. **Treatment goals** are **similar to DKA**; however, in HHS, caution should be used with aggressive fluid replacement to avoid fluid overload in elderly individuals.

IX. HYPOGLYCEMIA.

Hypoglycemia is the limiting factor for providing aggressive insulin therapy in individuals with T1DM or T2DM.

A. **Definition.** Hypoglycemia is difficult to define, but typically is represented by plasma glucose levels < 70 mg/dL. However, symptoms are the driving determinant rather than an absolute glycemic value since the threshold for the onset of symptoms varies among individuals.

B. **Symptoms** of mild hypoglycemia include sweating, shaking, vision changes, immediate hunger, confusion, and lack of coordination. Severe hypoglycemia occurs when an individual is unable to self-treat due to mental confusion, lethargy, or unconsciousness. Some individuals may have neuroglycopenia and present with symptoms of crying, argumentativeness, inappropriate giddiness, or euphoria.

C. **Causes** can include advanced age, poor nutrition, renal disease, excess of glucose-lowering agents (insulin or insulin secretagogues), or strenuous activity.

D. **Treatment**

1. Mild hypoglycemia: Individuals should check their blood glucose level prior to treating, if possible. If the blood glucose level is low, the person should **eat or drink 10 to 15 g of a fast-acting glucose source** (e.g., 4 oz of fruit juice or regular soda, 3 pieces of peppermint candy) to raise the plasma glucose level 30 to 45 mg/dL. If plasma glucose levels are < 50 mg/dL, treatment with 20 to 30 g of carbohydrate may be necessary. The blood glucose level **should be rechecked 15 to 20 mins after treatment**. If blood glucose levels are low, then hypoglycemia treatment can be repeated.
2. Severe hypoglycemia: Individuals able to swallow may be treated with glucose gel, syrup, or jelly placed inside the individual's check. If this is not possible, **glucagon**, which stimulates hepatic glucose production, may be given by SQ or IM injection. **Nausea and vomiting** are primary adverse effects of a glucagon injection, so the treated person may not immediately feel like consuming further carbohydrates. However, the glycemic response to glucagon is transient (approximately 1.5 hrs), so a small snack should be eaten when the individual is able.

E. **Other types of hypoglycemia**

1. **Pseudohypoglycemia occurs when the individual** perceives hypoglycemic symptoms, but the blood glucose level may be normal, or slightly above normal. Some literature states that there is no need to treat pseudohypoglycemia; however, providing 5 to 10 g of a rapid-acting glucose source can diminish the symptoms without causing significant elevations in blood glucose.
2. **Hypoglycemia unawareness** occurs when hormonal counterregulation and autonomic symptoms disappear. However, individuals do typically have select symptoms, such as those associated with neuroglycopenia, but they may be recognized too late to allow for timely treatment.

X. CHRONIC COMPLICATIONS

A. **Macrovascular complications** include three major types: **coronary artery**, **cerebral vascular, and peripheral vascular disease**. These events occur earlier and at a higher rate in those with diabetes than those who do not have diabetes. Attention to multiple risk factors (e.g., lipids, blood pressure, smoking cessation, and antiplatelet therapy) for prevention of these complications is paramount in the diabetes care plan.

1. **Dyslipidemia:** The **primary focus of lipid management is to lower LDL to < 100 mg/dL** in those without overt CVD and < 70 mg/dL in those individuals with overt CVD (optional

goal). However, the triglyceride value may be the primary target when it exceeds 400 mg/dL. When controlled, the focus should return to lowering the LDL levels. Statins are the drug of choice in lowering LDL levels and should be initiated in any patient with overt CVD and any patient over the age of 40 without overt CVD but with other CVD risk factors, regardless of baseline LDL. **Goals for HDL and triglycerides levels are > 40 mg/dL and < 150 mg/dL, respectively**. Of note, **correcting poor glycemic control will have positive impact on the triglyceride levels**.

2. **Hypertension:** Development of hypertension in persons with T1DM is often the result of nephropathy, whereas in T2DM, it is part of the conglomeration of cardiovascular risk factors. The goal blood pressure should be < 130/80 mm Hg, but this may require more than 2 agents at maximum doses in the individual with diabetes. Initial therapy should be with either an ACE-I or ARB; a thiazide diuretic can be added, if necessary, to meet the blood pressure goal. Lifestyle modifications should include reduction in sodium intake (< 1500 mg/day), weight loss (if appropriate), increased physical activity, and increased consumption of fresh fruits and vegetables.
3. **Smoking cessation** should be recommended at every visit for individuals who smoke because nicotine contributes significantly to the development of both macrovascular and microvascular complications of diabetes.
4. **Antiplatelet therapy:** Aspirin therapy has cardiovascular morbidity and mortality data when used as secondary prevention, but the benefits of aspirin for primary prevention is more controversial.
   a. **Aspirin (75 to 162 mg/day)** should be considered for primary prevention in those with T1DM or T2DM who are at increased cardiovascular risk (e.g., men > age 50 or women > age 60 with another CVD risk factor).
   b. Aspirin is currently not recommended for primary prevention in individuals with diabetes who are at low CVD risk because risks outweigh benefits.
   c. Aspirin should be used as secondary prevention in any individual with diabetes and a history of CVD. If aspirin cannot be tolerated, clopidogrel 75 mg/day should be used.

B. **Eye disease**, considered a microvascular complication, is 25 times more common in the individual with diabetes. In fact, diabetes is the leading cause of new blindness in the United States. Several significant diabetic eye complications can occur (e.g., vitreal hemorrhage, retinal detachment), but **diabetic retinopathy** is the most common.
1. **Cause:** Diabetic retinopathy occurs when damage occurs to the retinal blood vessels, resulting in leakage of blood components through the vessel walls.
2. **Classification:** Retinopathy may be classified as **proliferative diabetic retinopathy (PDR)** or **nonproliferative diabetic retinopathy (NPDR)**.
   a. PDR occurs in response to the lack of oxygen following capillary closure. New vessels are formed along the surface of the retina, but these new vessels are weak and prone to rupture, leading to vitreous hemorrhage and/or macular edema. Visual alteration can range from mild blurring of vision to severe visual obstruction.
   b. NPDR occurs prior to growth of new blood vessels along the retina and may remain asymptomatic for years. NPDR can range from mild to severe and is typically progressive.
3. **Prevention** measures include optimizing control of blood glucose and blood pressure, achieving lipid goals, and avoidance of nicotine-containing products. Routine dilated eye exams should occur within 5 years of diagnosis of T1DM and at diagnosis of T2DM and annually thereafter. Some individuals may be cleared to have eye exams performed at 2-year intervals, but the standard recommendation is an annual exam.
4. **Treatment:** NPDR management is by observation and modifying risk factors. PDR can be treated with panretinal photocoagulation to reduce severe vision loss.

C. **Diabetic nephropathy.** Approximately 20% to 40% of individuals with diabetes will develop diabetic nephropathy, which is the **leading cause of end-stage renal disease (ESRD)**. Markers of kidney damage (e.g., serum creatinine, urine microalbumin levels) are used to detect early stages of kidney disease.
1. **Assessment:** Persistent microalbuminuria is the earliest stage of kidney disease in individuals with T1DM and a marker for the future development in those with T2DM. Serum creatinine is

used to estimate the glomerular filtration rate (GFR) and stage the level of chronic kidney disease (CKD).

a. **Albumin-to-creatinine ratio** in random spot collection can be used to screen for microalbuminuria or macroalbuminuria.
   (1) Classification
      (a) Normal: < 30 μg/mg creatinine
      (b) **Microalbuminuria: 30 to 299 μg/mg creatinine**
      (c) **Macroalbuminuria : $>$ 300 μg/mg creatinine**
   (2) Interpreting results: At least **two positive screenings** should occur within a **3- to 6-month** period to classify an individual as having microalbuminuria or macroalbuminuria, due to the variability in urinary albumin excretion. Levels may be affected by exercise within 24 hrs, infection, fever, heart failure, or significant hyperglycemia or hypertension.

b. **Serum creatinine** should be measured at least annually, regardless of the albumin-to-creatinine ratio. Scr levels can then be used to determine an estimated GFR for staging chronic kidney disease, which ranges from Stage 1 (kidney damage with GFR $\geq$ 90 mL/min) to Stage 5 (kidney failure with GFR $<$ 15 mL/min or dialysis).

2. **Prevention:** attaining and maintaining glycemic and blood pressure control, dietary protein restriction, and the use of ACEI or ARB

3. **Treatment** for microalbuminuria or macroalbuminuria should be with an **ACE-I or ARB** to slow the progression of renal disease. ARBs have data to support their use in individuals with T2DM and macroalbuminuria.

D. **Diabetic neuropathies** include distal symmetric polyneuropathy (DPN) and autonomic neuropathy.

1. **Peripheral neuropathy**, also known as DPN, is a major pathophysiologic risk factor for foot ulceration and amputation.
   a. **Presentation:** DPN occurs at the most distal portions of the lower extremities in a **"stocking and glove" pattern**. Protective sensation is first diminished in the toes and feet, then in the fingers and hands. Affected individuals may complain of **burning**, **numbness**, **or tingling in the lower extremities**.
   b. **Screening** should occur at least **annually** with several simple clinical tests, including the vibration perception (using a 128-Hz tuning fork) and **10-g monofilament** pressure sensation.
   c. **Treatment** is for **symptomatic relief** and may include antidepressants, anticonvulsants, or opioids.

2. **Autonomic neuropathy** involves multiple systems throughout the body, including the cardiovascular, gastrointestinal, and genitourinary systems.
   a. Presentation: Clinical manifestations include resting tachycardia, exercise intolerance, orthostatic hypotension, constipation, gastroparesis, erectile dysfunction, and hypoglycemia unawareness.
   b. Treatment: Improve glycemic control; symptoms associated with the gastrointestinal and genitourinary tracts may be improved with pharmacologic agents, but progression of the disease will not be affected.

XI. PATIENT EDUCATION AND SELF-CARE.

Education and development of self-management goals should be provided for individuals diagnosed with diabetes and prediabetes. Self-care for diabetes typically involves significant lifestyle changes, including dietary changes and activity implementation. Lifestyle changes can often be difficult and therefore require positive reinforcement and involvement of the person with diabetes in the decision-making process.

A. **Medical Nutrition Therapy (MNT)** is nutrition care that provides assessment, education, goal setting, and evaluation of outcomes in an attempt to attain and maintain optimal metabolic control (e.g., glucose, lipid, and blood pressure goals). Exchanges, based on the amount of carbohydrates in different food groups, were previously recommended for regulating blood glucose levels. However, this strategy has been replaced by carbohydrate counting and the plate method.

1. **Carbohydrate counting:** Consistency in carbohydrate intake at meals and snacks is essential for achieving glycemic control, particularly for the postprandial blood glucose levels. Foods that contain a significant amount of carbohydrates (e.g., breads, milk, fruit, rice, beans, corn, and potatoes)

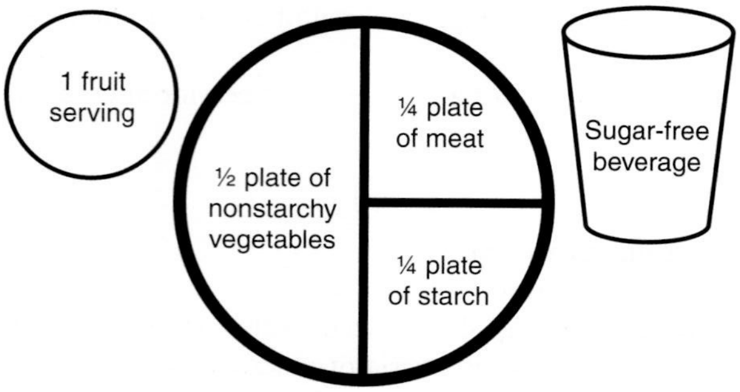

Figure 46-1. The plate method.

should not be eliminated from the meal plan, but incorporated at regularly scheduled intervals. Total carbohydrate intake should be the focus, but protein and fat intake should also be considered due to comorbid conditions (e.g., nephropathy, cardiovascular disease) associated with diabetes.

2. **The plate method** is a tool to provide portion control with healthier food group choices. The concept is to divide and fill a standard-sized dinner plate as follows: half of plate with nonstarchy vegetables (e.g., broccoli, salad, cabbage, collards); one-fourth of the plate with meat (3 oz, cooked); one-fourth of plate with starch (e.g., potatoes, beans, bread, noodles). A serving of fruit may also be combined with the meal in addition to the plate described (*Figure 46-1*).

B. **Physical activity** may be gradually incorporated into daily routines with the goal of at least 150 mins per week of moderate-intensity aerobic exercise. Muscle strengthening activities should be performed at least 2 or more days per week.

C. **Prevention, recognition, and treatment of acute hypoglycemic and hyperglycemic episodes** should be reviewed at every opportunity.

D. **Reduction of modifiable risk factors** to minimize or prevent the development of chronic complications
1. Achievement of glycemic, lipid, and blood pressure goals
2. Smoking cessation
3. Reduction in weight, if appropriate

E. **Pattern control** to determine effect of sickness, dietary choices, stress, and physical activity on ability to attain and maintain glycemic goals.

F. Implementation of **specific self-care measures**
1. **Foot care.** Peripheral neuropathy and peripheral vascular disease in individuals with T1DM or T2DM increase the likelihood of developing lower extremity complications and amputations. Proper foot care is essential to minimize these risks.
   a. The feet should be inspected daily, looking for abnormalities (e.g., cuts, sores, blisters, or irritated areas). Medical attention should be sought if abnormalities are present.
   b. Shoes should be properly fitted and free of foreign objects. Shoes should be worn at all times to avoid trauma to a bare foot.
   c. Toenails should be trimmed straight across with the edges filed.
   d. Lotions, creams, or ointments applied between the toes may lock in moisture, leading to maceration. Avoid applying these agents between the toes.
2. **Dental care.** A yearly dental exam is recommended. In the absence of teeth in the adult with diabetes, examination of the gums is essential due to the high prevalence of periodontal disease in this population.
3. **Eye care.** An annual dilated eye exam should be recommended, beginning 5 years after diagnosis of T1DM and at diagnosis of T2DM. Increased frequency of eye exams may be necessary, depending on the development and severity of eye disease.

XII. DEVICES FOR DIABETES

A. **Syringes**
1. **Barrel size:** Syringes for insulin administration are marked in units. Markings may differ based on size of insulin syringe barrel chosen. Barrel sizes include 0.25-, 0.3-, 0.5-, and 1.0-mL capacity.

The recommendation of a particular size of insulin syringe should be the smallest capacity size available for the prescribed dose of insulin:

   - **a.** up to 25 units of insulin: 0.25 cc (0.25-mL)
   - **b.** up to 30 units of insulin: 0.3 cc (0.30-mL)
   - **c.** up to 50 units of insulin:0.5 cc (0.50-mL)
   - **d.** up to 100 units of insulin: 1 cc (1.0 mL)

2. **Needle length:** available as original ½ inch (12.7 mm) and short 5/16 inch (8 mm)
3. **Needle gauge** simply refers to the **"thickness" of the needle** and is an **inverse relationship (i.e., the higher the gauge, the thinner the needle).** Typical gauges for insulin administration range from 28 to 31 gauge. Because higher gauge needles are thinner, they are also more fragile. Thus, higher gauge needles are typically shorter needles.

B. Insulin pens allow for enhanced portability and eliminate the need for coordination in drawing up a dose of insulin. Most devices are prefilled with insulin and are disposable. It is important to note that insulin pens are for **single-person use** to prevent the spread of blood-borne illnesses.

1. Devices
   - **a.** Solostar (Sanofi Aventis products): glargine (Lantus); glulisine (Apidra)
   - **b.** Flexpen (Novo Nordisk products): detemir (Levemir); aspart (Novolog); aspart mix (Novolog Mix 70/30)
   - **c.** Kwikpen (Eli Lilly products): lispro (Humalog); lispro mix (Humalog Mix 50/50, 75/25)
2. Pen needles are available in several lengths:
   - **a.** ½ inch (12.7 mm)
   - **b.** 5/16 inch (8 mm)
   - **c.** 3/16 inch (5 mm)
   - **d.** 5/32 inch (4 mm)

C. Home blood glucose monitors. A plethora of meters are available to patients today.

1. Meter selection: Some patients choose meter on size, others on cost, and still others on appearance of the meter. When recommending a meter for an elderly patient, the cost of the meter and the manual dexterity and vision of the individual should be kept in mind. Children usually do better with a meter that requires only a minimal amount of blood sample applied to the strip. Meter choices for the visually impaired have tactile markings on the strip or speech output on the meter.
2. Alternate site testing has become more prominent in all populations. However, it is not appropriate in all situations.
   - **a.** Conditions when alternate site testing may be appropriate include:
     - **(1)** In pre-meal or fasting state (> 2 hrs since last meal)
     - **(2)** 2 or more hours after taking insulin
     - **(3)** 2 or more hours after exercise
   - **b.** Alternate site testing should *not* be used if:
     - **(1)** The results from the alternate site do not match how the person feels
     - **(2)** Symptoms of hypoglycemia are present.

XIII. SIGNIFICANT DRUG INTERACTIONS AFFECTING GLYCEMIC CONTROL.

This is only a partial list of potential drug interactions that may affect glycemic control. Consult standard references or drug package inserts for more detailed information.

A. Potential hyperglycemia, as a dose-dependent, direct glucogenic effect. Corticosteroids, nicotinic acid, phenytoin, pentamidine (long-term effect), protease inhibitors, sympathomimetics, isoniazid, furosemide, thiazide diuretics

B. Potential hypoglycemia, as a direct hypoglycemic effect; monoamine oxidase (MAO) inhibitors, fluoxetine, salicylates (large doses), fenfluramine, alcohol, pentamidine (initial effect)

C. Prolonged hypoglycemia and masking of hypoglycemic symptoms. β-Blockers

D. Altered protein binding of, or other drug interaction with, sulfonylurea agents. Alcohol, salicylates, nonsteroidal anti-inflammatory drugs (NSAIDs), methyldopa, chloramphenicol, MAO inhibitors, clofibrate, probenecid

Study Questions

Directions: Each of the questions, statements, or incomplete statements in this section can be correctly answered or completed by **one** of the suggested answers or phrases. Choose the **best** answer.

1. Which patient meets the diagnostic criteria for diabetes, assuming tests were taken on separate visits?

(A) An elderly female with fasting blood glucose values of 102 mg/dL and 132 mg/dL.
(B) A teenage boy with a fasting blood glucose of 128 mg/dL and an A1c of 6.6%.
(C) A 10-year-old girl with a random blood glucose value of 180 mg/dL and 190 mg/dL.
(D) A morbidly obese male with a random blood glucose value of 102 mg/dL and an oral glucose tolerance test result of 160 mg/dL.

2. A 45-year-old obese female has just been diagnosed with diabetes. Otherwise, she is healthy with no other medical conditions. Her blood pressure today is 110/75 mm Hg; spot urine microalbumin < 30; TC 180; HDL 32; LDL 122; TG 150. Based on ADA guidelines, which should be started today?

(A) Aspirin 81 mg daily
(B) Pravastatin 10 mg daily
(C) Lisinopril 10 mg daily
(D) Irbesartan 150 mg daily

3. A patient is currently on a regimen of Humalog Mix 70/30, 24 units in the morning and 12 units in the evening. Based on the following averages obtained from his blood glucose meter, which would be the most appropriate recommendation for his glycemic control today?

Pre-Breakfast: 220 mg/dL
Pre-Lunch: 110 mg/dL
Pre-Supper: 90 mg/dL
Bedtime: 108 mg/dL
3 AM: 62 mg/dL

(A) Increase evening dose of Humalog Mix to 15 units
(B) Decrease evening dose of Humalog Mix to 10 units
(C) Continue current regimen without changes
(D) Increase morning dose of Humalog Mix to 28 units
(E) Decrease morning dose of Humalog Mix to 20 units

4. A 222-lb male presents to the diabetes care team for routine diabetes management. His fingerstick blood glucose value is 452 mg/dL (445 mg/dL on repeat) and his urine is negative for ketones. Per clinic protocol, he may be treated in the office for hyperglycemia. Which is the most appropriate treatment to bring his blood glucose to a target of 120 mg/dL?

(A) Glargine 20 units
(B) Lispro 60 units
(C) Aspart 30 units
(D) Glulisine 11 units
(E) Detemir 24 units

5. A 400-lb male has just been diagnosed with type 2 diabetes. His A1c is greater than 15% and his kidney and liver function are normal. Which would be the most appropriate initial agent for monotherapy?

(A) Metformin 850 mg q.d.
(B) Pioglitazone 30 mg q.d.
(C) Glargine 36 units q.d.
(D) Liraglutide 0.6 mg q.d.
(E) Glimepiride 4 mg q.d.

6. An individual with T2DM currently takes metformin XR 500 mg 2 b.i.d., pioglitazone 45 mg, and glimepiride 4 mg b.i.d. He takes his morning medications at 8 A.M. with breakfast and his evening medications at 6 P.M. with supper. He does not eat lunch. He brings in his log book and meter today, which reveal multiple hypoglycemic events (45 to 62 mg/dL) around 1 P.M. to 2 P.M. His A1c today is 6.0%. Which would be the most appropriate recommendation for glycemic control at this time?

(A) Discontinue morning dose of metformin
(B) Discontinue evening dose of metformin
(C) Discontinue daily dose of pioglitazone
(D) Discontinue morning dose of glimepiride
(E) Discontinue evening dose of glimepiride

7. A 64-year-old female is taking metformin, pioglitazone, and sitagliptin for T2DM. Her liver function tests were elevated (AST 132 u/L and ALT 140 u/L) and she tested positive for Hepatitis C. Which is the best recommendation at this time?

(A) Discontinue metformin only
(B) Discontinue pioglitazone only
(C) Discontinue sitagliptin only
(D) Discontinue metformin and pioglitazone
(E) Discontinue all agents for glycemic control

8. Which best describes the mechanism of action of repaglinide?

(A) Insulin secretagogue
(B) Insulin sensitizer
(C) DPP-IV inhibitor
(D) GLP-1 agonist
(E) α-glucosidase inhibitor

9. A patient has been hospitalized for the past 3 days following a severe asthma exacerbation, but is being discharged today. He weighs 228 lb, but he has no previous history of diabetes. Blood work today shows a random blood glucose of 320 mg/dL and an A1c of 5.2%. His current medication list includes albuterol nebules, prednisone, pulmicort, and oxygen. Which statement is most appropriate?

(A) The patient has diabetes and should be discharged on an insulin regimen.
(B) The patient has hyperglycemia induced by his inhaled corticosteroid.
(C) The patient has hyperglycemia induced by his β agonist.
(D) The patient has hyperglycemia induced by his oral glucocorticoid.

10. A patient currently takes Amaryl, Actos, Januvia, and Lantus. He presents to the clinic today concerned about the swelling in his lower extremities, significant weight gain, and shortness of breath. Which is the most likely cause of presenting symptoms?

(A) Amaryl
(B) Actos
(C) Januvia
(D) Lantus

11. A person newly diagnosed with T1DM will need to start an insulin regimen. Based on her weight of 100 lb, which would be the most appropriate *basal* regimen?

(A) Levemir 13 units daily
(B) Lantus 27 units daily
(C) Novolog 4 units three times daily
(D) NPH 15 units once daily
(E) U-500 1.5 mL twice daily

12. Which formulation is the best recommendation for a patient needing an intravenous insulin infusion?

(A) Regular insulin, U-500
(B) Regular insulin, U-100
(C) NPH insulin, U-100
(D) Aspart insulin, U-100
(E) Aspart insulin, U-400

13. A patient presents for treatment of his type 2 diabetes mellitus (T2DM). His A_{1C} is 7.2% and he has hepatitis C (AST = 150 units/L; ALT = 132 units/L), hypertension, dyslipidemia, rheumatoid arthritis, and mild renal impairment (SCr = 1.6). Which would be the best initial agent at this time?

(A) saxagliptin
(B) metformin
(C) pioglitazone
(D) glulisine

14. An obese woman (350 lb) has used metformin 1000 mg bid to control her T2DM for the past 2 years. Her A_{1C} today is 8%. Which would be the most appropriate recommendation to improve glycemic control without providing further weight gain?

(A) sulfonylurea
(B) thiazolidinedione
(C) GLP-1 agonist
(D) amylin agonist

15. All of the following are correct statements about metformin *except*

(A) metformin may cause renal impairment.
(B) metformin should not be used in patients who are alcoholic.
(C) metformin should be discontinued in women with a SCr > 1.4.
(D) metformin may cause vitamin B_{12} depletion.

16. A patient takes neutral protamine Hagedorn (NPH) 16 units bid and regular insulin 6 units bid. Based on her average blood glucose values below, what is the best recommendation for adjusting her insulin regimen?

(A) fasting: 82 mg/dL
(B) pre-lunch: 180 mg/dL
(C) pre-supper: 110 mg/dL
(D) bedtime: 98 mg/dL

17. A patient has been using continuous intravenous insulin infusion at 0.8 units/hr with steady control after being diagnosed with type 1 diabetes mellitus (T1DM). He is to be discharged from the hospital with prescriptions for detemir and glulisine. When is the most appropriate time to initiate the detemir?

(A) 30 minutes prior to discontinuing the continuous insulin infusion
(B) 1 hour prior to discontinuing the continuous insulin infusion
(C) 2 hours prior to discontinuing the continuous insulin infusion
(D) 1.5 hours after discontinuing the continuous insulin infusion
(E) 3 hours after discontinuing the continuous insulin infusion

Answers and Explanations

1. **The answer is B** *[see III.B]*.
Regardless of age or gender, diagnostic criteria for diabetes in the nonpregnant individual is a positive of at least two of the following values: random blood glucose > 200 mg/dL; fasting blood glucose ≥ 126 mg/dL; OGTT ≥ 200; A1c $\geq 6.5\%$.

2. **The answer is B** *[see X.A.1]*.
Based on ADA guidelines, aspirin should be initiated for primary prevention in women greater than age 60; statin therapy should be initiated in patients with overt CVD or any patient over the age of 40 without overt CVD, but with other CVD risk factors; ACEI and ARBs are recommended for blood pressure control if necessary (not needed here) and when urine microalbumin is > 30.

3. **The answer is B** *[see Table 46-2; V.A.8.b]*.
Increasing the morning dose will only lower the lunch and supper readings further. Increasing the evening dose will lower the 3 A.M. even more. This patient is most likely experiencing rebound hyperglycemia (Symogyi) as evidenced by the hypoglycemia at the 3 A.M. readings and elevated fasting readings pre-breakfast.

4. **The answer is D** *[see V.A.7.a]*.
The blood glucose needs to come down rapidly in-office, thus he would not choose glargine or detemir as agents due to their longer onset of action. Lispro, aspart, and glulisine would all be appropriate choices, but the dose should be based on the point-of-care correction equation ([Current blood glucose-Target blood glucose]/CF). Steps to solve:
    1. Weight in kg: Weight is 222lb = 101 kg
    2. Determine TDD: (101)(0.6) = 60
    3. Determine CF: 1800/60 = 30
    4. Plug into equation: (452–120)/30 = 11 units

5. **The answer is C** *[see VI.A.1.c]*.
Metformin would typically be the initial agent of choice in a patient diagnosed with type 2 diabetes. However, with this patient's A1c greater than 15%, insulin is the most appropriate choice. Metformin can be started in addition to the insulin, but not as monotherapy. Oral agents and non-insulin injections will bring the A1c down no greater than 1%.

6. **The answer is D** *[see V.B.1.a; Table 46-3]*.
The pharmacologic agent most responsible for causing hypoglycemia is the sulfonylurea (glimepiride), which is compounded by the fact that the patient does not eat lunch. The morning dose of glimepiride would peak around lunch time when food intake should be occurring. In the absence of lunch, hypoglycemia results.

7. **The answer is D** *[see V.C.3.b; V.D.3.a; V.F]*.
Metformin and pioglitazone should not be used in a patient with liver disease and elevated LFTs. Sitagliptin may be used in hepatic impairment. When the LFTs go back to a normal range, it can be considered to reinitiate metformin and pioglitazone.

8. **The answer is A** *[see V.B.1.b]*.
Repaglinide is a meglitinide, which works to produce a rapid burst of insulin secretion from the pancreas.

9. **The answer is D** *[see III.B; XIII.A]*.
Inhaled corticosteroids have no effect on the blood glucose of an individual without diabetes and β agonists have no effect. However, oral steroids, such as prednisone can induce significant hyperglycemia, particularly in the midafternoon when dosed in the morning.

10. **The answer is B** *[see V.D.6.a; Table 46-3]*.
Patients taking a TZD such as Actos should be monitored for peripheral edema, weight gain, and shortness of breath due to its propensity to cause or worsen heart failure.

11. **The answer is A** *[see V.A.6.a]*.
NovoLog is not a basal insulin and U-500 is reserved for patients with severe insulin resistance. NPH is dosed twice daily. Basal insulin should be initiated at 50% of TDD. TDD is 27 units, which gives 13.5 units as basal.

12. **The answer is B** *[see V.A.9.b]*.
Regular insulin, U-100 is the most logical choice for an IV infusion. Aspart may be given in an emergency preparedness situation, but should not be given routinely due to the additional cost above that of regular U-100 insulin.

13. **The answer is A** *[see V.F.2; VI.A.1.a]*.
Metformin and pioglitazone should not be used in liver impairment and metformin must be used cautiously in renal impairment. Rapid acting insulin would help with postprandial blood glucose values, but is not considered a standard recommendation for initial insulin therapy in T2DM. Saxagliptin may be used in patients with hepatic and renal impairment.

14. **The answer is C** *[see V.B.6.b; V.D.6.a; Table 46-3].*
Both sulfonylureas and TZDs have the potential to increase weight, whereas GLP-1 agonists and amylin agonists can provide weight loss. Amylin agonist is not appropriate because it should only be added after a basal and bolus insulin have been added.

15. **The answer is A** *[see V.C.3.a].*
Metformin should not be used in patients with renal disease, but the metformin itself does not cause renal impairment.

16. **The answer is B** *[see V.A.8; Table 46-2].*
Increasing morning NPH will cause further decrease of pre-supper reading. Increasing evening doses of insulin will cause fasting blood glucose to be too low.

17. **The answer is C** *[see V.A.9.b.(2)].*
Long-acting insulin should be injected 2 hours prior to discontinuation of a continuous insulin infusion to allow adequate onset time.

47 Thyroid Disease

ERIC C. NEMEC

I. DEFINITION

A. Thyroid disease consists of a multitude of disorders affecting the production or secretion of thyroid hormones resulting in an altered metabolic state. The clinical and biochemical syndromes resulting from too little or too much thyroid hormone production are called **hypothyroidism** and **hyperthyroidism**, respectively.

II. PHYSIOLOGY

A. **Thyroid hormone regulation**

1. The thyroid gland synthesizes, stores, and secretes **thyroxine (T_4)** and **triiodothyronine (T_3)** hormones that are important to growth, development, metabolic rate, as well as the maintenance of healthy, mature, central nervous and skeletal systems.
2. Thyroid hormone secretion and transport are controlled by **thyroid-stimulating hormone (thyrotropin; TSH)**. TSH is released by the anterior pituitary gland that is triggered by **thyrotropin-releasing hormone (TRH)**, secreted from the hypothalamus.
   a. Stimulation of the thyroid by TSH produces increased levels of thyroid hormone (circulating free T_4 and free T_3), which, in turn, signals the pituitary to stop releasing TSH (**negative feedback**).
   b. Conversely, low blood levels of free hormone trigger pituitary release of TSH, which stimulates the thyroid to secrete T_4 and T_3 until free hormone levels return to normal. At this point, the pituitary gland ceases to release TSH, which completes the feedback loop (*Figure 47-1*).
   c. This negative feedback mechanism attempts to maintain the level of circulating thyroid hormone within a narrow range.
3. The thyroid gland also secretes **calcitonin**, which plays a role in calcium homeostasis by reducing blood calcium ion concentration.

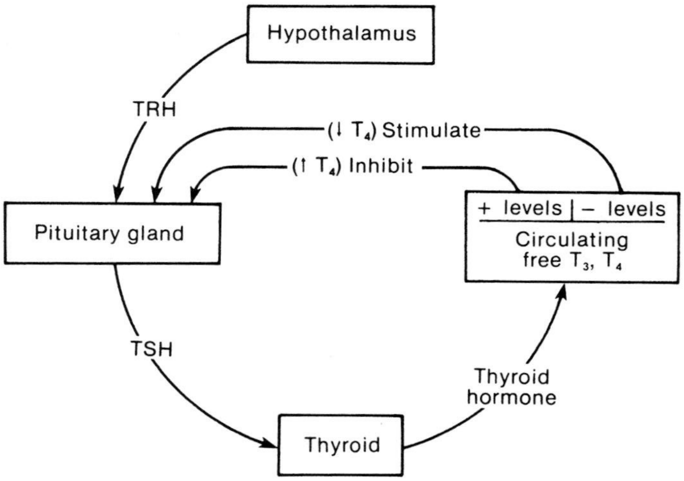

Figure 47-1. Thyroid hormone regulation loop. This carefully balanced hormone regulation system uses both positive (stimulating) and negative (inhibiting) feedback to maintain homeostasis. Disruption of any of these elements can produce serious consequences, such as myxedema crisis (under availability of thyroid hormone) or thyroid storm (overabundance of thyroid hormone). *T_3*, triiodothyronine; *T_4*, thyroxine; *TRH*, thyroid-releasing hormone; *TSH*, thyroid-stimulating hormone.

B. Biosynthesis (*Figure 47-2*)

1. Essential to synthesis of thyroid hormones is dietary iodine, reduced to **inorganic iodide**, which the thyroid actively extracts from the plasma through iodide trapping (**iodide pump**). Some of this iodide is stored within the colloid; some diffuses into the lumen of thyroid follicles.
2. Iodide is oxidized by thyroid peroxidase, and bound to tyrosine residues within the thyroglobulin molecule in the colloid via a process called **organification**.
   a. The oxidation of inorganic iodide to iodine and incorporation into tyrosine residues occurs within thyroglobulin molecules in the colloid, forming **monoiodotyrosine (MIT)**.
   b. **Diiodotyrosine (DIT)** results from the iodization of MIT.
   c. The combination of two DIT molecules forms **tetraiodothyronine (thyroxine, T_4)**, and the combination of MIT with DIT forms **triiodothyronine (T_3)**. These reactions are also catalyzed by thyroid peroxidase.

C. Hormone transport

1. After TSH stimulation of the thyroid gland, T_4 and T_3 are cleaved from thyroglobulin and released into the circulation.
2. When in the circulation, thyroid hormone is transported bound to several plasma proteins, a process that:
   a. Helps protect the hormone from premature metabolism and excretion
   b. Prolongs its half-life in the circulation
   c. Allows the thyroid hormone to reach its site of action
3. Most thyroid hormone is transported by **thyroxine-binding globulin (TBG)**. Transthyretin (TBPA, thyroxine-binding prealbumin) and **albumin** also serve as carriers.
4. T_4 and T_3 are lipophilic molecules and cross the cell membrane easily, however there are iodothyronine transporters that facilitate transportation.

D. Hormone metabolism

1. T_4 is solely a product of the thyroid gland, whereas T_3 is a product of both the thyroid as well as many other tissues; it is produced by deiodination of T_4.
2. Peripheral conversion of T_4 to T_3 occurs in the pituitary gland, liver, and kidneys and accounts for about 80% of T_3 generation.
3. **Deiodination** accounts for most thyroid hormone degradation. The major steps in this process are shown in *Figure 47-3*.
4. Deiodinated hormones are excreted in feces and urine.
5. Minor nondeiodination pathways of metabolism include conjugation with sulfate and glucuronide, deamination, and decarboxylation.

E. Hormone function

1. Although the effects of thyroid hormones are known, the basic mechanisms producing these effects elude precise definition; however, they seem to activate the messenger RNA (mRNA) transcription process, and can promote protein synthesis or (in excessive amounts) protein catabolism.
2. **Thyroid hormones** affect the following:
   a. Growth and development by regulating long bone growth and affecting protein synthesis
   b. Calorigenesis by increasing the rate of basal metabolism
   c. Cardiovascular system by increasing the metabolic rate, which increases blood flow, cardiac output, and heart rate (may be related in part to an increased tissue sensitivity to catecholamines)
   d. The central nervous system (CNS) by increasing or diminishing cerebration
   e. Musculature by causing a fine tremor
   f. Sleep by inducing wakefulness with hyperthyroidism or somnolence with hypothyroidism
   g. Lipid metabolism by stimulating lipid mobilization and degradation

F. Thyroid function studies (*Table 47-1*)

1. **Serum thyrotropin (TSH) assays**
   a. This test is the **most sensitive** test for detecting the hypothyroid state because the hypothalamic–pituitary axis compensates very quickly for even slight decreases in circulating free hormone by releasing more TSH. The TSH levels may be elevated even before low circulating levels of serum total T_4 are detectable by diagnostic testing.

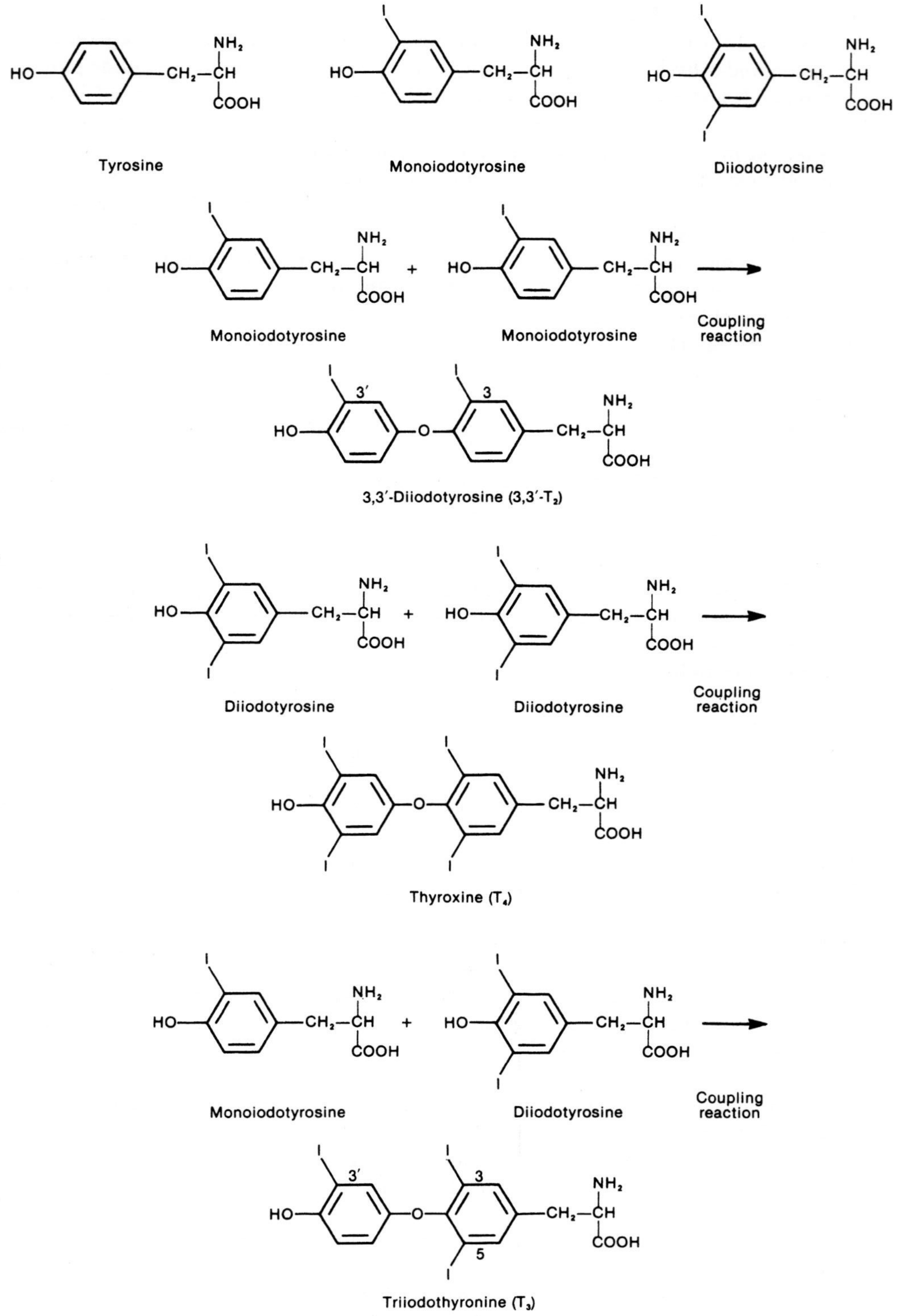

Figure 47-2. Biosynthesis of thyroid hormones. The major products are thyroxine (T_4) and triiodothyronine (T_3). These are formed in the follicle cells of the thyroid gland by iodination of tyrosine residues. Monoiodotyrosine and diiodotyrosine residues are formed first. These then react to form T_3 and T_4.

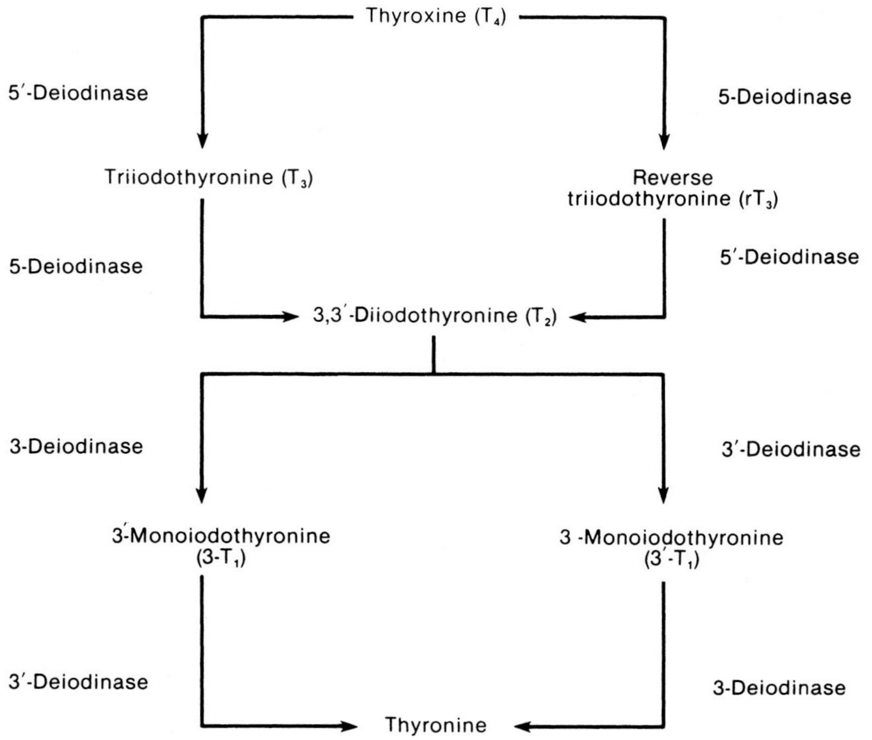

Figure 47-3. Thyroxine metabolism—major steps in the primary and alternative deiodination pathways.

b. The early TSH assay used radioimmunoassay (RIA) methodology. The sensitivity of the assay has improved since, moving to the use of monoclonal antibodies in the late 1980s. Nomenclature established by the American Thyroid Association (ATA) has classified the improvement in sensitivity based on the lower limit of detection. The new classification follows a generational format, as shown in *Table 47-3*.

c. The current (third-generation) serum TSH assay (level of detection 0.01 to 0.02 mIU/L) uses monoclonal antibodies referred to as immunoradiometric (IRMA) or immunometric (IMA) methodology (instead of the older RIA techniques), and demonstrates greater sensitivity in the detection of thyroid disease than older tests.

d. This assay is usually used to diagnose thyroid disease and monitor patients receiving replacement therapy to control overtreatment. Overtreatment—TSH < 0.4 mIU/L—may contribute to excessive bone demineralization (reduced bone density), electrocardiogram (ECG) changes, atrial fibrillation, or elevation of liver function tests.

Table 47-1 TEST RESULTS IN THYROID DISORDERS

Thyroid Function Test	Hypothyroidism	Hyperthyroidism
Serum resin triiodothyronine uptake (RT_3U)	↓ (< 35%)	↑ (> 45%)
Serum total thyroxine (TT_4)	↓ (< 5 μg/dL)	↑ (> 12 μg/dLl)
Serum total triiodothyronine (TT_3)	↓ (< 80 ng/dL)	↑ (> 180 ng/dLl)
Free thyroxine index (FTI)	↓ (< 5.5)	↑ (< 10.5)
Serum thyrotropin (TSH) assay[a]	↑ (> 4.5 μU/mL)	↓ (< 0.4 μU/mL)[b]

[a]In clinical practice the third-generation test is commonly used with sensitivity to detect 0.01–0.02 mIU/L.
[b]Fourth-generation assays detect 0.001–0.002 mIU/L.
↑, increased levels; ↓, decreased levels.

- **e.** The IMA technique is very sensitive. The fourth-generation IMA can detect TSH levels in the range of 0.001 to 0.002 mIU/L.
- **f.** The third-generation IMA assays may also detect subclinical thyroid disease (TSH = 0.1 to 0.45 mIU/L). Treatment of subclinical hypothyroidism is controversial because there is insufficient evidence to indicate a benefit.
- **g.** TSH levels may also be influenced by psychiatric illness. Some studies of hospitalized patients have reported abnormally high or low TSH levels in otherwise euthyroid patients. Current findings in HIV-positive patients are uncertain; however, autoimmune thyroid disease appears to be more prevalent in these patients.
- **h.** Effects of drugs on the serum TSH are shown in *Tables 47-2* and *47-4*.
- **i.** There is some controversy as to the appropriate upper limit of normal for serum TSH. Most laboratories use values of about 4.5 to 5.0 mIU/L.

2. Serum total thyroxine (TT_4)

- **a.** This test provides the most direct reflection of thyroid function by indicating hormone availability to tissues. It determines total (free and bound) T_4 by RIA, which is sensitive and rapid.
- **b.** Virtually all (99.97%) of serum T_4 is bound to TBG, TBPA, or albumin.
- **c.** Changes in thyroid globulin concentration, particularly TBG, which increases during pregnancy, alter the total concentration of T_4, and may produce a misleading high or low test result.
- **d.** However, these changes in TBG do not affect the concentration of free T_4. Therefore, to clarify thyroid function, either protein-binding (T_3 uptake test) or free T_4 must be measured.
- **e.** An elevated TT_4 level indicates hyperthyroidism; a decreased TT_4 level, hypothyroidism. However, the TT_4 level in a euthyroid patient can be altered by other factors, such as pregnancy or febrile illnesses (which elevate the TT_4), nephrotic syndrome or cirrhosis (which lower the TT_4), and various drugs (*Table 47-2*).
- **f.** Normal ranges vary among laboratories; a typical range is 4.6 to 11.2 mcg/dL

3. Serum total triiodothyronine (TT_3)

- **a.** This sensitive and highly specific test measures total (free and bound) T_3 via RIA.
- **b.** T_3 is less tightly bound to TBG and TBPA, but more tightly bound to albumin than T_4.
- **c.** Serum T_4 and T_3 usually rise and fall together; however, hyperthyroidism commonly causes a disproportionate rise in T_3, and the TT_3 can rise before the TT_4 level. Therefore, TT_3 is useful for early detection or to rule out hyperthyroidism. Many of the symptoms associated with hyperthyroidism are the result of the elevated TT_3.
- **d.** This test may not be diagnostically significant for hypothyroidism in which TT_3 levels may fall but stay within the normal range. The TT_3 may be low in only 50% of patients with hypothyroidism.
- **e.** If there is an abnormality in binding proteins, this test can yield the same misleading results as the TT_4 readings. Other factors affecting test results include pregnancy (which increases TT_3 levels), malnutrition or hepatic or renal disease (which lower TT_3 levels), or various drugs (*Table 47-2*).
- **f.** Normal ranges vary among laboratories; a typical range is 75 to 195 ng/dL.

4. Resin triiodothyronine uptake (RT_3U)

- **a.** This test clarifies whether abnormal T_4 levels are the result of a thyroid disorder or to abnormalities in the binding proteins because it evaluates the binding capacity of TBG.
- **b.** If an abnormal amount (high or low) of thyroid hormone is present in the blood, the RT_3U results **change in the same direction** as the altered level—elevated in hyperthyroidism, decreased in hypothyroidism.
- **c.** However, if there is an underlying abnormality in binding proteins the abnormal levels of TT_4, TT_3, or both, the RT_3U results **change in the opposite direction**—decreasing as TBG increases, increasing as TBG decreases.
- **d.** Several drugs can cause spurious changes in the RT_3U (*Table 47-2*).

5. Free thyroxine index (FTI)

- **a.** Free hormone represents only 0.03% of serum total T_4.
- **b.** The FTI has the advantage that the clinician is given both a total T_4 and a thyroid hormone binding ratio or index (THBI), making it clear when the patient has a potential binding protein abnormality.

$$\text{THBI} = RT_3U/\text{mean serum } RT_3U$$

Table 47-2 EFFECTS OF DRUGS ON THYROID FUNCTION TESTS

Drug	Serum T_4	Resin T_3 Uptake	Free Thyroxine Index	Serum T_3	Serum TSH	Comment
p-Aminosalicylic acid	↓	n/d	↓	n/d	↑[a]	Antithyroid effect, rarely, with long-term use
Aminoglutethimide (*Cytadren*)	↑	n/d	n/d	n/d	↑	
Amiodarone[b]	↑	n/d	n/d	↓	↑[q]	Inhibits peripheral conversion of T_4 to T_3
Anabolic steroids and androgens	↓	↑	0	↓[a]	n/d	Decreased serum TBG
Antithyroid drugs (propylthiouracil or methimazole)	↓	↓	↓	↑	0 or ↑	TSH may increase if patient becomes hypothyroid
Asparaginase (Elspar)	↑	↑	n/d	↑[a]	↑[a]	Decreased serum TBG
Barbiturates	↓[c]	n/d	↓	n/d	n/d	Stimulates T_4 metabolism
Calcium carbonate[d]	↓	n/d	n/d	0	↑	Subclinical signs of hypothyroidism; separate time of ingestion of calcium and levothyroxine
Ciprofloxacin[e]	↓	n/d	n/d	↓	↑	Clinical signs of hypothyroidism; separate administration by 6 hrs.
Contraceptives, oral	↑	↓	0	↑	0	TBG usually increased
Corticosteroids	0 or ↓	0 or ↑	0 or ↓	↓	↓	Usual doses decrease TBG; high doses may increase TBG
Danazol (Danocrine)	↓	↑	0[p]	↓	0 or ↓	Decreased serum TBG
Estrogens and SERMs[g]	↑	↓	0	↑	0	Increased serum TBG
Ethionamide (Trecator-SC)	↓	n/d	↓[a]	n/d	↑[a]	Antithyroid effect
Fluorouracil (Adrucil)	↑	↓	n/d	↑	0	Patients clinically euthyroid; TBG increased
Heparin, IV	↑[h]	0 or ↑	↑[a]	0	n/d	FTI is increased with some measures
Hypoglycemics (sulfonylureas)	0[i]	0[i]	0[i]	n/d	n/d	
Iodides, inorganic	0	0	0	n/d	n/d	
Iodides, organic	0	0	0	n/d	n/d	
Levodopa and levodopa-carbidopa (Sinemet, Parcopa)	0	0	0	0	↓[j]	
Levothyroxine (Levothroid, Levoxyl, Synthroid, Unithroid)	↑s[k,l]	↑ or 0 or ↓[k,l]	0 or ↑[k,l]	↑ or 0[k,l]	↑ or 0[k]	
Liothyronine (Cytomel)	↓[k]	0 or ↓[k]	↓[k]	↑ or ↓[k,l]	0[k]	
Liotrix (Thyrolar)	0[k] or ↓s	0[k]	0[k]	0[k,l]	0[k]	

(Continued on next page)

Table 47-2 Continued.

Drug	Serum T_4	Resin T_3 Uptake	Free Thyroxine Index	Serum T_3	Serum TSH	Comment
Lithium carbonate (Eskalith, Lithobid)	0 or ↓	0 or ↓	0 or ↓	0 or ↓	0 or ↑	
Methadone (Dolophine)	↑s	↓	0	↑	0	Increased serum TBG
Mitotane (Lysodren)	↓	0	0[a]	n/d	n/d	
Nitroprusside (Nitropress)	↓	n/d	n/d	n/d	n/d	Clinical hypothyroidism
Oxyphenbutazone and phenylbutazone (Butazolidin)	0 or ↓	↑	↓	n/d	↑[a]	May compete with T_4 for TBG binding, rarely, overt hypothyroidism and goiter may occur
Perphenazine (Trilafon)	↑	↓	↓	↑	0[a]	
Phenytoin (Dilantin)	↓	0 or ↑s	0 or ↓s	↓	0	Stimulates T_4 metabolism and may compete with T_4 for TBG binding
Propranolol (Inderal)	0 or ↑[m]	0[n]	n/d	↓[o]	0	
Raloxifene[g] (Evista)	↑	↓	0	↑	0	Increased serum TBG
Resorcinol (excessive topical use)	↓	↓	↓	↓	↑	
Salicylates (large doses)	↓	↑s	↓[a]	↓	0[a]	Compete with T_4 for TBG binding
Tamoxifen[g]	↑	↓	0	↑	0	Increased serum TBG

[a]Effect deduced, not based on reported clinical evidence.
[b]Data from Rae P, Farrar J, Beckett G, et al. Assessment of thyroid status in elderly people. *Br Med J.* 1993;307(6897):177–180.
[c]Patients requiring thyroid replacement therapy have decreased serum thyroxine when barbiturates are given.
[d]Data from Singh N, Singh PN, Hershman JM. Effect of calcium carbonate on the absorption of levothyroxine. *JAMA.* 2000;283(21):2822–2825.
[e]Data from Cooper JG, Harboe K, Frost SK, et al. Ciprofloxacin interacts with thyroid replacement therapy. *Br Med J.* 2005;330(7498):1002.
[f]May increase slightly but usually remains in the normal range.
[g]Data from Siraj ES, Gupta MK, Reddy SS. Raloxifene causing malabsorption of levothyroxine. *Arch Intern Med.* 2003;163(11):1367–1370.
[h]T_4 assay by competitive protein binding is spuriously increased, but T_4 radioimmunoassay is probably not affected. Free thyroxine measured by dialysis may be increased.
[i]May occasionally decrease serum T_4 and increase resin T_3 uptake.
[j]Slight decrease in euthyroid patients; but in long-standing hypothyroid patients, levodopa considerably decreases the elevated TSH.
[k]In a patient on adequate doses for thyroid replacement.
[l]Increased T_4, FTI, and T_3 tend to return to normal after several months of therapy with levothyroxine. After liothyronine, T_3 may be elevated 2 hrs after a dose and depressed 24 hrs after a dose.
[m]Increased T_4 levels are reported in one study, but not in others.
[n]With short-term propranolol in hyperthyroid patients.
[o]In euthyroid patients, the decreased serum T_3 returns to normal with continued propranolol therapy.
[p]Free thyroxine index may increase slightly but usually remains in the normal range.
[q]Data from Batcher EL, Tang XC, Singh BN, et al. Thyroid function abnormalities during amiodarone therapy for persistent atrial fibrillation. *Am J Med.* 2007;120(10):880–885.
FTI, free thyroxine index; *IV*, intravenous; *n/d*, no data; *s*, slight effect; *SC*, subcutaneous; *SERMs*, selective estrogen receptor modulators; T_3, triiodothyronine; T_4, thyroxine; *TBG*, thyroxine-binding globulin; *TSH*, thyroid-stimulating hormone; *0*, no effect; ↑, increased; ↓, decreased.

Table 47-3 SERUM THYROID-STIMULATING HORMONE ASSAY NOMENCLATURE

Generation	Lower Level of Detection
First (RIA method)	1–2 mIU/L
Second	0.1–0.2 mIU/L
Third	0.01–0.02 mIU/L
Fourth	0.001–0.002 mIU/L

RIA, radioimmunoassay

c. FTI is not a separate test but rather an estimation of the free T_4 level through a mathematical interpretation of the relationship between RT_3U and serum T_4 levels.

$$FTI = TT_4 \times RT_3U/\text{mean serum } RT_3U$$

d. FTI values are elevated in hyperthyroidism, when TBG is low, and decreased in hypothyroidism, when TBG is elevated.

e. Effects of drugs on FTI are shown in *Table 47-2*.

G. Strategies and cost considerations for testing

1. The ATA recommends a free thyroxine (FT_4) and a sensitive TSH assay as the primary laboratory tests for diagnosing thyroid disease (*Figure 47-4*).

2. Thyroid disease screening for the otherwise generally healthy population has been shown to **not be cost-effective** based on the rate of detection and cost associated with massive screening. However, with increased use and improvements in technology, costs have been falling (*Figure 47-5*).

3. Screening of asymptomatic individuals is controversial, and recommendations from major medical groups have been conflicting. The most appropriate **target population** for screening includes:

a. Women older than 60 years and others at high risk for thyroid dysfunction (history of autoimmune disease or type 1 diabetes)

b. Family history of thyroid disease

c. Patients with clinical symptoms of hypothyroidism/hyperthyroidism

d. Pregnant women or those hoping to become pregnant

4. The sensitive TSH assay is useful in detecting patients at risk of receiving an excess amount of thyroxine as replacement therapy.

III. HYPOTHYROIDISM

III. HYPOTHYROIDISM is the inability of the thyroid gland to supply sufficient thyroid hormone. There are varying degrees of hypothyroidism from mild, clinically insignificant forms to the life-threatening extreme, myxedema coma.

A. Classification

1. Primary hypothyroidism (> 90% of hypothyroidism cases)

a. Gland destruction or dysfunction caused by disease or medical therapies (e.g., radiation, surgical procedures)

b. Failure of the gland to develop or congenital incompetence (i.e., **cretinism**)

2. Secondary hypothyroidism

a. Result of a **pituitary** disorder that inhibits TSH secretion. The thyroid gland is normal but lacks appropriate stimulation by TSH.

3. Tertiary hypothyroidism

a. Refers to a condition in which the pituitary–thyroid axis is intact, but the **hypothalamus** lacks the ability to secrete TRH to stimulate the pituitary.

4. Subclinical hypothyroidism

a. Refers to patients without clinical symptoms, a normal FT_4, and elevated TSH levels. Currently, there is insufficient evidence to support treatment because consequences of nontreatment are minimal. However, pregnant women with subclinical hypothyroidism may benefit from T_4 replacement.

Table 47-4 MEDICATIONS INFLUENCING THYROID-STIMULATING HORMONE (TSH) LEVELS

Agent	Mechanisms	Potential Clinical Thyroid Effect(s)	Effect on TSH	Effect on Other Thyroid Function Tests	Comments
Amiodarone	Iodine effects (see Iodine below)	Clinical or subclinical detected hypothyroidism; subclinical hyperthyroidism infrequently	Hypothyroidism is usually during the first 3 months after starting therapy; continue to detect patients at 6 months. Overt hypothyroidism (TSH > 10 μU/mL) has been observed at 6 months. Mild elevations (TSH 4.5–10.0 μU/mL) have been observed at 12 months. Subclinical hyperthyroidism (TSH < 0.35 μU/mL) has been observed occasionally	Increased total T_4 levels	The large iodine load with the administration of amiodarone is the primary contributor to the drug interaction. Regions where patients have adequate intake of iodine in their diet have been associated with higher rates of hypothyroidism. Biochemical changes in thyroid function noted in a majority of patients on therapy, requiring frequent monitoring
	Direct inhibition of T_4 to T_3 conversion			Increased free T_4 levels	
	Direct toxic effects on thyroid			Increased reverse T_3 levels	
	Induction of thyroid autoimmunity	Hyperthyroidism		Decreased total and free T_3	
Calcium carbonate	Adsorption of levothyroxine to calcium in acid environment	Subclinical hypothyroidism	Elevation	Decrease free T_4 and total T_4	
Ciprofloxacin	Decreases absorption of levothyroxine	Hypothyroidism	Elevation	Decreased thyroid hormone levels	Clinical hypothyroidism detected
Corticosteroids	Central suppression of TSH release	Minimal or none	Suppression	Usually within normal range, although total T_4, free T_4, T_3 reduced, and reverse T_3 increased from baseline	Compensatory mechanisms lead to normalization of TSH levels with chronic exposure

	Reduction of thyroid iodine uptake				
	Inhibition of T_4 to T_3 conversion				
	Reduction of thyroid-binding globulin levels				
Dopamine and dopamine agonists	Central suppression of TSH release	Minimal or none	Suppression	Normal or decreased hormone levels	Prolonged use of dopamine in high doses may potentiate the low thyroxine state of critical illness
Dopamine antagonists	Release of central TSH inhibition	Minimal or none	Elevation	Usually normal	Effects not well characterized
Iodine	Inhibition of iodine uptake and organification	Clinical or subclinical hypothyroidism	Elevation	Decreased thyroid hormone levels	Clinical hypothyroidism most common in those with underlying organification defects, such as autoimmune thyroiditis or previous radioiodine therapy; iodine-induced hyperthyroidism is generally confined to those with iodine deficiency or autoimmune thyroid disease
	Impairment of thyroid hormone				
	Inhibition of T_4 to T_3 conversion	Hyperthyroidism	Suppression	Elevated thyroid hormone levels	
	Induction of thyroid autoimmunity				
Interferon	Unclear; likely owing to immunomodulating properties and stimulation of autoimmunity	Hypothyroidism (silent thyroiditis, Graves disease)	Elevation	Decreased thyroid hormone levels	No apparent direct influence on TSH secretion: pretreatment detectable antimicrosomal antibodies may represent a risk factor for interferon-induced thyroid disease
		Hyperthyroidism (with or without autoantibodies)	Suppression	Increased thyroid hormone levels	

(Continued on next page)

Table 47-4 Continued.

Agent	Mechanisms	Potential Clinical Thyroid Effect(s)	Effect on TSH	Effect on Other Thyroid Function Tests	Comments
Lithium salts	Inhibition of iodothyronine biosynthesis Reduction of thyroid iodine concentration Suppression of thyroid hormone release Induction of thyroid autoimmunity	Clinical or subclinical hypothyroidism	Elevation	Normal or decreased thyroid hormone levels	Some sources recommend thyroid function testing at 6-month intervals while on therapy
Radiographic contrast media	Iodine effects (See Iodine above) Direct inhibition of T_4 to T_3 conversion	Minimal or none	Elevation	Normal or decreased thyroid hormone levels Elevation of reverse T_3 levels	Alterations are maximal 3–4 days after administration and may persist for up to 2 weeks
Raloxifene	Malabsorption; mechanism unknown	Hypothyroidism	Elevation	Decreased thyroid hormone levels	Clinical hypothyroidism detected
Somatostatin and analogs	Central suppression of TSH release	Minimal or none	Suppression	Usually normal	Effects not well characterized

T_3, triiodothyronine; T_4, thyroxine.

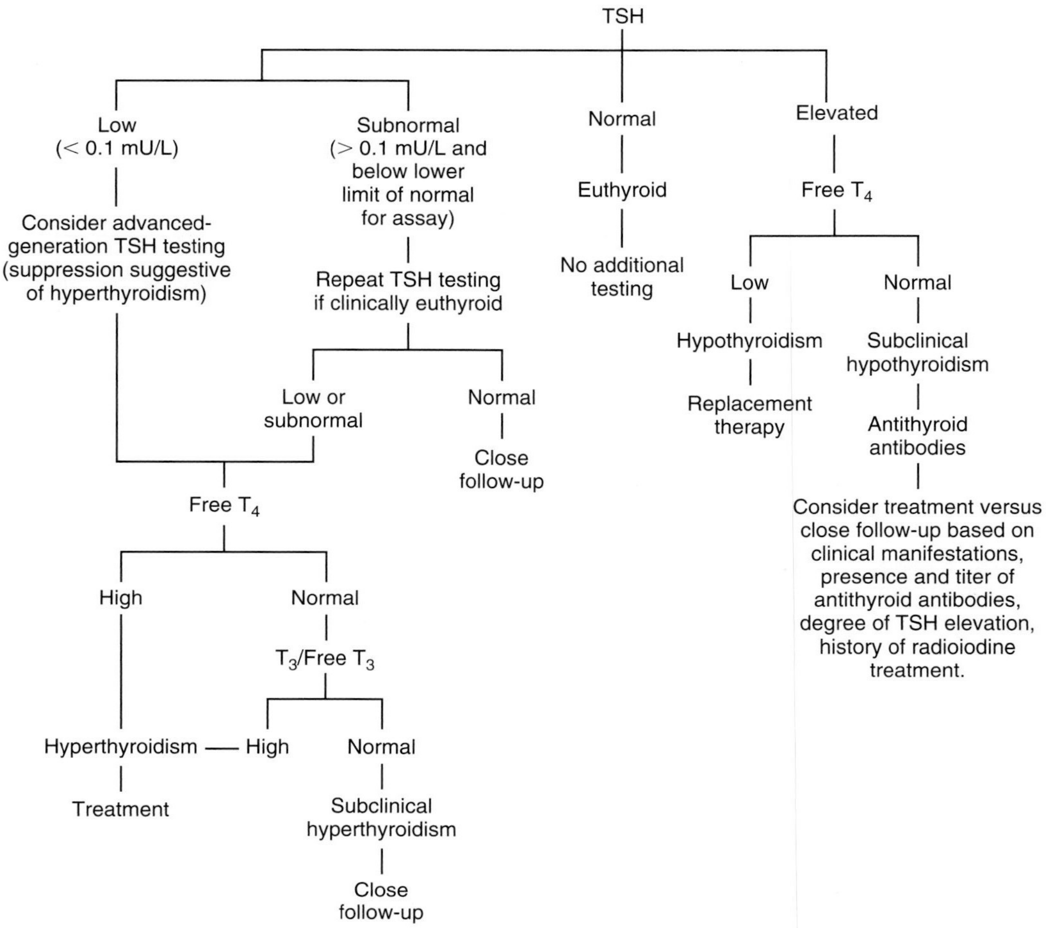

Figure 47-4. Algorithm for using a sensitive thyroid-stimulating hormone (TSH) assay as a single test of thyroid function. The algorithm assumes a clinically intact hypothalamic–pituitary axis, absence of medications known to influence TSH or other thyroid indices, and generally good physical and psychiatric health. The TSH assay should meet the American Thyroid Association criteria for a sensitive assay and/or have a known functional sensitivity limit at the second-generation (0.1 mIU/L) level or greater. *Close follow-up*, clinical observation for signs and symptoms of hyperthyroidism or hypothyroidism and repeated TSH determinations at intervals of 6 to 12 months. *T_3*, triiodothyronine; *T_4*, thyroxine.

B. Causes

1. **Hashimoto thyroiditis**, a chronic lymphocytic thyroiditis that is considered to be an autoimmune disorder
2. **Treatment of hyperthyroidism**, such as radioactive iodine therapy, subtotal thyroidectomy, or administration of antithyroid agents
3. **Surgical excision** of thyroid gland
4. **Goiter** (enlargement of the thyroid gland)
   a. **Endemic goiter** results from inadequate intake of dietary iodine. This is common in regions with iodine-depleted soil and in areas of endemic malnutrition.
   b. **Sporadic goiter** can follow ingestion of certain drugs or foods containing **progoitrin** (L-5-vinyl-2-thiooxazolidone), which is inactive and converted by hydrolysis to goitrin.
      (1) Goitrins inhibit oxidation of iodine to iodide and prevent iodide from binding to thyroglobulin, thereby decreasing thyroid hormone production.
      (2) Progoitrin has been isolated in cabbage, kale, peanuts, Brussels sprouts, mustard, rutabaga, kohlrabi, spinach, cauliflower, and horseradish.
      (3) **Goitrogenic drugs** include propylthiouracil (PTU), iodides, amiodarone, and lithium.

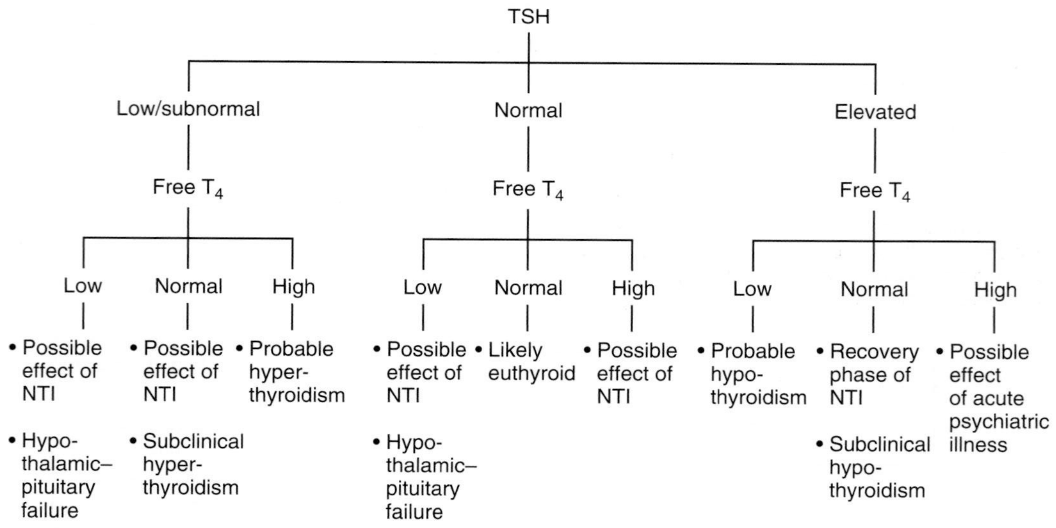

Figure 47-5. Algorithm for the use of sensitive thyroid-stimulating hormone (TSH) testing in patients with nonthyroidal illness (NTI). The TSH assay should meet the American Thyroid Association criteria for a sensitive assay and/or have a known functional sensitivity limit at the second-generation (0.1 mIU/L) level or greater. Medications known to alter TSH levels (i.e., corticosteroids, dopamine) must be considered when interpreting results.

c. **Less common causes** include acute (usually traumatic) and subacute thyroiditis, nodules, nodular goiter, and thyroid cancer.

5. **Amiodarone's** intrinsic drug effects as well as its high iodine content can cause thyroid dysfunction (both hypothyroidism and hyperthyroidism)
   a. It causes decreased T_3 production, T_3 receptor binding, and direct toxic effect on thyroid follicular cells.
   b. Amiodarone's iodine content has a direct toxic effect on the thyroid, and can cause both hypothyroidism and hyperthyroidism based on other underlying disease states.

C. **Signs and symptoms**
1. Early clinical features tend to be somewhat vague: lethargy, fatigue, depression, forgetfulness, sensitivity to cold, unexplained weight gain, and constipation.
2. Progressively, the characteristic features of myxedema emerge: dry, flaky, inelastic skin; coarse hair; slowed speech and thought; hoarseness; puffy face, hands, and feet; eyelid droop; hearing loss; menorrhagia; decreased libido; and slow return of deep tendon reflexes (especially in the Achilles tendon). If untreated, myxedema coma will develop.

D. **Laboratory findings** (*Table 47-1*)

E. **Treatment goal** is replacement therapy to mimic normal, physiologic levels and alleviate signs, symptoms, and biochemical abnormalities (*Table 47-5*).

F. **Therapeutic agents**
1. **Desiccated thyroid preparations**
   a. At one time the agent of choice, desiccated thyroid (Armour Thyroid, Westhroid) has fallen out of favor since standardized synthetic levothyroxine preparations have become available.
   b. Desiccated thyroid preparations are not considered bioequivalent; they have evidenced varying amounts of active substances. Although they met established *United States Pharmacopeia* (*USP*) criteria for iodine content, variation in hormonal content and activity was noted. The content assay, while specific for iodine, was unable to specify the ratio of T_3 to T_4, and this ratio varies with the animal source. Porcine gland preparations are most commonly used, and have a higher T_3 to T_4 ratio than those from ovine and bovine sources.
2. **Fixed-ratio liotrix (Thyrolar) preparations**. In an effort to standardize the T_3 to T_4 ratio, substances that mimic glandular content were developed. However, the T_3 component proved unnecessary (because T_4 is metabolized to T_3) and even disadvantageous because of T_3-induced **adverse effects** (e.g., tremor, headache, palpitations, diarrhea).

Table 47-5 THYROID REPLACEMENT PREPARATIONS

Preparation (Trade Names)	Advantage	Disadvantage	Comments	Source
Desiccated thyroid (Thyroid USP, Thyroid Strong, Armour Thyroid, Thyrar, S-P-T)	Low cost	Some preparations have unpredictable results; inconsistent T_3:T_4 ratio T_3 increases adverse effects	Contains T_3; some brands are standardized by iodine content[a]	Porcine, bovine, or ovine thyroid glands
Liothyronine (Cytomel)	Predictable results; useful for myxedema crisis	Lacks T_4	Usually reserved for myxedema crisis	Synthetic
Liotrix (Thyrolar)	Standardized formulation	T_3 increases adverse effects; expensive	Fixed T_3:T_4 ratio of 1:4; metabolism of T_4 to T_3 renders T_3 component unnecessary	Synthetic
Levothyroxine[b] (Levothroid, Synthroid, Levoxyl, Unithroid)	Predictable results, intravenous preparation available	Expensive	Agent of choice; does not contain T_3; all preparations may be interchangeable	Synthetic

[a]Iodine content and T_3:T_4 ratio vary with species.
[b]Generic formulations manufactured by Pharmaceuticals Basics for Geneva Generics and Rugby have been shown to be bioequivalent to Synthroid and Levoxyl.
T_3, triiodothyronine; T_4, thyroxine; USP, United States Pharmacopeia.
From Dong BJ, Hauck WW, Gambertoglio JG, et al. Bioequivalence of generic and brand-name levothyroxine products in the treatment of hypothyroidism. *JAMA*. 1997;277(15):1205–1213.

3. **Levothyroxine**
   a. Predictable results of the synthetic T_4 preparation and lack of T_3-induced side effects have made levothyroxine (Levothroid, Synthroid, and Levoxyl) the agent of choice.
   b. Levothyroxine preparations are generally considered bioequivalent despite significant controversy. However, when switching formulations, it is recommended to monitor the patient closely because there may be some individual patient variability among formulations (*Figure 47-6*).
   c. The **average adult maintenance** dose is 75 to 150 mcg/day. The dose range has been shown to be 1.5 to 1.7 mcg/kg/day or an average of 1.6 mcg/kg/day for otherwise healthy adults. Levothyroxine should be administered preferably on an empty stomach in the morning, before breakfast.
   d. **Elderly** or **chronically ill patients** require an average dose of 50 to 100 mcg/day, which is 25 to 50 mcg/day less than otherwise healthy adults of the same height and weight.
   e. Athyreotic **pregnant patients** may require a 25% to 50% increase in levothyroxine dosage when pregnancy is confirmed (FDA pregnancy category A). Prepregnancy dosage can be reinstated immediately following delivery.
   f. Thyroxine levels usually return to normal within a few weeks. Clinical improvement begins in 2 weeks with full resolution of signs and symptoms of hypothyroidism by 3 to 6 months of therapy.
   g. TSH levels begin to decrease after starting thyroid replacement. TSH remains elevated for some time after T_4 levels return to normal. Generally, TSH levels return to normal after a minimum of 6 to 8 weeks, but may continue to fall over 6 to 12 months (*Figure 47-6*).
4. **Liothyronine**
   a. Liothyronine (Cytomel) is the L-isomer of T_3
   b. **Average adult maintenance** is 25 to 75 mcg/day
   c. Liothyronine is generally not recommended for treating hypothyroidism. However, it may be useful treating patients with persistent clinical symptoms on levothyroxine. Assessment of this therapy requires measurement of serum T_3 and TSH, since liothyronine will not affect serum T_4.

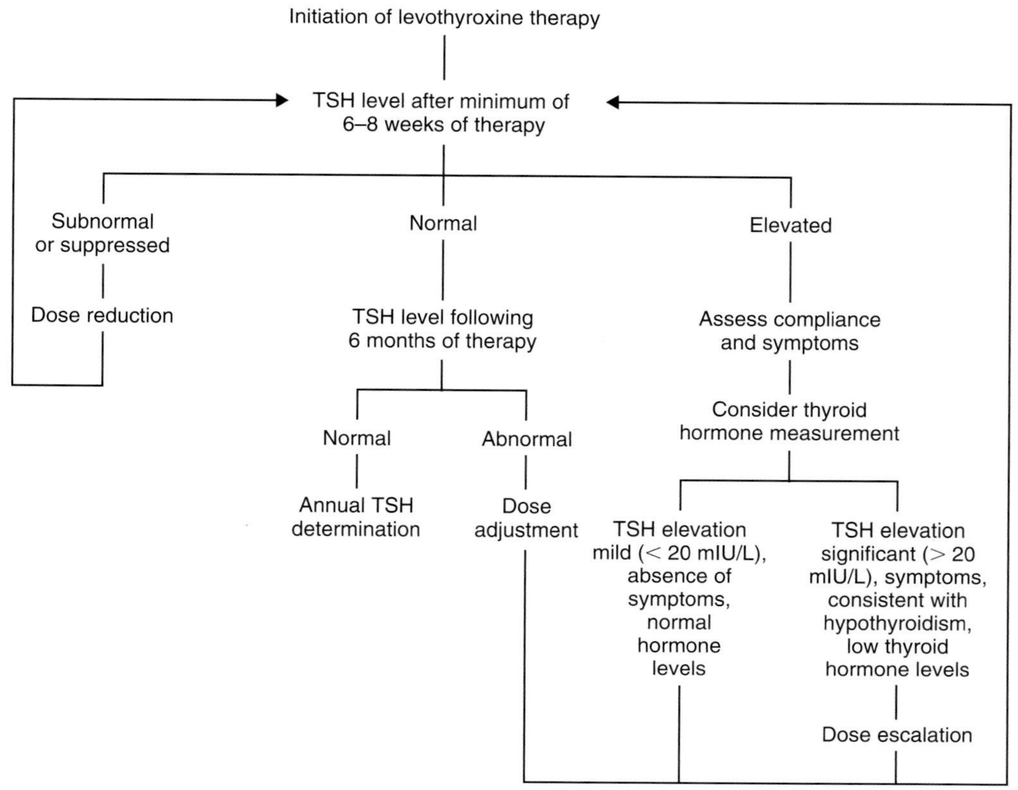

Figure 47-6. Algorithm for management of patients on levothyroxine therapy. *TSH*, thyroid-stimulating hormone.

G. **Precautions and monitoring effects**

1. Adult patients with a history of cardiac disease and elderly patients should begin therapy with lower doses (e.g., 25 mcg/day of levothyroxine). After 2 to 4 weeks, the dose should be increased gradually (12.5 to 25.0 mcg) to an individually adjusted maintenance dose (usually $<$ 100 mcg daily).
2. Patients should be observed on initiation of therapy for possible **cardiac complications**, such as angina, palpitations, or arrhythmias.
3. Serum thyroid levels should be monitored, particularly T_4, sensitive TSH and RT_3U levels, and the FTI. Serum thyroxine tests may remain elevated during the first few months of treatment even with the presence of clinical symptoms. Serum thyroxine tests do not predict the clinical state. Testing is unnecessary unless noncompliance is suspected.
4. It is recommended to monitor the sensitive TSH test 2 to 6 months after the last dose change. However, this test continues to change for up to 1 year. Testing early may result in overtreatment. Refer to *Figure 47-6* for the management of patients on levothyroxine therapy.
5. Levothyroxine administration, particularly long-term therapy, can induce thyrotoxicosis; T_4 levels can rise even though the dosage remains unchanged. Monitor for clinical signs of thyroid disease.
6. **Accelerated bone loss** has been associated with overtreatment. Patients receiving replacement therapy with low TSH values may have lower bone mineral density because excess hormone accelerates the rate of remodeling (rate of resorption $>$ rate of formation), and may contribute to an increased incidence of nontraumatic fracture.
7. **Drug interactions**
   a. **Cholestyramine (Questran) and colestipol (Colestid)**, bile acid sequestrants, can contribute to a decrease in **thyroxine** bioavailability when administered concomitantly. Bile acid sequestrants should be administered at least 6 hrs after oral thyroxine to reduce the potential for this clinically significant drug interaction.

b. **Calcium carbonate** (Os-Cal, Tums) can reduce thyroxine bioavailability by adsorption in an acid environment. These should be administered separately to avoid interaction.
c. **Estrogens** (Estrace, Premarin) and selective estrogen receptor modulators (SERMs) tamoxifen (Nolvadex) or raloxifene (Evista) may contribute to lower levels of FT_4 and elevated TSH levels, requiring an increase in levothyroxine dose.
d. **Raloxifene** has been shown to cause malabsorption of levothyroxine when coadministered resulting in hypothyroidism. Absorption studies demonstrated that separating administration times by ~12 hrs for the two medications prevents the interaction.
e. **Ciprofloxacin** (Cipro) has been reported to interact with levothyroxine when given together, resulting in elevated TSH and reduced FT_4 and FT_3 levels. Administration of the drugs separately, with a 6-hr interval, resulted in rapid normalization of the thyroid function tests.

8. **FDA black box warning**: Do not use thyroid hormones, including levothyroxine, either alone or with other therapeutic agents, for the treatment of obesity or for weight loss. They are ineffective for weight reduction in euthyroid patients, and may produce serious or even life-threatening manifestations of toxicity, particularly when given in association with sympathomimetic amines such as those used for their anorectic effects.
9. **Approximate oral dose equivalency**: Levothyroxine 100 mcg = Liothyronine 25 mcg = Thyrolar 1 grain = Desiccated Thyroid 1 grain

H. **Myxedema coma** is defined as severe hypothyroidism leading to decreased mental status, hypothermia, and other symptoms related to slowing of function in multiple organs. It is a life-threatening complication with a high mortality rate.

1. It is **most common** in elderly patients with preexisting, although usually undiagnosed, hypothyroidism.
2. **Precipitating factors** include alcohol, sedative hypnotic, or narcotic use; overuse of antithyroid agents; abrupt discontinuation of thyroid hormone therapy; infection; exposure to cold temperatures; and iatrogenic insult owing to radiation therapy or thyroid surgery.
3. The patient usually declines from profound lethargy to coma, hypothermia, and a significant decrease in respiratory rate, potentially leading to respiratory failure as the crisis progresses. Hypometabolism produces a fluid and electrolyte imbalance that leads to fluid retention and hyponatremia. **Cardiac effects** include decreased heart rate and contractility, decreasing cardiac output.
4. **Treatment** consists of rapid restoration of T_3 and T_4 levels to normal.
   a. A loading dose of levothyroxine 300 to 500 mcg is given as an intravenous (IV) bolus followed by a daily dose of 1.6 mcg/kg thereafter. Liothyronine, may be given simultaneously as a dose of 5 to 20 mcg, followed by 2.5 to 10.0 mcg given orally every 8 hrs.
   b. Treatment is continued until improvement is noted. Then liothyronine is discontinued, and levothyroxine is changed to the oral preparation. A maintenance dose is then determined (see III.F.3).

IV. HYPERTHYROIDISM

is the overabundance of thyroid hormone. **Thyrotoxicosis** is the general term applied to overactivity of the thyroid gland.

A. **Graves disease (diffuse toxic goiter)**

1. The **most common form** of hyperthyroidism, Graves disease occurs primarily, but not exclusively, in **young women**.
2. The basis of this disease is an **autoimmune disorder** in which antibodies (TSHR-Ab) bind to and activate TSH receptors, resulting in the overproduction of thyroid hormone.
   a. TSHR-Ab are termed **long-acting thyroid stimulators (LATSs)** because their duration of action extends beyond that of TSH. As TSH is only mimicked, not overabundant, neither testing for TSH nor attempts to influence it are productive.
   b. Antibody titers often are elevated in patients with Graves disease.
3. **Signs and symptoms** characteristic of Graves disease include:
   a. Diffusely enlarged nontender goiter
   b. Nervousness, irritability, anxiety, and insomnia
   c. Heat intolerance and profuse sweating
   d. Weight loss despite increased appetite
   e. Tremor and muscle weakness
   f. Palpitations and tachycardia

- **g.** Exophthalmos, stare, and lid lag (slow upper lid closing)
- **h.** Diarrhea
- **i.** Thrill or bruit over the thyroid
- **j.** Periorbital edema

B. Plummer disease (toxic nodular goiter)

1. This **form of thyrotoxicosis** is less common than Graves disease. Its underlying cause remains unknown, but its incidence is highest in patients > 50 years of age, and it arises usually from a long-standing nontoxic goiter.
2. The thyrotoxicosis is a result of one or more adenomatous nodules autonomously secreting excessive thyroid hormone, which suppresses the rest of the gland. Scanning confirms the diagnosis if it indicates that activity and iodine uptake are confined to the nodular mass, unless TSH is introduced.
3. **Signs and symptoms** are essentially the same as for Graves disease except that one or more nodular masses are found, rather than diffuse glandular enlargement, and ophthalmopathy is usually absent. **Cardiac abnormalities** (e.g., congestive heart failure [CHF], tachyarrhythmias) are commonly seen with Plummer disease.

C. Less common forms of hyperthyroidism

1. **Jod-Basedow phenomenon** is an overproduction of thyroid hormone following a sudden, large increase in iodine ingestion—through either a sudden reversal of an iodine-deficient diet or the introduction of iodide or iodine in contrast agents or drugs (e.g., the antiarrhythmic agent amiodarone).
2. **Factitious hyperthyroidism** occurs with abusive ingestion of thyroid-replacement agents, usually in a misguided effort to lose weight. Diagnosis is aided by the absence of glandular swelling and of exophthalmos and the lack of autoimmune activity found in Graves disease.
3. **Subclinical hyperthyroidism** refers to patients without clinical symptoms, a normal FT_4 and FT_3 and TSH levels below the lower limits of normal (< 0.4 mIU/L). Currently, there is insufficient evidence to support treatment because consequences of nontreatment are minimal.

D. Laboratory findings (*Table 47-1*)

E. Treatment goal. Symptomatic relief is provided until definitive treatment can be effected.

F. Therapeutic agents

1. **Antithyroid agents (thioamides)—PTU and methimazole (Tapazole)**
   - **a.** These agents may help attain remission through direct interference with thyroid hormone synthesis. Both agents inhibit iodide oxidation and iodothiouracil coupling. In addition, PTU (but not methimazole) diminishes peripheral deiodination of T_4 to T_3.
   - **b. Therapeutic uses** of these drugs include
     - (1) **Definitive treatment** in which remission is achieved
     - (2) **Adjunctive therapy** with radioactive iodine until the radiation takes effect
     - (3) **Preoperative preparation** to establish and maintain a euthyroid state until definitive surgery can be performed
   - **c. Dosages**
     - (1) **Propylthiouracil**
       - (a) For **adults**, the initial dose is 300 to 450 mg/day in three divided doses (i.e., 100 to 150 mg every 8 hrs). Adult patients with severe disease may require as much as 600 to 900 mg/day initially.
       - (b) The initial dose is continued for about 2 months; then a maintenance dose of 100 to 150 mg/day is given, as a single dose or divided into two doses.
       - (c) Maintenance therapy is continued for approximately 1 year, then gradually discontinued over 1 to 2 months while the patient is monitored for signs of recurrent hyperthyroidism. The patient may remain in remission for several years. A recurrent episode of hyperthyroidism is most likely to occur within 3 to 6 months of drug discontinuation.
       - (d) If hyperthyroidism recurs after drug therapy is stopped, the agent should be restarted, and alternative therapy should be considered (e.g., thyroid gland ablation or removal).
       - (e) **FDA black box warning**: Severe liver injury and acute liver failure, in some cases are fatal, have been reported in patients treated with PTU.
       - (f) A medication guide must be dispensed with this product.

(2) **Methimazole** (Tapazole, MMI)

(a) The initial dose range is 15 to 60 mg/day in three divided doses, depending on disease severity. After 2 months of therapy, a maintenance dose of 5 to 30 mg/day is initiated.

(b) Maintenance therapy is continued for approximately 1 year at which time the drug is gradually discontinued, usually over 1 to 2 months.

(c) **MMI** is generally preferred because of its longer duration of action, more rapid efficacy, and lower incidence of side effects. However, PTU may be the treatment of choice when therapy is indicated during or just prior to the first trimester of pregnancy due to risk of fetal abnormalities with MMI. MMI may be resumed during the second trimester.

d. Precautions and monitoring effects

(1) Serum thyroid levels and the FTI should be monitored for a return to normal. An elevated T_3 may indicate inadequate treatment, whereas an elevated TSH may indicate excessive antithyroid treatment.

(2) Goiter size should decrease with reduced hormone output.

(3) The **adverse effects** are similar for the two agents.

(a) The most bothersome are **dermatologic reactions** (e.g., rash, urticaria, pruritus, hair loss, skin pigmentation). Others include headache, drowsiness, paresthesia, nausea, vomiting, vertigo, neuritis, loss of taste, arthralgia, and myalgia.

(b) **Severe adverse effects**—agranulocytosis, granulocytopenia, thrombocytopenia, drug fever, hepatitis, and hypoprothrombinemia—occur less frequently. Patients receiving methimazole who are > 40 years old and are receiving doses above 40 mg/day are at increased risk of developing agranulocytosis. Patients receiving PTU who are > 40 years old are at increased risk of developing agranulocytosis, but no dose association has been established.

2. Radioactive iodine (RAI)

a. Action. The thyroid gland picks up the radioactive element iodine-131 (^{131}I) as it would regular iodine. The radioactivity subsequently destroys some of the cells that would otherwise concentrate iodine and produce T_4, thus decreasing thyroid hormone production.

b. Advantages

(1) **High cure rate**—almost 100% for patients with Graves disease and only slightly less for patients with Plummer disease

(2) **Avoids surgical risks**—such as adverse reaction to anesthetics, hypoparathyroidism, nerve palsy, bleeding, and hoarseness

(3) **Less expensive**—avoids cost of hospitalization

c. Disadvantages

(1) Risk of delayed hypothyroidism

(2) Slight, though undocumented, risk of genetic damage

(3) Multiple doses, which may be required, may delay therapeutic efficacy for a long period (many months or a year).

d. Usual dosage is 4 to 10 mCi administered orally. Toxic nodular goiter and other special situations will require the use of larger doses.

e. Precautions and monitoring effects

(1) Radioiodine is not typically used in patients younger than 30 years old especially women because effects on future offspring are not known.

(2) Response to ^{131}I is difficult to gauge, and patients must be monitored early for recurrence of hyperthyroidism, and later for hypothyroidism, which may develop even 20 years or more after therapy.

3. β-Adrenergic blocking agents

a. Propranolol (Inderal) usually dosed 20 to 40 mg four times daily reduces some of the thyrotoxic manifestations (e.g., tachycardia, sweating, severe tremor, nervousness) of hyperthyroidism.

b. In addition to providing symptomatic relief, propranolol at high doses (> 160 mg/day) inhibit the peripheral conversion of T_4 to T_3.

c. β-Blockers are primary adjunctive therapy to RAI

4. **Subtotal thyroidectomy**. Partial removal of the thyroid gland may be indicated if drug therapy fails or radioactive iodine is undesirable or contraindicated. This is a difficult procedure, but the success rate is high, and the cure is rapid. Risks include those mentioned in IV.F.2.b.(2), precipitating thyroid storm (see IV.G.2), and permanent postoperative hypothyroidism. The risk of inducing thyroid storm can be minimized by obtaining a euthyroid state through use of antithyroid agents (see IV.F.1) or propranolol (see IV.F.3).

G. **Complications**

1. **Hypothyroidism** may occur iatrogenically or, it has been proposed, as a natural sequel to Graves disease.
2. **Thyroid storm (thyrotoxic crisis)** is a sudden exacerbation of hyperthyroidism caused by rapid release (leakage) of thyroid hormone. It is invariably fatal if not treated rapidly. In this crisis, unchecked hypermetabolism leads ultimately to dehydration, shock, and death.
   a. **Precipitating factors** include thyroid trauma or surgery, RAI therapy, infection, severe emotional stress, and sudden discontinuation of antithyroid therapy.
   b. **Characterized** by a severe hyperpyrexia, tachycardia, agitation, delirium, psychosis, stupor, or coma
   c. **Treatment** is similar to that of uncomplicated hyperthyroidism; however, the doses are higher and given more frequently
      (1) Thioamide selection recommendations vary. **PTU**, in doses of 800 to 1200 mg/day given as 200 to 300 mg every 4 to 6 hrs, may provide additional benefits over MMI as it prevents peripheral deiodination of T_4 to T_3. However, **MMI** 20 to 25 mg every 6 hrs has a longer duration of action.
      (2) **Propranolol**, in doses of 60 to 80 mg every 4 hrs or 1 to 3 mg intravenously every 4 to 6 hrs, should be administered unless β-blockade is contraindicated (e.g., if the patient has CHF).
      (3) **Potassium iodide** (Lugol's solution, SSKI) Lugol's solution, 10 drops three times daily, or SSKI, five drops every 6 hrs, can be given after PTU to block thyroid hormone release.
      (4) Other supportive therapy includes rehydration, cooling, antibiotics, rest, and sedation.

Study Questions

Directions for questions 1–16: Each of the questions, statements, or incomplete statements in this section can be correctly answered or completed by **one** of the suggested answers or phrases. Choose the **best** answer.

1. What is the correct formula to use for calculating the FTI?
   (A) $T_4 \times RT_3U$/mean serum RT_3U
   (B) $T_3 \times T_3$/mean serum RT_3U
   (C) $T_3 \times RT_3U$/mean serum RT_3U
   (D) $T_4 \times RT_3U \times$ mean serum RT_3U
   (E) $T_3 \times RT_3U \times$ mean serum RT_3U

2. What is the necessary precursor besides dietary iodine required for thyroxine biosynthesis?
   (A) T_3
   (B) threonine
   (C) tyrosine
   (D) TSH
   (E) TBG

3. All of the following conditions are causes of hyperthyroidism *except*
   (A) Graves disease
   (B) Hashimoto thyroiditis
   (C) toxic multinodular goiter
   (D) triiodothyronine toxicosis
   (E) Plummer disease

4. Which of the following preparations is used to attain remission of thyrotoxicosis?
   (A) propranolol
   (B) liotrix
   (C) levothyroxine
   (D) PTU
   (E) desiccated thyroid

5. The thyroid gland normally secretes which of the following substances into the serum?
   (A) TRH
   (B) TSH
   (C) DIT
   (D) thyroglobulin
   (E) T_4

6. All of the following conditions are causes of hypothyroidism *except*
   (A) endemic goiter
   (B) surgical excision
   (C) Hashimoto thyroiditis
   (D) goitrin-induced iodine deficiency
   (E) Graves disease

7. Common tests to monitor patients receiving replacement therapy for hypothyroidism include all of the following *except*
   (A) TSH stimulation test
   (B) serum TSH assay
   (C) FTI
   (D) RT_3U
   (E) TT_4

8. The FTI allows the clinician to evaluate all of the following *except*?
   (A) TT_4
   (B) THBI
   (C) Estimated Free T_4
   (D) Exact Free T_4
   (E) RT_3U

9. The inhibition of pituitary thyrotropin secretion is controlled by which of the following?
   (A) free T_4
   (B) TRH
   (C) FTI
   (D) reverse triiodothyronine (rT_3)
   (E) TT_4

10. Which of the following agents has been shown to interact with oral T_4 replacement therapy?
    (A) PTU
    (B) Cholestyramine
    (C) Thyrotropin
    (D) Levothyroxine
    (E) Lovastatin

11. What laboratory tests are currently recommended by the ATA to diagnose thyroid disease?
    (A) RT_3U and TT_4
    (B) TSH and FTI
    (C) TT_4 and sensitive TSH assay
    (D) free T_4 and sensitive TSH assay
    (E) free T_4 and RT_3U

12. Which of the following patient populations should not routinely be screened for thyroid disease?
    (A) Pregnant women
    (B) Patients with type I diabetes
    (C) Patients with a family history of thyroid disease
    (D) College students
    (E) Women > 60 years old

13. What is the average replacement dose of levothyroxine for an otherwise healthy adult?
    (A) 25 to 50 mcg/day
    (B) 50 to 100 mcg/day
    (C) 75 to 150 mcg/day
    (D) 100 to 200 mcg/day
    (E) 200 to 400 mcg/day

14. What factors affect the optimal replacement dose of levothyroxine?
    (A) Age, height, and weight
    (B) Duration of hypothyroidism
    (C) Pretreatment TSH level
    (D) Presence of chronic illness
    (E) All of the above

15. Which of the values represents the lower level of detection for the fourth-generation sensitive TSH assay as established by the ATA?
    (A) 0.5 to 5.0 mIU/L
    (B) 1 to 2 mIU/L
    (C) 0.01 to 0.02 mIU/L
    (D) 0.001 to 0.002 mIU/L
    (E) 0.0001 to 0.0002 mIU/L

16. In which of the following clinical presentations should the TSH assay be used?
    (A) Population screening for thyroid disease
    (B) Screening hospitalized patients
    (C) Patients receiving thyroid replacement after 6 to 8 weeks of therapy
    (D) Patients who are HIV positive
    (E) Screening patients with psychiatric illness

Directions for question 17: The question in this section can be correctly answered or completed by **one or more** of the suggested answers. Choose the answer, **A–E**.

A If **I only** is correct
B If **III only** is correct
C If **I and II** are correct
D If **II and III** are correct
E If **I, II, and III** are correct

17. A 62-year-old woman with a 5-year history of well-managed hypothyroidism was recently started on raloxifene 60 mg daily in the morning for the prevention of postmenopausal osteoporosis. Her thyroid disease had been well-controlled on 150 mcg levothyroxine (Synthroid) daily in the morning. Her TSH has remained within the normal range while on treatment. Her most recent TSH of 2.5 mIU/L and normal FT_4 values where noted last year. She presents today with an elevated TSH 15.5 mIU/L after 4 months of raloxifene therapy and symptoms of hypothyroidism. What change in therapy would be best for this patient?

- **(I)** Repeat the TSH test and FT_4 Tests
- **(II)** Increase the dose of levothyroxine to 200 mcg daily
- **(III)** Switch the dosing of the raloxifene to the evening

Directions for question 18: The question in this section can be correctly answered by **one** of the suggested answers. Choose the **best** answer.

18. A 69-year-old woman with hypertension and hypothyroidism is being treated for a wound infection. In the past, she was maintained on 125 mcg levothyroxine (Levoxyl) daily with a normal TSH of 2.0 mIU/L. After 6 weeks of treatment with oral ciprofloxacin (500 mg twice a day) she complains of fatigue and sensitivity to cold. Her serum TSH level was 14 mIU/L and FT_4 was below normal. What is the best management for this patient.

- **(A)** Increase the dose of levothyroxine
- **(B)** Switch the patient from Levoxyl to Synthroid
- **(C)** Discontinue levothyroxine until the wound is healed
- **(D)** Continue therapy without any changes
- **(E)** Separate the administration of ciprofloxacin and levothyroxine by at least 6 hrs

Directions for question 19: The questions in this section can be correctly answered or completed by **one or more** of the suggested answers. Choose the answer, **A–E**.

- **(A)** If **I only** is correct
- **(B)** If **IV only** is correct
- **(C)** If **I and IV** are correct
- **(D)** If **I, II, III, and IV** are correct
- **(E)** If **II, III, and V** are correct

19. Which of the following agents have been shown to interact with oral T_4 replacement therapy?

- **I** Atenolol
- **II** Calcium carbonate
- **III** Ciprofloxacin
- **IV** Levothyroxine
- **V** Raloxifene

20. What is the effect of amiodarone therapy on thyroid function?

- **(A)** Patients with underlying thyroid dysfunction are at an increase risk of developing hypothyroidism within 6 months of therapy.
- **(B)** Patients without underlying thyroid dysfunction routinely develop subclinical hyperthyroidism with amiodarone therapy.
- **(C)** Amiodarone interacts directly with circulating serum thyrotropin.
- **(D)** Amiodarone has no effect on thyroid function.
- **(E)** None of the above.

21. A 33-year-old underweight woman presents to you. She is currently taking levothyroxine (Synthroid) 200 mcg daily. Her TSH level is reported to be 0.15 mIU/L. What would be the most appropriate change to make to her therapy?

- **(A)** Continue current therapy
- **(B)** Repeat TSH, continue levothyroxine 200 mcg daily
- **(C)** Decrease levothyroxine to 175 mcg daily and recheck TSH in 6 weeks
- **(D)** Decrease levothyroxine to 150 mcg daily, recheck TSH in 6 weeks
- **(E)** Repeat TSH, TT_4, continue levothyroxine 200 mcg daily

22. What is the correct formula to use for calculating THBI?

- **(A)** RT_3U/mean serum RT_3U
- **(B)** $RT_3U \times$ mean serum RT_3U
- **(C)** $TT_4 \times RT_3U$/mean serum RT_3U
- **(D)** $T_4 \times RT_3U \times$ mean serum RT_3U
- **(E)** $T_3 \times RT_3U \times$ mean serum RT_3U

Directions for question 23: The question in this section can be correctly answered or completed by **one or more** of the above suggested answers. Choose the answer, **A–E.**

- **(A)** If **I only** is correct
- **(B)** If **III only** is correct
- **(C)** If **I and II** are correct
- **(D)** If **II and III** are correct
- **(E)** If **I, II, and III** are correct

23. Which of the following drugs are possible treatment options for primary hypothyroidism?

- **I** Desiccated Thyroid (Armour Thyroid)
- **II** Levothyroxine (Levoxyl)
- **III** PTU

Questions 24 and 25 are based on the following case:

AB is a 58-year-old female with a history of Graves disease who has been suffering from severe emotion distress from a recent divorce. She began to develop heart palpitations, a fever, and delirium. She is transported to the emergency department where she admits to stopping her methimazole 2 weeks prior.

24. Which of the following disease states is most likely related to AB's clinical presentation?

(A) Hashimoto thyroiditis
(B) Thyrotoxic crisis
(C) Jod-Basedow phenomenon
(D) Factitious hyperthyroidism
(E) Plummer disease

25. Which of the following is part of the normal therapy for thyroid storm?

(A) Quetiapine to treat delirium
(B) A β-blocker like lisinopril
(C) PTU to inhibit the synthesis of thyroid hormones
(D) Levothyroxine to help augment the negative feedback mechanism and decrease production of thyroid hormone
(E) Methimazole because it is a thioamide and also prevents peripheral deiodination of T_4 to T_3

26. The FDA black box warning for thyroid hormone replacement therapy is:

(A) May cause life-threatening toxicity if used for weight loss
(B) Risk of hepatotoxicity
(C) Risk of nephrotoxicity
(D) May cause tendon ruptures
(E) May cause lactic acidosis

Answers and Explanations

1. The answer is A *[see II.F.5.c]*.
The FTI is a mathematical interpretation of the relationship between the rRT_3U and T_4 levels, compared to the mean population value for RT_3U. The FTI is calculated using reported values for TT_4 and RT_3U. The normal FTI value in euthyroid patients is 5.5 to 12.0.

2. The answer is C *[see II.B]*.
Biosynthesis of thyroid hormones begins with iodide binding to tyrosine, which forms MIT. MIT binds another iodide atom to form DIT. When MIT and DIT are formed, a coupling reaction occurs, which produces T_3, T_4, rT_3, and other by-products.

3. The answer is B *[see III.B.1; IV.A–B]*.
Hashimoto thyroiditis (chronic lymphocytic thyroiditis) is a cause of hypothyroidism. The incidence of Hashimoto thyroiditis is 1% to 2%, and it increases with age. It is more common in women than in men and more common in whites than in blacks. There may be a familial tendency. Patients with Hashimoto thyroiditis have elevated titers of antibodies to thyroglobulin: A titer $<$ 1:32 is seen in $>$ 85% of patients. Two variants of Hashimoto thyroiditis have been described: gland fibrosis and idiopathic thyroid atrophy, which is most likely an extension of Hashimoto thyroiditis.

4. The answer is D *[see IV.F.1–2]*.
In hyperthyroid patients, remission of thyrotoxicosis is achieved with PTU by two mechanisms: (1) interference of iodination of the tyrosyl residues, ultimately reducing production of T_4 and (2) inhibition of peripheral conversion of T_4 to T_3. Propranolol is commonly used as an adjunct to PTU for symptomatic management of hyperthyroidism.

5. The answer is E *[see II.A.1]*.
The major compounds secreted by the thyroid gland, after its stimulation by thyrotropin, are T_3 and T_4. When released from the thyroid, T_3 and T_4 are transported by plasma proteins—namely TBG and albumin.

6. The answer is E *[see III.B; IV.A.1]*.
Graves disease (diffuse toxic goiter) is the most common form of hyperthyroidism. It occurs most often in women in the third and fourth decades of life. There is a genetic and familial predisposition. The cause is linked to an autoimmune reaction between immunoglobulin G (IgG) and the thyroid.

7. The answer is A *[see III.G.3]*.
The TSH stimulation test measures thyroid tissue response to exogenous TSH. It is not commonly used to monitor thyroid replacement therapy. It may be useful in the initial diagnosis of hypothyroidism.

8. **The answer is D** *[see II.F.5.d]*.
The FTI is not an exact measure of free T_4 rather it is a mathematical interpretation between RT_3U and serum T_4 levels that estimates free T_4. The correct formula use would mean that a clinician has knowledge of TT_4, THBI, and estimated free T_4, RT_3U.

9. **The answer is A** *[see II.A.2.a]*.
An increase in the blood level of thyroid hormone (see circulating free T_4 and free T_3) signals the pituitary to stop releasing TSH. The free fraction of T_4 is available to bind at the pituitary receptors.

10. **The answer is B** *[see III.G.7.a]*.
Euthyroid patients receiving oral replacement therapy have become hypothyroid after concomitant administration of bile acid sequestrant therapy. It appears that bioavailability is reduced as a result of administering these agents at close dosing intervals. It is recommended that at least 6 hrs pass before administration of a bile acid sequestrant. It would be preferable to select another nonbile acid sequestrant when clinically possible.

11. **The answer is D** *[see II.G.1]*.
The free T_4 and the (third-generation) TSH assay should be used only for the diagnosis of patients most likely to have thyroid disease based on clinical presentation and relative risk (e.g., age, sex, family history), not for population screening. The third-generation TSH assay is also more commonly used to monitor replacement therapy, and to minimize overtreatment and the corresponding risk of accelerated bone loss.

12. **The answer is D** *[see II.G.3]*.
Cost versus benefit is critical to the decision of choosing to screen entire populations, and screening for thyroid disease has been shown to not be cost effective in the general healthy population. Screening recommendations from major medical groups has been conflicting; however, none of them recommend the routine screening of young, healthy adults.

13. **The answer is C** *[see III.F.3.c]*.
The average adult maintenance dose is 75 to 150 mcg/day, which has been shown to be 1.5 to 1.7 mcg/kg/day. The dose is usually adjusted in increments of 25 to 50 mcg/day every 4 weeks. The total daily dose used to be 100 to 200 mcg/day, which resulted in overtreatment after the introduction of the sensitive TSH assay. Elderly or chronically ill patients require an average dose of 50 to 100 mcg/day, which is 25 to 50 mcg/day less than otherwise healthy adults of the same height and weight.

14. **The answer is E** *[see III.F.3]*.
Elderly or chronically ill patients require an average dose of 50 to 100 mcg/day, which is 25 to 50 mcg/day less than otherwise healthy adults of the same height and weight. Because the average dose for replacement therapy is between 1.5 and 1.7 mcg/kg/day, weight affects the total daily dose.

15. **The answer is D** *[see II.F.1.b–f; Table 47-3]*.
The ATA has established standard nomenclature that indicates each technological improvement and the ability to detect lower levels of TSH using monoclonal antibodies. As the sensitivity of the assay improves, the lower level of detection is reported as a range in milli-International Units per liter. The most sensitive test is currently the fourth-generation IMA, with a reported lower level of detection of 0.001 to 0.002 mIU/L. In usual clinical practice the third-generation IMA is most commonly used, with sensitivity in the range of 0.01 to 0.02 mIU/L.

16. **The answer is C** *[see III.F.3.g; III.6; Figure 47-6]*.
The current third-generation TSH assay is not indicated for use in hospitalized patients who are not suspected to have thyroid disease. Studies have indicated that abnormally high or low TSH levels are detected in euthyroid hospitalized patients. Psychiatric illness may also influence TSH levels.

17. **The answer is B (IV)** *[see III.G.7; Tables 47-2 and 47-4]*.
The patient is most likely experiencing a drug interaction between raloxifene and levothyroxine. The best choice is to separate the medications by at least 12 hrs. A repeat of the TSH assay will only confirm the results, which are significantly elevated. Increasing the dose of levothyroxine may result in overtreatment.

18. **The answer is E** *[see III.G.7; Tables 47-2 and 47-4]*.
This patient is most likely experiencing a drug interaction between levothyroxine and ciprofloxacin when taken concomitantly. There is no benefit to switching to another brand of levothyroxine or increasing the dose. The best solution is to separate the doses of ciprofloxacin by 6 hrs.

19. **The answer is E (I, III, V)** *[see III.G.7; Tables 47-2 and 47-4]*.
Patients receiving oral replacement therapy who take calcium carbonate concomitantly have been shown to experience decreased free T_4 and total T_4 levels that resulted in an elevated TSH. The mechanism appears to be adsorption of levothyroxine to calcium carbonate at acid pH levels, which may reduce bioavailability. It is recommended to separate the time of ingestion of each product to reduce the chance of this interaction. Ciprofloxacin and raloxifene have also been shown to interact with levothyroxine when administered together. Separate administration times by 6 hrs for ciprofloxacin and by 12 hrs for raloxifene.

20. The answer is A *[see Tables 47-2 and 47-4].*
Patients receiving amiodarone therapy are at risk of developing hypothyroidism especially if there is underlying thyroid disease. Amiodarone delivers high levels of iodine to the system contributing to subclinical or clinical hypothyroidism more often. Subclinical hyperthyroidism has been observed rarely. Some patients without underlying thyroid disease may experience changes in thyroid function, while patients with underlying disease are more likely to present with hypothyroidism. Patients should be monitored closely for thyroid function when beginning amiodarone therapy.

21. The answer is C *[see II.G; III.F.3.c].*
The goal of levothyroxine therapy is to normalize TSH. Over replacement can result in symptoms of hyperthyroidism and lead to bone mineral density loss, osteoporosis, and palpitations. A suppressed TSH can identify excessive replacement. Serum T4 concentrations can be useful when nonadherence is suspected, but these concentrations are not routinely needed to monitor levothyroxine therapy. Dose adjustments to levothyroxine therapy should only be made in 12.5–25.0 mcg increments and the average adult dose is typically 75–150 mcg/day.

22. The answer is A *[see II.F.5.b].*
The thyroid hormone binding index (THBI) is a mathematical interpretation of the normalized T_3-resin uptake value (RT_3U). The THBI is calculated using the reported values from RT_3U: the patient's T_3 resin and the normal pool T_3 resin. The mean THBI is therefore by definition 1.00, with a normal range of approximately 0.83 to 1.16.

23. The answer is C *[see II.F; IV.F].*
Levothyroxine and desiccated thyroid are both oral thyroid hormone preparations that are indicated for primary hypothyroidism. PTU inhibits the synthesis of thyroid hormones by blocking the oxidation of iodine in the thyroid gland and is indicated in hyperthyroid disorders.

24. The answer is B *[see IV.G.2; IV.B].*
The most likely disease state is thyrotoxic crisis (thyroid storm). AB has many risk factors for developing a thyrotoxic crisis: Underlying Graves disease, severe emotional stress, and a sudden discontinuation of her antithyroid medication. Hashimoto thyroiditis is an autoimmune hypothyroid disorder and is unlikely as the patient already has a history of Graves hyperthyroidism. Jod-Basedow phenomenon is hyperthyroidism following ingestion of iodine or iodide, there is not anything in the patient's history to suggest iodine ingestion. Factitious hyperthyroidism is the result of an overdose of thyroid hormone, while the clinical symptoms may suggest this; her medical history rules it out. Plummer disease would be evident on physical exam.

25. The answer is C *[see IV.F.1; IV.G.2].*
PTU is a thioamide which inhibits the synthesis thyroid hormones which would be essential for the treatment of a hyperthyroid state like thyroid storm. β-Blockers are effective at controlling the symptoms induced by increased adrenergic tone, however, lisinopril is not a β-blocker. The addition of a synthetic thyroid hormone like levothyroxine has no place in thyroid storm; it will not induce negative feedback; on the contrary, it would contribute to the hyperthyroid state. Methimazole is a thioamide, however, only PTU prevents peripheral deiodination of T_4 to T_3. Delirium will resolve with the treatment of the underlying disease, quetiapine may actually increase TSH, and is not warranted in thyroid storm.

26. The answer is A *[see III.G.8].*
FDA black box warning: Do not use thyroid hormones, including levothyroxine, either alone or with other therapeutic agents, for the treatment of obesity or for weight loss. They are ineffective for weight reduction in euthyroid patients and may produce serious or even life-threatening manifestations of toxicity, particularly when given in association with sympathomimetic amines such as those used for their anorectic effects.

48 Renal Disorders

HEATHER A. SWEENEY

I. ACUTE RENAL FAILURE

A. **Definition.** Acute renal failure (ARF) is the sudden, potentially reversible interruption of kidney function, resulting in retention of nitrogenous waste products in body fluids.

B. **Classification and etiology.** ARF is classified according to its cause.

1. **Prerenal ARF** stems from impaired renal perfusion, which may result from
   a. reduced arterial blood volume (e.g., dehydration, hemorrhage, vomiting, diarrhea, other gastrointestinal [GI] fluid loss).
   b. urinary losses from excessive diuresis.
   c. decreased cardiac output (e.g., from congestive heart failure [CHF] or pericardial tamponade).
   d. renal vascular obstruction (e.g., stenosis).
   e. severe hypotension.
2. **Intrinsic ARF (intrarenal or parenchymal ARF)** reflects structural kidney damage resulting from any of the following conditions.
   a. **Acute tubular necrosis (ATN)**, the leading cause of ARF, may be associated with
      (1) exposure to nephrotoxic aminoglycosides, anesthetics, pesticides, organic metals, and radiopaque contrast materials.
      (2) ischemic injury (e.g., surgery, circulatory collapse, severe hypotension).
      (3) pigment (e.g., hemolysis, myoglobinuria).
   b. Acute glomerulonephritis
   c. Tubular obstruction, as from hemolytic reactions or uric acid crystals
   d. Acute inflammation (e.g., acute tubulointerstitial nephritis, papillary necrosis)
   e. Renal vasculitis
   f. Malignant hypertension
   g. Radiation nephritis
3. **Postrenal ARF** results from obstruction of urine flow anywhere along the urinary tract including:
   a. Ureteral obstruction, as from calculi, uric acid crystals, or thrombi
   b. Bladder obstruction, as from calculi, thrombi, tumors, or infection
   c. Urethral obstruction, as from strictures, tumors, or prostatic hypertrophy
   d. Extrinsic obstruction, as from hematoma, inflammatory bowel disease, or accidental surgical ligation

C. **Pathophysiology.** ARF progresses in three phases.

1. **Initiating phase**
   a. The initiating phase is defined as the time between the renal insult and the point at which extrarenal factors no longer reverse the damage caused by the obstruction or other cause of ARF. This phase may not be well defined clinically and may escape notice or diagnosis.
   b. **Urine output** may drop markedly to 400 mL/day or less **(oliguria)**. In some patients, urine output falls below 100 mL/day **(anuria)**. Oliguria may last only hours or as long as 4 to 6 weeks. However, it has been shown that 40% to 50% of ARF patients are not oliguric or anuric.
   c. **Nitrogenous waste products** accumulate in the blood.
      (1) **Azotemia** reflects urea accumulation due to impaired glomerular filtration and concentrating capacity.
      (2) Serum creatinine concentration, sulfate, phosphate, and organic acid levels climb rapidly.

d. The **serum sodium concentration** falls below normal from intracellular fluid shifting and dilution.
e. **Hyperkalemia** occurs due to the accumulation of organic acids (metabolic acidosis). If potassium intake is not restricted or body potassium is not removed, hyperkalemia results. Without treatment, hyperkalemia may lead to neuromuscular depression and paralysis, impaired cardiac conduction, arrhythmias, respiratory muscle paralysis, cardiac arrest, and ultimately death.

2. **Maintenance phase**
   a. This phase begins when urine output rises above 500 mL/day—typically after several days of oliguria. A rise in urine output or a "diuretic response" may not be seen in non-oliguric patients. Increased urinary output does not signal recovery of renal function.
   b. Urine output rises in increments of several milliliters to 300 to 500 mL/day. Urine output may double from day-to-day in the initial recovery period.
   c. Azotemia and associated laboratory findings may persist until urine output reaches 1000 to 2000 mL/day.
   d. The maintenance phase carries a risk of fluid and electrolyte abnormalities, GI bleeding, infection, and respiratory failure.
3. **Recovery phase**. During the recovery phase, renal function gradually returns to normal. Most recovered renal function appears in the first 2 weeks; however, recovery of renal function may continue for a year. Residual impairment may persist indefinitely.

D. **Clinical evaluation**

1. **Physical findings**. Initially, ARF causes azotemia and, in 50% to 60% of cases, oliguria. Later, electrolyte abnormalities and other severe systemic effects occur.
   a. **Urine output** typically is **low**, from 20 to 500 mL/day. Complete anuria is rare.
   b. **Signs** and **symptoms of hyperkalemia**, resulting from metabolic acidosis and reduced potassium excretion by impaired kidneys, include:
      (1) neuromuscular depression (e.g., paresthesias, muscle weakness, paralysis)
      (2) diarrhea and abdominal distention
      (3) slow or irregular pulse
      (4) electrocardiographic changes with potential cardiac arrest
   c. **Uremia**, caused by excessive nitrogenous waste retention, leads to nausea, vomiting, diarrhea, edema, confusion, fatigue, neuromuscular irritability, and coma.
   d. **Metabolic acidosis**, a common complication of ARF, is evidenced by:
      (1) deterioration of mental status, obtundation, coma, and lethargy.
      (2) depressed cardiac contractility and decreased vascular resistance, leading to hypotension, pulmonary edema, and ventricular fibrillation.
      (3) nausea and vomiting
      (4) respiratory abnormalities (e.g., hyperventilation, Kussmaul's respiration)
   e. **Hyperphosphatemia** arises from decreased phosphate excretion. It is generally not seen in ARF.
      (1) As serum phosphate rises, hypocalcemia results from the formation of insoluble calcium phosphate complexes.
      (2) The signs and symptoms relate to resultant hypocalcemia and metastatic soft tissue calcification.
      (3) Manifestations of hypocalcemia include:
         (a) neuromuscular irritability, cramps, spasms, and tetany.
         (b) hypotension.
         (c) soft tissue calcification.
         (d) mental status changes (e.g., confusion, mood changes, loss of intellect and memory).
         (e) hyperactive deep-tendon reflexes, and Trousseau's and Chvostek's signs.
         (f) abdominal cramps.
         (g) stridor and dyspnea.
   f. **Hyponatremia** results from dilution and intravascular fluid shifts during the diuretic phase of ARF. Physical findings include lethargy, weakness, seizures, cognitive impairment, and possible reduction in level of consciousness.

g. **Intravascular volume depletion**, suggesting **prerenal failure**, may cause:
  (1) flat jugular venous pulses when the patient lies supine.
  (2) orthostatic changes in blood pressure and pulse.
  (3) poor skin turgor and dry mucous membranes.

h. **Other findings** suggesting **prerenal failure** include:
  (1) an abdominal bruit, possibly indicating renal artery stenosis.
  (2) increased paradoxus, suggesting pericardial tamponade.
  (3) increased jugular venous pressure, pulmonary rales, and a third heart sound, signaling CHF.

i. **Postrenal failure** caused by obstructed urinary flow may manifest itself in:
  (1) a suprapubic or flank mass.
  (2) bladder distention.
  (3) costovertebral angle tenderness.
  (4) prostate enlargement.

2. **Diagnostic test results**

a. **Urinalysis** includes an examination of sediment; identification of proteins, glucose, ketones, blood, and nitrites; and measurement of urinary pH and urine specific gravity (concentration) or osmolality (dilution). Prior administration of fluids, diuretics, and changes in urinary pH may confound accurate diagnosis, using urinalysis.
  (1) **Urinary sediment examination**
    (a) Few casts and formed elements are found in prerenal ARF.
    (b) Pigmented cellular casts and renal tubular epithelial cells appear with ATN.
    (c) Red blood cell and white blood cell casts generally reflect inflammatory disease.
    (d) Large numbers of broad white cell casts suggest chronic renal failure.
  (2) The presence of blood in the urine **(hematuria)** or proteins **(proteinuria)** indicates renal dysfunction.
  (3) **Urine-specific gravity** ranges from 1.010 to 1.016 in ARF.
  (4) **Urine osmolality** typically rises in prerenal ARF due to increased secretion of antidiuretic hormone.

b. **Measurement of urine sodium** and **creatinine levels** can help classify ARF.
  (1) In **prerenal** ARF, the urine creatinine concentration **increases** and urine sodium level **decreases.**
  (2) In **intrinsic** ARF resulting from ATN, the urine creatinine concentration **decreases** and the urine sodium level **increases.**

c. **Creatinine clearance**, an index of the **glomerular filtration rate (GFR)**, allows estimation of the number of functioning nephrons; decreased creatinine clearance indicates renal dysfunction. A timed urine collection should be used to calculate GFR in acute renal failure.

d. **Blood chemistry** provides an index of renal excretory function and body chemistry status. Findings typical of ARF include:
  (1) increased blood urea nitrogen (BUN).
  (2) increased serum creatinine concentration.
  (3) possible increase in hemoglobin and hematocrit values due to dehydration.
  (4) abnormal serum electrolyte values.
    (a) Serum potassium level above 5 mEq/L
    (b) Serum phosphate level above 2.6 mEq/L (4.8 mg/dL)
    (c) Serum calcium level below 4 mEq/L (8.5 mg/dL), reflecting hypocalcemia. (The serum calcium level must be correlated with the serum albumin level. Each rise or fall of 1 g/dL of serum albumin beyond its normal range is responsible for a corresponding increase or decrease in serum calcium of approximately 0.8 mg/dL. A below-normal serum albumin level may result in a deceptively low serum calcium level.)
    (d) Serum sodium level below 135 mEq/L, reflecting hyponatremia
  (5) Abnormal arterial blood gas values (pH below 7.35, bicarbonate concentration [$HCO^{-}3$] below 22), reflecting metabolic acidosis

e. **Renal failure index (RFI)** is the ratio of urine sodium concentration to the urine-to-serum creatinine ratio. The RFI helps determine the etiology of ARF. Typically, the RFI is less than 1 in prerenal ARF or acute glomerulonephritis (a cause of intrinsic ARF). The RFI is greater than 2 in postrenal ARF and in other intrarenal causes of ARF.

f. **Electrocardiography (ECG)** may show evidence of hyperkalemia—that is, tall, peaked T waves; widening QRS complexes; prolonged PR interval, progressing to decreased amplitude and disappearing P waves; and, ultimately, ventricular fibrillation and cardiac arrest.

g. **Radiographic findings**
   (1) **Ultrasound** may detect upper urinary tract obstruction.
   (2) **Kidney**, **ureter**, or **bladder radiography** may reveal:
      (a) urinary tract calculi.
      (b) enlarged kidneys, suggesting ATN.
      (c) asymmetrical kidneys, suggesting unilateral renal artery disease, ureteral obstruction, or chronic pyelonephritis.
   (3) **Radionuclide scan** may reveal:
      (a) bilateral differences in renal perfusion, suggesting serious renal disease.
      (b) bilateral differences in dye excretion, suggesting parenchymal disease or obstruction as the cause of ARF.
      (c) diffuse, slow, dense radionuclide uptake, suggesting ATN.
      (d) patchy or absent radionuclide uptake, possibly indicating severe, acute glomerulonephritis.
   (4) **Computed tomography (CT) scan** may provide better visualization of an obstruction.

h. **Renal biopsy** may be performed in selected patients when other test results are inconclusive.

E. **Treatment objectives**

1. Correct reversible causes of ARF, preventing or minimizing further renal damage or complications.
   a. Discontinue nephrotoxic drugs; remove other nephrotoxins through dialysis or gastric lavage for poisonings.
   b. Treat underlying infection.
   c. Remove any urinary tract obstructions.
2. Correct and maintain proper fluid and electrolyte balance. Match fluid, electrolyte, and nitrogen intakes to urine output.
3. Treat body chemistry alterations, especially hyperkalemia and metabolic acidosis, when present. Treatment may include renal dialysis.
4. Improve urine output.
5. Treat systemic manifestations of ARF.

F. **Therapy**

1. **Conservative management** alone may suffice in uncomplicated ARF.
   a. **Fluid management**
      (1) Fluid intake should match fluid losses. **Sensible losses** (i.e., urine, stool, tube drainage) and **insensible losses** (i.e., skin, respiratory tract) of 500 to 1000 mL/day should be included in fluid balance calculations.
      (2) Volume overload should be avoided to minimize the risk of hypertension and CHF.
      (3) The patient should be weighed daily to determine fluid volume status.
   b. **Dietary measures**
      (1) Because catabolism accompanies renal failure, the patient should receive a **high-calorie, low-protein diet**. Such a diet helps to
         (a) reduce renal workload by decreasing production of end products of protein catabolism that the kidneys cannot excrete.
         (b) prevent ketoacidosis.
         (c) alleviate manifestations of uremia (e.g., nausea, vomiting, confusion, fatigue).
      (2) If edema or hypertension is present, sodium intake should be restricted.
      (3) Potassium intake must be limited in most patients. Fruits, vegetables, and salt substitutes containing potassium should be limited or avoided.
2. **Management of body chemistry alterations**
   a. **Treatment of hyperkalemia**
      (1) **Dialysis** may be used to treat acute, life-threatening hyperkalemia (see *II.F.7*).
      (2) **Calcium chloride or calcium gluconate**
         (a) **Mechanism of action and therapeutic effects.** Calcium chloride or calcium gluconate replaces and maintains body calcium, counteracting the cardiac effects of acute hyperkalemia.

(b) **Administration and dosage**. When used to reverse hyperkalemia-induced cardiotoxicity, calcium chloride is given intravenously, as 5 to 10 mL of a 10% solution (1.4 mEq Ca^{2+}/mL) administered over 2 mins. Doses of up to 20 mL of a 10% solution are safe when given slowly. Another 10 to 20 mL of a 10% solution placed in a larger fluid volume and administered slowly may follow the initial dose. Calcium gluconate is administered as 10 mL of a 10% solution (1 g) for 2 to 5 mins. This may be repeated a second time.

(c) **Precautions and monitoring effects**

(i) Intravenous (IV) calcium is contraindicated in patients with ventricular fibrillation or renal calculi.

(ii) The infusion rate should not exceed 0.5 mL/min. Patients should remain recumbent for about 15 mins after infusion.

(iii) The ECG should be monitored during calcium gluconate therapy.

(iv) Calcium gluconate should not be mixed with solutions containing sodium bicarbonate because this can lead to precipitation.

(v) **Adverse effects** include hypotension, tingling sensations, and renal calculus formation.

(d) **Significant interactions**. Calcium may cause increased digitalis toxicity when administered concurrently with digitalis preparations.

(3) **Sodium bicarbonate** may be given as an emergency measure for severe hyperkalemia or metabolic acidosis.

(a) **Mechanism of action and therapeutic effect**. IV sodium bicarbonate restores bicarbonate that the renal tubules cannot reabsorb from the glomerular filtrate and increases arterial pH. This results in a shift of potassium into cells and reduces serum potassium concentration.

(b) **Onset of action** is 15 to 30 mins.

(c) **Administration and dosage**

(i) Sodium bicarbonate is administered intravenously.

(ii) The dosage is calculated as follows:

$$[50\% \text{ of body weight (kg)}] \times [\text{desired arterial bicarbonate } (HCO^{-}3) - \text{actual } HCO^{-}3]$$

One ampule (50 mEq) may be given intravenously for 5 mins.

(d) **Precautions and monitoring effects**

(i) To avoid sodium and fluid overload, sodium bicarbonate must be given cautiously. Half of the patient's bicarbonate deficit is replaced over the first 12 hrs of therapy.

(ii) Sodium bicarbonate may precipitate calcium salts in IV solutions and should not be mixed in the same infusion fluid.

(iii) Arterial blood gas values and serum electrolyte levels should be monitored closely during sodium bicarbonate therapy.

(4) **Regular insulin with dextrose**

(a) **Mechanism of action and therapeutic effect**. The insulin causes an intracellular shift of potassium. The combination of insulin with dextrose deposits potassium with glycogen in the liver, reducing the serum potassium.

(b) **Onset of action** is 15 to 30 mins.

(c) **Administration and dosage**. Regular insulin (10 units in 500 mL of 10% dextrose) is administered intravenously for 60 mins.

(d) **Precautions and monitoring effects**

(i) The serum glucose level should be monitored during therapy.

(ii) The patient should be assessed for signs and symptoms of fluid overload.

(5) **Sodium polystyrene sulfonate (SPS) (Kayexalate®)**

(a) **Mechanism of action**. SPS is a potassium-removing resin that exchanges sodium ions for potassium ions in the intestine (1 g of SPS exchanges 0.5 to 1 mEq/L of potassium). The SPS is distributed throughout the intestines and excreted in the feces.

(b) **Therapeutic effect**. Administered as an adjunctive treatment for hyperkalemia, SPS reduces potassium levels in the serum and other body fluids.

(c) **Onset of action** of orally administered SPS is 2 hrs; effects are seen in 1 hr when SPS is administered as a retention enema.

(d) **Administration and dosage**

(i) SPS is usually administered orally, although it may be given through a nasogastric tube. The oral dose is 15 to 30 g in a suspension of 70% sorbitol, administered every 4 to 6 hrs until the desired therapeutic effect is achieved.

(ii) When oral or nasogastric administration is not possible due to nausea, vomiting, or paralytic ileus, SPS may be given by retention enema. The rectal dose is 30 to 50 g in 100 mL of sorbitol as a warm emulsion, administered deep into the sigmoid colon every 6 hrs. Administration may be done with a rubber tube that is taped in place or via a Foley catheter with a balloon inflated distal to the anal sphincter.

(e) **Precautions and monitoring effects**

(i) The patient's serum electrolyte levels should be monitored closely during SPS therapy. Sodium, chloride, bicarbonate, and pH should be monitored in addition to potassium.

(ii) SPS therapy usually continues until the serum potassium level drops to between 4 and 5 mEq/L.

(iii) The patient should be assessed regularly for signs of potassium depletion, including irritability, confusion, cardiac arrhythmias, ECG changes, and muscle weakness.

(iv) SPS exchanges sodium for potassium, so sodium overload may occur during therapy. Patients with hypertension or CHF should be closely monitored.

(v) For oral administration, SPS should be mixed only with water or sorbitol. Orange juice, which has a high potassium content, should not be used because it decreases the effectiveness of the SPS. For rectal administration, SPS should be mixed only with water and sorbitol, never with mineral oil.

(vi) **Adverse effects** of SPS include constipation, fecal impaction with rectal administration, nausea, vomiting, and diarrhea.

(vii) SPS should not be used as the sole agent in the treatment of severe hyperkalemia; other agents or therapies should be used in conjunction with this agent.

(f) **Significant interactions**. Magnesium hydroxide and other nonabsorbable cation-donating laxatives and antacids may decrease the effectiveness of potassium exchange by SPS and may cause systemic alkalosis.

b. Treatment of metabolic acidosis. Sodium bicarbonate may be given if the arterial pH is below 7.35.

c. Treatment of hyperphosphatemia

(1) **IV calcium** is first-line therapy for severe life-threatening hyperphosphatemia. Calcium reduces the serum phosphorus concentration by chelation.

(2) **Oral calcium salts** bind dietary phosphorus in the GI tract.

(3) **Sevelamer (Renagel®)** is a non ionic polymer that binds dietary phosphorus in the GI tract.

(4) **Dialysis** may be used to treat acute, life-threatening hyperphosphatemia accompanied by acute hypocalcemia. It is also performed when volume overload is present.

(5) **Aluminum hydroxide (AlternaGel®)** (an aluminum-containing antacid)

(a) **Mechanism of action and therapeutic effect**. Aluminum binds excess phosphate in the intestine, thereby reducing phosphate concentration.

(b) **Onset of action** is 6 to 12 hrs.

(c) **Administration and dosage**. Aluminum hydroxide is administered orally as a tablet or suspension. For the treatment of hyperphosphatemia, 0.5 to 2.0 or 15 to 30 mL of suspension is administered three or four times daily with meals.

(d) **Precautions and monitoring effects**

(i) Aluminum hydroxide may cause constipation and anorexia.

(ii) Serum phosphate levels should be monitored because aluminum hydroxide can cause phosphate depletion.

(iii) Aluminum hydroxide can cause calcium resorption and bone demineralization.

d. **Treatment of hypocalcemia**. Immediate treatment is necessary if the patient has severe hypocalcemia, as evidenced by tetany.

(1) **Calcium gluconate**

(a) **Mechanism of action and therapeutic effect**. This drug replaces and maintains body calcium, raising the serum calcium level immediately.

(b) **Administration and dosage**. When used to reverse hypocalcemia, calcium gluconate is administered intravenously in a dosage of 1 to 2 g for a period of 10 mins, followed by a slow infusion (for 6 to 8 hrs) of an additional 1 g.

(c) **Precautions, monitoring effects, and significant interactions**

(i) Frequent determinations of serum (or ionized in the critically ill patient) calcium concentrations should be performed.

(ii) Serum calcium concentrations usually should not be allowed to exceed 12 mg/dL.

(iii) Avoid administration of IV calcium in patients taking digoxin as inotropic and toxic effects are synergistic and arrhythmias can occur.

(2) **Oral calcium salts**. Calcium carbonate, chloride, gluconate, or lactate may be given by mouth when oral intake is permitted or if the patient has relatively mild hypocalcemia. The usual adult dosage is 4 to 6 g/day given in three or four divided doses.

e. **Treatment of hyponatremia**

(1) Moderate or asymptomatic hyponatremia may require only **fluid restriction**.

(2) **Sodium chloride** may be given for severe symptomatic hyponatremia (i.e., a serum sodium level below 120 mEq/L).

(a) **Mechanism of action and therapeutic effect**. Sodium chloride replaces and maintains sodium and chloride concentration, thereby increasing extracellular tonicity.

(b) **Administration and dosage**

(i) A 3% or 5% sodium chloride solution may be administered by slow IV infusion. The amount of solution needed is calculated from the following equation:

(Normal serum sodium level − actual serum sodium level) total body water

(ii) Typically, 400 mL or less is administered.

(c) **Precautions and monitoring effects**

(i) Hypertonic sodium chloride must be administered very slowly to avoid circulatory overload, pulmonary edema, or central pontine demyelination.

(ii) Serum electrolyte levels must be monitored frequently during therapy.

(iii) Excessive infusion may cause hypernatremia and other serious electrolyte abnormalities and may worsen existing acidosis. Infusion rates should not exceed 0.5 mEq/kg/hr.

3. **Management of systemic manifestations**

a. **Treatment of fluid overload and edema**. As water and sodium accumulate in extracellular fluid during ARF, fluid overload and edema may occur. **Diuretics** and dopamine may be given to reduce fluid volume excess and edema. Treatment should be initiated as soon as possible after oliguria begins. **Mannitol** or a **loop diuretic** may be used; thiazide diuretics are avoided in renal failure because they are ineffective when creatinine clearance is less than 25 mL/min, and they may worsen the patient's clinical status.

(1) **Step 1. Loop (high-ceiling) diuretics**. These agents include **furosemide (Lasix®)**, **bumetanide (Bumex®)**, **torsemide (Demadex®)**, and **ethacrynic acid (Edecrin®)**. Loop diuretics are more potent and faster acting than thiazide diuretics.

(a) **Mechanism of action and therapeutic effects**. Loop diuretics inhibit sodium and chloride reabsorption at the loop of Henle, promoting water excretion.

(b) **Onset of action** for an oral dose is 1 hr; several minutes for an IV dose. Duration of action for an oral dose is 6 to 8 hrs; 2 to 3 hrs for an IV dose.

(c) **Administration and dosage**

(i) **Furosemide**, the **most commonly used** loop diuretic, usually is administered intravenously in patients with ARF to hasten the therapeutic effect. The dose is titrated to the patient's needs; the usual initial dose is 1.0 to 1.5 mg/kg. If the first dose does not produce a urine output of 10 to 15 mL within 20 to

30 mins, a dose of 2 to 3 mg/kg is administered; if the desired response still does not occur, a dose of 3 to 6 mg/kg is administered 20 to 30 mins after the second dose.

(ii) Bumetanide may be given to patients who are unresponsive or allergic to furosemide. The usual dosage, administered intravenously or intramuscularly in the treatment of ARF, is 0.5 to 1.0 mg/day; however, some patients may require up to 20 mg/day. A second or third dose may be given at intervals of 2 to 3 hrs. When bumetanide is given orally, the dosage is 0.5 to 2.0 mg/day, repeated up to two times, if necessary, at intervals of 2 to 3 hrs.

(iii) Ethacrynic acid is **less commonly used** to treat ARF because ototoxicity (sometimes irreversible) is associated with its use. It may be given intravenously (slowly for several minutes) in a dose of 50 to 100 mg. The usual oral dosage is 50 to 200 mg/day; some patients may require up to 200 mg twice daily. Ethacrynic acid can be safely given to patients who may have a sulfonamide allergy, which would preclude them from therapy with furosemide or torsemide.

(iv) Torsemide may also be given to patients unresponsive to or allergic to furosemide. The usual dose is 20 mg, administered intravenously. Doses may be increased by doubling up to 200 mg; 10 to 20 mg of torsemide is equipotent to 40 mg of furosemide or 1 mg bumetanide. Torsemide offers better bioavailability compared to other loop diuretics; however, it is considerably more expensive.

(d) Precautions and monitoring effects

(i) Loop diuretics must be used cautiously because they may cause overdiuresis leading to orthostatic hypotension and fluid and electrolyte abnormalities, including volume depletion and dehydration, hypocalcemia, hypokalemia, hypochloremia, hyponatremia, hypomagnesemia, and transient ototoxicity, especially with rapid IV injection.

(ii) Serum electrolyte levels should be monitored frequently and the patient assessed regularly for signs and symptoms of electrolyte abnormalities.

(iii) Blood pressure and pulse rate should be assessed during diuretic therapy.

(iv) GI reactions include abdominal pain and discomfort, diarrhea (with furosemide and ethacrynic acid), and nausea (with bumetanide).

(v) Blood glucose levels should be monitored in diabetic patients receiving loop diuretics because these agents may cause hyperglycemia and impaired glucose tolerance.

(vi) Patients who are allergic to sulfonamides may be hypersensitive to bumetanide and furosemide.

(vii) Furosemide and ethacrynic acid may cause agranulocytosis.

(e) Significant interactions

(i) Aminoglycoside antibiotics may potentiate ototoxicity when administered with any loop diuretic.

(ii) Nonsteroidal anti-inflammatory drugs (NSAIDs) may hamper the diuretic response to furosemide and bumetanide; **probenecid** may hamper the diuretic response to bumetanide.

(iii) Ethacrynic acid may potentiate the anticoagulant effects of **warfarin (Coumadin®)**.

(2) Step 2. Mannitol, an osmotic diuretic, is a non-reabsorbable polysaccharide.

(a) Mechanism of action and therapeutic effect. Mannitol increases the osmotic pressure of the glomerular filtrate; fluid from interstitial spaces is drawn into blood vessels, expanding plasma volume and maintaining or increasing the urine flow. This drug may be given to prevent ARF in high-risk patients, such as those undergoing surgery or suffering from severe trauma or hemolytic transfusion reactions.

(b) Onset of action is 15 to 30 mins. Duration of action is 3 to 4 hrs.

(c) Administration and dosage. Mannitol is available in solutions ranging from 5% to 25%. For the treatment of oliguric ARF or the prevention of ARF, the usual initial dose is 12.5 to 25.0 g, administered intravenously; the maximum daily dosage is 100 g, administered intravenously. The exact concentration of the solution is determined by the patient's fluid requirements.

(d) **Precautions and monitoring effects**

(i) Mannitol is contraindicated in patients with anuria, pulmonary edema or congestion, severe dehydration, and intracranial hemorrhage (except during craniotomy).

(ii) Mannitol may cause or worsen pulmonary edema and circulatory overload. If signs and symptoms of these problems develop, the infusion should be stopped.

(iii) Other adverse effects of mannitol include fluid and electrolyte abnormalities, water intoxication, headache, confusion, blurred vision, thirst, nausea, and vomiting.

(iv) Vital signs, urine output, daily weight, cardiopulmonary status, and serum and urine sodium and potassium levels should be monitored during mannitol therapy.

(v) Mannitol solutions with undissolved crystals should not be administered.

4. **Dialysis**. If the previously mentioned strategies fail, hemodialysis or peritoneal dialysis may be necessary in ARF patients who develop anuria, acute fluid overload, severe hyperkalemia, metabolic acidosis, or a BUN level above 100 mg/dL.

II. CHRONIC KIDNEY DISEASE

A. **Definition.** Chronic kidney disease (CKD) is the progressive, irreversible deterioration of renal function. Usually resulting from long-standing disease, CKD sometimes derives from ARF that does not respond to treatment.

B. **Classification and pathophysiology**

1. CKD is defined as kidney damage or GFR < 60 mL/min/1.73 m^2 for ≥ 3 months. Kidney damage is defined as pathological abnormalities or markers of damage, including abnormalities in blood or urine tests or imaging studies. CKD has recently been reclassified as stages I to V to denote the severity of renal impairment. Generally, CKD, if left untreated, progresses at a predictable, steady rate from stage I through stage V.

   a. **Stage I** is defined as kidney damage with a normal or increased GFR. The corresponding GFR in stage I CKD is usually > 90 mL/min/1.73 m^2.

   b. **Stage II** is defined as kidney damage or a mildly decreased GFR (60 to 89 mL/min/1.73 m^2).

   c. **Stage III** signifies moderate reductions in GFR (30 to 59 mL/min/1.73 m^2).

   d. **Stage IV** connotes a GFR of 15 to 29 mL/min/1.73 m^2.

   e. **Stage V** is kidney failure or a GFR of < 15 mL/min/1.73 m^2.

2. As CKD progresses, nephron destruction worsens, leading to deterioration in the kidneys' filtration, reabsorption, and endocrine functions.

3. Renal function typically does not diminish until about 75% of kidney tissue is damaged. Ultimately, the kidneys become shrunken, fibrotic masses.

C. **Etiology**. **Causes of CKD in adults**

1. Diabetic nephropathy
2. Hypertension
3. Glomerulonephritis
4. Polycystic kidney disease
5. Long-standing vascular disease (e.g., renal artery stenosis)
6. Long-standing obstructive uropathy (e.g., renal calculi)
7. Exposure to nephrotoxic agents

D. **Clinical evaluation**

1. **Physical findings.** Signs and symptoms, which vary widely, do not appear until renal insufficiency progresses to renal failure.

   a. **Metabolic abnormalities** include loss of the ability to maintain sodium, potassium, and water homeostasis, leading to hyponatremia or hypernatremia, based on relative sodium or water intake. Hyperkalemia is uncommon until end-stage disease. Fluid overload, edema, and CHF may become a problem unless fluid intake is closely managed. As renal failure progresses, the inability to excrete acid and maintain buffer capacity leads to metabolic acidosis (see *I.D.1.b, d, g, h*). Calcium and phosphate metabolism is altered due to hyperparathyroidism.

   b. **Neurological manifestations** include short attention span, loss of memory, and listlessness. As CKD progresses, these advance to confusion, stupor, seizures, and coma. Neuromuscular findings include peripheral neuropathy and pain, itching, and a burning sensation, particularly in the feet and legs. Patients may appear intoxicated. If dialysis is not started after these abnormalities occur, motor involvement begins, including loss of deep-tendon reflexes, weakness, and finally, quadriplegia.

c. **Cardiovascular problems** include arterial hypertension, peripheral edema, CHF, and pulmonary edema. Uremic pericarditis is now increasingly infrequent as a result of early dialysis.

d. **GI manifestations** include hiccups, anorexia, nausea, vomiting, constipation, stomatitis, and an unpleasant taste in the mouth. CKD patients have an increased incidence of ulcers, pancreatitis, and diverticulosis.

e. **Respiratory problems** include dyspnea when CHF is present, pulmonary edema, pleuritic pain, and uremic pleuritis.

f. **Integumentary findings** typically include pale yellowish, dry, scaly skin; severe itching; uremic frost; ecchymoses; purpura; and brittle nails and hair.

g. **Musculoskeletal changes** range from muscle and bone pain to pathological fractures and calcifications in the brain, heart, eyes, joints, and vessels. Soft tissue calcification and renal osteodystrophy may occur.

h. **Hematological disturbances** include anemia. The signs and symptoms of anemia arise from lack of epoetin alfa and reduced life span of red blood cells, including

(1) pallor of the skin, nail beds, palms, conjunctivae, and mucosa.

(2) abnormal bruising or ecchymoses, and uremic bleeding due to platelet inactivation.

(3) dyspnea and angina pectoris.

(4) extreme fatigue.

2. **Diagnostic test results**

a. **Creatinine clearance** may range from 0 to 90 mL/min, reflecting renal impairment.

b. **Blood tests** typically show

(1) elevated BUN and serum creatinine concentration.

(2) reduced arterial pH and bicarbonate concentration.

(3) reduced serum calcium level.

(4) increased serum potassium and phosphate levels.

(5) possible reduction in the serum sodium level.

(6) normochromic, normocytic anemia (hematocrit 20% to 30%).

c. **Urinalysis** may reveal glycosuria, proteinuria, erythrocytes, leukocytes, and casts. Specific gravity is fixed at 1.010.

d. **Radiographic findings**. Kidney, ureter, and bladder radiography, IV pyelography, renal scan, renal arteriography, and nephrotomography may be performed. Typically, these tests reveal small kidneys (less than 8 cm in length).

E. **Treatment objectives**

1. Improve patient comfort and prolong life.
2. Treat systemic manifestations of CKD.
3. Correct body chemistry abnormalities.

F. **Therapy.** Management of the CKD patient is generally conservative. Dietary measures and fluid restriction relieve some symptoms of CKD and may increase patient comfort and prolong life until dialysis or renal transplantation is required or available.

1. **Treatment of edema. Angiotensin-converting enzyme (ACE) inhibitors** and **diuretics** may be given to manage edema and CHF and to increase urine output.

a. **ACE inhibitors—captopril (Capoten®), enalapril (Vasotec®), lisinopril (Prinivil®, Zestril®), fosinopril (Monopril®)**—are widely used to delay progression of CKD because they help preserve renal function and typically cause fewer adverse effects than other antihypertensive agents. They also decrease proteinuria and nephrotic syndrome.

b. **Diuretics**. An osmotic diuretic, a loop diuretic, or a thiazide-like diuretic may be given.

(1) **Osmotic and loop diuretics**. See I.F.3.a.(1), (2) for information on the use of these drugs in renal failure.

(2) **Thiazide-like diuretics**. **Metolazone (Zaroxolyn®)** is the most commonly used thiazide diuretic in CKD.

(a) **Mechanism of action and therapeutic effect**. Metolazone reduces the body's fluid and sodium volume by decreasing sodium reabsorption in the distal convoluted tubule, thereby increasing urinary excretion of fluid and sodium.

(b) **Administration and dosage**. Metolazone is given orally at 5 to 20 mg/day; the dose is titrated to the patient's needs. Due to its long half-life, metolazone may be given every other day. Furosemide and metolazone act synergistically. Combination use is common, and metolazone should be administered 30 mins before furosemide to achieve the optimal diuretic effect.

(c) **Precautions and monitoring effects**

(i) Metolazone should not be given to patients with hypersensitivity to sulfonamide derivatives, including thiazides.

(ii) To avoid nocturia, the daily dose should be given in the morning.

(iii) Metolazone may cause hematological reactions, such as agranulocytosis, aplastic anemia, and thrombocytopenia.

(iv) Fluid volume depletion, hypokalemia, hyperuricemia, hyperglycemia, and impaired glucose tolerance may occur during metolazone therapy.

(v) Metolazone may cause hypersensitivity reactions, including vasculitis and pneumonitis.

(d) **Significant interactions**

(i) **Diazoxide** may potentiate the antihypertensive, hyperglycemic, and hyperuricemic effects of metolazone.

(ii) **Colestipol** and **cholestyramine** decrease the absorption of metolazone.

2. **Treatment of hypertension. Antihypertensive agents** may be needed if blood pressure becomes dangerously high as a result of edema and the high renin levels that occur in CKD. Antihypertensive therapy should be initiated in the lowest effective dose and titrated according to the patient's needs.

a. **ACE inhibitors—captopril, enalapril, lisinopril, fosinopril**—as mentioned in II.F.1.a.

b. **Dihydropyridine calcium-channel blockers**, including **amlodipine (Norvasc®)** and **felodipine (Plendil®)**, have similar effects and may be used instead of ACE inhibitors.

c. **β-Adrenergic blockers**, including **propranolol (Inderal®)** and **atenolol (Tenormin®)**, reduce blood pressure through various mechanisms.

d. **Other antihypertensive agents** are sometimes used in the treatment of CKD, including α-adrenergic drugs, **clonidine (Catapres®)**, and vasodilators, such as **hydralazine (Apresoline®)**.

3. **Treatment of hyperphosphatemia** involves administration of a phosphate binder, such as aluminum hydroxide or calcium carbonate (see *I.F.2.c*).

4. **Treatment of hypocalcemia**

a. **Oral calcium salts** [see *I.F.2.d.(2)*]

b. **Vitamin D**

(1) **Mechanism of action and therapeutic effect**. Vitamin D promotes intestinal calcium and phosphate absorption and utilization and, thus, increases the serum calcium concentration.

(2) **Choice of agent**. For the treatment of hypocalcemia in CKD and other renal disorders, **calcitriol (Rocaltrol®)** (vitamin D_3, the active form of vitamin D) is the preferred vitamin D supplement because of its greater efficacy and relatively short duration of action. Other single-entity preparations include dihydrotachysterol, ergocalciferol (Calciferol®), doxercalciferol (Hectorol®) and paricalcitol (Zemplar®).

(3) **Administration and dosage**. Calcitriol is given orally or via IV; the dose is titrated to the patient's needs (0.5 to 1.0 mg/day may be effective).

(4) **Precautions and monitoring effects**

(a) Vitamin D administration may be dangerous in patients with renal failure and must be used with extreme caution.

(b) Vitamin D toxicity may cause a wide range of signs and symptoms, including headache, dizziness, ataxia, convulsions, psychosis, soft tissue calcification, conjunctivitis, photophobia, tinnitus, nausea, diarrhea, pruritus, and muscle and bone pain.

(c) Vitamin D has a narrow therapeutic index, necessitating frequent measurement of BUN and serum urine calcium and potassium levels.

5. **Treatment of other systemic manifestations of CKD**
   a. **Treatment of anemia** includes administration of iron (e.g., ferrous sulfate), folate supplements, and epoetin alfa.
      (1) Severe anemia may warrant transfusion with packed red blood cells.
      (2) Epoetin alfa (Procrit®, Epogen®) stimulates the production of red cell progenitors and the production of hemoglobin. It also accelerates the release of reticulocytes from the bone marrow.
         (a) An initial dose of epoetin alfa is 50 to 100 U/kg intravenously or subcutaneously three times a week. The dose may be adjusted upward to elicit the desired response.
         (b) Epoetin alfa works best in patients with a hematocrit below 30%. During the initial treatment, the hematocrit increases 1.0% to 3.5% in a 2-week period. The target hematocrit is 33% to 35%. Maintenance doses are titrated based on hematocrit after this level is reached.
         (c) Epoetin alfa therapy should be temporarily stopped if hematocrit exceeds 36%. Additional side effects include hypertension in up to 25% of patients. Headache and malaise have been reported.
         (d) The effects of epoetin alfa are dependent on a ready supply of iron for hemoglobin synthesis. Patients who do not respond should have iron stores checked. This includes serum iron, total iron-binding capacity, transferrin saturation, and serum ferritin. Iron supplementation should be increased as indicated.
      (3) Darbepoetin (Aranesp®) is an epoetin alfa analogue. Its advantage is a prolonged plasma half-life, thus allowing it to be administered once weekly or biweekly.
      (4) Intravenous iron products may be given to replete iron stores. This route is preferred to oral supplementation due to low oral bioavailability and GI intolerance. Iron dextran is commonly used; however, it is associated with hypotension and anaphylaxis. Newer iron products include sodium ferric gluconate and iron sucrose, which are better tolerated and can be infused more rapidly compared to iron dextran. Patients with severe iron deficiency may receive up to a total of 1 g of an iron preparation over several days. The rate of infusion depends on the preparation used.
   b. **Treatment of GI disturbances**
      (1) Antiemetics help control nausea and vomiting.
      (2) Docusate sodium or methylcellulose may be used to prevent constipation.
      (3) Enemas may be given to remove blood from the GI tract.
   c. **Treatment of skin problems**. An antipruritic agent, such as diphenhydramine (Benadryl®), may be used to alleviate itching.
6. **Management of body chemistry abnormalities** (see *I.F.2*)
7. **Dialysis**. When CKD progresses to end-stage renal disease and no longer responds to conservative measures, long-term dialysis or renal transplantation is necessary to prolong life.
   a. **Hemodialysis** is the preferred dialysis method for patients with a reduced peritoneal membrane, hypercatabolism, or acute hyperkalemia.
      (1) This technique involves shunting of the patient's blood through a dialysis membrane-containing unit for diffusion, osmosis, and ultrafiltration. The blood is then returned to the patient's circulation.
      (2) Vascular access may be obtained via an arteriovenous fistula or an external shunt.
      (3) The procedure takes only 3 to 8 hrs; most patients need three treatments a week. With proper training, patients can perform hemodialysis at home.
      (4) The patient receives heparin during hemodialysis to prevent clotting.
      (5) Various complications may arise, including clotting of the hemofilter, hemorrhage, hepatitis, anemia, septicemia, cardiovascular problems, air embolism, rapid shifts in fluid and electrolyte balance, itching, nausea, vomiting, headache, seizures, and aluminum osteodystrophy.
   b. **Peritoneal dialysis** is the preferred dialysis method for patients with bleeding disorders and cardiovascular disease.
      (1) The peritoneum is used as a semipermeable membrane. A plastic catheter inserted into the peritoneum provides access for the dialysate, which draws fluids, wastes, and electrolytes across the peritoneal membrane by osmosis and diffusion.

(2) Peritoneal dialysis can be carried out in three different modes.

(a) **Intermittent peritoneal dialysis** is an automatic cycling mode lasting 8 to 10 hrs, performed three times a week. This mode allows nighttime treatment and is appropriate for working patients.

(b) **Continuous ambulatory peritoneal dialysis** is performed daily for 24 hrs with four exchanges daily. The patient can remain active during the treatment.

(c) **Continuous cyclic peritoneal dialysis** may be used if the other two modes fail to improve creatinine clearance. Dialysis takes place at night; the last exchange is retained in the peritoneal cavity during the day, then drained that evening.

(3) **Advantages** of peritoneal dialysis include a lack of serious complications, retention of normal fluid and electrolyte balance, simplicity, reduced cost, patient independence, and a reduced need (or no need) for heparin administration.

(4) **Complications** of peritoneal dialysis include hyperglycemia, constipation, and inflammation or infection at the catheter site. Also, this method carries a high risk of peritonitis.

8. **Renal transplantation**. This surgical procedure allows some patients with end-stage renal disease to live normal and, in many cases, longer lives.

a. **Histocompatibility** must be tested to minimize the risk of transplant rejection and failure. Human leukocyte antigen (HLA) type, mixed lymphocyte reactivity, and blood group types are determined to assess histocompatibility.

b. Renal transplant material may be obtained from a living donor or a cadaver.

c. **Three types of graft rejection** can occur.

(1) **Hyperacute (immediate) rejection** results in graft loss within minutes to hours after transplantation.

(a) Acute urine flow cessation and bluish or mottled kidney discoloration are intraoperative signs of hyperacute rejection.

(b) Postoperative manifestations include kidney enlargement, fever, anuria, local pain, sodium retention, and hypertension.

(c) Treatment for hyperacute rejection is immediate nephrectomy.

(2) **Acute rejection** may occur 4 to 60 days after transplantation.

(3) **Chronic rejection** occurs more than 60 days after transplantation.

(a) Signs and symptoms include low-grade fever, increased proteinuria, azotemia, hypertension, oliguria, weight gain, and edema.

(b) Treatment may include alkylating agents, cyclosporine, antilymphocyte globulin, and corticosteroids. In some cases, nephrectomy is necessary.

d. **Complications** include

(1) infection, diabetes, hepatitis, and leukopenia, resulting from immunosuppressive therapy.

(2) hypertension, resulting from various causes.

(3) cancer (e.g., lymphoma, cutaneous malignancies, head and neck cancer, leukemia, colon cancer).

(4) pancreatitis and mental and emotional disorders (e.g., suicidal tendencies, severe depression, brought on by steroid therapy).

Study Questions

1. Severe hypotension may result in what type of acute renal failure?

(A) Prerenal
(B) Intrarenal
(C) Postrenal
(D) Intrinsic
(E) Parenchymal

2. Why might sodium polystyrene sulfonate (SPS) be utilized in ARF?

(A) It reduces calcium levels in the serum.
(B) It increases calcium levels in the serum.
(C) It increases potassium levels.
(D) It reduces potassium levels in the serum.
(E) It elevates glucose levels.

3. Why are thiazide diuretics avoided in patients with renal failure?
   (A) Overdiuresis may occur.
   (B) Patients are often allergic to furosemide.
   (C) They are ineffective when creatinine clearance is less than 25 mL/min.
   (D) They are too costly.
   (E) Sodium and potassium are already depleted.

4. The following are causes of chronic kidney disease *except*
   (A) diabetic nephropathy.
   (B) hypertension.
   (C) glomerulonephritis.
   (D) long-term exposure to acetaminophen.
   (E) polycystic kidney disease.

5. What is the major difference between epoetin alfa and darbepoetin?
   (A) Epoetin alfa has a longer plasma half-life.
   (B) Darbepoetin has a longer plasma half-life.
   (C) Epoetin alfa does not require adequate iron stores.
   (D) Darbepoetin does not require adequate iron stores.
   (E) Epoetin alfa is a newer agent.

Answers and Explanations

1. **The answer is A** *[see I.B.1.e]*.
   Prerenal ARF stems from impaired renal perfusion, which may result from reduced arterial volume, urinary losses from excessive dieresis, decreased cardiac output, renal vascular obstruction, and severe hypotension.

2. **The answer is D** *[see I.F.2.a.(5).(b)]*.
   SPS is a potassium-removing resin that exchanges sodium ions for potassium ions in the intestine (1 g of SPS exchanges 0.5 to 1.0 mEq/L of potassium). The SPS is distributed throughout the intestines and excreted in the feces. It is administered as an adjunctive treatment for hyperkalemia since SPS reduces potassium levels in the serum and other body fluids.

3. **The answer is C** *[see I.F.3.a]*.
   Thiazide diuretics are avoided in renal failure because they are ineffective when creatinine clearance is less than 25 mL/min and they may worsen the patient's clinical status.

4. **The answer is D** *[see II.C]*.
   Long-term exposure to acetaminophen (APAP) has not been shown to be a cause of chronic kidney disease. APAP can lead to chronic hepatic disorders such as chronic liver failure. The other listed conditions have been shown to lead to chronic kidney disease.

5. **The answer is B** *[see II.F.5.a.(3)]*.
   Darbepoetin is an epoetin analogue that has a prolonged plasma half-life that allows for once weekly or biweekly dosing compared to a three times a week regimen with epoetin alfa.

49 Hepatic Disorders

HEATHER A. SWEENEY

I. ACUTE LIVER FAILURE (ALF)

A. General information

1. ALF is a rare condition. The United States approximates 2000 cases a year.
2. It is classified by a rapid deterioration (less than 26 weeks) of liver function, which results in jaundice, coagulopathy (international normalized ratio [INR] greater than 1.5), and hepatic encephalopathy in previously normal individuals.
3. The most common causes of ALF are drug-induced liver injury, viral hepatitis, autoimmune liver disease, and hypoperfusion.

B. Signs and symptoms

1. Right upper quadrant tenderness
2. Nausea, vomiting
3. Jaundice

C. Diagnosis

1. All patients with clinical or laboratory evidence of moderate-to-severe acute hepatitis should have a measurement of prothrombin time.
2. If the prothrombin time is prolonged by ~4 to 6 secs or more (INR $\geq$ 1.5) and there is evidence of altered sensorium, the diagnosis of ALF is established and hospital admission is mandatory.
3. Since ALF may progress rapidly, early transfer to the ICU is recommended once the diagnosis of ALF is made.
4. Seek specific cause of ALF.

D. Treatment

1. Admit patient to ICU.
2. Specific treatment is dependent on etiology of ALF.
3. Consider need for liver transplantation.

II. ACETAMINOPHEN HEPATOTOXICITY

A. General information

1. In the United States, acetaminophen (APAP) is the leading cause of acute liver failure.
2. APAP is a dose-related toxin. To cause toxicity, an acute overdose usually totals $\geq$ 150 mg/kg (about 7.5 g in adults) within 24 hrs.
3. The main toxic metabolite of APAP is *N*-acetyl-*p*-benzoquinone imine (NAPQI), which is produced by the hepatic P450 system. Glutathione in the liver normally detoxifies NAPQI. An acute overdose of APAP depletes glutathione stores which results in an accumulation of NAPQI that causes hepatocellular necrosis.
4. Likelihood and severity of hepatotoxicity from an acute APAP ingestion is predicted by the serum APAP level.

B. Signs, symptoms, and labs (Postingestion times)

1. Stage I (0 to 24 hrs): anorexia, nausea, vomiting
2. Stage II (24 to 72 hrs): right upper quadrant pain, elevated aspartate aminotransferase (AST) and alanine aminotransferase (ALT), possible elevation of bilirubin and prothrombin time (PT)
3. Stage III (72 to 96 hrs): vomiting, peaking of AST, ALT, bilirubin, and INR
4. Stage IV (greater than 5 days): resolution of hepatotoxicity or progression to multiple organ failure

C. Treatment

1. Administer activated charcoal
   a. Ideally give within 1 hr of ingestion. It may be of benefit as long as 3 to 4 hrs after ingestion.
   b. Adult oral dose: 25 to 100 g as a single dose; if multiple doses are needed, additional doses may be given as 12.5 g/hr.
2. Administer *N*-acetylcysteine (Acetadote®)
   a. *N*-acetylcysteine is a precursor for glutathione and decreases APAP toxicity by increasing glutathione hepatic stores. It does not reverse damage to liver cells that have already been injured.
   b. Ideally begin treatment within 8 hrs of ingestion. It may be of value 48 hrs or more after ingestion.
   c. Adult oral dose: 140 mg/kg, followed by 70 mg/kg every 4 hrs times 17 doses.
   d. Adult IV dose: 150 mg/kg infused over 60 mins, followed by 50 mg/kg infused over 4 hrs, followed by 100 mg/kg infused over 16 hrs.

D. Chronic APAP toxicity

1. Chronic excessive use or repeated overdoses of APAP can lead to chronic APAP poisoning. Often patients are treating pain with high doses of APAP from multiple or single source products.
2. Symptoms may be similar to those symptoms listed with acute ingestion or may be absent.
3. Labs
   a. If AST and ALT are normal and APAP level is less than 10 mcg/mL, significant hepatotoxicity is unlikely.
   b. If AST and ALT are normal and APAP level is greater than 10 mcg/mL, significant hepatotoxicity is possible.
   c. If initial AST and ALT are initially high regardless of APAP levels, significant hepatotoxicity is assumed.
4. Sometimes *N*-acetylcysteine is used, but its role is unclear in the treatment of chronic APAP toxicity.

III. HEPATITIS: INFLAMMATION OF THE LIVER

A. Hepatitis A

1. General information
   a. The primary means of hepatitis A virus (HAV) transmission in the United States is via the fecal–oral route.
   b. Hepatitis A does not become chronic.
   c. Most persons with acute disease recover with no lasting liver damage.
   d. Incubation period is 15 to 50 days (average: 28 days).
2. Persons at risk
   a. Travelers to regions with high or intermediate hepatitis A
   b. Sex contacts of infected persons
   c. Household members or caregivers of infected persons
   d. Men who have sex with men
   e. Users of certain illegal drugs
   f. Persons with clotting-factor disorders
3. Prevention
   a. Vaccination with the full, two-dose series of hepatitis A vaccine (Havrix®, Vaqta®) given 6 months apart
   b. Immune globulin administered intramuscularly is available for short-term protection (~3 months) against hepatitis A both preexposure and postexposure
   c. Good hygiene (e.g., hand washing)
4. Signs and symptoms
   a. Some patients are asymptomatic, particularly young children.
   b. Symptoms occur abruptly and can include fever, fatigue, jaundice, nausea, vomiting, abdominal pain, loss of appetite, and dark urine.
   c. Symptoms usually last less than 2 months.
5. Serologic tests
   a. Acute—IgM anti-HAV
   b. Chronic—not applicable

6. Treatment
- **a.** Postexposure prophylaxis
  - **(1)** Healthy persons 12 months to 40 years: hepatitis A vaccine
  - **(2)** People older than 40 years: IM immune globulin
  - **(3)** Children younger than 12 months, immunocompromised, people with chronic liver disease: IM immune globulin
- **b.** Confirmed infection
  - **(1)** No specific antivirals are available.
  - **(2)** Supportive treatment is recommended.

B. Hepatitis B

1. General information
- **a.** Hepatitis B virus (HBV) is transmitted by contact with infectious blood, semen, and other body fluids.
- **b.** Among unimmunized persons, chronic infection occurs in 6% to 10% of adults. In chronically infected persons, 15% to 25% of people will develop chronic liver disease including cirrhosis, liver failure, or liver cancer.
- **c.** Most persons with acute disease recover with no lasting liver damage.
- **d.** The incubation period is 45 to 160 days (average: 120 days).

2. Persons at risk
- **a.** Infants born to infected mothers
- **b.** Sex partners of infected persons
- **c.** Persons with multiple sex partners
- **d.** Injectable drug users
- **e.** Health care workers exposed to blood
- **f.** Hemodialysis patients

3. Prevention
- **a.** Vaccination with hepatitis B vaccine (Recombivax HB®, Engerix-B®)
  - **(1)** Infants and children: 3 to 4 doses given over a 6- to 18-month period depending on vaccine type and schedule
  - **(2)** Adults: 3 doses given over a 6-month period
- **b.** Passive immunization is obtained with hepatitis B immune globulin (HBIG), which provides temporary protection for about 3 to 6 months.

4. Signs and symptoms
- **a.** Fever, fatigue
- **b.** Nausea, vomiting
- **c.** Abdominal pain
- **d.** Jaundice
- **e.** Joint pain

5. Serologic tests
- **a.** HBsAg in acute and chronic infection
- **b.** IgM anti-HBc is positive in acute infection only

6. Treatment
- **a.** Acute
  - **(1)** No medication is available
  - **(2)** Provide supportive care
- **b.** Chronic
  - **(1)** Goal of treatment is amelioration of hepatic dysfunction and seroconversion of HBsAg-positive (surface antigen) to HBsAg-negative and production of HBs antibodies.
  - **(2)** Treatment is indicated for chronic HBV infection with high pretreatment ALT level, detectable serum HBV DNA, and moderately active necroinflammation with or without fibrosis on liver biopsy.
  - **(3)** First-line drugs
    - **(a)** Pegylated interferon-alfa 2a (Pegasys®)
      - **(i)** Class: Interferon
      - **(ii)** Dose: 180 mcg SQ weekly
      - **(iii)** Duration: 48 weeks

(b) Entecavir (Baraclude®)
(i) Class: reverse transcriptase inhibitor (nucleoside)
(ii) Dose: 0.5 mg daily
(iii) Duration for HBeAg+(antigen is a marker for active replication): treat for more than 1 year until HBeAg seroconversion and undetectable serum HBV DNA; continue treatment for more than 6 months after HBeAg seroconversion
(iv) Duration for HBeAg negative: treat for more than 1 year until HBsAg (surface antigen) clearance
(c) Tenofovir (Viread®)
(i) Class: Reverse transcriptase inhibitor (nucleotide)
(ii) Dose: 300 mg daily
(iii) Duration for HBeAg+: treat for more than 1 year until HBeAg seroconversion and undetectable serum HBV DNA; continue treatment for more than 6 months after HBeAg seroconversion
(iv) Duration for HBeAg negative: treat for more than 1 year until HBsAg clearance.

C. Hepatitis C

1. General information
   a. Hepatitis C virus (HCV) is transmitted by contact with blood of an infected person.
   b. Of people newly infected, 75% to 85% develop a chronic infection. Of these chronically infected persons, 60% to 70% will develop chronic liver disease such as cirrhosis or liver cancer.
   c. The incubation period is 14 to 180 days (average: 45 days).
2. Persons at risk
   a. Current or former injectable drug users
   b. Recipients of clotting factor concentrates before 1987
   c. Recipients of blood transfusions before 1992
   d. Long-term hemodialysis patients
   e. Health care workers after needle sticks
   f. HIV-infected persons
   g. Babies born to infected mothers
3. Prevention
   a. No vaccines are available.
   b. Don't reuse needles.
4. Signs and symptoms
   a. Fever, fatigue
   b. Nausea, vomiting
   c. Abdominal pain
   d. Jaundice
   e. Joint pain
5. Serologic tests
   a. Acute—no serologic markers
   b. Chronic
      (1) Screening assay for anti-HCV
      (2) Verification by a specific assay for HCV RNA
6. Treatment
   a. Acute
      (1) There is no specific treatment for acute exposure until viremia is established.
      (2) Typically, a period of at least 12 weeks is observed to see if the HCV will spontaneously clear. If it does not clear, then the patient should be treated.
      (3) Pegylated interferon monotherapy can cure recent HCV infection in approximately 90% of the patients.
   b. Chronic
      (1) All patients with chronic hepatitis C are potential candidates for antiviral therapy with combination pegylated interferon and ribavirin. For patients with chronic HCV genotype 1 who are candidates for therapy, it is recommended that they receive triple therapy with pegylated interferon, ribavirin, and one protease inhibitor (telaprevir or boceprevir).

(2) The actual duration of treatment is determined in part by viral response. Viral load should be monitored throughout therapy.

(3) Medications for HCV genotype 1

(a) Pegylated interferon-alfa 2a (Pegasys®)

(i) Class: Interferon

(ii) Dose: 180 mcg SQ weekly

(iii) Duration: 48 weeks

(b) Ribavirin (Copegus®) - weight based dosing

(i) Class: Antiviral

(ii) Dose: if weight is less than or equal to 75 kg, then 1000 mg per day divided into two doses or if weight is greater than 75 kg, then 1200 mg per day divided into two doses

(iii) Duration: 48 weeks

(c) Boceprevir (Victrelis®)

(i) Class: Antiviral; protease inhibitor

(ii) Dose: 800 mg TID

(iii) Duration: After 4 weeks of lead-in treatment with pegylated interferon-alfa and ribavirin only, boceprevir is combined with pegylated interferon-alfa and ribavirin for 24 to 44 weeks

(d) Telaprevir (Incivek®)

(i) Class: Antiviral; protease inhibitor

(ii) Dose: 750 mg TID

(iii) Duration: Together with pegylated interferon-alfa and ribavirin for 12 weeks followed by an additional 12 to 36 weeks of pegylated interferon-alfa and ribavirin only

(4) Medications for HCV genotypes 2, 3, and 4

(a) Pegylated interferon-alfa 2a (Pegasys®)

(i) Class: Interferon

(ii) Dose: 180 mcg SQ weekly

(iii) Duration genotype 2 or 3: 24 weeks

(iv) Duration genotype 4: 48 weeks

(b) Ribavirin (Copegus®)

(i) Class: Antiviral

(ii) Dose genotype 2 or 3: 800 mg per day divided into two doses

(iii) Duration genotype 2 or 3: 24 weeks

(iv) Dose genotype 4: if weight is less than or equal to 75 kg, then 1000 mg per day divided into two doses or if weight is greater than 75 kg, then 1200 mg per day divided into two doses

(v) Duration genotype 4: 48 weeks

D. Hepatitis D

1. General information
   - a. Hepatitis D virus (HDV) is transmitted through percutaneous or mucosal contact with infectious blood.
   - b. HDV is an incomplete virus that requires the helper function of HBV to replicate and only occurs in people infected with HBV.
   - c. HDV is uncommon in the United States.
2. Persons at risk
   - a. Persons infected with HBV
   - b. Injectable drug users
3. Prevention
   - a. There is no vaccine for HDV.
   - b. Give hepatitis B vaccine to prevent infection with HBV.
4. Signs and symptoms
   - a. Fever, fatigue
   - b. Nausea, vomiting
   - c. Abdominal pain

d. Jaundice
e. Joint pain
5. Serologic tests
a. Acute
(1) IgM anti-HDV
(2) HDAg
b. Chronic—HDAg
6. Treatment—pegylated interferon-alfa

E. Hepatitis E
1. General information
a. Hepatitis E virus (HEV) is spread by the fecal–oral route.
b. HEV usually results in a self-limited, acute illness.
c. HEV is uncommon in the United States.
2. Persons at risk are those who travel to developing countries.
3. Prevention
a. Good sanitation
b. Clean drinking water
4. Signs and symptoms
a. Fever, fatigue
b. Nausea, vomiting
c. Abdominal pain
d. Jaundice
e. Joint pain
5. Treatment
a. Hepatitis E usually resolves on its own.
b. Treatment is supportive (e.g., rest, fluids)

IV. ALCOHOL-INDUCED LIVER DISEASE

A. General information
1. The cause of alcoholic liver disease (ALD) is chronic, heavy alcohol ingestion.
a. About 40 to 80 g per day in men for 10 to 12 years
b. About 20 to 40 g per day in women for 10 to 12 years
2. Prevalence in the United States is estimated at greater than 2 million people.

B. Stages of liver damage
1. Fatty liver
a. It is represented by a fatty infiltration in the liver.
b. Clinical findings include hepatomegaly and mild liver enzyme abnormalities.
c. The condition is potentially reversible if alcohol is stopped and nutrition maintained.
2. Alcoholic hepatitis
a. It is characterized by hepatic inflammation with necrosis.
b. Clinical features include fever, abdominal pain, anorexia, nausea, and weight loss.
3. Cirrhosis
a. It is marked by severe hepatic fibrosis.
b. ALD is the most common cause of cirrhosis.

C. Signs and symptoms
1. Fatigue
2. Anorexia, weight loss
3. Nausea, vomiting
4. Jaundice
5. Right upper abdominal pain

D. Liver-related labs
1. In ALD patients, the AST is almost always elevated.
2. The classic ratio AST/ALT greater than 2 is seen in 70% of the cases.
3. ALT and AST may be in the normal range in patients with advanced cirrhosis due to the lack of viable hepatocytes left to produce transaminases.

E. Treatment

1. No approved pharmacotherapy
2. Alcohol abstinence
3. Optimal nutrition
4. Consideration for liver transplantation in patients with end-stage ALD

V. CIRRHOSIS

A. General information

1. Cirrhosis describes a diseased liver characterized by fibrosis usually due to many years of continuous injury.
2. The most common causes of cirrhosis are:
   - **a.** Long-standing alcohol abuse
   - **b.** Chronic hepatitis B or C
   - **c.** Nonalcoholic steatohepatitis
3. Cirrhosis has no cure.

B. Classification

1. Compensated cirrhosis
   - **a.** Cirrhosis present
   - **b.** Preservation of hepatic synthetic function
   - **c.** No evidence of complications related to portal hypertension, hepatic encephalopathy, and/or jaundice
2. Decompensated cirrhosis
   - **a.** Cirrhosis present
   - **b.** Reduced hepatic synthetic function
   - **c.** Portal hypertension including ascites, gastroesophageal varices, and variceal bleeding
   - **d.** Hepatic encephalopathy
   - **e.** Jaundice

C. Signs and symptoms

1. Fatigue
2. Jaundice
3. Varices
4. Ascites
5. Edema
6. Hepatic encephalopathy

D. Treatment

1. Treat underlying causative condition (e.g., hepatitis B, hepatitis C)
2. Avoid substances that injure the liver (e.g., alcohol, high-dose APAP)
3. Treat complications
   - **a.** Ascites—the most common complication
     - **(1)** Dietary sodium restriction: less than 2 g per day
     - **(2)** Diuretics
       - **(a)** Combination of spironolactone (Aldactone®) and furosemide (Lasix®) is the usual diuretic regimen.
       - **(b)** Starting doses are usually 100 mg spironolactone and 40 mg furosemide.
       - **(c)** Doses can be increased every 3 to 5 days with typical maximal doses of 400 mg per day of spironolactone and 160 mg per day of furosemide.
     - **(3)** Avoid non-steroidal anti-inflammatory drugs (NSAIDs)
   - **b.** Refractory ascites
     - **(1)** This condition is defined as fluid overload that is unresponsive to a sodium-restricted diet and high-dose diuretic treatment or recurs rapidly after therapeutic paracentesis.
     - **(2)** Options
       - **(a)** Large-volume paracentesis (LVP) and albumin replacement
       - **(b)** Transjugular intrahepatic portosystemic shunt (TIPS)
       - **(c)** Consideration for liver transplantation

c. Esophageal varices
   (1) Acute bleeding in a cirrhotic patient
      (a) Admit patient to intensive care unit (ICU) for resuscitation and management.
      (b) Maintain hemoglobin at ~8 g/dL.
      (c) Administer short-term prophylactic antibiotics
         (i) Shown to increase survival rate
         (ii) Norfloxacin (Noroxin®) 400 mg bid orally or ceftriaxone (Rocephin®) 1 g daily IV
      (d) Initiate octreotide (Sandostatin®) at 50 mcg IV bolus followed by 50 mcg/hr continuous infusion for 3 to 5 days for vasoconstriction.
      (e) Use sclerotherapy or endoscopic variceal ligation (EVL) to control hemorrhage.
      (f) Balloon tamponade can be used to temporarily control bleeding by applying pressure to the bleeding sites.
      (g) If the above measures fail, then a shunt (e.g., TIPS) is indicated.
   (2) Ongoing prevention
      (a) Initiate a nonselective β-blocker (e.g., nadolol [Corgard®], propranolol [Inderal®]).
      (b) Conduct an EVL.
      (c) If the aforementioned therapy fails, a shunt (e.g., TIPS) should be considered.
d. Hepatic encephalopathy
   (1) Encompasses a spectrum of neuropsychiatric abnormalities as a result of liver dysfunction
      (a) Cognitive deficits
      (b) Extrapyramidal alterations
      (c) Sleep disturbances
   (2) Ammonia has been implicated as a neurotoxin in the pathogenesis of this condition.
      (a) Ammonia is a by-product of protein metabolism and is normally metabolized by the liver to urea (blood urea nitrogen [BUN]), which is renally eliminated.
      (b) Cirrhosis impairs hepatic blood flow and metabolism, which can result in increased levels of ammonia in the central nervous system (CNS).
   (3) Treatment options
      (a) Correct precipitating factors (e.g., excessive protein intake, infection)
      (b) Reduce nitrogenous load
         (i) Reduce protein intake.
         (ii) Administer lactulose (Enulose®) 20 to 30 g (30 to 45 mL) three to four times a day. Lactulose results in acidification of the colon, which converts ammonia into a less readily absorbed ammonium ion.

Study Questions

Directions: Each of the questions, statements, or incomplete statements in this section can be correctly answered or completed by **one** of the suggested answers or phrases. Choose the **best** answer.

1. What is the toxic metabolite that builds up with an acute acetaminophen overdose?
   (A) Glutathione
   (B) NAPQI
   (C) HBV
   (D) ALD
   (E) *N*-acetylcysteine

2. What are the three first-line drugs for the treatment of chronic Hepatitis B?
   (A) Lamivudine, telbivudine, entecavir
   (B) Pegylated interferon-alfa, lamivudine, acyclovir
   (C) Adefovir, telbivudine, tenofovir
   (D) Pegylated interferon-alfa, entecavir, tenofovir
   (E) Entecavir, acyclovir, telbivudine

3. What medication is administered to patients with hepatic encephalopathy to decrease nitrogenous load?
   - **(A)** Lactulose
   - **(B)** Furosemide
   - **(C)** Spironolactone
   - **(D)** Propranolol
   - **(E)** Norfloxacin

4. What medication is administered to patients to decrease APAP toxicity?
   - **(A)** Naloxone
   - **(B)** Interferon-alfa
   - **(C)** Tenofovir
   - **(D)** Neomycin
   - **(E)** *N*-acetylcysteine

5. Which types of viral hepatitis have vaccines available?
   - **(A)** Hepatitis A, B, and C
   - **(B)** Hepatitis A and B
   - **(C)** Hepatitis B and C
   - **(D)** Hepatitis A and C
   - **(E)** Hepatitis A, B, and D

6. What is the most common cause of cirrhosis?
   - **(A)** APAP toxicity
   - **(B)** Hepatitis A
   - **(C)** Hepatitis E
   - **(D)** Alcoholic liver disease
   - **(E)** Renal dysfunction

7. What medication maybe used to treat bleeding of esophageal varices by causing vasoconstriction?
   - **(A)** Propranolol
   - **(B)** Spironolactone
   - **(C)** Ribavirin
   - **(D)** Diphenhydramine
   - **(E)** Octreotide

Answers and Explanations

1. **The answer is B** *[see II.A.3].*
   The main toxic metabolite of APAP metabolism is NAPQI. Normally, glutathione in the liver detoxifies NAPQI, but an acute overdose of APAP depletes glutathione stores, which results in accumulation of NAPQI, which causes hepatic necrosis.

2. **The answer is D** *[see III.B.6.b.(3)].*
   The American Association for the Study of Liver Diseases (AASLD) has stated that the first-line drugs for the treatment of chronic Hepatitis B are pegylated interferon-alfa, entecavir, and tenofovir. In choosing which antiviral agent to use as the first-line therapy, consideration should be given to the safety and efficacy of the treatment, risks of drug resistance, and costs.

3. **The answer is A** *[see V.D.3.d.(3).(b).(ii)].*
   Lactulose (Enulose®) 20 to 30 g (30 to 45 mL) administered three to four times a day is given to patients with hepatic encephalopathy. Lactulose results in acidification of the colon, which converts ammonia into a less readily absorbed ammonium ion, therefore decreasing the nitrogenous load.

4. **The answer is E** *[see II.C.2].*
   N-acetylcysteine is a precursor for glutathione and decreases APAP toxicity by increasing glutathione hepatic stores. It does not reverse damage to liver cells that have already been injured. Ideally begin treatment within 8 hrs of ingestion. It may be of value 48 hrs or more after ingestion.

5. **The answer is B** *[see III.A.3.a; III.B.3.a].*
   Hepatitis A can be prevented with the full, two-dose series of hepatitis A vaccine given 6 months apart in adults. Hepatitis B can be prevented with a three-dose series of hepatitis B vaccine given over a period of 6 months in adults.

6. **The answer is D** *[see IV.B.3.b].*
   Alcoholic liver disease is the most common cause of cirrhosis in the United States. Alcohol is metabolized in the liver and oxidative stress promotes hepatocyte necrosis and severe hepatic fibrosis develops.

7. **The answer is E** *[see V.D.3.c.(1).(d)].*
   Pharmacologic therapy such as octreotide should be initiated as soon as variceal hemorrhage is suspected, and continued for 3 to 5 days. The vasoconstrictive action of octreotide helps to control bleeding.

Cancer Chemotherapy

50

BROOKE BERNHARDT

I. PRINCIPLES OF ONCOLOGY.

The term *cancer* refers to a heterogeneous group of diseases caused by an impairment of the normal functioning of genes, which leads to genetic damage.

A. **Characteristics of cancer cells.** Cancer cells are also referred to as tumors or neoplasms. Tumors are thought to arise from a single abnormal cell, which continues to divide indefinitely. Uncontrolled growth, the ability to invade local tissues, and the ability to spread, or **metastasize**, are unique characteristics of cancer cells.

1. **Carcinogenesis.** The mechanism of how many cancers occur is thought to be a multistage, multifactorial process that involves both genetic and environmental factors.
   a. **Initiation.** The first step involves the exposure of normal cells to a carcinogen, producing genetic damage to a cell.
   b. **Promotion.** The environment becomes altered to allow preferential growth of mutated cells over normal cells. The mutated cells become cancerous.
   c. **Progression.** Increased proliferation of cancer cells allows for invasion into local tissue and metastasis.
2. **Types of cancer.** Tumors can be benign or malignant. **Benign** tumors are generally slow growing, resemble normal cells, are localized, and are not harmful. **Malignant** tumors often proliferate more rapidly, have an atypical appearance, invade and destroy surrounding tissues, and are harmful if left untreated. Malignant cancers are further categorized by the location from where the tumor cells arise.
   a. **Solid tumors. Carcinomas** are tumors of epithelial cells. These include specific tissue cancers (e.g., lung, colon, breast). **Sarcomas** include tumors of connective tissue such as bone (e.g., osteosarcoma) or muscle (e.g., leiomyosarcoma).
   b. **Hematological malignancies. Lymphomas** are tumors of the lymphatic system and include Hodgkin and non-Hodgkin lymphomas. **Leukemias** are tumors of blood-forming elements and are classified as acute or chronic and myeloid or lymphoid.

B. **Incidence.** Cancer is the **second leading cause of death** in the United States. The most common cancers are breast, prostate, and colorectal. The leading cause of cancer death is lung cancer.

C. **Cause.** Many factors have been implicated in the origin of cancer. Some of these factors are as follows:

1. **Viruses**, including Epstein-Barr virus (EBV), hepatitis B virus (HBV), and human papillomavirus (HPV)
2. **Environmental and occupational exposures**, such as ionizing and ultraviolet radiation and exposure to chemicals, including vinyl chloride, benzene, and asbestos
3. **Lifestyle factors**, such as high-fat, low-fiber diets and tobacco and ethanol use
4. **Medications**, including alkylating agents and immunosuppressants
5. **Genetic factors**, including inherited mutations, cancer-causing genes (oncogenes), and defective tumor-suppressor genes

D. **Detection** and **diagnosis** are critical for the appropriate treatment of cancer. Earlier detection may improve response to treatment.

1. **Warning signs** of cancer have been outlined by the American Cancer Society. General signs and symptoms of cancer may include unexplained weight loss, fever, fatigue, pain, and skin changes. Signs and symptoms of specific types of cancer can include changes in bowel habits or bladder

function, a sore that does not heal, white patches or spots in the mouth or on the tongue, unusual bleeding or discharge, thickening or lump in the breast or other body part, indigestion or difficulty swallowing, a recent change in a wart or mole, other skin changes, or a nagging cough or hoarseness.

2. **Guidelines for screening** asymptomatic people for the presence of cancer have been established by the American Cancer Society, the National Cancer Institute, and the U.S. Preventive Health Services Task Force, among others. Because many cancers do not produce signs or symptoms until they have become large, the goal of screening is to detect cancers early, when the disease may be more likely to be curable, thus potentially reducing cancer-related mortality. The different sets of guidelines vary slightly in their recommendations for age and frequency of screening procedures.
3. **Tumor markers** are biochemical indicators of the presence of neoplastic proliferation detected in serum, plasma, or other body fluids. These tumor markers may be used initially as screening tests, to reveal further information after abnormal test results, or to monitor the efficacy of therapy. Elevated levels of these markers are not definitive for the presence of cancer because levels can be elevated in other benign and malignant conditions, and false-positive results do occur. Examples of some commonly used markers include the following:
   - **a.** Carcinoembryonic antigen (CEA) for colorectal cancer
   - **b.** α-Fetoprotein (AFP) for hepatocellular carcinoma or hepatoblastoma
   - **c.** Prostate-specific antigen (PSA) for prostate cancer
4. **Tumor biopsy.** The definitive test for the presence of cancerous cells is a biopsy and pathological examination of the biopsy specimen. Several types of procedures are used in the pathological analysis of tumors, including evaluating the morphological features of the tissue and cells (via pathologic evaluation), looking for cell-surface markers (via flow cytometry), and cytogenetic evaluation for specific chromosomal abnormalities (via fluorescence in situ hybridization).
5. **Imaging studies**, such as radiograph, CT scans, MRI, and positron emission tomography (PET), may be used to aid in the diagnosis or location of a tumor and to monitor response to treatment.
6. **Other laboratory tests** commonly used for cancer diagnosis include complete blood counts (CBCs) and blood chemistries. A CBC measures the levels of the three basic blood cells—white cells, red cells, and platelets.
   - **a.** The CBC will often include an absolute neutrophil count (ANC), which measures the absolute number of neutrophils in a person's white blood count. The ANC is calculated by multiplying the white blood count (WBC) × total neutrophils (segmented neutrophils percent + segmented bands percent) = ANC. Segmented neutrophils are often listed as "polys" and segmented bands are immature "polys."

E. **Staging** is the categorizing of patients according to the extent of their disease. The stage of the disease is used to determine prognosis and treatment. In adult patients with cancer, two different staging systems are widely employed for the staging of neoplasms.

1. **TNM classification**
   - **a.** *T* indicates tumor size and is classified from 0 to 4, with 0 indicating the absence of tumor.
   - **b.** *N* indicates the presence and extent of regional lymph node spread and is classified from 0 to 3, with 0 indicating no regional lymph node involvement and 3 indicating extensive involvement.
   - **c.** *M* indicates the presence of distant metastases and is classified as 0 (for absence) or 1 (for presence of distant metastases).
   - **d.** For example, T2N1M0 indicates a moderate-size tumor with limited nodal disease and no distant metastases.
2. **AJCC** staging, developed by the American Joint Committee on Cancer, classifies cancers as stages 0 to IV. An assigned TNM translates into a stage. A high number indicates larger tumors with extensive nodal involvement and/or metastasis. Generally, high numbers also indicate a worse prognosis. There are specific staging criteria for each tumor type.

F. **Survival** depends on the tumor type, the extent of disease, and the therapy received. Although some patients are free of all detectable disease, not all patients are cured. The terms **complete response** and **remission** are used to indicate that the patient has no evidence of disease after treatment. This is not a synonym for *cure*, as several patients who have achieved complete remission may **relapse**. Other markers used to describe disease response or survival include partial response (PR), very good partial response (VGPR), stable disease (SD), progressive disease (PD), time to progression (TTP), and progression-free survival (PFS).

II. CELL LIFE CYCLE.

Knowledge of the cell life cycle and cell cycle kinetics is essential to the understanding of the activity of chemotherapy agents in the treatment of cancer (*Figure 50-1*).

A. **Phases of the cell cycle**
   1. **M phase**, or **mitosis**, is the phase in which the cell divides into two daughter cells.
   2. **G_1 phase**, or **postmitotic gap**, is when RNA and the proteins required for the specialized functions of the cell are synthesized in preparation for DNA synthesis.
   3. **S phase** is the phase in which DNA synthesis and replication occurs.
   4. **G_2 phase**, or the **premitotic** or **postsynthetic gap**, is the phase in which RNA and the enzymes topoisomerase I and II are produced to prepare for duplication of the cell.
   5. **G_0 phase**, or **resting phase**, is the phase in which the cell is not committed to division. Cells in this phase are generally not sensitive to chemotherapy. Some of these cells may reenter the actively dividing cell cycle. In a process called **recruitment**, some chemotherapy regimens are designed to enhance this reentry by killing a large number of actively dividing cells.

B. **Cell growth kinetics.** Several terms describe cell growth kinetics.
   1. **Cell growth fraction** is the proportion of cells in the tumor dividing or preparing to divide. As the tumor enlarges, the cell growth fraction decreases because a larger proportion of cells may not be able to obtain adequate nutrients and blood supply for replication.
   2. **Cell cycle time** is the average time for a cell that has just completed mitosis to grow and again divide and again pass through mitosis. Cell cycle time is specific for each individual tumor.
   3. **Tumor doubling time** is the time for the tumor to double in size. As the tumor gets larger, its doubling time gets longer because it contains a smaller proportion of actively dividing cells owing to restrictions of space, nutrient availability, and blood supply.
   4. The **gompertzian growth curve** illustrates these cell growth concepts (*Figure 50-2*).

C. **Tumor cell burden** is the number of tumor cells in the body.
   1. Because a large number of cells is required to produce symptoms and be clinically detectable (approximately 10^9 cells), the tumor may be in the plateau phase of the growth curve by the time it is discovered.
   2. The **cell kill hypothesis** states that a certain percentage of tumor cells will be killed with each course of cancer chemotherapy.
      a. As tumor cells are killed, cells in **G_0** may be recruited into **G_1**, resulting in tumor regrowth.
      b. Thus, repeated cycles of chemotherapy are required to achieve a complete response or remission (*Figure 50-3*).
      c. The percentage of cells killed depends on the chemotherapy dose.
   3. In theory, the tumor burden would never reach absolute zero because only a percentage of cells are killed with each cycle. Less than 10^4 cells may depend on elimination by the host's immune system.

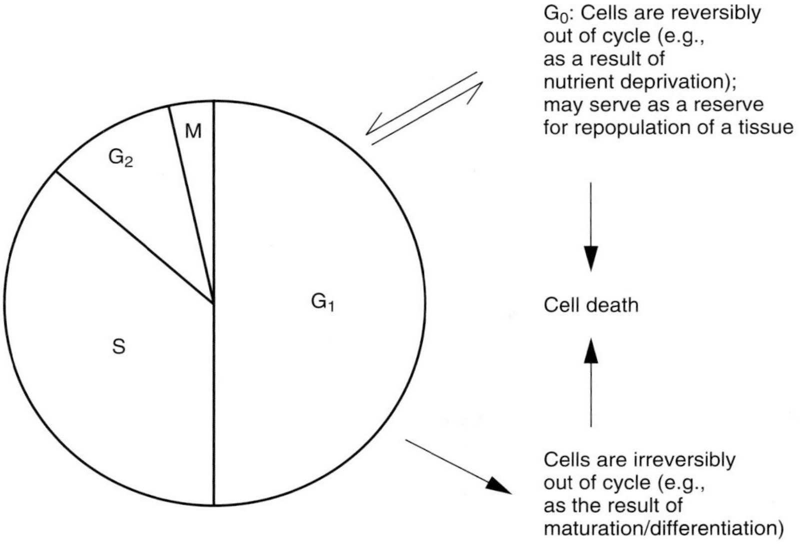
G0: Cells are reversibly out of cycle (e.g., as a result of nutrient deprivation); may serve as a reserve for repopulation of a tissue
M
G2
G1
S
Cell death
Cells are irreversibly out of cycle (e.g., as the result of maturation/differentiation)

Figure 50-1. The cell cycle. The cell growth cycle, emphasizing the relationship between proliferating cell populations. (Reprinted with permission from Lenhard RE Jr, Osteen RT, Gansler T, eds. *The American Cancer Society's Clinical Oncology*. Atlanta, GA: American Cancer Society; 2001.)

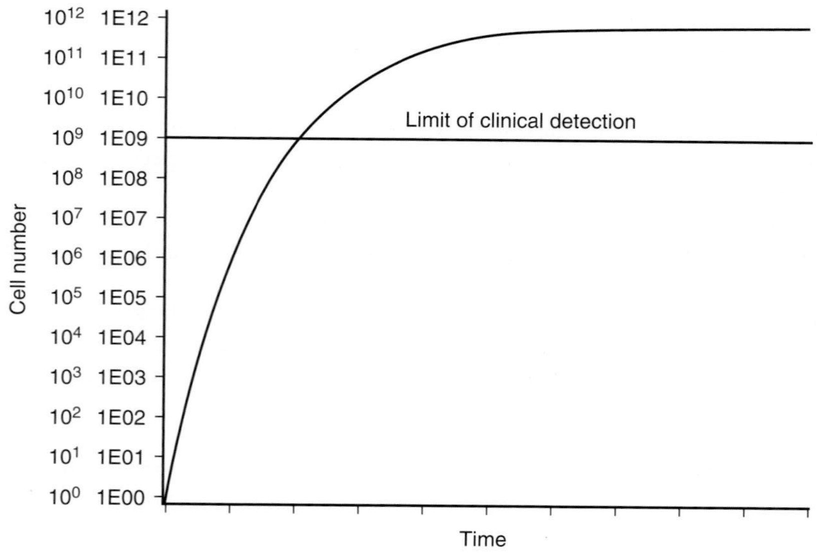

Figure 50-2. The gompertzian growth curve. During the early stages of its development, a tumor grows exponentially. But as a tumor enlarges, its growth slows. By the time a tumor becomes large enough to cause symptoms and be clinically detectable, the majority of its growth has already occurred and is no longer exponential. (Reprinted with permission from Lenhard RE Jr, Osteen RT, Gansler T, eds. *The American Cancer Society's Clinical Oncology*. Atlanta, GA: American Cancer Society; 2001.)

D. Chemotherapeutic agents may be classified according to their **reliance on cell cycle kinetics** for their cytotoxic effect. Combinations of chemotherapy agents that are active in different phases of the cell cycle may result in a greater cell kill. A cell cycle classification of some commonly used chemotherapeutic agents is given in II.D.1.a–d.

1. **Phase-specific agents** are most active against cells that are in a specific phase of the cell cycle. These agents are most effective against tumors with a high growth fraction. Theoretically, administering these agents as continuous intravenous infusions or by multiple repeated doses may increase the likelihood of hitting the majority of cells in the specific phase at any one time. Therefore, these agents are also considered schedule-dependent agents. Examples are as follows:
   - **a.** M phase: mitotic inhibitors (e.g., vinca alkaloids, taxanes)
   - **b.** G_1 phase: asparaginase, prednisone
   - **c.** S phase: antimetabolites
   - **d.** G_2 phase: bleomycin, etoposide

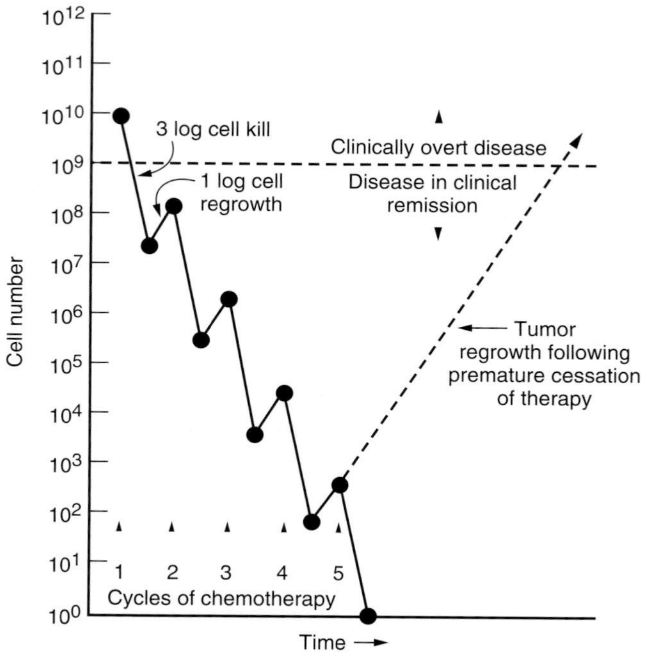

Figure 50-3. Chemotherapy and tumor cell survival. Relationship between tumor cell survival and chemotherapy administration. The exponential relationship between chemotherapy drug dose and tumor cell survival dictates that a constant proportion, not number, of tumor cells is killed with each cycle of treatment. In this example, each cycle of drug administration results in 99.9% (3 log) cell kill, and 1 log of cell regrowth occurs between cycles. The broken line indicates what would occur if the last cycle of therapy were omitted. Despite complete clinical remission of disease, the tumor would ultimately recur. (Reprinted with permission from Lenhard RE Jr, Osteen RT, Gansler T, eds. *The American Cancer Society's Clinical Oncology*. Atlanta, GA: American Cancer Society; 2001.)

2. **Phase-nonspecific agents** are effective while cells are in the active cycle but do not require that the cell be in a particular phase. These agents generally show more activity against slow-growing tumors. They may be administered as single bolus doses because their activity is independent of the cell cycle. These drugs are also considered dose-dependent agents. Examples are alkylating agents and antitumor antibiotics.
3. **Cell cycle–nonspecific agents** are effective in all phases, including $\mathbf{G_0}$. Examples are carmustine and lomustine. Radiation therapy is also considered cell cycle nonspecific.

III. CHEMOTHERAPY

A. **Objectives of chemotherapy**
1. **For cancers like leukemias and lymphomas, several phases of chemotherapy are necessary**. A **cure** may be sought with aggressive therapy for a prolonged period to eradicate all disease. For leukemias, this curative approach may consist of the following components:
   a. **Remission induction**: therapy given with the intent of maximizing cell kill.
   b. **Consolidation** (also known as intensification or post-remission therapy): therapy to eradicate any clinically undetectable disease and to lower the tumor cell burden below 10^3, at which level host immunological defenses may keep the cells in control.
   c. **Maintenance**: therapy given in lower doses with the aim of maintaining or prolonging a remission.
2. For solid tumors, one or more approaches to chemotherapy may be used when seeking a cure based on the known utility of chemotherapy in line with other modalities, such as surgery or radiation.
   a. **Adjuvant** chemotherapy is given after more definitive therapy, such as surgery, to eliminate any remaining disease or undetected micrometastasis.
   b. **Neoadjuvant** chemotherapy is given to decrease the tumor burden before definitive therapy, such as surgery or radiation.
4. **Palliative** therapy is usually given when complete eradication of the tumor is considered unlikely or the patient refuses aggressive therapy. Palliative chemotherapy may be given to decrease the tumor size, control growth, and reduce symptoms.
5. **Salvage** chemotherapy is given as an attempt to get a patient into remission, after previous therapies have failed.

B. **Chemotherapy dosing** may be based on body **weight**, body surface area (**BSA**), or area under the concentration versus time curve (**AUC**). BSA is most frequently used because it provides an accurate comparison of activity and toxicity across species, making it easier to translate preclinical dosing into clinical trials and practice in humans. In addition, BSA correlates with cardiac output, which determines renal and hepatic blood flow and thus affects drug elimination. In very young or very small patients (e.g., infants less than a year of age or less than 10 to 12 kg of body weight), the BSA is not a good measure for calculating the dose as it can overestimate the patient's size and lead to overdosing of chemotherapeutic agents, resulting in excessive toxicities. In this patient population, dosing chemotherapy based on body weight (in kilograms) is often a more frequently employed technique.

C. **Dosing adjustments** may be required for kidney or liver dysfunction to prevent toxicity. For some agents, dose adjustments are also made based on hematologic or non-hematologic toxicities. Very little is known about dosing chemotherapy in the obese population.

D. **Combination chemotherapy** is usually more effective than single-agent therapy.
1. When combining chemotherapy agents, factors to consider include
   a. Antitumor activity
   b. Different mechanisms of action
   c. Minimally overlapping toxicities
2. The reasons for administering combination chemotherapy include
   a. Overcoming or preventing resistance
   b. Cytotoxicity to resting and dividing cells
   c. Biochemical enhancement of effect
   d. Rescue of normal cells
3. **Dosing** and **scheduling** of combination regimens are important because they are designed to allow recovery of normal cells. These regimens generally are given as short courses of therapy in cycles.

4. **Acronyms** often are used to designate chemotherapy regimens. For example, CMF refers to a combination of cyclophosphamide, methotrexate, and fluorouracil used in the treatment of breast cancer.

E. **Administration**

1. **Routes** of administration vary depending on the agent and the disease state. Although intravenous (IV) administration is most commonly employed, oral administration of chemotherapy is becoming increasingly more common.
2. Other administration techniques include oral, subcutaneous, intrathecal, intra-arterial, intraperitoneal, intravesical, continuous IV infusion, bolus IV infusion, and hepatic artery infusion.
3. Drugs that may be given **intrathecally** include methotrexate, cytarabine, and hydrocortisone. Drugs should not be administered by the intrathecal route without specific information supporting intrathecal administration. **Inadvertent administration of vinca alkaloids (e.g., vincristine) by the intrathecal route results in ascending paralysis and death**. The U.S. Food and Drug Administration (FDA) requires that specific wording alerting the provider to this error must be included on the packaging of each dose of vincristine. They also recommend that safety measures are employed in the preparation and delivery of vinca alkaloids.
4. Products with different formulations, including liposomal or pegylated agents (e.g., liposomal doxorubicin, pegfilgrastim), are being used to decrease frequency of administration and/or reduce toxicities.

F. **Response to chemotherapy** is defined in several ways and does not always correlate with patient survival.

1. **Complete response** (**CR**) indicates disappearance of all clinical, gross, and microscopic disease.
2. **PR** indicates a greater than 50% reduction in tumor size, lasting a reasonable period. Some evidence of disease remains after therapy.
3. **Response rate** (**RR**) is defined as CR + PR.
4. **SD** indicates tumor that neither grows nor shrinks significantly (less than 25% change in size).
5. **PD** or **no response** after therapy is defined by a greater than 25% increase in tumor size or the appearance of new lesions.

G. **Factors affecting response to chemotherapy**

1. **Tumor cell heterogeneity**. Large tumors have completed multiple cell divisions, resulting in several mutations and genetically diverse cells.
2. **Drug resistance**. The **Goldie-Coldman hypothesis** states that genetic changes are associated with drug resistance, and the probability of resistance increases as tumor size increases. The hypothesis assumes that at the time of diagnosis, most tumors possess resistant clones. A well-studied mechanism of resistance involves the multidrug resistance (*mdr*) gene, which codes for membrane-bound P-glycoprotein. P-glycoprotein serves as a channel through which cellular toxins (i.e., chemotherapeutic agents) may be excreted from the cell.
3. **Dose intensity** is defined as a specific dose delivered over a specific period. Occasionally, the full dose cannot be given or a cycle is delayed owing to complications or toxicities. Suboptimal doses have resulted in reduced response rates and survival. **Dose density** involves shortening the usual interval between doses to maximize the drug effects on the tumor growth kinetics.
4. **Patient-specific factors** such as poor functional status, impaired organ function, or concomitant diseases may compromise how a chemotherapy regimen is given and affect how the patient responds to treatment.

IV. CLASSIFICATION OF CHEMOTHERAPEUTIC AGENTS

A. Examples of the following agents and their toxicities are listed in *Table 50-1*.

B. **Alkylating agents** were the first group of antineoplastic agents. The prototype of this class is mechlorethamine, or **nitrogen mustard**, which was researched as a chemical warfare agent. Alkylating agents cause cross-linking and abnormal base pairing of DNA strands, which inhibit replication of the DNA. This mechanism is known as **alkylation**. These are phase-nonspecific agents.

C. Most of the **antitumor antibiotics** are obtained from organisms of the *Streptomyces* genus. These agents may act by either alkylation (mitomycin) or **intercalation**. Intercalation is the process by which the drug slides between DNA base pairs and inhibits DNA synthesis. These are phase-nonspecific agents.

D. **Antimetabolites** are structural analogs of naturally occurring substrates for biochemical reactions. They inhibit DNA synthesis by acting as false substitutions in the production of nucleic

Table 50-1 CANCER CHEMOTHERAPEUTIC AGENTS BY MECHANISM OF ACTION AND TOXICITIES

Drug	Toxicities
Alkylating agents	
Altretamine (hexamethylmelamine)	Nausea and vomiting, myelosuppression, paresthesias, CNS toxicity
Busulfan	Myelosuppression, pulmonary fibrosis, aplastic anemia, skin hyperpigmentation
Carmustine	Delayed myelosuppression, nausea and vomiting, hepatotoxicity
Chlorambucil	Myelosuppression, pulmonary fibrosis, hyperuricemia
Carboplatin	Myelosuppression, nausea and vomiting, peripheral neuropathy, ototoxicity
Cisplatin	Nephrotoxicity, nausea and vomiting, peripheral neuropathy, myelosuppression, ototoxicity
Cyclophosphamide	Myelosuppression, hemorrhagic cystitis, immunosuppression, alopecia, stomatitis, SIADH
Dacarbazine	Myelosuppression, nausea and vomiting, flulike syndrome, hepatotoxicity, alopecia, flushing
Estramustine	Myelosuppression, ischemic heart disease, thrombophlebitis, hepatotoxicity, nausea and vomiting
Ifosfamide	Myelosuppression, hemorrhagic cystitis, somnolence, confusion
Lomustine	Delayed myelosuppression, nausea and vomiting, hepatotoxicity, neurotoxicity
Mechlorethamine	Myelosuppression, nausea and vomiting, phlebitis, gonadal dysfunction
Melphalan	Myelosuppression, anorexia, nausea and vomiting, gonadal dysfunction
Oxaliplatin	Sensory peripheral neuropathy, nausea and vomiting, diarrhea, mucositis, transaminase elevations, alopecia
Procarbazine	Myelosuppression, nausea and vomiting, lethargy, depression, paresthesias, headache, flulike syndrome
Streptozocin	Renal toxicity, nausea and vomiting, diarrhea, altered glucose metabolism, liver dysfunction
Temozolomide	Myelosuppression, nausea and vomiting, fatigue, headache, peripheral edema
Thiotepa	Myelosuppression, nausea and vomiting, mucositis, skin rashes
Antitumor antibiotics	
Bleomycin	Pneumonitis, pulmonary fibrosis, fever, anaphylaxis, hyperpigmentation, alopecia
Dactinomycin	Stomatitis, myelosuppression, anorexia, nausea and vomiting, diarrhea, alopecia
Daunorubicin	Myelosuppression, cardiotoxicity, stomatitis, alopecia, nausea and vomiting
Doxorubicin	Myelosuppression, cardiotoxicity, stomatitis, alopecia, nausea and vomiting
Epirubicin	Myelosuppression, nausea and vomiting, cardiotoxicity, alopecia
Idarubicin	Myelosuppression, nausea and vomiting, stomatitis, alopecia, cardiotoxicity
Mitomycin C	Myelosuppression, nausea and vomiting, anorexia, alopecia, stomatitis
Mitoxantrone	Myelosuppression, cardiotoxicity, alopecia, stomatitis, nausea and vomiting
Valrubicin	Urinary frequency, dysuria, hematuria, bladder spasm, incontinence, cystitis (For intravesical bladder administration)
Antimetabolites	
Azacytidine	Myelosuppression, nausea and vomiting, diarrhea, constipation, injection site pain, muscle aches, fatigue, edema, dizziness
Capecitabine	Diarrhea, stomatitis, nausea and vomiting, hand–foot syndrome, myelosuppression
Cladribine	Myelosuppression, fever, rash
Clofarabine	Tachycardia, hypotension, headache, fever, chills, fatigue, pruritis, rash, nausea, vomiting, transaminitis, hyperbilirubinemia
Cytarabine	Myelosuppression, nausea and vomiting, diarrhea, stomatitis, hepatotoxicity, fever, conjunctivitis, CNS toxicity

(Continued on next page)

Table 50-1 Continued.

Drug	Toxicities
Decitabine	Myelosuppression, petechiae, fatigue, diarrhea, constipation, hyperglycemia, myalgias/arthralgias, rash, edema
Fludarabine	Myelosuppression, nausea and vomiting, fever, malaise, pulmonary infiltrates
Floxuridine	Hepatotoxicity, gastritis, mucositis
Fluorouracil	Stomatitis, myelosuppression, diarrhea, nausea and vomiting, cerebellar ataxia
Gemcitabine	Myelosuppression, fever, flu-like syndrome, rash, mild nausea and vomiting
Hydroxyurea	Myelosuppression, mild nausea and vomiting, rash
Mercaptopurine	Myelosuppression, nausea and vomiting, anorexia, diarrhea, cholestasis
Methotrexate	Mucositis, myelosuppression, pulmonary fibrosis, hepatotoxicity, nephrotoxicity, diarrhea, skin erythema
Nelarabine	Neurologic toxicities, somnolence, hypoesthesia, seizures, thrombocytopenia, anemia, and neutropenia, fatigue, and nausea
Pemetrexed	Myelosuppression, edema, fatigue, nausea and vomiting, diarrhea, mucositis, skin rash
Pentostatin	Nephrotoxicity, CNS depression, myelosuppression, nausea and vomiting, conjunctivitis
Thioguanine	Myelosuppression, hepatotoxicity, stomatitis
Mitotic inhibitors	
Docetaxel	Myelosuppression, fluid retention, hypersensitivity, paresthesias, rash alopecia
Ixabepilone	Peripheral sensory neuropathy, neutropenia, fatigue, myalgia, arthralgia, stomatitis, hypersensitivity reactions, anorexia
Paclitaxel	Myelosuppression, peripheral neuropathy, alopecia, mucositis, anaphylaxis, dyspnea
Vinblastine	Myelosuppression, paralytic ileus, alopecia, nausea, stomatitis
Vincristine	Peripheral neuropathy, paralytic ileus, SIADH
Vinorelbine	Peripheral neuropathy, myelosuppression, nausea and vomiting, hepatic dysfunction
Topoisomerase inhibitors	
Etoposide	Myelosuppression, nausea and vomiting, diarrhea, fever, hypotension with infusion, alopecia
Irinotecan	Myelosuppression, diarrhea, nausea and vomiting, anorexia
Teniposide	Myelosuppression, nausea and vomiting, alopecia, hepatotoxicity, hypotension with infusion
Topotecan	Myelosuppression, fever, flulike syndrome, nausea and vomiting
Enzymes	
Asparaginase	Allergic reactions, nausea and vomiting, liver dysfunction, CNS depression, hyperglycemia
Pegaspargase	Hypersensitivity reactions, hepatotoxicity, fever, nausea and vomiting
Protein tyrosine kinase inhibitors	
Dasatinib (Sprycel)	Pleural and pericardial effusions, diarrhea, myelosuppression, gastrointestinal hemorrhage, rash
Erlotinib (Tarceva)	Acneiform rash, diarrhea, nausea, pruritus, fatigue, eye irritation
Imatinib mesylate (Gleevec)	Myelosuppression, hepatotoxicity, fluid retention, nausea, diarrhea
Lapatinib (Tykerb)	Diarrhea, rash, nausea, fatigue, anemia, left ventricular and liver dysfunction
Nilotinib (Tasigna)	Rash, headache, nausea, fatigue, thrombocytopenia, neutropenia
Sorafenib (Nexavar)	Hand-and-foot syndrome, fatigue, hypertension, rash/desquamation, diarrhea
Sunitinib (Sutent)	Hand-and-foot syndrome, skin and hair discoloration, fatigue, diarrhea, hypothyroidism, hypertension, left ventricular dysfunction, mucositis/stomatitis, nausea
mTOR kinase inhibitors	
Temsirolimus (Torisel)	Hyperglycemia, hypophosphatemia, anemia, hypertriglyceridemia, rash, diarrhea, mucositis/stomatitis

Table 50-1 Continued.

Drug	Toxicities
Histone deacetylase inhibitors	
Vorinostat (Zolinza)	Thrombocytopenia, anemia, diarrhea, nausea/vomiting, hyperglycemia
Miscellaneous	
Arsenic trioxide	Arrhythmias, hyperleukocytosis, nausea and vomiting, diarrhea, abdominal pain, APL differentiation syndrome (fever, dyspnea, weight gain, pulmonary infiltrates)
Bexarotene (Targretin)	Hyperlipidemia, pancreatitis, hypothyroidism, hypercalcemia, leukopenia, peripheral edema, rash
Bortezomib (Velcade)	Fatigue, peripheral neuropathy, myelosuppression, hypotension, arthralgias, diarrhea, nausea and vomiting, headache, fever
Isotretinoin (13-cis-retinoic acid, Accutane)	Dry skin and mucous membranes epistaxis, chelitis, photosensitivity, back pain, arthralgias, hypertriglyceridemia, hypercalcemia, major fetal toxicity
Tretinoin (all-trans-retinoic acid, ATRA; Vesanoid)	Leukocytosis, arrhythmias, headache, nausea and vomiting, scaling of skin, ATRA syndrome (fever, dyspnea, weight gain, pulmonary infiltrates)
Lenalidomide	Myelosuppression, thromboembolic events, bacterial infection, fatigue, diarrhea
Thalidomide	Fatigue; headache; numbness in hands, feet, arms, and legs; constipation; increased risk for thrombotic events major fetal toxicities
Hormonal agents	
Adrenocorticoids Dexamethasone Methylprednisolone Prednisone	Fluid retention, hyperglycemia, hypertension, infection
Estrogens Estradiol	Fluid retention, feminization, uterine bleeding, nausea and vomiting, thrombophlebitis
Progestins Medroxyprogesterone Megestrol acetate	Weight gain, fluid retention, feminization, cardiovascular effects
Antiestrogens Fulvestrant Tamoxifen Toremifene	Hot flashes, nausea and vomiting, altered menses
Estrogen agonist/antagonist Raloxifene	Hot flashes, arthralgias, flu-like syndrome
Aromatase inhibitors Aminoglutethimide Anastrozole Exemestane Letrozole	Rash, electrolytes disturbance, drowsiness, nausea, anorexia
Androgens Testosterone Methyltestosterone Fluoxymesterone	Masculinization, amenorrhea, gynecomastia, nausea, water retention, changes in libido, skin hypersensitivity, hepatotoxicity
Antiandrogens Bicalutamide Flutamide Nilutamide	Hot flashes, decreased libido, impotence, diarrhea, nausea and vomiting, gynecomastia, hepatotoxicity
LHRH analogs Leuprolide Goserelin	Hot flashes, menstrual irregularity, sexual dysfunction, edema
LHRH antagonist Abarelix	Hypersensitivity reactions, hypotension, syncope, hot flashes, breast enlargement, prolongation of QT interval

APL, acute promyelocytic leukemia; *ATRA*, all-*trans*-retinoic acid; *CNS*, central nervous system; *LHRH*, luteinizing hormone-releasing hormone; *SIADH*, syndrome of inappropriate antidiuretic hormone.

acids. These are S phase–specific agents. Unique features involving the use of antimetabolites are as follows:

1. **Leucovorin rescue** must be given following with high-dose methotrexate administration to rescue normal, healthy cells from the cytotoxicity of methotrexate. Leucovorin serves as a reduced folate (i.e., folinic acid) that enters the folic acid synthesis pathway downstream of the site of effect of methotrexate. Timing and dosing of leucovorin is critical to ensure the maximal benefit with the least risk of reversing the cytotoxic effects of methotrexate.
2. **Polymorphisms of thiopurine methyltransferase** (**TPMT**) may produce excessive toxicity in patients receiving mercaptopurine. Dose reductions may be necessary in some patients.

E. **Mitotic inhibitors.** The vinca alkaloids arrest cell division by preventing microtubule formation. The taxanes promote microtubule assembly and stabilization, thus prohibiting cell division. These are M phase–specific agents.

F. **Topoisomerase inhibitors** inhibit the enzymes topoisomerase I or II. The topoisomerases are necessary for DNA replication and RNA transcription. These are **G_2** phase–specific agents.

G. **Enzymes.** Asparaginase is an enzyme that causes the degradation of the amino acid asparagine to aspartic acid and ammonia. Unlike normal cells, tumor cells lack the ability to synthesize asparagine. This is a **G_1** phase–specific agent.

H. **Protein tyrosine kinase inhibitors.** These agents are also known as targeted agents because they affect specific receptors to induce cancer cell death.

1. Imatinib, dasatinib, and nilotinib are selective tyrosine kinase inhibitor that causes apoptosis or arrest of growth in cells expressing the Bcr-Abl oncoprotein. Bcr-Abl is the product of a specific chromosomal abnormality (Philadelphia chromosome), which is present in virtually all patients with chronic myelogenous leukemia (CML).
2. Erlotinib is a selective inhibitor of epidermal growth factor receptor (EGFR) tyrosine kinase. EGFR is a cell surface receptor that is overexpressed in certain solid tumors. The binding of the EGFR receptor to its ligand activates tyrosine kinase, which then stimulates cell proliferation and growth of the tumor. Erlotinib blocks the tyrosine kinase signaling cascade and inhibits cancer cell growth.

I. Various **miscellaneous** agents have a critical role in the treatment of specific cancers.

1. **Retinoid derivatives**
   a. **Tretinoin** (all-*trans*-retinoic acid; ATRA) is a retinoic acid derivative that is used in the treatment of a specific type of acute myelogenous leukemia, known as acute promyelocytic leukemia (APL), to help cells differentiate into functionally mature cells.
   b. **Isotretinoin** (13-*cis*-retinoic acid; 13-CRA) is a retinoic acid derivative that is used in the treatment of neuroblastoma, a type of solid tumor seen in young children.
   c. **Bexarotene** is a selective retinoid X receptor (RXR) ligand used for cutaneous T-cell lymphoma. Activation of the retinoid receptors leads to regulation of gene expression and apoptosis.
2. **Arsenic trioxide** is an antineoplastic compound used in the treatment of APL that may induce selective apoptosis of APL cells.
3. **Bortezomib** is a proteosome inhibitor currently used in patients with multiple myeloma and under investigation for the treatment of several other types of cancer.
   a. Proteosomes are enzyme complexes that are responsible for degrading proteins that control the cell cycle.
   b. Bortezomib is specific in that it interferes with the degradation of nuclear factor κβ (NF-κβ). NF-κβ is released from its inhibitory partner protein and moves to the nucleus. When the inhibitory partner does not degrade because of the action of bortezomib, NF-κβ is prevented from transcribing the genes that promote cancer growth.
4. **Thalidomide and lenalidomide** are immunomodulatory agents with various mechanisms of action. They work as angiogenesis inhibitors by interfering with the growth of new blood vessels needed for tumor growth and survival. They inhibit the production of tumor necrosis factor α (TNF-α) production, induce oxidative damage to DNA, and help stimulate human T cells. They can be used as treatment for multiple myeloma in combination with dexamethasone.

J. **Hormones** are a class of heterogeneous compounds that have various effects on cells.

K. **Biological response modifiers** alter or enhance the patient's immune system to fight cancer or to lessen the side effects of the cancer treatment. Examples are given in *Table 50-2*.

1. **Cytokines** are soluble factors secreted or released by cells that affect the activity of other cells and/or the secreting cell itself. These agents generally act as regulatory or hematopoietic growth factors.

Table 50-2 BIOLOGICAL AGENTS USED IN ONCOLOGY

Agent	Indications	Toxicity
Cytokine		
Interferon-α -2a, -2b (Intron A)	Malignant melanoma, chronic myelogenous leukemia, hairy cell leukemia, Kaposi sarcoma, chronic hepatitis B and C, follicular lymphoma	Flulike syndrome, anorexia, depression, fatigue
Interleukin 2 (aldesleukin, Proleukin)	Renal cell carcinoma, malignant melanoma	Chills, fever, dyspnea, pulmonary congestion, edema, nephrotoxicity, hypotension, mental status changes, anemia, thrombocytopenia, diarrhea, nausea and vomiting
Interleukin 11 (oprelvekin, Neumega)	Thrombocytopenia	Fluid retention, peripheral edema, dyspnea, tachycardia, atrial arrhythmias, dizziness, blurred vision
Filgrastim (G-CSF, Neupogen)	Decrease incidence/duration of neutropenia, hematopoietic stem cell mobilization	Bone pain, fever, malaise
Pegfilgrastim (Neulasta)	Decrease incidence/duration of neutropenia	Bone pain, fever, malaise
Sargramostim (GM-CSF, Leukine)	Acceleration of myeloid recovery, BMT failure or engraftment delay, induction for acute myelogenous leukemia, hematopoietic stem cell mobilization, myeloid reconstitution after BMT	Bone pain, arthralgia/myalgia, chills, fever, rash, first-dose reaction (hypotension, tachycardia, dyspnea)
Epoetin α (erythropoietin, Epogen, Procrit)	Anemia associated with chronic renal failure, cancer chemotherapy or HIV treatments, reduction of blood transfusions in surgery patients	Hypertension, headache, arthralgias
Darbepoetin α (Aranesp)	Anemia associated with chronic renal failure, chronic renal insufficiency, cancer- and chemotherapy-associated anemia	Hypertension, myalgia, headache, fever, tachycardia, nausea
Monoclonal antibody		
Alemtuzumab (Campath)	B-cell chronic lymphocytic leukemia	Infusion-related fevers, chills, rash, hypotension, shortness of breath, nausea and vomiting, opportunistic infections, neutropenia, thrombocytopenia
Bevacizumab (Avastin)	Metastatic colorectal cancer, non-small cell lung cancer (nonsquamous)	Hypertension, proteinuria, GI perforation, thrombotic events, impaired wound healing
Cetuximab (Erbitux)	Metastatic colorectal cancer	Acneiform rash, infusion-related reactions, fatigue, nausea and vomiting, diarrhea
Ibritumomab tiuxetan (Zevalin)	Non-Hodgkin lymphoma	Infusion-related fevers, chills, rigors, hypersensitivity, hypotension, myelosuppression
Panitumumab	EGFR-expressing, metastatic colorectal carcinoma with disease progression on or following fluoropyrimidine-, oxaliplatin-, and irinotecan-containing chemotherapy regimens.	Transient acneiform skin rash, erythema, dry skin, skin fissures/exfoliation, diarrhea
Rituximab (Rituxan)	Non-Hodgkin lymphoma	Hypersensitivity, infusion-related fevers, chills, rigors, hypotension
Tositumomab (Bexxar)	Non-Hodgkin lymphoma	Hypersensitivity reactions, fever, chills, myelosuppression, especially thrombocytopenia, rash, nausea and vomiting, diarrhea

(Continued on next page)

Table 50-2 Continued.

Agent	Indications	Toxicity
Trastuzumab (Herceptin)	Breast cancer	Infusion-related fevers, chills, cardiac dysfunction including dyspnea, cough, peripheral edema, nausea and vomiting, hypersensitivity, hypotension, diarrhea
Immunotoxin		
Denileukin diftitox (Ontak)	Cutaneous T-cell lymphoma	Acute hypersensitivity, including hypotension, dyspnea, rash, chest pain, tachycardia, vascular leak syndrome, dizziness, nausea and vomiting, diarrhea

BMT, bone marrow transplant; *EGFR*, epidermal growth factor receptor; *G-CSF*, granulocyte colony-stimulating factor; *GI*, gastrointestinal; *GM-CSF*, granulocyte-macrophage colony-stimulating factor.

2. **Monoclonal antibodies** are recombinant antibodies designed to identify cancer-specific antigens, bind to the antigens on the patient's cancer cells, and allow the patient's immune system to eliminate those cells.
   a. Some monoclonal antibodies have been conjugated to radioisotopes (e.g., ibritumomab tiuxetan) to help target cytotoxic therapy to the tumor cells.
   b. Bevacizumab (Avastin) is a chimeric monoclonal antibody that targets and inhibits vascular endothelial growth factor (VEGF). VEGF is an important regulator of the growth and survival of blood vessels, known as angiogenesis. Bevacizumab works by inhibiting angiogenesis and, therefore, inhibiting the blood supply to the tumor.
   c. Trastuzumab (Herceptin) is a humanized monoclonal antibody that binds to the HER2/neu (ErbB2) receptor. This receptor is overexpressed in many patients with breast cancer. Trastuzumab has several proposed mechanisms, including antibody-dependent cell-mediated cytotoxicity, downregulation of the HER2/neu receptors resulting in disruption of downstream signaling, cell cycle arrest in the G1 phase, and suppression of angiogenesis.
   d. Other monoclonal antibodies are listed in *Table 50-2*.
3. **Immunotoxins.** Denileukin diftitox is a fusion protein composed of diphtheria toxin and interleukin 2 (IL-2). It is designed to direct the cytocidal action of diphtheria toxin to cells with the IL-2 receptor on their surface. This form of therapy is able to bypass the need for a functioning immune system, which may be defective in many cancer patients.
4. **Tumor vaccines.** Sipuleucel-T (Provenge) is a therapeutic, patient-specific cancer vaccine. It was the first therapeutic cancer vaccine to demonstrate a survival advantage in phase III clinical trials.

V. TOXICITIES OF CHEMOTHERAPY AGENTS.

Chemotherapeutic agents are most toxic to rapidly proliferating cells, including mucous membranes, skin, hair, gastrointestinal (GI) tract, and bone marrow.

A. **Bone marrow suppression** is the **most common** dose-limiting **side effect** of cancer therapy and may be one of the most life threatening.
   1. **Complications**
      a. **Infections.** White blood cells are most affected due to their short life span (6 to 12 hrs).
         (1) A significant decrease in the white blood cell count, particularly a neutrophil count less than $500/mm^3$ (**neutropenia**), predisposes the patient to development of serious infections.
         (2) The usual signs and symptoms of infection may be absent, and fever may be the only indicator (**febrile neutropenia**).
         (3) **Colony-stimulating factors**—for example, granulocyte colony-stimulating factor (**G-CSF**) and granulocyte-macrophage colony-stimulating factor (**GM-CSF**)—may be used to stimulate neutrophil production and lessen the degree and duration of neutropenia.

b. **Bleeding.** Platelets have an intermediate life span of 5 to 10 days. Decreased platelets (**thrombocytopenia**) can also occur from chemotherapy, which can lead to bleeding and may require platelet transfusions. Oprelvekin (interleukin-11, IL-11) has been used with the goal of stimulating platelet production; however, its use is not routine in clinical practice.

c. **Anemia** and **fatigue** secondary to cancer chemotherapy may also occur. It generally does not occur as quickly as other bone marrow toxicities because of the long life span of red blood cells (about 120 days). **Human recombinant erythropoietin** (e.g., epoetin α, darbepoetin α) may be used to increase hemoglobin, decrease transfusion requirements, and decrease fatigue. Recent data suggests that the risks (i.e., tumor progression and thrombosis) associated with the use of these agents (erythropoietin-stimulating agents, or ESAs) in patients with cancer can outweigh their benefits. A FDA-required REMS program has been implemented for the use of these agents in patients with cancer.

2. The **time course** of myelosuppression varies with the chemotherapy regimen. In general, the onset of myelosuppression is 7 to 10 days after the chemotherapy has been administered. The lowest point of the counts, called the **nadir**, is usually reached in 10 to 14 days, though for some agents this can be much longer. Recovery of counts usually occurs in 2 to 3 weeks.

3. The **depth and duration** of myelosuppression is related to the chemotherapy agents used and doses given.

   a. Drugs that can cause severe myelosuppression include carmustine, cytarabine, daunorubicin, doxorubicin, and paclitaxel.

   b. Some chemotherapy agents cause little or no myelosuppression. These include asparaginase, bleomycin, and vincristine.

   c. Sufficient **count recovery** is typically required before receiving subsequent chemotherapy cycles. Requirements vary based on the treatment protocol and the agents to be administered. Some protocols include requirements such as an ANC more than 1000/mm^3 and platelets more than 100,000/mm^3 prior to the administration of additional chemotherapy.

B. **Dermatological toxicity**

1. **Alopecia** is the loss of hair associated with chemotherapy. Not all agents cause alopecia, and hair loss may be partial or complete. Chemotherapy agents that commonly cause alopecia include cyclophosphamide, doxorubicin, mechlorethamine, and paclitaxel.

2. Drugs associated with necrosis of tissue are called **vesicants**. Local tissue necrosis may result from **extravasation** of vesicant chemotherapeutic agents outside the vein and into the subcutaneous tissue during administration.

   a. Most vesicant extravasations produce immediate pain or burning. However, a delayed reaction may occur hours to weeks later. Significant tissue injury, including ulceration or necrosis, may require plastic surgery intervention.

   b. The treatment of extravasations varies, depending on the vesicant. Heat or cold packs and chemicals such as hyaluronidase or dexrazoxane (Totect) may be used.

   c. Examples of vesicant agents include dactinomycin, daunorubicin, doxorubicin, idarubicin, mechlorethamine, mitomycin, vinblastine, vincristine, and vinorelbine.

   d. Some agents are classified as **irritants** (e.g., etoposide) and can cause irritation but not necessarily necrosis when extravasated.

3. The EGFR inhibitors have been associated with a **papulopustular**, **acneiform-like skin rash**. The development of this rash may be associated with a greater success in treating specific types of cancers.

4. Cancer chemotherapy can cause other **skin changes** such as **dryness and photosensitivity**. Examples are fluorouracil and methotrexate.

C. **GI toxicities** are frequently experienced by patients receiving chemotherapy.

1. **Nausea** and **vomiting** are often among the most distressing toxicities from the patient's perspective. However, this side effect can generally be prevented or controlled with the use of currently available antiemetics.

   a. Nausea and vomiting may be classified as **acute**, **delayed**, **anticipatory**, **or breakthrough** in nature. Antiemetics should be used prophylactically to prevent the occurrence of nausea and vomiting, particularly with chemotherapeutic agents that have a high emetogenic risk. Various clinical guidelines have been created to guide the use of antiemetics in patients receiving chemotherapy.

b. Severe vomiting can result in dehydration, electrolyte imbalances, and esophageal tears and may result in interruptions in therapy or therapy discontinuation.
c. *Table 50-3* lists **commonly used chemotherapeutic agents** and their emetogenic potential on a scale of 1 to 5.
   (1) The emetogenic potential of combinations of chemotherapy agents can be estimated by identifying the most emetogenic agent in the combination.
   (2) The contribution of the other agents can then be evaluated by using the following guidelines:
      (a) Level 1 agents do not contribute to the emetogenicity of the regimen.
      (b) Adding one or more level 2 agents increases the emetogenicity to one level higher than the most emetogenic agent in the combination.
      (b) Adding level 3 or 4 agents increases the level of emetogenicity by one level per agent.
d. The occurrence of nausea and vomiting is influenced by the emetogenicity of the chemotherapeutic agent or combination of agents, the chemotherapeutic dose, the method of administration, and individual patient characteristics.

2. **Stomatitis** is a generalized inflammation of the oral mucosa or other areas of the GI tract. Because of the rapid turnover of epithelial cells in the GI tract, this is a common site of toxicity.
   a. **Signs** and **symptoms** include erythema, pain, dryness of the mouth, burning or tingling of the lips, ulcerations, and bleeding.
   b. Chemotherapy agents commonly associated with stomatitis include capecitabine, fluorouracil, and methotrexate.
   c. **Time course.** Stomatitis usually appears within a week after the offending agent is administered and resolves in 10 to 14 days.
   d. **Consequences** of stomatitis include infection of the ulcerated areas, inability to eat, pain requiring opioid analgesics, and subsequent decreases in chemotherapy doses.

Table 50-3 EMETOGENIC POTENTIAL OF CANCER CHEMOTHERAPEUTIC AGENTS

Level 5: Very Highly Emetogenic	Level 4: Highly Emetogenic	Level 3: Moderately Emetogenic	Level 2: Low Emetic Risk	Level 1: Very Low Emetic Risk
Carmustine > 250 mg/m^2	Carmustine ≤ 250 mg/m^2	Carboplatin	Docetaxel	Asparaginase
Cisplatin ≥ 50 mg/m^2	Cisplatin < 50 mg/m^2	Cyclophosphamide ≤ 750 mg/m^2	Etoposide	Bleomycin
Cyclophosphamide ≥ 1500 mg/m^2	Cyclophosphamide 750–1500 mg/m^2	Cytarabine < 1000 mg/m^2	Fluorouracil	Capecitabine
Dacarbazine	Cytarabine > 1000 mg/m^2	Daunorubicin	Gemcitabine	Chlorambucil
Mechlorethamine	Dactinomycin	Doxorubicin ≤ 60 mg/m^2	Irinotecan	Dasatinib
Streptozocin	Doxorubicin > 60 mg/m^2	Idarubicin	Methotrexate 50–250 mg/m^2	Decitabine
	Lomustine	Ifosfamide	Mitomycin	Erlotinib
	Melphalan (intravenous > 50 mg/m^2)	Methotrexate 250–1000 mg/m^2	Paclitaxel	Gemtuzumab
	Methotrexate > 1000 mg/m^2	Mitoxantrone	Thiotepa < 15 mg/m^2	Hydroxyurea
	Procarbazine	Temozolamide	Topotecan	Lenalidomide
	Temozolomide	Melphalan > 50 mg/m^2	Pemetrexed	Methotrexate ≤ 50 mg/m^2
	Thiotepa ≥ 15 mg/m^2			Melphalan (oral)
				Nelarabine
				Rituximab
				Sorafenib
				Sunitinib
				Thalidomide
				Thioguanine
				Trastuzumab
				Vinblastine
				Vincristine
				Vinorelbine

e. **Topical and local analgesics** in the form of mouth rinses are commonly used and can help with mouth and throat pain.

3. Other GI toxicities include **diarrhea** (e.g., irinotecan, fluorouracil), **constipation** (e.g., vincristine), **anorexia**, and **taste changes**.

D. **Tumor lysis syndrome** (**TLS**) may occur in hematological malignancies such as leukemia and lymphoma in which there is a high tumor cell burden or rapidly growing tumors. Owing to the spontaneous lysis of cells from treatment with chemotherapy, cell lysis causes release of intracellular products, including uric acid, potassium, and phosphate, which can lead to renal failure and cardiac arrhythmias. This may be prevented by giving intravenous hydration, by alkalinizing the urine, and by giving agents such as **allopurinol** or **rasburicase** (Elitek) to decrease uric acid.

E. **Hypercalcemia** may occur in patients with solid or hematologic malignancies and can often be the presenting sign of malignancy. The major cause of hypercalcemia is increased osteoclastic bone resorption, which is generally caused by the release of parathyroid hormone-related protein (PTHrP) by the tumor cells. Common presenting symptoms include mental status changes, fatigue and muscle weakness, polyuria, polydipsia, nausea, and vomiting. Treatment includes aggressive hydration with normal saline; calciuric therapy, which consists of calcitonin; and bisphosphonates such as pamidronate (Aredia) or zoledronic acid (Zometa).

F. **Chills** and **fever** may occur after the administration of some chemotherapy and biological agents. This fever generally can be differentiated from fever owing to infection because of its temporal relationship to chemotherapy administration. This reaction is commonly associated with bleomycin, cytarabine, monoclonal antibodies, and IL-2.

G. **Pulmonary toxicity** is generally irreversible and may be fatal.

1. **Signs** and **symptoms** are shortness of breath, nonproductive cough, and low-grade fever. In some cases, the risk of pulmonary toxicity increases as the cumulative dose of the drug increases (e.g., bleomycin).
2. Chemotherapeutic agents associated with pulmonary toxicity include bleomycin, busulfan, carmustine, and mitomycin.

H. **Cardiac toxicity** may manifest as an acute or chronic problem.

1. **Acute changes** are generally transient electrocardiograph abnormalities that may not be clinically significant.
2. **Chronic cardiac toxicity** presents as irreversible, left-sided heart failure. **Risk factors** include chest irradiation and high cumulative doses of cardiotoxic chemotherapy.
3. Chemotherapy agents that are associated with chronic cardiotoxicity include daunorubicin, doxorubicin, epirubicin, idarubicin, and mitoxantrone. **Dexrazoxane** is a cardioprotective agent that may be used with doxorubicin to help prevent or lessen its toxic effects to the heart.

I. **Hypersensitivity reactions** may occur with any chemotherapy agent. Life-threatening reactions, including anaphylaxis, appear to be more common with asparaginase, carboplatin, cisplatin, etoposide, paclitaxel, and teniposide.

J. **Neurotoxicity** may occur with systemic or intrathecal chemotherapy.

1. Vincristine is associated with **autonomic** and **peripheral** neuropathies. Patients may experience gait disturbances, numbness and tingling of hands and feet, and loss of deep-tendon reflexes. Inadvertent intrathecal administration of vincristine results in fatal neurotoxicity.
2. **Peripheral neuropathy** and **ototoxicity** are common dose-limiting toxicities of cisplatin. **Sensory** neuropathies, including tingling or numbing of the hands and feet, may be associated with capecitabine, oxaliplatin, and paclitaxel.
3. **Cerebellar toxicity** has been reported with high doses of cytarabine and it manifests initially as loss of eye–hand coordination and may progress to coma.
4. **Arachnoiditis** has been associated with intrathecal administration of cytarabine and methotrexate.
5. **Encephalopathy** has been reported in patients receiving ifosfamide. Patient-related risk factors have been identified with this adverse event and include high serum creatinine, low serum albumin, and the presence of pelvic disease.

K. **Hemorrhagic cystitis** is a bladder toxicity that is seen most commonly after administration of cyclophosphamide and ifosfamide. **Acrolein**, a metabolite of these agents, is thought to cause a chemical irritation of the bladder mucosa, resulting in bleeding. Preventive measures include aggressive hydration with subsequent frequent urination, and the administration of the uroprotectant mesna. **Mesna** acts by binding to acrolein and preventing it from contacting the bladder mucosa.

L. **Renal toxicity** may manifest by elevations in serum creatinine and blood urea nitrogen (BUN) as well as electrolyte abnormalities. Nephrotoxicity is associated with cisplatin, ifosfamide, methotrexate, and streptozocin. Intravenous hydration is used to protect the kidneys from the nephrotoxic effects of cisplatin. Osmotic diuresis with mannitol may help reduce the incidence of cisplatin nephrotoxicity.

M. **Hepatotoxicity** may manifest as elevated liver function tests, jaundice, or hepatitis. Asparaginase, cytarabine, mercaptopurine, and methotrexate are known to cause hepatic toxicity.

N. **Secondary malignancies**, such as solid tumors, lymphomas, and leukemias, may occur many years after chemotherapy or radiation. Antineoplastic agents known to possess a high carcinogenic risk include cyclophosphamide, etoposide, melphalan, and mechlorethamine.

O. Chemotherapy may cause **infertility**, which may be temporary or permanent. Cyclophosphamide, chlorambucil, mechlorethamine, melphalan, and procarbazine are associated with a significant incidence of infertility in males and females.

VI. OTHER THERAPEUTIC MODALITIES

A. **Surgery** may be diagnostic (biopsy, exploratory laparotomy, second look) or therapeutic (tumor debulking or removal). Surgery is often combined with chemotherapy and/or radiation.

B. **Radiation therapy** involves high doses of ionizing radiation directed at the cancerous tissue. Radiation may be combined with surgery and/or chemotherapy. **Adverse reactions** vary based on the area of the body being irradiated and may include stomatitis, nausea and vomiting, diarrhea, and myelosuppression. In patients who have received anthracyclines, **radiation recall dermatitis** may occur resulting in skin inflammation in the area of previously received radiation.

C. **Hematopoietic stem cell transplantation** involves intravenous infusion of stem cells from a compatible donor to a recipient following high-dose chemotherapy. It is used for treatment of diseases involving the bone marrow or immune system and to allow for administration of high-dose chemotherapy or radiation for tumors resistant to standard doses. Stem cells can be obtained from bone marrow or peripheral blood.

1. In **autologous** transplants, stem cells are obtained from the patient, preserved, and later reinfused into the same patient. **Allogeneic** transplants involve two separate individuals. Cells are obtained from a matched donor and then infused into a separate patient. A **syngeneic** transplant occurs when both the donor and recipient are identical twins.
2. Transplant-related complications include hepatic veno-occlusive disease (VOD), acute and chronic graft versus host disease (GVHD), infection, and pulmonary complications.

Study Questions

Directions for questions 1–14: Each of the questions, statements, or incomplete statements in this section can be correctly answered or completed by **one** of the suggested answers or phrases. Choose the **best** answer.

1. Body surface area (BSA) is used in calculating chemotherapy doses because
   (A) BSA is an indicator of tumor cell mass.
   (B) BSA correlates with cardiac output.
   (C) BSA correlates with gastrointestinal transit time.
   (D) the National Cancer Institute requires that BSA be used.
   (E) the U.S. Food and Drug Administration (FDA) requires that BSA be used.

2. The rationale for combination chemotherapy includes all of the following *except*
   (A) biochemical enhancement of effect.
   (B) rescue of normal cells.
   (C) overcoming or preventing resistance.
   (D) biochemical nullification of effect.
   (E) cytotoxic to both resting and dividing cells.

3. All of the following chemotherapy agents can be administered intrathecally *except*
   (A) methotrexate.
   (B) cytarabine.
   (C) hydrocortisone.
   (D) thiotepa.
   (E) vincristine.

4. Hypersensitivity reactions have been commonly associated with all of the following agents *except*
   (A) asparaginase.
   (B) busulfan.
   (C) carboplatin.
   (D) etoposide.
   (E) paclitaxel.

5. Which of these supportive agents may have a greater risk than benefit in patients with cancer when the goal is cure due to the potential increased risk of tumor progression?
   (A) Antiemetics
   (B) Colony-stimulating factors
   (C) Corticosteroids
   (D) Erythropoietin-stimulating agents
   (E) Oprelvekin (IL-11)

6. How do antimetabolites exert their cytotoxic effect?
   (A) Inhibiting DNA synthesis by sliding between DNA base pairs
   (B) Inhibiting RNA synthesis by sliding between RNA base pairs
   (C) Acting as false metabolites in the microtubules
   (D) Acting as false substitutions in the production of nucleic acids
   (E) Promoting microtubule assembly and stabilization

7. All of the following chemotherapy agents work through affecting microtubule function *except*
   (A) docetaxel.
   (B) vinblastine.
   (C) mitoxantrone.
   (D) vincristine.
   (E) vinorelbine.

8. When does the neutrophil nadir associated with chemotherapy agents generally occur?
   (A) During administration of the chemotherapy
   (B) 1 to 2 days after therapy
   (C) 10 to 14 days after therapy
   (D) 1 month after therapy
   (E) When the platelet count begins to rise

9. Which of the following statements describes hemorrhagic cystitis?
   (A) It is caused by excretion of tumor cell breakdown products.
   (B) It is associated with ifosfamide or cyclophosphamide administration.
   (C) It is caused by the administration of mesna.
   (D) It can be prevented or treated with acrolein.
   (E) It can be treated with granulocyte colony-stimulating factor (G-CSF).

10. All of the following chemotherapy agents are vesicants *except*
   (A) doxorubicin.
   (B) mechlorethamine.
   (C) vincristine.
   (D) methotrexate.
   (E) idarubicin.

Directions for questions 11–15: Each agent in this section is most closely associated with **one** of the following adverse effects. Each effect is used only **once**. Choose the **best** answer, **A–E**.

   (A) Cardiotoxicity
   (B) Conjunctivitis
   (C) Diarrhea
   (D) Pulmonary fibrosis
   (E) Constipation

11. Vincristine

12. Irinotecan

13. Doxorubicin

14. Cytarabine

15. Bleomycin

Answers and Explanations

1. **The answer is B** *[see III.B]*.
BSA correlates with cardiac output, which determines renal and hepatic blood flow and thus affects drug elimination.

2. **The answer is D** *[see III.D.2]*.
Combination chemotherapy has been developed to have maximal cytotoxicity to tumor cells and minimal toxicity to normal cells. The drugs are dosed and scheduled such that maximal cell kill occurs, while sparing normal cells as much as possible. Combination regimens often contain agents with different spectrums of toxicity.

3. **The answer is E** *[see III.E.3]*.
Intrathecally administered vincristine is fatal. All syringes of vincristine must be labeled "Fatal if given intrathecally. For intravenous use only."

4. **The answer is B** *[see V.I]*.
Hypersensitivity reactions have been commonly associated with asparaginase, carboplatin, etoposide, and paclitaxel. Busulfan is not commonly associated with hypersensitivity reaction.

5. **The answer is D** *[see V.A.1.c]*.
Erythropoietin-stimulating agents (ESAs) have been found to increase the likelihood of tumor progression in certain patient populations and therefore should not be used in patients with cancer when the goal is cure.

6. **The answer is D** *[see IV.D]*.
Antimetabolites are structural analogs of naturally occurring substrates for biochemical reactions. They inhibit DNA synthesis by acting as false substitutions in the production of DNA.

7. **The answer is C** *[see IV.E]*.
Docetaxel is a taxane, which works by promoting microtubule assembly and stabilization, resulting in inhibition of cell division. Vincristine, vinblastine, and vinorelbine are vinca alkaloids, which work by preventing microtubule formation. Mitoxantrone is an antitumor antibiotic, which works by DNA intercalation.

8. **The answer is C** *[see V.A.2]*.
Bone marrow suppression, particularly of the neutrophils, usually is the most profound 10–14 days after chemotherapy.

9. **The answer is B** *[see V.K]*.
Hemorrhagic cystitis results from irritation of the lining of the bladder by acrolein, a metabolite of ifosfamide and cyclophosphamide. Mesna may be used to inactivate the acrolein, thus preventing hemorrhagic cystitis.

10. **The answer is D** *[see V.B.2]*.
Vesicant chemotherapy agents may cause local necrosis if extravasated outside the vein. Doxorubicin, idarubicin, mechlorethamine, and vincristine are all classified as vesicants.

11. **The answer is E** *[see V.C.3; V.E.–G]*.
Severe constipation and paralytic ileus is associated with the use of vincristine.

12. **The answer is C** *[see V.C.3; V.E.–G]*.
Severe diarrhea, requiring treatment with atropine and/or loperamide, is associated with irinotecan.

13. **The answer is A** *[see V.C.3; V.E.–G]*.
Cardiotoxicity is associated with cumulative doses of doxorubicin and other antitumor antibiotics.

14. **The answer is B** *[see V.C.3; V.E.–G]*.
Conjunctivitis occurs with high-dose cytarabine; patients receiving high-dose cytarabine should receive prophylaxis with steroid eye drops.

15. **The answer is D** *[see V.C.3; V.E.–G]*.
Pulmonary toxicity, including fibrosis, is associated with cumulative doses of bleomycin.

Pain Management

51

ALAN F. KAUL

I. INTRODUCTION

A. **Definitions**

1. **Pain** is an unpleasant sensory and emotional experience that is associated with actual or potential tissue damage or described in terms of such damage. It is a subjective, individual experience that has physical, psychological, and social determinants. There is no objective measurement of pain. In the United States alone, recurrent or persistent pain is experienced by more than 75 million individuals.
2. **Acute pain** lasts 30 days longer than the usual healing process for that type of injury, and occurs after muscle strains and tissue injury, such as trauma or surgery. The pain is usually self-limiting, decreasing with time as the injury heals. It is described as a linear process, with a beginning and an end. Increased autonomic nervous system activity often accompanies acute pain, causing tachycardia, tachypnea, hypertension, diaphoresis, and mydriasis. Increased anxiety also may occur.
3. **Chronic pain** is persistent or episodic pain of a duration or intensity that adversely affects the function or well-being of the patient and can persist after the resolution of an injury. Some define it as lasting more than 6 months.
   a. **Chronic nonmalignant pain** may be a complication of acute injury in which the healing process does not occur as expected or may be caused by a disease such as a rheumatological disorder (e.g., osteoarthritis, rheumatoid arthritis, fibromyalgia).
   b. The elderly are more likely to experience chronic pain because of the increased prevalence of degenerative disorders in this age group.
   c. The pain is constant, does not improve with time, and is described as a cyclic process (vicious circle).
   d. Compared to acute pain, there is no longer autonomic nervous system stimulation, so the patient may not appear to be in pain. Instead, the patient may be depressed; suffer insomnia, weight loss, and sexual dysfunction; and may not be able to cope with the normal activities of daily living, including family and job-related activities.
4. **Chronic cancer pain** occurs in 60% to 90% of patients with cancer. Its characteristics are similar to those of chronic nonmalignant pain. In addition to depression, prominent characteristics are fear, anger, and agony. The cause of chronic cancer pain can be related to the tumor or cancer therapy or can be idiosyncratic. Tumor causes of pain include bone metastasis, compression of nerve structures, occlusion of blood vessels, obstruction of bowel, or infiltration of soft tissue.
5. **Breakthrough pain** is the intermittent, transitory increase in pain that occurs at a greater intensity over baseline chronic pain. It may have temporal characteristics, precipitating factors, and predictability.
6. **Neuropathic pain** is a result of an injury or malfunction of the nervous system. Excluding patients with a progressive peripheral neuropathy or neuropathic pain associated with a cancer lesion, tissue damage is not ongoing. Neuropathic pain is described as aching, throbbing, burning, shooting, stinging, and tenderness or sensitivity of the skin.
7. **Migraine pain** is characterized by a severe headache generally associated with nausea and light and sound sensitivity. Migraine is a common disorder with a 1 year prevalence rate in Americans of approximately 13% ranging from 6% to 7% of men and 18% of women.

B. Principles of management

1. **Comprehensive pain assessment** should determine the characteristics of the patient's pain complaint, clinical status, and pain management history.
   - **a.** Assessment of the pain complaint should include chronology and symptomatology of the presenting complaint such as information about onset, location, intensity, duration, quality, distribution, provocative factors, temporal qualities, severity, and pain history.
   - **b.** Assessment of clinical status should include the extent of underlying trauma or disease. Also, the patient's physical, psychological, and social conditions should be determined.
   - **c.** Assessment of pain management history includes drug allergies, analgesic response, onset, duration, and side effects.
2. **Appropriate pain management targets** should be established.
   - **a.** The primary pain management goal is to improve patient comfort.
   - **b.** For acute pain management, improved comfort can aid the healing and rehabilitation process.
   - **c.** For chronic pain, the specific objectives are to break the pain cycle (i.e., erase pain memory) and minimize breakthrough pain.
   - **d.** Other targets for chronic pain management include improvement of general well-being, sleep, outlook, self-esteem, activities of daily living, support, and mobility.
3. **Individualized pain management regimens** should be determined and initiated promptly.
   - **a.** The optimal analgesic regimen, including dose, dosing interval, and mode of administration, should be selected.
   - **b.** Additional pharmacological adjuncts and nonpharmacological therapies should be added if needed.
   - **c.** The most common regimens for acute pain include intermittent (as needed) dosing, patient-controlled analgesia (PCA), or epidural infusions with narcotic or nonnarcotic agents.
   - **d.** Nonnarcotic analgesics and nonpharmacological management usually are maximized. Narcotic use may be appropriate for certain patients being treated for chronic nonmalignant pain. Pain management specialists often include these agents in their plans.
   - **e.** For chronic cancer pain, an individualized around-the-clock analgesic regimen is established, using a long-acting analgesic. An intermittent, as-needed regimen for breakthrough pain, using a short-acting analgesic, is also determined.
4. **Monitoring** the pain management regimen and **reassessment** of the patient's pain should occur on a continuous, timely basis. Any changes in analgesic, dose, dosing interval, or method of administration should be noted in the patient's medical record and carried out in a timely fashion.

II. ANALGESICS

A. Nonnarcotic analgesics include aspirin, other salicylates, acetaminophen, nonsteroidal anti-inflammatory drugs (NSAIDs), selective cyclooxygenase 2 (COX-2) inhibitors, disease-modifying antirheumatic drugs (DMARDs), and tumor necrosis factor α (TNF-α) inhibitors (*Table 51-1*). Aspirin products, acetaminophen, and some low-dose NSAIDs such as ibuprofen, ketoprofen, and naproxen sodium are available as over-the-counter (OTC) products.

1. **Mechanism of action.** Salicylates and NSAIDs are prostaglandin inhibitors and prevent peripheral nociception by vasoactive substances such as prostaglandins and bradykinins. Most NSAIDs inhibit both COX-1, which produces prostaglandins that are believed to be cytoprotective of the stomach lining, and COX-2, which produces prostaglandins responsible for pain and inflammation. Selective COX-2 inhibitors like celecoxib do not inhibit COX-1.

   Adalimumab, etanercept, and infliximab act by binding or capturing excess TNF-α, one of the dominant cytokines, or proteins, that play an important role in the inflammatory response. The exact mechanism of action of leflunomide, a novel drug used to treat rheumatoid arthritis, is not completely known but it is thought to inhibit pyrimidine synthesis.
2. **Therapeutic effects**
   - **a.** The peripherally acting, nonnarcotic analgesics have several effects in common. These effects distinguish these agents from narcotic analgesics.
     - **(1)** They are antipyretic.
     - **(2)** They are anti-inflammatory (except acetaminophen).
     - **(3)** There is a ceiling effect to the analgesia.

Table 51-1 NONNARCOTIC ORAL ANALGESICS AND NONSTEROIDAL ANTI-INFLAMMATORY DRUGS (NSAIDs)

Drug	Adult Dose Range (mg)	Dosing Interval (hr)	Maximum Dose/Day (mg)
Para-aminophenol derivatives			
Acetaminophen (Tylenol)	325–1000	4–6	4000
Salicylates			
Aspirin	325–1000	4–6	4000
Choline magnesium trisalicylate (Trilisate)	1000–1500	12	3000
Diflunisal (Dolobid)	250–1000	8–12	1500
Salsalate (Disalcid)	500–1000	8	3000
Arylpropionic acid derivatives			
Fenoprofen (Nalfon)	200	4–6	3200
Flurbiprofen (Ansaid)	50–100	6–12	300
Ibuprofen (Motrin)	300–800	6–8	3200
Ketoprofen (Orudis)	12.5–75.0	6–8	300
Naproxen (Naprosyn)	200–500	12	1250
Naproxen sodium (Anaprox)	275–550	12	1375
Oxaprozin (Daypro)	600–1200	12	1200
Heteroaryl acetic acid derivatives			
Diclofenac (Voltaren)	25–75	6–12	200
Ketorolac (intramuscular) (Toradol)	15–60	6	120
Ketorolac (oral)	10	4–6	40
Tolmetin (Tolectin)	200–600	6–8	1800
Indole and indene acetic acid derivatives			
Etodolac (Lodine)	200–400	6–12	1200
Indomethacin (Indocin)	25–50	8–12	200
Sulindac (Clinoril)	150–200	12	400
Anthranilic acid derivatives (fenamates)			
Meclofenamate	50–100	4–6	400
Mefenamic acid (Ponstel)	250	6	1000
Alkanone derivatives			
Nabumetone (Relafen)	1000	12–24	2000
Enolic acid derivatives (oxicams)			
Piroxicam (Feldene)	20	24	20
Cyclooxygenase 2 (COX-2) selective inhibitors			
Celecoxib (Celebrex)	100–200	12–24	400
Disease-modifying antirheumatic drugs (DMARDs)			
Leflunomide (Arava)	20	24	20[a]
Anakinra (Kineret)	100 mg SC	24	
Abatacept (Orencia)	500 mg for patients weighing less than 60 kg, 750 mg for patients weighing 60 to 100 kg, or 1 g for patients weighing over 100 kg	2 to 4 weeks after the first and then every 4 weeks	

(Continued on next page)

Table 51-1 Continued.

Drug	Adult Dose Range (mg)	Dosing Interval (hr)	Maximum Dose/Day (mg)
Biological response modifiers (tumor necrosis factor α inhibitors)			
Adalimumab (Humira)	40 SC injection	Every other week	TBD
Etanercept (Enbrel)	25 SC injection	Once weekly	50 SC injection
Infliximab (Remicade)	3/kg IV infusion	Every 4 to 6 weeks	10/kg
Certolizumab (Cimzia)	200 mg SC	Every 2 weeks	
Adalimumab (Humira)	40 mg SC	Every other week	
Golimumab (Simponi)	50 mg SC (give with methotrexate)	Every month	
Others			
Tocilizumab (Actemra)	4 mg/kg IV infusion over 1 hr Max = 800 mg/infusion	Every 4 weeks	
Rituximab (Rituxan)	1000 mg IV (give with methotrexate)	Every 2 weeks × 2 doses	

[a]Excludes loading dose of 100 mg/day for 3 days.
IV, intravenous; *SC*, subcutaneous; *TBD*, to be determined.

(4) They do not cause tolerance.
(5) They do not cause physical or psychological dependence.

b. The efficacy of nonnarcotics is compared to aspirin. Most drugs are comparable to aspirin; however, several NSAIDs have shown a superior effect to 650 mg of aspirin.
(1) Diflunisal (500 mg)
(2) Ibuprofen (200 to 400 mg)
(3) Naproxen sodium (550 mg)
(4) Ketoprofen (25 to 50 mg)

c. The newer classes of drugs, in general, have not been compared to aspirin.

3. Clinical use

a. Generally, the nonnarcotic analgesics are used orally to manage mild to moderate pain.
(1) They are particularly suited for acute pain of skeletal muscle (orthopedic) or oral (dental) origin.
(2) They are used to treat pain and inflammation associated with osteoarthritis and rheumatoid arthritis.
(3) They are used in chronic pain and can have an additive effect with narcotic analgesics.
(4) They also may be effective in managing pain owing to bone metastases.
(5) They are used for mild to moderate migraine pain.

b. The NSAID ketorolac is administered intramuscularly and is useful in moderate-to-severe pain, particularly in cases in which narcotics are undesirable (e.g., with drug addicts, excessive narcotic sedation, respiratory depression).

c. The NSAID diclofenac epolamine is available as a topical patch (Flector Patch®) for treatment of strains, sprains, and contusions. One patch is applied to the most painful area twice a day (should not be applied to damaged or nonintact skin).

d. Patients may vary in their response and tolerance to nonnarcotic analgesics. If a patient does not respond to the maximum therapeutic dose, then an alternate NSAID should be tried. Likewise, if a patient experiences side effects with one drug, then another agent should be tried.

e. Several drugs (e.g., diflunisal, choline magnesium trisalicylate, naproxen, celecoxib, leflunomide, etanercept, infliximab, adalimumab) have long half-lives and, therefore, may be administered less frequently.

f. The cost of nonnarcotic analgesics is highly variable and should be considered when an agent is selected. Pharmacotherapy with the COX-2 inhibitor celecoxib, the newer DMARDs like leflunomide or TNF-α inhibitors is significantly more expensive than older agents.

4. Adverse effects

a. **Gastrointestinal (GI) effects.** Most nonnarcotic analgesics cause GI symptoms secondary to prostaglandin inhibition. At normal doses, acetaminophen and choline magnesium trisalicylate produce minimal GI upset. Because of their mechanism of action, the COX-2 inhibitors have a GI toxicity similar to placebo. Adalimumab, etanercept, infliximab, and leflunomide have been associated with GI side effects including nausea, abdominal pain, dyspepsia, constipation, vomiting, hematochezia, intestinal obduction, intestinal perforation, pancreatitis, peritonitis, peptic ulcer, and diarrhea.

(1) The most common GI symptom is dyspepsia, but ulceration, bleeding, or perforation can occur.

(2) Patients most predisposed to severe GI effects include the elderly, patients with a history of ulcers or chronic disease, and those who smoke or use alcohol.

(3) To minimize GI effects, the lowest possible analgesic dose should be used. Aspirin, available as enteric-coated products, may minimize GI upset. Combination therapy with a GI "protectant" (e.g., antacid, H_2-antagonist, sucralfate, misoprostol) may be needed.

b. **Hematological effects.** Most nonnarcotic analgesics inhibit platelet aggregation. The effect is produced by reversible inhibition of prostaglandin synthetase. Aspirin is an irreversible inhibitor. Acetaminophen and choline magnesium trisalicylate lack antiplatelet effects. TNF-α inhibitors have been associated with anemia, aplastic anemia, leukopenia, neutropenia, pancytopenia, and thrombocytopenia. Leflunomide has been associated with anemia and ecchymosis.

(1) The effect of the NSAIDs correlates to the presence of an effective serum concentration.

(2) Use of anticoagulants (e.g., heparin, warfarin [Coumadin]) is relatively contraindicated in combination with aspirin or NSAIDs.

c. **Renal effects.** NSAIDs can produce renal dysfunction. Etanercept has not been shown to affect renal function.

(1) The mechanism of NSAID-induced renal dysfunction includes prostaglandin inhibition, interstitial nephritis, impaired renin secretion, and enhanced tubular water/sodium reabsorption.

(2) Many risk factors have been implicated, including congestive heart failure (CHF), chronic renal failure (CRF), cirrhosis, dehydration, diuretic use, and atherosclerotic disease in elderly patients.

(3) Renal dysfunction is commonly manifested as abrupt onset oliguria with sodium/water retention. The effect reverses after discontinuation of the NSAID.

d. **Malignancies and lymphoproliferative disorders.** Agents that block TNF-α may affect host defenses against malignancies because TNF-α mediates inflammation and modulates cellular immune response. Lymphomas have occurred more frequently in patients receiving TNF-α-blocking agents than in controls.

e. **Infections.** Opportunistic and serious infections leading to sepsis and death have been associated with leflunomide and the TNF-α-blocking agents.

f. **Miscellaneous effects**

(1) Even in normal doses, acetaminophen can cause hepatotoxicity in patients with liver disease or chronic alcoholism. Hepatotoxicity has also been reported with the use of all NSAIDs, including the COX-2 selective inhibitors. Leflunomide and infliximab have also been shown to cause transient elevations in liver function tests such as aspartate aminotransferase (AST)—serum glutamic-oxaloacetic transaminase (SGOT)—and alanine aminotransferase (ALT)—serum glutamic pyruvic transaminase (SGPT).

(2) Some patients exhibit acute hypersensitivity reactions to aspirin. Manifestations include either a rhinitis or asthma presentation or a true allergic reaction (e.g., urticaria, wheals, hypotension, shock, syncope). A cross-sensitivity to other NSAIDs may develop.

(3) Some NSAIDs produce central nervous system (CNS) effects, including impaired mentation, headaches, and attention deficit disorder.

(4) Leflunomide has received a **black box warning** because of its Category X pregnancy warning. It has also been associated with weight loss, alopecia, rash, and anemia.

(5) TNF-α-blocking agents have been associated with reactions at the injection site and autoantibody production.

(6) Celecoxib, a selective COX-2 inhibitor, has a **black box warning** U.S. Food and Drug Administration (FDA) warning from the because if its link to an increased risk for

cardiovascular events (heart attack and stroke). This increased risk has been demonstrated to be a drug class effect for all NSAIDs, excluding aspirin. Celecoxib is also contraindicated in patients with sulfonamide allergy.

NSAIDs for short- or long-term use are not advised in patients with established cardiovascular disease, particularly in those who have had a myocardial infarction (MI). A nationwide cohort study in patients $>$ 30 years of age who were hospitalized with their first-time MI from 1997 to 2006 found that even short-term treatment with most NSAIDs was associated with an increased risk of death and recurrent MI. Among the NSAIDs studied, diclofenac was associated with the highest risk.

5. **Drug interactions.** Salicylates have two clinically significant drug interactions.
   a. **Oral anticoagulants.** Aspirin should be carefully monitored, if used, in anticoagulated patients because it inhibits platelet function and can cause gastric mucosal damage. This can significantly increase the risk of bleeding in anticoagulated patients. Also, doses of $>$ 3 g/day of aspirin produces hypoprothrombinemia. Choline magnesium trisalicylate or acetaminophen can be used if a nonnarcotic is needed in an anticoagulated patient.
   b. **Methotrexate.** Salicylates may enhance the toxicity of methotrexate. The primary mechanism is blockage of methotrexate renal tubular secretion by salicylates. The resultant methotrexate toxicity has been reported as pancytopenia or hepatotoxicity. Salicylates should be avoided in patients receiving methotrexate.
   c. **TNF-α-blocking agents.** Anakinra (Kineret), a recombinant interleukin-1 (IL-1) receptor antagonist, has been observed to cause an increased risk of serious infections as neutropenia when used concomitantly with etanercept in patients with rheumatoid arthritis. Consequently, its use is not recommended concomitantly with any TNF-α-blocking agent.

B. **Narcotic analgesics** include the opioid drugs (*Table 51-2*). Because of their abuse potential, opioids are classified as controlled drugs. Special regulations control their prescribing.
   1. **Mechanism of action**
      a. Endogenous opiates afford the body self–pain-relieving mechanisms. These endogenous peptides include the endorphins, enkephalins, and dynorphins.

Table 51-2 SOME COMMONLY USED OPIOID ANALGESICS

Drug	Parenteral Dose (mg)[a]	Oral Dose (mg)[a]	Duration (hr)
Morphine	10	60	4–7
Morphine (CR) (MS Contin)	n/a	n/a	12–24
Hydromorphone (Dilaudid)	1.3	7.5	4–6
Oxymorphone (Numorphan)	1	—	4–6
Levorphanol (Levo-Dromoran)	2	4	4–7
Methadone (Dolophine)	10	20	4–6
Meperidine (Demerol)	75	300	3–6
Fentanyl (Sublimaze)	0.1	—	1–2
Fentanyl transdermal (Duragesic)	n/a	n/a	48–72
Codeine	130	200	4–6
Hydrocodone[b]	—	5–10	4–5
Hydromorphone ER (Exalgo)	—	16	24
Dihydrocodeine[b]	—	32	4–5
Oxycodone[b]	—	5–10	4–5
Oxycodone (CR) (OxyContin)	—	n/a	12–24
Nalbuphine (Nubain)	10	—	4–6
Butorphanol (Stadol)	2	—	4–6
Dezocine (Dalgan)	10	—	4–7
Buprenorphine	—	n/a	168

[a]Doses equivalent to 10 mg intramuscular or subcutaneous morphine.
[b]Doses for moderate pain not necessarily equivalent to 10 mg morphine.
CR, controlled release; *n/a*, not applicable, *ER*, extended-release.

b. Exogenous opiates are classified as agonists (stimulate opiate receptors), antagonists (displace agonists from opiate receptors), and mixed opiates (agonist–antagonist or partial agonist actions).

c. Opiate receptors are located in the brain and spinal cord. Several types of opiate receptors have been identified, including μ, κ, δ, σ, and ϵ.

d. Stimulation of μ-receptors produces the characteristic narcotic (morphine-like) effects.

(1) Analgesia
(2) Miosis
(3) Euphoria
(4) Respiratory depression
(5) Sedation
(6) Physical dependence
(7) Bradycardia

e. The specific mechanism (central and spinal) of opiate agonist is alteration of the effects of nociceptive neurotransmitters, possibly norepinephrine or serotonin.

2. Clinical use

a. Opioid analgesics are used for the management of moderate-to-severe pain (acute or chronic pain) of somatic or visceral origin.

b. The use of narcotics should be individualized for each patient. The optimal analgesic dose varies from patient to patient. Each analgesic regimen should be titrated by increasing the dose up to the appearance of limiting adverse effects. Changing to another analgesic should occur only after an adequate therapeutic trial.

c. The appropriate route of administration should be selected for each patient.

(1) Oral administration is the preferred route, particularly for patients with chronic, stable pain. Controlled-release morphine and oxycodone tablets are available for convenience in controlling continuous pain, particularly in those patients with cancer.

(2) Intramuscular and subcutaneous administration are very commonly used in the postoperative period. Fluctuations in absorption may occur, particularly in elderly or cachectic patients.

(3) Intravenous (IV) bolus administration has the most rapid, predictable onset of effect.

(4) IV infusion is used to titrate pain relief rapidly, particularly in patients with unstable chronic pain. Morphine is most commonly used, often with supplemental IV bolus doses for breakthrough pain. A mechanical infusion device is necessary.

(5) IV PCA is most often used for acute postoperative pain. It produces prompt analgesia with minimal side effects because small doses (e.g., 1 to 2 mg morphine) are delivered at frequent intervals (e.g., every 10 mins). It allows patient control of pain management. Morphine and meperidine are the most commonly used agents. A mechanical infusion device and properly trained patient and staff are necessary.

(6) Epidural and **intrathecal administration** are used for acute postoperative pain and early management of chronic cancer pain. All drugs used epidurally or intrathecally must be preservative-free because of the neurotoxicity of parabens and benzyl alcohol when administered via these routes. Intrathecal doses are generally 1/10 of the corresponding drug's epidural dose.

(a) Low opiate doses stimulate spinal opiate receptors and reduce the amount of narcotic reaching the brain. This results in delayed or minimal effects such as sedation, nausea, and respiratory depression. The opiate distribution that causes such effects depends on the site of spinal injection, water solubility of the opiate, and volume infused. For example, after lumbar administration of a more water-soluble opiate (morphine), severe respiratory depression can be observed 12 to 24 hrs after initial dosing.

(b) Local side effects of intrathecal opiate administration are itching and urinary retention. Depending on the opiate used and the type of pain being treated, intermittent doses or continuous infusions (via a mechanical infusion device) can be used (*Tables 51-3* and *51-4*).

(7) Rectal administration is an alternative for patients unable to take oral narcotics. Generally, poor absorption results in an unreliable analgesic response. It is an unacceptable route of administration for many patients.

Table 51-3 EPIDURALLY ADMINISTERED PRESERVATIVE-FREE OPIOIDS: INTERMITTENT DOSING

Drug	Dose (mg)	Onset of Action (min)	Time to Peak Effect (min)	Duration (hr)
Morphine	5–10	25	60	12–24
Fentanyl	0.1	5–10	20	6
Meperidine	50–100	5–10	15–30	7
Hydromorphone	1.0	10–15	20	12
Buprenorphine	0.3	30	40–60	8–9

(8) **Transdermal administration** is an alternative for patients with chronic pain who are unable to take oral narcotics. A controlled-release patch is available for fentanyl. Slow onset requires additional analgesia when starting treatment. The duration of analgesia is 48 to 72 hrs per patch. A slow reduction of effect follows removal of the patch and requires 24 to 36 hrs of monitoring.

d. Patients who have chronic pain or acute pain that is constant throughout the day should receive regularly scheduled (around-the-clock) doses of narcotics.

(1) Long-acting opiates (e.g., controlled-release morphine and oxycodone) are preferable.

(2) A supplement given as needed may be necessary to manage breakthrough pain, for which short-acting opiates (e.g., immediate-release morphine, hydromorphone) are preferable. If frequent supplements are required, then the around-the-clock regimen should be adjusted based on morphine equivalents (*Table 51-2*).

e. Although the analgesia and side effects of opiates are qualitatively similar, individual patients may respond differently. Analgesic selection is based on:

(1) Patient's past analgesia experience

(2) Need for a rapid onset of effect

(3) Preference for a long (or short) duration of action

(4) Preference for a particular mode of delivery

(5) Preference for a particular dosage form

(a) Controlled-release morphine or oxycodone for a long duration of action (8 to 12 hrs) may be preferable to opiates with long half-lives (e.g., methadone, levorphanol), which can accumulate and cause overdose symptoms (e.g., respiratory depression).

(b) Transdermal fentanyl can be used for patients who are unable to swallow.

(c) Rectal suppositories can be used for patients who are unable to swallow. They are available for morphine, hydromorphone, and oxymorphone.

(d) Concentrated hydromorphone injection (10 mg/mL) can be used for cachectic patients who require subcutaneous injections and in patients whose injection volumes must be minimized.

Table 51-4 EPIDURALLY ADMINISTERED PRESERVATIVE-FREE OPIOIDS: CONTINUOUS INFUSION

Drug	Initial Bolus Dose (mg)	Infusion Concentration (mg/mL)	Rate (mg/hr)
Morphine	2	0.05–0.25	0.2–1.5
Fentanyl	0.05–0.10	0.005–0.025	0.02–0.15
Meperidine	50–100	10–20	5–20
Hydromorphone	0.5–1.0	0.02–0.05	0.15–0.30

(6) Individual sensitivity to side effects, which includes nausea, euphoria, sedation, and respiratory depression

(a) Partial agonists or mixed agonist–antagonists may be preferable for acute pain management in patients at risk for respiratory depression secondary to opiate agonists. These agents should not be used in patients who have received chronic doses of opiates because withdrawal symptoms will occur.

(b) Epidural administration may be preferable for critically ill patients at risk for respiratory depression secondary to systemic narcotic administration.

3. **Adverse effects.** All narcotics can produce a variety of side effects that range from bothersome to life threatening.

a. **Constipation** occurs as a result of decreased intestinal tone and peristalsis. There is a patient variability, but generally most patients experience constipation after several days of therapy. Constipation may be more bothersome with certain types of opiates (e.g., codeine). It may occur sooner and be more problematic in hospitalized or bedridden patients or in patients who have received anesthesia or drugs with anticholinergic effects. Prophylaxis with a laxative/stool softener combination (e.g., bisacodyl/docusate [Gentlax-S]) and dietary counseling are warranted for patients who need chronic opiate therapy.

b. **Nausea** and **vomiting** occur owing to central stimulation of the chemoreceptor trigger zone. It is more problematic with one-time or intermittent parenteral dosing for acute pain. Occasionally, patients require concomitant therapy with an antiemetic (e.g., hydroxyzine, prochlorperazine); however, these agents may add to the sedative effects of opiates.

c. **Sedation** is a dose-related effect but sometimes is enhanced by concomitant use of other drugs with sedating effects (e.g., benzodiazepines, antiemetics). Most chronic pain patients become tolerant to this effect, but occasionally the addition of a CNS stimulant, such as dextroamphetamine or methylphenidate, is needed.

(1) Patients starting therapy with narcotics should be warned about driving or operating machinery.

(2) Sedation may be a sign of excessive dosing or accumulation. However, sedation should not be confused with physiological sleep in patients who have pain control difficulties. Patients in pain often develop insomnia. When pain is brought under control by appropriate narcotic titration, the patient initially may sleep for several hours.

d. **Respiratory depression** is the most serious adverse effect accompanying narcotic overdose. Respiratory depression may be a sign of an excessive dose, accumulation of long half-lived opiates (e.g., methadone, levorphanol), or accumulation of active morphine metabolites in renal failure patients.

(1) Respiratory rate should be carefully monitored in patients receiving IV or epidural opiates, in neonates, in elderly patients, and in patients receiving other drugs that cause respiratory depression.

(2) The opiate antagonists, naloxone and nalmefene, are administered intravenously to reverse life-threatening respiratory depression. Use of naloxone or nalmefene (Revex) in an opiate-dependent patient (e.g., a chronic cancer pain patient) can precipitate opiate withdrawal.

e. **Anticholinergic effects**, such as dry mouth and urinary retention, can be bothersome for some patients.

f. **Hypersensitivity** reactions, such as itching owing to histamine release, can occur secondary to opiate use, particularly with epidural or intrathecal administration. Wheals sometimes occur at the site of morphine injection. These reactions do not represent true allergy.

g. **CNS excitation**, such as myoclonus and other seizure-like activity, can be produced with the use of meperidine in renal failure. These symptoms have also been observed in patients with normal renal functions who receive high doses of meperidine (e.g., $<$ 800 mg/day of intramuscular meperidine). The accumulation of the metabolite normeperidine is the cause.

4. **Drug interactions**

a. Narcotics have additive CNS depressant effects when used in combination with other drugs that also are CNS depressants (e.g., alcohol, anesthetics, antidepressants, antihistamines, barbiturates, benzodiazepines, phenothiazines).

b. Narcotics, particularly meperidine, can cause severe reactions such as excitation, sweating, rigidity, and hypertension in patients receiving monoamine oxidase (MAO) inhibitors. Meperidine should be avoided and other narcotics started at lower doses in patients being treated with MAO inhibitors.

5. Tolerance means that increasing doses of opiate are needed to maintain analgesia. Tolerance usually develops to the analgesic, sedative, and euphoric effects of opioids, but not to the pupillary-constricting and constipating effects. This is usually observed as a decreasing duration of analgesia in chronic pain patients. The addition of an NSAID may help delay or provide adequate analgesia in tolerant patients.

6. Dependence. The use of opiates for chronic pain may result in physical dependence, such that the abrupt discontinuation of the opiate results in the development of withdrawal symptoms.

a. Withdrawal symptoms include anxiety, irritability, insomnia, chills, salivation, rhinorrhea, diaphoresis, nausea, vomiting, GI cramping and diarrhea, and piloerection.

(1) The appearance and intensity of withdrawal symptoms vary according to the half-life of the opiate. For example, the withdrawal symptoms after discontinuation of chronic methadone may take several days to develop and may be less intense than those of withdrawal from morphine owing to its shorter half-life.

(2) The development of tolerance may be associated with withdrawal symptoms.

(3) The use of naloxone or a partial agonist–antagonist such as pentazocine in a patient receiving chronic opiate therapy produces acute withdrawal.

b. The development of physical dependence seen in chronic pain patients is not the same as psychological dependence or addiction. Also, the drug-seeking behavior observed in many acute pain patients (i.e., from postoperative pain) is not a sign of addiction, but rather a need for adequate pain relief. Studies suggest that the addictive rates for long-term treatment of noncancer pain are low in patients without a prior history of addiction. The analgesic needs of this type of patient should be reassessed and usually necessitates increasing the dose of opiate, changing to a longer duration drug, changing to a PCA, or adding an analgesic adjunct.

C. Adjuvant analgesics and miscellaneous analgesics. Adjuvant analgesics are drugs whose initial FDA-approved indication was for a condition other than pain. Other classes of drugs affect nonopiate pain pathways and may be useful in certain types of pain (e.g., neuropathic pain). These drugs often are used with other analgesics, and some may help manage narcotic side effects (*Table 51-5*).

1. Neuropathic pain agents include anticonvulsants (e.g., gabapentin, pregabalin, lamotrigine, carbamazepine), systemic local anesthetic agents—for example, 5% lidocaine (Lidoderm) patch—and tricyclic antidepressants—such as amitriptyline, nortriptyline, and desipramine. Gabapentin and systemic local anesthetic agents are considered first-line therapy in treating polyneuropathies. Anticonvulsant can be used for lancinating neurogenic pain (e.g., trigeminal neuralgia, phantom limb pain, posttrauma neurogenic pain). Tricyclic antidepressant and anticonvulsants are also used to treat migraine pain.

a. Mechanism of action

(1) Gabapentin and pregabalin may relieve neuropathic pain by the presynaptic binding of the α-2-δ subunit of voltage-sensitive calcium channels.

(2) Pregabalin may also modulate the release of the sensory neuropeptide substance P.

(3) Lamotrigine and carbamazepine are believed to block sodium channels at the site of ectopic discharge of damaged nerves.

(4) The use of local anesthetics allows for local pain relief without systemic toxicity, specifically by binding to the sodium channels in the damaged nerves.

(5) It is hypothesized that TCAs obtain their analgesic effects as a result of sodium channel blockade at the site of ectopic discharge in the peripheral nerves.

(6) All of these agents are recommended to aid in the reduction of neuronal hyperexcitability, whether it is peripherally or centrally.

b. Clinical use

(1) Data are available to give guidance on which agents to use to treat neuropathic pain, but they do not predict which agent will provide relief for each individual patient's pain.

Table 51-5 ANALGESIC ADJUNCTS AND MISCELLANEOUS ANALGESICS

Drugs	Dose	Maximum	Indications/Comments
Tricyclic Antidepressants			
Amitriptyline Nortriptyline Doxepin Clomipramine Desipramine	10 mg/day 10 mg/day 10 mg/day 10 mg/day 10 mg/day	250 mg/day 125 mg/day 250 mg/day 250 mg/day 200 mg/day	Used at bedtime and started at low dose. Contraindicated in patients with urinary retention, glaucoma, and bundle branch block; severe anticholinergic effects and weight gain can be limited.
Anticonvulsants			
Valproate	250 mg b.i.d.	500 mg t.i.d./q.i.d.	High teratogenicity incidence
Gabapentin	100 mg t.i.d. or 300 mg q.h.s.	300–1200 mg t.i.d.	No blood monitoring required
Pregabalin	100 mg t.i.d.	300 mg/day	This dose is for neuropathic pain.
Topiramate	25 mg/day	100 mg/day	Slow titration minimizes adverse events. Weight loss and metabolic acidosis are common.
Phenytoin	300 mg/day		Cosmetic side effects
Carbamazepine	100 mg/day	200–600 mg t.i.d.	Needs to monitor complete blood count (CBC) and liver function tests (LFTs)
Neuroleptics			
Fluphenazine Prochlorperazine Haloperidol	2–20 mg 5–10 mg t.i.d./q.i.d. 0.5–5.0 mg q 2–12 hrs	30 mg/day 10 mg q.i.d. 30 mg/day	Refractory neurogenic pain; pain complicated by delirium or nausea (prochlorperazine)
Corticosteroids			
Dexamethasone	1–4 mg b.i.d./q.i.d.	24 mg/day	From neural infiltration; pain associated with bony metastases
Antihistamines			
Hydroxyzine	25–100 mg q 4–6 hrs		Pain complicated by anxiety or nausea
Benzodiazepines			
Alprazolam Lorazepam Clonazepam	0.25–2.00 mg t.i.d./q.i.d. 0.5–2.0 mg t.i.d./q.i.d. 0.5–2.0 mg b.i.d./q.i.d.	4 mg/day 10 mg/day 4 mg/day	Pain complicated by anxiety or muscle spasm
Amphetamines and Amphetamine-Like Agents			
Dextroamphetamine Methylphenidate	15 mg b.i.d./t.i.d. 5 mg–20 mg b.i.d./t.i.d.	5–60 mg/day 65 mg	For excessive opiate-induced sedation in chronic pain patients

(2) Typically, a **treatment algorithm** may recommend:
(a) **First line**
(i) Gabapentin
(ii) Pregabalin
(iii) 5% lidocaine patches
(iv) TCAs
(b) **Second line**
(i) Other anticonvulsants (lamotrigine or carbamazepine)
(ii) Other antidepressants (bupropion, citalopram, paroxetine, venlafaxine, imipramine)
(c) **Other**
(i) Capsaicin, clonidine

c. **Adverse effects.** The most common adverse events associated with anticonvulsants are dizziness, headaches, and drowsiness. Lamotrigine has been associated with the development of Stevens–Johnson syndrome (SJS). It is recommended that lamotrigine be titrated up every 2 weeks to minimize the occurrence of SJS.

2. **Tramadol (Ultram)** is an oral, centrally acting analgesic with weak opiate activity. It has not been placed in a controlled drug schedule.

a. **Mechanism of action**
(1) Tramadol is a synthetic aminocyclohexanol that binds to opiate receptors, inhibiting norepinephrine and serotonin.
(2) The analgesic effects are partially antagonized by naloxone.

b. **Clinical use**
(1) Tramadol is used for moderate to moderately severe pain.
(2) The recommended dosage is 50 to 100 mg every 4 to 6 hrs, up to a maximum of 400 mg/day. The extended-release formulation (Ultram ER) is given at a dose of 100 to 300 mg/day.
(3) At maximum dosage, tramadol appears no more effective than acetaminophen–codeine combinations.

c. **Adverse effects**
(1) **GI effects** include nausea, constipation, and dry mouth.
(2) **CNS effects** include dizziness, headache, sedation, and seizures (overdose).
(3) **Diaphoresis**

d. **Drug interactions**
(1) Tramadol can increase the sedative effect of alcohol and hypnotics.
(2) Tramadol inhibits monoamine uptake and should not be used with MAO inhibitors.
(3) Tramadol used with selective serotonin reuptake inhibitors (SSRIs) and other agents that increase serotonergic activity can cause "serotonin syndrome," which is characterized by irritability, anxiety, CNS excitation, and myoclonus.

D. **Agents used to treat migraine (*see Table 51-6*)**

1. **Triptans** include sumatriptan, zolmitriptan, naratriptan, rizatriptan, almotriptan, eletriptan, and frovatriptan.

a. **Mechanism of action.** Triptans are 5-hydroxytryptamine (5-HT [1B/1D]) receptor agonists. One hypothesis for the efficacy of triptans in migraine is that activating 5-HT (1B/1D) receptors can lead intracranial blood vessels constriction.

b. **Clinical use.** Triptans are effective for acute treatment of migraine but not used as a prophylaxis treatment. Triptans should be used as soon as possible after onset of migraine attack.

c. **Adverse effects**
(1) Cardiovascular (CV) effects include: rare but serious transient myocardial attack, coronary artery vasospasm, myocardial infarction, and atrial and ventricular arrhythmia.
(2) Minor adverse events of sumatriptan injection: irritation at the injection site. However, orally administered triptans can cause paresthesias, flushing, feeling of pressure, tightness or pain in the chest, neck, and jaw.
(3) Zolmitriptan has an incidence of recurrent headache similar to that seen with oral sumatriptan.
(4) Naratriptan may have a lower risk of headache recurrence than other oral triptans, and has a lower incidence of side effects than sumatriptan and most other oral triptans.

Table 51-6 AGENTS USED TO TREAT MIGRAINE

Drug	Initial Dose	Daily Maximum Dose	Comments
Serotonin Agonists (Triptan)			
Sumatriptan (subcutaneous)	6 mg SC	12 mg/day	• May repeat after 1 hr • Useful when non-oral route of administration is needed
Sumatriptan (oral)	25–100 mg PO	200 mg/day	• May repeat after 2 hrs • Maximum recommended monthly dose for migraine is 18 tablets (50 mg) or an equal amount.
Sumatriptan (nasal)	20 mg nasally	40 mg/day	• May repeat after 2 hrs • Similar speed of action and effectiveness to oral sumatriptan
Zolmitriptan	2.5 mg/day	10 mg/day	• Maximum monthly dose is 18 tablets (5 mg) each or equal amount.
Naratriptan	1.0–2.5 mg/day	5 mg/day	• Only triptan not contraindicated with MAO inhibitors
Rizatriptan	5–10 mg/day	30 mg/day	• Propranolol increase serum concentration of rizatriptan, which result in bradycardia; then use 5-mg dose; max = 15 mg/day
Almotriptan	6.25 or 12.5 mg/day	Two doses in 24 hrs	
Frovatriptan	2.5 mg/day	7.5 mg in 24 hrs	
β-Blockers			
Propranolol	60 mg/day	320 mg/day	• Benefits may lag 3 to 4 weeks.
Nadolol	40 mg/day	240 mg/day	
Timolol	10 mg/day	40 mg/day	
Atenolol	50 mg/day	150 mg/day	
Metoprolol	50 mg/day	300 mg/day	
Calcium-Channel Blockers			
Verapamil	120 mg/day	720 mg/day	• Widely used but weak evidence for efficacy • Benefits may be noted after 3–4 weeks on therapeutic dose.
Nifedipine	30 mg/day	180 mg/day	
Diltiazem	60 mg/day	360 mg/day	
Nimodipine	20 mg/day	60 mg/day	
Angiotensin-Converting Enzyme Inhibitors			
Lisinopril	10 mg/day for 1 week then 20 mg/day	40 mg/day	

d. Contraindications

(1) Triptans should be avoided in patients with familial hemiplegic migraine, basilar migraine, ischemic stroke, uncontrolled hypertension, ischemic heart disease, Prinzmetal angina, ischemic complications, cerebrovascular or peripheral vascular disease, and renal or hepatic disease.

e. Drug interactions: Triptans are contraindicated in patients with near-term prior exposure to ergots alkaloid or other 5-HT agonists. Triptans, excluding eletriptan, frovatriptan, and naratriptan, are contraindicated in combination with monoamine oxidase inhibitors (MAOIs). Because eletriptan is metabolized by cytochrome P450 3A4 enzyme (CYP3A4), it should not be used within 72 hrs of treatment with potent CYP3A4 inhibitors such as ketoconazole, itraconazole, nefazodone, troleandomycin, clarithromycin, nelfinavir, and ritonavir.

2. **β-Blockers.** Using β-blockers for prevention is effective in 60% to 80% of patients in reducing the severity and frequency of migraine attack by 50%. It is unclear how β-blockers prevent migraine, but their action is most likely related to inhibition of β1 receptors with secondary effects on serotonin. As serotonin plays an important role in the pathogenesis of migraine. β-Blockers with intrinsic sympathomimetic activity (ISA), such as pindolol and acebutolol, are less effective in the treatment of migraine. β-Blockers should not be used as initial therapy for migraine prophylaxis in patients over age 60 and in smokers. The use of β-blockers may be limited in patients with erectile dysfunction, peripheral vascular disease, Raynaud syndrome or disease, and in patients with baseline bradycardia or low blood pressure. They must be used cautiously in patients with diabetes mellitus, asthma, and those with cardiac conduction disturbances or sinus node dysfunction.
3. **Calcium-channel blockers (CCBs).** In treating migraines, CCBs are used prophylactically. They decrease the frequency of the attack, have minimal effect on headache severity and are, generally, not as effective as other agents. Also, the vasodilatory action of some calcium-channel blockers may induce or worsen migraine attacks. Their mechanism of action is unclear, but excessive levels of intracellular calcium under ischemic condition can cause neuronal damage and cell death. Among these agents, verapamil is frequently the first choice for prophylactic therapy because of ease of use and a favorable side effect profile. After 8 weeks of successful therapy with CCBs, tolerance may develop that can be overcome by increasing the dose or by switching to a different CCB. CCBs are contraindicated in patients with heart block, hypotension, heart failure, and atrial flutter and fibrillation.
4. **Angiotensin-converting enzyme inhibitors (ACEi) and angiotensin receptor blockers (ARBs).** Based on a double-blind, placebo-controlled, crossover study in patients with two to six migraine episodes, lisinopril (10 mg/day for 1 week, then 20 mg/day) significantly reduced the headache severity. ARB such as candesartan had similar results. ACE inhibitors are contraindicated in idiopathic and hereditary angioedema and hypersensitivity to lisinopril.
5. **Ergot (Ergotamine and Dihydroergotamine [DHE]).** Ergotamine and DHE bind to serotonin (5-HT 1B/1D) receptors similar to triptans. Various ergotamine preparations are available alone or in combination with caffeine and other analgesics for oral, sublingual, and rectal use, whereas DHE is available for intravenous, intramuscular, subcutaneous, and intranasal use. Based on clinical trials, oral ergotamine alone failed to show efficacy in migraine relief. Ergotamine tartrate can cause pruritus, muscle weakness, paresthesia, visual disturbance, vascular spasm, and cardiovascular system disorder (angina, MI, arrhythmia). In addition, ergotamine may worsen nausea and vomiting that associated with migraine. As a result, ergotamine is used in relatively few patients because issue of efficacy and side effects. It is used in patients with prolonged duration of attacks (e.g., greater than 48 hrs), and possibly frequent headache recurrence. Besides being a potent 5-HT (1B/1D) receptor agonist, DHE 45 is an alpha blocker that is a weaker arterial vasoconstrictor and more potent venoconstrictor than ergotamine tartrate. Also, it has fewer side effects than ergotamine tartrate. DHE is given intravenously for acute migraine in combination with antiemetic. Parenteral DHE 45 should not be used as monotherapy.

E. **Miscellaneous agents**

1. **Capsaicin**, a component of red peppers, causes the release of substance P from sensory nerve fibers, resulting in prolonged cutaneous pain transmission, histamine release, and erythema because of reflex vasodilation. Repeated local application depletes the peripheral sensory C-nerve fiber of substance P, resulting in pain inhibition. Topical capsaicin cream 0.025% or 0.075% has been shown to be useful in treating joint pain and tenderness in patients with arthritis. Other uses may include treating diabetic neuralgia, reflex sympathetic dystrophy, trigeminal neuralgia, notalgia paresthetica, psoriasis and psoralen (P), and long-wave ultraviolet radiation (UVA) induced skin pain, and postherpetic neuralgia. Local toxicity may include burning, stinging, erythema, pruritus, and superficial skin ulcers. Capsaicin 8% patch (Qutenza) administered for 1 hr can provide 3 months of relief for pain associated with postherpetic neuralgia. Significant dermal reactions have been associated with this formulation.
2. **Glucosamine sulfate and chondroitin sulfate** have been used with increasing frequency in the treatment of degenerative joint disease. Glucosamine sulfate appears to act as a substrate for and stimulant

to the biosynthesis of glycosaminoglycans and hyaluronic acid for forming proteoglycans found in the structural matrix of joints. Chondroitin sulfate provides additional substrates for the formation of healthy joint matrix. Short-term side effects associated with glucosamine include GI problems, drowsiness, skin reactions, and headache. Further research is needed to validate their roles.

F. **Nonpharmacological pain management.** Other therapeutic modalities for pain management include cognitive behavioral interventions and physical methods. These modalities are appropriate for interested patients, patients experiencing anxiety with their pain, patients who have incomplete relief from analgesic therapy, and patients who need to avoid or reduce analgesic use (e.g., those with chronic nonmalignant pain).
   1. **Cognitive behavioral interventions** include education and instruction, simple relaxation, biofeedback, and hypnosis.
   2. **Physical methods** include acupuncture, physical therapy, compression gloves, orthotic devices, heat and cold applications, massage, exercise, rest, immobilization, and transcutaneous electrical nerve stimulation (TENS).

Study Questions

Directions for questions 1–7: Each of the questions, statements, or incomplete statements in this section can be correctly answered or completed by **one** of the suggested answers or phrases. Choose the **best** answer.

1. An emaciated 69-year-old man with advanced inoperable throat cancer is hospitalized for pain management. He is receiving a morphine solution (40 mg orally) every 3 hrs for pain. He complains of dysphagia and the frequency with which he must take morphine. An appropriate analgesic alternative for this patient would be
   (A) changing to a controlled-release oral morphine.
   (B) increasing the dose of the oral morphine solution.
   (C) changing to intramuscular methadone.
   (D) changing to transdermal fentanyl.
   (E) decreasing the frequency of oral morphine administration.

For questions 2–3: A 52-year-old woman with a diagnosis of ovarian cancer presents with complaints of pain. Her pain was reasonably well-controlled with two capsules of oxycodone every 4 hrs until 2 weeks ago, at which point she was hospitalized for pain control. She was placed on meperidine (75 mg) every 3 hrs but still complained about pain. Her meperidine dosage was increased to 100 mg every 2 hrs.

2. At this dosage of meperidine, the patient is likely to experience
   (A) excellent pain relief.
   (B) respiratory depression.
   (C) worsening renal function.
   (D) myoclonic seizures.
   (E) excessive sedation.

3. An appropriate next step in this patient's therapy would be to
   (A) add an NSAID.
   (B) discontinue the meperidine and convert her to a controlled-release oral morphine or oxycodone.
   (C) continue the present meperidine dosage because she will eventually get relief.
   (D) decrease the meperidine dose to avoid side effects.
   (E) consider hypnosis or relaxation techniques.

4. A 20-year-old victim of a motor vehicle accident is 3 days postsurgery for orthopedic and internal injuries. He has been in severe pain, and was placed on a regimen of intramuscular morphine (5 to 10 mg) every 4 hrs as needed for pain. A pain consultant starts the patient with a 20-mg intravenous morphine loading dose, and then begins a continuous intravenous morphine infusion with as-needed morphine boosters. About 2 hrs after this regimen is started, the patient is asleep. The nurse is concerned and calls the physician. The physician should
   (A) call for a psychiatric consult.
   (B) administer naloxone.
   (C) examine the patient, and reconfirm the dosage and monitoring parameters.
   (D) add an injectable NSAID.
   (E) add an amphetamine.

5. Potential adverse effects associated with aspirin include all of the following *except*
   (A) gastrointestinal ulceration.
   (B) renal dysfunction.
   (C) enhanced methotrexate toxicity.
   (D) cardiac arrhythmias.
   (E) hypersensitivity asthma.

6. All of the following facts are true about NSAIDs *except* which one?
   (A) They are antipyretic.
   (B) There is a ceiling effect to their analgesia.
   (C) They can cause tolerance.
   (D) They do not cause dependence.
   (E) They are anti-inflammatory.

7. Which of the following narcotics has the longest duration of effect?
   (A) Methadone
   (B) Controlled-release morphine
   (C) Levorphanol
   (D) Transdermal fentanyl
   (E) Dihydromorphone

Directions for questions 8–13: The questions and incomplete statements in this section can be correctly answered or completed by **one or more** of the suggested answers. Choose the answer, **A–E.**

(A) if **I only** is correct
(B) if **III only** is correct
(C) if **I and II** are correct
(D) if **II and III** are correct
(E) if **I, II, and III** are correct

8. Agents that are safe to use in a patient with bleeding problems include
   (I) choline magnesium trisalicylate.
   (II) acetaminophen.
   (III) ketorolac.

9. Which of the following drugs bind or capture excess TNF-α?
   (I) Adalimumab
   (II) Etanercept
   (III) Leflunomide

10. Leflunomide has been associated with
    (I) diarrhea.
    (II) alopecia.
    (III) anemia.

11. Which of the following agents needs to be administered with: Dihydroergotamine (DHE 45):
    (A) Ibuprofen.
    (B) IV metoclopramide.
    (C) Sumatriptan.
    (D) Acetaminophen.
    (E) Rizatriptan.

12. Which of the following should be done when eletriptan is administered with ketoconazole:
    (A) Eletriptan should not be administered within 72 hrs of treatment with ketoconazole.
    (B) Eletriptan should be used at the same time of ketoconazole administration time.
    (C) Eletriptan should be administered within 2 hrs of ketoconazole administration time.
    (D) None of the above.

Answers and Explanations

1. **The answer is D** *[see II.B.2.c.(8)].*
   Patients with throat cancer often cannot take oral analgesics. The patient described in the question is also having pain difficulties with an every 3-hr regimen. Transdermal fentanyl is a good alternative because, after titration, excellent analgesia can be produced without using oral or parenteral agents. Also, the frequency of analgesic use may be decreased when titration has occurred.

2. **The answer is D** *[see II.B.3.g].*

3. **The answer is B** *[see II.B.2.c.(1); II.B.2.d.(1)].*
   Myoclonic seizures can occur after frequent, high-dose meperidine owing to the accumulation of the metabolite, normeperidine. Both oxycodone and meperidine have short durations of effect. In the chronic pain patient, an around-the-clock regimen, using a controlled-released oral morphine, would be an appropriate alternative. With titration, the patient should have good pain relief with an every 8- to 12-hr regimen.

4. **The answer is C** *[see II.B.3.c].*
   A patient suffering from pain cannot sleep properly. When the pain is adequately controlled, the patient may sleep initially for many hours. This usually is not oversedation owing to the narcotic. These patients should be monitored closely (e.g., respiratory rate), and other sedating drugs should be eliminated. Usually, no other intervention is needed.

5. **The answer is D** *[see II.A.4].*
   Aspirin has several adverse effects and drug interactions. However, cardiac arrhythmias are not induced by aspirin.

6. **The answer is C** *[see II.A.2].*
   Unlike the opiates, NSAID use is not associated with the development of tolerance.

7. **The answer is D** *[see Table 51-2].*
   Transdermal fentanyl is a controlled-release dosage form that is effective for up to a 72-hr period. All of the other drugs listed in the question are effective for periods of 1 to 8 hrs.

8. **The answer is C (I, II)** *[see II.A.4.b].*
Unlike aspirin and NSAIDs, acetaminophen and choline magnesium trisalicylate lack antiplatelet effects. Therefore, they are safe to use for patients with bleeding problems.

9. **The answer is C (I, II)** *[see II.A.1].*
Adalimumab, etanercept, and infliximab act by binding or capturing excess TNF-α, one of the dominant cytokines or proteins that play an important role in the inflammatory response. The exact mechanism of action of leflunomide, a novel drug used to treat rheumatoid arthritis, is not completely known, but it is thought to inhibit pyrimidine synthesis.

10. **The answer is E (I, II, III)** *[see II.A.4.a; II.A.4.f.(4)].*
Leflunomide has been associated with weight loss, diarrhea, nausea, alopecia, rash, anemia, and transient elevations in liver function tests.

11. **The answer is B** *[see II.D.5].*
Dihydroergotamine can cause nausea and vomiting. It needs to be administered with IV antiemetic. DHE 45 should not be used as monotherapy.

12. **The answer is A** *[see II.D.1.e].*
Because eletriptan is metabolized by cytochrome P450 enzyme CYP3A4, it should not be used within 72 hrs of treatment with potent CYP3A4 inhibitors such as ketoconazole, itraconazole, nefazodone, troleandomycin, clarithromycin, nelfinavir, and ritonavir.

52 Nutrition and the Hospitalized Patient

ROBERT A. QUERCIA, KEVIN P. KEATING

I. NUTRITIONAL PROBLEMS IN HOSPITALIZED PATIENTS

A. **Incidence.** It has been estimated that 30% to 50% of patients admitted to hospitals have some degree of malnutrition. As many as 75% of patients undergo a deterioration of nutritional status while hospitalized.

B. **Definitions**

1. **Malnutrition** is a pathological state, resulting from a relative or absolute deficiency or excess of one or more essential nutrients.
2. **Marasmus** is a chronic disease that develops over months or years as a result of a deficiency in total caloric intake. Depletion of fat stores and skeletal protein occurs to meet metabolic needs. Marasmic patients are generally not hypermetabolic and are able to preserve their visceral protein compartment as determined by measurements of serum albumin, prealbumin, and transferrin.
    - **a.** Marasmus is a well-adapted form of malnutrition, and despite a cachectic appearance, immunocompetence, wound healing, and the ability to handle short-term stress are generally well preserved.
    - **b.** Nutritional support in these patients should be initiated cautiously because aggressive repletion can result in severe metabolic disturbances, such as hypokalemia and hypophosphatemia.
3. **Kwashiorkor** is an acute process that can develop within weeks and is associated with visceral protein depletion and impaired immune function. It is the result of poor protein intake with adequate to slightly inadequate caloric intake; thus, patients usually appear well nourished. A hypermetabolic state (e.g., trauma, infection) combined with protein deprivation can rapidly develop into a severe kwashiorkor malnutrition characterized by hypoalbuminemia, edema, and impaired cellular immune function.
    - **a.** In hospitalized patients, the development of kwashiorkor has been implicated in poor wound healing, gastrointestinal (GI) bleeding, and sepsis.
    - **b.** Aggressive nutritional support to replete protein stores and decrease morbidity and mortality is indicated when the diagnosis of kwashiorkor is made.
4. **Mixed marasmic kwashiorkor** is a severe form of protein–calorie malnutrition that usually develops when a marasmic patient is subjected to an acute hypermetabolic stress, such as trauma, surgery, or infection.
    - **a.** This condition results in depletion of fat stores, skeletal muscle protein, and visceral protein.
    - **b.** Because of the marked immune dysfunction that develops in this state, vigorous nutritional support is indicated.

II. NUTRITIONAL ASSESSMENT AND METABOLIC REQUIREMENTS

A. **Nutritional assessment.** The most commonly used tools for nutritional assessment are as follows:

1. **Subjective global assessment (SGA)** relies heavily on the patient's history.
    - **a.** SGA takes into account:
        - (1) Recent weight change
        - (2) Diet history

(3) Type and length of symptoms affecting nutritional status (e.g., nausea, vomiting, diarrhea)
(4) Functional status
(5) Metabolic demands of the current disease process
(6) Gross physical signs
(a) Status of subcutaneous fat
(b) Evidence of muscle wasting
(c) Presence or absence of edema and ascites

b. Patients are then classified as being well nourished or moderately or severely malnourished.

2. **Mini Nutritional Assessment (MNA)** similar to the SGA, validated in elderly patients
a. MNA takes into account:
(1) Loss of appetite
(2) Weight loss
(3) Mobility
(4) Psychological/physical stress
(5) Neuropsychological problems
(6) Body mass index (BMI)
b. Patient is then assessed as being at no or increased nutritional risk. If at increased risk, a full nutritional assessment is undertaken

3. **Nutritional Risk Index (NRI) similar to SGA and MNA**
a. 16-item questionnaire
b. A modification exists for geriatric patients

4. **Malnutrition Universal Screening Tool (MUST) uses standardized tables to score the following:**
a. Calculated BMI
b. Unplanned weight loss
c. Acute disease effect
d. Add scores from a, b, and c and establish nutrition risk

5. **Nutritional Risk Score (NRS) similar to the MUST, scores are assigned to the following:**
a. Weight loss
b. Severity of disease
c. Age
d. Scores are totaled and nutritional risk assigned

6. **Visceral Protein Markers (VPM)** can be indicators of protein depletion if results are subnormal.
a. Most commonly used VPM are:
(1) Albumin
(2) Prealbumin (transthyretin)
(3) Transferrin
(4) Retinol-binding protein

7. **Total lymphocyte count**—an indicator of immune competence—subnormal levels can be an indicator of malnutrition.

8. **Anthropomorphics**—skinfold measurements
a. Values $<$ 5th percentile can be indicators of fat and protein depletion
b. Most commonly used:
(1) Triceps
(2) Biceps
(3) Subscapular
(4) Suprailiac

9. **Multifactorial prognostic indicators**
a. Prognostic Nutritional Index (PNI) is derived from a formula that attempts to quantify a patient's risk of developing operative complications based on various markers of nutritional status, including:
(1) Visceral protein markers
(2) Anthropomorphics
(3) Immune competence
b. Prognostic Inflammatory Nutritional Index (PINI) is similar to the PNI but adds the inflammatory markers alpha 1 acid glycoprotein and c-reactive protein.

10. **Body composition analysis** assesses nutritional status by measuring and comparing the ratios of various body compartments.
   a. **Bioelectrical impedance.** The resistance to an electrical current is used to calculate lean body mass. The equipment is relatively inexpensive and easy to use. The results are inaccurate in critically ill patients and patients with fluid and electrolyte abnormalities.
   b. **Dual-energy x-ray absorptiometry (DEXA).** The differential attenuation of x-rays is used to measure fat and lean body mass. The equipment is expensive, and results are affected by hydration status.
   c. **Total body potassium** estimates lean body mass by using a whole body counter to measure a potassium isotope concentrated in lean tissue. This method of body composition analysis is impractical and available at only a few centers.
   d. **Total body water** estimates lean body mass from deuterium total body water measurements. This technique is clinically impractical.
   e. **In vivo neutron activation analysis.** Unlike other techniques, this analysis divides the body into several compartments. This technique requires a significant dose of radiation and is available at only a few research centers.
11. **Tests of physiological function** attempt to quantitate malnutrition based on the decrease in muscle strength caused by amino acid mobilization.
   a. **Maximum voluntary grip strength** is measured with isokinetic dynamometry. The results correlate well to total body protein. This test requires patient cooperation.
   b. **Electrical stimulation of the ulnar nerve** measures contractile function of the adductor pollicis muscle. This technique does not require voluntary patient effort and is inexpensive and easy to do. Its prognostic reliability is still under evaluation.

B. **Metabolic requirements**

1. **Energy requirements** are determined as **nonprotein calories (NPCs)**. It is important to avoid excess calories to minimize complications of nutrient delivery and to optimize nutrient metabolism. Energy requirements can be determined by the following three methods:
   a. **Indirect calorimetry or measured energy expenditure (MEE)** is the most accurate method of determining caloric requirements.
      (1) Oxygen (O_2) consumption and carbon dioxide (CO_2) production are measured directly.
      (2) Energy expenditure is related directly to oxygen consumption and is calculated from these measurements.
      (3) A respiratory quotient (RQ) can also be obtained from an MEE and is defined as the ratio of the amount of CO_2 produced to that of O_2 consumed during the course of oxidation of body fuels. The oxidation of carbohydrate results in an RQ of 1.0—that is, as much CO_2 is produced as O_2 is consumed. The oxidation of fat produces significantly less CO_2 and results in an RQ of 0.7. Normal mixed substrate oxidation results in an RQ of 0.8 to 0.9.
      (4) The provision of excess carbohydrate calories causes their conversion to fat (lipogenesis). Lipogenesis produces significantly more carbon dioxide than oxidation does. This can result in an RQ > 1.0, which is consistent with overfeeding. The determination of RQ can, therefore, indicate patterns of substrate use.
   b. **Estimated energy expenditure (EEE)** first requires the calculation of the **basal energy expenditure (BEE)** from the **Harris-Benedict equation**; the BEE is then multiplied by appropriate stress and activity factors.
      (1) **Men:** $BEE = 66.5 + [13.8 \times \text{weight (kg)}] + [5 \times \text{height (cm)}] - [6.8 \times \text{age (years)}]$
      (2) **Women:** $BEE = 65.5 + [9.6 \times \text{weight (kg)}] + [1.8 \times \text{height (cm)}] - [4.7 \times \text{age (years)}]$
      (3) **Stress factors:** uncomplicated surgery 1.00 to 1.05, peritonitis 1.05 to 1.25, and sepsis or multiple trauma 1.25 to 1.50
      (4) **Activity factors:** bed rest 0.95 to 1.10 and ambulation 1.10 to 1.30
   c. **Simple nomogram.** The least accurate method of estimating caloric requirements, this technique is based on the patient's weight in kilograms. It is useful when the other methods cannot be used. Patients with mild to moderate degrees of stress require approximately 25 to 30 kcal/kg/day, whereas the severely stressed patient (e.g., a patient with major burns) may require 35 kcal/kg/day or more.

2. **Protein (nitrogen) requirements** can be determined by several techniques, but nitrogen balance determinations and nomograms appear to be the most practical.
   a. **Nitrogen balance techniques.** The practitioner determines the patient's nitrogen output and develops a nutritional support program in which the protein administered results in a nitrogen input that exceeds losses.
      (1) Nitrogen balance = 24-hr nitrogen intake − 24-hr nitrogen output.
      (2) A 24-hr nitrogen intake = 24-hr total protein intake ÷ 6.25 (approximately 16% of protein is composed of nitrogen).
      (3) A 24-hr nitrogen output = [24-hr urine urea nitrogen (UUN) × 1.25 + 2, where 1.25 accounts for non-UUN losses (e.g., ammonia, creatinine) and two accounts for non-urine nitrogen losses (e.g., skin, feces). Total urinary nitrogen (TUN) determinations are currently available in some centers. Because TUN is a more accurate method of assessing urinary nitrogen losses, it should be used when available in place of a 24-hr UUN × 1.25 when calculating a nitrogen balance.
      (4) A positive nitrogen balance of 3 to 6 g is the goal.
      (5) This method cannot be used in renally impaired patients.
   b. **Nomogram method.** This method estimates protein needs based on lean body weight. Protein requirements are 1.5 to 2.0 g protein/kg/day for hospitalized patients.
   c. **Nonprotein calorie to nitrogen (NPC:N) ratio.** An NPC:N ratio of 125 to 150:1 generally has been recommended for the mildly to moderately stressed patient to achieve optimal nitrogen retention and protein synthesis. In the severely stressed patient, some studies indicate that ratios as low as 85:1 may be effective.
3. **Essential fatty acids (EFAs)** are those polyunsaturated fatty acids that cannot be synthesized by humans. EFAs affect immune responses by influencing energy production, eicosanoid synthesis, and cell membrane fluidity. They also affect levels of arachidonic acid in lymphocytes—especially monocytes, macrophages, and polymorphonuclear neutrophils (PMNs). Linoleic acid, an omega-6 polyunsaturated fatty acid (PUFA), is the principal EFA for humans. α-Linolenic acid, an omega-3 PUFA, also cannot be synthesized in vivo; its metabolic significance in humans continues to be investigated. It might be a conditionally essential fatty acid.
   a. Deficiency states of **linoleic acid** are characterized by diarrhea, dermatitis, and hair loss.
   b. The currently available lipid emulsions have a high linoleic acid content.
   c. Providing 4% to 7% of a patient's caloric requirements as linoleic acid from lipid emulsion prevents the development of essential fatty acid deficiency.
4. **Vitamins** are essential for proper substrate metabolism. Accepted daily allowances for oral administration have been established.
   a. **Vitamin A** (fat soluble). Normal stores can last up to 1 year but are rapidly depleted by stress. Vitamin A has essential functions in vision, growth, and reproduction. Recommended oral intake is 2500 to 5000 IU/day. **The recommended requirement is 3300 IU/day in parenteral nutrition (PN) formulations.**
   b. **Vitamin D** (fat soluble). In conjunction with parathormone and calcitonin, vitamin D helps regulate calcium and phosphorus homeostasis. Recommended oral intake is 100 to 400 IU/day. **The PN requirement is 200 IU/day.**
   c. **Vitamin E** (fat soluble) appears to function as an antioxidant, inhibiting the oxidation of free unsaturated fatty acids. Recommended daily oral allowances are 12 to 15 IU/day. **The requirement in PN formulations is 10 IU/day.** The presence of polyunsaturated fatty acids increases the requirement for vitamin E, which needs to be considered with the use of lipid system PN.
   d. **Vitamin K** (fat soluble) plays an essential role in the synthesis of clotting factors. The suggested oral intake is 0.7 to 2.0 mg/day. **The recommended PN requirement is 150 μg/day.**
   e. **Vitamin B_1 (thiamine**; water soluble) functions as a coenzyme in the phosphogluconate pathway and as a structural component of nervous system membranes. The development of its deficiency state (i.e., acute pernicious beriberi with high output cardiac failure) is well described in patients on PN receiving inadequate thiamine replacement. A prolonged deficiency state can cause Wernicke encephalopathy. Recommended doses are 0.5 mg/1000 oral calories/day and **6 mg/day in PN formulations**.

f. **Vitamin B_2 (riboflavin**; water soluble) functions as a coenzyme in oxidative phosphorylation. Essentially, no intracellular stores are maintained. Oral requirements are 1.3 to 1.7 mg/day. **The requirement in PN formulations is 3.6 mg/day.**

g. **Vitamin B_3 (niacin**; water soluble) functions as a coenzyme in oxidative phosphorylation and biosynthetic pathways. Pellagra is the well-described deficiency state. Oral requirements are 14.5 to 19.8 mg/day. **The recommended PN requirement is 40 mg/day.**

h. **Vitamin B_5 (pantothenic acid**; water soluble). The functional form of vitamin B_5 is coenzyme A, which is essential to all acylation reactions. Oral requirements are 5 to 10 mg/day. Intravenous (IV) requirements are 10 to 29 mg/day.

i. **Vitamin B_6 (pyridoxine**; water soluble) functions as a coenzyme in various enzymatic pathways. Deficiency states are accentuated by some medications, including isoniazid, penicillamine, and cycloserine. Oral requirements are 1.5 to 2.0 mg/day. **The recommended PN requirement is 6.0 mg/day.**

j. **Vitamin B_7 (biotin**; water soluble) functions in carboxylation reactions. It is synthesized by intestinal flora; therefore, deficiency states are rare. **The requirement in PN formulations is 60 μg/day.**

k. **Vitamin B_9 (folic acid**; water soluble) is involved in various biosynthetic reactions and amino acid conversions. Folate cofactors are necessary for purine and pyrimidine (DNA) synthesis. Stores usually last 3 to 6 months; however, rapid depletion is seen with metabolic stress. Deficiency of vitamin B_{12} causes deficiency in folate. A megaloblastic anemia is classic in the deficiency state. Deficiency of folic acid in a pregnant mother can cause neural tube defects in the fetus. Oral requirements are 200 to 400 μg/day. **The recommended requirement in PN formulations is 600 μg/day.**

l. **Vitamin B_{12} (cyanocobalamin**; water soluble) has various metabolic and biosynthetic functions. Because of large stores, deficiency states can take years to develop. Megaloblastic (pernicious) anemia is one manifestation of deficiency. Another manifestation of deficiency is peripheral neuropathy because B_{12} is responsible for biosynthesis of the insulation sheet on nerves called myelin. Oral requirements are 2.0 μg/day. **The requirement in PN formulations is 5.0 μg/day.**

5. **Trace mineral deficiency** may develop during PN because of reduced intake, increased use, decreased plasma binding, or increased excretion.

   a. **Iron** is necessary for hemoglobin and myoglobin production and is a necessary cofactor in various enzymatic reactions. Deficiency is classically demonstrated by a hypochromic, microcytic anemia as well as by the development of immune deficiency. Oral requirements are 16 to 18 mg/day. IV requirements are 0.5 to 1.0 mg/day.

   b. **Zinc** is necessary for DNA and RNA synthesis and is a necessary cofactor in various enzymatic reactions. Zinc deficiency results in impaired wound healing, growth retardation, hair loss, dermatitis, diarrhea, anorexia, and glucose intolerance. Patients at high risk for developing zinc deficiency are those with long-term steroid therapy, malabsorption syndromes, fistulas, sepsis, and major surgery. Oral requirements are 10 to 15 mg/day. IV requirements are **3.0 to 5.0 mg/day.**

   c. **Copper** is necessary for heme synthesis, electron transport, and wound healing. Deficiency that develops during PN usually manifests as anemia, leukopenia, and neutropenia. Oral requirements are 30 μg/kg/day. **IV requirements are 0.5 to 1.5 mg/day.**

   d. **Manganese** is involved in protein synthesis and possibly glucose use. Oral requirements are 0.7 to 22.0 mg/day. **IV requirements are 150 to 300 μg/day.**

   e. **Selenium** is important in antioxidant reactions. Deficiency during PN has been associated with muscle pain and cardiomyopathy. **IV** requirements are **40 to 60 μg/day.**

   f. **Iodine** is a component of the thyroid hormones. Deficiency manifests as a goiter. Recommended intake is 1 μg/kg/day.

   g. **Chromium** is important in glucose use and potentiates the effect of insulin. Signs of deficiency include hyperglycemia and abnormal glucose tolerance. Oral requirements are 70 to 80 μg/day. IV maintenance requirements are 0.14 to 0.20 μg/kg/day (10 to 15 μg/day). **Suggested IV requirements for deficiency and severe glucose intolerance are 150 to 200 μg/day.**

   h. **Molybdenum** is essential to xanthine oxidase. Oral requirements are 2.0 μg/kg/day.

III. METHODS OF SUPPORT

A. PN is also called **total parenteral nutrition (TPN)** and **hyperalimentation**. It is used to meet the patient's nutritional requirements when the enteral route cannot accomplish this.

1. **Indications.** When the enteral route cannot be used because of dysfunction or disease states (e.g., acute pancreatitis, inflammatory bowel disease, complete bowel obstruction), PN is instituted.
2. **Initiation** of PN should be undertaken within 1 to 3 days in moderately to severely malnourished patients when the inadequacy of enteral support is anticipated for more than 5 to 7 days. In healthy or mildly malnourished patients, PN should be initiated within 5 to 7 days if enteral support has not been initiated.
3. **Routes of administration**
   a. **A central venous route** is used with hypertonic PN formulations (i.e., dextrose concentrations > 10%). Most commonly, dextrose concentrations of 25% are used centrally, and the osmolarity exceeds 2000 mOsm/L. Such highly osmolar solutions must be infused into a large-diameter central vein (e.g., superior vena cava), where they are rapidly diluted by high flow rates.
   b. **A peripheral venous route** can be used when the dextrose concentration is 10% or less.
      (1) Solutions with 10% dextrose, amino acids, electrolytes, and trace minerals have a resulting osmolarity of 900 to 1000 mOsm/L. Higher osmolarity is associated with a higher incidence of thrombophlebitis.
      (2) The major reason for use of the central venous PN rather than the peripheral route is the development of thrombophlebitis. Maintaining the osmolality of the peripheral PN solution < 900 mOsm/kg and preferably between 600 and 800 mOsm/kg with IV lipid emulsion administered concurrently over 24 hrs minimizes the incidence of thrombophlebitis. Also, the development of new peripheral fine-bore catheters made from polyurethane or silicone has been shown to be significantly less thrombogenic. In addition, the use of low-dose heparin (1 unit/mL) and hydrocortisone (5 mg/L) delivered in the PN solutions has been shown to protect against thrombophlebitis.
      (3) **Glyceryl trinitrate** patches (5 mg), when applied over the area where the tip of the catheter is expected to lie, have been shown to significantly reduce peripheral PN infusion failure caused by phlebitis. With the use of this new catheter technology and new techniques for infusion, it is now feasible to administer peripheral PN in selected patients for short-term therapy (7 to 10 days) with a low incidence of peripheral vein thrombophlebitis.
4. **NPC sources**
   a. **Dextrose monohydrate** is the form of dextrose used for parenteral administration. It yields 3.4 kcal/g. It is the component in PN formulas that contributes the most to osmolarity. It is available commercially in concentrations up to 70%.
   b. **IV lipids** are commercially available as 10% or 20% emulsions derived from soybean oil (intralipid) or a combination of soybean oil and safflower oil (Liposyn II).
      (1) Both the 10% and 20% emulsions are isotonic (280 and 340 mOsm/L, respectively) and can be administered via the peripheral vein with a low incidence of phlebitis; these emulsions provide 1.1 and 2.0 kcal/mL, respectively. They contain 1.2% egg yolk phospholipids as the emulsifying agent and 2.25% to 2.50% glycerol to make the emulsions isosmotic.
      (2) Lipid emulsions can be given as part of the daily NPC requirement or two to three times per week to prevent essential fatty acid deficiency. Both types of lipid emulsion contain particles of 0.4 to 0.5 μm, which prevents the use of 0.22 μm bacterial retention filters.
5. **Protein (nitrogen) source. Synthetic crystalline amino acids** are currently used as the nitrogen source in PN formulations.
   a. **These formulations are available commercially without electrolytes and dextrose in concentrations of 5.5% (Travasol), 8.5% (Travasol), 10% (Aminosyn II, Travasol), 15% (Aminosyn II, Clinisol), and 20% (Prosol).**
   b. These formulations yield 4 kcal/g.
   c. These solutions generally contain a mixture of free essential and nonessential L-amino acids.
   d. Specialized amino acid formulations are available for specific disease states.

6. Systems of PN

a. Glucose system PN

(1) Definition. The glucose system PN is a parenteral formulation in which dextrose is used exclusively as the NPC source. Nitrogen is provided as crystalline amino acids. Electrolytes, vitamins, and trace minerals are added to the formulation as needed.

(2) Administration. The glucose system PN formulations usually have dextrose concentrations of 25% or greater and must be administered by the central venous route. These formulations are also referred to as two-in-one formulations because the dextrose and amino acids are usually mixed in one container with electrolytes, vitamins, and trace minerals.

(a) Because of the high dextrose concentration, initial administration should be at low hourly rates (e.g., 50 mL/hr) and increased gradually over 24 hrs to avoid hyperglycemia ($>$ 200 mg/dL).

(b) To avoid reactive hypoglycemia ($<$ 70 mg/dL), discontinuation should be gradual over several hours.

(c) Lipid emulsions should be administered for **essential fatty acid replacement** in a dose that provides 4% to 7% of required calories as linoleic acid. This can be accomplished by the administration of 250 mL of 20% or 500 mL of 10% emulsion, two to three times weekly.

b. Lipid system PN

(1) Definition. The lipid system PN is a parenteral formulation in which lipid is administered daily to provide a substantial proportion of the NPC. Nitrogen is provided as crystalline amino acids. Electrolytes, vitamins, and trace minerals are added to the formulation as needed.

(2) Administration. The lipid system PN is administered peripherally when the dextrose concentration is less than or equal to 10% and centrally when the dextrose concentration is more than 10%.

(a) Piggyback method. The solution with amino acids, dextrose, electrolytes, trace minerals, and vitamins is infused concurrently with a separate bottle of lipid emulsion through a Y site on the intravenous administration set.

(b) Total nutrient admixture (TNA) method—three-in-one, all-in-one. Lipids, amino acids, dextrose, electrolytes, trace minerals, and vitamins are mixed in one container and administered by the central or peripheral route, depending on dextrose concentration.

(i) Advantages include simplification of administration and decreased training time for home PN patients.

(ii) Disadvantages include the inability to inspect for particulate matter in the opaque admixture, the inability to use 0.22-μm bacterial retention filters, and stability problems.

(iii) Because the presence of lipid emulsion in TNAs obscure the presence of a precipitate and may present a life-threatening hazard to patients, the U.S. Food and Drug Administration (FDA) suggests that the piggyback method be used to administer lipid emulsion. If a TNA is deemed medically necessary, then specific admixture guidelines recommended by the FDA should be followed. Also, a particle filter (i.e., 1.2 μ) should be used with TNA administration.

(c) Lipid dosage

(i) Lipid calories should not exceed 60% of total daily calories, including protein calories.

(ii) Maximum dosage of lipids for adults is 2.5 g/kg/day.

(iii) Baseline and weekly serum triglycerides must be monitored in patients on lipid system PN.

(3) Adverse effects of lipids are uncommon. The most frequent adverse effects include fever, chills, sensation of warmth, chest pain, back pain, vomiting, and urticaria (overall incidence $<$ 1%). Severe hypoxemia has been reported with rapid infusion of lipid emulsion.

7. **Additives**
   a. **Electrolytes.** PN formulations must include adequate amounts of sodium, magnesium, calcium, chloride, potassium, phosphorus, and acetate. The intracellular "anabolic" electrolytes—potassium, magnesium, and phosphate—are essential for protein synthesis. Requirements vary widely, depending on a patient's fluid and electrolyte losses; renal, hepatic, and endocrine status; acid–base balance; metabolic rate; and type of PN formula used. The electrolyte composition of the PN formula must be adjusted to meet the needs of the individual patient.
   b. **Vitamins and trace minerals.** Vitamins are usually added to PN solutions in the form of commercially available multivitamin preparations. The current adult multiple vitamin infusion formula available (Infuvite Adult, MVI-Adult) meets the amended requirements of the FDA for adult parenteral multivitamins.
      (1) The new FDA requirements are based on the prior multivitamin formulation recommended by the Nutrition Advisory Group of the Department of Foods and Nutrition of the American Medical Association (NAG-AMA) but with increased dosages of vitamins B_1, B_6, C, and folic acid and the addition of vitamin K.
      (2) The FDA also approved the same multivitamin formulation without vitamin K (MVI-12; multivitamin infusion without vitamin K) for those patients who receive warfarin-type anticoagulant therapy. Because of stability problems, one vial of Infuvite Adult and MVI-Adult contains vitamins A, D, E, B_1, B_2, B_3, B_5, B_6, and K. MVI-12 contains the same vitamins in one vial without vitamin K. The second vial for both preparations contains vitamins B_{12}, biotin, and folic acid.
      (3) Trace minerals may be added individually or as a commercially available multielement preparation. Precise requirements for trace minerals have yet to be determined.
   c. **Insulin** may be required for patients receiving PN formulations (especially glucose system PN) to maintain blood glucose levels < 200 mg/dL. If insulin is required, it is best provided by the addition of an appropriate amount of regular insulin to the PN formulation at the time of admixture. Although a small amount of insulin (5 to 10 U per bag) may be adsorbed to the container and tubing, such losses can be overcome by appropriate titration of the dose. The addition of insulin to the PN formulation has the advantage of changes in the rate of PN infusion being automatically accompanied by appropriate changes in the rate of insulin infusion.
   d. **Miscellaneous drugs.** Several medications have been successfully admixed with PN formulations for continuous infusion. The H_2-receptor antagonists are the most common drugs used in this way. The routine addition of medications to PN formulations remains controversial because of:
      (1) **Questions of stability** over the wide range of PN component concentrations
      (2) Possible **therapeutic inadequacy** or toxicity secondary to PN rate changes and loss of peak and trough levels
      (3) Increased **potential for waste** with dose changes
8. **Complications** with the use of PN can be serious and potentially life threatening but can be avoided by careful management. Complications can be divided into mechanical, infectious, and metabolic.
   a. **Mechanical** complications generally relate to the central venous catheter or its placement and include pneumothorax, catheter occlusion, and venous thrombosis.
   b. **Infectious** complications usually are related to the central venous catheter. This line-related sepsis is secondary to multiple catheter manipulations, contamination during insertion, or contamination during routine maintenance. Hyperglycemia and IV lipids also have been implicated. Maintaining blood sugars < 200 mg/dL has been shown to significantly reduce septic complications in certain subsets of patients.
   c. **Metabolic** complications are the most common. These include hyperglycemia, hypoglycemia, hypokalemia, hypomagnesemia, hypophosphatemia, metabolic acidosis, respiratory acidosis, prerenal azotemia, and zinc deficiency. A transient self-limited hepatic dysfunction is also seen with long-term PN.

B. **Enteral nutrition (EN).** Use of the GI tract to achieve total nutritional support or partial support in combination with the parenteral route should be attempted whenever possible in the face of inadequate oral intake. Theoretical advantages include maintenance of normal digestion, absorption, and gut mucosal barrier function.
   1. **Contraindications** to EN include complete intestinal obstruction, high-output intestinal fistulas, severe acute pancreatitis, severe acute inflammatory bowel disease, and severe diarrhea.

2. **Routes of administration.** Tube feedings can be administered via nasogastric, nasoduodenal, nasojejunal, gastrostomy, and jejunostomy tubes.
3. **EN formulations** can be classified as being standard (complete) or modular.
   a. **Standard formulas** generally contain carbohydrates, fats, vitamins, trace minerals, and a nitrogen source. They are further classified according to their nitrogen source.
      (1) **Monomeric** formulas contain crystalline amino acids as their nitrogen source. These formulas are usually marketed commercially for specific indications (e.g., ileus, pancreatitis, hepatic coma).
      (2) **Short-chain peptide** formulas contain dipeptides and tripeptides from hydrolyzed protein or de novo synthesis as their nitrogen source. They are currently marketed for the metabolically stressed patient.
      (3) **Polymeric** formulas contain either intact proteins or protein hydrolysates as their nitrogen source. Most patients can be managed with these formulas.
   b. **Modular formulas** consist of separate modules of specific nutrients that can be combined or administered separately. They are used for supplemental use or to custom design an EN formula to meet a specific clinical situation.
      (1) **Carbohydrate** modules differ in the type of carbohydrate present (e.g., polysaccharides, disaccharides, monosaccharides).
      (2) **Protein** modules contain either intact protein, hydrolyzed protein, or crystalline amino acids.
      (3) **Fat** modules contain either long-chain triglycerides (LCTs) prepared from vegetable oils or medium-chain triglycerides (MCTs) prepared from coconut oil. MCTs are more water soluble and more easily absorbed than LCTs. (Bypassing the intestinal lacteal and lymphatic system, MCTs are transported directly to the portal system.) MCTs are, however, relatively expensive and contain no essential fatty acids.
4. **Complications.** The two **most common** complications of EN are diarrhea and improper tube placement.
   a. **Diarrhea** in patients receiving EN is usually secondary to concomitant administration of medication (e.g., antibiotics and sorbitol-containing liquids). Infectious causes should be eliminated (e.g., *Clostridium difficile*), after which antidiarrheal medications may be beneficial. Reducing the rate or concentration may also be effective.
   b. A **feeding tube improperly placed** into the tracheobronchial tree can have disastrous consequences. Tube feedings should never be initiated without radiological verification of tube position.
   c. **Aspiration**

IV. MONITORING SUPPORT

A. **PN.** In addition to appropriate general medical and nursing care, patients receiving PN initially require daily and weekly laboratory monitoring to assess nutritional progress and metabolic status.
   1. **Electrolytes**
      a. Initially, **potassium**, **sodium**, and **chloride** should be determined daily. Potassium is used intracellularly; thus, hypokalemia is not an uncommon finding.
      b. **Calcium**, **magnesium**, and **phosphate** are primarily intracellular electrolytes, serum levels of which become depleted during protein synthesis. Serum levels generally do not fall as rapidly as potassium; therefore, monitoring two to three times a week is recommended initially until the patient is stabilized, then weekly thereafter.
      c. **Bicarbonate** should be monitored to assess acid–base balance. Hyperchloremic metabolic acidosis may develop in patients on PN. This imbalance can be corrected by providing the potassium and sodium as acetate (converted to bicarbonate in the serum) rather than as the chloride salt. After initial correction, provision of one-half the sodium and potassium requirements as the acetate salt and one-half as the chloride salt may be beneficial.
   2. **Serum glucose** should be monitored daily, particularly in central glucose systems. Maintaining a blood glucose concentration between 100 to 200 mg/dL is generally recommended.
   3. **Weights** obtained on a daily or every other day basis track optimum lean body weight gain of 0.25 to 0.50 lb/day. Weight gain in excess of 0.5 lb/day generally indicates fluid overload or fat deposition.

4. **Visceral proteins** (e.g., albumin, prealbumin, transferrin) are important indicators of the adequacy of nutritional support.
   a. **Albumin** is useful in the initial assessment of nutritional status, but its long half-life (18 to 21 days) limits its utility as a short-term marker of nutritional repletion.
   b. **Prealbumin** has a short half-life (2 to 3 days) and is a more sensitive and early indicator of the adequacy of nutritional support. Its serum value is falsely elevated in renal failure.
   c. **Transferrin** has an intermediate half-life (7 to 10 days), which makes weekly monitoring useful. Transferrin may be falsely elevated in iron-deficiency states.
   d. **Retinol-binding protein** has an ultrashort half-life (12 hrs). Values are affected by injury and metabolic stress.
5. **Serum creatinine** and **blood urea nitrogen (BUN)** should be obtained at least weekly. Evidence of renal impairment may require modification of the PN formula. Elevation of the BUN in the absence of renal impairment may be secondary to the PN formula (e.g., excess nitrogen, low NPC:N ratio) and appropriate adjustments need to be made.
6. **Liver function tests**—aspartate aminotransferase (AST), alanine aminotransferase (ALT), alkaline phosphatase, lactate dehydrogenase (LDH), and bilirubin—require baseline and periodic monitoring because of potential toxicity from the PN formulation (i.e., fatty infiltration of the liver). Abnormal liver function studies may necessitate changes in the PN formulation.
7. **Serum triglycerides** should be measured for a baseline and weekly thereafter for patients on lipid system PN. It is not necessary to monitor triglycerides on a weekly basis for patients receiving lipids two to three times per week for essential fatty acid replacement.
8. **A 24-hr UUN** should be obtained weekly to determine nitrogen balance for patients in whom nitrogen requirements are uncertain. These are usually highly stressed, severely ill, or injured patients in an intensive care unit (ICU) setting.
9. **Serum iron** levels should be obtained weekly to determine deficiency and to allow appropriate interpretation of serum transferrin levels.

B. **EN** generally requires less intense laboratory monitoring. Specific laboratory guidelines for monitoring EN support vary from institution to institution.

V. SUPPORT OF SPECIFIC STATES

A. **Conditionally essential nutrients**

1. **Glutamine.** Because of its instability, glutamine is currently not a component of commercially available standard PN amino acid solutions and is found in free form in relatively few EN formulas. A relative deficiency has been shown to occur in critical illness. It is known to be used as a primary fuel source by enterocytes and may exert a trophic effect on the gut mucosa. It is most widely used as a PN component for bone marrow transplant patients and short gut syndrome. Glutamine-containing dipeptides that are stable and highly soluble are being investigated as a source of glutamine in PN. At present, glutamine must be added to the PN solution at the time of compounding. Increasing evidence supports glutamine supplementation in critical illness.
2. **Arginine** has been shown experimentally and clinically to enhance immune function. EN formulas enriched with arginine are available commercially. Recently, the efficacy of exogenously administered arginine to subsets of critically ill patients, specifically septic patients, has come into question.
3. **Antioxidant formulations.** Oxidant production occurs as part of the normal inflammatory response and has been implicated in reperfusion injury. The body also produces antioxidant defenses to limit oxidant damage to healthy tissue. These defenses rely on adequate intake of dietary nutrients, such as the sulfur-containing amino acids, vitamin E, vitamin C, selenium, and zinc.
4. **Tyrosine**, **cysteine**, and **taurine** are either absent or present in low concentrations in commercially available PN formulas. They are believed to be conditionally essential amino acids by some investigators.
5. **Omega-3 polyunsaturated fatty acids** are derived from fish oils and are currently found in some EN formulations. These fatty acids have been shown experimentally to enhance immune response, protect against tumor growth, and inhibit some of the proinflammatory effects of omega-6 fatty acids. In addition, they have been shown to lower cardiovascular risk factors by decreasing platelet activation, lowering blood pressure, and reducing triglycerides.

6. Commercially available enteral formulas supplemented with various combinations of the aforementioned agents are advocated for appropriate patient populations, i.e., major elective surgery, trauma, burns, head and neck cancer, and critically ill patients on mechanical ventilation. In particular, patients on mechanical ventilation with adult respiratory distress syndrome (ARDS) should be given an enteral formula rich in omega-3 polyunsaturated fatty acids and antioxidants.

B. **Nutritional support for renal failure.** The goal of nutritional support in acute renal failure (ARF) is to meet the patient's NPC requirements while minimizing volume, protein load, and potential electrolyte imbalance.

1. **PN formulations** used in ARF are low-nitrogen, high-caloric density formulas (e.g., 2% amino acid/47% dextrose), resulting in NPC:N ratios of approximately 500:1.
2. **Commercial renal failure formulations** (e.g., NephrAmine, Aminosyn RF) containing primarily essential amino acids have shown no clinical advantage over less expensive, low-concentration standard amino acid formulations.
3. **Standard glucose system formulations** (4.25% amino acid/25% dextrose) can generally be used in renal failure patients receiving hemodialysis or continuous renal replacement therapy (CRRT) on a regular basis. This formulation is particularly useful in critically ill ICU patients because it can provide adequate protein to attain positive nitrogen balance, which is not possible with renal failure PN. ICU patients with ARF almost always have preexisting comorbidities and other complications and should be provided adequate protein to attain positive nitrogen balance. Dialysis therapy should not be avoided or delayed to provide these patients adequate protein doses of 1.5 to 2.5 g/kg/day to achieve positive nitrogen balance.
4. **Monitoring transferrin** is a more sensitive and accurate visceral protein marker compared to albumin and prealbumin for assessing nutritional progress in these patients.
5. **Enteral formulations** that are low in nitrogen and calorie dense (1.7 to 2.0 NPC/mL) are available for patients with renal failure.

C. **Nutritional support for hepatic failure.** Patients with hepatic failure have altered protein metabolism, resulting in decreased serum levels of branched-chain amino acids (i.e., leucine, isoleucine, valine) and increased levels of aromatic amino acids (i.e., phenylalanine, tyrosine, tryptophan), methionine, and glutamine. A similar amino acid profile can exist in the cerebrospinal fluid (CSF) and is thought to contribute to hepatic encephalopathy. Fluid and electrolyte disturbances are frequently associated with hepatic failure as well.

1. **PN and EN formulations** enriched in branched-chain amino acids and low in aromatic amino acids (e.g., HepatAmine, Hepatic-Aid 11) have been **used to improve** mental status in patients with altered serum amino acid profiles and hepatic encephalopathy. However, studies have not demonstrated definitive clinical differences in morbidity and mortality with these more expensive formulations compared to standard formulas. These enriched branched-chain amino acid formulations should be reserved for the rare encephalopathic patient who is refractory to standard treatment with luminal acting antibiotics and lactulose.
2. EN is recommended whenever feasible as the optimal route of nutrient delivery for ICU patients with acute and/or chronic liver disease. EN has been shown to improve nutritional status, reduce complications, and prolong survival in liver disease patients.
3. Protein requirements in ICU patients should not be restricted as a clinical management strategy to reduce the risk of developing hepatic encephalopathy. The protein dose should be determined in the same manner as the general ICU patient. In patients with encephalopathy, a protein intake of 0.8 to 1.2 g/kg/day is warranted.

D. **Nutritional support for respiratory failure.** The type and amount of substrate administered as NPC can have an effect on a patient's ventilatory status. Overfeeding with resultant lipogenesis and increased carbon dioxide production can be a cause of respiratory acidosis and/or increased minute ventilation and therefore should be avoided. Even in the presence of appropriate amounts of NPC administered as carbohydrate, the normal carbon dioxide load generated by glycolysis may be excessive for the patient with underlying pulmonary dysfunction—for example, chronic obstructive pulmonary disease (COPD).

1. **PN lipid system formulations** (e.g., 4.25% amino acid/15% dextrose with daily lipid emulsion), where the lipid component constitutes 40% to 50% of the total NPC, may be beneficial in reducing the ventilatory demands in respiratory failure patients because lipolysis generates less carbon dioxide than glycolysis.

2. **EN formulations** containing similar amounts of fat can be prepared from standard EN formulas with the use of lipid modules (i.e., MCT oil, corn oil). More expensive commercial pulmonary formulas are also available.
3. **Oxepa**, a low-carbohydrate enteral formula containing antioxidants, eicosapentaenoic acid, and γ-linolenic acid, is currently available for adult respiratory distress syndrome (ARDS). It modulates the phospholipid fatty acid composition of inflammatory cell membranes, decreases the synthesis of the proinflammatory eicosanoids of lung injury, and attenuates endotoxin-induced increases in pulmonary microvascular protein permeability.

E. **Nutritional support for cardiac failure.** The goal in these patients is to meet metabolic needs while restricting fluid and sodium intake.
1. **PN formulations** that provide protein and calories in as high a concentration as possible is the goal of nutritional therapy. This can be accomplished with both central glucose and lipid system PN formulations (e.g., 5% amino acid/35% dextrose; 7% amino acid/21% dextrose/20% lipid emulsion).
2. **Serum electrolyte monitoring** and **adjustment** are imperative in cardiac failure patients receiving PN, particularly when potent diuretics are used concurrently.
3. **EN formulations** with high nutrient density are available for oral supplementation or tube feedings. Infusion of enteral tube feedings should begin at one-third to one-half the strength, with a gradual increase in concentration, while maintaining a slow infusion rate (30 to 50 mL/hr) to avoid rapid increases in fluid load, cardiac output, heart rate, and myocardial oxygen consumption.

F. **Nutritional support in pancreatitis.** Severe acute pancreatitis is a hypercatabolic state that without nutritional support renders the patient a poor surgical candidate and at increased risk of infection.
1. Early initiation of enteral feeding via the gastric or jejunal route is advocated for these patients. Elemental or small peptide-based formulas that are nearly fat-free or contain medium chain triglycerides are well tolerated. If intolerance to gastric feeds occurs, more distal feeding should be attempted.
2. PN should be reserved for the patient with severe acute pancreatitis who is intolerant to enteral feeding.

G. Thermal injury is one of the most hypermetabolic conditions observed in the critical care setting.
1. Methods for estimating the calorie requirements in this patient population are conflicting owing to differences in bias and precision. One of the more accurate unbiased methods reported for estimating energy requirements in thermal injury is

$$\text{Kcal} = (1000\ \text{kcal} \times \text{BSA}) + (25 \times \%\text{BSAB})$$

where BSA is body surface area and BSAB is body surface area burned.
2. Protein requirements in thermally injured patients are high at 2.0 to 2.5 g/kg/day because of the significant degree of catabolism associated with this injury.
3. The increased dermal losses of nitrogen from their burn wounds renders the use of the conventional nitrogen balance formulas less accurate in assessing nitrogen requirements, especially with thermal injuries $>$ 40% of BSA. The UUN plus the insensible loss factor can differ significantly from total nitrogen losses in this patient population.

H. **Hyperglycemia** and **insulin resistance** are common occurrences in critically ill patients. Previous recommendations in critically ill ICU patients were to provide intensive insulin therapy (IIT) to maintain blood glucose levels between 80 to 110 mg/dL to reduce morbidity and mortality in this patient population. Based on the results of a recent systematic evidence review of the literature on ITT in hospitalized patients, the American College of Physicians (ACP) provided the following practice guideline for the management of glycemic control in medical intensive care unit (MICU) and surgical intensive care unit (SICU) patients.
1. ACP recommends not using IIT to normalize glucose in SICU/MICU patients with or without diabetes mellitus
2. ACP recommends a target blood glucose level of 140 to 200 mg/dL if insulin therapy is used in SICU/MICU patients.
3. The ACP also noted the following clinical considerations:
   a. Critically ill medical and surgical patients who are hyperglycemic have a higher mortality rate.
   b. Most clinicians agree that prevention of hyperglycemia is an important intervention.

c. The range of optimal glucose level is controversial. A few studies show that IIT improves mortality, whereas most have shown that patients who receive IIT have no reduction in mortality and have a significantly increased risk for severe hypoglycemia.

I. **Nutritional support in pregnancy.** Nutritional support in pregnancy can have a significant effect on fetal outcome. Weight gain throughout pregnancy is the primary indicator of the adequacy of the nutritional state of mother and child. A weight gain of 11.5 to 16.0 kg should be the desired goal in women with normal prepregnancy BMI. PN and EN have both been used successfully during pregnancy, with both modalities demonstrating adequate maternal weight gain, appropriate fetal growth, and term delivery. The calories required to achieve appropriate weight gain throughout the entire pregnancy per the World Health Organization recommendations are an additional 300 kcal/day above the estimated basal energy expenditure (based on the pregravid weight) during all trimesters. The recommended daily protein intake during a normal pregnancy is approximately 1 g/kg/day. This amount represents the normal recommended daily allowance for females plus an additional 10 g/day. In pregnant patients with moderate-to-severe stress, both calories and protein requirements need to be adjusted in the same manner as for other hypermetabolic nonpregnant patients.

1. PN glucose system and lipid system formulations can both be used successfully to meet the nutrient requirements of pregnant patients. PN is most commonly used during pregnancy in patients with severe hyperemesis gravidarum.
2. Essential fatty acids (EFAs) are required by both mother and fetus. They are necessary for prostaglandin synthesis and normal fetal lipid development. The provision of at least 4.5% to 7.0% of calorie requirements as EFAs has been estimated to meet the minimum requirements during pregnancy.
3. The **daily vitamin requirements** in a normal pregnancy based on the 1999 dietary reference intakes (DRIs) can be met with the parenteral vitamin infusion Infuvite Adult and MVI-Adult. If MVI-12 is used as the parenteral vitamin preparation, an additional 65 μg of vitamin K needs to be added to the daily PN formulation to meet the daily DRI requirements.
4. Prealbumin appears to be the preferred biochemical marker to assess protein status in pregnancy, because albumin is falsely depressed and transferrin is falsely elevated in pregnant patients.
5. EN may be useful during pregnancy for patients with less severe hyperemesis gravidarum. The composition of polymeric formulas should be adequate for meeting the nutritional requirements of most pregnant patients.
6. Blood glucose levels should be kept at approximately 100 mg/dL during prolonged continuous PN or EN infusion because chronically elevated maternal glucose levels can result in fetal anomalies, increased risk of miscarriages, and stillbirth.

J. **Nutritional support in inflammatory bowel disease (IBD).** IBD is associated with weight loss, hypoalbuminemia, anemia, electrolyte imbalance, and vitamin/mineral deficiencies (especially zinc)

1. PN has no role as primary therapy.
2. PN has a role with high-output fistulae.
3. Polymeric and elemental enteral formulas seem equally tolerated.

K. **Nutritional support in short bowel syndrome (SBS).** A loss of bowel from resection or dysfunction can result in reduced absorption of fluid, electrolytes, macronutrients and micronutrients. Specific deficiencies are related to the regions of lost absorption (e.g., free water and iron deficiency are associated with jejunal loss, vitamin B_{12}, bile salt, and fat-soluble vitamin deficiency are associated with ileal loss). Complications include dehydration; weight loss; deficiencies of electrolytes, mineral, and trace elements; metabolic bone disease; cholelithiasis; nephrolithiasis; gastric acid hypersecretion and D-lactic acidosis. Intestinal adaptation begins to occur after resection and is promoted by enteral feeding.

1. PN is not uncommonly required for the short-term and is usually required for the long-term in massive small bowel resection.
2. Hypersecretion of gastric acid should be treated with H2-blockers.
3. D-lactic acidosis is caused by fermentation of an increased carbohydrate load delivered to the colon. Treatment is aimed at decreasing enteral carbohydrates.
4. Fat-soluble vitamins should be monitored and replaced.
5. Stool volume should be monitored and treated with antidiarrheal agents if greater than 2 L/day.
6. Oral calcium and magnesium supplementation needed when enteral feeding achieved.

7. Intestinal adaptation in patients with massive resection may be hastened/improved by the provision of glutamine (enteral and/or parenteral) recombinant human growth hormone and high-carbohydrate, low-fat feeds.

L. **Nutritional support in bariatric surgery.** Bariatric surgeries are divided into restrictive (vertical banded gastroplasties and silastic ring vertical gastroplasties), restrictive/malabsorptive (Roux-en-Y gastric bypass), and malabsorptive procedures (biliopancreatic diversion). Since restrictive procedures retain the use of the entire GI tract, nutritional deficiencies are less common than in malabsorptive procedures. The primary nutrients affected by bariatric surgery include:

1. Iron—one of the most frequent deficiencies after bariatric surgery. Occurs in both restrictive and malabsorptive procedures. Deficiency is secondary to reduced areas of absorption in the small bowel with malabsorptive procedures and reduced production of hydrochloric acid in the stomach for both types of bariatric procedures. The result is a reduction in iron reduced to the absorbable ferrous state. Prevention/treatment is with oral iron supplementation combined with ascorbic acid to acidify the stomach and facilitate absorption.
2. Vitamin B_{12} deficiency—common after gastric bypass surgery. Absorption is dependent on intrinsic factor produced in the parietal cells of the stomach, and hydrochloric acid is required to cleave vitamin B_{12} from protein foodstuffs in the stomach. Prevalence after Roux-en-Y procedure is estimated at 12% to 33%. Prevention/treatment: oral B_{12} formulations of 350 to 1000 mcg/day or monthly injections of 2000 mcg in those patients who do not respond to the oral supplements.
3. Folate deficiency—less frequent than B_{12} deficiency. Folate absorption occurs preferentially in the proximal intestines, but with adaptation after gastric bypass surgery, absorption can occur throughout the small bowel. Prevention/treatment: 1 mg folate PO/day.
4. Thiamine deficiency—uncommon. Seen with postoperative hyperemesis syndromes. Prevention: 50 to 100 mg IV or IM thiamine at 6 weeks postop in patients with hyperemesis.
5. Zinc—depends on fat absorption. Deficiency observed with malabsorptive surgery. Standard daily supplementation of zinc is recommended after malabsorptive surgery.
6. Selenium deficiency and a life-threatening cardiomyopathy have been reported in patients after malabsorptive surgery. Supplementation of selenium at 40 to 80 mcg/day is recommended in patients undergoing malabsorptive bariatric surgery.
7. Fat-soluble vitamins (A, D, E, K)—malabsorptive bariatric surgery results in a high incidence of vitamin A, D, and K deficiency with altered calcium metabolism (vitamin E, to a lesser extent). Patients undergoing malabsorptive surgery require long-term annual measurements of fat-soluble nutrients. There is no proven regimen for vitamin supplementation after malabsorptive surgery, but lifelong daily supplementation of fat-soluble vitamins has been recommended at the following dosages: 10,000 IU vitamin A; 1200 IU vitamin D; 300 mcg vitamin K, and 1800 mg calcium citrate.

VI. TECHNICAL ASPECTS OF PN PREPARATIONS

A. PN formula preparation is performed **aseptically** in the pharmacy under a laminar flow hood that filters the air, removing airborne particles and microorganisms. PN is especially at risk of contamination because it is a mixture of multiple additives and is an excellent growth medium for microorganisms. An expert committee of the *United States Pharmacopeia* (*USP*) developed Chapter <797>, the first official monograph containing medication standards that must be followed and are enforceable by regulatory agencies concerning the procedures and requirements for pharmacy prepared sterile products. The *USP* Chapter <797> provides evidence-based instructions for pharmacy design, washing, garbing, quality assurance, and personnel training and evaluation to improve compounding practices for sterile products including PN. PN is classified as a medium-risk level compounded sterile product (CSP) when it is prepared from injectable amino acids, dextrose, lipid emulsions, electrolytes, trace elements, and sterile water. When PN is compounded using powdered amino acids, it is classified as a "high-level" CSP because its preparation involves the use of nonsterile ingredients and carries the highest risk for contamination by microbial, chemical, or physical matter. PN solutions prepared for inpatient administration have a beyond-use date of 30 hrs based on storage at room temperature and a medium risk level. In the home care setting, the beyond-use date can be extended to 9 days, but the PN admixture must be stored under refrigeration at 36° to 46°F until use. The 30-hr time limit still applies once PN is initiated.

B. **Compatibility** of the various components of PN formulations is determined by several factors, including their concentration, solution pH, temperature, and the order of admixture. The **most common** compatibility concern is in regard to the addition of calcium and phosphate salts to PN solutions. Dibasic calcium phosphate is very insoluble, whereas monobasic calcium phosphate is relatively soluble. At low pH, a greater amount of monobasic calcium phosphate predominates. The pH of the PN solutions is determined primarily by the concentration and type (brand) of amino acids. PN solutions containing higher concentrations of amino acids have a lower pH that allows for greater solubility of calcium and phosphate. The type (brand) of amino acid solutions commercially available differ in their pH. Thus, the choice of amino acid preparation as well as the concentration of amino acids may allow for more or less calcium and phosphate to be administered in PN solutions. An increase in the temperature of PN solutions increases the dissociation of calcium. This increases the amount of calcium ion available to complex with phosphate and results in a decrease in calcium and phosphate solubility. Therefore, lower PN solution temperatures may allow for a greater amount of calcium and phosphate to be solubilized. The order of calcium and phosphate addition to PN solutions can also affect the solubility of these electrolytes. It is recommended that phosphate be added and diluted in the PN solution prior to the addition of calcium.

C. After admixture of the various components, the PN solution should be **visually inspected** for precipitate or particulate matter. After labeling and final checking, the PN solution should be refrigerated until delivery to the nursing unit.

D. A statistically valid, continuous **sterility testing program** should be an essential component of quality control in preparing PN solutions.

VII. HOME PARENTERAL NUTRITION (HPN).

HPN has become a widely accepted and useful technique for provision of complete nutritional requirements in the home setting. When used appropriately, this modality benefits the patient medically and psychologically, with a decreased cost to the health care system.

A. **Indications** for HPN include SBS, severe IBD, radiation enteritis, enterocutaneous fistulae, and selected malignancies.

B. **Candidate selection** requires a multidisciplinary approach to determine if the patient and family can assume the responsibility and training needed for safe and successful HPN.

C. **Administration.** HPN is infused through a central venous silastic catheter (e.g., Hickman, Broviac), which allows for prolonged PN with low clotting and infection rates. The PN solution is generally infused over a 12- to 15-hr period at night. This type of cycling program allows the patient to be free from the infusion pump during the day, allowing for a more normal lifestyle.

D. **Clinical monitoring** and follow-up are done periodically, depending on the needs of the individual patient. Long-term HPN patients generally are seen by the physician on a monthly basis after initial stabilization.

VIII. MISCELLANEOUS

A. **Soluble fiber** is present in some commercially available EN formulas. This fiber is fermented by normal large intestinal flora to short chain fatty acids that are used by colonocytes as a fuel source. These short chain fatty acids also seem to have a trophic effect on the large intestinal mucosa.

B. **Growth factors.** The use of recombinant human growth hormone, insulin-like growth factor, and anabolic steroids, in combination with nutritional support to improve nitrogen balance and reduce hospital length of stay in select patient populations, is currently under investigation. To date, recombinant growth hormone (Humatrope) is available for nutritional support in children with cystic fibrosis, sickle-cell anemia, and thalassemia and in adults with AIDS-related cachexia. Oxandrolone is a synthetic anabolic steroid with FDA approval for increasing weight gain in patients with chronic infection, major surgery, and severe trauma. It also has established efficacy in alcoholic cirrhosis (improved survival and liver function), burns (improved nitrogen balance, wound healing, and weight gain), and in AIDS cachexia (improved weight gain). Usual dose is 2.5 to 20.0 mg orally (80 mg in alcoholic cirrhosis) in divided doses daily for up to 4 weeks.

Study Questions

Directions: Each of the questions, statements, or incomplete statements in this section can be correctly answered or completed by **one** of the suggested answers or phrases. Choose the **best** answer.

1. A 32-year-old, well-nourished man involved in a motor vehicle accident was admitted to the surgical intensive care unit with multiple long bone fractures and abdominal injuries with no nutritional support for 4 days. This patient is most likely
   (A) suffering from moderate-to-severe kwashiorkor malnutrition.
   (B) at low risk for hospital-acquired infection and other complications.
   (C) not suffering from protein or calorie malnutrition.
   (D) suffering from severe marasmus malnutrition.
   (E) not a candidate for aggressive nutritional support.

2. A patient in the ICU on a ventilator was placed on a glucose system PN formulation providing 2040 kcal/day and 98 g protein/day. A measured energy expenditure (MEE) of 2038 kcal and RQ of 1.1 were subsequently obtained. Which of the following is correct based on this information?
   (A) The patient is receiving adequate glucose calories, and an adjustment in the program is not necessary.
   (B) The daily protein intake has to be decreased to reduce the patient's RQ.
   (C) The PN formulation should be switched to a lipid system formulation to reduce the carbon dioxide load.
   (D) The patient is retaining oxygen from the glucose calories in the PN formulation.
   (E) Lipid emulsion should be added to the current PN formulation to enhance lipogenesis.

3. Total nutrient admixture (TNA)
   (A) is more complicated to administer for home parenteral nutrition patients.
   (B) should be filtered with a 1.2-μ filter.
   (C) consists of glucose, amino acids, electrolytes, and trace minerals mixed in one container.
   (D) is the method recommended by the FDA to administer lipid system PN.
   (E) can be visualized for particulate matter.

4. The calorie requirements of a moderately hypermetabolic hospitalized patient are best estimated by using the
   (A) nomogram method.
   (B) nitrogen balance method.
   (C) (EEE) method.
   (D) PNI.
   (E) SGA method.

5. Lipid system PN
   (A) can be administered by peripheral vein if the glucose concentration is less than 15%.
   (B) requires daily serum triglyceride monitoring.
   (C) is contraindicated in patients with elevated carbon dioxide levels.
   (D) requires daily lipid administration to provide a portion of the patient's nonprotein calorie requirements.
   (E) can be administered with a maximum lipid dosage of 4.5 g/kg/day.

6. Commercial PN formulations for hypermetabolic critically ill patients
   (A) are enriched in branched-chain amino acids and contain low concentrations of aromatic amino acids.
   (B) contain primarily essential amino acids.
   (C) have not demonstrated a positive clinical outcome benefit in this patient population.
   (D) are the preferred PN formulation used in this clinical setting.
   (E) are enriched with arginine to enhance immune function.

7. Which of the following methods of parenteral nutritional support would be most appropriate in a severely protein calorie malnourished patient with acute renal failure?
   (A) 2% amino acid/47% dextrose.
   (B) 4.25% amino acid/25% dextrose.
   (C) 4% essential amino acid/47% dextrose.
   (D) 4.25% amino acid/25% dextrose with dialysis on a regular basis.
   (E) 2% amino acid/47% dextrose/20% lipid emulsion.

8. Which of the following statements regarding the monitoring of nutritional support is true?

(A) Prealbumin is not the optimal marker to follow for short-term nutritional progress.
(B) Transferrin is falsely depressed in patients with iron deficiency.
(C) Albumin is falsely elevated in renal failure.
(D) A positive nitrogen balance of 3 to 6 g of nitrogen daily is optimal.
(E) A weight gain of 1.5 to 2.0 lb/day indicates optimal lean body weight gain.

9. Patients with end-stage liver disease

(A) generally have increased levels of branched-chain amino acids and decreased levels of aromatic amino acids.
(B) should be placed on a low-branched chain, high-aromatic amino acid PN solution.
(C) should not have their protein restricted in the ICU as a clinical management strategy to reduce the risk of developing hepatic encephalopathy.
(D) require glutamine-enriched amino acid solutions.
(E) can tolerate standard glucose system formulations 4.25% amino acid/25% dextrose with regular dialysis.

For questions 10–12: A 67-year-old white female presented to the attending physician with a 3-month history of progressive difficulty swallowing and a 10-kg weight loss. She is currently 160 cm tall and weighs 50 kg. She has just undergone a distal esophagectomy and proximal gastrectomy for distal esophageal cancer. At the time of surgery, she had a feeding jejunostomy tube inserted.

10. The dieticians who are adept at using the Harris-Benedict equation have gone home for the day, and the surgeon calls you for your best guess at what the hourly goal rate for this patient should be using isotonic enteral formula, which provides 0.85 nonprotein calories (NPCs)/mL. Your answer should be

(A) 65 mL/hr.
(B) 75 mL/hr.
(C) 85 mL/hr.
(D) 95 mL/hr.
(E) 50 mL/hr.

11. The enteral formulation the surgeon has selected is enriched with fish oils. He is hoping this additive will

(A) prevent diarrhea.
(B) prevent dermatitis.
(C) prevent hyperglycemia.
(D) improve immune function.
(E) improve neurological function.

12. On the 5th postoperative day, the feeding jejunostomy tube becomes clogged and unusable. The patient will be NPO an additional 5 days to ensure the integrity of her surgical anastomosis. The most appropriate course at this time is

(A) start the patient on a lipid-based peripheral PN program.
(B) keep the patient NPO and without PN support.
(C) have a central venous catheter inserted, and initiate a lipid-based PN program.
(D) start the patient on a glucose-based peripheral PN program.
(E) have a central venous catheter inserted, and start the patient on a high branched-chain amino acid parenteral program.

For questions 13–14: RJ is a 28-year-old pregnant woman. She is in the 9th week of her pregnancy and is diagnosed with hyperemesis gravidarum. Her pregravid weight was 57 kg, and her height is 5 ft., 5 in. She has lost 7 kg (12.3%) during her pregnancy. She was placed on a central glucose PN program.

13. Which one of the following represents the best estimate of her daily caloric requirements?

(A) 1675 kcal
(B) 1790 kcal
(C) 2261 kcal
(D) 2062 kcal
(E) 1925 kcal

14. MVI-12 is used as the parenteral vitamin preparation in the PN formulation. Which of the following vitamin(s) need to be supplemented in the daily PN formulation to meet the daily requirements during pregnancy?

(A) Vitamin K
(B) Thiamine (B_1)
(C) Folic acid
(D) A and C
(E) Pyridoxine (B_6)

For questions 15–17: A 55-year-old male with multiple traumatic injuries and type II diabetes was admitted to the surgical ICU. He was placed on mechanical ventilation and initiated on glucose system PN. After 3 days of PN therapy his blood glucose levels have ranged from 250 to 285 mg/dL over the past 24 hrs with 80 U of insulin/L in his PN formulation. He is on no other insulin supplementation at this time.

15. The nutritional support service recommends an insulin drip with the goal of achieving a blood glucose level of

(A) 180 to 225 mg/dL.
(B) 200 to 215 mg/dL.
(C) 140 to 200 mg/dL.
(D) 65 to 100 mg/dL.
(E) 70 to 105 mg/dL.

16. What parenteral trace mineral therapy may be an effective adjunct if the insulin drip fails to achieve the glucose level goal?

(A) 20 to 40 mg zinc/day
(B) 150 to 200 μg chromium/day
(C) 0.5 to 1.5 mg copper/day
(D) 150 to 400 mcg manganese/day
(E) 40 to 60 μg selenium/day

17. The recommended ACP guideline for management of glucose levels in this patient population has shown that:

(A) The range of optimal glucose level is definitive.
(B) Hyperglycemia results in decreased duration of PN therapy.
(C) Most patients receiving intensive insulin therapy have no reduction in mortality but have a significantly increased risk for severe hypoglycemia.
(D) Length of time on the ventilator is decreased.
(E) A & C.

For questions 18–19: A 35-year-old female with severe morbid obesity (BMI = 51 kg/m^2) of more than 12 years duration and refractory to conventional obesity treatment was entered into a bariatric surgery program. The patient underwent a Roux-en-Y procedure without any major postoperative complications.

18. The patient was readmitted to the hospital 3 months after discharge with intolerance to solid and liquid foods and persistent hyperemesis. She also presented with generalized paresthesia, ataxis, and mental confusion. Which of the following nutrients is most likely deficient in this patient?

(A) Selenium
(B) Vitamin D
(C) Calcium
(D) Thiamine
(E) Vitamin E

19. This patient should be placed on which of the following nutrient supplementations to prevent potential cardiomyopathy?

(A) Folate (1 mg/day)
(B) Vitamin B_{12} (350 to 1000 mcg/day)
(C) Selenium (40 to 80 mcg/day)
(D) Vitamin A (10,000 IU/day)
(E) Vitamin K (300 mcg/day)

For questions 20–22: A pharmacist managing the PN department of an IV home infusion company decided to review all technical aspects of PN preparation with the pharmacy staff in an effort to update procedures and educate pharmacy staff on current standards of PN admixtures.

20. There is some confusion among the staff as to where to obtain the most current document on medication standards for pharmacy prepared sterile products that provides evidence-based instructions for pharmacy design, quality assurance, washing, garbing, and personnel training and evaluation to improve compounding practice for PN admixtures. The most appropriate source to obtain this information is the

(A) ASHP 2015 Initiative.
(B) ASPEN Practice Guidelines.
(C) *USP* Chapter <797> Monograph.
(D) National IV Therapy Association.
(E) FDA Intravenous Compounding Guidelines.

21. In reviewing their procedures for storage of prepared PN admixtures, they found a beyond-use date of 14 days under refrigeration until PN is initiated in the home setting. Based upon the most current standards for pharmacy prepared sterile products, which one of the following is the correct beyond-use date for storage of PN admixtures prepared for home use?

(A) 30 hrs under refrigeration
(B) 3 days under refrigeration
(C) 14 days under refrigeration
(D) 24 hrs at room temperature
(E) 9 days under refrigeration

22. In compounding PN for home patients, there are several patients with SBS for whom physicians are prescribing the addition of the amino acid glutamine to the PN formulation. The pharmacists must use nonsterile glutamine powder to compound these PN formulations. In updating their procedure manual, what would be the risk-level for compounding these specialty PN formulations based on the most current document on medication standards for pharmacy prepared sterile products?

(A) Intermediate-risk level
(B) High-risk level
(C) Low-risk level
(D) Medium-risk level
(E) Minimum-risk level

For questions 23–24: A 28-year-old white male involved in a motor vehicle accident was admitted to the SICU with severe abdominal and head injuries. The patient is fluid restricted because of his head injury and was subsequently placed on a concentrated glucose system PN. His calcium and phosphate serum levels are quite low and because of his fluid restriction, they want to add as much calcium and phosphate to the PN formulation to correct these electrolyte deficiencies.

23. Which of the following strategies would allow for the best calcium and phosphate solubility?
   (A) Use a brand of amino acids that has the lowest pH.
   (B) Calcium should be added and diluted in the PN prior to the addition of phosphate.
   (C) The amino acid concentration should be kept as low as possible.
   (D) The temperature of the PN solution should be kept as high as tolerable.
   (E) The pH of the PN solution should be increased by the addition of 0.1N sodium hydroxide.

24. The form of calcium phosphate that is most soluble in PN solutions is
   (A) dibasic.
   (B) divalent.
   (C) monobasic.
   (D) trivalent.
   (E) tribasic.

Answers and Explanations

1. **The answer is A** *[see I.B.3]*.
A hypermetabolic state (e.g., trauma, infection) combined with protein deprivation can rapidly develop into a severe kwashiorkor malnutrition characterized by hypoalbuminemia, edema, and impaired cellular immune function.

2. **The answer is C** *[see V.D.1]*.
Even in the presence of appropriate amounts of NPCs administered as carbohydrate, the normal carbon dioxide load generated by glycolysis may be excessive for the patient with underlying pulmonary dysfunction. PN lipid system formulations, in which the lipid component constitutes 40% to 50% of the total NPCs, may be beneficial in reducing the ventilatory demands in respiratory failure patients because lipolysis generates less carbon dioxide than glycolysis.

3. **The answer is B** *[see III.A.6.b.(2).(b).(iii)]*.
A particle filter (i.e., 1.2 μ) should be used with TNA administration.

4. **The answer is C** *[see II.B.1]*.
Energy requirements are determined as nonprotein calories by indirect calorimetry, estimated energy expenditure, and the simple nomogram method. The nomogram method is the least accurate method of estimating caloric requirements.

5. **The answer is D** *[see III.A.6.b.(1)]*.
The lipid system PN is a formulation in which lipid is administered daily to provide a substantial portion of the NPCs.

6. **The answer is C** *[see V.C.1]*.
PN formulations enriched in branched-chain amino acids have been made available with the rationale that, being the preferred fuel source in this patient population, it would enhance protein synthesis, decrease protein catabolism, and improve the patient's clinical outcome. However, these more expensive branched-chain amino acid formulations have not been shown to favorably influence clinical outcomes in critically ill patients.

7. **The answer is D** *[see V.B.3]*.
Standard glucose system formulations (4.25% amino acid/25% dextrose) can generally be used in renal failure patients who are being dialyzed on a regular basis. This formulation is particularly useful in severely malnourished patients because it can provide adequate protein to attain positive nitrogen balance, which is not possible with renal failure PN.

8. **The answer is D** *[see II.B.2.a.(4)]*.
A positive nitrogen balance of 3 to 6 g is the goal.

9. **The answer is C** *[see V.C.3]*.
Protein requirements in ICU patients should not be restricted as a clinical management strategy to reduce the risk of developing hepatic encephalopathy.

10. **The answer is B** *[see II.B.1.c]*.
Use the nomogram of 30 kcal/kg to determine the NPCs/day, and divide that by the NPCs/mL of the enteral formula to determine the volume of formula per day, which is divided by 24 hrs to yield the hourly goal rate.

11. **The answer is D** *[see V.A.5]*.
Omega-3 polyunsaturated fatty acids are derived from fish oils and are currently found in some enteral formulations. These fatty acids have been shown experimentally to enhance immune response.

12. **The answer is A** *[see III.A.3.b]*.
With the use of new catheter technology and new techniques for infusion, it is now feasible to administer peripheral PN in selected patients for short-term therapy (7 to 10 days) with a low incidence of peripheral vein thrombophlebitis. This method of PN administration avoids the potential of more serious complications associated with central venous route administration.

13. **The answer is A** *[see V.I]*.
The estimated basal energy expenditure is calculated using the pregravid weight in the Harris-Benedict equation. An additional 300 kcal/day is added to the basal energy expenditure to provide the required calories per day during pregnancy.

14. **The answer is A** *[see V.I.3]*.
An additional 65 μg of vitamin K needs to be added to the daily PN formulation when MVI-12 is used as the parenteral vitamin preparation to meet the daily requirements during pregnancy.

15. **The answer is C** *[see V.H.2]*.
ACP recommends a target blood glucose level of 140 to 200 mg/dL if insulin therapy is used in SICU/MICU patients

16. **The answer is B** *[see II.B.5.g]*.
Suggested IV requirements of chromium for deficiency and severe glucose intolerance are 150 to 200 μg/day.

17. **The answer is C** *[see V.H.3.c]*.
A few studies show that IIT improves mortality, whereas most have shown that patients who receive IIT have no reduction in mortality and have a significantly increased risk for severe hypoglycemia.

18. **The answer is D** *[see V.L.4]*.
Thiamine deficiency is not common after bariatric surgery but is seen in patients with postoperative hyperemesis syndromes.

19. **The answer is C** *[see V.L.6]*.
Selenium deficiency and a life-threatening cardiomyopathy have been reported in patients after malabsorptive surgery. Supplementation of selenium at 40 to 80 mcg/day is recommended in patients undergoing malabsorptive surgery.

20. **The answer is C** *[see VI.A]*.
The *USP* Chapter <797> provides evidence-based instructions for pharmacy design, washing, garbing, quality assurance, and personnel training and evaluation to improve compounding practices for sterile products, including PN.

21. **The answer is E** *[see VI.A]*.
In the home care setting, the beyond-use date can be extended to 9 days, but the PN admixture must be stored under refrigeration at 36° to 46° F until use.

22. **The answer is B** *[see VI.A]*.
When PN is compounded using powdered amino acids, it is classified as a "high-level" CSP because its preparation involves the use of nonsterile ingredients and carries the highest risk for contamination by microbial, chemical, or physical matter.

23. **The answer is A** *[see VI.B]*.
The pH of the PN solutions is determined primarily by the concentration and type (brand) of amino acids. PN solutions containing higher concentrations of amino acids have a lower pH that allows for greater solubility of calcium and phosphate. The type (brand) of amino acid solutions commercially available differ in their pH.

24. **The answer is C** *[see VI.B]*.
Dibasic calcium phosphate is very insoluble, whereas monobasic calcium phosphate is relatively soluble.

53 Immunosuppressive Agents in Organ Transplantation

DAVID I. MIN

I. ORGAN TRANSPLANTATION

A. **Definition.** Replacement of a diseased vital organ with a viable organ from a living or deceased donor. Solid organ transplantation has become the therapy of choice for many patients with end-organ failure (i.e., heart, liver, lung, and kidney disease). However, it generally requires immunosuppression to overcome the immunological barrier between donor and recipient, except in syngeneic (i.e., identical twins) or autologous transplantation.

B. **Classification**

1. **Solid organ transplantation**
    a. **Life-saving transplantation** (e.g., heart, heart–lung, lung, and liver transplantation). There is no alternative life-sustaining method available.
    b. **Non–life-saving transplantation** (i.e., kidney, pancreas, face, hand, and cornea transplantation). There are alternative life-sustaining methods available, such as dialysis or external insulin injection. In these cases, transplantation will improve the patient's quality of life or long-term survival significantly.
2. **Hematopoietic stem cell (bone marrow) transplantation** is used mainly for hematological malignancy or aplastic anemia.

II. GRAFT REJECTION

A. **Transplant immunology** (see *Chapter 56*)

1. **Graft rejection.** The body's immune system recognizes the allograft (transplanted organ) as a foreign antigen, and it initiates the immune response to remove or destroy the transplanted graft. This reaction is called "rejection." The degree of the reaction depends on the genetic similarities or differences between the organ of the donor and the immune system of the recipient.
2. **Histocompatibility.** The antigen determining the compatibility between the donor and the recipient is called a **histocompatibility antigen**, the gene being located on chromosome 6. In many transplants (e.g., bone marrow or kidney transplant), this histocompatibility matching is an important factor for determining the long-term survival of the graft. However, more selective, potent immunosuppression may alleviate the importance of tissue matching between donor and recipient (exception: in hematopoietic stem cell transplantation, the tissue matching is still important).
3. **Other factors.** Another group of substances that also plays an important role is the **ABO blood group system** of red blood cells. The donor and recipient must be ABO-compatible; otherwise, immediate graft destruction occurs. Some patients may have preformed antibody for unspecified donors because of multiple blood transfusions or other reason. In this case, patients may destroy the transplanted organ immediately. To detect the preformed antibody, the recipient's serum will be tested immediately before the transplantation (cross-match).

B. **Types of graft rejection**

1. **Types of graft rejection according to the time course**

a. **Hyperacute rejection.** Immediate destruction (within minutes or hours) of the transplant organ by a preformed antibody or complement system. Today, this is extremely rare. It occurs only in an ABO-mismatched organ or a cross-match positive (preformed antibody) organ. There is no adequate treatment available.

b. **Acute rejection** occurs within a few days to several months after transplantation. It is mediated mainly by T lymphocyte (acute cellular rejection), but occasionally, it is mediated by antibody (antibody-mediated rejection) and this rejection can be reversible by steroids or antibody therapy such as muromonab/CD3 or antithymocyte globulin (acute cellular rejection) or intravenous immunoglobulin (IVIG; antibody-mediated rejection).

c. **Chronic rejection** occurs several months to several years after transplantation. The exact mechanism of this reaction is unknown, but it is thought to be mediated by B lymphocyte (antibody), and there is no adequate treatment available.

2. **Graft versus host, host versus graft.** In most solid organ transplants, rejection occurs as the host immune system rejects or attacks the transplant organ (host vs. graft). However, in hematopoietic stem cell (bone marrow) transplant, the host is generally immune deficient and the transplanted graft is immune competent and attacks host tissues (graft vs. host).

III. PROPHYLAXIS AND TREATMENT OF GRAFT REJECTION (*Table 53-1*)

A. **Calcineurin inhibitors**

1. **Cyclosporine (Neoral®, Sandimmune®, Gengraf®, others)**

a. **Mechanism of action.** Cyclosporine binds an intracellular receptor, cyclophilin. This complex inhibits calcineurin, an intracellular phosphatase that involves activation of the promoter region for the gene-encoding cytokine, such as interleukin-2. This results in inhibiting T-cell activation in the early stage of immune response to a foreign antigen such as a graft.

b. **Dosing and monitoring.** Cyclosporine pharmacokinetics is unpredictable, and many factors such as age, time after transplant, different oral formulation (Neoral® or Sandimmune®), or drugs affect it. Oral bioavailability is about 30%. Generally, 8 mg/kg/day of oral cyclosporine as two divided doses is used in solid organ transplantation and adjusted according to the blood levels. Serum creatinine should be monitored with the blood levels of cyclosporine. The blood levels are useful in the clinical monitoring.

c. **Side effects. Nephrotoxicity** is the major side effect. Neurotoxicity and hepatotoxicity are also common. Hirsutism and gingival hyperplasia are also cumbersome side effects. Numerous drug interactions have been reported (*Table 53-2*).

2. **Tacrolimus (Prograf®, and generics)**

a. **Mechanism of action.** It is very similar to cyclosporine (*III.A.1.a*).

b. **Dosing and monitoring.** Tacrolimus pharmacokinetics is also variable, and oral bioavailability is about 25%. Blood levels are useful in clinical monitoring.

c. **Side effects. Nephrotoxicity** is the major side effect. Neurotoxicity and posttransplant diabetes are more common than with cyclosporine. Hair loss is also a common side effect.

B. **Antimetabolites**

1. **Azathioprine (Imuran®)**

a. **Mechanism of action.** It is converted to 6-mercaptopurine in the body and is a non-specific purine synthesis inhibitor. It interferes with DNA and RNA synthesis so that it may reduce both cell-mediated and humoral immune responses.

b. **Dosage and monitoring.** An initial dose of 3 to 5 mg/kg/day is administered preoperatively. Immediately after transplantation, the dose is usually tapered to a maintenance dose of 1 to 3 mg/kg/day or titrated to the patient's white blood cell (WBC) count. The WBC count is generally maintained greater than 3000/mm^3.

c. **Side effects. Bone marrow suppression** (leukopenia, thrombocytopenia) is the major side effect. In addition, a xanthine oxidase inhibitor, allopurinol, inhibits azathioprine metabolism. When these drugs are used concurrently, the azathioprine dose should be reduced by 80%. Otherwise, the patient may develop severe leukopenia due to azathioprine overdose.

Table 53-1 CURRENT IMMUNOSUPPRESSIVE AGENTS USED IN ORGAN TRANSPLANTATION

Classification	Drug	Usual Initial Dose	Major Side Effects	Monitoring
Calcineurin inhibitors	Cyclosporine (Neoral, Sandimmune, Gengraf)	10 mg/kg/day	Nephrotoxicity	Blood concentrations and serum creatinine concentrations monitoring
	Tacrolimus (Prograf and others)	0.1–0.3 mg/kg/day	Neurotoxicity	
Antimetabolites	Azathioprine (Imuran)	1.5–3.0 mg/kg/day	Bone marrow suppression	WBC count monitoring
	Mycophenolate mofetil (CellCept)	1 g twice daily	Bone marrow suppression and GI side effects	WBC monitoring and GI symptoms
	Mycophenolate sodium (Myfortic)	720 mg twice daily	Same as above	Same as above
	Methotrexate	15 mg/m^2 on day 1; 10 mg/m^2/day on days 3, 6, and 11	Same as above	Same as above
mTOR inhibitor	Sirolimus (Rapamune)	6–15 mg loading dose and 2–5 mg once daily	Hyperlipidemia, leukopenia, and thrombocytopenia	Blood trough concentrations and WBC, platelet, and lipid profile monitoring
	Everolimus (Zortress)	0.75 mg twice daily	Same as above	Blood trough concentrations and WBC, platelet, and lipid profile monitoring
Alkylating agent	Cyclophosphamide (various)	3–4 mg/kg/day for 4 days, followed by reduction to 1 mg/kg/day for treatment of rejection	Hemorrhagic cystitis	WBC count
Antibody products	Thymoglobulin	1.5 mg/kg/day for 7–14 days	Leukopenia and thrombocytopenia	T-cell count
	Antithymocyte globulin (Atgam)	15–20 mg/kg/day for 7–14 days	Same as above	Same as above
	Basiliximab (Simulect)	For adults, two doses of 20 mg each (day 0 and day 4)	No significant side effects reported	No special monitoring required
Corticosteroids	Prednisone (Deltasone or others) or methylprednisolone (Solumedrol)	500 mg IV on the day of surgery and rapidly tapering to 10 mg daily at 1 month	Fluid retention, psychosis, cataracts, osteonecrosis	Signs and symptoms

GI, gastrointestinal; *IV*, intravenous; *mTOR*, mammalian target of rapamycin; *WBC*, white blood cell.

Table 53-2 MAJOR DRUG INTERACTIONS OF CYCLOSPORINE, TACROLIMUS, SIROLIMUS, OR EVEROLIMUS WITH OTHER DRUGS AND THEIR MANAGEMENT

Drugs	Mechanism	Effects	Management
Antiepileptic drugs Phenytoin Phenobarbital Carbamazepine	Increased metabolism by inducing cytochrome P450 enzyme	Cyclosporine or tacrolimus trough levels drop within 48 hrs after initiation of these drugs	Increase cyclosporine dose or tacrolimus with frequent monitoring of blood levels
Rifampin or isoniazid	Same as above	Same as above	Same as above
Azole antifungal agents Ketoconazole Fluconazole Itraconazole	Inhibition of liver cytochrome P450 enzyme by these drugs	Significant increase of cyclosporine or tacrolimus levels	Reduce cyclosporine or tacrolimus dose with frequent monitoring of levels
Macrolide antibiotics Erythromycin	Inhibition of liver and GI cytochrome P450 enzyme	Increase AUC (× 2) and cyclosporine or tacrolimus trough levels (× 2–3)	Same as above
Calcium-channel blockers Verapamil Diltiazem Nicardipine	Same as above	Same as above	Reduce cyclosporine or tacrolimus dose or use nifedipine, isradipine
Antiviral agents Indinavir Ritonavir Saquinavir	Same as above	Same as above	Reduce cyclosporine or tacrolimus dose or use nifedipine, isradipine
Grapefruit juice	Inhibition of GI cytochrome P450 enzyme	Increase AUC and peak concentrations of cyclosporine and possibly tacrolimus and increase variability of blood levels	Avoid grapefruit juice

AUC, area under the curve, *G.I.*,gastrointestinal.

2. **Mycophenolic acid (CellCept® and generics, Myfortic®)**
   a. **Mechanism of action.** Two forms are available. Mycophenolate mofetil (CellCept®) is a prodrug that is converted to mycophenolic acid in the body, which is the active form. Myfortic® is an enteric formulation of mycophenolic acid. In the body, mycophenolic acid inhibits *de novo* purine synthesis pathway by inhibiting inosine monophosphate dehydrogenase. As a result, it inhibits DNA and RNA synthesis in immune cells such as lymphocytes.
   b. **Dosing and monitoring.** A dose of 2 g/day (CellCept®) or 1440 mg/day (Myfortic®) is administered as two divided doses. The WBC and GI symptoms should be monitored.
   c. **Side effects. Bone marrow suppression** (leukopenia, thrombocytopenia) is the major side effect, as in azathioprine. In addition, GI side effects such as nausea, gastric pain, or diarrhea are more common than with azathioprine.
3. **Methotrexate.** This agent is used mainly in autoimmune disease and preventing graft versus host disease in hematopoietic stem cell transplant patients.
   a. **Mechanism of action.** It prevents dihydrofolic acid from converting to tetrahydrofolic acid by inhibiting the enzyme dihydrofolate reductase. As a result, DNA and protein synthesis are inhibited.
   b. **Dosing and monitoring.** Dosage regimens in BMT patients usually consist of 15 mg/m^2/day on day 1 after transplant and 10 mg/m^2/day on days 3, 6, and 11 with other agents such as cyclosporine.
   c. **Side effects. Bone marrow suppression** (leukopenia, thrombocytopenia) is the major side effect as in azathioprine. In addition, diarrhea and mucositis are common.

C. **mTOR (mammarian Target of Rapamycin) inhibitors** are specific for inhibiting a kinase called mammarian target of rapamycin, resulting in halting cell proliferation.
   1. **Sirolimus (Rapamune®)**
      a. **Mechanism of action.** Sirolimus binds intracellular receptor, FKBP-12 (FK binding protein-12). This complex inhibits the mTOR, which is a key regulatory kinase. This results

in inhibiting T-cell activation in a later stage of immune response to foreign antigens, such as a graft.

b. **Dosing and monitoring.** A dose of 2 to 10 mg/day is administered as a once-daily dose. Usually, a loading dose of 6 to 15 mg with a maintenance dose of 2 to 5 mg once daily is used. Blood levels are useful in clinical monitoring. The serum lipid profile, WBC count, and GI symptoms should be monitored.

c. **Side effects. Hyperlipidemia** is the major side effect. In addition, leukopenia, thrombocytopenia, and GI side effects are common.

2. **Everolimus (Zortress®)**

a. **Mechanism of action.** Similar to sirolimus, but it has a short half-life.

b. **Dosing and monitoring.** A dose of 1.5 mg/day is administered as two divided doses. Usually, without loading dose, 0.75 mg twice daily is given and after 4 to 5 days, the dose should be adjusted according to the blood levels. Blood levels are useful in clinical monitoring and 3 to 8 ng/mL of trough level is a therapeutic target. The serum lipid profile, WBC count, and GI symptoms should be monitored.

c. **Side effects. Hyperlipidemia** is the major side effect. In addition, anemia, leukopenia, thrombocytopenia, and GI side effects are common.

D. **Alkylating agent. Cyclophosphamide** is the alkylating agent mainly used for hematopoietic stem cell transplant patients. Rarely, it is used as a substitute agent for azathioprine in solid organ transplantation.

1. **Mechanism of action.** It is converted to the active metabolite, phosphoramide mustard in the liver, which inhibits the cross-linking of DNA, leading to cell death.

2. **Dosing and monitoring.** Doses of cyclophosphamide up to 3 to 4 mg/kg/day for 4 days followed by a reduction to 1 mg/kg/day to treat graft rejection. The dosage should be titrated to maintain a WBC count greater than 4000/mm^3.

3. **Side effects. Hemorrhagic cystitis** and **bone marrow suppression** (leukopenia, thrombocytopenia). In addition, nausea, vomiting, and diarrhea are common.

E. **Antibody products**

1. **Antithymocyte globulin (Thymoglobulin®, Atgam®)**

a. **Mechanism of action.** It is a purified polyclonal immunoglobulin from rabbits (Thymoglobulin®) or horses (Atgam®) that binds to the human T cells. However, it may have cross-reactivity against the red blood cells, platelets, and granulocytes.

b. **Dosing and monitoring.** The dosage is 1.5 mg/kg (Thymoglobulin®) or 15 to 20 mg/kg (Atgam®) infusion daily through a central line for 7 to 14 days for prevention or treatment of rejection. The T-lymphocyte counts are monitored and maintained less than 100/mm^3. Generally, premedications such as acetaminophen, diphenhydramine, and corticosteroid are required to reduce the infusion-related side effects (e.g., fever, chills). For the infusion of these drugs, the central venous line is a preferred route, rather than a peripheral vein.

c. **Side effects.** Antithymocyte globulin may cause fever, chills, erythema, leukopenia, thrombocytopenia, and anaphylactic reaction or serum sickness.

2. **Basiliximab (Simulect®)**

a. **Mechanism of action.** It is a chimeric (murine/human) monoclonal antibody (IgG1), produced by recombinant DNA technology, that binds to block the interleukin-2 receptor on the surface of activated T lymphocytes, and as a result, it prevents T-lymphocyte activation, thus preventing acute rejections.

b. **Dosing and monitoring.** It is indicated only for the prevention of acute rejection. The usual recommended dosage for the adult patient is two doses of 20 mg each at day 0 and day 4 after kidney transplantation. No special monitoring is required.

c. **Side effects.** Based on results of clinical trials, no cytokine release syndromes have been noticed.

3. **Other antibody agents**

Alemtuzumab (Campath®) or rituximab (Rituxan®) are indicated for hematologic malignancy and not approved for the organ transplantation, but are occasionally used in the organ transplantation for prevention of acute rejection or intractable antibody-mediated rejection.

F. **Corticosteroids. Prednisone** (Deltasone®) and **methylprednisolone** (Solumedrol®) are the major corticosteroid products used for transplant patients.

1. **Mechanisms of action.** Corticosteroids have multiple pharmacological effects in various cells. Corticosteroids bind with intracellular glucocorticoid receptors, which results in altering DNA

and RNA translation. As a result, corticosteroids cause a rapid and profound drop in circulating T lymphocytes. They have potent anti-inflammatory effects by inhibiting arachidonic acid release and macrophage phagocytosis.

2. **Dosing and monitoring.** They are used in both preventing and treating graft rejection and acute graft versus host disease. In general, prophylactic doses in solid organ transplantation are in the range of 1 to 2 mg/kg/day and tapered over months to 0.1 to 0.3 mg/kg/day. In the case of treatment, the dosage is 500 mg of methylprednisolone IV for 3 to 5 days or 1 to 2 mg/kg/day of oral prednisone, which should be tapered rapidly.
3. **Side effects.** In the long-term, corticosteroids cause more troubling side effects. They include psychological disturbances (i.e., euphoria, depression), adrenal axis suppression, hypertension, sodium and water retention, myopathy, impaired wound healing, increased appetite, osteoporosis, hyperglycemia, and cataracts.

IV. COMPLICATIONS OF IMMUNOSUPPRESSION

A. **Infections**

1. **Risk.** Transplant patients have a high risk of acquiring an infection due to patient factors such as diabetes mellitus, hepatitis, or uremia. In addition, immunosuppressive agents can cause various effects, such as leukopenia, lymphopenia, or T-cell dysfunction, that inhibit adequate immune response to the infection.
2. **Time course.** The risk of infection is greatest during the first 3 months after transplantation, when higher doses of immunosuppression are used, and again after a rejection episode is treated. This risk correlates with the overall level of immunosuppression.
3. **Types of infections** include bacterial, fungal, viral, and protozoan.
4. **Prevention**
   a. **Trimethoprim-sulfamethoxazole** (Bactrim® and others). One single- or double-strength tablet daily for 6 months significantly reduces *Pneumocystis carinii* pneumonia and bacterial urinary tract infection. After 6 months, three times a week is effective.
   b. **Herpes and cytomegalovirus (CMV) infection.** Oral acyclovir (200 mg b.i.d. for normal renal function, with doses adjusted according to renal function) for herpes prophylaxis. For CMV prophylaxis, various prophylaxes can be used. High doses of acyclovir (800 mg q.i.d for normal renal function, with doses adjusted according to renal function), valganciclovir (Valcyte®) 450 mg to 900 mg daily, or high-titer CMV immunoglobulin are effective in reducing the incidence of CMV infection and invasive CMV disease.
   c. **Polyoma virus infection.** In kidney transplant patients, polyoma virus infections such as BK virus nephropathy can be an important cause of kidney dysfunction or graft loss after transplantation. In many cases, reactivation of polyomavirus after transplantation causes kidney dysfunction and reduction of immunosuppression and leflunomide (Arava®) therapy shows some effectiveness.
   d. **Nystatin solution, clotrimazole troche, or fluconazole** reduces oral candidiasis (thrush).

B. **Increased risk of malignancy**

1. **Cause.** Continuous immunosuppression interferes with normal immune surveillance and function for malignancy. In addition, some of the immunosuppressive drugs may be directly carcinogenic or activate oncogenic virus, such as Epstein–Barr virus (EBV).
2. **Characteristics.** Cancers that occur most frequently in the general population (e.g., lung, breast, colon) are not increased among transplant patients. However, various cancers uncommon in the general population are often more prevalent in transplant patients: lymphomas, squamous cell carcinomas of the lip and skin, Kaposi's sarcoma, and other sarcoma.
3. **Posttransplant lymphoproliferative diseases (PTLDs).** The incidence of lymphoma appears to correlate with the intensity of immunosuppression. It is especially well documented that T-cell specific agents, including OKT3, cyclosporine, and tacrolimus, increase the incidence of lymphoproliferative diseases.
4. **Treatment.** In case of nonvital organ transplant, immunosuppression should be reduced or stopped. If EBV-related lymphoma occurs, acyclovir or ganciclovir therapy appears to be effective; the B-cell–specific monoclonal antibody, rituximab (Rituxan®), is also used.

C. Hypertension. Many immunosuppressive agents cause hypertension. Cyclosporine and tacrolimus clearly increase the arterial blood pressure, and steroids may exacerbate hypertension after transplantation from fluid and sodium retention. Treatment usually requires the use of multiple agents, including diuretics and calcium-channel blockers.

D. Posttransplant diabetes mellitus. Many immunosuppressive agents increase blood glucose levels. Corticosteroids, cyclosporine, and tacrolimus increase blood glucose. Some patients develop a new onset of diabetes after transplantation, which increases morbidity and mortality and reduces graft and patient survivals. Careful monitoring of blood glucose and patient counseling are essential.

Study Questions

Directions: Each of the numbered items 1–6 is based on the case. The remaining questions (7–10) are based on the statement, not based on the case. Select the **one** lettered answer or completion that is **best** in each question.

Case: A 28-year-old white female patient was admitted to the hospital for a kidney transplant from a deceased donor who had died 12 hrs earlier. She had a history of type I diabetes mellitus since 8 years old. She started chronic hemodialysis 2 years ago. She was blood typed and the final cross-match was negative. She underwent a successful renal transplant.

Lab at admission: Na 130 mEq/L (135–145), K 5.1 mEq/L (3.5–5.0), Cl 99 mEq/L (98–110), CO_2 18 mEq/L (22–28), Cr 9.5 mg/dL (0.8–1.2), BUN 65 mg/dL (5–15), hemoglobin 9.5 gm/dL (13–15), and glucose 185 mg/dL (60–100).

Virus serology: CMV and EBV titer negative and donor positive for CMV and EBV, Hepatitis A, B, & C serology negative.

Vital signs: BP 150/90 mm Hg, pulse 65/min, RR 12/min, Temp. 98.6°F.

Physical exam: Pale, slightly edematous.

Allergy: no known allergy

Medications on admission: Human NPH/regular insulin, 35/10 units in the morning and 10/5 units in the evening; calcium carbonate 1250 mg t.i.d., calcitriol 0.5 mcg orally daily, enalapril 5 mg b.i.d., metoclopramide 10 mg q.i.d., and erythropoietin 10,000 units sq per week

1. The patient received Simulect® with cyclosporine, mycophenolate, and prednisone. The nurse asked about Simulect®. Which of the following is an appropriate response?

(A) Simulect® is useful, but patient's weight gain should be less than 3% from the dry weight before therapy.
(B) Simulect® is useful agent to treat rejection, but chest x-ray and monitoring of patient's fluid status are required before this therapy.
(C) Simulect® is a chimeric IgG with specificity against IL-2 receptor, and it is useful for prevention acute cellular rejection.
(D) Simulect® is a humanized IgG product against IL-2 receptor, and it is useful in preventing acute humeral rejection.
(E) Simulect® is a rabbit serum against human T cells, and it is useful for prevention and treatment of rejection.

2. On day 7, her serum creatinine was 1.4 mg/dL and BUN 28 mg/dL. Her urine output was excellent and her blood cyclosporine level was 250 ng/mL (200–300). She was discharged to her home. Several days later, she developed a worsening hypertension of 170/105 mm Hg. Which of the following medication(s) she is taking worsened her hypertension?

I. Cyclosporine
II. Prednisone
III. Mycophenolate

(A) **I** only
(B) **III** only
(C) **I** and **II**
(D) **II** and **III**
(E) **I, II,** and **III**

3. Due to her worsening hypertension, her local physician wants to start Cardizem® CD 240 mg daily. What is your advice for this hypertension therapy?

(A) Cardizem® CD will decrease cyclosporine metabolism, so please reduce the cyclosporine dose by 25% and check cyclosporine level twice a week.
(B) Cardizem® CD will decrease cyclosporine metabolism, so please increase cyclosporine dose by 25% and check cyclosporine level twice a week.
(C) Cardizem® CD will increase cyclosporine metabolism, so please switch cyclosporine to tacrolimus.
(D) Cardizem® CD will decrease cyclosporine metabolism, so please switch cyclosporine to tacrolimus.
(E) Cardizem® CD will increase cyclosporine metabolism, so please switch cyclosporine to azathioprine.

4. Which of the following is most appropriate regarding prophylactic regimen for her infections?

I. Co-trimoxazole s.s. daily for PCP prophylaxis
II. Nystatin for prophylaxis of fungal infection
III. Valcyte® for CMV disease

(A) I only
(B) III only
(C) I and II
(D) II and III
(E) I, II, and III

5. Which of the following is correct regarding Myfortic®?

I. It is an enteric-coated formulation of mycophenolic acid.
II. Its major side effect is leukopenia.
III. It causes severe hyperlipidemia.

(A) I only
(B) III only
(C) I and II
(D) II and III
(E) I, II, and III

6. The patient's urine output decreased, her creatinine rose to 2.2 mg/dL (baseline: 1.4 mg/dL) and her feet had +2 edema. Her cyclosporine dose was 150 mg twice daily and her trough level was 450 ng/mL (200 to 300). She felt shaky and subsequent physical exam revealed a mild hand tremor. Acute rejection was ruled out by kidney biopsy. Which of the following is the appropriate adjustment of her immunosuppression?

(A) Increase cyclosporine dose to 175 mg b.i.d. and prednisone 10 mg q.d.
(B) Reduce cyclosporine dose to 125 mg b.i.d. and monitor cyclosporine trough level.
(C) Increase prednisone from 10 mg to 20 mg daily.
(D) Switch cyclosporine to tacrolimus.
(E) Stop cyclosporine and start thymoglobulin.

End of the case

7. A 38-year-old woman came to your clinic and complained of hair loss and did not want to take an immunosuppressant anymore. Which of the following is an appropriate advice for her problem?

(A) Switch mycophenolate mofetil to sirolimus
(B) Stop her prednisone and add methylprednisolone
(C) Switch her tacrolimus to cyclosporine
(D) Switch her mycophenolate mofetil to Myfortic
(E) Add azathioprine to her regimen

8. Which of the following is *not* a side effect of corticosteroid therapy?

(A) Osteoporosis
(B) Leukopenia
(C) Moon faces
(D) Poor wound healing
(E) Hypercalcemia

9. Which of the following is likely to decrease tacrolimus blood concentration when it is used concomitantly?

(A) Grapefruit juice
(B) Erythromycin
(C) St. John's wort
(D) Voriconazole
(E) Verapamil

Answers and Explanations

1. The answer is C *[see III.E.2]*.
Simulect® (basiliximab) is a chimeric monoclonal antibody against the Interleukin-2 receptor. This drug can be used as prevention of an acute cellular rejection. The dose for rejection treatment is 20 mg on day 0 and day 4. It occasionally causes mild fever, but it does not cause any serious side effects. (A) Orthoclone (OK3) requires < 3% weight gain. (B) Simulect® does not require for monitoring fluid status by x-ray. (D) Simulect® does not prevent acute humeral rejection. (E) Simulect® is used only for prevention of rejection, not for the treatment of rejection.

2. **The answer is C** *[see III.A.1; III.F]*.
Cyclosporine and prednisone increase the blood pressure. Cyclosporine (Neoral®) promotes the vasoconstriction and causes renal dysfunction, which contributes to hypertension. Prednisone (Deltasone®) increases fluid and sodium retention, which contributes to hypertension. Mycophenolate mofetil (CellCept®) is an antimetabolite inhibiting DNA synthesis and cell proliferation. Its side effects include leukopenia and thrombocytopenia, and it does not cause hypertension.

3. **The answer is C** *[see Table 53-2]*.
Cardizem® CD (diltiazem) CD is a cytochrome P450 enzyme inhibitor that decreases cyclosporine metabolism. When cyclosporine is used concurrently with diltiazem, it is necessary to decrease cyclosporine dose by 25% in order to prevent the toxicity. Frequent monitoring of cyclosporine blood levels and the cyclosporine dose adjustment should be made based on the blood levels.

4. **The answer is E** *[see IV.A]*.
All of these drugs are required for posttransplant infection prophylaxis. Co-trimoxazole (Bactrim) single strength (s.s.) once daily for pneumonitis jirovecci, nystatin 5 mL swish and swallow four times daily for fungal infection, and valganciclovir (Valcyte) 450 to 900 mg daily for CMV are important prophylactic regimen.

5. **The answer is C** *[see III.B.2.a]*.
Myfortic® is an enteric-coated formulation of mycophenolate sodium that inhibits inosine monophosphate dehydrogenase. Its major side effects include gastrointestinal side effects (e.g., nausea, vomiting, or diarrhea) and leukopenia. It does not cause hyperlipidemia, but sirolimus does.

6. **The answer is B** *[see III.A.1]*.
This is a typical symptom of cyclosporine toxicity, which is confirmed by her high blood level (therapeutic level, 200 to 300 ng/mL) with tremor, acute renal dysfunction (serum creatinine 2.2 mg/dL from baseline 1.4 mg/dL), and +2 edema. The dose of cyclosporine should be reduced by 25 mg (There are 25 mg and 100 mg capsules), and the blood levels as well as signs and symptoms should be closely monitored.

7. **The answer is C** *[see III.A.2]*.
Tacrolimus causes alopecia (hair loss) and cyclosporine causes hirsutism.

8. **The answer is E** *[see III.F]*.
All of the above are side effects of corticosteroid therapy except hypercalcemia. The corticosteroid use causes calcium loss by kidney resulting in hypocalcemia.

9. **The answer is C** *[see Table 53-2]*.
All of the above except St. John's wort are CYP3A inhibitors, which increase tacrolimus blood concentrations. St. John's wort is a CYP3A inducer, which decreases tacrolimus levels.

54

Outcomes Research and Pharmacoeconomics

ALAN H. MUTNICK

I. GENERAL CONCEPTS

A. **Outcomes research (OR)** is used to describe the study of health care interventions (treatment modalities such as drug therapies, surgery, and palliative therapy), care delivery processes, and health care quality that are evaluated to measure the extent to which optimal and desirable outcomes can be reached. Generally speaking, OR is research: it evaluates effectiveness as compared to efficacy; utilizes observational studies that balance generalizability with confounding/bias; is used to supplement rather than replace randomized, controlled clinical trials; and is more extensive than "pharmacoeconomics."

1. The **Economic, Clinical, Humanistic Outcome (ECHO) model** provides a framework for comprehensive evaluation of outcomes. Three areas of outcomes identified by Kozma and Reeder (1998) are economic outcomes, clinical outcomes, and humanistic outcomes.
2. **Outcomes research methodologies** include retrospective chart review, prospective clinical trials, meta-analysis, observational studies, and computer modeling studies.
3. **Examples of outcomes measures**
   a. **Economic outcomes** include acquisition costs associated with care, labor costs associated with care, costs to treat adverse drug reactions, costs of treatment failure, costs of hospital readmission, and costs of emergency room and clinic visits.
   b. **Clinical outcomes** include length of hospital stay, adverse drug reactions, hospital readmission costs, emergency room/clinic costs, and death.
   c. **Humanistic outcomes** include patient satisfaction, functional status as measured by a validated instrument, and quality-of-life assessment.

B. **Pharmacoeconomics (PE)**, a division of health economics, is designed to provide decision makers with information about the value of the different pharmacotherapies. Pharmacoeconomics balances the costs with the consequences or outcomes of pharmaceutical therapies and services.

II. COST

A. **Definitions**

1. **Total cost.** All expenses directly and indirectly necessary to provide a product or service
2. **Average cost.** The average cost per unit of output (total cost divided by quantity)
3. **Fixed cost.** Costs that do not vary with the quantity of output for a short-run production (e.g., rent, fixtures, fixed salary, depreciation, administrative costs)
4. **Variable cost.** Costs that vary with the level of output (e.g., wages, supplies)
5. **Marginal cost.** The extra cost of producing *one extra* unit of output
6. **Incremental cost.** Additional costs when comparing one alternative to another

7. **Direct cost.** Costs directly related to producing/providing a specific quantity of services or output (e.g., salary, drug cost, supply cost for the provision of pharmacy services)
8. **Indirect cost.** Costs that are allocated to the area(s) that produce/provide a specific quantity of services or output (e.g., overhead cost)
9. **Allowable cost.** A cost that is eligible to claim for purposes of reimbursement as necessary and relevant to the delivery of a unit of output
10. **Opportunity cost.** The cost of the benefit of pursuing an alternative course of action
11. **Operating cost.** Any cost that supports the operations to provide the output

B. **Cost and charge**

1. The meaning of the term *cost* depends on the perspective for the analysis. The following examples show differing perspectives.
2. Providers may include hospitals, physician offices, or ambulatory surgery centers, and the term *cost* means the total costs for providing the specific service(s).
3. Payors may include third-party providers such as insurance companies, Medicare, or Medicaid, and the term *cost* means the price that they have to pay to obtain the service (i.e., charges by providers).
4. Charges do not equal the payment to providers. Depending on the contractual terms, many providers receive only a percentage of the charges for payment. These are called discounted charges. Many providers today receive a lump-sum amount of dollars for each episode of care, for example, diagnosis-related groups (DRGs) or case rate payment. This may also apply to both inpatient and outpatient treatments.
5. During recent years, reimbursement for various health-related services have transitioned from the more traditional "fee for service" to a more "prospective reimbursement" process, where rates are established through contracts prior to patients needing such services. This change has resulted in the need to minimize additional consequences of health care services because reimbursement is not necessarily increased due to such consequences, and providers may actually be rewarded financially for "improvements" of the quality of services being provided.
6. Contractual terms are rarely reviewed and vary with different insurance carriers. This creates additional confusion as to the costs associated for various services or therapies.
7. A recognizable way to resolve these hurdles is to use the cost to charge (RCC) ratio for the cost estimation. Multiply the RCC by the patient's charge to yield the estimated cost. RCC can be obtained from the individual hospital's Centers for Medicare and Medicaid Services (CMS) yearly cost report.

C. **Basic steps in assessing cost**

1. Define the units of service or output
2. Determine the number of service or output units provided
3. Determine cost drivers of these units of service or output
4. Calculate total costs, direct or indirect, related to the provision of this output or service
5. Calculate the average cost and incremental cost

III. ELEMENTS OF A GOOD STUDY

A. **Sound objective(s).** The study has well-defined objective(s) and answerable question(s).

B. **Perspective(s).** There is a defined perspective for analysis (e.g., patient, payer, provider, society). In many cases, study perspective determines the cost-effectiveness of an intervention. Most of the published PE guidelines suggest that societal perspective be considered as an additional perspective for analysis.

C. **Patient population** chosen must be within the scope of analysis. Patient selection criteria that are too stringent pose a threat to external validity. Patient selection criteria that are too liberal are a threat to internal validity. Consideration is also given to comorbidity and multiple treatment modalities.

D. **Possible comparators and their effectiveness.** All relevant alternatives for comparison are identified. Chosen comparator(s) should be reasonable and is the current preferred standard treatment. In some instances, no treatment (placebo) is considered as an alternative.

E. **Metrics for costs and consequences.** Measures chosen for costs and consequences can affect the results of the analysis. Biases can be introduced into the analysis if units of measures are not clearly defined. This may pose a problem with a multi country study in the aggregation of the final costs and consequences because currency exchange rates may fluctuate from time to time.

F. **Inclusion of relevant costs and consequences in the analysis** are based on the perspective chosen. The computation of costs and consequences should be transparent to readers. The key is reproducibility. Readers should be able to use the published computation methods with the local data to validate the findings.

G. **A valid data source.** Depending on the design of the study, data can come from clinical trials, observational studies, health care claim databases, chart reviews, and epidemiological data. Each of the sources of these data was designed for some other purpose than economic analysis. Limitations are listed in VIII.

H. **Discounting for costs and consequences.** Much discussion has been devoted to the appropriateness of discounting costs and consequences as well as the discount rate. The consensus at this time is to discount both costs and consequences. The discount rate normally is the opportunity cost of using resources. Many researchers have used the government bond rate. Regardless, the researcher must offer the justification for the chosen discount rate(s).

I. **Incremental analysis** provides an insight on the comparison for cost generated from one alternative to another alternative, and the additional benefit yielded from the increased cost.

J. **Sensitivity analysis** should include all the plausible values and their justification for the key parameters.

K. **Time horizon of the analysis** covers the full duration of treatment for the disease process. For example, the time horizon for the cholesterol-lowering agent's treatment should be the life span from the start day of treatment to the end of life.

L. **Appropriateness and comprehensiveness of presentation and discussion of the study results.** Similar to clinical studies, the presentation of study results should not be biased. Interventional alternatives and study limitations must be addressed. Generalizability and applicability are also discussed.

IV. PHARMACOECONOMIC METHODOLOGIES

A. **Cost of illness (COI)** is the evaluation and assessment of the resources used in treating an illness. This technique is used to obtain the baseline cost information before the introduction of a new intervention. Costs are measured in terms of dollars. Like any PE analysis, the evaluator needs to define the analysis perspective. A different perspective will change the cost structure. For example, from a patient's perspective, the cost of illness will include the transportation to and from the treatment site. Time duration of the disease can be critical in determining the cost and may be a source of bias. No comparison is made in this type of analysis.

B. **Cost-benefit analysis (CBA)** is a tool used to determine priority for the resource allocation. The technique can be applied to the comparison of health care programs and with non-health care programs, such as social welfare programs. For example, one can compare the costs and benefits of a coronary risk factor reduction program and the childhood immunization program and the domestic violence prevention program. This technique consists of identifying all of the benefits that accrue from the program and converting them into dollars in the year that they accrue. The stream of costs and benefits are then discounted to present value at the selected discount rate. Net benefit is computed for each program and can then be compared with other programs.

C. **Cost-minimization analysis (CMA).** The underlying assumption for this type of analysis assumes that consequences are equivalent. Therefore, only cost is compared. The cheapest intervention will be chosen for implementation. Equivalent outcomes may not necessarily be equal. One needs to determine the key outcome of each comparator. For example, two drugs may have the equivalent therapeutic value but different side effect profiles. In such cases, consequences may not be equivalent, and this technique is not appropriate. CEA should be used instead.

D. **Cost-effectiveness analysis (CEA)** is a technique to assist the decision maker in identifying a preferred choice among possible alternatives within similar consequences (e.g., same therapeutic category) in terms of health improvement created (e.g., life year gained, clinical cures). It is not to be used to compare different consequences for each alternative, such as blood pressure reduction to degree of cholesterol lowering. Consequences can be intermediate outcomes or surrogate outcomes such as the reperfusion time of the vessel after thrombolytic therapy. Generally, the incremental cost of a program or an intervention from a specified perspective is compared to the incremental health effects. An example is the cost per unit of blood pressure reduction with each antihypertensive agent compared. The results of the analysis normally are stated in terms of cost per unit of effectiveness.

E. **Cost-utility analysis (CUA).** Unlike CEA, CUA measures the consequences in terms of the quality-adjusted life year (QALY) gained. The results of the analysis are normally expressed as a cost per QALY. The metric of QALY incorporates both the improvement in quantity of life, quality of life, and the preference (utility value) of the health state. There are three sources of obtaining utility values for health states in CUA: judgment to estimate the utility values, values from the literature, or values elicited from a sample of subjects. Common techniques for eliciting utility values are rating scale (visual analog scale), standard gamble, and time trade-off. Five circumstances have been summarized that detail when CUA may be the appropriate technique to apply.

1. When quality of life is the only outcome
2. When quality and quantity of life are health outcomes
3. When the intervention affects both mortality and morbidity and a combined unit of outcome is desired
4. When the intervention being compared has a wide range of potential outcomes and a common unit of outcome is needed
5. When the objective is to compare a gold standard intervention that already has the cost per QALY. QALY is calculated by multiplying the utility values obtained for the specific health state with the quantity of life years spent in that specific health state. Comparison can then be made for the program and intervention.

F. **Multiattribute utility theory (MAUT) or analysis (MAUA)** is another technique available in assessing utilities. In this situation, several attributes can be included, such as clinical, financial, and quality of life. It is possible to preferentially weigh the decision based on what the priorities are for the decision maker, and then apply the weights to identify the most preferable therapy, service, and so on. As evidenced from the following three examples, the individual's perspective will have a major effect on the final decision made, based on the levels of priority chosen for evaluation.

1. A physician may view clinical outcome to represent 70% of his or her decision, followed by patient's quality of life (20%), and last being therapy costs (10%).
2. A hospital administrator may view the financial outcomes (70%) as a major priority, followed by the clinical outcome (20%), and last, the quality of life (10%).
3. A patient with health insurance might view the clinical outcome (45%) and quality of life (45%) as the top priorities and have minimal concern for the financial outcomes (10%) of such a decision, especially with adequate insurance coverage.

G. **Willingness to pay (WTP)** technique is used to assess the perceived value or benefit of a product and service. The WTP values can be obtained through two approaches:

1. Indirect measurement, which examines in actual payments previous real-world decisions that involve trade-offs between money and expected outcomes.
2. Direct measurement, which uses survey methods to elicit stated dollar on the perceived benefits. In this second approach, researchers are seeking to provide sufficient background information to create within the respondent's mind a hypothetical market in which the person provides a judgment of the value of the proposed service.
3. The challenge of using contingent valuation is to present within the questionnaire sufficient, clearly organized information to allow this judgment to occur. Basic facts need to be given at the appropriate time. Unlike CBA, WTP takes into consideration the psychological aspects of the illness as well as the physical deterioration. The use of WTP as an outcome measure is theoretically consistent with welfare economics. It also provides a means to assign dollar values to health outcomes.

V. DECISION ANALYSIS.

Is a systematic approach to decision making under conditions of uncertainty. It is a tool for helping the decision makers identify options that are available, predict the consequences and value of each option based on the probabilities assigned to each option, and choose the option that has the best payoff. Decision analysis can be incorporated into a pharmacoeconomics evaluation. Steps in performing a decision analysis are as follows:

A. **Identify and bound the decision.** All the ground rules such as analysis perspective, comparators selection, time span, and decision rules are identified and clarified.

B. **Develop a decision tree** (*Figure 54-1*). The decision maker will structure the decision in the form of a tree with branches from left to right. Each branch is a segment of a path that leads to an outcome.

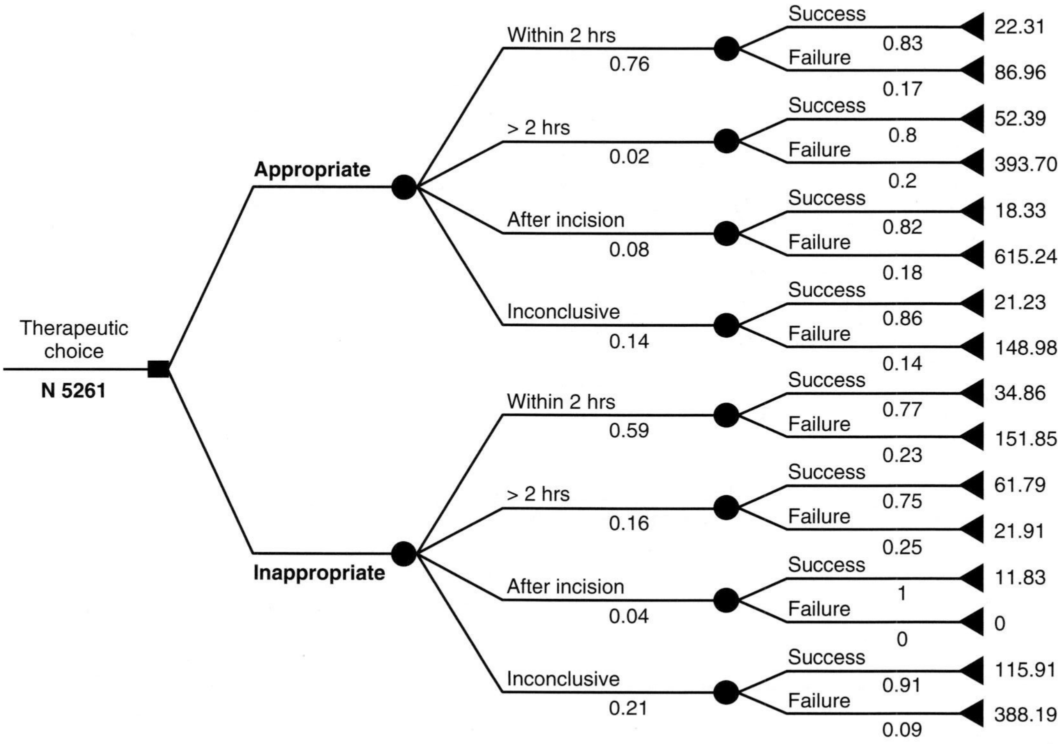

Figure 54-1. Decision tree with probabilities included.

The process of setting up the tree helps the decision maker put thoughts on paper and provides an evaluation for each option that occurs.

C. **Assess and assign probabilities.** Probability related to each branch is assessed and assigned. Probabilities can be obtained from the published literature, an expert panel, or clinical trials.
D. **Value outcomes.** For each of the outcome possibilities, assign a value. This can be in the form of monetary or utility values.
E. **Calculate the expected value.** Using the averaging-out and folding-back method, start from the right and work backward to the left, and calculate the expected value by multiplying the outcome value to each assigned probability (*Figure 54-2*).
F. **Choose the preferred course of action.** Depending on the ground rules set in the beginning of either optimization or minimization, choose the best course of action.
G. **Perform a sensitivity analysis.** Assign different values to all plausible outcomes and resolve the decision tree to identify the robustness of the data and/or results.

VI. PATIENT-REPORTED OUTCOMES (PRO).

PRO refers to any outcomes based on data provided by patient or patient proxy. It includes health-related quality of life data. PRO data can be collected during the clinical trial. Examples of PRO data include patient satisfaction with treatment and providers, functional status, psychosocial well-being, treatment compliance/adherence, and disease symptoms. There is a growing amount of interest in adding PRO data into the drug review and evaluation process.

A. **Health-related quality of life (HRQOL).** Although quality of life focuses on all aspects of life, HRQOL focuses only on a patient's nonclinical information such as functional status, well-being, perception of health, return to work from an illness, and other health outcomes that are directly affect by health status. Standardized questionnaires are used to capture HRQOL data in various research settings. Data are obtained either by telephone interview, self-administration, personal face-to-face interview, observation, or mail-in survey. Such standardized questionnaires can also be divided into general health status instruments—for example, Short-Form 36 (SF-36), Short-Form 12, SF-10 for Children, SF-8 Health Surveys, sickness impact profiles (SIPs)—or disease-specific instrument

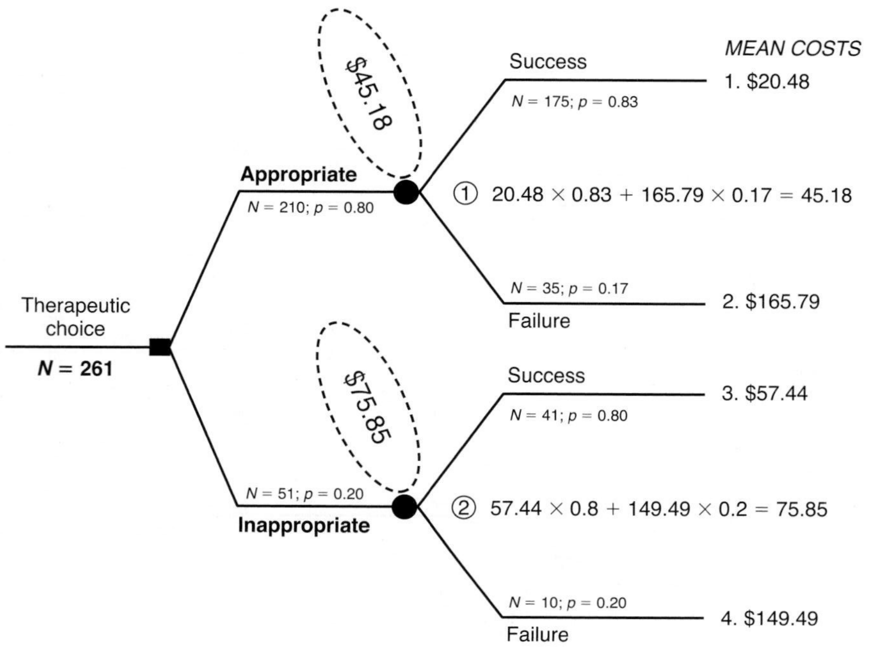

Figure 54-2. Completed decision tree after averaging out and folding back.

(e.g., McGill Pain Inventory, Beck Depression Scale, Functional Living Index—Cancer). The general health status instruments measure the global health status, whereas the disease-specific instruments target the disease-specific issues.

B. Short form surveys are the most frequently used general health status instruments. There are a variety of dimensions available, depending on the chosen short form instrument. The original SF-36 includes physical functions, social functions, emotional role, physical role, bodily pain, mental health, general health, and vitality. Other survey instruments may contain only some of these dimensions. Interested readers can explore the following Web site: http://www.qualitymetric.com for more information.

C. At the time of this update, the entire set of rules and regulations of the recently approved, Patient Protection and Affordable Care Act (PPACA) have not been finalized. However, a key aspect of the act besides working to ensure health care for all U.S. citizens is to begin creating a venue where "quality-performing" health care providers and institutions will be able to recapture health care dollars by demonstrating improvements in patient outcomes. This will include patient satisfaction with the services received and quality clinical therapies provided as a way to improve outcomes (β-blockers after myocardial infarctions, correct antibiotics for designated infections, appropriate surgical procedures to minimize negative outcomes, etc.). Health care providers will become incentivized to improve in quality as a way to capture maximal amounts of reimbursements. Bad performances will result in poor reimbursements.

D. Psychometric properties. Before using any instrument, the researcher must understand the psychometric properties of the chosen instrument. The psychometric properties consist of the reliability and validity information of the instrument. In addition, the sensitivity and specificity of the instrument are also important.

1. **Reliability** is a measure of consistency. Can we reproduce the same score under the same conditions with the same individual? Statistical methods of measuring reliability are Cronbach's α, Pearson's r coefficient, and the κ statistic.
2. **Validity** is a measure of accuracy. Is the instrument measuring what it is supposed to measure? Types of validity are content validity, construct validity, criterion validity, and convergent/divergent validity.
3. **Use of the instrument.** The psychometric properties preclude "mixing and matching" sections of established questionnaires or selection of a section of an established questionnaire for administration without recalibrating the instrument's psychometric properties.

VII. MODELING STUDIES.

Mathematical modeling is widely used today in the economic evaluation of medications and health care technologies.

A. The goal for modeling is to assemble evidence of costs and outcomes in a form that can project long-term consequences. Model-based evaluations are great tools for health care decision makers.

B. Mathematical models provide the cost-consequence estimates that cannot be revealed by randomized control trials or epidemiological studies because of the duration required for long-term studies (10 to 20 years).

C. Results derived from modeling assist decision makers in making informed decisions. However, the quality of the decision is based completely on the truthfulness of the projected results, which in turn depends on the input information and assumptions imposed for each model.

D. The International Society of Pharmacoeconomics and Outcomes Research (ISPOR) recommends the following criteria for assessing the quality of models: model structure, data used as inputs for the model, and model validation.[1]

VIII. 1997 FDA MODERNIZATION ACT, SECTION 114, HEALTH CARE ECONOMIC INFORMATION

A. "Health care economic information provided to a formulary committee, or other similar entity, in the course of the committee or entity carrying out its responsibilities for the selection of drugs for managed care or other similar organizations, shall not be considered to be false or misleading under this paragraph if the health care economic information directly relates to an indication approved . . . for such drug and is based on competent and reliable scientific evidence." (From the FDA's Modernization Act of 1997, http://www.fda.gov/cder/guidance/s830enr.txt)

B. Health economic information means any analysis that identifies, measures, or compares the economic consequences including the costs of the represented health outcomes, or the use of a drug to the use of another drug, or to another health care intervention, or to no intervention.

C. Key concepts of the act

1. A venue for the pharmaceutical industry to provide OR and/or PE research studies to decision makers
2. Economic information can be provided in the form of CMA, CBA, CUA, COI, and cost quality of life.
3. Competent and reliable scientific information pertaining to an approved indication
4. Standard of competent and reliable scientific information has not been addressed.

IX. PRACTICAL ISSUES IN INTERPRETING OUTCOMES RESEARCH AND PHARMACOECONOMIC STUDIES

A. Comparisons between economic study and randomized clinical trials (RCTs)

1. Economic studies are carried out in an observational environment, whereas RCTs depend on rigorous experimental design with strict inclusion/exclusion criteria.
2. RCTs rely on highly controlled and artificial clinical settings to demonstrate clinical efficacy. Clinical and economic end points of the study may not be the same. In addition, RCTs tend to have additional protocol costs (e.g., extra tests) and inflated benefits (e.g., medication compliance, appropriateness of utilization).
3. Economic studies have large sample sizes, whereas RCTs are limited to a relatively small sample size.
4. Economic studies are generalizable to the broader patient population, whereas RCTs are limited to those included within the stringent entry criteria, which might not represent the typical patient receiving the tested therapy.
5. Economic studies are usually involved in evaluating "effectiveness" as compared to RCTs, which evaluate "efficacy."

B. Multiple countries' OR and PE studies

1. There are significant differences in physician practice patterns and care delivery systems among different countries.

[1]Weinstein MC, O'Brien B, Hornberger J, et al. ISPOR Task Force on Good Research Practices. Principles of good practice for decision analytic modeling in health-care evaluation. *Value Health*. 2003;6(1):9–17.

2. Different methods of funding health care and allocating health expenditures make it almost impossible to calculate costs.
3. Patients' concerns and beliefs are different.

C. **Budgetary constraints.** Decision making should not be solely based on the information from the PE analysis because most published PE studies do not impose budgetary constraint as part of the analysis. *Cost-effective* does not equal *affordable.* In addition, one should also consider the implementation costs of the program. In many instances, implementation costs may exceed the benefits or effectiveness of the program.

D. **Reproducibility**
1. Often, owing to journal space limitation, lengthy cost computations are eliminated from the published article. Such practice creates an impossible auditing mechanism for the derivation and computation of costs. Critical assessment of this section of the published article is necessary to ensure the validity and reliability of the results.
2. Modeling is an appropriate method when the disease and treatment in question has a lengthy time span and ethical dilemma of withdrawing treatment. However, assumptions and input values to these models are not transparent to readers.
3. Both issues make it almost impossible to reproduce the study results using the local data.

E. **Limitations of claim data studies.** Claim data studies are designed for billing purposes. There is no differentiation between comorbid conditions and complications in coding data. This can pose a problem in quality benchmark studies. In addition, coding practice may be different from one institution to another, a threat to reliability.

Study Questions

Directions: Each of the questions, statements, or incomplete statements in this section can be correctly answered or completed by **one** of the suggested answers or phrases. Choose the **best** answer.

1. The underlying assumption of cost-minimization analysis (CMA) is
   (A) calculation of cost minimization ratio.
   (B) consequences or outcomes are equivalent.
   (C) costs are equivalent.
   (D) patient satisfaction is equivalent
   (E) no more than two comparators in any analysis.

2. Which one of these statements is *not* true for the differences between economic studies and randomized clinical trials (RCTs)?
   (A) Generalizability and applicability of the results differ between economic studies and RCTs.
   (B) Clinical end point and economic end point are identical.
   (C) RCTs tend to have inflated benefits and additional protocol-driven costs.
   (D) Sample size of the economic study is normally larger than in the RCT.
   (E) Clinical efficacy assessment through the RCTs as compared to clinical effectiveness through the economic study.

3. In choosing an instrument to measure the health-related quality of life (HRQOL), which of the following is *not* a key component of the assessment?
   (A) Reliability as a sign of consistency for the instrument.
   (B) Validity of the instrument in order to assure its accuracy.
   (C) Incorporate similar questionnaires into a single instrument after calibration.
   (D) Sensitivity and specificity of the instrument.
   (E) Length of the instrument.

4. In choosing a study perspective, the current pharmacoeconomic guidelines have suggested which one of the following perspectives to be included?
   (A) Society
   (B) Payers
   (C) Patients
   (D) Providers
   (E) Practitioners

Directions for questions: The questions and incomplete statements for questions 5–6 in this section can be correctly answered or completed by **one or more** of the suggested answers. Choose the answer, **A–E.**

(A) if **I only** is correct
(B) if **III only** is correct
(C) if **I and II** are correct
(D) if **II and III** are correct
(E) if **I, II, and III** are correct

5. When interpreting outcomes research amongst multiple countries, what issues needs special attention?
   (I) Cost computations
   (II) Health care funding and cost-allocating mechanisms
   (III) Patients' variations and beliefs

6. Which one of these pharmacoeconomic techniques does not address both cost and consequences?
   (I) Cost-benefit analysis
   (II) Cost-effectiveness analysis
   (III) Cost of illness

7. Which of the following is an example of a clinical outcome indicator?
   (A) Dollars spent treating acute myocardial infarction
   (B) Resources used in diagnosing the presence of medical errors
   (C) Duration of hospitalization and mortality versus discharge rate for ventricular fibrillation patients treated with amiodarone
   (D) Functional capacity of patients treated with ramipril in the presence of cardiovascular risk factors
   (E) Patient satisfaction survey upon discharge

Answers and Explanations

1. **The answer is B** *[see IV.C]*.
   CMA assumes all consequences compared are equivalent. Patient satisfaction would represent a humanistic outcome and is not considered in a CMA. For this reason, only the cost of each alternative is compared with the least expensive alternative being chosen.

2. **The answer is B** *[see IX.A]*.
   Clinical and economic end points are generally not equal. In the sequence of the study events, efficacy should come before effectiveness and is routinely a key outcome associated with the RCTs as compared to effectiveness being associated with the economic or outcomes study.

3. **The answer is C** *[see VI.D.1–3]*.
   A key process involved in each instrument used to assess quality of life is the need to "calibrate" and "recalibrate" the psychometric properties in order to make sure it is adequately assessing the instrument's intention. This would be of paramount concern when one incorporates items from one satisfactory instrument to that of another similar instrument. Both instruments on their own might meet all necessary purposes. However, when combining them, the process of recalibration is again necessary to adequately assure the reconfigured instrument's value.

4. **The answer is A** *[see III.B]*.
   The societal perspective must be included. It is critical in the health care environment to identify the perspective from which a decision is being made because that perspective directly affects the final decision. The decision to add a high-cost, moderately effective therapy for the treatment of hospitalized patient might be different if viewed from a hospital formulary committee (in-house budgetary concerns) than from the local community, national government (saving lives at whatever expense).

5. **The answer is E** *[see IX.B.1–3]*.
   All of the issues stated need special attention and play a major role in developing multinational economic evaluations to avoid carrying out a study that when completed cannot be generalized to the broad patient population.

6. **The answer is B** *[see IV.A]*.
   The cost of illness methodology is carried out as an assessment of the necessary resources that will be used to treat a designated illness. Resources are measured in terms of dollars, and there are no comparator groups in the evaluation.

7. **The answer is C** *[see I.A.3]*.
   Clinical outcomes include the following: length of hospital stay, adverse drug reactions, hospital readmission, and death. These are definable measures of a patient's response to a given treatment, such as amiodarone used for the treatment of ventricular fibrillation.

Index

Page numbers in italic type indicate items found in the supplemental online chapters and page numbers followed by an *f* or *t* denotes figures and tables respectively.